EMERGENCY PEDIATRICS

A Guide to Ambulatory Care

EMERGENCY PEDIATRICS
A Guide to Ambulatory Care

Editor

ROGER M. BARKIN, M.D., M.P.H., F.A.A.P., F.A.C.E.P.

Vice President for Pediatric and Newborn Programs
Vice President of Medical Services
HealthONE
Professor of Surgery, Division of Emergency Medicine
University of Colorado Health Sciences Center
Denver, Colorado

Associate Editor

PETER ROSEN, M.D., F.A.C.E.P.

Associate Professor, Harvard University
Boston, Massachusetts;
Visiting Professor, University of Arizona
Tucson, Arizona;
Professor Emeritus, University of California, San Diego
San Diego, California;
Attending Physician, Department of Emergency Medicine
Beth Israel Deaconess Medical Center
Boson, Massachusetts;
Attending Physician, Department of Emergency Medicine
St. John's Hospital
Jackson, Wyoming

SIXTH EDITION

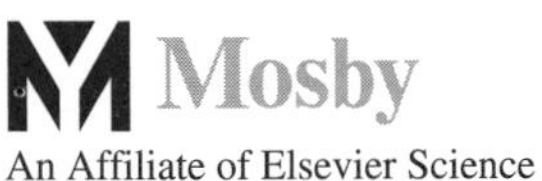

An Affiliate of Elsevier Science

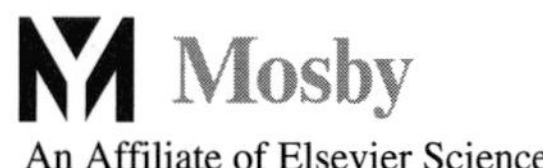

An Affiliate of Elsevier Science

The Curtis Center
Independence Square West
Philadelphia, Pennsylvania 19106

EMERGENCY PEDIATRICS: A GUIDE TO AMBULATORY CARE 0-323-01901-3

NOTICE

Medicine is an ever-changing field. Standard safety precautions must be followed, but as new research and clinical experience broaden our knowledge, changes in treatment and drug therapy may become necessary or appropriate. Readers are advised to check the most current product information provided by the manufacturer of each drug to be administered to verify the recommended dose, the method and duration of administration, and contraindications. It is the responsibility of the licensed prescriber, relying on experience and knowledge of the patient, to determine dosages and the best treatment for each individual patient. Neither the publisher nor the author assumes any liability for any injury and/or damage to persons or property arising from this publication.

Previous editions copyrighted 1984, 1986, 1990, 1994, 1999

Library of Congress Cataloging-in-Publication Data

Emergency pediatrics: a guide to ambulatory care / editor, Roger Barkin; associate editor, Peter Rosen.—6th ed.
p. ; cm.
Includes bibliographical references and index.
ISBN 0-323-01901-3
1. Pediatric emergencies. I. Barkin, Roger M. II. Rosen, Peter, 1935-[DNLM: 1. Emergencies—Child. 2. Emergencies—Infant. 3. Ambulatory Care—Child. 4. Ambulatory Care—Infant. WS 200 E53 2003]
RJ370.E44 2003
618.92'0025—dc21

2002045157

Acquisitions Editor: Todd Hummel
Developmental Editor: Kim J. Davis
Publishing Services Manager: Patricia Tannian
Project Manager: Sarah Wunderly
Designer: Gail Morey Hudson
Cover Design: Liz Rohne Rudder

Printed in United States of America

Last digit is the print number: 9 8 7 6 5 4 3 2 1

Contributors

Adam Z. Barkin, M.D.
Resident
Harvard Affiliated Emergency Medicine Residency;
Department of Emergency Medicine
Beth Israel Deaconess Medical Center
Boston, Massachusetts

Suzanne Z. Barkin, M.D.
Associate Professor, Department of Radiology
University of Colorado Health Sciences Center;
Subsection Chief, Pediatric Radiology
Denver Health Medical Center
Denver, Colorado

Gary K. Belanger, D.D.S.
Associate Professor, Pediatric Dentistry
University of Colorado School of Dentistry
Department of Pediatric Dentistry
Children's Hospital
Denver, Colorado

Joseph T. Flynn, M.D.
Associate Professor of Clinical Pediatrics
Department of Pediatrics
Albert Einstein College of Medicine;
Director, Pediatric Hypertension Program
Division of Pediatric Nephrology
Children's Hospital at Montefiore
Bronx, New York

Benjamin Honigman, M.D.
Professor of Surgery
Division of Emergency Medicine, Department of Surgery
University of Colorado;
Staff Physician
Department of Emergency Medicine
University of Colorado Health Sciences Center
Denver, Colorado

Mark A. Hostetler, M.D., M.P.H., F.A.C.E.P., F.A.A.P.
Assistant Professor
Chief, Section of Emergency Medicine, Department of Pediatrics
Medical Director, Pediatric Emergency Department
University of Chicago
Chicago, Illinois

Kenneth W. Kulig, M.D.
Associate Clinical Professor
Division of Emergency Medicine, Department of Surgery
University of Colorado Health Sciences Center
Denver, Colorado

Vincent J. Markovchick, M.D., F.A.A.E.M.
Professor of Surgery
Division of Emergency Medicine, Department of Surgery
University of Colorado Health Sciences Center;
Director, Emergency Medical Services
Denver Health Medical Center
Denver, Colorado

James C. Mitchiner, M.D., M.P.H.
Clinical Assistant Professor
Department of Emergency Medicine
University of Michigan Medical School;
Attending Physician, Department of Emergency Medicine
St. Joseph Mercy Hospital
Ann Arbor, Michigan

Anthony F. Philipps, M.D.
Professor and Chair, Department of Pediatrics
University of California Davis Medical Center
Sacramento, California

Peter T. Pons, M.D.
Professor of Surgery
Division of Emergency Medicine, Department of Surgery
University of Colorado Health Sciences Center;
Emergency Physician
Department of Emergency Medicine
Denver Health Medical Center
Denver, Colorado

Francis R. Poulain, M.D.
Associate Professor
University of California Davis Medical Center;
Department of Neonatology
University of California Children's Hospital
Sacramento, California

Thomas J. Smith, M.D.
Pediatric Hematologist-Oncologist
Childhood Hematology-Oncology Associates
Mother and Child Hospital
Presbyterian/St. Luke's Medical Center
Denver, Colorado

Reginald L. Washington, M.D.
Associate Professor of Pediatrics
University of Colorado School of Medicine;
Past Chairman, Department of Pediatrics
Mother and Child Hospital
Presbyterian/St. Luke's Medical Center
Denver, Colorado

Lynne M. Yancey, M.D.
Assistant Professor
Division of Emergency Medicine, Department of Surgery
University of Colorado Health Sciences Center;
Attending Physician
Emergency Department
The Children's Hospital
Denver, Colorado

Rochelle A. Yanofsky, M.D., F.R.C.P.C.
Associate Professor of Pediatrics
Department of Pediatrics and Child Health
Section of Pediatric Hematology/Oncology/BMT
University of Manitoba;
Pediatric Hematologist/Oncologist
Children's Hospital of Winnipeg;
Pediatric Hematologist/Oncologist
Department of Hematology/Oncology/BMT
CancerCare Manitoba
Winnipeg, Manitoba, Canada

Julie D. Zimbelman, M.D.
Pediatric Hematologist-Oncologist
Childhood Hematology-Oncology Associates
Mother and Child Hospital
Presbyterian/St. Luke's Medical Center
Denver, Colorado

To

our colleagues and **patients**

in the hope that the delineation of the practice of
pediatric emergency medicine will help reduce
anxiety and suffering and prevent untimely death

To

Physicians, nurses, and **prehospital** and **other health professionals**

who practice pediatric emergency medicine and ensure the
highest quality of prehospital and hospital-based care for children

To

Suzanne

who continues to provide the needed insight and understanding
while serving as a model of professionalism

To

Adam

who represents the new generation of emergency physicians and
brings commitment, knowledge, and sensitivity to his practice
while maintaining perspective

To

Michael

who provides balance and a view of the
larger world beyond medicine

To

children

who will continue to be our partners in learning and whose needs
will be better served through the application of the principles,
guidelines, and information contained in this book to the
clinical practice of emergency pediatrics

R.M.B.

Foreword

Note: The foreword remains as an integral part of ***Emergency Pediatrics*** *because of the insights and perspective it conveys. It is truly timeless and provides an essential message for all physicians caring for pediatric emergencies.*

Over the past 36 years, a great number of medical students and some residents have told me something like the following: "I am afraid I cannot handle medicine as a career. Last night I worked in the emergency department, and a desperately ill accident victim was brought in for treatment. My only thought was to flee out the back door, and I was in a panic." I have always replied that I was so pleased to hear that because only people devoid of conscience will run toward such acute disasters with joy; to be scared is to be honest as well as intelligent.

The unprepared student soon acquires experience by working alongside senior role models, nurses, paramedics, and other physicians—learning that team care is essential. All emergencies require more than one set of hands. Practitioners must be well trained and intellectually as well as emotionally prepared to deal with anything that comes through the door. I always urge practicing physicians, residents, and students to "play" at situations in which a mother rushes her child to the office or to the emergency department or in which an urgent call comes from a ward and the immediate needs for survival must be practiced: an airway established, breathing ensured, and the vascular bed brought back to a capacity to carry oxygen to all organs. The entire team must maintain its competency to maximize each patient's chances. The ability to tell a four-star from a one-star emergency is learned with time.

Often the patient's history is obtained while urgent care for life support is given. It isn't easy to do both at the same time, yet both are required. This is no moment for textbooks or lengthy dissertations; ready access to a broad range of diagnostic and therapeutic information is needed. The basics are crucial and must be learned by heart. What are vital medications? Where is a working laryngoscope? Who will assist the primary members of the team? What are the most important drug dosages, fluids, and electrolytes? Practice, expertise, organization, and cooperation make the components flow smoothly.

Emergency care is always a bit scary, and it should be! It needs the best kind of quick and broadly based diagnostic thought and action. Yet, regardless of where the emergency is treated—even in the best-equipped and trained units—some patients will die. This is always a very bad time for all who have worked so hard to pull a youngster through. Recriminations between parents and relatives abound.

Among the members of the health care team, there are similar frustrations, anger, and sorrow, and the temptation to "scapegoat" somebody must be avoided at all costs. It is best to lock the door, pick up, clean the dead child, and have the provisional rites of baptism administered to a Catholic child.* Important too is taking a few minutes to calm down before talking to the parents in a quiet place and with plenty of time. The response to "I am

* Note that any person of any faith can administer provisional baptism: "I baptize you in the name of the Father, the Son, and the Holy Spirit. Amen."

sorry we lost your baby" is often disbelief. Properly run emergency departments will already have seen that a supportive relative or a minister is in the waiting room. Relatives usually want to see the child, and they will remember these next moments forever.

Then follows the time of questioning. It is simply bad medicine to blame anyone, tempting though it may be. It is useless to tell a mother that she should have brought the child in 2 hours earlier or that the child's regular doctor should have diagnosed the problem better and sooner, even though that may be true. A devastated family needs compassion and support, wherever it can be found. In my experience, when families have been treated with respect and kindness, permission for diagnostic autopsies is routinely given.

The field of emergency care is continuing to expand rapidly and well. Recent technical advances have made for better survival rates, and greater understanding of physiology has led to new and better medications. Thus emergency medicine has become a new and highly sophisticated specialty. Yet all physicians are expected to perform basic life support procedures in any setting and, sometimes, without any help or tools.

This book addresses the field of pediatric emergencies in a comprehensive and readily accessible format, focusing on information that is immediately required. It contains these priority items, as well as those many conditions that permit more thought and time. It prepares the conscientious physician, resident, student, and other members of the team to overcome and thus lessen the anxiety that signifies a good conscience while capably performing all that is needed in an outwardly calm manner. In this field, experience allows rapid growth in building the confidence that management will be proficient.

I shall always trust and admire the competent, yet honestly frightened, practitioner.

The late **C. Henry Kempe, M.D.** (1922-1984)
Former Professor of Pediatrics and Microbiology
University of Colorado Health Sciences Center
Denver, Colorado

Preface

The sixth edition of *Emergency Pediatrics: A Guide to Ambulatory Care* reflects an evolving specialty with a redefined biology: pathophysiologic principles and research applied to the pediatric patients. The escalation of knowledge generates controversy; concurrently, it stimulates searching, discovery, and analysis.

Children present a unique challenge and a rare opportunity. Although medical and traumatic illnesses progress rapidly, the vast majority are expected to leave the child without sequelae and with a full life ahead.

The child is often frightened or nonverbal; the history may be available only from parents. Data are frequently nonspecific, and frustration may be encountered in gaining cooperation and performing examinations, procedures, and tests.

Caregivers must be sensitive to the concerns, fears, anxieties, and grief of families whose youngsters are experiencing major illness. Children are constantly looking for support from parents, who simultaneously are seeking small reassurances from a child, such as an infrequent smile or nod. This mutual dependency is exaggerated during illness.

Emergency physicians are unique in their need to solve problems within the time constraints of an acute illness, frequently modified by field considerations as well as the logistical demands of concurrent priorities and patients. In emergency medicine perhaps more than any other area of medicine, when the database conflicts with the clinical assessment, the clinician must often go with judgment and "gestalt"; it is often too easy to endow laboratory numbers with infallibility and ignore pertinent clinical findings.

This book brings together, in an accessible format, all that is immediately required for the care of the acutely ill child by the health care provider, whether that individual is a pediatrician, emergency medicine physician, nurse practitioner, emergency medicine technician, or student of medicine. *Emergency Pediatrics* is a resource for the clinician to consult, analyze, alter, and add to as experience dictates but certainly not to leave on the bookshelf for leisure reading.

The sixth edition reflects the rapid expansion of available pharmacologic agents, changing recommendations for advanced life support, evolving clinical entities, and broadened scientific and clinical literature. Emergency departments have increasingly become community clinics for children without routine sources of primary care; this development is reflected in the scope of this book.

The initial sections of this book emphasize nontraumatic and traumatic conditions that may be life threatening, presenting strategies and diagnostic considerations crucial to stabilization. Resuscitation of the newborn and child reflects the latest in our knowledge base.

Throughout the book, diagnostic categories are organized alphabetically. Differential diagnoses are encompassed within the mnemonic "INDICATIVE":

*i*nfection/*i*nflammation
*n*eoplasm
*d*egenerative/*d*eficiency
*i*ntoxication
*c*ongenital
*a*utoimmune/*a*llergy
*t*rauma
*i*ntrapsychic
*v*ascular
*e*ndocrine

Tables are used extensively to facilitate access to material; commonly encountered conditions are set in **boldface type** for ease of identification.

Diagnostic entities are the focus of a major section. The systems approach provides a resource for the vast majority of children's problems seen at any ambulatory facility. Specific attention is given to parental education, follow-up, and prevention. Appendixes are intended to provide a database for the practitioner.

I hope that this text will continue to serve the clinician by facilitating the synthesis of experience, reason, and data in our care of children.

Roger M. Barkin

Acknowledgments

This book is a synthesis of the contributions of many dedicated individuals whose knowledge, experience, concerns, and sensitivities in patient care in general, and the care of children in particular, serve as models for all of us.

We are grateful to HealthONE and the Department of Surgery at the University of Colorado Health Sciences Center for their ongoing support.

A host of dedicated professionals have produced this book through encouragement and continuous attention to detail. The authors and editors have made it happen and kept it on schedule. Kathi Thompson facilitated and watched over the many administrative and organizational aspects of the production of this book. We especially want to thank Todd Hummel, Patricia Tannian, Sarah Wunderly, Gail Hudson, Kim Davis, and Kavitha Kuttikan who have been there throughout the process of revising this book.

We would also like to thank our readers, who we hope will take this book with them to the front lines and use it with expertise and confidence in caring for pediatric patients, to whom all our efforts are dedicated.

Note: The indications for and dosages of medications recommended conform to practices at present; clinician judgment may alter management of a specific patient. References to specific products are incorporated to serve only as guidelines; they are not meant to exclude a practitioner's choice of other, comparable drugs. Many oral medications may be given with more scheduling flexibility than implied by the specific time intervals noted. Individual drug sensitivity and allergies must be considered in drug selection. Adult dosages are provided as a gauge of the maximum dosage commonly used.

Every attempt has been made to ensure accuracy and appropriateness. New investigations and broader experience may alter present dosage schedules, and it is recommended that the package insert of each drug be consulted before administration. Often there is limited experience with established drugs for neonates and young children. Furthermore, new drugs may be introduced, and indications for use may change. This rapid evolution is particularly noticeable in the use of antibiotics and cardiopulmonary resuscitation. The clinician is encouraged to maintain expertise concerning appropriate medications for specific conditions.

Contents

I

Pediatric Care in the Emergency Department

1 Approaching the Pediatric Patient

Each encounter is an opportunity to observe a child and speak with parents. Unless the condition is life threatening, the clinician should initially focus on reducing anxiety by being friendly and interacting with them before undertaking threatening or painful aspects of the evaluation. In the approach to children, it is useful to assess their growth and development and provide counsel and assistance as appropriate and needed. Gleaning information about prior behavior, family and environmental issues, and unusual stress and pressures may point toward a functional rather than organic basis for a sign or symptom.

Understanding behavior may make the visit go more smoothly and allow the clinician to influence many aspects of care. Parental presence and participation during the encounter usually ease the process. Occasionally it is necessary to redirect a child's activity and redefine appropriate limits; consistency must be the basis for all such efforts. Expectations and limits should be appropriate for the child's development. Two-year-old children should not be asked to sit still and be "angels" while their parents speak to the physician. Anxiety is probably tremendous for everyone involved and may escalate "acting-out behaviors."

THE DEVELOPING CHILD

Understanding the growth and development of children during their early years provides tremendous insight into pediatric care. Babies are unique, and during the first 2 years of life, children gain skills with a rapidity that is astounding. Each day new things are learned, new behaviors are evident, and new sounds and responses are present. Part of the excitement is that all children develop on somewhat different timetables. Although the pattern and general framework are consistent, the variability makes child development fun and full of surprises (see Denver Development Screening Test, Appendix B-6).

Normal development provides insights into behavior and disease mechanisms and allows for a more thoughtful, age-specific evaluation of the child in the emergency department (ED). Children adopt behaviors that may occasionally be frustrating but are usually a part of normal development. Independence, separation anxiety, and jealousy are recurrent themes that form the basis for many developmental changes that affect behavior. Most behaviors that pose problems are actually exaggerations of normal development and may be a reflection of the variability that exists among children in acquiring new skills. It is essential to recognize this fact in encouraging children to take age-appropriate risks and challenges that allow them to explore and experiment. Supporting and encouraging a child's growth and the expansion of horizons lead to self-confidence.

Newborn

Babies arrive to anticipation and fanfare but create unexpected stress and time demands. Although babies have little control of muscles and can barely (if at all) hold their heads up, they have an amazing ability to look at their environment and respond to people, sounds, colors, and shapes. Babies' eyes follow to the midline, and infants enjoy looking at faces and occasionally interact with bright, shiny moving objects. They should be talked to, played with, and entertained.

The early weeks are ones of bonding with mother, father, and siblings. Time demands are intense: feedings to give, diapers to change, and laundry to do. These tasks fill the time between enjoying the baby and ensuring that other children are included and that spouses are not forgotten. Everyone must be part of the excitement and get pleasure from the new arrival while some semblance of family functioning is maintained.

The stress and sibling rivalry may lead to somatization in older children.

Six Weeks

Children by 6 weeks are increasingly able to do things and respond in a more positive and animated way to sounds, faces, actions, and so on. Even as newborns, babies are taking everything in; they are just not responding. By age 6 weeks some children are making some sounds and smile in response to faces. Their eyes now follow past the midline.

Interactive playing is essential. Babies follow brightly colored objects better than dull objects and even make early attempts at grabbing things. However, they do not hold them or play with them in a consistent manner.

Babies sleep continuously but they now show greater responsiveness and make more noises; part of this behavior becomes a response to the actions of others. They feed with somewhat more purpose and are less passive in terms of position and demands.

Four Months

By age 4 months, the infant is sociable and responds with an exciting array of facial expressions, sounds, and motions to every word. The baby constantly makes sounds, such as squeals, coos, and babbles, because he or she either gets pleasure from the noise or provokes a response from someone. Babies now respond to most people who are willing to play, crawl, squeal, or make funny faces. Smiling becomes more common.

Muscle control improves, and physical interaction with the environment is more frequent. Children look at their hands and grab for things and are able to grasp an object with a wide swing of the arms and hands. They slowly develop the ability to support themselves while in someone's arms or in an infant seat. One of the most exciting events is when a child finally turns over. Often the baby does not understand what has just happened and begins to cry after this tremendous feat. Some evidence also exists that babies enjoy being held in a standing position. All of this increased control allows children to entertain themselves and keep track of what is going on in a more active fashion. Their interest is still primarily in people.

Six Months

Children at 6 months are constantly exploring. Eyes, fingers, hands, and mouth become essential parts of this process. Everything is new and needs to be looked at, held, tasted, and chewed. Objects can now be grabbed with more skill and even transferred from one hand to another. Cubes are common play toys. All of a sudden children become social beings, making sounds for themselves or anyone who will respond. Sitting becomes an important landmark at this age, and it may happen suddenly. Children are in constant motion, but crawling is limited by the inability to keep the stomach off the floor.

Nine Months

Increasingly, the baby's interaction with the world becomes more sophisticated. Body movements become more purposeful, usually in moving toward something that appears attractive. They can stand if they hold on to something. Babies reach out to learn about things, places, and people. Picking up objects and touching everything become common. The index finger and thumb can now work together in an efficient pincer action, and the baby's world is thereby expanded immeasurably.

For the baby, being included in everything is essential; games such as peek-a-boo are fun.

The tone of "no" is understood. Sounds are made in a meaningful fashion, and "Dada" and "Mama," as well as imitation sounds, become incorporated into the language pattern. Children listen to readings of books with pictures for longer periods. Stranger anxiety becomes a dominant force. Parents are clearly preferred to everyone else, and children who a month earlier loved for anyone to hold them and pay attention now cry whenever someone else picks them up. There is tremendous variability in this stage, and it will pass. It is part of the development toward being a healthy, independent person.

Sitting is now perfected; children also scoot or crawl, permitting mobility that is astounding. Many children never crawl much if they can scoot efficiently. One must remember that the object is to get from one place to another, not necessarily to acquire skills that are not needed. Children enjoy standing up while holding on to some object.

Twelve Months

The first birthday is a landmark, and walking is the big achievement; children may not become efficient walkers for a few more months. The pincer grasp has improved, and playing with cubes and other objects is more sophisticated.

Communication skills have escalated and single words, especially "Mama" and "Dada," are clearly understood. Simple directions are understood, and limit setting becomes a reality. Children are much more responsive, waving goodbye and wanting to do things by themselves. They now have the ability to ambulate and find things; feeding requires compromise because children want to hold the spoon while combining, smearing, and spilling foods. Dependency is still paramount. Although they like to do things by themselves, separation is still difficult. The security of the favorite blanket is essential, and parents often need to stay by the crib for a few minutes until the child goes to sleep.

Mobility is fundamental and becomes a part of the child's desire to explore and be independent, but the child still always wants the security of a loved one around. Providing an area that is safe to explore is helpful in assisting in this growth.

Eighteen Months

The 18-month-old child is an explorer whose world has expanded over the last few months. Walking has opened a whole new world and, when combined with crawling, leaves no place safe from the curiosity and initiative of the youngster. The child has a tremendous sense of independence and a much greater focus on what he or she really wants. Separation from parents is now more acceptable, but frequent checks for eye contact are reassuring.

Behavior becomes somewhat inconsistent; children may develop fears of certain things, such as baths or loud noises. "No" becomes an important part of an expanded vocabulary, particularly when the child's desires are not met. Children often demonstrate their temper and displeasure with these limits. Diverting attention to more acceptable activities is usually easy at this age. At this time consistency is important to help children internalize appropriate behavior patterns.

Vocabulary has increased to several single words, and there is constant babbling. Words are imitated, and usually one or more body parts are incorporated into normal play. Playing with friends is now more fun, although it is often done in parallel, with minimal interaction with peers. Often children become frustrated when they cannot do something; diverting their attention may be useful. Children can turn pages by themselves and they like to draw and scribble. They can partially undress themselves at this time.

Two Years

Independence is the hallmark of the 2-year-old child, who is trying to build new skills and competencies. Two-year-old children want to do everything themselves and have everything exactly their way. They want choices, and these should be given when appropriate (e.g., a choice of what clothes to wear but not a choice about when to go to bed or eat). The 2-year-old child has emblazoned the word "No" on all communications. Periodically, these intense feelings of independence do give way to a need to be held, praised, and supported; parents should enjoy these moments while they last.

Obviously, children can now move around with tremendous skill, even using tricycles. Balls can be kicked, steps climbed, and objects jumped. Vocabulary becomes increasingly sophisticated, and sentences can be understood and words combined. Pictures can often be named and body parts identified. Cooperative play and sharing remain limited. Listening to stories is a favorite activity, as is helping with housework.

Three Years

Three-year-old children can pedal a tricycle and go up stairs using alternate steps. They enjoy playing with blocks and can even stack them. Balls can usually be thrown overhand a small distance. Copying drawings is tremendous fun. Speech is more understandable, and children can describe pictures by combining different objects and describing the action within the story. Play is more interactive. Masturbation may occur.

Four Years

Hopping is a favorite activity, and sense of balance greatly improves at age 4 years. People increasingly become the subject of their drawings, and they still love to copy and imitate pictures. Speech is totally understandable, and naming opposites is a favorite game. "Why," "how," and "when" are constantly included in all questions and should be recognized as important parts of the learning process.

Children can usually dress themselves with help, and many are toilet trained. Separation from parents is easier, and playgroups work cooperatively.

Five to Eight Years

Balancing is possible at 5 to 8 years, and the child plays with a bouncing ball with better eye-hand coordination and speed. Drawings of people are more complicated, including multiple body parts. Exploring is constant. More control of their environment is expected and self-reliance is observed. The child increasingly requests group activities, sports, and diversions.

Language is tremendously important and children know body parts; vocabulary is expanded and counting improves. Children can dress themselves at this age.

Older Children

With more years, children develop enhanced and increasing independence. The ED encounter can be less frightening if the clinician directs particular attention to communicating with and relieving anxiety in the child and parents. Parents increasingly become allies in this process. With this growth also comes greater experimentation, which on occasion may lead to "acting out" and other behaviors that raise the risk of injury. The rationality of this age group should be considered but not overestimated. Children's fears, anxiety, and concern about body image must be respected.

Children and adolescents are developing and responding to their environment. Being responsive to the behavioral, physical, familial, and environmental stresses and problems gives the clinician better focus in the care of the pediatric patient in the ED.

The ED clinician must understand the growth and development of children. An awareness of these patterns provides unique challenges and delights for all those involved in patient care and allows greater sensitivity in approaching children and their families during times of stress.

II

Advanced Cardiac Life Support

2 Emergency Department Environment

The expansion of emergency services is a response to a growing demand for accessible, efficient, and superior health care facilities. The pediatric patient is seen in a variety of emergency department (ED) settings. Often the patient is integrated into a general ED with a specific environment and staff for children; equipment, supplies, and expertise must be available. More and more EDs are developing separate physical areas for children, providing personnel, equipment, and space conducive to caring for youngsters, but integrating major resuscitation activities with the expertise and responsiveness of the entire staff. Children's hospitals with EDs have provided for the needs of children through triage, evaluation, and treatment systems. The growth of pediatric emergency medicine fellowships has broadened the cadre of physicians with a specific pediatric focus.

Approximately 25% to 35% of patients in the general ED are children or adolescents, presenting problems ranging from benign and self limited to life threatening. Fewer than 5% require admission, a statistic that emphasizes the noncritical nature of most encounters. Parents take children to the ED for a variety of reasons. Many who have private health care providers have been frustrated in their attempts to schedule an appointment with their primary care provider (PCP) and believe that their children require immediate attention to relieve discomfort. Others prefer the anonymity of the emergency facility and use it as their primary source of health care. A significant number of patients have been directed to the emergency facility by health care professionals.

The ED is a major focus of pediatric health care in the United States and a central component of the emergency medical services system. In balancing the medical, nursing, and related needs of pediatric patients, it is essential to ensure that EDs reflect the unique medical and nursing care requirements of this age group. Whether the child is seen in an area that treats only children or one that treats patients of all ages, certain aspects must be addressed prospectively to ensure family-oriented, high-quality, effective care.

CLINICAL ASPECTS

Traditional components of triage, history, physical examination, laboratory assessment, and management are essential (Box 2-1). Children who require emergent care should be treated, irrespective of formal consent. Adults generally cannot make decisions that significantly jeopardize the health of a child through the refusal of care. Emancipated minors are those who live apart from their parents, are self-supporting, and are not subject to parental control as well as those individuals who are married, pregnant, or members of the armed forces. Many states have special provisions related to venereal disease, pregnancy, and drug-related problems.

Federal regulations—Emergency Medical Treatment and Labor Act (EMTALA) and Consolidated Omnibus Budget Reconciliation Act (COBRA)—require a screening examination for all patients presenting to an ED and establish specific guidelines for consideration in transferring patients, particularly those who might be considered unstable.

Box 2-1

INITIAL NURSING ASSESSMENT OF PEDIATRIC PATIENTS

1. Age
2. Chief complaint: history of present illness (brief), recent interventions, and contacts with health professionals/facilities
3. Previous medical history
4. Weight
5. Medications
6. Allergies
7. Immunizations: identify any deficiencies and encourage parent to make health maintenance appointment at usual health care facility
8. Source of routine care

Note:

Vital signs and laboratory tests must be individualized for each patient. Oximetry is generally done in all patients with altered mental status/behavior, abnormal vital signs, or respiratory signs/symptoms.

If abnormalities in pulse, respiration, oximetry, or blood pressure are recorded, notify MD immediately.

Antipyretic should be initiated in children with temperatures about 39° C if none has been given in the past 2-4 hr (e.g., acetaminophen 15 mg/kg/dose PO or ibuprofen 10/mg/kg dose PO).

Any patient seen at a health care facility earlier in the day and brought back within a few hours is a source of concern. Notify MD.

Document concerns about parenting and home environment, if any.

In the pediatric arena, the most common basis for liability claims is "failure to diagnose." Claims related to a missed diagnosis of meningitis, fracture, or appendicitis are most common.

Beyond the traditional clinical components of the evaluation, it is essential to respond to the relatively transient nature of the interface between patients and health professionals. This requires some specific attention to routine health maintenance in children, including identifying a PCP and determining immunization status. Although the issue is controversial, many believe that actively utilizing the ED to update immunizations is ineffective because of the inability to ascertain status and parental refusal to accept immunizations in the ED. Follow-up is improved when the PCP is notified in a timely manner of the ED visit. Among many factors, noncompliance is associated with a parental belief that the child was not seriously ill and with ED visits for which laboratory tests were not performed.

Ongoing quality improvement programs should be initiated specific to diagnostic categories and evaluations of children.

DESIGN

Physical constraints are often produced by waiting areas, room design, and layout. Pediatric patients should be cared for in well-defined areas, ideally with some physical separation. Space should be provided to facilitate parental presence during procedures; parental presence has not been documented to negatively affect the ability to perform a procedure. Observation and monitoring capacity should be incorporated into the structure. A variety of observation unit structures within either the ED area or the inpatient unit have been established. It is estimated that approximately 150 patients per 10,000 pediatric ED visits could benefit from an observation unit whereby patients are discharged within 24 hours of admission. Play areas, toys, and other mechanisms for distracting anxious children should be provided. Waiting times should be monitored because perception of parents is often inaccurate and is a central issue in achieving patient and parental satisfaction.

EQUIPMENT

Special age-specific equipment must be available in an organized fashion. Oximetry equipment, overhead warmers, and other relevant supplies should be present.

PERSONNEL

Staff must be trained and competent in the care of pediatric patients. Pediatric advanced life support training has provided a mechanism for preparing health professionals to care for children.

Physicians must ensure that the patient with a life-threatening problem who expresses only nonspecific complaints is readily identified. The nurse complements the physician's unique clinical skills with a broad psychosocial base that facilitates early evaluation.

Emergency physicians and pediatric emergency physicians should staff the ED, with appropriate pediatric and surgical expertise

TABLE 2-1 Major Pediatric Triage Categories*

Emergent

ABNORMAL VITAL SIGNS

Age	Systolic BP (mm Hg)	Pulse (beats/min)	Respirations (breaths/min)
0-2 yr	<60	<80	<15 or >40
2-5 yr	<70	<60	<10 or >30
>5 yr	<90	<50	<5 or >25

RESPIRATIONS
- Irregular
- Labored

PULSE
- Irregular
- Dysrhythmia

COMA (ALTERED MENTAL STATUS)

CYANOSIS

STATUS EPILEPTICUS

MULTIPLE OR MAJOR TRAUMA
- Head
  - Loss of consciousness
  - Altered mental status
  - Changing or asymmetric neurologic findings
  - Cerebrospinal fluid leak
  - Depressed fracture
- Neck or spinal injury
- Chest
- Abdomen
- Orthopedic
  - Two or more long bone fractures
  - Pelvic fracture
  - Potential neurovascular compromise
  - Amputation

MAJOR BURN

BLEEDING: ACUTE AND SIGNIFICANT

Urgent†
- Abuse, child
- Abuse, sexual
- Acute symptoms in child <2-3 mo
- ALTE or near-SIDS
- Behavioral alteration
- Bite, poisonous snake
- Bleeding, moderate
- Burn, moderate
- Dehydration
- Drowning (near)
- Eye: alkali, acid, or chemical burn
- Fever >40° C
- GI hemorrhage
- Headache: acute and severe
- History of apnea
- Hypertension
- Hyperthermia
- Hypothermia
- Neck pain or stiffness
- Pain: acute and severe
- Poisoning
- Rash (isolate patient)

ALTE, Apparent life-threatening event; *SIDS,* sudden infant death syndrome.

* If none of these emergent or urgent problems is present, the patient should be appropriately screened and treated according to normal facility flow patterns unless there is a complicating condition.

† May be emergent, depending on patient's condition. Repeat visits or very anxious parents may require that the visit be categorized as urgent.

readily available. The certification of pediatric emergency medicine physicians and the expanded pediatric training based on emergency medicine residencies provide greater expertise in the stabilization of children.

Support staff from radiology, laboratory, respiratory therapy, and other departments should be oriented to the care of the pediatric patient.

Personnel must function independently and interdependently. Communication is vital for all members of the health care team. It provides the basis for team functioning and ensures a coordinated effort.

PROTOCOLS

Protocols specific for the pediatric patient should be developed, or a book such as this one should be readily available for reference. A triage system needs to be established. Decisions must be made on the basis of a short history, vital signs, and brief physical assessment. Tables 2-1 and 2-2 provide a foundation for triage and effective screening that may serve as a basis for formalizing this

TABLE 2-2 Initial Nursing Assessment: Pediatric Patients

	PROCEDURES							
Condition	**Temp**	**Resp**	**Pulse**	**BP**	**CBC**	**UA**	**Other**	**Comments**
Abdominal pain	+		+	±O	±	+	± β-hCG	
Anemia			+	±O	+		Oximetry	Do reticulocyte count, assess diet
Asthma	+	+	+	+			Oximetry	Assess medications; nebulizer
Behavioral alteration	+	+	+	+	±	+	Glucose,* electrolytes, ± LP	Exhaustive work-up required, monitor, oximetry
Burn	+	+	+	+	±	+	± Electrolytes	Notify MD if >5%
Child abuse	+	+	+	+		+	Growth parameters	Reassure, observe
Communicable disease	+	+	+	+				Isolate patient
Cough	+	+					Oximetry	
Croup	+	+					Oximetry	Notify MD, ±IV,
Diabetic ketoacidosis	+	+	+	+O		+	Glucose,* acetone	electrolytes, pH
Diarrhea	+	+	+	±O	±	+	± Electrolytes, capillary refill	Assess hydration; also hematuria or proteinuria
Dysuria (painful urination)	+			+		+ and urine culture		
Earache	+	+	+					
Eye infection	+	+						
Eye injury								Screen vision
Fever <2 mo old	+	+	+		+	+	Oximetry	Notify MD
>2-3 mo old	+	+	+			+	Oximetry	+ Antipyretics
Head injury		+	+	+			Oximetry	Do brief neurologic examination

process. Obviously, many of the management approaches outlined in *Emergency Pediatrics*, 6th edition, must be individualized for a specific institution. Referral, transport, and follow-up protocols should be established.

Emergency medical services for children (EMS-C) should be organized within the emergency medical services system to ensure appropriate ED preparation. Prevention, access, prehospital care, ED care, inpatient services, and rehabilitation are all central components that must be considered as protocols and systems are developed. The growth of children who have special needs or are technologically dependent adds a further challenge to the entire EMS-C. Emergency information forms for children with special needs are available online (*www.aap.org* or *www.acep.org*). Transport considerations for all children are discussed in Chapter 3. A coordinated approach for children will improve care and ensure access to an efficient and high-quality level of emergency care during times of stress and tremendous need. Within this environment, sharing, communication, and trust can ensure optimal patient care.

TABLE 2-2 Initial Nursing Assessment: Pediatric Patients—cont'd

	PROCEDURES							
Condition	**Temp**	**Resp**	**Pulse**	**BP**	**CBC**	**UA**	**Other**	**Comments**
Headache	+		+	+				Do brief neurologic examination; ± vision screen
Ingestion		+	+	+		+	± Toxicology screen, oximetry	Obtain history, do neurologic examination, ± ipecac/lavage, ± charcoal/cathartic, prevention talk
Laceration			+	±O				Clean; ± apply pressure
Nosebleed			+	±O	±			Apply pressure
Rash	+							± Isolate patient
Seizure	+	+	+	+			Glucose*, oximetry	Give O_2, maintain airway, monitor, ± IV, ± antipyretics, do neurologic examination
Sore throat	+	+					± Throat culture	± Rapid strep screen
Sprain/fracture			±	±O			X-ray study	
Vaginal bleeding		+	+	±O	+		β-hCG	± Ultrasound
Vomiting	+	+	+	±O	±	+	± Electrolytes, capillary refill	Assess hydration

The initial assessment steps noted for a specific condition are the minimal required database. Generally, temperature, pulse, and respiratory rate are obtained on all patients. Oximetry, capillary refill, and blood pressure are individualized in some settings. The patient's presentation, history, and level of toxicity may suggest the need for additional initial nursing evaluation.
+, Perform procedure; *±,* perform if indicated by patient's condition; *O,* obtain orthostatic BP if appropriate; *BP,* blood pressure; *CBC,* complete blood count; *UA,* urinalysis.
* May be performed initially by bedside techniques (Dextrostix or Chemstrip).

BIBLIOGRAPHY

American Academy of Pediatrics, Committee on Pediatric Emergency Medicine and American College of Emergency Medicine: Care of children in the emergency department: guidelines for preparedness *Pediatrics* 707:777, 2001.

Baker DW, Stevens CD, Brook RH: Determinants of emergency department use by ambulatory patients at an urban public hospital, *Ann Emerg Med* 25:311, 1995.

Baucher H, Vinci R, Bak S et al: Parents and procedures: a randomized controlled trial, *Pediatrics* 98:861, 1996.

Boie ET, Moore GP, Brummett C et al: Do parents want to be present during invasive procedures on their children in the emergency department? *Ann Emerg Med* 34:70, 1999.

Bond GR, Wiegand CB: Estimated use of a pediatric emergency department observation unit, *Ann Emerg Med* 29:739, 1997.

Emergency Medical Services, National Task Force on Children with Special Health Care Needs: EMS for children: recommendations for coordinating care for children with special health care needs, *Ann Emerg Med* 30:274, 1997.

Foltin GL, Tunik MG: Emergency medical services for children: organizational and operational principles. In Barkin RM, editor: *Pediatric emergency medicine: concepts and clinical practice,* ed 2, St Louis, 1997, Mosby.

Gausche M, Rutherford M, Lewis RL: Emergency department quality assurance/improvement practices for the pediatric patient, *Ann Emerg Med* 25:804, 1995.

Goodman DC, Fisher ES, Gittelsohn A et al: When are children hospitalized? The role of non-clinical factors in pediatric hospitalization, *Pediatrics* 93:896, 1994.

King C, Nilsen GJ, Henretig FM et al: Proposed fellowship training program in pediatric emergency medicine for emergency medicine graduates, *Ann Emerg Med* 22:542, 1993.

Leffler S, Hayes M: Analysis of parental estimates of children's weights in the ED, *Ann Emerg Med* 30:167, 1997.

Mower WR, Sachs C, Nickline EL et al: Pulse oximetry as a fifth pediatric vital sign, *Pediatrics* 99:681, 1997.

Robinson PE, Gausche M, Gerardi MJ et al: Immunization of the pediatric patients in the emergency department, *Ann Emerg Med* 28:334, 1996.

Rodewald LE, Szilagyi PG, Humiston SG et al: Effect of emergency department immunization rates and subsequent primary care visits, *Arch Pediatr Adolesc Med* 150:1271, 1996.

Sacchetti A, Lichenstein R, Carracaio CA et al: Family member presence during pediatric emergency department procedures, *Pediatr Emerg Care* 12:2688, 1996.

Scarfone RJ, Jaffe MD, Wiley JF et al: Noncompliance with scheduled revisits to a pediatric emergency department, *Arch Pediatr Adolesc Med* 150:948, 1996.

Storgion SA: Care of the technology-dependent child, *Pediatr Ann* 25:677, 1996.

Thompson DA, Yarnold PR, Adams SL et al: How accurate are waiting time perceptions of patients in the emergency department? *Ann Emerg Med* 28:652, 1996.

Weinberg JA, Medearis DN: Emergency medical services for children: the report of the Institute of Medicine, *Pediatrics* 93:821, 1994.

Zimmerman DR, McCarten-Gibbs KA, DeNoble DH et al: Repeat pediatric visits to a general emergency department, *Ann Emerg Med* 28:467, 1996.

3 Transport of the Pediatric Patient

Systems for pediatric care in the emergency department (ED) must be established to provide for prehospital stabilization and transport of patients as well as for interhospital transport to ensure appropriate care within the emergency medical services system. Children account for 5% to 10% of all ambulance runs; 0.3% to 0.5% of transported children need tertiary care, and 5% of cases involve potentially life-threatening problems. Younger children often have medical problems, whereas children older than 2 years have predominantly traumatic conditions.

Pediatric patients in the prehospital setting are often a source of inordinate anxiety, primarily because of the inexperience of prehospital care providers with this age group. However, the principles of resuscitation and management that are used every day for older patients parallel those used for the younger patient. Judgment forms the basis for management of emergency situations.

The prehospital care provider enters the patient's environment. Paramedics and emergency medical technicians develop "street sense," an ability to create order out of chaos: to "read" the scene, the people, and the emotions, and then to intervene. Personnel, education and training, and equipment must be provided. Management strategies and protocols must be established. The concept of "pick up and run" is not uniformly appropriate, given the current sophistication of prehospital care. Each action must be individualized to the particular circumstances, patient's stability, anticipated length of transport, and so on, and close coordination with the base station and receiving hospital is essential. The expansion of technology, such as the development of ventilators that facilitate home care, enhances the complexity of patients encountered in the prehospital setting. A warm and safe environment must be provided. Aggressive management should be maintained throughout the transport.

Field triage, using specific criteria, has been developed and may be useful in communication with the base station and in assessment of outcome. Trauma scores such as the Champion and Pediatric Trauma Scores are discussed in Chapter 56, and the Glasgow Coma Scale in Chapter 57.

The prehospital setting presents additional unique difficulties when the death of a child is involved. Controversy abounds regarding the best approach when death seems apparent, but many believe that the standard should be to initiate all-out resuscitative efforts and to expedite transport to an ED. This resuscitation can obviously be modified by the base station in circumstances involving major trauma, nonaccidental injuries, sudden infant death syndrome (SIDS), the family's acceptance of the outcome, or an obviously nonviable child.

INTERHOSPITAL TRANSPORT

Patients' conditions may be stabilized at an institution that does not have adequate staff and equipment to deal with the acute or long-term medical problems of a child. Transfer becomes a priority. The Emergency Medical Treatment and Labor Act has established specific guidelines for transport of the unstable patient.

Before transport can be considered, resuscitation must be initiated and immediate therapy instituted. The airway must be assessed and stabilized; adequate ventilation must be ensured, often through administration of oxygen and active airway management. An intravenous line (or lines) should be started to permit fluid resuscitation and administration of lifesaving medications.

An urgent evaluation is appropriate. The physical examination should be completed, baseline laboratory values obtained, and x-ray examinations performed as indicated by the apparent medical or traumatic condition. Early pharmacologic therapy, including administration of antibiotics, anticonvulsants, β-adrenergic agents, and bronchodilators, should be initiated as necessary. Traumatic injuries may require surgical, neurosurgical, or orthopedic intervention before transport.

Once stabilization has been achieved, the physician must carefully analyze facilities that can adequately care for the child in terms of personnel, equipment, and distance. Special needs such as dialysis, intensive care, and cardiac catheterization programs should be considered. The institution selected should be contacted, and transport discussed and arranged. It is imperative that communication at this time be adequate between the physicians and nursing staffs at the two hospitals to ensure a smooth transfer of the patient. Specific transfer forms must be completed and signed, including a clear delineation of the risks and benefits of transfer, and documentation of communication with the receiving institution.

The mechanism of transfer should be a joint decision of the referring and receiving institutions, focusing on equipment, speed, distance, weather, traffic patterns, and level of expertise of medical personnel required to care for the child. Many communities have access to formal ground (ambulance) or air (helicopter or airplane) transport systems that are particularly useful for critically ill patients who will be admitted to an intensive care unit on arrival at the receiving hospital or who may experience respiratory, cardiovascular, or neurologic deterioration during transport. Clinicians should know how to arrange for transport through these systems.

Active management of the patient must continue until transfer of care to the receiving hospital or transport team. Concurrently, charts, x-ray films, laboratory results, and past records should be duplicated and readied for transport with the patient. Intravenous lines and tubes should be secured and fractures stabilized to prevent disruption.

Parents and patients should be involved throughout the resuscitation and stabilization processes to help them feel comfortable with the transfer and understand its benefits.

BIBLIOGRAPHY

Baker MD, Ludwig S: Pediatric emergency transport and the private practitioner, *Pediatrics* 88:691, 1991.

Day S, McCloskey K, Orr R et al: Pediatric interhospital critical care transport: consensus of a national leadership conference, *Pediatrics* 88:696, 1991.

Dernocoeur K: *Streetsense*, Bowie, Md, 1985, Brady Communication.

McCloskey KA, Orr RA: Interhospital transport. In Barkin RM, editor: *Pediatric emergency medicine: concepts and clinical practice*, ed 2, St Louis, 1997, Mosby.

Woodward GA, Insoft RM, Pearson-Shaver AL et al: The state of pediatric interfacility transport: consensus of the second National Pediatric and Neonatal Interfacility Transport Medicine Leadership Conference, *Pediatr Emerg Care* 18:38, 2002.

4 Cardiopulmonary Arrest

Also See Chapters 5 (Shock), 6 (Dysrhythmias), 7 (Dehydration), 9 (Resuscitation in the Delivery Room)

ALERT Cardiopulmonary arrest in children is commonly respiratory in origin, emphasizing the importance of stabilization of the airway, breathing, and then circulation (the ABCs). The coordinated effort of a team of professionals is required for optimal care.

The outcome of cardiopulmonary arrests in children is poor, reaching a 90% mortality rate in some studies. Most of the patients (87%) have an underlying disease. In contrast, respiratory arrest has been associated with a mortality rate of 25% to 33%; most affected children are younger than 1 year. Mortality is affected by whether the arrest occurs in the prehospital or hospital setting. Survival is better in the emergency department (ED) than in the prehospital setting but worse than in an inpatient arrest. Out-of-hospital cardiac arrests in children younger than 18 years are commonly a result of sudden infant death syndrome (SIDS), drowning, and respiratory arrest, and they occur most commonly in children less than 1 year. In survivors, 70% of patients with arrest had good neurologic outcomes, those experiencing a respiratory arrest having a better outcome (88%).

ANTICIPATING CARDIOPULMONARY ARREST

Progressive deterioration of respiratory and ultimately circulatory function may lead to cardiopulmonary arrest in infants and children. The underlying condition is usually ***respiratory*** in origin, stemming from obstruction and hypoxia, secondarily leading to cardiac arrest. Hypoxia may be acute or chronic, resulting from either an acquired or underlying disease. Respiratory arrest and hypoxia almost always precede cardiac standstill; with careful observation, signs of these two conditions can be recognized, and the progression prevented.

Respiratory failure is recognizable in the compensated state. Prevention can be facilitated by noting abnormal respirations characterized by tachypnea, bradypnea, apnea, or increased work of breathing.

Decompensation of ***cardiac*** function leads to a shock state associated with impaired cardiac output. Excessive output from stool or vomitus or inadequate intake is often contributory. Tachycardia, hypotension (note orthostatic changes), and poor peripheral circulation are present. Ultimately, impaired perfusion causes delayed capillary refill time (>2 seconds), mottling, cyanosis, cool skin, altered level of consciousness, poor muscle tone, and finally, decreased urine output.

Recognizing this typical pattern may prevent dysfunction from progressing to failure and arrest. Intervention can then be initiated in a timely and effective manner.

Etiology

The precipitating causes of a catastrophic event can often be identified and prevented:

1. Respiratory disease (see Chapters 20 and 84)

   a. Upper airway obstruction: croup, epiglottitis, foreign body, suffocation, strangulation, and trauma
   b. Lower airway disease: pneumonia, asthma, bronchiolitis, foreign body aspiration, near-drowning, smoke inhalation, and pulmonary edema
2. Infection: sepsis and meningitis (infection may be the underlying process leading to respiratory or circulatory compromise)
3. Intoxication: narcotic depressants, sedatives, and antidysrhythmics (see Chapter 54)
4. Cardiac disorders: congenital heart disease, myocarditis, pericarditis, and dysrhythmias, often associated with congestive heart failure and pulmonary edema
5. Shock: cardiogenic, hypovolemic, or distributive (see Chapter 5)
6. Central nervous system: meningitis, encephalitis, head trauma, anoxia, and other causes of hypoventilation (see Chapter 81)
7. Trauma or environment: multiple organ failure, child abuse, hypothermia or hyperthermia, and near-drowning
8. Metabolic: hypoglycemia, hypocalcemia, and hyperkalemia
9. Near-SIDS or apparent life-threatening event (ALTE) (see Chapter 22)

The causes of cardiopulmonary arrest in children may also be divided according to age group. *Newborn* causes primarily are prematurity, uteroplacental insufficiency, congenital malformations, sepsis, and nuchal cord. Problems in *infancy* include SIDS, child abuse, pulmonary or congenital heart disease, ingestions, congenital malformations, and sepsis. *Adolescents* experience cardiopulmonary arrest primarily from trauma, drug overdose, dysrhythmias, and congenital heart disease.

TEAM APPROACH

The management of cardiorespiratory arrest in children requires the combined efforts of several professionals working as a team. The team captain must be immediately identifiable and must provide direction, expertise, and coordination in a precise way. This individual must be responsible for ensuring that everything gets done; he or she should delegate responsibilities rather than assuming them single-handedly. Beyond dealing with the immediate logistics of procedures and medication and monitoring their effects, the leader must also be able to delineate issues that are crucial to the outcome and that may alter management:

1. Etiology
   a. What condition(s) preceded the arrest?
   b. What process caused the arrest (i.e., hypoxia, hypovolemia)?
   c. Why is the patient in shock (hypovolemic, distributive, or cardiogenic)?
   d. Why are we having difficulty oxygenating or ventilating the patient?
   e. Have we considered reversible causes:
      4H's: *H*ypoxemia, *h*ypovolemia, *h*ypothermia, *h*yper/hypokalemia and metabolic (hypoglycemia)
      4T's: *T*amponade, *t*ension pneumothorax, *t*oxins/poisons/drugs, *t*hromboembolism (pulmonary)
2. Time
   a. How long have we been treating the patient?
   b. How much time has elapsed since cardiopulmonary resuscitation (CPR) was initiated, and how long was the patient in arrest before CPR was begun?
3. End point: When do we stop, and what criteria do we have for stopping?
4. Evaluation
   a. Can we learn about our performance from this resuscitation?
   b. How can we improve techniques, equipment, personnel training, and team functioning?

BASIC LIFE SUPPORT (Table 4-1)

Basic life support of the child provides immediate intervention until additional capabilities are available. The basic principles parallel those evolved for adults. The importance of the elements known as the ABCs cannot be overemphasized. These elements are stabilizing the ***airway,*** establishing adequate ***breathing,*** and facilitating ***circulation.*** Basic CPR using the ABCs should be interrupted only for defibrillation or intubation. Following is a list of the skills and procedures of the ABCs. They require practice and repetition.

1. Establish unresponsiveness or respiratory difficulty. Gently shake the patient; if conscious, he or she should display motor activity.
2. Position the patient supine, on a firm, flat surface. Do not subject the patient to further injury.
3. Open the airway using the head tilt–chin lift method (place hand closer to child's head on forehead and gently tilt head back into a "sniffing" position).
4. Assess breathing to ensure air movement by demonstrating movement of the chest or abdomen with ventilation, by feeling air moving through the mouth, or by hearing noise during expiration. Look, feel, and listen. Assess use of accessory muscles.
5. If the patient is an infant who is not breathing, cover both the mouth and the nose (mouth to nose and mouth) and establish a seal. If the child is too large, cover the child's mouth (mouth to mouth) while pinching the nose.
6. Give two slow breaths, using enough volume to cause the chest to rise. If air enters freely, the airway is clear. If air does not enter, the airway is obstructed (see item number 12).
7. Begin rescue breathing if breathing is not noted.
8. Assess for cardiac function. Lay rescuers should check for signs of circulation, which include normal breathing, coughing, and movement in response to

TABLE 4-1 Basic Life Support Procedures

	Infant (<1 yr)	Child (1-8 yr)	Adult
AIRWAY	Head tilt-chin lift (if trauma present, use jaw thrust)		
BREATHING	Initially, 2 breaths at 1.0-1.5 sec (adult 2 sec)/breath, then		
	20 breaths/min	20 breaths/min	12 breaths/min
CIRCULATION			
Pulse check†	Brachial	Carotid	Carotid
Site of compression over sternum	1 fingerwidth below intermammary line	Lower half	Lower half
Mechanism	2-3 fingers*	Heel of hand	Two hands
Rate/min	At least 100	100	100
COMPRESSION: VENTILATION RATIO‡			
	5:1	5:1	15:2
FOREIGN BODY OBSTRUCTION			
	Back blow-chest thrust	Abdominal thrust	Abdominal thrust

* Two thumbs encircling for two-rescuer CPR.
† Lay rescuer should check for signs of circulation.
‡ Pause for ventilation.

the 2 rescue breaths. Health care providers may assess the brachial or femoral arteries in infants less than 1 year old. The carotid artery should be used in older children.

9. Begin chest compressions if no pulse is present.
   a. In infants less than 1 year old, thoracic squeeze using two-thumb chest compression is performed with 2-rescuer CPR. Compress one fingerbreadth below the imaginary line between the nipples on the sternum.
   b. In older children, compress over the lower half of the sternum.
   c. Some clinicians have suggested that the compression rate be increased to more than 100 per min to improve coronary perfusion pressure.
10. In children younger than 8 years, the lone rescuer should call for help "fast" because respiratory problems are likely.
11. Coordinate compressions and breathing. In the infant, a 5:1 compression/ventilation ratio is maintained; in older victims the ratio should be 15:2.
12. Upper airway foreign body may be present; if so, urgent intervention is required (p. 808).
   a. In the infant (<1 year), do five back blows with the child straddled over the rescuer's arm. Then do five chest thrusts at the location described for chest compressions. Repeat until obstruction is relieved.
   b. If the conscious child is more than 1 year, perform a Heimlich maneuver or abdominal thrust. Repeat until obstruction is relieved.
   c. In the unconscious child, visible obstructing objects should be removed and standard CPR initiated by lay rescuers. If ventilation is unsuccessful, reposition the head and resume efforts. Blind finger sweeps should not be done by lay rescuers.

ADVANCED LIFE SUPPORT

Basic life support must be initiated immediately and followed by advanced life support and more sophisticated intervention on the basis of stabilization of the airway, breathing, and circulation.

Specific components of the resuscitation that must be emphasized and are unique to children include the following:

1. Children usually respond to initial airway, ventilation, and fluid therapy; additional interventions should be individualized.
2. All drugs, medications, invasive catheters, and tubes must be age and weight specific. Children should be monitored aggressively as appropriate. The Broselow tape facilitates determination of appropriate medication doses and equipment sizes on the basis of body length as a proxy for weight.
3. Fluid resuscitation must reflect the child's size and volume. Intravascular fluid is about 80 ml/kg. Laboratory studies requiring extensive blood samples should be minimized.
4. Children are developing physically and psychologically, and the team must be responsive to the needs of the child and family.
5. Iatrogenic injuries may occur in as many as 3% of patients undergoing CPR, including retroperitoneal hemorrhage and pneumothorax.

Airway

Anatomic differences between children and adults may be considered in approaching stabilization of the child's airway.

1. The child's head and occiput are proportionately larger, causing neck flexion and airway obstruction when the child is supine. Moderate extension is necessary.
2. The tongue is relatively larger with less muscle tone.
3. The epiglottis is shorter, narrower, more horizontal, and softer.

4. The larynx is more anterior and higher (cephalad), located at the C2 level in children but at the C6 level in adults.
5. The trachea is shorter, raising the enhanced risk of a right main stem intubation.
6. The airway is narrower, increasing airway resistance. The cricoid is the narrowest portion.
7. Lymphoid tissue is hypertrophied.

It is useful to recognize a "difficult" airway early. This is particularly important when induction agents and neuromuscular blockade are being considered. The physical examination may be predictive:

1. Mouth: limited opening, small, short mandible, large tongue, prominent central incisors
2. Short neck
3. Cervical spine immobility (immobilization, trauma, congenital)
4. Obese child
5. Laryngeal edema
6. Mandibular, midface, or facial trauma

An airway should be established to ensure patency, facilitate suctioning, prevent aspiration, or administer drugs. Patency should be established by one of the techniques outlined. The options are restricted if there is a question of neck trauma.

The following adjuncts to airway management may be used in conjunction with appropriate barrier devices and universal precautions:

1. Oxygen: administered by hood, mask, or cannula: 3 to 6 L/min by mask or cannula produces a forced inspiratory oxygen (FiO_2) of 40% to 50%. To achieve higher oxygen (O_2) concentrations, a mask with reservoir is required (100% or nonrebreathing bag).
2. Oropharyngeal airway: a semicircular apparatus of plastic curved to fit over the back of the tongue and inserted into the lower posterior pharynx. It is introduced into the mouth backward and rotated as it approaches the posterior wall of the pharynx near the back of the tongue (poorly tolerated in conscious patients).
3. Nasopharyngeal airway: a soft rubber or plastic tube inserted into the nose close to the midline along the floor of the nostril and into the posterior pharynx behind the tongue (tolerated fairly well in conscious patients).
4. Self-inflating bag-valve ventilation is usually effective (see p. 24). Studies have demonstrated that outcomes of out-of-hospital bag-valve-mask ventilation are equivalent to those of endotracheal (ET) intubation.
   a. Neonatal size (250 ml) for premature infants. May be inadequate for full-term neonates and infants, who may require a minimum value of 450 ml.
   b. Infant size (450 ml) for full-term neonates, infants, and children.
   c. Adult size (1600 ml). When large bags are used, care must be taken to use only that force and tidal volume necessary to produce effective chest expansion.
   d. If a pop-off valve is present, it should usually be bypassed because pressures required for adequate ventilation during CPR may exceed the pop-off limit. This is especially true in patients with poor lung compliance.
   e. Self-inflating bag delivers 21% unless supplemental oxygen is provided. A reservoir permits delivery of concentrations of 60% to 95% at a flow of 10% to 15% oxygen.
   f. Two hands are needed, one to create a tight seal between the mask and face and the other to compress the bag.
5. Laryngeal mask airway (LMA): The LMA has a wide-bore tube with a 15-mm adapter at the proximal end for connection to a breathing circuit. At the distal end is an elliptical mask that is inflated through a pilot balloon and conforms to the shape of the larynx. It potentially fills

the gap between self-inflating bag-valve-mask and ET intubation. Available in six sizes, the LMA is passed without visualization into the hypopharynx. It is not useful when there is high airway resistance, pharyngeal disease, low pulmonary compliance, an intact gag reflex, or a small mouth. The LMA also carries a potential risk for aspiration and damage to facial or pharyngeal structures. Drugs may not be administered through the LMA.

6. Endotracheal intubation: provides and protects a stable airway for more efficient ventilation. The size of the ET tube varies with the age and size of the child but may be estimated by selecting a tube that approximates the diameter of the patient's little (fifth) finger. An estimate also may be made by adding 16 to the child's age in years (up to 16 years) and dividing this total by 4 ([Age + 16]/4). In children younger than 7 or 8 years, uncuffed tubes are used because the airway is narrowest at the cricoid in this age group; cuffed tubes are used in older children. Cuffed tubes must be treated as if they were 0.5 mm larger in size (e.g., 6.0 mm cuffed = 6.5 mm uncuffed tube). Although patient-to-patient variability exists, the following guidelines may be useful in estimating the correct tube size (see Appendix B-2):

Age	Tube Size (mm)	Suction Catheter (Fr)
Newborn	3.0	6
1 mo	3.5	8
6 mo	3.5	8
1 yr	4.0	8
2-3 yr	4.5	8
4-5 yr	5.0	10
6-8 yr	6.0	10
10-12 yr	6.5	12
16 yr	7.0	12
Adult female	7.0-8.0	12
Adult male	7.5-8.5	14

a. Prepare by checking the laryngoscope to ensure adequate functioning and light source. Be certain that suction is available. In the newborn, a DeLee trap suction may be helpful. If a stylet is used, it should not protrude beyond the tip of the ET tube. Lighted stylets and endoscopic laryngoscopes are available.

b. Oxygenate the patient and attach a heart monitor. Position the patient in sniffing position.

c. Visualize the esophagus, epiglottis, and cords. Laryngeal pressure may be helpful.

d. Whether intubating the patient orally or nasotracheally, watch the tube pass through the cords, and pass it 1 to 2 cm beyond.

e. If the patient becomes bradycardic or cyanotic, abort the procedure, administer oxygen, and ventilate. Start again once signs have stabilized.

f. Gastric inflation can be reduced by cricoid pressure (Sellick maneuver).

g. Check the position of the tube by listening on both sides of upper chest and stomach. Make sure the tube is not in the right stem bronchus or esophagus. Confirm by x-ray film, if possible. The tip should be at the T2 to T3 vertebral level or at the level of the lower edge of the medial aspect of the clavicle. Further confirmation can be achieved by using end-tidal CO_2 detectors. Colorimetric, semi-quantitative monitors are available.

h. Stabilize the tube with adhesive tape or other device. The skin to which adhesive tape is to be affixed should be cleansed and dried, followed by an application of tincture of benzoin.

i. Blind nasotracheal intubation is relatively safe in the hypoventilating patient. The tube may also be introduced under direct visualization.

j. Common causes of emergencies in children with an artificial airway include **D**isplacement of the tube, **O**bstruction of the tube, **P**neumothorax, or **E**quipment failure. Mnemonic is **DOPE**.

7. Cricothyroidotomy is indicated as a temporizing measure in children more than 3 years old when acute upper airway obstruction cannot otherwise be relieved. It is rarely needed, however.
8. If unable to ventilate on an emergent basis with intubation, bag and mask, or cricothyroidotomy (not readily available as alternative), a 14-gauge catheter over the needle may be inserted into the cricothyroid membrane. The adapter from a 3 Fr nasotracheal or ET tube may be inserted into the Luer adapter of the catheter for application of oxygen and positive pressure for a limited time.
9. Patients with pure respiratory arrest not associated with trauma often respond rapidly to bag-and-mask or mouth-to-mouth (or mouth-to-mouth and nose) ventilation. However, if no response is seen, intubation should be considered. Respiratory arrests complicated by such findings as cyanosis and hypotension usually require intubation.
10. Prophylactic intubation of nontraumatized patients in the ED setting is rarely indicated because of a concern about depression of respirations resulting from pharmacologic management of diseases such as seizures with diazepam (Valium), lorazepam (Ativan), or phenobarbital and of agitation with sedatives. Flumazenil (Mazicon) may be a useful agent to reverse the effects of benzodiazepine overdose. Intubate when necessary.
11. Although judgment ultimately becomes the prime determinant of a patient's need for intubation, each situation must be individualized to consider the patient's condition, the progression of disease, potential therapeutic maneuvers, and availability of personnel and equipment.

Muscle Relaxants. Muscle relaxants may be required to achieve intubation; this is sometimes the case in patients with excessive muscle tone, as seen with seizures, tetanus, or neurologic disease. Obviously, the problems inherent in using such agents relate to the inability to further evaluate the patient neurologically and the potential inability to intubate the patient after relaxation, aspiration, and dysrhythmias.

Neuromuscular blocking agents may either cause or prevent depolarizing of the end-plate (if a nondepolarizing or competitive agent is used).

Succinylcholine is the classic depolarizing agent and is contraindicated in patients with hyperkalemia, burns, glaucoma, penetrating ocular injury, and increased intracranial pressure.

The patient's anatomy is initially evaluated with a search for oral or dental abnormalities, trauma to the neck or face, and systemic abnormalities. Equipment is checked.

One suggested protocol for controlled intubation with paralysis or rapid sequence intubation is as follows:

1. The patient is preoxygenated. If the patient is hypoventilating, hyperventilate while the Sellick maneuver is performed. Place a towel under the head of an adolescent or adult to elevate it about 10 cm off the bed.
2. Administer vecuronium (Norcuron), 0.01 mg/kg IV (adults: 1 mg IV), to reduce fasciculations. It is a nondepolarizing agent. Allow 3 to 5 minutes before proceeding with succinylcholine. This step is *not* necessary in children younger than 5 years.
3. Atropine, 0.01 to 0.02 mg/kg IV (minimum 0.10 mg/dose), may be given to children less than 5 years old to reduce bradycardia or if succinylcholine is used. In the presence of significant head injury, administer lidocaine, 1.0 to 1.5 mg/kg IV,

and allow 2 minutes before giving succinylcholine.

4. Sedate patient with thiopental, 3 to 5 mg/kg IV, if he or she is not hypotensive or in status asthmaticus.

Alternatives are as follows:

Normotensive	Midazolam, etomidate, thiopental, propofol
Hypotensive/hypovolemic	
Mild	Etomidate, ketamine, midazolam
Severe	Etomidate, ketamine, none
Head injury or status epilepticus	
Normotensive	Etomidate, thiopental, propofol
Hypotensive	Etomidate or low dose thiopental
Status asthmaticus	Ketamine or midazolam

5. Give succinylcholine, 1 to 1.5 mg/kg IV to adults and 2 mg/kg IV to children weighing less than 10 kg. Allow 45 to 60 seconds for muscle relaxation. Cricoid pressure should be maintained. Other choices of agents are vecuronium (0.1 mg/kg IV) or rocuronium (0.6-1.2 mg/kg IV).
6. Lidocaine (1 mg/kg IV) is commonly given to patients with head injuries prior to intubation.
7. Orally intubate the patient, verify position, and release cricoid pressure. When paralysis wears off, pancuronium, up to 0.1 mg/kg IV, may be used if needed.

Obviously, this procedure should be performed with tremendous caution if there is any concern about inability to intubate the patient.

Breathing

Breathing is demonstrated by detecting movement of the chest or abdomen with ventilation, by feeling air moving through the mouth, or by hearing noise during expiration.

1. Limit ventilation to the amount of air needed to cause the chest to rise (excessive volumes exacerbate gastric distension and increase the risk of pneumothorax).
2. Use a self-inflating bag-valve-mask ventilation system whenever possible, optimally with a pop-off valve or in-line manometer to override the pop-off valve. An oxygen reservoir is useful in increasing the oxygen concentration. Bags are available for neonates (stroke volume of 250-300 ml), infants and children (stroke volume of 550 to 600 ml), and adults (stroke volume of 1-1.5 L). Neonatal bags are usually inadequate for full-term neonates and infants; infant size should be used in these children. Tidal volume should be about 10 ml/kg. An oxygen reservoir should be used to enhance the oxygen concentration achieved:

Flow Rate (L/min)	Adult Bag FIO_2	Pediatric Bag FIO_2	Infant Bag FIO_2
5	—	59%	75%
10	67%	85%	94%
15	78%	95%	95%

Masks are available in infant, child, and adult sizes.

Circulation

Circulation is assessed by checking brachial, femoral, or carotid pulses, blood pressure, heart rate, and capillary refilling (normally <2 seconds).

All patients should be monitored, if possible.

1. Initiate external chest compressions if there is no effective pulse as described previously. Monitor pulse and blood pressure during compression. Children older than 1 year must be placed on a hard surface.
2. Intravenous cannulation for fluid and drug administration is achieved by a variety of peripheral modalities; most common is the catheter over the needle. The butterfly or scalp vein type of needle is helpful but less commonly used in the resuscitation setting. The size and type of catheter depend on the clinician's level of comfort and the availability of sites;

engineered needle devices are increasingly being used because of enhanced safety for the care provider. If access is difficult, rapid consideration of a cutdown or central line may be appropriate (Box 4-1).

3. Intraosseous infusion of crystalloid solution can be used as an alternative route for establishing venous access in children of any age. However, it is indicated only in life-threatening or potentially life-threatening situations in which intravenous cannulation is not achieved in a timely fashion.

   Insert a bone marrow needle or special intraosseous needle (less desirable alternative is a spinal needle or other similar device with a stylet) into the anterior tibia (midline flat surface of the tibia) 2 to 3 cm below the tibial tuberosity. Under aseptic conditions insert the needle perpendicular to the skin or directed inferiorly, away from the epiphysis.

   The needle is in the marrow when a lack of resistance is felt and the needle stands up by itself, bone marrow can be aspirated, and fluid runs in safely. The procedure is safe for infusion of crystalloid and a large number of drugs (see Appendix A-3).

4. *Atropine, epinephrine, lidocaine,* and *naloxone* can be administered by ET tube. Although the exact dosing by this route has not been established, it is suggested that the dose of epinephrine be larger than the initial IV dose. Instill the dose as deeply as possible into the tracheobronchial tree by using a catheter or feeding tube inserted beyond the distal tip of the ET tube. Dilution of the drug in 1 to 2 ml of saline solution may assist delivery.

5. Central venous catheters, preferably inserted into the internal jugular or femoral vein, may be used by the experienced practitioner for infusion or monitoring. Because most children have normal renal and cardiac function and respond rapidly to resuscitation, such monitoring is rarely required. If central venous pressure (CVP) monitoring is appropriate, the middle approach to the internal jugular cannulation is preferred but still carries a risk of lung puncture. Insert a guide wire and then a larger catheter (see Appendix A-3).

6. If there is any question of hypovolemia, give a rapid infusion of normal saline or lactated Ringer's solution at 20 ml/kg over 10 to 20 minutes; this may be repeated. If no response is seen, initiate further evaluation of fluid status on the basis of underlying conditions, the nature of the acute insult, and hemodynamic indications such as CVP, heart rate, blood pressure, and capillary refill. If the patient is considered normovolemic and shock persists, start dopamine, 5 to 20 µg/kg/min IV, and begin a rapid evaluation for shock (see Chapter 5).

Box 4-1

PRIORITIES FOR VASCULAR ACCESS

Attempt peripheral venous access. If not successful in timely fashion, consider alternative route.

FOR DRUGS

If endotracheal (ET) tube present, may give atropine, epinephrine, lidocaine, or naloxone. If no ET tube, consider intraosseous or central lines.

FOR CRYSTALLOID AND OTHER FLUIDS

Consider intraosseous, central, or surgical access.

Essential Medications and Measures

First-line drugs are given to virtually all patients who have a cardiopulmonary arrest that does

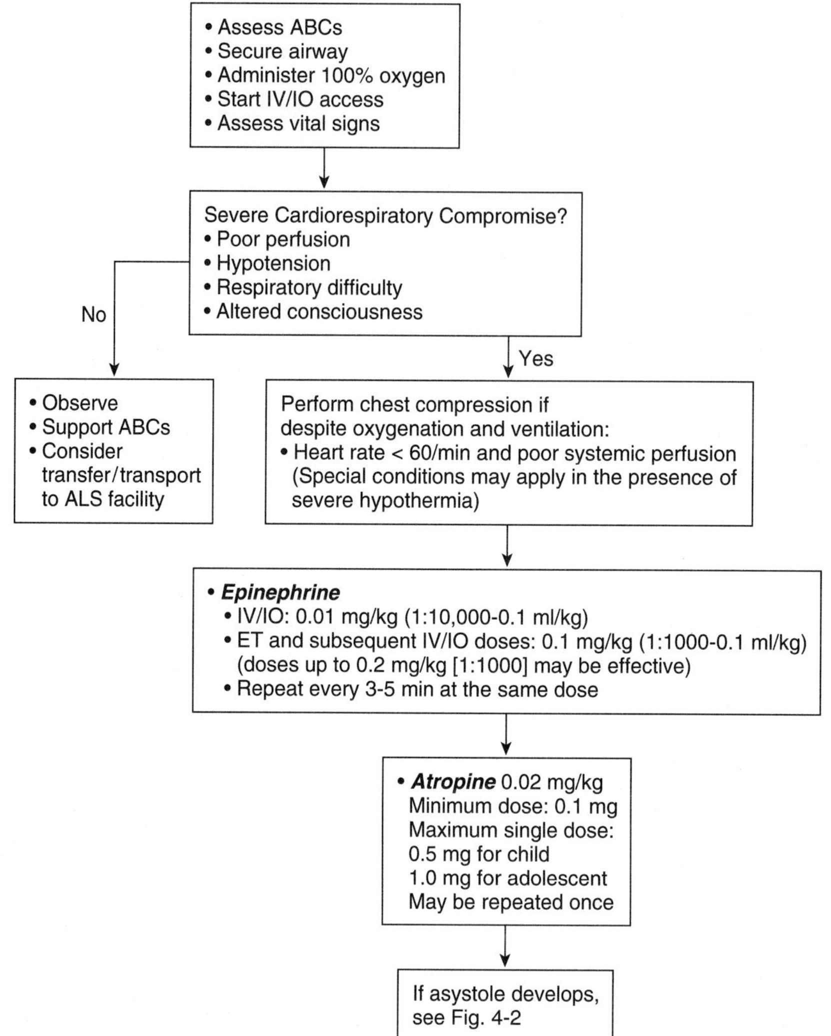

Fig. 4-1 Bradycardia decision tree. *ABC*, Airway, breathing, and circulation; *ALS*, Advanced life support; *ET*, endotracheal; *IO*, intraosseous; *IV*, intravenous.

(Modified from *JAMA* 268:2171, 1992. Copyright 1992, American Medical Association.)

not respond to initial airway and ventilatory intervention and support, as shown in Figs. 4-1 and 4-2. The recommendation of the International Liaison Committee on Resuscitation (ILCR) varies slightly in suggesting that 2 to 4 J/kg be used for the second and third shocks. Furthermore, lidocaine is not used with epinephrine, and the ILCR recommends up to three shocks. Although the guidelines outlined in these figures are standard protocols, working groups continue to develop consensus on these and other issues.

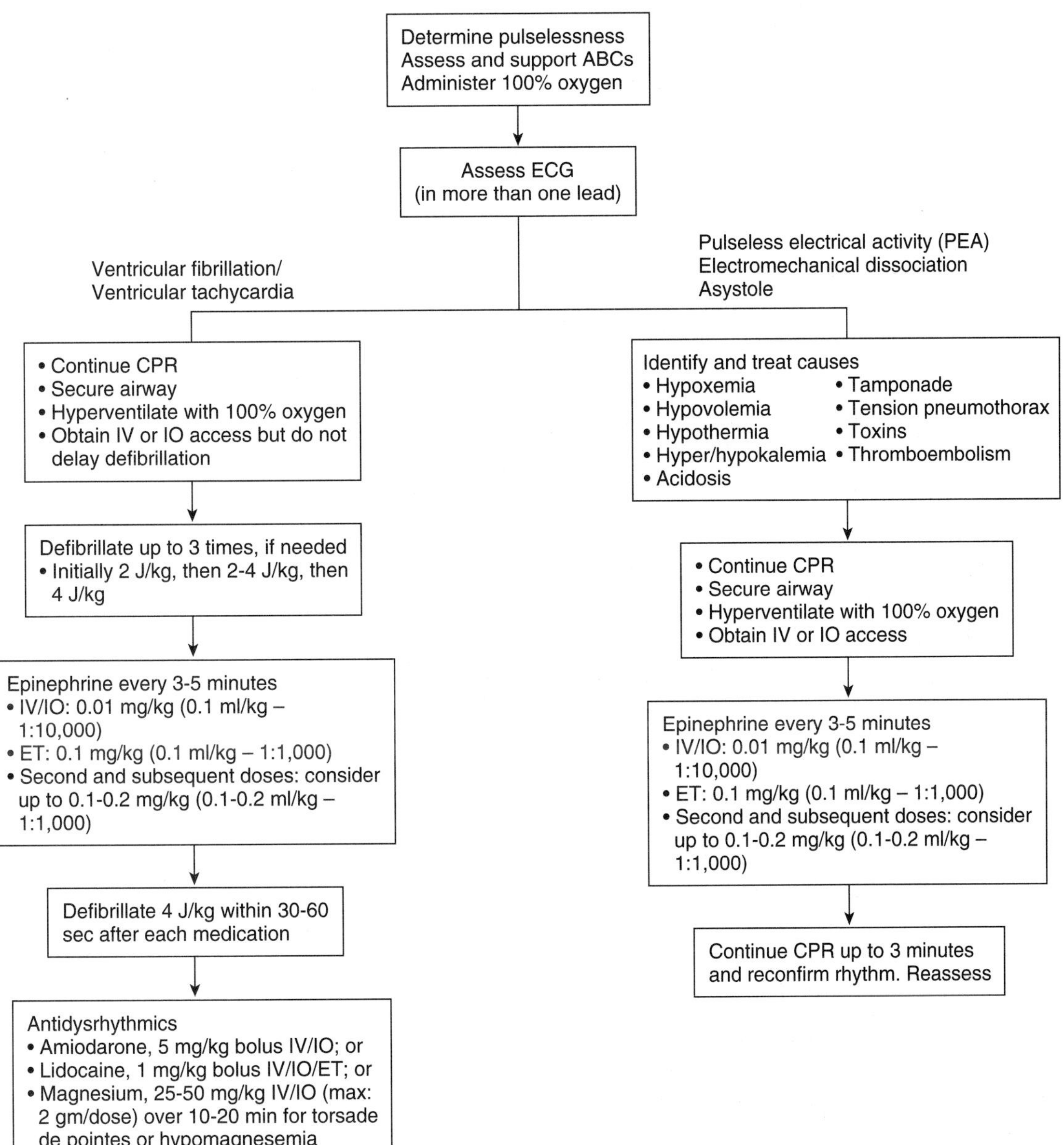

Fig. 4-2 Asystole and pulseless arrest decision tree. *CPR,* Cardiopulmonary resuscitation; *ET,* endotracheal; *IO,* intraosseous; *IV,* intravenous.

(From *JAMA* 268:2171, 1992. Copyright 1992, American Medical Association.)

The patient is given the following agents:

1. Oxygen.
2. Epinephrine. The recommended initial dose for asystolic and pulseless arrest is 0.01 mg/kg (0.1 ml/kg of 1:10,000 solution) given IV or intraosseously. If it is given ET, the initial dose is 0.1 mg/kg (0.1 ml/kg of 1:1000 solution [10 times the initial IV dose]). Further doses of epinephrine (0.1 mg/kg [0.1 ml/kg of 1:1000 solution]) are recommended every 3 to 5 minutes for ongoing arrest. The same dose of epinephrine is recommended for second and subsequent doses for unresponsive asystolic and pulseless arrest, although higher doses of epinephrine (0.1-0.2 mg/kg) by any intravascular route may be considered.

If asystolic or pulseless arrest continues, a continuous infusion of epinephrine at 0.1 to 1 μg/kg/min may be used until effective pulses are noted, at which time an infusion may be used. Low-dose infusions (<0.3 μg/kg/min) produce β-adrenergic effects; larger doses result in α-adrenergic vasoconstriction.

The measures and medications for resuscitation are summarized in Table 4-2.

Blood pressure, pulse, and heart rhythm must be monitored constantly throughout the resuscitation to ensure that therapeutic measures are appropriate and effective. Additional steps may include treatment of the following conditions:

1. Acidosis. Acidosis is pathophysiologically undesirable because it depresses myocardial contractility, decreases the threshold for ventricular fibrillation, impairs normal cardiac automaticity, and blocks the cardioaccelerator and vasopressor action of catecholamines. Acidosis in children is primarily a problem of ventilation and oxygenation.

   The benefits of bicarbonate therapy in the arrest situation are unsupported; furthermore, this type of therapy does not improve the ability to defibrillate. It causes oxygen to bind more tightly to oxyhemoglobin, and it may lead to hyperosmolality and hypernatremia. Bicarbonate therapy also worsens the mixed venous acidosis and inactivates simultaneously administered catecholamines. Bicarbonate administration may be initiated after resuscitation efforts have been tried for some time (usually 10 minutes) and ventilation is effective. Further doses ideally are administered in response to arterial blood gas (ABG) determinations.
2. EMD or PEA. The role of calcium blockers in cerebral resuscitation is under investigation. Calcium salts may not be beneficial in EMD or PEA, and their use should be restricted to circumstances in which a benefit is documented (hyperkalemia, hypocalcemia, calcium channel blocker overdose, fluoride poisoning, and hypermagnesemia). Reversible causes of EMD or PEA should be sought, including hypovolemia, tension pneumothorax, pericardial tamponade, and severe acidosis.
3. Dysrhythmias (see Chapter 6 and Figs. 4-1 and 4-2).
4. Congestive heart failure (see Chapter 16).
5. Seizure (see Chapter 21).
6. Malignant hypertension (see Chapter 18).
7. Increased intracranial pressure (see Chapter 57).
8. Glucose support and correction of electrolyte abnormalities. Hypoglycemia has been found in as many as 18% of children requiring resuscitation.
9. Temperature stabilization. Hypothermia may occur, requiring close monitoring and expectant management.
10. Recovery from cortical blindness after cardiac arrest is usually good if the neurologic status returns.

Text continued on p. 34

TABLE 4-2 Common Primary and Secondary Measures in Resuscitation

Drug Availability	Dose/Route	Indications	Adverse Reactions	Comments
Adenosine (Adenocard) Vial: 3 mg/ml	0.1 mg/kg IV bolus as rapidly as possible; may double and repeat in 2 min; adult: 6 mg IV, if no response in 2 min, give 12 mg IV	Supraventricular tachycardia	Flushing, shortness of breath	Rapid half-life (10 sec); do not use for 2nd or 3rd degree AV block (unless pacemaker present) or sick sinus syndrome
Albuterol (Proventil, Ventolin) soln (inhalation) (0.5%-5 mg/ml)	Inhalation 0.03 ml/kg/dose (maximum: 1.0 ml/dose) diluted in 2 ml saline; repeat as necessary	Bronchoconstriction	Tachycardia, nausea	β_2 agonist; also available as MDI (90 µg/dose); available as levalbuterol
Amiodarone (Cordarone) (50 mg/ml)	Pulseless ventricular fibrillation or ventricular tachycardia: 5 mg/kg IV rapidly (maximum: 15 mg/kg/24 hr IV) Perfusing tachycardia; Load: 5 mg/kg IV over 20-60 min (maximum: 15 mg/kg/24 hr)	Tachydysrhythmias	Hypotension, dysrhythmia (increased risk with $\downarrow K^+$, $\downarrow Mg^{++}$) myocardial depression, CHF	Avoid combination with drugs prolonging QT interval
Atropine (0.1, 0.4, 1.0 mg/ml)	0.02 mg/kg/dose (minimum: 0.1 mg/dose) (adult: 0.6-1.0 mg/dose; maximum 2 mg) q5min prn IV, ET, IO	Bradycardia, asystole, ↑ vagal tone Heart block (temporary); increases AV node conduction	Tachycardia, dysrhythmias, anticholinergic	Parasympatholytic (Table 6-4); use 2-3 times dose for ET
Bicarbonate, sodium ($NaHCO_3$) (8.4%-50 mEq/50 ml) (7.5%-44.5 mEq/50 ml)	1 mEq/kg/dose q10min prn IV	Metabolic acidosis Hyperkalemia	Metabolic alkalosis, hyperosmolality, hypernatremia	Incompatible with calcium, catecholamine infusion; monitor ABG
Calcium chloride (10%-100 mg/ml) (1.36 mEq Ca^{++}/ml)	20-30 mg (0.2-0.3 ml)/kg/dose (maximum: 500 mg/dose) q10min prn IV slowly	Hyperkalemia Calcium channel blocker OD	Rapid infusion causes bradycardia, hypotension Extravasation-necrosis	Inotropic; monitor; use caution with digitalized patient; probably no benefit in asystole or electromechanical dissociation
Crystalloid 0.9% NS, LR, D5W 0.9% NS, D5WLR	20 ml/kg over 20-30 min IV; repeat as necessary	Hypovolemia	Fluid overdose and pulmonary edema	Monitor volume status; see Chapter 5

IV drugs may generally be given intraosseously (IO).

Continued

TABLE 4-2 Common Primary and Secondary Measures in Resuscitation—cont'd

Drug Availability	Dose/Route	Indications	Adverse Reactions	Comments
Defibrillation	2 J/kg (adult: 200 J sec)	Ventricular fibrillation Ventricular tachycardia		Use correct paddle size and paste; if initial dose is unsuccessful, use 2-4 J/kg, which may be repeated once; if still unresponsive, give 4 J/kg after lidocaine; *synchronized cardioversion* (0.5-1.0 J/kg)
Dexamethasone (Decadron) (4, 24 mg/ml)	0.15-0.60 mg/kg/dose IM, IV	Croup, asthma, meningitis	Hypoglycemia	Delayed onset
Diazepam (Valium) (5 mg/ml)	0.2-0.3 mg/kg/dose (maximum: 10 mg/dose) IV	Status epilepticus	Respiratory depression	Also begin maintenance medication (Table 81-6); may give higher dose rectally (0.5 mg/kg PR)
Diazoxide (Hyperstat) (15 mg/ml)	1-3 mg/kg q4-24hr IV	Hypertension	Hypotension, hyperglycemia	Monitor (very prompt onset) (Table 18-2)
Digoxin (0.1, 0.25 mg/ml)	Preemie: 0.01-0.02 mg/kg TDD IV 2 wk-2 yr: 0.03-0.05 mg/kg TDD IV Newborn and >2 yr: 0.04 mg/kg TDD IV ½ TDD initially, then ¼ q4-8hr IV × 2	Congestive heart failure Supraventricular tachycardia	Dysrhythmia, heart block, vomiting	Monitor ECG; may also load PO in stable, nonurgent situation; if mild CHF, may give PO without loading (Table 16-2)
Dobutamine (Dobutrex) (vial: 250 mg)	2-20 μg/kg/min IV	Cardiogenic shock	Tachycardia, dysrhythmia, hypotension or hypertension	β Adrenergic; positive inotropic; may be synergistic with dopamine or isoproterenol (Table 5-2)
Dopamine (200 mg/5 ml)	Low: 2-5 μg/kg/min IV Mod: 5-20 μg/kg/min IV High: >20 μg/kg/min IV	Cardiogenic shock (moderate dose) Maintain renal perfusion Septic shock	Tachycardia, bradycardia, vasoconstriction (increases with higher doses)	β Adrenergic; avoid in hypovolemic shock; may use in combination with isoproterenol or levarterenol (norepinephrine) (Table 5-2)

Epinephrine (1:10,000) (0.1 mg/ml)	0.01 mg/kg (or 0.1 ml/kg of 1:10,000 solution) IV or IO q3-5min; *subsequent doses* may be as high as 0.1-0.2 mg/kg (0.1-0.2 ml/kg of 1:1000 solution)	Ventricular standstill Ventricular fibrillation (fine) Anaphylaxis Hemodynamically significant bradycardia	Tachycardia, dysrhythmia, hypertension, decreased renal and splanchnic blood flow	α and β Adrenergic; inotropic; not effective if acidotic (Table 5-2); endotracheal dose is 0.1 mg/kg (0.1 ml/kg of 1:1000 solution) initially; epinephrine infusion: initiate at 0.1 μg/kg/min IV; titrate to desired effect up to 1 μg/kg/min IV
Epinephrine (1:1000) (1 mg/ml)	0.01 ml/kg/dose SC (max: 0.35 ml/dose) q10-20min SC × 3 prn	Reactive airway disease	Tachycardia, headache, nausea	Rarely used; albuterol preferred
Epinephrine racemic (Vaponefrin) (2.25% solution)	0.25-0.75 ml/dose in 2.5 ml saline by inhalation	Croup	Tachycardia, rebound stridor	Observe, concurrent steroids
Fentanyl (Sublimaze, Innovar) 50 μg/ml	1-5 μg/kg/dose IV, IM	Analgesia	Respiratory depression, muscle rigidity	Monitor
Flumazenil (Romazicon) (0.1 mg/ml)	10 μg/kg IV for 2 doses (adult: 0.2 mg, 0.3 mg, then 0.5 mg separated by 30 sec up to a total of 3 mg)	Benzodiazepine overdose		
Furosemide (Lasix) (10 mg/ml)	1 mg/kg/dose q6-12hr IV up to 6 mg/kg/dose; may repeat q2hr prn	Fluid overload, pulmonary edema, cerebral edema	Hypokalemia, hyponatremia, prerenal azotemia	Reduce dosage in newborn to q12hr; if no response in urine output in 30 min, repeat; do not use if hypovolemic (Table 16-3)
Glucagon 1 mg (1 unit)/ml	0.03-0.1 mg/kg/dose q20min prn IV, SC, IM	β-Blocker overdose, hypoglycemia		Not adequate as only glucose support in neonate, inotropic
Glucose (D50W-0.5 g/ml)	0.5-1.0 g (2-4 ml D25W or 1-2 ml D50W)/kg/dose IV	Hypoglycemia, with coma or seizure	Hyperglycemia	Draw glucose; if possible use D25W
Hydralazine (Apresoline) (20 mg/ml)	0.1-0.4 mg/kg/dose q4-6hr IV/IM	Hypertension	Tachycardia, tachyphylaxis	Prompt onset (Table 18-2); may also be given as 1.5 μg/kg/min IV infusion; limited availability
Hydrocortisone (Solu-Cortef) (100, 250, 500 mg)	Asthma: 4-5 mg/kg/dose q6hr IV	Adrenal failure Asthma		May be detrimental in shock (controversial) (Table 74-2)

TDD, Total digitalizing dose.

Continued

TABLE 4-2 Common Primary and Secondary Measures in Resuscitation—cont'd

Drug Availability	Dose/Route	Indications	Adverse Reactions	Comments
Isoproterenol (1 mg/5 ml)	0.05-1.5 μg/kg/min Begin at 0.1 μg/kg/min and increase q5-10min prn	Bradycardia or heart block (S/P atropine)	Tachyrhythmias	β Adrenergic; avoid in hypovolemic shock; do not use with digoxin (Table 5-2)
Lidocaine (1%-10 mg/ml) (2%-20 mg/ml)	1 mg/kg/dose q5-10min IV, ET up to 5 mg/kg, then 20-50 μg/kg/min	Ventricular dysrhythmias Cardiac arrest caused by ventricular fibrillation	Hypotension, bradycardia with block, seizures	↓ automaticity and ectopic pacemaker (Table 6-4); for ET administration give 1:1 dilution, with 2-3 times IV dose
Lorazepam (Ativan) (2, 4 mg/ml)	0.05-0.10 mg/kg/dose (maximum: 4 mg/dose) IV; may repeat	Status epilepticus	Respiratory depression	Longer acting than diazepam
Magnesium sulfate (500 mg/ml)	25-50 mg/kg/dose IV over 10-20 min (maximum: 2 g/dose)	Torsades de pointe, hypomagnesemia, unresponsive asthma		Also useful for seizures associated with preeclampsia
Methylprednisolone (Solu-Medrol) (40, 125, 500, 1000 mg)	Asthma: 1-2 mg/kg/dose q6hr IV; usual maximum is 12.5-25 mg/dose	Adrenal failure Asthma	Hypoglycemia	May be detrimental in shock (controversial) (Table 74-2)
Midazolam (Versed) (1, 5 mg/ml)	0.05-0.1 mg/kg/dose (maximum: 5 mg/dose IV)	Sedation	Respiratory depression, hypotension	Monitor, must be prepared to manage airway
Morphine (8, 10, 15 mg/ml)	0.1-0.2 mg/kg/dose (maximum: 15 mg/dose) q2-4hr IV	Pulmonary edema Tetralogy spell Reduce preload and afterload	Hypotension, respiratory depression	Antidote: naloxone (Narcan)
Naloxone (Narcan) (0.4, 1 mg/ml)	0.1 mg/kg/dose (minimum: 0.4 mg/dose; maximum: 2.0 mg/dose) IV, ET	Narcotic overdose; (see p. 390); septic shock (unproven)		Give empirically in suspected opiate overdose; may be given ET; higher dosage may be used for unresponsive overdose
Nitroglycerin (Nitrostat, Nitro-Bid) (0.5, 0.8, 5, 10 mg/ml)	IV 0.5-10 μg/kg/min	Pulmonary edema, angina pectoris, perioperative hypertension	Hypotension, headache, nausea, vomiting, palpitations	Contraindicated with hypotension, increased ICP, hypovolemia, cardiac tamponade, pericarditis, inadequate cerebral circulation

Nitroprusside (50 mg/vial)	0.5-10 µg (average: 3 µg)/kg/min IV	Hypertensive emergency Afterload reduction	Hypotension, cyanide poisoning	Monitor closely; light sensitive (Table 18-2); thiocyanate toxicity in patient with impaired renal function
Oxygen	100% mask, ET	Hypoxia Major injury	Toxicity not a problem with acute short-term use	Use high flow (3-6 L/min); monitor ABG, oximetry
Pancuronium (Pavulon) (1, 2 mg/ml)	0.04-0.1 mg/kg/dose IV; may repeat 0.01-0.02 mg/kg/dose q20-40min IV prn	Muscle relaxation	Tachycardia	Rapid onset; support respirations; lower dose in newborn
Phenobarbital (65 mg/ml)	15-20 mg/kg load IV/IM (adult: 100 mg/dose q20min prn × 3), then 5 mg/kg/24 hr PO, IV, IM	Seizures	Sedation	If not controlled after load, repeat 10 mg/kg/dose IV; administer <1 mg/kg/min IV; IM erratically absorbed (Table 81-6)
Phenytoin (Dilantin) (50 mg/ml)	10-20 mg/kg load IV slowly, then 5-10 mg/kg/24 hr q12-24hr PO, IV 5 mg/kg/dose IV q5-20min × 2 prn	Seizures Dysrhythmia	Hypotension, bradycardia when given too fast; cerebral disturbance	Do not give faster than 0.5 mg/kg/min; dilute in normal saline (Table 81-6); fosphenytoin (Cerebyx) (50 mg/ml) is available for IV or IM administration with less toxicity and local reaction
Succinylcholine (20 mg/ml)	1-2 mg/kg/dose IV (larger dose in children <20 kg)	Muscle relaxation	Dysrhythmia, hypotension	Must be able to control ventilation
Vecuronium (Norcuron) (10 mg/ml)	0.08-0.1 mg/kg/dose IV	Nondepolarizing muscle blockade	Profound skeletal muscle weakness; respiratory arrest	Monitor; to be used only by persons with advanced airway skills

Ancillary Data and Measures

Laboratory tests and other procedures beyond those required for evaluation of the patient's underlying disease must be performed:

1. Complete blood count with hematocrit measured in ED
2. Chemical evaluations: electrolytes, blood urea nitrogen, creatinine, sugar, calcium, phosphorus levels
3. ABG levels and oximetry
4. X-ray film: chest x-ray study for underlying disease, placement of ET and nasogastric (NG) tubes, and monitoring of potential complications
5. Ultrasonography: assess cardiac function and exclude pneumothorax and tamponade
6. Electrocardiogram and ongoing cardiac monitoring
7. Type and cross-match of blood, if appropriate
8. NG tube insertion: determine nature of aspirate and output monitoring
9. Urinary catheter: urinalysis and output monitoring

Disposition-Termination

If resuscitation is successful, ongoing support and monitoring are mandatory. Patients seen in the ED in arrest despite prehospital intervention usually have a poor outcome.

Potentially reversible causes of cardiopulmonary arrest that need to be considered are as follows (4 **H**'s and 4 **T**'s):

Hypoxemia, **H**ypovolemia, **H**ypothermia, **H**yper/hypokalemia and other metabolic disorder (acidosis, etc.)

Tamponade, **T**ension pneumothorax, **T**oxins, poisons, or drugs, **T**hromboembolism

Efforts should be terminated if obvious brain death has not occurred; the clinician should recall that the brain of the infant or child is relatively resistant to hypoxic damage. Useful clinical evidence includes the oculocephalic reflex (doll's eyes reflex), oculovestibular reflex (calorics), absence of a corneal reflex, and fixed, dilated pupils. Resuscitation should be continued if evidence of drug depression or hypothermia is present. Underlying disease may modify the aggressiveness of resuscitation.

Psychologic Support

Support of the child and the entire family is essential throughout the resuscitation period. The child is separated from the parents and in a strange environment, surrounded by unfamiliar nurses and physicians. If the resuscitation is successful and vital signs and consciousness are restored, time should be taken to reassure and calm the child.

1. A member of the health care team should be assigned to give the family information, explanations, and emotional support. Health professionals must recognize their own personal feelings while being available to and allowing parents to verbalize their feelings and emotions.
2. The decision whether to allow parents to stay with a child must be individualized on the basis of the child's medical condition and level of consciousness and the family's emotional state. Family members often find it reassuring to be in the resuscitation room, even if the outcome is poor. Parents should participate in the decision about their presence. They should also be asked whether relatives or clergy should be called to give them support.
3. If the child dies, support and compassion are needed along with an attempt to relieve the family of feelings of guilt and facilitate the normal grieving process. Most parents will want to touch and hold their child after the youngster has been made as presentable as possible (see Foreword). Some parents have found it useful to have a lock of the child's hair or a footprint (using nursery's print pad identification system) taken at this time. Arrangements should be made for support of the family during the next days and weeks to ensure that appropriate

resources have been mobilized to assist them.

When faced with the sudden death of a child, all concerned experience grief at the loss. It is essential that support be provided not only to the family but also to the entire health care team.

BIBLIOGRAPHY

Ahrens W, Hart R, Maruyama N: Pediatric death: the aftermath in the emergency department, *J Emerg Med* 15:601, 1997.

American Academy of Pediatrics and American College of Physicians: *APLS—the pediatric emergency medicine course*, ed 2, Dallas, 1993, The College.

American Academy of Pediatrics and American Heart Association: *Pediatric advanced life support (PALS) provider manual*, Dallas, 2002, American Heart Association.

American Heart Association: Guidelines 2000 for cardiopulmonary resuscitation (CPR) and emergency cardiovascular care, *Circulation* 102:I1-I384.

Bhendi MS, Thompson AE: Evaluation of an end-tidal CO_2 detector during pediatric cardiopulmonary resuscitation, *Pediatrics* 95:395, 1995.

Bush CM, Jones JS, Cohle SD et al: Pediatric injuries from cardiopulmonary resuscitation, *Ann Emerg Med* 28:40, 1996.

Cook RT, Moglia BB, Consevage MW et al: The use of Beck Airway Airflow Monitor for verifying intratracheal endotracheal tube placement in patients in the pediatric emergency department and intensive care unit, *Pediatr Emerg Care* 12:331, 1996.

Cerardi MJ, Sacchetti AD, Cantor RM et al: Rapid sequence intubation of the pediatric patient, *Ann Emerg Med* 28:55, 1996.

Dorfsman ML, Menegazzi JJ, Wadas RJ et al: Two-thumb versus two-finger chest compression in an infant model of prolonged cardiopulmonary resuscitation, *Acad Emerg Med* 7:1077, 2001.

Gausche M, Lewis RJ, Stratton SJ et al: Effect of out-of-hospital pediatric endotracheal intubation on survival and neurological outcome: a controlled clinical trial, *JAMA* 283:783, 2001.

Halperin HR, Chandra NC, Levin HR et al: Newer methods of improving blood flow during CPR, *Ann Emerg Med* 27:553, 1996.

Hickey RW, Kochanek FM, Ferimer H et al: Hypothermia and hyperthermia in children after resuscitation from cardiac arrest, *Pediatrics* 106:118, 2000.

Hooker EA, Danzl DF, Brueggmeyer M et al: Respiratory rate in pediatric emergency patients, *J Emerg Med* 10:407, 1992.

Johnston C: Endotracheal drug delivery, *Pediatr Emerg Care* 8:94, 1992.

King BR, Baker MD, Braitman LE et al: Endotracheal tube selection in children: a comparison of four methods, *Ann Emerg Med* 22:530, 1993.

Lefkowitz W: Oxygen and resuscitation: beyond the myth, *Pediatrics* 109:517, 2002.

Losek JD: Hypoglycemia and the ABC'S (sugar) of pediatric resuscitation, *Ann Emerg Med* 35:43, 2000.

Luten RC, Wears RL, Broselow J et al: Length-based endotracheal tube and emergency equipment selection in pediatrics, *Ann Emerg Med* 21:900, 1992.

Mendex DR, Goto CS, Abrama TJ et al: Safety and efficacy of rocuronium for controlled intubation with paralytics in the pediatric emergency department, *Pediatr Emerg Care* 17:233, 2001.

Peak DA, Roy S: Needle cricothyroidotomy revisited, *Pediatr Emerg Care* 15:224, 1999.

Pollack CV: The laryngeal mask airway: a comprehensive review for the emergency physician, *J Emerg Med* 20:53, 2001.

Schindler MB, Bohn D, Cox PN et al: Out of hospital cardiac arrest, *N Engl J Med* 335:1473, 1995.

Schlessel JS, Rappa HA, Lesser M et al: CPR knowledge, self-efficacy and anticipated anxiety as functions of infant/child CPR training, *Ann Emerg Med* 25:618, 1995.

Sirbaugh PE, Pepe PE, Shookk JE et al: A prospective, population based study of the demographics, epidemiology, management and outcome of out-of-hospital pediatric cardiopulmonary arrest, *Ann Emerg Med* 33:174, 1999.

Sokolove PE, Price DO, Okada P: The safety of etomidate for emergency rapid sequence intubation of pediatric patients, *Pediatr Emerg Care* 16:18, 2000.

Sullivan KJ, Kisson N: Securing the child's airway in the emergency department, *Pediatr Emerg Care* 18:108, 2002.

Teach SJ, Moore PE, Fleisher CR: Death and resuscitation in the pediatric emergency department, *Ann Emerg Med* 25:799, 1995.

Young KD, Seidel JS: Pediatric cardiopulmonary resuscitation: a collective review, *Ann Emerg Med* 33:195, 1999.

Zaritsky A, Nadharni V, Hazinshi MR et al: Recommended guidelines for uniform reporting of pediatric advanced life support: pediatric resuscitation pharmacology, *Ann Emerg Med* 26:487, 1993.

Zideman D, Zaritsky A, Carol W et al: Airways in pediatric and newborn resuscitation, *Ann Emerg Med* 37:S126, 2001.

5 Shock

Also See Chapters 4 (Cardiopulmonary Arrest) and 7 (Dehydration)

After the airway and ventilation are stabilized, it is essential, in the approach to the cardiovascular system, to determine the type and stage of shock. Blood pressure (often including orthostatic vital signs), heart rate, capillary perfusion, and organ function (especially central nervous system and kidney) must be assessed. Fluids and, rarely, pharmacologic agents (if normovolemic) may be required.

Shock occurs when acute circulatory dysfunction is marked by progressive impairment of blood flow to the skin, muscles, kidneys, mesentery, lungs, heart, and brain. Patients in shock have diminished perfusion manifested by decreased blood pressure, tachycardia, poor capillary refill, decreased skin temperature, altered mental status, diminished urinary output, and ultimately multiple system failure. In children, hypovolemia is the most common cause. Compensatory mechanisms initially prevent functional deterioration, but with progression, cellular metabolic changes are marked by anaerobic metabolism, leading to further injury and eventually cell death and release of proteolytic enzymes and cellular byproducts.

Blood pressure reflects cardiac output (rate and filling volume) and peripheral resistance. Normal blood pressure and pulse values are summarized in Appendix B-2. Normal systolic blood pressures in individuals 1 to 20 years of age can be estimated by adding twice the age in years to 80. Diastolic blood pressure is usually two thirds of systolic blood pressure.

Normal blood volume is averaged as 80 ml/kg; age-specific volumes are as follows:

Preterm infant	90-105 ml/kg
Term newborn	85 ml/kg
>1 mo	75 ml/kg
>1 yr	67-75 ml/kg
Adult	55-75 ml/kg

STAGES OF SHOCK AND DIAGNOSTIC FINDINGS

Compensated Shock

Vital organ functions are maintained by intrinsic compensatory mechanisms that stabilize vital signs. As fluid loss progresses, compensation causes venous capacitance to decrease by 10% to 25%, fluid to shift from interstitial to intravascular compartments, and arteriolar constriction to increase. With compensation the central venous pressure (CVP) is decreased, as are stroke volume and urine output; heart rate and systemic vascular resistance increase. Perfusion to the periphery (skin and muscles) and to the kidneys and intestine may be compromised, even without major alterations in blood pressure. Decreased skin perfusion may produce diminished skin temperature, delayed capillary refill (>2 seconds), and a pale, blue, or mottled appearance. Poor central nervous system (CNS) perfusion ultimately leads to impaired mentation and poor responsiveness.

Capillary refill is measured in the fingernail bed after application of just the amount of pressure necessary to blanch the nail bed. In children 2 to 24 months of age, a refill time shorter than 1.5 seconds is consistent with a less than 5% deficit, 1.5 to 3 seconds with a 5% to 10% deficit, and longer than 3 seconds with a greater than 10% deficit. Other factors that prolong the capillary refill are hyponatremia, hypothermia, and congestive heart failure. Capillary refill time is a less reliable measurement in patients with edema or malnutrition.

Ultimately, the efficacy of compensatory mechanisms depends on the patient's preexisting cardiac and pulmonary status and the rate and volume of fluid loss.

Diagnostic Findings. Orthostatic changes (systolic blood pressure decreases >15 mm Hg or pulse increases >20 beats/min with change from supine to seated or erect position) reflect primarily intravascular volume but are difficult to delineate in the child younger than 5 years.

1. An **acute** volume deficit of 10% may be marked by a rise in pulse rate of 20 beats/min. A 20% deficit has an associated heart rate increase of 30 beats/min, with a variable decrease in blood pressure. Larger volume deficits have a consistent blood pressure decrease (>15 mm Hg) and pulse rate increase (>30 beats/min).
2. A 10% to 15% **gradual** volume loss produces minimal physiologic change. On the other hand, a 20% to 30% gradual volume deficit is marked by compensation, but no related hypotension is present. Progressive hypotension is noted with gradual volume loss of 30% to 50%.

In acute blood loss, *supine* blood pressure may remain normal with a 20% or greater deficit. Orthostatic changes *must* be measured. Acidosis, which may be the most sensitive indicator of inadequate perfusion, must also be monitored closely.

Uncompensated Shock

Cardiovascular dysfunction and impairment of microvascular perfusion lead to lowered perfusion pressures, increased precapillary arteriolar resistance, and further contraction of venous capacitance; with progressive blood stagnation, anaerobic metabolism and release of proteolytic enzymes and vasoactive substances occur. These events exacerbate myocardial depression. Platelet aggregation and release of tissue thromboplastin produce hypercoagulability and disseminated intravascular coagulation (DIC).

Diagnostic Findings. Hypotension, tachycardia, decreased cardiac output, and variable CVP values are observed. Multiple organ system failure occurs with adult respiratory distress syndrome (ARDS), liver and pancreatic failure, coagulopathies with DIC, oliguria and renal failure, gastrointestinal (GI) bleeding, impaired mental status, acidosis, abnormal calcium and phosphorus homeostasis, and ongoing cellular damage. Although variability does exist, the observations listed in Table 5-1 may be useful.

The traditional distinction between "early" and "late" shock has not proved to be clinically useful on a consistent basis.

TABLE 5-1 Presentation of Shock

	TYPE OF SHOCK		
	Hypovolemic	**Cardiogenic**	**Distributive**
Pulse	Tachycardic, thready	Markedly tachycardic, thready	Tachycardic: Early (bounding) Late (thready)
Respirations	Tachypnea	Marked tachypnea, increased effort	Tachypnea, variable effort
Skin perfusion	Cool, clammy, pale, usually delayed capillary refill	Mottled (gray or blue), cool, delayed capillary refill	Warm, dry, flushed, progressing to cool, clammy, delayed capillary refill
Neck veins	Flat	Bulging	Variable
Mental status	Normal to lethargy	Lethargy to coma	Lethargy, confused to coma

Box 5-1

ETIOLOGIC CLASSIFICATION OF SHOCK

HYPOVOLEMIC

1. Hemorrhage
   - **a.** External: laceration
   - **b.** Internal: ruptured spleen or liver, vascular injury, fracture (neonate: intracerebral/intraventricular hemorrhage)
   - **c.** Gastrointestinal: bleeding ulcer, ruptured viscus, mesenteric hemorrhage
2. Plasma loss
   - **a.** Burn
   - **b.** Inflammation or sepsis; leaky capillary syndrome
   - **c.** Nephrotic syndrome
   - **d.** Third spacing: intestinal obstruction, pancreatitis, peritonitis
3. Fluid and electrolyte loss
   - **a.** Acute gastroenteritis
   - **b.** Excessive sweating (cystic fibrosis)
   - **c.** Renal disorder
4. Endocrine
   - **a.** Adrenal insufficiency, adrenal-genital syndrome
   - **b.** Diabetes mellitus
   - **c.** Diabetes insipidus
   - **d.** Hypothyroidism (myxedema coma)

CARDIOGENIC

1. Myocardial insufficiency
   - **a.** Dysrhythmia: bradycardia, atrioventricular (AV) block, ventricular tachycardia, supraventricular tachycardia
   - **b.** Cardiomyopathy: myocarditis, ischemia, hypoxia, hypoglycemia, acidosis
   - **c.** Drug intoxication
   - **d.** Hypothermia
   - **e.** Myocardial depressant effects of shock
   - **f.** Postoperative cardiac surgery
2. Filling or outflow obstruction
   - **a.** Pericardial tamponade
   - **b.** Pneumopericardium
   - **c.** Tension pneumothorax
   - **d.** Pulmonary embolism
   - **e.** Congenital heart disease, including patent ductus arteriosus (PDA)—dependent lesion such as coarctation of the aorta or critical pulmonary stenosis

DISTRIBUTIVE (VASOGENIC)

1. High or normal resistance (increased venous capacitance)
   - **a.** Septic shock
   - **b.** Anaphylaxis
   - **c.** Barbiturate intoxication
2. Low resistance, vasodilation: CNS injury (i.e., spinal cord transection)

Terminal Shock

Irreversible damage to the heart and brain as a result of altered perfusion and metabolism ultimately leads to death.

ETIOLOGY AND DIAGNOSTIC FINDINGS

The clinical presentation and progression of findings partially reflect the underlying condition and the stage and classification of shock (Box 5-1). Patients demonstrate altered vital signs associated with tachycardia; poor capillary refill (abnormal if >2 seconds); cool, mottled, and pale skin; and altered mental status. They may show evidence of impaired cardiac function. Blood pressure changes may develop, often preceded by orthostatic changes. Respiratory alkalosis and metabolic acidosis are common.

Specific focus must be directed to defining the underlying disease and its specific sequelae and complications as well as to understanding the pathophysiology of the disease process.

Hypovolemic Shock

Reduction in circulating blood volume from volume loss produces progressive dysfunction:

1. Decreased preload through capillary pooling and leakage accompanied by extrinsic and intrinsic losses of intravascular volume and decreased cardiac output

2. Increased afterload secondary to arteriolar constriction
3. Myocardial ischemia resulting from impairment of subendocardial blood flow and decreased supply of oxygen to myocardium; concurrently, a greater myocardial oxygen requirement is associated with tachycardia, increased afterload, and cardiac distension
4. Excessive aldosterone secretion with sodium and water retention, leading to pulmonary edema and further hypoxia

Compensatory homeostasis is achieved at the expense of regional blood flow initially to the skin and muscles and then to the kidneys, mesentery, lungs, heart, and brain. Because children have highly reactive vascular beds, an adequate blood pressure can be maintained even in the presence of significant intravascular volume depletion; when hypotension does develop, it is profound and rapid.

Cardiogenic Shock

Dysfunction of the heart caused by depressed cardiac output may result from myocardial insufficiency (dysrhythmia, cardiomyopathy, etc.) or mechanical obstruction of the flow of blood into and out of the heart (tamponade, tension pneumothorax, congenital heart disease, etc.). Inadequate preload, with accompanying hypovolemia, capillary injury, vascular instability, decreased cardiac output, and tissue perfusion, produces a rapid downhill spiral of microcirculatory failure. Children rarely go through a prolonged compensated phase before decompensation because of their excellent compensatory mechanisms.

Hemodynamic signs are decreased cardiac output and elevations of CVP, pulmonary wedge pressure, and systemic vascular resistance. These may be the terminal physiologic events associated with primary shock of other origin (Fig. 5-1).

Distributive or Vasogenic Shock

Distributive or vasogenic shock is associated with an abnormality in the distribution of blood flow, initially resulting from acute arteriolar dilation (spinal cord injury) and increased venous capacitance (septic shock, anaphylaxis) accompanied by decreased intravascular volume secondary to leaky capillaries. Although a clear progression is uncommon in children, an early hyperdynamic phase associated with decreased afterload may be followed by diminished cardiac output and increased systemic vascular resistance secondary to hypoxemia, acidosis, and increased venous capacitance. Warm, dry, flushed skin may be noted initially, followed by rapid progression to a vasoconstrictive phase.

A distinct evolution from systemic inflammatory response syndrome through shock and severe shock to septic shock is common. In septic shock the endotoxin inhibits platelet function while injuring the endothelium and activating intrinsic clotting factors, with subsequent DIC.

The initial hyperdynamic phase is rare in children, but when present it may respond to volume therapy. With progression of shock, volume administration must be rapidly combined with agents that decrease peripheral resistance (alpha effect), whereas cardiac function is improved with positive inotropic agents (β_1).

Complications

Complications are common, reflecting stage of shock, rapidity of response, underlying disease process, and problems secondary to therapy:

1. ARDS (p. 41)
2. Acute tubular necrosis (ATN) with renal failure (p. 828)
3. Myocardial dysfunction with failure (p. 149)
4. Stress ulcers, GI bleeding, ileus

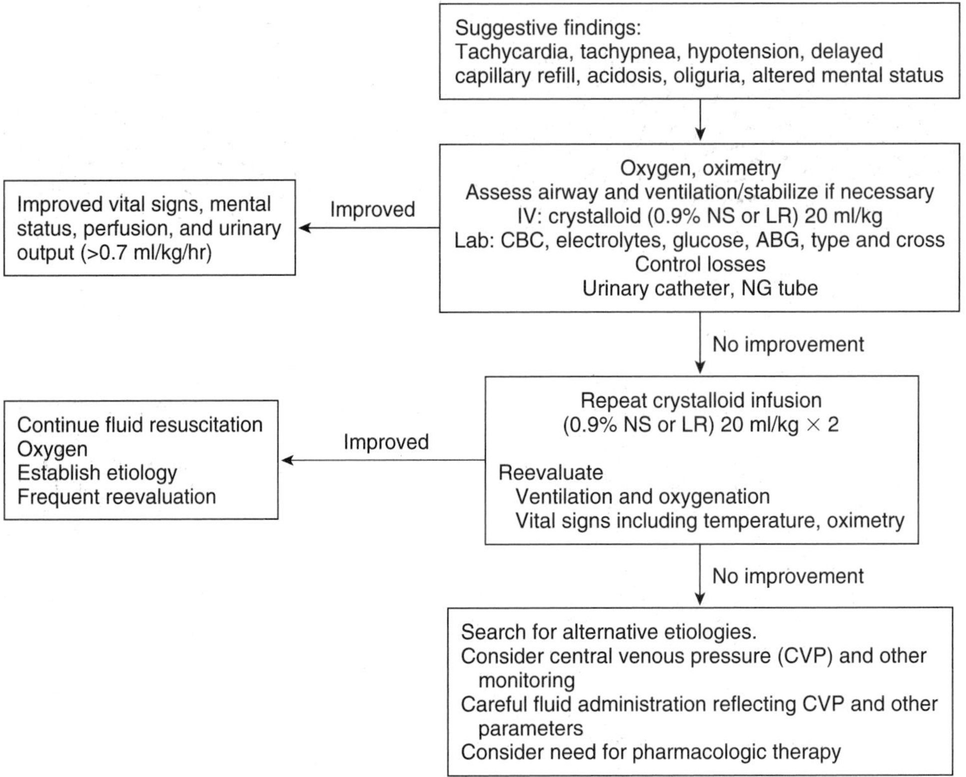

Fig. 5-1 Approach to hypovolemic shock.

Ancillary Data

1. Chest radiographic studies for all patients to evaluate for cardiac size, pneumothorax, pneumonia, and pulmonary edema.
2. Arterial blood gas (ABG) level to monitor progression of acidosis and diffusion and ventilation problems associated with respiratory distress syndrome.
3. Electrocardiography (ECG) and consideration of echocardiography to evaluate cardiac function, exclude dysrhythmias, monitor preload, and exclude effusion.
4. Chemical studies: electrolytes, blood urea nitrogen, creatinine, glucose, liver functions, calcium, phosphorus, cardiac enzymes, as indicated.
5. Hematologic evaluation: complete blood count, platelets, coagulation (prothrombin time, partial thromboplastin time), and screening for DIC (fibrinogen, fibrin split products) (p. 694). Hemoglobin (Hb) and hematocrit (Hct) values may be artificially normal for several hours in the presence of a rapid decrease in intravascular volume and must be measured on a continuing basis.
6. Type and cross-match of blood because of the potential for hemorrhage, DIC, and intravascular hemolysis, which are common.
7. Urinalysis to exclude hematuria, proteinuria, and infection; output must be continuously monitored.
8. Cultures of blood and urine. Spinal fluid as indicated. Counterimmunoelectrophoresis (CIE) and other antigen

detection or DNA amplification techniques such as polymerase chain reaction (PCR) may be useful when culture results are negative.

MANAGEMENT

Initial resuscitation must be followed by a systematic approach to fluid therapy, pharmacologic support, and diagnostic evaluation. It is imperative to monitor perfusion constantly through hemodynamic measures, including blood pressure, heart rate and capillary refill, urine output, acid-base status, and mental alertness. If one approach is not effective, the fluid and pharmacologic intervention must be adjusted on an empiric basis. Intervention must also be individualized to reflect underlying and preexisting conditions.

After stabilization of the airway and ventilation and initiation of resuscitation of the cardiovascular system, the underlying disease process requires urgent attention.

Airway and Ventilation

1. Administer oxygen at 3 to 6 L/min by cannula or mask (see Chapter 4).
2. Determine need for intubation and mechanical ventilation. The indications for intubation include the following:
   a. Arterial oxygen tension (PaO_2) less than 50 mm Hg (sea level) when oxygen is administered with FiO_2 of 50%
   b. Arterial carbon dioxide tension ($PaCO_2$) greater than 50 mm Hg (unless caused by compensation from a prolonged condition such as bronchopulmonary dysplasia or cystic fibrosis)
   c. Decreasing vital capacity, increasing respiratory rate, or rapidly progressive disease
   d. Severe metabolic acidosis
   e. Inability to protect airway
   f. Severe pulmonary edema or marked respiratory distress after near-drowning or a similar accident requiring positive end-expiratory pressure (PEEP)

ARDS may develop with increased extravascular pulmonary water, thereby increasing both the work of breathing and permeability secondary to damage of the alveolar epithelium and the pulmonary capillary endothelium (alveolar-capillary membrane). This syndrome is not a single disease but a group of disorders with similar clinical, pathologic, and pathophysiologic findings. No one mediator can explain every case, and for a given insult, more than one pathogenic process can occur simultaneously.

As a result of the cellular injury, the pulmonary capillaries become permeable, and proteinaceous fluid leaks into the interstitial space and alveoli. This development is characterized by progressive hypoxemia, hypercapnia, respiratory alkalosis, increased shunting, and decreased compliance.

Ventilation with early introduction of PEEP is essential if PaO_2 does not respond to PEEP alone or if other indications for intubation are present. A PEEP of 3 to 6 cm H_2O should be used at first; the pressure should be raised gradually until an adequate PaO_2 is achieved without decreasing cardiac output. Chest radiographs and ABGs should be monitored.

NOTE: PEEP may increase intrapulmonary shunting, with a potential to decrease cardiac output and delivery of oxygen to the tissues. This usually does not occur until PEEP exceeds 15 cm H_2O.

Intravenous Fluids

Fluids should be administered after insertion of one or two large-bore intravenous (IV) lines (see p. 403 and Appendix A-3). When administering IV fluids, the clinician must remember the relationship between preload and stroke volume described by the Frank-Starling curve; giving excessive fluids may actually impair cardiac function, emphasizing the importance of monitoring the CVP or pulmonary capillary wedge pressure (PCWP) in hemodynamically unstable patients.

Hypovolemic Shock (see Fig. 5-1)

1. Administer 0.9% normal saline solution (NS) at a rate of 20 ml/kg over 20 minutes. D5W (5% dextrose in water) in 0.9% NS may be used if the cause is gastroenteritis and low blood glucose levels are anticipated. Monitor urine output, pulse, perfusion, blood pressure, and glucose level.
2. If no response, repeat the infusion of 0.9% NS with ongoing evaluation of ventilatory status, temperature, electrolytes, glucose, ABGs, and ECG.
3. Place a CVP line if there is no response after 2 to 3 infusions and hemodynamic instability persists. Observe CVP or PCWP for 10 minutes after fluid challenge.
   a. If either pressure value is elevated (>10 mm Hg CVP* or >12 mm Hg PCWP), consider other causes, including tension pneumothorax, pericardial tamponade, myocardial insufficiency, congestive heart failure, patent ductus arteriosus (PDA) dependent lesion with closing of PDA (coarctation of aorta in newborn), and myocarditis.
   b. If pressure values are decreased (<10 mm Hg CVP or <12 mm Hg PCWP), administer crystalloid (0.9% NS) in increments of 5 to 10 ml/kg over 20 to 30 minutes while monitoring CVP response. Observe response for at least 10 minutes after infusion. If CVP returns to within 3 mm Hg of the preinfusion value, continue infusion and repeat until either hemodynamic measurements are corrected or the CVP persistently exceeds the initial value by 3 mm Hg.
   c. CVP may not reflect left ventricular function. PCWP may be needed, particularly if positive-pressure ventilation is used, pulmonary disease or mitral stenosis is present, or there is evidence of failure of either the left or right side of the heart.
4. If hemorrhage is the cause of hypovolemia, type-specific or cross-matched blood should be considered after an initial crystalloid resuscitation. Once 40 to 50 ml/kg of crystalloid has been infused, it is increasingly important to administer blood. Whole blood is particularly useful for massive ongoing acute bleeding; however, packed red blood cells may be appropriate after the infusion of large amounts of crystalloid in an acute situation or in a more chronic process (Table 5-2).
   a. If completely cross-matched blood is not available, administer type-specific blood. It is usually available within 10 to 15 minutes after delivery of a clot to the blood bank. O-negative blood should be reserved for patients in profound shock secondary to hypovolemia who have no response to crystalloid or who are in cardiac arrest after trauma.
   b. Fresh frozen plasma and platelets are often indicated to correct coagulation defects rapidly. Coagulation status should be monitored.
   c. Massive blood transfusions (equivalent to one blood volume of 80 ml/kg) require the use of blood warmers and micropore filters.
5. If hypovolemia exists concurrently with hypoproteinemia, use of 5% *albumin* in 0.9% NS (Plasmanate) or fresh frozen plasma at 5 to 10 ml/kg over 30 minutes with careful monitoring may be considered as an adjunct to crystalloid. This infusion may be repeated until the patient is hemodynamically stable or the CVP rises.
6. The role of *colloid* in severe shock or capillary leak syndromes is controversial. There may be a role for 5% albumin or products like 6% hetastarch combined

* 0.75 mm Hg = 1 cm H_2O.

TABLE 5-2 Pediatric Blood Component Therapy

Problem	"Classic" Coagulation Panel Abnormalities	Blood Component	Quantity
Acute blood loss	Hct <40 (infants) <30 (children)	Whole blood* P-RBCs	To replace loss or 10-20 ml/kg 10 ml/kg should raise Hct 10 points
Chronic anemia	Hct <15% to 20% Hemoglobin <5-7 g/dl Patient symptomatic	P-RBCs If frequent or multiple transfusions are required, or history of febrile reactions, consider leukocyte-poor RBCs (buffy coat removed to prevent reactions with white blood cells)	Administer *slowly* if clinically unstable: 3 ml/kg/hr (consider diuretics)
Anemia in child with T-cell immune deficiency	Hct <40 (infants) <30 (children) (consider patient baseline)	If time and patient stability allows, consider irradiated blood cells	As above (see acute blood loss)
Thrombocytopenia	↓ platelets (isolated) ↑ template bleeding time Clot formation but lack of clot retraction	Platelets	1 U/5 kg (maximum: 10 U)
Thrombocytopathia	Normal or only slightly decreased platelet count, template bleeding time	Platelets	1 U/5 kg (maximum: 10 U)
Disseminated intravascular coagulation (DIC)	↓ fibrinogen and platelets (lower than expected) ↑ PT, PTT ↑ fibrin split products	Treat cause If fibrinogen <50, cryoprecipitate plus FFP should be given; if fibrinogen >50, FFP alone may be effective	FFP: 10 ml/kg Cryoprecipitate: 1 bag/5 kg Titrate to achieve improvement in fibrinogen and platelet count
DIC with purpura fulminans	As above with evidence of peripheral embolic phenomena	Administer FFP to restore levels of antithrombin III, then heparin	FFP: 10 ml/kg Heparin: Load: 50 U/kg IV: 10-25 U/kg/hr Titrate to achieve rise in fibrinogen and platelet count and fall in PTT
Hemophilia A (Table 79-2)	Bleeding ↓ factor VIII activity	Purified factor VIII	Severe life-threatening bleeding or major surgery: up to 50 U/kg or continuous infusion of 2 U/kg/hr to maintain factor VIII activity at 100% Minor bleeding: up to 25 U/kg

Continued

TABLE 5-2 Pediatric Blood Component Therapy—cont'd

Problem	"Classic" Coagulation Panel Abnormalities	Blood Component	Quantity
Lack of coagulation factors in general†	↑ PT, PTT, thrombin time ↓ fibrinogen Slow clot formation	FFP	10 ml/kg
Heparin excess‡	↑ ↑ PTT, thrombin time, and template bleeding time PT may be slightly ↑ Platelet count normal (initially) Slow clot formation	Protamine sulfate (titrated to correct thrombin time)	1 mg/kg (slowly): 1 mg IV each 100 U heparin given concurrently; 0.5 mg IV each 100 U heparin given in previous 30 min, and so on; maximum: 50 mg/dose (slowly)
Protamine sulfate excess‡	↑ ↑ PTT, thrombin time, and template bleeding time PT may be slightly ↑ Platelet count normal (initially) Slow clot formation	When protamine is titrated and thrombin time does not improve, heparin may be administered	Heparin IV: 50 U/kg Infusion: 10-15 U/kg/hr
Effects of aspirin (ASA)	↑ template bleeding time	Platelets	1 U/5 kg (maximum: 10 U)

From Hazinski MF: Cardiovascular disorders. In Hazinski MF, editor: *Nursing care of the critically ill child*, ed 2, St Louis, 1992, Mosby.

FFP, Fresh frozen plasma; *Hct*, hematocrit; *P-RBC*, packed red blood cells; *PT*, prothrombin time; *PTT*, partial thromboplastin time.

* Generally unavailable; largely replaced by P-RBC.

† Usually, this condition results from a complex function of dilution and lack of replacement during surgery, inability of the liver to compensate, and occasionally from excessive loss of plasma protein (large proteins) via chest tubes.

‡ The only way to distinguish between these two problems is through protamine sulfate titration.

with crystalloid to improve intravascular blood flow, but these have not been consistently demonstrated to be superior to crystalloid. Colloid is not used for initial burn therapy.

Cardiogenic Shock

1. A fluid push may improve cardiac output by increasing filling pressure in accordance with the Frank-Starling curve, particularly if the CVP is less than 15 mm Hg. The PCWP is a more reliable measure of the response to fluid challenge in cardiogenic shock and should be measured if possible; insertion of a Swan-Ganz catheter should not delay aggressive stabilization, however. At 5 ml/kg over 30 minutes, 0.9% NS may be administered with careful monitoring of response.
2. Pressor agents (Table 5-3) are usually necessary if the response to IV fluid challenge is inadequate. Ultimately, inotropic and vasodilating drugs may be needed to normalize blood pressure.
3. Evaluation of the adequacy of preload (by CVP or PCWP measurements) and afterload is essential in monitoring the efficacy of therapy. Monitoring by echocardiography in consultation with a cardiologist is extremely important.

Distributive (Vasogenic) Shock

1. Septic shock. Intravenous fluids do not usually improve vital signs because cardiac output actually diminishes when preload is increased. Pressor agents are commonly required after adequate preload has been established and documented. Filling

TABLE 5-3 Commonly Used Drugs for Shock*

Drug	Dose (IV)	Comments
Isoproterenol (Isuprel)	0.05-1.5 μg/kg/min	Positive inotropic and chronotropic effect; peripheral vasodilation; increased cardiac oxygen requirement; relatively large increase in cardiac output; decreased coronary blood flow Use: decreased cardiac contractility; bradycardia and third-degree atrioventricular (AV) block
Dopamine (Inotropin)	Low: 2-5 μg/kg/min Mod: 5-20 μg/kg/min High: >20 μg/kg/min	Low: increased renal and mesenteric blood flow, little effect on heart (dopaminergic effect) Mod: increased renal blood flow, heart rate, cardiac contractility, and cardiac output High: systemic vasoconstriction May be used synergistically with isoproterenol or dobutamine
Dobutamine (Dobutrex)	2-20 μg/kg/min (usually 10-15 μg/kg/min)	Positive inotropic effect with minimal chronotropic; minimal β_2; useful in cardiogenic shock; may use with low-dose dopamine
Norepinephrine (Levophed)	0.1-1.0 μg/kg/min	Positive inotropic; intense alpha vasoconstrictor, with compromised peripheral tissue and organ perfusion Useful in cardiogenic shock caused by myocardial insufficiency; seldom used without an α blocker
Milrinone	Load: 50-75 μg/kg IV over several minutes Infusion: 0.5-0.75 μg/kg/min IV	Hypotension; risk of ventricular dysrhythmia
Epinephrine (Adrenalin)	0.1-1.0 μg/kg/min	Use only when isoproterenol and dopamine are ineffective; positive inotropic and chronotropic effects; renal and mesenteric ischemia; tachyrhythmia; increased cardiac oxygen requirements; intense alpha effect if >0.3 μg/kg/min
Sodium nitroprusside (Nipride)	0.5-10 μg/kg/min (average: 3 μg/kg/min)	Arterial and venous dilator; afterload reduction; rapid response, short duration
Phentolamine (Regitine)	0.05-0.1 mg/kg/dose q1-4hr IV prn	Counteracts vasoconstriction (alpha antagonist); useful for high CVP or in combination with vasoconstrictive drug; rapid onset, short activity; may also be given by continuous infusion
Naloxone (Narcan)	0.1 mg/kg/dose (0.8-2.0 mg/dose) IV q3-5min × 2 prn	May have role in septic shock (unproven); endorphin antagonist; alternative regimen: bolus of 0.03 mg/kg, then 0.03 mg/kg/hr IV infusion
Calcium chloride	0.2 ml/kg/dose q10 min prn IV slowly (20 mg/kg/dose) (maximum: 0.5 gm)	Positive inotropic and chronotropic effects; may cause bradycardia; controversial and unproven role

* Inotropic agents are not useful in the initial management of hypovolemic shock; volume replacement is required to achieve normovolemia.

pressure should be kept at the lowest level consistent with adequate tissue perfusion.

2. Anaphylaxis (see Chapter 12).
3. Head and spinal cord trauma (see Chapters 57 and 61). Pressor agents are usually required after adequate preload has been established and documented.

Cardiac Function

1. Treatment of dysrhythmias (see Chapters 4 and 6). Bradycardia, atrioventricular block, and tachyrhythmias are particularly detrimental to cardiac output. Predisposing conditions include electrolyte abnormalities, acidosis, alkalosis, drugs, fever, and pericardial disease as well as ischemic or hypoxic damage.
2. Inotropic agents (see Table 5-3). Although optimally the adequacy of preload should be evaluated by echocardiography, CVP, or PCWP before pharmacologic support is initiated, the evaluation must not delay aggressive stabilization. The efficacy of the agent can then be measured. Inotropic agents have no role in hypovolemic shock until normovolemia is achieved. They are fundamental components of therapy for cardiogenic and distributive shock.
   a. Classification of inotropic agents

	Mechanism/Effect		
Effector Organ	α-Adrenergic	β_1-Adrenergic	β_2-Adrenergic
Heart			
Rate		Increase	Increase
Contractility		Increase	
Conduction velocity		Increase	
Arterioles	Constrict		Dilate
Veins	Constrict		Dilate
Lung-bronchiolar smooth muscles	Constrict		Dilate

   b. If local infiltration of an agent with significant alpha effects (vasoconstriction) occurs during infusion, a significant risk of skin necrosis and ulceration exists. To minimize this when infiltration occurs, phentolamine (alpha antagonist), 1 to 5 mg diluted in 1 to 5 ml of 0.9% NS depending on the size of the child, is infiltrated locally.
   c. Often a combination of pressor agents is required to maximize the clinical effect. A typical combination consists of dopamine in low dosages (0.5-3 μg/kg/min) as one drug to maintain renal perfusion by dilating the splanchnic and renal vascular beds and a second drug such as dobutamine (5-15 μg/kg/min). Continuous infusions of isoproterenol and epinephrine may be used in severe, unresponsive situations.
3. Vasodilators
   a. If possible, the adequacy of preload and cardiac function should be evaluated by echocardiography and CVP or PCWP measurement before pharmacologic therapy is initiated, with careful monitoring of improvement of function with intervention.
   b. In cardiogenic shock, vasodilators such as nitroprusside (0.5-10 μg/kg/min IV) (p. 49) may be helpful for pulmonary congestion. Vasodilators are useful when peripheral hypoperfusion is present and when the patient is hypervolemic or has a major outflow obstruction secondary to arteriolar vasoconstriction. Vasodilators are usually used in combination with an inotropic drug. Because these agents may simultaneously reduce the preload, volume repletion may be required.

Hypovolemic Shock. Inotropic agents are not indicated for hypovolemic shock.

Cardiogenic Shock

1. Inotropic agents (e.g., dopamine, dobutamine) should be initiated if there is poor peripheral perfusion after an initial infusion of fluids to improve cardiac function. Periodically during inotropic therapy, a fluid challenge should be administered to reassess intravascular volume.
2. If pulmonary congestion exists or there is peripheral hypoperfusion in hypervolemic patients, vasodilators (e.g., nitroprusside) may be useful adjunctive therapy.

Distributive Shock. Primary therapy is to initiate positive inotropic agents while maintaining intravascular volume. In the early hyperdynamic phase (rare in children), there is a decreased afterload requiring volume administration. Later, with the decreased cardiac output and increased systemic vascular resistance secondary to hypoxemia and acidosis, isoproterenol (0.05-1.5 μg/kg/min) is particularly useful because it decreases peripheral resistance and has a positive inotropic effect.

Ancillary Procedures

These procedures require appropriate priority in the initial evaluation and stabilization concurrent with specific attention to the ABCs.

1. Elevate the legs unless respiratory distress or pulmonary edema is present.
2. Place a urinary catheter to monitor renal output and evaluate renal injury.
3. Insert a nasogastric tube to initiate decompression and provide information about GI bleeding.
4. Normalize temperature (see Chapters 50 and 51).
5. Consider and perform CT scan to exclude peritoneal blood loss (see Chapter 63) after trauma or, if appropriate, in the patient with ascites.
6. Insert a CVP catheter. This measure is particularly important in hypovolemic shock if positive-pressure ventilation is required or there is significant pulmonary, renal, or cardiac disease. A Swan-Ganz catheter permits measurement of the PCWP, which is particularly useful in cardiogenic or distributive shock.
7. Perform either pericardiocentesis (see Appendix A-5) to exclude pericardial tamponade or thoracentesis (see Appendix A-8) to treat tension pneumothorax if specific indications are present. Ultrasound may be helpful.

Other Considerations

1. Electrolyte and acid-base abnormalities must be corrected because they impair ventilation, depress the myocardium, predispose to dysrhythmias, and alter response to catecholamines. All corrections require frequent monitoring of response.
   a. Acidosis is a consistent finding, which must be at least partially corrected if the pH is less than 7.1. Early treatment of a pattern of deteriorating acid-base status may prevent complications. However, administration of bicarbonate causes oxygen to bind more tightly to oxyhemoglobin and may lead to hyperosmolality and hypernatremia. If acidosis is due to hypoventilation, consider active airway management. If the cause is metabolic, give 1 to 2 mEq/kg sodium bicarbonate ($NaHCO_3$) over 5 minutes IV. Repeat according to ABG levels. Correct pH only to 7.25, but monitor closely while ensuring good ventilation. Calculation: deficit mEq HCO_3^- = weight (kg) × base excess × 0.3.
   b. Hypocalcemia develops with a decrease in serum ionized calcium level; it is associated with impaired tissue perfusion. Hypocalcemia depresses myocardial function, as does hypophosphatemia. Give $CaCl_2$ 10% 10 to 20 mg/kg (0.1-0.2 ml/kg) IV slowly, optimally through a central venous line, while monitoring vital signs. Simultaneously check phosphorus level, treating a deficit with potassium phosphate, 5 to10 mg/kg slowly if K^+ is normal. If phosphorus level is high, care must be exercised in administering calcium.
2. Urine output is optimally maintained at 1 to 2 ml/kg/hr. Pharmacologic agents may be required to supplement volume repletion in the maintenance of urine flow. The choice of regimen must be individualized, reflecting the experience

of the clinician and the response to one or more of the agents. Oliguria is a common finding in prerenal failure and ATN (p. 828). The clinician must know the intravascular volume before initiating pharmacologic therapy. Treatment options in addition to fluid therapy include the following:

- **a.** Furosemide (Lasix), 1 mg/kg/dose up to 6 mg/kg/dose q2-6hr IV as needed.
- **b.** Mannitol, 0.25-1 g/kg/dose q4-6hr IV.
- **c.** Low-dose dopamine, 0.5-3 μg/kg/min IV continuous infusion.
- **d.** Monitoring input and output meticulously and replacing urine output milliliter by milliliter.
- **e.** Dialysis, which is required in unresponsive hyperkalemia, acidosis, or hypervolemia.

3. *Antibiotics* are appropriate because of the nonspecific nature of the clinical presentation. The critically ill child with shock from unknown cause is thus treated empirically. Ideally antibiotics are initiated after at least one blood culture result, and optimally all other relevant culture findings, has been obtained. Broad-spectrum antibiotics should be used initially to cover all potential pathogens, and the choice of antibiotic should be modified to reflect the results of culture and sensitivity testing.

- **a.** Cefotaxime, 50 to 150 mg/kg/24 hr q6-8hr IV (or ceftriaxone, 50-100 mg/kg/24 hr q12hr IV; or cefuroxime, 100-200 mg/kg/24 hr q6-8hr IV). In the newborn, ampicillin should be added and the dose altered.

  Other antibiotics should be used if there is a specific clinical indication, such as a perforated abdominal organ or toxic shock syndrome. Immunocompromised patients should receive coverage for *Pseudomonas aeruginosa* as well as more common pathogens.

4. *Corticosteroids* use in shock continues to be debated. The use of steroids in the treatment of gram-negative sepsis is probably detrimental. Administration of corticosteroids may be lifesaving, however, if a patient has adrenal cortical insufficiency. The exact role of these agents in patients in whom shock develops remains unclarified.

5. *Coagulopathy* may occur after shock of any cause. DIC is common (p. 694). With many coagulopathies associated with shock, the use of fresh frozen plasma is a rapid approach to correcting abnormalities and additionally provides volume expansion.

6. Mediator-specific therapy, including antiendotoxin and anti–tumor necrosis factor agents and LI-1 receptor antagonists, has been found to be effective in selected models. Recombinant human activated protein C (drotrecogin alfa) has antithrombotic, antiinflammatory, and profibrinolytic properties that have proven to reduce mortality in patients with severe sepsis. The role of such therapy in pediatric septic shock remains experimental.

7. Nitric oxide synthase inhibitors have been studied in animal models, leading to ongoing human investigations.

8. Extracorporeal membrane oxygenation (ECMO) has become an adjunct in the management of unresponsive septic shock progressing to multisystem organ dysfunction syndrome.

9. Anaphylactic shock is discussed in Chapter 12.

10. Patients who show no response to resuscitation efforts must be rapidly reevaluated to identify other coexisting causes. Consultation is mandatory. Factors that must be considered include the following:

- **a.** Multiple organ failure.

b. Myocardial injury, ischemia, or other damage as well as coronary artery disease.
c. Outflow or filling obstruction, such as tension pneumothorax or pericardial tamponade.
d. Coagulopathy and DIC.
e. Renal failure.
f. Respiratory failure.
g. Uncontrolled sepsis.
h. Ongoing blood loss.

DISPOSITION

All patients with shock must be admitted immediately to an intensive care unit. Cardiac, pulmonary, and infectious disease consultations should be requested immediately.

BIBLIOGRAPHY

Bernard GR, Vincent JL, Laterre PF et al: Efficacy and safety of recombinant human activated protein C for severe sepsis, *N Engl J Med* 244:699, 2001.

Bone RC: Sepsis and its complications: the clinical problem, *Crit Care Med* 22:88, 1994.

Hazinski MF, Barkin RM: Shock. In Barkin RM, editor: *Pediatric emergency medicine: concepts and clinical practice,* ed 2, St Louis, 1997, Mosby.

Royall JA, Levin DL: Adult respiratory distress syndrome in pediatric patients, *J Pediatr* 112:169, 335, 1988.

Saavedra JM, Harris GD, Li S et al: Capillary refilling (skin turgor) in the assessment of dehydration, *Am J Dis Child* 145:296, 1991.

Seffredini AF: Current prospects for the treatment of clinical sepsis, *Crit Care Med* 22:821, 1994.

Shapiro NI, Zimmer GD, Barkin AZ: Sepsis syndrome. In Marx JA, Hockberger RS, Walls RM et al, editors: *Rosen's Emergency Medicine: concepts and clinical practice,* ed 5, St Louis, 2002, Mosby.

6 Dysrhythmias

Dysrhythmias are uncommon in pediatric patients. Because of the differences in causes, particularly in infants and children, and the absence of ischemic heart disease, only a few types of disturbances are seen with any frequency.

The most common clinically significant dysrhythmias by age are as follows:

<1 yr	Bradycardia, atrial fibrillation, ventricular fibrillation
1-5 yr	Supraventricular tachycardia, bradycardia, atrial flutter
6-12 yr	Nonspecific dysrhythmia (NSD), supraventricular tachycardia, atrial flutter
13-18 yr	NSD, atrial fibrillation

Cardiac stimuli arise in specialized neuromuscular tissues within the heart, consisting of the sinus (sinoatrial) node, AV (atrioventricular) junction, bundle of His, right and left branches, and Purkinje fibers. The primary pacemaker is the sinus node. When this node is suppressed or fails to propagate impulses, a secondary pacemaker sets the cardiac rate. The stimuli become progressively slower as the site becomes more distal. The sympathetic and vagal fibers modify stimuli through the sinus node and AV junction. The sympathetic nervous system stimulates the heart, and the vagal or parasympathetic system has a suppressive effect, mostly on the sinus node and AV junction. Increased heart rate may result from greater sympathetic activity or diminished vagal tone; bradycardia is commonly caused by increased vagal tone, often secondary to myocardial hypoxia.

Dysrhythmias are caused by abnormal impulse formation or conduction or by a combined mechanism. *Automaticity* occurs when myocardial tissue independently depolarizes, reaches threshold, and fires. Automaticity is increased by hypokalemia, hypercalcemia, catecholamines, drugs (e.g., digitalis), and ischemia.

Reentry dysrhythmias occur when some areas of the heart are repolarized but other areas are not. Reentry can occur only when two pathways are connected proximally and distally.

Triggered automaticity occurs as a result of instability of the resting membrane potential after myocardial ischemia, fibrosis, or administration of a drug (e.g., calcium, digitalis).

Tachyrhythmias in children result from increased sympathetic activity, decreased vagal tone, ectopic pacemakers, or reentrant pathways that often involve abnormal or accessory connections. Accessory pathways produce preexcitation syndromes such as Wolff-Parkinson-White (WPW), which predisposes to paroxysmal atrial tachycardia, or supraventricular tachycardia (SVT).

Therapy is focused on interruption of the reentry or prevention of premature beats that trigger the cycle. Ectopic pacemakers are treated by suppression of the focus. Adenosine, an endogenous nucleoside, causes a temporary block through the AV node and interrupts the reentry circuit in stable patients with SVT; the dosage is 0.1 mg/kg IV (rapid). The adult dose is 6 mg initially, which may be doubled if there is no effect. Lidocaine is indicated in hemodynamically stable patients with ventricular dysrhythmias.

Bradyrhythmias are usually caused by slowing of the intrinsic pacemaker, which is often due to increased vagal tone or a conduction abnormality. The block in conduction may be complete, in which circumstance a more distal, slower pacemaker controls the rate, or it may be incomplete, allowing only a few impulses to pass (Tables 6-1 and 6-2).

Children at risk of dysrhythmias may have congenital or acquired heart disease, systemic disease, intoxication, or acute hemodynamic alterations.

Assessment requires a careful history and physical examination that focus on the vital signs, cardiac evaluation, and evidence of systemic disease. Prompt analysis of the electrocardiogram (ECG) and hemodynamic measurements is imperative.

Symptomatic patients may show evidence of congestive heart failure (see Chapter 16), including pallor, irritability, poor eating, dyspnea, decreased cerebral blood flow associated with syncope and altered behavior, decreased coronary blood flow and anginal pain, or a perception of a rhythm disturbance marked by palpitations or missed beats.

Newborns and infants with SVT commonly have tachypnea, lethargy, decreased feeding, and respiratory distress that may progress to hypotension and shock. Older children have chest discomfort or pain, palpitations, faintness, and occasionally syncope or cardiac arrest.

ANALYSIS OF ELECTROCARDIOGRAM
(see Appendix B-3)

1. Rate
   a. Rate (beats/min) is age dependent (newborn: 100 to 160, infant: 120 to 160, toddler: 80 to 150, child older than 6 years: 60 to 120).
   b. Each small box on the ECG represents 0.04 seconds, and the time between vertical lines at top of the strip is 3 seconds. Determine heart rate by multiplying number of complexes between two vertical lines by 20.
2. Axis: Axis is age specific, also reflecting hypertrophy or conduction defects.
3. Rhythm
   a. Regularity or irregularity.
   b. Voltage (low with myocarditis or effusion).
4. P wave
   a. Presence implies atrial activity, although it may be buried in QRS interval, ST segment, or T wave. Seen best in leads II, III, and aVF.
   b. Enlarged or biphasic (V_1) (atrial hypertrophy); normal: 0.08 to 0.1 second.
   c. Configuration (normal versus ectopic foci).
5. PR interval
   a. A fixed relationship between the P wave and QRS interval implies that the rhythm is supraventricular in origin.
   b. Interval is age and rate dependent, ranging from 0.1 to 0.2 second.
   c. Prolongation occurs with first-degree block, hyperkalemia, digitalis, propranolol, verapamil, adenosine, quinidine, and carditis (acute rheumatic fever).
   d. Short in WPW syndrome, it also has delta wave.
6. QRS complex
   a. Duration is normally less than 0.1 second.
   b. Prolongation occurs with conduction defect, ventricular focus, severe hyperkalemia, and quinidine.
   c. Abnormal configuration demonstrates that the focus is ventricular in origin or that there is a conduction defect.
   d. High voltage implies hypertrophy or overload pattern.
7. ST segment
   a. Elevated with transmural injury, pericarditis, ventricular aneurysm.
   b. Depressed with subendocardial injury, digitalis, systolic overload, and strain.
8. T wave
   a. Peaks in hyperkalemia (if severe, QRS interval is also widened); flat with hypokalemia.

TABLE 6-1 Characteristics of Common Dysrhythmias

Dysrhythmia	Rate/min (>6 yr old)	Rhythm	P Wave (atrial)	QRS Complex	AV Conduction	Response to Vagotonic Maneuver	Comments
BRADYRHYTHMIAS							
Sinus bradycardia	<60	Regular	Upright I, II, aVF	WNL	WNL	None	Found in athletes, hypothyroidism, increased intracranial pressure, with drugs (propranolol or digitalis); if no symptoms, no treatment; if serious, use atropine, pacemaker; rate is age specific
Sinus dysrhythmia	60-120	Irregular	Upright I, II, aVF	WNL	WNL	Transient slowing	Normal variation with respiration and varying vagal tone; reassurance needed
SUPRAVENTRICULAR TACHYRHYTHMIAS							
Sinus tachycardia	120-200	Regular	Upright I, II, aVF	WNL	WNL	Transient slowing	Secondary to fever, exercise, anemia, shock, hyperthyroidism; treat condition
Premature atrial complex (PAC)	60-120	Irregular	Variable	WNL	WNL, may be first-degree block	Slows	Stimulants (caffeine, smoking, alcohol), digitalis toxicity, early congestive heart failure (CHF), hypoxia; if infrequent, no treatment; avoid stimulants; if frequent, treat condition; rarely need propranolol or quinidine
Paroxysmal supraventricular tachycardia (SVT)	150-250	Regular	Buried; nonsinus, variably retrograde	WNL	WNL	None or converts	Most common significant dysrhythmia in children (reentry); children <5 yr: infection, fever, congenital heart disease; older children: WPW (short PR segment, ± prolonged QRS complex,

							delta wave); may cause cardiac decompensation secondary to inadequate filling time; occurs with digitalis toxicity, particularly with block
Junctional premature contraction	NA	Irregular	Retrograde, often obscured	WNL or aberrant	Variable	None	Same as PAC
Atrial flutter	100-300 (atrial: 200-300)	Regular	Flutter (saw toothed) waves II, III, aVF	WNL	Variable block	None	Heart disease, thyrotoxicosis, pulmonary embolism, myocarditis, chest trauma
Atrial fibrillation	60-190 (atrial: 400-700)	Irregularly irregular	No P waves; fibrillation waves	WNL	Variable block	Transient slowing	As above (atrial flutter); severe valvular disease (mitral stenosis, tricuspid insufficiency, aortic stenosis), WPW and without heart disease
VENTRICULAR TACHYRHYTHMIAS							
Premature ventricular complex (PVC)	NA	Irregular	Usually obscured	≥ 0.12 sec, premature, bizarre	Compensatory pause, variable retrograde	None	ST segment and T wave opposite in polarity to QRS complex; variably significant if >6/min, multifocal, occurs near T wave, increases with exercise, or occurs in bigeminy or trigeminy; associated with cardiac ischemia, digitalis toxicity, ↓ K^+, hypoxia, alkalosis
Ventricular tachycardia	150-220	Regular or slightly irregular	Usually not recog-nizable	≥ 0.12 sec, bizarre	None	None	ST segment and T wave opposite in polarity to QRS complex; may cause hemodynamic compromise requiring immediate treatment
Ventricular fibrillation	Indeter-minate	None	Not recog-nizable	Irregular undulation	None	None	Disorganized, ineffective cardiac activity without pulse or blood pressure; medical emergency: defibrillate

WNL, Within normal limits; *NA*, not applicable.

TABLE 6-2 Characteristics of Conduction Disturbances*

Type	Atrial Rate	Ventricle Rate	PR Interval	Ventricular Rhythm	P-QRS Relation	QRS Complex	Comment
First degree	Unaffected	Same as atrial	Prolonged for age	Same as atrial	Consistent 1 : 1	Unaffected	Delay anywhere from AV node to bundle branches; may be caused by digitalis; no therapy necessary
Second degree (Wenckebach Mobitz I)	Unaffected	Slower than atrial	Progressive increase until P wave is dropped	Irregular	Variable† (recurring)	Narrow; constant; irregular	Delay at AV node; may be caused by digitalis or quinidine; therapy rarely needed; do not give potassium
Second degree (Mobitz II)	Unaffected	Slower than atrial	Normal or prolonged; constant	Irregular or regular	Fixed†	Usually wide; constant	Delay at bundle of His or below; may be precursor to complete block; pacemaker needed; temporize with atropine or isoproterenol
Third degree	Unaffected	Slower than atrial	Variable	Regular	None†	Constant; regular	Delay is anywhere from AV node to bundle branches; life threatening; pacemaker; temporize with atropine or isoproterenol

* May be idiopathic, acquired (nonsurgical), postoperative, or congenital.
† More Ps than QRSs.

   b. Inverted with conduction defect or ischemia.
9. QT segment
   a. Duration is rate dependent but with correction (QTc) should be less than 0.42 second.
   b. Prolonged with quinidine, procainamide, overdose of cyclic antidepressants, hypokalemia, hypocalcemia, hypomagnesemia, and hypothermia.

ANCILLARY DATA

1. The patient's response to vagotonic maneuvers should be evaluated. Vagotonic maneuvers include massage of the carotid (unilateral), Valsalva's maneuver, brisk application of cold water to the face, deep inspiration, coughing, drinking cold water, and gagging. The resulting increased vagal tone should cause at least a transient slowing of the heart rate if the rhythm is supraventricular. Do not perform eyeball compression or simultaneous, bilateral carotid massage.
2. Continuous monitoring is essential. In the hospital setting the patient should be moved to a monitored unit. After discharge transtelephonic electrocardiography has been useful in defining dysrhythmias and monitoring the efficacy of drug and pacemaker therapy.
3. Electrophysiologic studies may be indicated.
   a. Tachydysrhythmias. Supraventricular (preexcitation WPW) with syncope and frequent episodes of SVT unresponsive to vagotonic maneuvers or medication. Ventricular dysrhythmias requiring study include patients with associated heart disease and those with cardiac tumors, myocarditis, or metabolic disorders.
4. Bradydysrhythmias requiring investigation are sick sinus syndrome and AV conduction defects.

MANAGEMENT (Tables 6-3, 6-4, and 6-5)

Once a dysrhythmia has been identified, the clinician must determine whether there is any compromise in cardiac output or hemodynamic parameters and whether the rhythm is potentially life threatening. Six questions must be addressed:

1. Does the patient truly have a dysrhythmia?
2. Is the heart rate fast or slow?
3. If the heart rate is fast, is the QRS complex wide (>0.08 second) or narrow?
4. Does the patient require therapy (i.e., how stable is the patient)?
5. How soon is therapy required?
6. What is the most effective and safest therapy?

TABLE 6-3 Overview of Dysrhythmia Pharmacologic Management*

	HEMODYNAMIC STABILITY	
Heart Rate/ QRS	**Unstable**	**Stable**
SLOW		
(See Fig. 4-2)	Epinephrine† Atropine Isoproterenol Pacing	Oxygen Ventilation Atropine
FAST		
Narrow QRS	Cardioversion Adenosine‡	Adenosine
Wide QRS	Cardioversion Consider amiodarone, procainamide, or lidocaine	Amiodarone, procainamide, or lidocaine Cardioversion§
ABSENT		
Ventricular fibrillation	Defibrillation (see Fig. 4-3)	
Asystole	See Fig. 4-3	
PEA	See Fig. 4-3	

* Assumes resuscitation efforts are ongoing.
† Give atropine first for bradycardia caused by suspected increased vagal tone or primary AV block.
‡ If vascular access and medication are immediately available.
§ Cardioversion or medication may be appropriate.

TABLE 6-4 Common Antidysrhythmic Drugs

			BLOOD LEVEL		DOSAGE		
Drug	**ECG Effect**	**Half-life**	**Therapeutic**	**Toxic**	**Initial**	**Maintenance**	**Adverse Reactions**
Digoxin (Table 16-2)	Prolongs PR	24 hr	1-3.5 μg/ml	>3.5 μg/ml (variable)	TDD premature infant: 0.01-0.02 mg/kg IV TDD 2 wk-2 yr: 0.03-0.05 mg/kg IV TDD newborn and >2 yr: 0.04 mg/kg IV; ½ TDD initially, then ¼ q4-8hr IV × 2	¼-⅓ TDD q12-24hr PO, or IV	Ventricular ectopy, tachycardia, fibrillation, atrial tachycardia, AV block, vomiting; slow onset
Lidocaine	Shortens QT	5 hr	1-5 μg/ml	>10 μg/ml	1 mg/kg/dose IV (may repeat in 10 min) to max 5 mg/kg	20-50 μg/kg/min IV (adult: 2-4 mg/min)	Seizure, drowsiness, euphoria, muscle twitching; may give ET (dilute 1:1)
Quinidine	Prolongs QRS, QT, ± PR	6 hr	2-6 μg/ml	>9 μg/ml	15-60 mg/kg/24 hr q6hr PO (adult: 300-400 mg q6hr PO)	Same	GI symptoms, PVC, syncope, hypotension, anemia
Procainamide	Prolongs QRS, QT, ± PR	3-4 hr	4-10 μg/ml	>10 μg/ml	2-6 mg/kg/dose IV slowly (adult: 100 mg/dose IV q10min prn or 25-50 mg/min, and titrate up to total dose of 1 g)	20-80 μg/kg/min IV (adult: 1-3 mg/min IV) 15-50 mg/kg/24 hr q4-6hr PO (adult: 250-500 mg/dose q4-6hr PO up to 4 g/24 hr)	Hypotension, lupuslike syndrome, urticaria, GI symptoms

Amiodarone (Cordarone)	Prolongs PR	20-47 days	Not useful		VF/VT: 5 mg/kg IV over 5-10 min; may repeat in 30 min PSVT: 5 mg/kg over 20-60 min	10-15 mg/kg/24 hr IV or 5 μg/kg/min IV	Bradycardia, myocardial depression, CHF, dysrhythmia (increased risk with ↓K^+, ↓Mg^{++}
Propranolol	Prolongs PR, shortens QT	2-4 hr	20-150 μg/ml	NA	0.01-0.1 mg/kg/dose IV over 10 min (adult: 1 mg/dose IV q5min up to 5 mg)	0.5-1.0 mg/kg/24 hr q6hr PO (adult: 10-80 mg/dose q6-8hr PO)	Bradycardia, hypotension, cardiac failure, asthma, hypoglycemia; do not give to patient with asthma; overdose treated with glucagon 0.1 mg/kg/dose IV
Verapamil	Shortens QT, prolongs PR	3-7 hr (variable)			0.1 mg/kg/dose IV over 1-2 min repeated in 10-30 min prn (adult: 5-10 mg/dose IV)	NA	Bradycardia, hypotension, apnea, AV block, negative inotropic agent; do not use in children <1 yr or if patient is taking β blocker; adenosine usually preferred

±, Variable effect; *NA*, not applicable; *TDD*, total digitalizing dose.

Continued

TABLE 6-4 Common Antidysrhythmic Drugs—cont'd

			BLOOD LEVEL		DOSAGE		
Drug	**ECG Effect**	**Half-life**	**Therapeutic**	**Toxic**	**Initial**	**Maintenance**	**Adverse Reactions**
Adenosine	Slows AV nodal conduction	10 sec	NA	NA	0.1 mg/kg IV as rapidly as possible; may double and repeat in 2 min; adult: 6 mg IV (rapid) and if no response in 2 min give 12 mg IV (rapid)	NA	Transient AV block; half-life is 10 sec
Phenytoin (Dilantin)	Shortens QT	20-26 hr	10-20 μg/ml	>20 μg/ml	5 mg/kg/dose IV over 5 min (<0.5 mg/kg/min) (adult: 100 mg/dose IV q5 min up to 1 g)	6 mg/kg/24 hr q12hr PO (adult: 300 mg/24 hr PO)	Ataxia, nystagmus, hypotension; new formulation available to reduce adverse reaction
Atropine	Increases rate	<5 min	NA	NA	0.02 mg/kg/dose IV; repeat q2-5 min × 2 prn	NA	Tachycardia, mydriasis, dry mouth
Isoproterenol	Increases rate	<5 min	NA	NA	0.05-1.5 μg/kg/min IV; begin 0.1 μg/kg/min and increase q5-10 min (adult: 2-20 μg/min/IV)	NA	Tachycardia, PVC

TABLE 6-5 Acute Treatment of Common Dysrhythmias*

Dysrhythmia	Treatment	Comments
SUPRAVENTRICULAR TACHYRHYTHMIA (FAST HEART RATE; NARROW QRS)		
Supraventricular tachycardia (SVT)	Vagotonic maneuvers (iced water to face, Valsalva's maneuver, etc.)	Attempt in all patients first: carotid sinus massage, Valsalva's maneuver
With critical hemodynamic compromise	DC-synchronized cardioversion (0.5-1.0 J/kg) Adenosine	
Without critical hemodynamic compromise	Adenosine Digoxin Edrophonium	Do not use digoxin if any question of WPW; adenosine may be used with WPW
Atrial flutter	Digoxin DC-synchronized cardioversion (0.5-1.0 J/kg) Propranolol	Do not use digoxin with WPW; cardioversion if hemodynamic compromise occurs; potentially unstable
Atrial fibrillation	Same as atrial flutter	Same as atrial flutter; considered anticoagulation with prolonged atrial fibrillation
VENTRICULAR TACHYRHYTHMIA (FAST HEART RATE; WIDE QRS)		
Premature ventricular contractions (PVC)	Amiodarone Procainamide Lidocaine	Quinidine, procainamide, propranolol, or phenytoin for long-term suppression
Ventricular tachycardia		
With critical hemodynamic compromise	DC-synchronized cardioversion (0.5-1.0 J/kg) Amiodarone Procainamide Lidocaine	Administer bolus simultaneously with cardioversion; maintenance therapy includes quinidine or procainamide
Without critical hemodynamic compromise	Amiodarone Procainamide Lidocaine DC-synchronized cardioversion (0.5-1.0 J/kg)	Same as above
Ventricular fibrillation	DC defibrillation (2-4 J/kg) Amiodarone Lidocaine	May also give epinephrine if defibrillation ineffective
BRADYRHYTHMIA (SLOW HEART RATE)		
Sinus bradycardia	Ventilation Oxygen Epinephrine Atropine	Hypoxia is most common cause; give atropine first for bradycardia caused by suspected increased vagal tone or primary atrioventricular block; therapy if unstable
Atrioventricular block	Atropine Isoproterenol (temporize) Pacemaker	Therapy if unstable; be certain not digoxin induced

Continued

TABLE 6-5 Acute Treatment of Common Dysrhythmias*—cont'd

Dysrhythmia	Treatment	Comments
DIGITALIS-INDUCED		
Paroxysmal atrial tachycardia (PAT) with block	Potassium chloride (40 mEq/L peripheral IV or 0.5-1.0 mEq/kg/hr central IV) Phenytoin	Stop drug, self-limited; avoid cardioversion, propranolol; worsened by ↓ K^+ ↓ Mg^{++}, ↑ Ca^{++}
PVC or ventricular tachycardia	Potassium chloride Phenytoin Lidocaine	Avoid cardioversion; see above

* Oxygen, CPR, and other supportive treatments may be required. Cardiology consultation should be requested. (See also Figs. 4-1 and 4-2.)

Management must focus on prevention, control of the underlying condition, and specific therapy for the dysrhythmia.

1. Administer oxygen during stabilization of the airway, ventilation, and circulation. Treatment of the underlying condition, which often causes hypoxia, may adequately resolve the dysrhythmia.
2. Usually, one medication is initiated until the therapeutic effect is achieved or toxicity is noted (see Figs. 4-1 and 4-2). If the agent has no effect, additional medications should be used. Adenosine in an initial dose of 0.1 mg/kg IV (given as rapidly as possible) is generally preferred in children with SVT. Amiodarone is good for life-threatening refractory atrial flutter, ventricular tachyrhythmias, and SVTs. For pulseless ventricular fibrillation (VF) or ventricular tachycardia, an initial dosage is 5 mg/kg IV (given as rapidly as possible), whereas for perfusing tachycardias, a loading dose of 5 mg/kg IV over 20 to 60 min should be used.
3. Electrical conversion is used to treat ventricular fibrillation and symptomatic tachyrhythmias that are unresponsive to pharmacologic therapy or are accompanied by hemodynamic compromise. Sedation is often advantageous before this procedure. Children can usually tolerate tachyrhythmias for long periods before cardiac decompensation occurs.
   a. Defibrillation is the untimed depolarization used to convert ventricular fibrillation. Synchronized cardioversion is a timed depolarization that prevents stimulation of the heart during the vulnerable part of the cardiac cycle, thereby avoiding the initiation of lethal ventricular dysrhythmias. Cardioversion is useful in conversion of ventricular tachyrhythmias.
   b. Direct current defibrillators are used; it is crucial that the low joule (J) range be appropriately calibrated. Paddle size should ensure full contact with the chest. Many models have a "quick-look" feature, allowing immediate assessment of the rhythm.

      Transthoracic impedance can be minimized by using an adult-sized paddle (8-10 cm in diameter) for a child if the chest is large enough to permit electrode-to-chest contact over the entire paddle surface, usually by 1 year or 10 kg. Smaller pediatric paddles should be used for infants less than 10 kg.
   c. The paddles are placed on the anterior chest, one to the right of the sternum at the second intercostal space and the other to the left of the midclavicular

line at the level of the xiphoid. Electrode cream or paste is applied to the paddles before they are placed on the chest.

d. Defibrillation uses 2 J/kg initially. This shock may be repeated if the first attempt is unsuccessful, and then repeated with double the dose. If still unsuccessful, apply another shock at 4 J/kg. The International Liaison Committee on Resuscitation suggests that 2 to 4 J/kg be used for the second and third shocks. If the third administration is unsuccessful, lidocaine is administered with oxygen and correction of the acid-base status and temperature abnormalities. Epinephrine should also be considered. Defibrillation is then repeated, if necessary, at 4 J/kg.

e. Cardioversion is useful for tachyrhythmias. Commonly, 0.5 J/kg is administered with the synchronizer circuit; if unsuccessful, the dose is doubled. Hypoxia, acidosis, hypoglycemia, and hyperthermia should be corrected.

4. Pacemakers are the definitive therapeutic modality in the treatment of bradyrhythmias and AV conduction abnormalities associated with hemodynamic compromise. External, transcutaneous, temporary transvenous, and permanent pacemakers are available. Transesophageal pacing may be effective for cardioversion of atrial flutter and SVTs, but experience in children is limited.

5. Radiofrequency ablation may emerge as a primary therapy for dysrhythmia in the future.

DISPOSITION

Cardiology consultation is usually indicated in recurrent or unresponsive dysrhythmias as well as in those that cause hemodynamic compromise. These principles should also determine the need for hospitalization and the urgency of initiating therapy. It is imperative not only to treat the dysrhythmia but also to institute a program to prevent recurrence. Caffeine and other stimulants should be avoided.

BIBLIOGRAPHY

American Heart Association: Guidelines for cardiopulmonary resuscitation (CPR) and emergency cardiac care, *Circulation* 102:I1-I384, 2000.

Atkins DL, Sirna S, Kieso R: Pediatric defibrillation: importance of paddle size in determining transthoracic impedance, *Pediatrics* 82:914, 1988.

Binder LS, Boeche R, Atkinson D: Evaluation and management of supraventricular tachycardia in children, *Ann Emerg Med* 20:51, 1991.

Chameides L: Dysrhythmias. In Barkin RM, editor: *Pediatric emergency medicine: concepts and clinical practice,* ed 2, St Louis, 1997, Mosby.

Etheridge SP and Craig J: Amiodarone is safe and highly effective as primary therapy for tachycardia in infancy, *Pediatrics* 104:675, 1999.

Losek JD, Endom E, Dietrich A et al: Adenosine and pediatric supraventricular tachycardia in the emergency department: multicenter study and review, *Ann Emerg Med* 33:185, 1999.

Magayzel C, Quan Land, Graves JC et al: Out-of-hospital ventricular fibrillation in children and adolescents: causes and outcomes, *Ann Emerg Med* 25:484, 1995.

Reyes G, Stanton R, Galvis AG: Adenosine in the treatment of paroxysmal supraventricular tachycardia in children, *Ann Emerg Med* 21:1499, 1992.

Sacchetti A, Moyer V, Baricella R et al: Primary cardiac arrhythmia in children, *Pediatr Emerg Care* 15:95, 1999.

Truong JH, Rosen P: Current concepts in electrical defibrillation, *J Emerg Med* 15:331, 1997.

III

Fluid and Electrolyte Balance

Management of the pediatric patient with fluid and electrolyte disturbance requires an understanding of maintenance requirements and of the sources of abnormal losses. It is imperative to correlate history, physical, and laboratory data in patient management.

7 Dehydration

Also See Chapter 5 (Shock)

DIAGNOSTIC FINDINGS

Clinical assessment combined with ancillary laboratory data determines the urgency and type of therapy required for dehydration.

Degree of Dehydration

	Mild (<5%)	Moderate (5-10%)	Severe (10-15%)
Signs and symptoms			
Dry mucous membrane	±	+	+
Reduced skin turgor	–	±	+
Depressed anterior fontanel	–	±	+
Mental status	Alert	Irritable	Lethargic
Sunken eyeballs	–	+	+
Hyperpnea	–	±	+
Hypotension (orthostatic)	–	±	+
Increased pulse	–	+	+
Capillary refill	≤2 sec	≥2 sec	>2 sec
Laboratory findings			
Urine			
Volume	Small	Oliguria	Oliguria/anuria
Specific gravity*	≤1.020†	>1.030	>1.035
Blood urea nitrogen (BUN)†	Within normal limits	Elevated	Very high
pH†	7.40-7.30	7.30-7.00	<7.10

+, Present; –, absent; ±, variable.
* Specific gravity value can confirm the physical assessment.
† Not usually indicated in mild or moderate dehydration.

In the child with only very mild dehydration (2% to 3%), a slight decrease in mucosal membrane moisture and the relative dryness and prominence of the papillae of the tongue may be all that are noted on physical examination. A useful guide to hydration status in the younger child is to determine the number of diapers changed and their dampness in the preceding 6 to 8 hours.

Beyond the measurements just indicated, the percentage of dehydration may be estimated with the following calculation, assuming weights are available:

$$\%\ \text{Dehydration} = 1 - \left(\frac{\text{Present weight}}{\text{Recent known weight}}\right) \times 100\%$$

Orthostatic vital signs should be assessed in older children. When the patient rises from a lying to a standing (or sitting) position, a decrease in blood pressure of 15 to 20 mm Hg or an increase in pulse of 20 beats/min after 2 or 3 minutes is significant. These changes may be seen in children without hypovolemia.

Children can often compensate for fluid losses because of their ability to constrict peripheral blood vessels and redistribute blood flow centrally. With uncompensated shock, vital organ functions are maintained. Perfusion to the peripheral (skin and muscle) blood vessels may be compromised, causing prolonged capillary refill (>2 seconds) and a pale, blue, or mottled appearance. Poor central nervous system perfusion may impair mental activity. An acute volume deficit of 10% may produce a minimal pulse increase, but progressive changes occur with further fluid deficit. Gradual volume losses are better tolerated.

The amount of fluid deficit can be calculated by multiplying the percentage of dehydration (e.g., 3%, 5%, 10%) by the weight of the child in kilograms (e.g., a 10-kg child who is 10% dehydrated has a total deficit of 1000 ml or 100 ml/kg). Clinical assessment combined with a HCO_3^- level less than 17 mEq/L is useful in predicting dehydration of more than 5%. The electrolyte composition of this fluid deficit depends on the rapidity of progression of dehydration (normally 60% extracellular fluid [ECF] and 40% intracellular fluid [ICF]). In general, the percentage of loss from ECF is larger with a more acute progression and smaller with more chronic loss. The electrolyte composition of these compartments may be simplified as follows: ECF, 140 mEq Na^+/L, and ICF, 150 mEq K^+/L.

Types of Dehydration

The types of dehydration are based on serum sodium concentration, reflecting osmolality in the moderately or severely dehydrated patient. Clinical assessment of the patient with hypernatremia tends to underestimate the severity of dehydration because perfusion is preserved longer in this condition.

	Isotonic	Hypotonic	Hypertonic
Serum sodium level (mEq/L)	130-150	<130	>150
Physical signs			
Skin			
Color	Gray	Gray	Gray
Temperature	Cold	Cold	Cold
Turgor	Poor	Very poor	Fair
Feel	Dry	Clammy	Thick, doughy
Mucous membrane	Dry	Dry	Parched
Sunken eyeballs	+	+	+
Depressed anterior fontanel	+	+	+
Mental status	Lethargic	Comatose/seizure	Irritable/seizure
Increased pulse	++	++	+
Decreased blood pressure	++	+++	+

+, ++, +++, Relative prominence of finding.

Complications

Complications of dehydration are shock (see Chapter 5) and acute tubular necrosis (p. 828).

Ancillary Data

The following laboratory findings to assess hydration status are always indicated for children who are moderately or severely dehydrated but only rarely for those with only a mild hydration deficit.

1. Serum electrolyte and glucose levels.
2. BUN level: often elevated; with appropriate rehydration, will drop by 50% over first 24 hours. If drop does not occur, consider hemolytic-uremic syndrome as a cause (p. 819). If intake is poor or the child is malnourished, BUN level may be low because of low protein.

3. Specific gravity of urine to confirm physical findings.
4. Complete blood count to assess risk of infection.
5. Other studies as indicated by underlying condition.

MANAGEMENT OF SEVERE AND MODERATE DEHYDRATION

Restoration of Vascular Volume: Phase I

Immediate infusion of fluids is needed, particularly in patients with abnormal vital signs. If possible, orthostatic blood pressure and pulse should be measured in the recumbent position on older patients with normal vital signs. While the patient changes from a lying to a standing (or sitting) position, a decrease of 15 mm Hg in blood pressure or an increase of 20 beats/min in pulse after 2 to 3 minutes is considered significant. These changes may be seen in the absence of hypovolemia and therefore require clinical correlations.

Fluid Therapy

1. In the moderately or severely dehydrated child, 0.9% NS (normal saline) solution or lactated Ringer's (LR) solution should be given at 20 ml/kg (adult = 1-2 L) over 20 minutes.
2. If a poor therapeutic response is noted, but renal and cardiac functions are normal, the initial infusion should be followed by an additional 10 to 20 ml/kg (adult: 0.5-1 L) over 20 to 30 minutes.
3. If a poor therapeutic response is noted in the severely dehydrated child after two or three fluid pushes (i.e., no urine, continued abnormal vital signs, poor perfusion) with ongoing losses or with suspected cardiac or renal disease, more aggressive assessment and monitoring may be indicated (see Chapter 5).
4. Glucose infusion with crystalloid as 5% dextrose in water (D5W) 0.9% NS or D5WLR may be used for the initial bolus in children who have experienced prolonged vomiting, diarrhea, or inadequate intake and in whom a low blood glucose level is anticipated. Blood glucose levels should be checked and monitored.
5. The initial phase I bolus of 20 to 50 ml/kg to restore vascular volume is not routinely included in phase II and III water deficit and maintenance corrections.

Specific Therapeutic Plans: Phases II and III

Case examples of the three major categories of dehydration (isotonic, hypotonic, and hypertonic) provide a basis for fluid management. Maintenance requirements are summarized in Chapter 8. Patients with ongoing abnormal losses need additional replacement therapy based on either approximations (see Chapter 8) or direct determination of the electrolyte composition of fluid losses. Vital signs, intake and output, and ancillary data (electrolyte, BUN, and glucose levels) must be monitored constantly. These patients require hospital observation and, often, admission.

Isotonic Volume Depletion: Management of Moderate to Severe Dehydration

In children, the most common form of dehydration is isotonic. Box 7-1 reflects a sample management plan for such children.

Oral rehydration has been recommended in specific circumstances for children who can tolerate oral fluids and who have no contraindications, including shock, intractable vomiting, voluminous diarrhea that cannot be matched with oral intake, intestinal obstruction, or short bowel syndrome. *This is generally most useful for mild to moderate deficits in cooperative children.*

Oral glucose facilitates the absorption of sodium and water across the mucosal cells of the small intestine, an osmolality in the range of 250 mOsm/L being preferable to a higher osmolality. Current

Box 7-1

ISOTONIC VOLUME DEPLETION: MANAGEMENT OF MODERATE TO SEVERE DEFICITS

INITIAL FINDINGS

Pre-illness weight: 10 kg (1-yr-old child)
Degree of volume depletion: Moderate (10%)
Body weight on admission: 9 kg
Electrolyte levels:

Na^+: 135 mEq/L	K^+: 5 mEq/L	Cl^-: 115 mEq/L	HCO_3^-: 12 mEq/L

SUMMARY OF FLUID REQUIREMENTS

	H_2O (ml)	Na^+ (mEq)	K^+ (mEq)
Maintenance	1000 (100 ml/kg)	30 (3 mEq/kg)	20 (2 mEq/kg)
Deficit (100 ml/kg)			
ECF (60%)	600	84 (140 mEq/L × 0.6)	
ICF (40%)	400	—	30 (150 mEq/L × 0.4 × 50% correction)
TOTAL	1000 ml	84 mEq	30 mEq
Rescuscitation fluids	200 ml	28 mEq	
Net total deficit	800 ml	56 mEq	30 mEq

FLUID SCHEDULE

Phase	Calculation	Fluids Administered
I (0–½ hr)	20 ml/kg	200 ml 0.9% NS or LR over 20-30 min
II (½–9 hr)	½ net deficit: 400 ml D5W with 28 mEq NaCl and 15 mEq KCl ⅓ maintenance: 333 ml D5W with 10 mEq NaCl and 7 mEq KCl TOTAL: 733 ml with 38 mEq NaCl and 22 mEq KCl	733 ml (~90 ml/hr) of D5W 0.45% NS with 22 mEq KCl (~30 mEq KCl) (this approximation facilitates care)
III (9–25 hr)	½ deficit ⅔ maintenance	1067 ml (~67 ml/hr) of D5W 0.45% NS with 28 mEq KCl (~26 mEq/L) (this approximation facilitates care)

NOTES:

1. Fluid resuscitation is critical during phase I. If initial response is poor, additional infusion(s) is warranted. Generally, the initial emergency fluid bolus should be included as part of the deficit replacement.
2. Blood glucose level should be assessed early, especially in children with prolonged vomiting, diarrhea, or inadequate intake. Early glucose infusion may be warranted.
3. In general, after a bolus of normal saline solution, D5W 0.45% NS with KCl 20 mEq/L is the appropriate fluid, infused at a rate reflecting both deficit and maintenance requirements.
4. If a patient is acidotic with HCO_3^- level of ≤10 mEq/L or a pH <7.1 on the basis of metabolic acidosis, one third of the sodium may be administered as $NaHCO_3$.
5. In the presence of acidosis, serum potassium level does not reflect total body deficit.
6. Should be adjusted for fever: (10% should be added for each 1° C over 37° C), stool loss (5 ml/kg), or vomiting (volume for volume).

recommendations in young children distinguish between fluids used for initial oral rehydration under close supervision and careful monitoring followed by maintenance solutions:

Component	Rehydration Solution (for treatment of acute dehydration)	Maintenance Solution
Sodium	70-90 mEq/L	40-60 mEq/L
Potassium	20-30 mEq/L	20 mEq/L
Glucose	2-2.5 g/dl	2-2.5 g/dl

In infants, Rehydralyte is an excellent rehydration solution, whereas Pedialyte and Infalyte are excellent liquids for maintenance.

Management using oral hydration may be performed as follows:

a. 100 ml/kg over 4 hours *or*
b. Twice the deficit volume over 6 to 12 hours *or*
c. Deficit volume plus 12 hours of maintenance fluids over 12 hours *or*
d. Ad lib feedings to a maximum of 200 ml/kg/24 hr

If the patient has vomited, increase the feeding aliquots in 5- to 10-ml increments. Small amounts of vomiting are not a contraindication to enteral therapy. For each diarrhea stool seen in the emergency department, 10 ml/kg of fluids should be added. As soon as children are rehydrated, they should be fed age-appropriate diets.

If the child refuses to feed actively, passive enteral therapy can be instituted with a nasogastric (NG) tube or with repeated 2- to 5-ml syringe boluses to the back of the mouth. A systematic study of nasogastric rehydration, utilizing standard oral rehydrating solutions (Pedialyte was used in the study) found delivery of 50 ml/kg over 3 hours to be efficacious. Obviously, if these are unsuccessful, parenteral therapy should be considered.

Hypotonic Volume Depletion: Management of Moderate to Severe Dehydration

In children the most common form of hyponatremia also is associated with hypovolemia (decreased total body water [TBW]) (p. 75) caused by abnormal gastrointestinal losses. Initial efforts should ensure hemodynamic stability through phase I expansion of intravascular volume. Blood glucose level should be monitored. A sample management protocol is outlined in Box 7-2.

In patients with increased TBW, whether associated with normal or slightly high total body sodium level, fluid restriction is usually necessary. Excess water may be calculated as follows:

$$\text{Present TBW (L)} = \text{Weight (kg)} \times 0.6$$
$$\text{Desired TBW (L)} = \frac{\text{Weight (kg)} \times 0.6 \times \text{Measured Na}^+ \text{ (mEq/L)}}{\text{Desired Na}^+ \text{ (mEq/L)}}$$
$$\text{Water excess (L)} = \text{Present TBW} - \text{Desired TBW}$$

NOTE: Sodium level is usually corrected to 125 mEq/L.

In addition, in the moderately symptomatic patient, furosemide (Lasix), 1 mg/kg/dose IV, may be administered. During the subsequent diuresis, urinary sodium, potassium, and chloride levels should be measured and losses should be replaced milliequivalent for milliequivalent with 3% saline solution and supplemental potassium chloride (beginning with 20 mEq of KCl per L). Demeclocycline may be useful in patients more than 8 years old with chronic severe syndrome of inappropriate antidiuretic hormone in whom water restriction is inadequate to correct the abnormality.

Box 7-2

HYPOTONIC VOLUME DEPLETION: MANAGEMENT OF MODERATE TO SEVERE DEFICITS

INITIAL FINDINGS

Pre-illness weight: 10 kg (a 1-yr-old)
Degree of volume depletion, moderate (10%)
Body weight on admission: 9 kg
Electrolytes:

Na^+ 110 mEq/L	K^+ 5 mEq/L	Cl^- 90 mEq/L	HCO_3^- 12 mEq/L

SUMMARY OF FLUID REQUIREMENTS

	H_2O (ml)	**Na^+ (mEq)**	**K^+ (mEq)**
Maintenance	1000 (100 ml/kg)	30 (3 mEq/kg)	20 (2 mEq/kg)
Deficit (100 ml/kg)			
ECF (60%)	600	84 (140 mEq × 0.6)	
ICF (40%)	400		30 (150 mEq × 0.4 × 50% correction)
Sodium deficit*		125	
TOTAL	1000 ml	209 mEq	30 mEq
Resuscitation fluids	200 ml	28 mEq	
Net total deficit	800 ml	181 mEq	30 mEq

FLUID SCHEDULE

Phase	**Calculation**	**Fluids Administered**
I (0-½ hr)	20 ml/kg	200 ml 0.9% NS or LR over 20-30 min.
II (½-9 hr)	½ net deficit: 400 ml D5W with 90 mEq NaCl and 15 mEq KCl ⅓ maintenance: 333 ml D5W with 10 mEq NaCl and 7 mEq KCl TOTAL: 733 ml with 100 mEq NaCl and 22 mEq KCl	733 ml (~90 ml/hr) of D5W 0.9% NS with 22 mEq KCl (~30 mEq/L) (this approximation facilitates care)
III (9-25 hr)	½ deficit ⅔ maintenance	1067 ml (~67 ml/hr) of D5W 0.9% NS with 28 mEq KCl (~26 mEq/L) (this approximation facilitates care)

Hypernatremic Volume Depletion

Most patients have a deficit of free water, but rapid rehydration often results in serious neurologic complications, including seizures. The level of hydration is difficult to assess.

If a patient has hypotension, phase I stabilization is used to expand the intravascular volume, beginning with 20 ml/kg of 0.9% NS or LR over the first hour. The blood glucose level should be checked and monitored. A protocol for the management of a child with hypertonic dehydration is presented in Box 7-3.

The underlying emphasis of therapy must be a slow and deliberate schedule designed to correct deficits over 48 hours. Guidelines are as follows:

1. If the serum sodium concentration is 175 mEq/L or greater, the deficit therapy should decrease serum sodium concentration by 15 mEq/L/24 hr.
2. If the serum sodium concentration is less than 175 mEq/L, the deficit therapy should decrease the serum sodium half the way to normal in the first day of therapy.
3. If the loss is primarily water, some suggest that the water deficit is 50 ml/kg if the Na^+ is 150 mEq/L, 90 ml/kg if 160 mEq/L, and 140 ml/kg if 170 mEq/L.

Box 7-2

HYPOTONIC VOLUME DEPLETION: MANAGEMENT OF MODERATE TO SEVERE DEFICITS —cont'd

NOTES

1. Fluid resuscitation is crucial during phase I. If initial response is poor, additional infusion(s) is warranted. Generally, the initial emergency fluid bolus should be included as part of the deficit replacement.
2. If a patient is acidotic with HCO_3^- of ≤10 mEq/L or a pH ≤7.1 on the basis of metabolic acidosis, one third of the sodium may be administered as $NaHCO_3$.
3. In the presence of severe hyponatremia with decreased TBW in symptomatic patients, hypertonic 3% saline must be given to raise the serum sodium level to 125 mEq/L. A 3% saline solution contains approximately 0.5 mEq Na^+/ml. Patients may be given 3% saline 4 ml/kg IV over 10 minutes, and the response monitored. Once seizures have stopped, half of the deficit may be corrected over the next 8 hours as outlined in the fluid schedule.
4. If excess water load is the cause, furosemide (Lasix) 1 mg/kg/dose IV may be used. During the subsequent diuresis, urinary sodium, potassium, and chloride levels should be measured and replaced milliequivalent for milliequivalent with 3% saline and supplemental potassium chloride.
5. Blood glucose level should be assessed early, especially in children with prolonged vomiting, diarrhea, or inadequate intake. Early glucose infusion may be warranted.
6. In general, after a bolus of normal saline solution, D5W 0.9% NS with KCl 20 mEq/L is the appropriate fluid, infused at a rate reflecting both deficit and maintenance requirements.
7. In the presence of acidosis, serum potassium level does not reflect total body deficit.
8. Should be adjusted for fever: (10% should be added for each 1°C over 37°C), stool loss (5 ml/kg), or vomiting (volume for volume).

---

* Sodium deficit calculation:
A is Na^+ required to correct to 135 mEq/L: 135 mEq/L – 110 mEq/L (observed Na^+) = 25 mEq/L
B is Total body water (TBW): 0.6 L/kg (pre-illness TBW) – 0.1 L/kg (water loss) = 0.5 L/kg
C is pre-illness weight: 10 kg
Sodium deficit = A × B × C = 25 mEq/L × 0.5 L/kg × 10 kg = 125 mEq

Other recommendations are:

1. Fluid to be used should be D5W 0.2% NS after hemodynamic stabilization. If altered mental status or seizures are present, higher sodium concentration may be needed.
2. The volume of free water needed to lower a serum sodium concentration above 145 mEq/L is about 4 ml/kg of free water for each 1 mEq/L evenly distributed over 48 hours.
3. Maintenance fluids should be continued.

Ongoing Management: Phases IV and V

1. After parenteral hydration, oral fluids should be initiated slowly. Lytren or Pedialyte should be given first, and then advanced slowly in both volume and composition.
2. If the dehydration has followed an episode of several days of gastroenteritis, a lactase deficiency is commonly present, and a lactose-free formula may be used.
3. After severe, prolonged diarrhea, an elemental formula such as Pregestimil or Alimentum may be necessary. A deliberate, conservative approach is needed in such cases, which may necessitate continuous NG feeding of dilute formula (one-fourth to one-half strength) and slow advancement to bolus feeding, with subsequent increase in volume and finally osmolality (p. 75).

Box 7-3
HYPERTONIC VOLUME DEPLETION

A 2-week-old infant presents to the ED with a history of 1 day of poor breast milk intake. Weight yesterday at a well-baby visit was 4 kg: today the child weighs 3.4 kg. Laboratory studies include serum Na^+–155 mEq/L: K^+–4.5 mEq/L: HCO_3^-–13 mEq/L.

Maintenance therapy:
100 ml/day for first 10 kg = 400 ml
Na^+ requirements = 3 mEq/kg × 4 kg = 12 mEq
K^+ requirements = 2 mEq/kg × 4 kg = 8 mEq
Total fluid deficit = 4.0 – 3.4 = 0.6 L
Free water deficits = [observed Na^+– ideal Na^+ (145 mEq/L)] × 4 ml/kg × wt (kg) = (155–145) × 4 ml/kg × 4 kg = 160 ml
Na^+ deficit (Duration of illness is less than 3 days. Therefore the fluid lost is 75% from the ECF and 25% from the ICF. Primary sodium reservoir is ECF.)
Na^+ loss = (ECF Na^+ concentration) × (75% of solute fluid deficit*) = (140 mEq/L) × (0.75 × 0.440 L) = 46 mEq
NOTE: Solute containing deficit = Total fluid deficit – free water deficit = 600 ml – 160 ml = 440 ml
K^+ deficit (primary potassium reservoir is ICF):
K^+ loss = (ICF K^+ concentration) × (25% of solute fluid deficit) = (150 mEq/L) × (0.25 × 0.440 L) = 16 mEq
48-hour requirements = maintenance + deficits
Total deficits: Fluid (ml) = (400 × 2) ml + 160 ml (free) + 440 (solute) = 1400 ml
Sodium (mEq) = 24 + 46 = 70 mEq
Potassium (mEq) = 16 + 16 = 32 mEq
Fluid schedule:
The fluid is administered in a step-wise fashion over 48 hours.
One half the deficit is given in the first 24 hours and then the remainder in the next 24 hours.
First day fluids = Maintenance + ½ deficits
First day fluids = (400 ml + 12 mEq Na^+ + 8 mEq K^+) + ½ (600 ml + 46 mEq Na^+ + 16 mEq K^+)
First day fluids = 700 ml D5W + 35 mEq Na^+ + 16 mEq K^+
In practice (and after the calculations are done), the usual fluid that is required to rehydrate the child with hypertonic dehydration is either D5W 0.2% NS or D5W 0.45% NS because it would appear that the *rate* not the type of fluid is most important. The volume of free water needed to lower a serum sodium concentration above 145 mEq/L is about 4 ml/kg of free water for each 1 mEq/L over 48 hours. Studies demonstrate that D5W, D5W 0.2% NS, or D5W 0.45% NS are all acceptable if infused at a conservative rate, correcting deficits over 48 hours.

* (600 ml fluid deficit – 160 free water deficit)

Phases of Response

Phase	Therapeutic Plan	Pattern of Response
I. Up to ½ hr Restoration of vascular volume	20 ml/kg 0.9% NS or LR over 20-30 min; may repeat 10-20 ml/kg	Improved vital signs Increased urine flow Improved state of consciousness
II. ½-9 hr Partial restoration of ECF deficit and acid-base status	⅓ maintenance daily fluids ½ deficit fluids	Gain in body weight Stabilization of vital signs Improved urine flow Partial restoration of normal acid-base status
III. 9-25 hr Restoration of ECF, ICF, and acid-base status	⅔ maintenance daily fluids ½ deficit fluids	Sustained gain in body weight Fall in BUN level (50% in 24 hr) Sustained urine flow Improved electrolytes

IV. 25-48 hr Total correction of acid-base and K^+ status	Ongoing parenteral ± oral hydration Maintenance fluids and replacement of ongoing losses	Sustained gain in body weight Normal electrolytes
V. 2-14 days Restoration of caloric and protein deficits	Ongoing oral support	Steady gain in weight Plasma constituents normal

MANAGEMENT OF MILD DEHYDRATION (<5%)

1. Oral hydration is usually adequate in the child who is less than 5% dehydrated *if that patient can tolerate oral intake.* An approach to oral rehydration is outlined on p. 68. If the patient cannot tolerate oral fluid, fluids may be administered by NG tube, usually beginning as 10 to 20 ml/kg/hr by continuous NG infusion.
2. If oral fluids are not retained, parenteral fluids should be given. Many children can tolerate fluids after the initial phase I flush of 20 ml/kg of 0.9% NS or LR over 30 to 45 minutes. However, if fluids continue to be vomited, observation and calculation of fluids as previously outlined are needed.
3. Intake, output, and weight must be monitored carefully. Laboratory data are rarely necessary.
4. Clear fluids (Table 7-1) should be pushed, although slowly in the child who is vomiting. Do not use rice water, tea, or boiled milk. Many fruit juices (especially apple juice) are hyperosmolar and may draw water into the intestinal lumen, worsening diarrhea.
5. In infants it is particularly important to provide adequate electrolytes while minimizing potential errors in formulation of solutions. Therefore fluids such as Rehydralyte are recommended during initial rehydration, followed by Lytren or Pedialyte.
6. Once ongoing losses have slowed, the diet may be advanced. There is no clear evidence that clinicians need to prescribe elaborate dietary manipulations after an episode of diarrhea in previously healthy children. For children who have had prolonged (>7 days) gastroenteritis, many suggest a lactose-free product initially, although this issue is controversial.
7. Applesauce, rice, dry toast, and bananas have been found useful in advancing the diet to solids. Attention should be given to caloric intake to facilitate mucosal healing.

TABLE 7-1 Common Oral Hydrating Solutions

Solution	Na^+ (mEq/L)	K^+ (mEq/L)	HCO_3^-/Citrate (mEq/L)	Glucose* (gm/dl)	mOsm/L
REHYDRATION					
Rehydrate	75	20	30	2.5	270
WHO solution	90	20	10	2.0	310
MAINTENANCE					
Pedialyte	45	20	30	2.5	270
Infalyte	50	25	30	1.9	200
CLEAR LIQUIDS					
Gatorade	20	3		2.1	
Cola	3	0.1-0.9	7-13	10.0	

* May be long-chain oligosaccharide subject to hydrolysis.

Disposition

Patients with mild dehydration who tolerate fluids may be discharged when close follow-up observation and good compliance are ensured and no underlying medical conditions necessitate early intervention (e.g., diabetes and sickle cell disease).

Parental Education

1. Give only clear liquids; give as much as your child wants.
   a. Children younger than 2 years should be given a maintenance electrolyte solution, such as Pedialyte or Infalyte.
   b. Children older than 2 years of age may be given other clear fluids, such as decarbonated sodas, Gatorade, or clear soups.
2. If your child is vomiting, give clear liquids (as above) in small frequent volumes initially and increasing to normal volumes for the child's age as tolerated. It may be necessary to use teaspoons, cups, syringes, or ladles to administer the small volumes. Fluid can be administered beginning 5 to 10 minutes after an episode of vomiting and should be continued despite the persistence of some minimal vomiting.
3. The child's diet may be advanced as soon as the vomiting has stopped and the child can tolerate fluids without vomiting. It is reasonable to wait 2 to 4 hours after the last episode of vomiting to resume feeding.
   a. Formula-fed or breast-fed infants should be given their regular formula or should resume breast-feeding.
   b. Older children should be given bland starch-containing foods (bananas, rice, applesauce, and toast are historically the popular routine) in small quantities first, moving to larger quantities and more complex items as the child's appetite returns.
4. The child may return to a regular diet as soon as the appetite returns and foods are desired.
5. Many foods may worsen diarrhea: pectin-containing foods such as fruits and fruit juices are not recommended until the diarrhea resolves.
6. Reduce cow's milk products until the diarrhea has lessened.
7. Do not use boiled milk. Kool-Aid and soda are not ideal liquids, particularly for younger infants, because they contain few electrolytes.
8. Call your physician if:
   a. The diarrhea or vomiting is increasing in frequency or amount.
   b. The diarrhea does not improve after 24 hours of clear liquids or does not resolve entirely after 3 to 4 days.
   c. Vomiting continues for more than 24 hours.
   d. The stool has blood or the vomited material contains blood or turns green.
   e. Signs of dehydration, including decreased urination, less moisture in diapers, dry mouth, no tears, weight loss, lethargy, and irritability, develop.

8 Maintenance Requirements and Abnormalities

MAINTENANCE FLUIDS AND ELECTROLYTES

Fluids

Fluid balance is closely regulated. Intake of water is controlled by the hypothalamic regulation of thirst, whereas absorption is largely a reflection of the gastrointestinal (GI) tract. Excretion occurs via the lungs, skin, GI tract, and kidneys. An antidiuretic hormone (ADH) regulates urinary volume and concentration.

Normal maintenance fluids reflect the necessity to replace daily water and electrolyte losses from the skin and the respiratory, urinary, and GI tracts. These losses may be divided into insensible, urinary, and fecal components; they amount to 100 ml/kg/24 hr up to age 1 year and decrease thereafter.

Insensible losses (30 ml/kg/24 hr) occur through the skin and respiratory tract. Water loss is affected by humidity, body temperature, respiratory rate, and ambient temperature. Fever increases insensible water loss by 7 ml/kg/24 hr for each degree rise in temperature above 37.2° C (99° F).

Urinary losses (60 ml/kg/24 hr) reflect the solute load and obligate excretion and urine concentration. Normal fecal water losses (10 ml/kg/24 hr) are small and, in older children, insignificant.

Water Requirements

Children <10 kg	100 ml/kg/24 hr
Children 11-20 kg	1000 ml plus 50 ml/kg/24 hr for each kilogram over 10 kg
Children >20 kg	1500 ml plus 20 ml/kg/24 hr for each kilogram over 20 kg
Adults	2000-2400 ml/24 hr

Beyond the newborn period, total body water (TBW) makes up about 60% of body weight; 40% is intracellular fluid (ICF) and the remaining 20% is extracellular fluid (ECF). The intravascular volume represents 5% of the ECF in adults and is as much as 8% (80 ml/kg) in younger children.

Electrolytes

Cation	Daily Requirement			Compartment
	0-10 kg	**10-20 kg**	**>20 kg**	
Na^+	3 mEq/kg	30 mEq + 1.5 mEq/kg for each kg >10 kg	45 mEq + 0.6 mEq/kg for each kg >20 kg	ECF (includes intravascular
K^+	2 mEq/kg	20 mEq + 1 mEq/kg for each kg >10 kg	30 mEq + 0.4 mEq/kg for each kg >20 kg	ICF

Osmolality

Osmolality is regulated by osmoreceptors in the hypothalamus. When a receptor detects increased ECF osmolality, ADH release is stimulated. Because cell membranes are permeable to water and osmotic equilibrium is homeostatically maintained, the volume of ICF is determined by the tonicity of ECF. The osmolality of plasma and therefore ICF can be approximated as follows:

$$\text{Plasma osmolality} = 2 \times (Na^+) + \frac{(\text{Glucose})}{18} + \frac{\text{BUN}}{2.8}$$

Plasma osmolality normally ranges between 280 and 295 mOsm/kg water.

If the measured osmolality is normal but the calculated osmolality is low, the difference is most likely caused by a decrease in serum water content. This can occur in hyperglobulinemia, triglyceridemia, and hyperglycemia.

Acid-Base Balance

Compensatory Mechanisms. The relationship between pH and bicarbonate–carbonic acid concentration is best expressed by the Henderson-Hasselbalch equation:

$$pH + pK + \log \frac{(HCO_3^-)^{Renal}}{(H_2CO_3)_{Respiratory}}$$

$$H_2CO_3 = H_2O + \text{Dissolved } (CO_2)$$

The renal and respiratory compensatory systems determine acid-base balance.

1. *Respiratory* systems can provide a *rapid* alteration in pH by changing the respiratory rate and tidal volume. The classic example is Kussmaul's pattern breathing in diabetic ketoacidosis. Respiratory alkalosis may be due to central nervous system (CNS) (increased intracranial pressure [ICP], anxiety, encephalitis or meningitis), hypotension, sepsis, or liver toxic (salicylates) conditions.
2. *Kidneys* provide a *slow* response, balancing the excretion of HCO_3^- and the secretion of H^+, primarily by the distal nephron.

Anion Gap

In addition to determining pH, P_{CO_2}, and HCO_3^- as reflections of acid-base balance, the anion gap should be calculated in considering potential causes:

$$\text{Anion gap} = Na^+ + K^+ - (Cl^- + HCO_3^-)$$

The normal anion gap is 8-12 mEq/L, comprising primarily phosphates, sulfates, and organic acids. The gap is usually normal in metabolic acidosis resulting from diarrhea, in which there is a loss of bicarbonate ion through the GI tract and kidneys. It is increased with excessive production of organic acids (ketones), lactic acid (shock, sepsis, congestive heart failure [CHF]), and toxins (salicylates), and in renal failure. A useful mnemonic for remembering entities that produce a metabolic acidosis with a large anion gap is MUDPILES: *m*ethanol, *u*remia, *d*iabetic ketoacidosis, *p*araldehyde overdose, *i*soniazid or iron overdose, *l*actic acidosis, *e*thanol or ethylene glycol, and *s*alicylate overdose or starvation.

ELECTROLYTE AND ACID-BASE ABNORMALITIES

The two major cations, sodium and potassium, are the primary determinants of the distribution of water between the ECF and ICF spaces. These compartments depend on active transport of potassium into the cells and sodium out of the cells by an energy-requiring process.

Sodium

Sodium regulation is a balance of intake, TBW, and excretion through urine, sweat, and feces. Disorders can result in hyponatremia or hypernatremia, both significantly affecting plasma osmolality.

1. *Hyponatremia.* Clinical presentation is variable, reflecting the rapidity of progression and severity of hyponatremia. Early signs include apathy, difficulty in concentrating, and agitation, with progression to confusion, irritability, coma, and seizures. Nausea, vomiting, muscle weakness and cramps, myoclonus, and decreased deep tendon reflexes may be noted. Several mechanisms may produce hyponatremia, reflecting the balance between TBW and total body sodium.
   a. Decreased TBW (hypovolemia) and decreased total body sodium. Examples: renal salt loss (diuretics, adrenal insufficiency, renal tubular acidosis), extrarenal salt loss (severe sweating, cystic fibrosis, GI losses, vomiting, diarrhea), and third spacing (burns,

peritonitis, pancreatitis). Urine sodium level is usually less than 20 mEq/L.

b. Increased TBW and normal total body sodium. Examples: syndrome of inappropriate antidiuretic hormone (SIADH) (pulmonary disease, CNS trauma, and drugs such as hypoglycemic agents, antineoplastic drugs, tricyclic antidepressants, and thiazide diuretics), hypothyroidism, severe potassium depletion, and psychogenic water drinking. Urine sodium level is usually more than 20 mEq/L.

c. Increased TBW (hypervolemia) relatively greater than increased total body sodium. Examples: CHF, renal or hepatic failure, nephrosis, and hypoproteinemia.

d. Pseudohyponatremia. Examples: hyperproteinemia, and hyperlipidemia.

NOTE: Serum sodium level decreases 1.6 mEq/L for each increment of 100 mg/dl in serum glucose level.

2. *Hypernatremia.* Symptoms of altered mental status, irritability, seizures, and coma may develop, with associated skeletal muscle rigidity and hyperactive reflexes. This condition may occur through one of two mechanisms:

   a. Decreased TBW and normal total body sodium (dehydration). Examples: increased insensible or renal water loss, excessive solute loss (mannitol, urea), abnormal water loss (diarrhea), and diabetes insipidus.

   b. Normal TBW and increased total body sodium. Examples: salt poisoning, rehydration with boiled milk, and CNS disease affecting hypothalamus. Urine sodium level is more than 20 mEq/L.

Potassium

Potassium is of central importance in the maintenance of ICF osmolality. Only 1.5% to 2.0% of the total body potassium is in the ECF, as reflected by serum measurements.

During metabolic acidosis, renal secretion of hydrogen ions is increased while that of potassium is decreased. For every 0.1 decrease in pH level, serum potassium increases by about 0.5 mEq/L, with a similar reverse relationship.

To alkalinize the urine as required in treatment of barbiturate or aspirin ingestions, adequate amounts of potassium must be administered to facilitate renal excretion of sodium bicarbonate.

1. *Hypokalemia.* Patients may have muscle weakness, abdominal distension, and decreased bowel sounds (ileus), impaired renal concentrating ability, and hypochloremic alkalosis. Delayed ventricular depolarization is noted, with a relatively flat T wave on electrocardiogram (ECG). Decreased potassium level commonly results from excessive loss of potassium from the GI tract (diarrhea, vomiting, or nasogastric [NG] suction), kidneys (diuretic, renal tubular acidosis), drug ingestion, and insulin or glucose therapy. It is often accompanied by hypomagnesemia. Significant hypokalemia (serum potassium level 3.0 mEq/L), especially in patients taking digoxin or in those with myocarditis, should be treated cautiously. Such patients may receive 0.1 to 0.2 mEq/kg infusions of KCl every 4 to 6 hours while their serum levels are monitored. Larger boluses (K^+ 0.2-0.3 mEq/kg/hr) ideally should be given through a central line.
2. *Hyperkalemia.* The primary toxicity of cardiac conduction is common. A peaked T wave progresses to a widened QRS complex and ventricular dysrhythmias, and muscle weakness is often noted. Renal or metabolic disease may be present as well as acidosis or excessive intake. Hemolysis of red blood cells during heelstick or venipuncture may artificially elevate the measured serum potassium level. Management is discussed on p. 832.

Calcium

Ninety percent of calcium is in the skeletal system. About 40% is bound to protein, primarily albumin.

1. *Hypocalcemia.* Patients may be symptomatic, with neuromuscular findings of tetany, presence of Chvostek's and Trousseau signs, laryngospasm, and seizures. Vitamin D and nutritional deficiency, malabsorption or abnormal metabolism of vitamin D, parathyroid disease, magnesium deficiency, and pancreatitis may be causative.

   Treatment of symptomatic patients begins with a dose of 0.5 to 1 ml/kg of 10% calcium gluconate IV over 5 minutes. Ongoing management comprises a combination of parenteral (5-8 ml/kg/24 hr 10% calcium gluconate given in four to six doses IV) and oral calcium gluconate (200-500 mg/kg/dose q6hr PO) as needed. Magnesium level should be monitored and supplemented as needed. Cardiac monitoring is essential.
2. *Hypercalcemia.* Calcium level may be higher than 11 mg/dl. Headache, irritability, lethargy, weakness, seizures, or coma may develop. Anorexia, dehydration, polydipsia, and polyuria may be noted. Hyperparathyroidism, vitamin D toxicity, immobilization, and malignancies may be contributory. Management focuses on hydration and intermittent furosemide (1 mg/kg/dose q6hr IV). Treatment of malignancies must include mithramycin.

Acid-Base Status

Alterations in acid-base status, which represent a balance of compensatory mechanisms (p. 76), may be summarized as follows:

	pH	P_{CO_2}	HCO_3^-
Metabolic acidosis	↓	↓	↓*
Metabolic alkalosis	↑	↑	↑*
Respiratory acidosis	↓	↑*	↑
Respiratory alkalosis	↑	↓*	↓

* Indicates primary abnormality.

NOTE: Mixed metabolic and respiratory disorders are common. In a simple disturbance without compensatory reaction, abnormalities in both Pa_{CO_2} and HCO_3^- level are in the same direction.

1. *Metabolic acidosis.* Initially accompanied by compensatory tachypnea and may be associated with cardiac dysrhythmias and cellular dysfunction. Initially, the Pa_{CO_2} level decreases, with the drop 1 to 1.5 times the reduction in the HCO_3^- level. Specific correction of the underlying condition requires treatment (often correction of intravascular volume); supplemental HCO_3^- therapy may also be needed. If the HCO_3^- level is less than 10 mEq/L in acute conditions, it should be corrected to at least 12 to 15 mEq/L. The initial correction should replace a maximum of *about one third* of the deficit:

$$\text{Deficit mEq } HCO_3^- = \text{Weight (kg)} \times \text{Base deficit (mEq/L desired} - \text{mEq/L observed)} \times 0.6 \times 0.5$$

2. *Metabolic alkalosis.* May be accompanied by muscle cramps, weakness, paresthesias, seizures, hyperreflexia, tetany, and dysrhythmias. The Pa_{CO_2} level increases 0.5 to 1.0 mm Hg for each mEq/L increase in HCO_3^-. Primary treatment of the causative condition often requires restoration of intravascular volume or discontinuation of diuretics as appropriate. If alkalosis is severe, with a pH of 7.7 (lower if symptomatic), treatment options include the following:
   1. Acetazolamide (Diamox), 5 mg/kg/24 hr q6-24hr (adult: 250-375 mg/24 hr) PO, IV; use only if K^+ level is normal; *or*
   2. Ammonium chloride (NH_4Cl), 150-300 mg/kg/24 hr q6hr (adult: 8-12 gm/24 hr) PO.

ELECTROLYTE COMPOSITION OF BODY FLUIDS

Knowing the electrolyte composition of body fluids (Table 8-1) may be useful in

TABLE 8-1 Electrolyte Composition of Body Fluids

Fluid	Na^+ (mEq/L)	K^+ (mEq/L)	Cl^- (mEq/L)	H^+ (mEq/L)	HCO_3^- (mEq/L)
Sweat	10-30	3-10	10-35		
Gastric	20-80	5-20	100-150	90	
Pancreas	120-140	5-40	50-120		90
Small Intestine	100-140	15-40	90-130		25
Diarrhea	10-90	10-80	10-110		45

delineating potential abnormalities associated with fluid loss.

BIBLIOGRAPHY

American Academy of Pediatrics, Provisional Committee on Quality Improvement, Subcommittee on Acute Gastroenteritis: Practice parameters: management of acute gastroenteritis in young children, *Pediatrics* 97:424, 1996.

Cohen MB, Mezoff AC, Laney DW et al: Use of a single solution or oral rehydration and maintenance therapy of infants with diarrhea and mild to moderate dehydration, *Pediatrics* 95:639, 1995.

MacKenzie A, Barnes G, Shann F: Clinical signs of dehydration in children, *Lancet* 2:605, 1989.

Moritz ML, Ayus JC: The changing pattern of hypernatremia in hospitalized children, *Pediatrics* 104:435, 1999.

Nager AL, Wang VJ: Comparison of nasogastric and intravenous methods of rehydration of pediatric patients with acute dehydration, *Pediatrics* 109:566, 2002.

Ozuah PO, Avner JR, Stein REK: Oral rehydration, emergency physicians, and practice parameters: a national survey, *Pediatrics* 109:259, 2002.

Pizzaro D, Posada G, Sandi L et al: Rice-based oral electrolyte solutions for the management of infantile diarrhea, *N Engl J Med* 324:517, 1991.

Santosham M, Fayad I, Zikri MA et al: A double blind clinical trial comparing World Health Organization oral rehydration solution with a reduced osmolality solution containing equal amounts of sodium and glucose, *J Pediatr* 128:45, 1996.

Vega RM, Avner JR: A prospective study of the usefulness of clinical and laboratory parameters for predicting the percentage of dehydration in children, *Pediatr Emerg Care* 13:179, 1997.

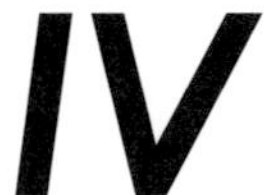

Newborn Emergencies

FRANCIS R. POULAIN and ANTHONY F. PHILIPPS

Care providers faced with a distressed newborn in the delivery room or emergency department may be forced to make rapid therapeutic decisions without an adequate patient database. Under such conditions, standardized guidelines for resuscitation, diagnosis, and management provide a basis for intervention.

9 Resuscitation in the Delivery Room

Also See Chapter 4 (Cardiopulmonary Arrest)

A number of maternal and fetal risk factors have been associated with poor outcome for the newborn. Their presence should alert neonatal care providers to the potential need for specific resuscitation strategies, with mobilization of additional personnel and equipment as appropriate.

1. *Factors related to maternal condition:*
   - **a.** Maternal diabetes, hypertension, anemia, isoimmunization, infection
   - **b.** Cardiac, pulmonary, renal, thyroid, or neurologic disease
   - **c.** Teen (<16 yr) or advanced (>35 yr) maternal age
   - **d.** History of fetal or prenatal loss
2. *Factors inherent to pregnancy:*
   - **a.** Presence of fetal malformations, multiple gestation, size-date discrepancy
   - **b.** Polyhydramnios or oligohydramnios
   - **c.** Preterm labor
   - **d.** Second- or third-trimester bleeding
   - **e.** Prolonged (>18 hr) rupture of membranes
   - **f.** Chorioamnionitis
   - **g.** Maternal drugs: lithium, magnesium, adrenergic-blocking agents
   - **h.** Maternal substance abuse
   - **i.** Absence of prenatal care
3. *Factors related to labor and delivery:*
   - **a.** Premature (<37 wk) or postterm (>41 wk) delivery
   - **b.** Abnormal fetal presentation
   - **c.** Prolonged or precipitous labor, uterine tetany
   - **d.** Meconium-stained amniotic fluid
   - **e.** Placenta previa, abruptio placentae
   - **f.** Fetal distress: abnormal biophysical profile, nonreassuring fetal heart rate patterns, fetal bradycardia
   - **g.** Emergent cesarean delivery, vacuum or forceps-assisted delivery
   - **h.** General anesthesia, narcotics administered to mother within 4 hours of delivery
   - **i.** Prolapsed cord

Equipment

Adequate preparation is essential. The following equipment should be available:

1. Temperature: radiant warmer present and preheated. Warm linens or special wraps (e.g., Thinsulate [3M]).
2. Suction equipment: bulb syringe, suction trap (adapters are available for use with low wall suction), suction catheters (5, 6, 8, and 10 French [Fr]), meconium aspirator.
3. Ventilation equipment: (see Chapter 4 and Table 9-1): oxygen, face masks (newborn and premature sizes), endotracheal (ET) tubes (2.5, 3, 3.5, and 4 mm ID), malleable stylet [sterile]), laryngoscope, laryngoscope blades (straight No. 0 and No. 1), extra batteries and bulbs, a resuscitation bag (non–self-inflating, able to deliver 90% to 100% oxygen, adaptable with a manometer and positive end-expiratory pressure [PEEP] valve). Although less optimal, standard self-inflating (750-ml) resuscitation bags may also be used.

TABLE 9-1 Intubation Equipment

Weight (kg)	ET Tube (mm)	Suction Catheter (French)	Laryngoscope Blade
1	2.5	5	0
2	3.0	6	0
3	3.5	8	0-1
4	3.5-4.0	8	1

Several types of disposable infant resuscitation bags that include an adjustable PEEP valve and adapter for a manometer may be used. A sterile, disposable end-tidal CO_2 device is commercially available for use in conjunction with neonatal or infant intubation as an adjunct to confirm ET tube placement (Pedi-cap, Nellcor Puritan Bennett, Pleasanton, CA).

4. Medications (Table 9-2): epinephrine (1:10,000, 0.1 mg/ml), sodium bicarbonate (dilute 1:1 to 4.2%, 0.5 mEq/ml), volume expander (normal saline or lactated Ringer's solution), dextrose (10%), and naloxone (0.4 mg/ml).
5. Equipment to initiate administration of parenteral fluids: normal equipment plus umbilical catheterization supplies, including catheters (3.5 F and 5 F), three-way stopcock, and sterile umbilical vessel catheterization tray containing towels, gauze pads, scissors, hemostats, curved iris forceps, scalpels, syringes, and umbilical tape.
6. Clock and stethoscope.
7. Obstetric (OB) kit and cord-cutting material.
8. Gloves and other protective devices.

Personnel

A team approach is absolutely necessary for resuscitation of the depressed neonate. This approach calls for close cooperation among physicians, nurses, nurse practitioners, and other health care providers in the delivery room setting. A team leader must direct efforts of the resuscitation. Periodic practice drills are strongly recommended.

Optimally, this team should be very familiar with the principles of resuscitation and management of neonatal asphyxia, including the practical uses of bag-and-mask ventilation, ET intubation, chest massage, drug administration, and umbilical vein and artery catheterization. Completion of the Neonatal Resuscitation Program (NRP) curriculum or equivalent is essential for personnel involved in delivery room care of the neonate.

ROUTINE NEWBORN CARE

Most term newborns are vigorous at birth and have no risk factors. Such infants need not be separated from their mothers in order to initiate the following routine measures:

1. Maintain temperature. Minimize heat loss by towel drying and placing the infant under a radiant warmer (avoid overheating) or in warm blankets.
2. Assess respiratory pattern and rate visually. Heart rate may be determined

TABLE 9-2 Drugs Used in Resuscitation of Newborns

Drug	Availability	Indications	Dosage/Route
Epinephrine	1:10,000	Bradycardia	0.1-0.3 ml/kg IV, ET
Sodium bicarbonate	4.2% (0.5 mEq/ml)	Metabolic acidosis	1-2 mEq/kg IV
Dextrose (glucose)	10%	Hypoglycemia	2 ml/kg IV
Normal saline	0.9%	Hypovolemic shock	10-20 ml/kg IV
Naloxone (Narcan)	0.4, 1 mg/ml	Narcotic-induced respiratory depression	0.1 mg/kg IV, ET

rapidly by either auscultation or palpation of the umbilical cord (pulsations). Determining capillary refill time after gentle pressure over the midsternum (<2-3 seconds for refill time after the release is the norm) is the best way to assess perfusion. Visually inspect the patient quickly to detect any major external anomalies (e.g., myelomeningocele, omphalocele).

3. Calculate Apgar score (Table 9-3) at 1 minute and 5 minutes, evaluating *a*ppearance (color), *p*ulse, *g*rimace (reflex irritability), *a*ctivity (muscle tone), and *r*espirations. The score is a useful indicator of the infant's overall condition and response to resuscitation. It is recommended that observation be continued at intervals until an Apgar score of 7 or higher is achieved for up to 20 minutes. Optimally, someone who is not directly involved in the resuscitation efforts should assign the score. These scores should not be used to determinate appropriate resuscitative actions.

After stabilization, several other routine steps are carried out:

1. Prophylaxis against ophthalmia neonatorum is performed with silver nitrate (1%) drops or erythromycin (0.5%) or tetracycline (1%) ophthalmic ointment.
2. Vitamin K (0.5-1 mg phytonadione) is administered IM to prevent vitamin K–dependent hemorrhagic disease of the newborn. (Oral administration of parenteral vitamin K preparations to the newborn, in lieu of parenteral injection, is not efficacious).

RESUSCITATION MEASURES

See Chapters 4 and 5 and Fig. 9-1.

Initial Evaluation

Evaluation of the newborn should begin immediately after birth. Normal newborn response to the extrauterine environment leads to vigorous crying, movements of all extremities, and pink skin color. If no meconium is present on the skin or in the amniotic fluid (see later section on meconium-stained amniotic fluid), and the infant is full term and vigorous, routine care is usually adequate. In other cases further assessment is needed, with focus on the status of respirations, heart rate, and color of the infant as described in Fig. 9-1.

1. *Respirations:* should be regular and sufficient to improve color and maintain heart rate above 100 beats/min. Apnea or gasping indicates the need to initiate resuscitative efforts.
2. *Heart rate:* is measured by palpating the base of the umbilical cord or listening to precordium with a stethoscope. The rate should be sustained above 100 beats/min. A rate lower than 100 beats/min is an indication for intervention. The presence of tachycardia, however, may indicate other disease and requires further evaluation.

TABLE 9-3 Apgar Score

	SCORE		
Sign	**0**	**1**	**2**
Muscle tone (activity)	Limp	Some flexion	Active, good flexion
Pulse	Absent	<100/min	>100/min
Reflex irritability* (grimace)	No response	Some grimace or avoidance	Cough, cry, or sneeze
Color (appearance)	Blue, pale	Pink body, blue hands/feet	Pink
Respirations	Absent	Slow, irregular, ineffective	Crying, rhythmic, effective

* Nasal or oral suction catheter stimulus.

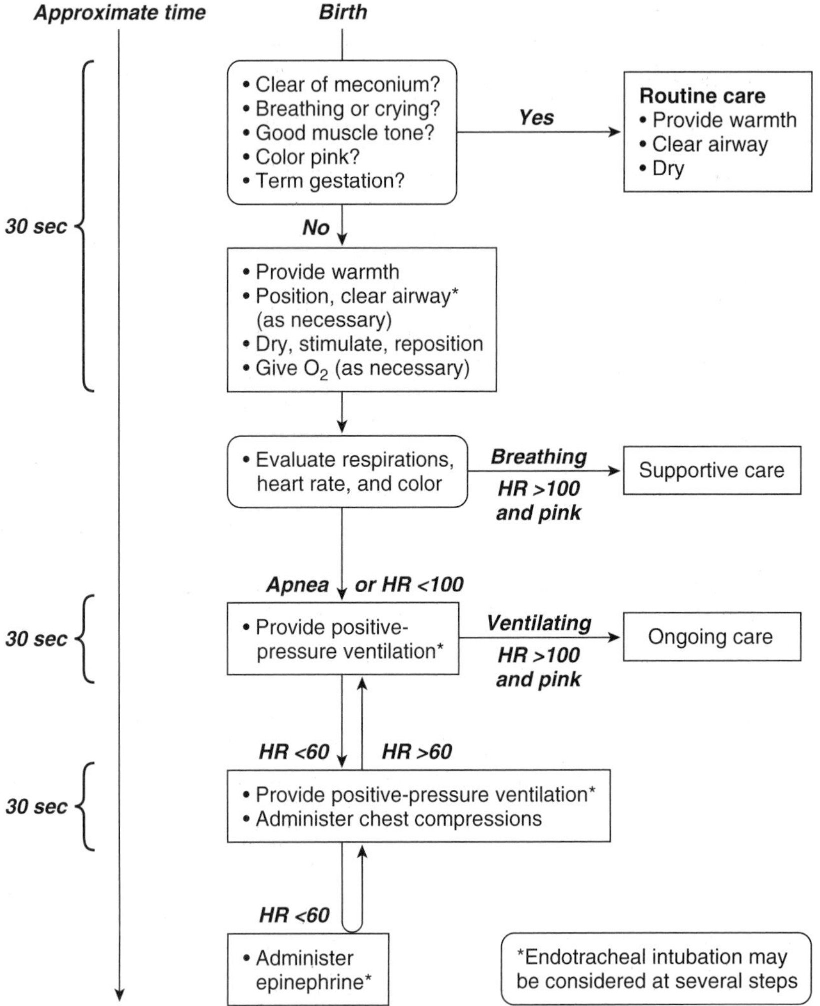

Fig. 9-1 International guidelines for neonatal resuscitation.
(From *Pediatrics,* 106:e29, 2000. Figure 3, Copyright 2000.)

3. *Color:* The infant should be able to acquire and maintain pink *color* of the mucous membranes. Blue discoloration of the face and trunk or mucous membranes indicates cyanosis and is abnormal. Acrocyanosis (cyanosis of the hands and feet) is usually a normal finding at birth.

Resuscitation Techniques

Resuscitation techniques are applied to infants who do not appear vigorous, remain cyanotic, or are preterm. The quality of the response to each measure or group of measures dictates the need for additional procedures.

1. *Basic steps of resuscitation* are drying the infant with warm linens, positioning the infant supine with the head in a neutral position, clearing the airway of secretions (suctioning of nares and mouth with bulb syringe or suction catheter), and oxygen administration. Gentle rubbing or flicking of the soles of the feet may

provide further stimulation. These measures are often enough to overcome primary apnea and trigger the onset of regular respirations. Oxygen should be administered if cyanosis persists or if the initial measures fail to improve the infant's condition. The oxygen source should deliver at least 5 L/min. Oxygen may be delivered through a facemask, an oxygen mask, or a hand cupped around oxygen tubing.

2. *Ventilation*: If the infant remains apneic or cyanotic or the heart rate stays below 100 beats/min, positive-pressure ventilation (PPV) must be administered. Adequate ventilation is key to successful resuscitation, and most newborns can be adequately ventilated with a bag and mask. A proper technique is critical to successful ventilation and requires a proper positioning of the head (in neutral position or slightly extended), clearing of secretions from the oropharynx, and an effective seal of the ventilation mask over the face. The inflating pressure to be used varies with the infant's condition, but indications of adequate ventilation include visible chest expansion, increase in heart rate above 100 beats/min, and improvement of color. Inadequate head position, presence of secretions, a closed mouth, or an inadequate seal between the face and mask may lead to a lack of response to ventilation and should be remedied before increased inflating pressures are considered.

   Gastric distension may result from prolonged bag-and-mask ventilation and can be relieved by insertion of an 8 F orogastric tube. After 30 seconds of adequate ventilation with 100% oxygen, spontaneous breathing, heart rate, and color should be evaluated again. If spontaneous breathing is present and the heart rate is sustained above 100 beats/min, PPV can be progressively discontinued. If breathing is inadequate or the heart rate remains below 100 beats/min, PPV must be continued, and ET intubation considered. If the heart rate is below 60 beats/min, chest compressions should be started.

3. *Endotracheal intubation:* ET intubation is indicated when tracheal suctioning is required (see section on meconium-stained amniotic fluid), when previous resuscitation measures, including bag-mask ventilation, have failed to improve the infant's condition, or in the presence of special circumstances (e.g., severe lung lesion such as congenital diaphragmatic hernia [CDH] or body weight less than 1000 g). ET intubation needs to be performed by the most experienced personnel available. Refer to Table 9-1 for a list of the equipment needed according to weight group. Appropriate placement of an ET tube should result in equal breath sounds with ventilation.

   An estimate of the depth of ET tube insertion from the upper lip can be calculated by adding 6 cm to the weight of the infant expressed in kilograms. If the infant's trachea is to remain intubated beyond the initial period of resuscitation, placement of the tube must be checked on a chest radiograph.

4. *Chest compressions:* If HR remains below 60 beats/min after 30 seconds of PPV with 100% oxygen, closed-chest massage is indicated. In the term newborn, one can accomplish closed-chest massage best by either (1) encircling the chest with both hands, placing the thumbs over the lower third of the sternum and the tips of fingers over the spine, or (2) placing the tips of the middle two fingers over the lower sternum region. The sternum is then compressed approximately one third of the depth of the chest, in a ratio of three compressions/breath at a compression rate of approximately 90/min, until

spontaneous HR rises above 60 beats/min.

5. *Medications* (see Table 9-2): Medications are usually unnecessary for the neonate with perinatal depression unless there is advanced vascular collapse or decreased cardiac output that has not responded to previous resuscitative measures. The drug most commonly used as a cardiac stimulant in the delivery room is epinephrine, which can be given through the ET tube before vascular access is established. Such access can be achieved easily in the emergency setting, however, via the umbilical vein (see p. 89). Specific drugs and volume expanders can also be administered.

   Volume resuscitation is rarely indicated because many depressed babies have normal blood volume. Volume expanders may be appropriate, however, if there are signs of shock (pallor, poor perfusion, or weak pulses). Hypovolemia is most commonly associated with placenta previa or abruptio placentae, but can also be noted after twin-to-twin or fetomaternal transfusion. Rupture of membranes with relative oligohydramnios may produce umbilical cord compression during labor, probably a common, as well as occult, cause of fetal blood loss (fetal-placental transfusion). Isotonic saline or lactated Ringer's solution (10 ml/kg over 5-10 minutes) is now recommended over albumin-containing solutions for volume expansion, but administration of O-negative red blood cells may be indicated for replacement of a large blood loss.

   The use of IV bicarbonate after perinatal asphyxia remains controversial and its administration is best deferred until after blood gas levels are known. Sodium bicarbonate should never be given via the intratracheal route. Naloxone hydrochloride is specifically indicated in cases of respiratory depression secondary to maternal narcotics within 4 hours of delivery. Its usage is no substitute, however, for proper ventilation of the depressed neonate and should be avoided in infants whose mothers have a long-term narcotic abuse history.

Factors that should be considered when resuscitation efforts are unsuccessful include equipment failure, ET tube malposition, pneumothorax, and congenital anomalies such as congenital heart disease (CHD) and pulmonary hypoplasia. Under some circumstances, such as extreme prematurity (<24 weeks, birth weight <500 g) or severe congenital anomaly (trisomy 13 or 18, anencephaly), withholding resuscitation may be reasonable. In addition, discontinuation of resuscitative efforts may also be appropriate for prolonged lack of response to aggressive intervention and absence of vital signs. As much information should be made available to the practitioner and family as possible to help with these difficult decisions. Several national and local standards are available, but in some cases continuing resuscitation may be the most practical approach because it does not preclude later discontinuation of support once more information (and discussion with family members) is available. Partial resuscitation efforts are to be discouraged.

Umbilical Catheterization

In an emergency the umbilical cord provides easy access for administration of intravascular drugs and fluid. Catheterization of the umbilical cord is performed as follows:

1. Restrain the extremities, prepare the abdomen and cord with antiseptic solution (surgical scrub), and drape the lower abdomen and legs with sterile towels.
2. After placing loosely knotted umbilical tape around the base of the cord, trim the umbilical cord to 1 to 2 cm above the skin surface (vertical traction with hemostats controls venous bleeding).
3. Identify the umbilical vein (single, thin wall, large-diameter lumen) and

umbilical artery (normally paired, thick wall, small-diameter lumen).

Umbilical Venous Catheterization. The umbilical venous catheterization technique is easier and more practical in the delivery room. This vessel can often be catheterized in the first 4 to 5 days after birth as well.

1. With caudal countertraction on the umbilical cord, insert a 3.5 Fr to 5 Fr end-hole catheter (previously filled with saline solution and attached to a three-way stopcock and syringe) into the lumen. Gently pass the catheter cephalad in the direction of the liver 1 to 2 cm or until blood return is noted. If resistance to passage is encountered once the catheter has gone beyond the peritoneal fascia, the tip is probably in a portal vein tributary; pull the catheter back until blood can be withdrawn smoothly. Infusion of hypertonic or vasoactive substances in the liver is dangerous and contraindicated.

Occasionally (e.g., in severe congenital heart disease, hydrops, septic shock), it may be helpful to catheterize a central vein. If no resistance is encountered, it may be possible (roughly 50% chance) to pass this catheter above the ductus venosus to a position near the right atrium (8-10 cm in the term newborn) (Fig. 9-2). However, for most simple resuscitations the more shallow position is adequate. In both situations great

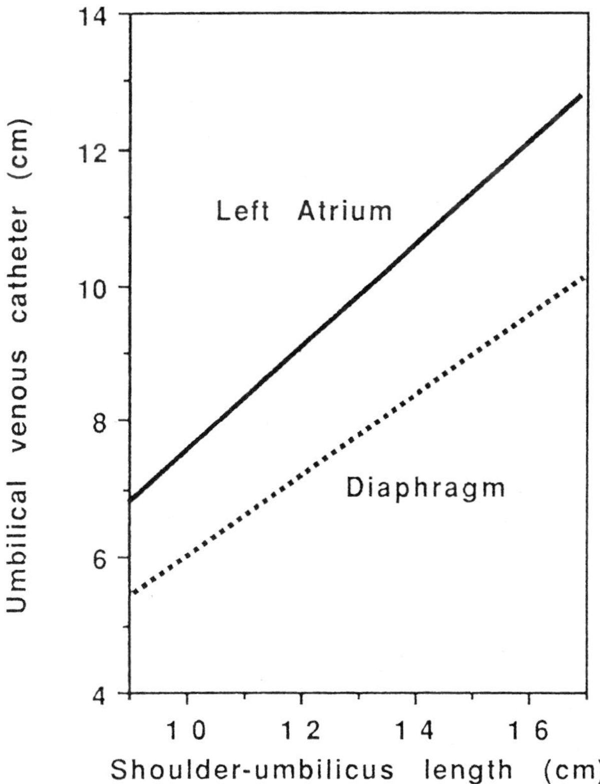

Fig. 9-2 Nomogram for estimation of proper length of insertion of umbilical venous catheter (distance from lateral end of clavicle to umbilicus versus length of catheter to reach designated level).

(From *Arch Dis Child* 41:69,1966.)

care should be taken to prevent IV injection of air and prevent injury of vessels within the liver caused by too forceful advancement of the catheter tip. If a central catheter is deemed necessary, radiographic confirmation of catheter tip's location should be obtained; optimal placement is at the diaphragm near the entrance to the right atrium.

2. Remove the catheter only when resuscitation is completed and patient is stable. If it is deemed necessary to continue IV fluid or drug therapy, the central catheter should be removed only after stable peripheral venous access has been achieved. Prolonged maintenance of indwelling umbilical venous catheters may be associated with neonatal bacteremia and portal vein thrombosis.

Umbilical Arterial Catheterization. Umbilical arterial catheterization requires more time than umbilical venous catheterization and may not be appropriate for achieving vascular access in an emergency. Arterial access for blood sampling and hemodynamic monitoring is very useful to complex resuscitations.

1. Gently dilate the vessel with an iris forceps. Avoid trauma to the vessel wall.
2. Insert a 3.5 F to 5 Fr end-hole catheter (previously filled with saline solution and attached to a three-way stopcock and syringe) into the lumen until blood return is noted. Advance the catheter so it is at the diaphragm or aortic bifurcation. The catheter should be angled slightly caudad to conform with the direction of the umbilical arteries. The length of catheter required for proper insertion may be estimated from Fig. 9-3.
3. Resistance to passage of the catheter is caused by vasoconstriction and can usually be overcome by gentle, steady pressure. Reposition or replace the catheter if resistance persists. Observe the extremities and buttocks for evidence of circulatory compromise.

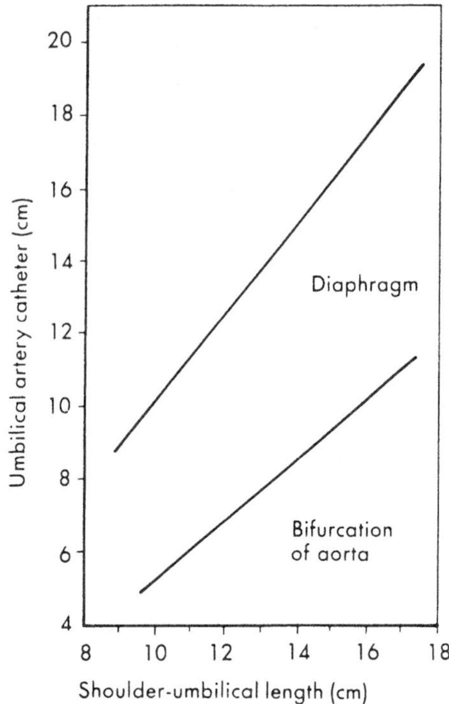

Fig. 9-3 Nomogram for estimation of proper length of umbilical artery catheter (distance from lateral end of clavicle to umbilicus versus length of catheter to reach designated level).

4. If the catheter is to be left in place after the resuscitation, check the position of its tip with an abdominal radiograph. The optimal position above the diaphragm is at T6 to T9, and below the diaphragm, at the aortic bifurcation (L4 to L5). A catheter tip facing caudad or in a lateral position must be removed. Secure the catheter with a 3-0 silk pursestring suture through the cord.
5. Infuse parenteral solutions at a rate of at least 2 to 3 ml/hr IV. Hyperosmolar solutions infused through the catheter may cause significant ischemic reactions and should be avoided.

MECONIUM-STAINED AMNIOTIC FLUID

Meconium staining of the amniotic fluid, which complicates 10% to 15% of all pregnancies, predominantly in term or post-term infants, is usually benign, particularly when the meconium is noted to be thin and nonparticulate. However, in some cases passage of meconium into the amniotic fluid may be associated with intrapartum asphyxia. Under these circumstances fetal distress may promote gasping, allowing meconium to pass below the vocal cords.

Fetal distress or depression at birth is more likely if the meconium is thick or particulate. Meconium aspiration syndrome (MAS) (see Chapter 11) may result, with significant morbidity and mortality rates. Management at delivery depends on the presence or absence of significant neonatal depression.

Diagnostic Findings

Meconium staining of cord and skin and perinatal depression may or may not be present.

Management

In all babies who have passed meconium in utero, clear the mouth and pharynx of meconium with a suction device before delivery of the thorax from the perineum or hysterotomy site.

If thick or particulate meconium was present in amniotic fluid, management consists of the following:

1. If the infant appears vigorous and has an energetic cry, normal tone, and a heart rate above 100 beats/min, only routine measures are indicated: drying, clearing of secretions, positioning, continued observation.
2. If the infant does not cry, gasps, or appears weak, or if the heart rate does not rise above 100 beats/min, ET intubation and suction are indicated. Adapters may be used to attach a suction apparatus to the ET hub. While applying continuous suction, withdraw the ET tube slowly. This procedure may be repeated until little or no meconium is retrieved or the infant's heart rate warrants immediate resuscitation. An alternative (less efficient) method is to pass a suction catheter through the ET tube for suctioning of the airway. Other resuscitation measures may be required after tracheal intubation.

Considerable judgment must be used. Symptomatic meconium aspiration has occurred in nondepressed term infants. Rapid and efficient intubation of these babies is often indicated, with care taken to minimize airway trauma. Attempts to remove residual meconium via tracheal intubation should probably be limited to two to three before PPV is started, if required.

10 Distress at Birth

Several diagnostic entities may be associated with distress or depression of the newborn immediately after birth.

INTRAPARTUM ASPHYXIA

Etiology

Decreased transplacental gas exchange with resultant fetal hypoxemia, acidosis, and ischemia lead to intrapartum asphyxia.

Diagnostic Findings

Diagnostic findings in intrapartum asphyxia consist of pallor or cyanosis, bradycardia, apnea, and flaccidity.

Management

Resuscitation is given as described in Chapter 9.

MECONIUM ASPIRATION

See Chapters 9 and 11.

MATERNAL DRUGS

Narcotics, sedatives, and magnesium sulfate may cause depression of the newborn.

Etiology

Drugs given to the mother may pass transplacentally to the fetus, with subsequent central or neuromuscular depression.

Diagnostic Findings

Diagnostic findings in a newborn depressed by maternal drugs are apnea and decreased muscle tone.

Management

1. If depression is believed to be the result of narcotics, administer naloxone (Narcan), 0.1 mg/kg/dose q3-5min prn intramuscularly, intravenously (IV), or by endotracheal (ET) tube and provide support. Naloxone is contraindicated in babies exposed in utero to opiates, including methadone, because it may induce convulsions.
2. If magnesium sulfate is suspected as a cause of depression, calcium gluconate, 100 mg/kg/dose IV, should be given slowly with cardiac monitoring. Improvement in clinical status may be temporary and patients must be monitored closely. In addition, the potential risk of calcium extravasation may make repetitive doses impractical and potentially dangerous. In premature infants, temporary mechanical ventilation may be required. The negative effects of hypermagnesemia as well as the therapeutic role of calcium are usually temporary; routine intervention should be limited.

CONGENITAL ANOMALIES

See also Chapter 20.

Upper Airway Disorders

Etiology. Choanal atresia or stenosis, micrognathia, and macroglossia are the most common upper airway disorders in the newborn. Other causes are anterior nasal stenosis, laryngomalacia, laryngeal atresia, cyst, or web, vascular ring, goiter, cystic hygroma, vocal cord paralysis, and tracheal anomalies.

Diagnostic Findings. Substernal and intercostal retractions, cyanosis, apnea, and inspiratory stridor are observed. A neck mass or hypoplastic mandible may also be noted.

Passage of feeding tube or suction catheter through the nasopharynx is impossible in choanal atresia.

Management

1. Oxygen and oral airway. Prone position, with micrognathia.
2. Tracheal intubation if obstruction is unrelieved or apnea develops. Laryngoscopy may reveal the cause of obstruction.
3. Surgical consultation as needed.

Lower Airway and Pulmonary Disorders

Etiology. The most common lower airway and pulmonary disorders in newborns are diaphragmatic hernia, tracheoesophageal fistula (TEF), and Potter's syndrome (oligohydramnios, lung hypoplasia, and characteristic facies). Less commonly observed are neonatal chylothorax, congenital pneumonia, cystic adenomatoid malformation of the lung, and lobar emphysema. Some of these abnormalities may be identified prenatally.

Diagnostic Findings

1. Severe respiratory distress with poor air entry and cyanosis.
   a. Scaphoid abdomen is occasionally prominent in diaphragmatic hernia.
   b. TEF is suggested by excessive mucus production, crowing respirations, hoarse cry, and inability to place a nasogastric (NG) tube in stomach. TEF is associated with esophageal atresia in its commonest form.
   c. Potter's syndrome is suggested by resistance to lung inflation, early pneumothorax, flattened facies, redundant skin folds, renal dysgenesis, and history of oligohydramnios.
2. Characteristic radiographic findings.
   a. Diaphragmatic hernia: unilateral lung hypoplasia with multiple bowel loops in the chest, tip of stomach tube in chest if left-sided hernia.
   b. TEF: NG tube coiled in air-filled esophageal pouch.
   c. Potter's syndrome: lung hypoplasia often with pneumothorax.
3. Strong suspicion is important, particularly if oligohydramnios, scaphoid abdomen, or early respiratory distress is present in a full-term infant.

Management

1. Oxygen, tracheal intubation, and ventilatory support as indicated. Bag-and-mask ventilation in diaphragmatic hernia is contraindicated because it will inflate the intrathoracic stomach and bowel, compromising ventilation further. In all cases of lung malformation, allowing for a certain degree of hypercapnia may be wise, so as to minimize risks of further lung injury.
2. Early insertion of a large (e.g., 8 F-10 Fr) NG tube and suction for decompression.
3. Portable ultrasonography to identify kidneys, cystic tumors, or pleural fluid (chylothorax or hydrops presentation).
4. Appropriate surgical consultation.

NEUROMUSCULAR DISORDERS

Etiology

Although individually, neuromuscular orders are rare entities, they have a common presentation. Neonatal myotonic dystrophy, congenital fiber-type disproportion, muscular dystrophy, spinal muscular atrophy, and a number of other relatively rare entities should be considered.

Diagnostic Findings

Diagnostic findings are flaccidity and a paucity to absence of spontaneous respirations, spontaneous movements, and swallowing efforts. Breech presentation and polyhydramnios are also intrauterine clues to diagnosis. Family history may be useful, but neuromuscular disorders often occur as sporadic events. Muscle and nerve biopsies may be indicated with neurologic consultation.

Management

Management should be supportive once initial resuscitative efforts have been carried out.

Infants with neuromuscular disorders often pose difficult diagnostic dilemmas because postpartum hypoxia may obscure the clinical picture. Consultation with a neurologist is essential.

OTHER CAUSES

More common abnormalities, such as sepsis, respiratory distress syndrome, and shock, may manifest symptoms while the patient is still in the delivery room setting. These disorders are discussed in Chapter 11.

11 Postnatal Emergencies

Cardiovascular Disorders

CONGENITAL HEART DISEASE

Congenital heart disease (CHD) is the most common major birth defect, affecting approximately 8 of every 1000 newborns. It is more common in infants of mothers with insulin-dependent diabetes, in infants with chromosomal disorders (e.g., trisomy) and certain genetic syndromes, in the setting of a history of CHD in siblings or parents, or after the use of specific drugs in the first trimester of pregnancy (e.g., lithium). Surgical treatment of cardiac defects has greatly improved the prognosis. This progress has made it imperative that all neonatal care providers be familiar with early recognition of CHD and have established consultation lines with a tertiary care center specializing in the diagnosis and surgical treatment of neonatal cardiac disease, for rapid referral if indicated.

Some cardiac lesions manifest immediately after birth and may constitute a true surgical emergency—for example, total anomalous pulmonary venous return (TAPVR) with obstruction of the veins, transposition of great arteries (TGA), or hypoplastic left heart syndrome (HLHS) with restrictive atrial septum. Others, however, may become symptomatic only after physiologic postnatal changes take place (decrease in pulmonary vascular resistance, ductal constriction). Table 11-1 shows the most common cardiovascular diagnoses encountered in the first 4 weeks of life.

The number and variety of all possible lesions is large (see Table 16-1), making each case unique, but the pattern of presentations usually includes one or more of the following symptoms: cyanosis, congestive heart failure or shock, abnormal heart murmur, and dysrhythmia. The presence of these symptoms alerts the practitioner to the possibility of CHD and in large part dictates the ensuing steps of evaluation and initial management. The evaluation for CHD should include a complete physical examination (in particular to look for associated birth defects), four-limb (BP) measurements, chest radiograph, electrocardiogram (ECG), hyperoxia test if cyanosis is present, and, when possible, an echocardiogram.

CYANOSIS (see Chapter 17)

Although CHD is not the only cause of neonatal cyanosis, it must be considered in the differential diagnosis. Neonates who present with cyanosis and in whom CHD is suspected should undergo a hyperoxia test. In this test samples for arterial blood gas (ABG) are obtained preductally (right radial artery in most cases) with the patient breathing room air and then with the patient breathing 100% oxygen. The magnitude of the Pao_2 change is useful in defining whether the cyanosis is likely to be secondary to cyanotic CHD. CHD is probably the cause of the observed cyanosis if the rise in Pao_2 is less than 20 mm Hg, there is no overt respiratory distress (normal work of breathing and $Paco_2$), and the chest radiograph shows decreased vascular markings but no evidence of parenchymal disease. Lung disease may be the cause of cyanosis if the Pao_2 rises by more than 200 mm Hg or if there is respiratory distress and the chest radiograph shows signs of parenchymal disease (e.g., respiratory distress syndrome [RDS], meconium aspiration syndrome [MAS], pneumonia, air leak). However, both congestive

TABLE 11-1 Frequency Distribution of Congenital Heart Disease Lesions in the First Month of Life

Age on Admission (number of patients)	0-6 days (537)	7-13 days (195)	14-28 days (177)
DIAGNOSIS (FREQUENCY)	D-TGA (19%) HLHS (14%) TOF (8%) CoA (7%) VSD (3%) Others (49%)	CoA (16%) VSD (14%) HLHS (8%) D-TGA (7%) TOF (7%) Others (48%)	VSD (16%) CoA (12%) TOF (7%) D-TGA (7%) PDA (5%) Others (53%)

CoA, Coarctation of the aorta; *D-TGA*, D-transposition of the great arteries; *HLHS*, hypoplastic left heart syndrome; *PDA*, patent ductus arteriosus; *TOF*, tetralogy of Fallot; *VSD*, ventricular septum defect.
Modified from Flanagan MF, Fyler DC: Cardiac Disease. In Avery GB, Fletcher MA, MacDonald M, editors: *Neonatology: pathophysiology and management of the newborn*, Philadelphia, 1994, JB Lippincott.

heart failure and pulmonary venous obstruction can manifest as signs of pulmonary edema, making the differentiation between lung and cardiac diseases more difficult. In the end, echocardiographic examination of the newborn is generally needed to delineate CHD.

Infants with persistent cyanosis who do not appear to have pulmonary lung disease to explain their condition should be started on an intravenous (IV) infusion of prostaglandin E_1 (PGE_1) in preparation for transfer to a tertiary care center. Starting dose of PGE_1 infusion is 0.05 μg/kg/min, which may be increased to 0.1 μg/kg/min. Respiratory depression is a common complication of PGE_1 administration and patients may need to be started on assisted ventilation and, at the very least, carefully monitored.

CONGESTIVE HEART FAILURE (see Chapter 16)

In the premature infant, the most common cause of congestive heart failure (CHF) is the presence of a PDA, often during recovery from hyaline membrane disease (HMD). In the term infant, causes of CHF include left-sided obstructive lesions (e.g., coarctation of the aorta, other aortic arch anomalies, critical aortic stenosis, TAPVR, cor triatriatum); large intracardiac or extracardiac shunts (e.g., single ventricle and large ventricular septal defect [VSD], truncus arteriosus, arteriovenous [AV] fistulas); dysrhythmias (see later section); and causes of myocardial dysfunction, either extrinsic (e.g., infectious, metabolic) or intrinsic (e.g., cardiomyopathy).

Management should be directed at minimizing energy consumption (neutral thermal environment; assisted ventilation, sedation, and neuromuscular blockade if necessary) and improving oxygen delivery (optimize hematocrit [Hct]; administer supplemental oxygen and cardiotonics when indicated). In cases of left-sided outflow tract obstruction, ductal patency should be maintained with IV PGE_1. Most neonates with CHF must be referred to a tertiary care center for evaluation and management.

DYSRHYTHMIAS (see Chapter 6)

The most common dysrhythmias of the neonate are *premature atrial or ventricular beats,* which are generally transient and benign. A 12-lead ECG and a review of current drugs given to the patient or the mother are usually sufficient precautions. If the manifestations persist, evaluation of the patient for possible structural heart disease and consultation with a pediatric cardiologist are indicated. *Neonatal tachycardia* may be due to the presence of an accessory pathway (reentry tachycardia as in Wolff-Parkinson-White syndrome, atrial flutter) or to increased automaticity (e.g., paroxysmal atrial tachycardia, junctional ectopic tachycardia).

Supraventricular tachycardias may need to be treated if they persist for more than 1 hour or if there is associated hemodynamic compromise (e.g., respiratory distress, oxygen requirement, shock, poor feeding). Treatment should be undertaken in consultation with a pediatric cardiologist, if at all practical. Cardiac monitoring with a chart recorder should be available. Management consists of the following:

1. Adenosine is an effective therapeutic and diagnostic tool. Give 100 μg/kg IV, followed immediately with a 2 to 3 ml normal saline (NS) rapid IV push, at the same IV site and using a three-way stopcock apparatus, to flush the small amount of adenosine into the circulation. This dose may be repeated one time with 100 to 200 μg/kg in 10 to 15 minutes if there is no response to the first dose. A brief but significant bradycardia may ensue. For diagnostic purposes it is very useful to record a six-lead (bipolar leads only) ECG during adenosine administration because the pattern of tachycardia termination and recurrence helps differentiate between types of tachycardia and therefore may dictate long-term therapy, if indicated.
2. Other therapies are β-blockers (esmolol or propranolol), class I antiarrhythmic agents (e.g., procainamide, flecainide), digoxin, or class III antiarrhythmic agents (e.g., amiodarone or sotalol). They should be used only under the supervision of a pediatric cardiologist. The use of verapamil is contraindicated in infants.
3. In general, avoid vagal stimulation. However, application of iced water (small bag with half ice, half water) centered over the bridge of the nose for 15 to 20 seconds can be effective in some circumstances. This maneuver may be repeated two or three times at most. Do *not* perform ocular or rectal pressure maneuvers in the newborn.
4. If the patient's condition deteriorates (acidosis, impending shock), synchronized cardioversion at 0.5 to 2 Joules (J)/kg is indicated.

Congenital heart block: The uncommon dysrhythmia of congenital heart block may be due to either major congenital heart malformations (e.g, left TGA [L-TGA], endocardial cushion defect) or an underlying maternal collagen vascular disease (anti–Ro/SSA and anti–La/SSB antibodies). If associated with a malformation, congenital heart block is often fatal. In situations without associated CHF (ascites, pleural effusions, anasarca), no emergent therapy may be necessary. The condition is often recognized prenatally and, in some cases, has resulted in emergency delivery because of the mistaken interpretation of fetal distress. Management includes the following:

1. Make the diagnosis with an ECG, which usually shows evidence of normal atrial rate (120-150 beats/min) and dissociated ventricular rate (50-60 beats/min).
2. Establish venous access (see Chapter 9).
3. Evaluate for respiratory and circulatory insufficiency.
4. Consult with a pediatric cardiologist and consider pacemaker placement.
5. In the presence of CHF or with evidence of tissue hypoxia (significant metabolic acidosis), pacing (transcutaneous, esophageal, or transvenous) is necessary. Infusion of isoproterenol, 0.05 to 0.5 μg/kg/min, or epinephrine, 0.05 to 0.5 μg/kg/min IV in 5% dextrose solution, may be helpful as a temporizing measure.

HYPERTENSION (see Chapter 18)

In the term newborn, a systolic BP reading consistently above 100 mm Hg is considered elevated and warrants therapy. The most common conditions associated with neonatal hypertension are RDS and asphyxia. Often the cause is never determined. However, renovascular disease (anomalies, injury such as incurred from catheterization, renal vein thrombosis), coarctation of the aorta, and intracranial hemorrhage have been noted as proven causes of hypertension, so this condition warrants investigation. Therapy should be initiated under close monitoring and consultation.

PERSISTENT PULMONARY HYPERTENSION OF THE NEWBORN

Persistent pulmonary hypertension of the newborn (PPHN) is commonly seen in term or near-term neonates, in newborns with significant intrapartum asphyxia, and in infants delivered after due date. PPHN is occasionally associated with polycythemia or diaphragmatic hernia. It also may complicate pulmonary disease, such as RDS, MAS, or bacterial pneumonia. PPHN is presumed to be caused in many instances by failure of vasodilation of the pulmonary arteriolar bed as well as by a hyperreactive pulmonary arteriolar medial muscle mass, with resultant continued pulmonary hypertension and right-to-left shunting through fetal channels (ductus arteriosus and foramen ovale).

Diagnostic Findings

Cyanosis with quiet but persistent tachypnea occurs in the first 12 hours of life. If PPHN is associated with pulmonary disease (e.g., MAS or diaphragmatic hernias), there may be significant dyspnea with chest wall retractions.

Ancillary Data

1. Radiographic findings are often normal or may show a nonspecific pattern much milder than the clinical presentation would indicate. Decreased pulmonary vascular markings may be suggested. In PPHN with associated pulmonary disease, there may be associated typical findings (e.g., aspiration pattern in MAS or ground-glass appearance in HMD).
2. ECG shows nonspecific right ventricular hypertrophy.
3. Pulse oximeter saturation is usually below 85% and often below 75% in room air. Right upper extremity saturation is often 5% to 10% above lower extremity saturation, suggesting right-to-left ductal shunting.
4. ABG results usually demonstrate hypoxemia in room air with little or only transient response to oxygen administration. When pulmonary disease is present, the $PaCO_2$ level may be elevated. Radial artery PaO_2 is often 15 mm Hg higher than umbilical artery PaO_2, suggesting ductal shunting.

Management

1. Consultation with a tertiary care facility and a pediatric cardiologist should be obtained. Cyanotic congenital heart disease cannot be excluded without further evaluation.
2. Some cases respond to increased ambient oxygen alone. Inducement of metabolic alkalosis, through the use of bicarbonate infusion, or of moderate respiratory alkalosis, achieved by ventilator-assisted hyperventilation, may be useful. Both conventional and high-frequency ventilation strategies are now commonly applied in babies with severe PPHN. However, excessive alkalosis, especially ventilation-induced, has been associated with an increased risk of neurologic sequelae.
3. Other drugs may be useful in the management of PPHN. For example, cardiotonic agents such as dopamine and dobutamine may improve cardiac output and enhance pulmonary blood flow significantly. These drugs should not be administered if the diagnosis is uncertain or without the support of a tertiary care center because of the lability of patients with PPHN and the systemic side effects encountered with drug therapy. Similarly, surfactant administered by endotracheal (ET) tube may also be of benefit in selected patients with lung disease (those with significant alveolar collapse) but

should be given only by individuals with significant experience in use of surfactants and management of ventilated newborns.

4. Inhaled nitric oxide (iNO), a selective pulmonary vasodilator, has now been approved as therapy for PPHN. It has been shown to reduce mortality and/or the need for more invasive therapies (e.g, extracorporeal membrane oxygenation [ECMO]) and is most successful in patients with little or no parenchymal lung disease. Abrupt discontinuation of iNO may lead to worsening of oxygenation, and its administration requires devices approved for such use by the U.S. Food and Drug Administration (FDA) and ready access to ECMO for possible rescue.
5. ECMO is a heroic but occasionally lifesaving modality available for affected term or near-term neonates in a number of specialized centers. The adjunct of new therapies (iNO) and improvement in ventilation strategies has led to a decrease in the use of ECMO for PPHN.

Endocrine and Metabolic Disorders

HYPOGLYCEMIA

The definition of clinically significant hypoglycemia remains one of the most contentious issues in contemporary neonatology. The currently recommended operational threshold for intervention is a serum glucose concentration of 45 mg/dl (2.5 mmol/L) in symptomatic neonates. In the absence of symptoms, a serum glucose concentration lower than 35 mg/dl (2 mmol/L) is an indication for treatment. Healthy term infants born after a normal pregnancy do not need to undergo serum glucose monitoring if they remain asymptomatic.

Etiology

1. Hypoglycemia is most commonly caused by decreased availability of mobilizable substrates, as in intrauterine growth restriction (IUGR), postdate birth, asphyxia, cold stress, sepsis, polycythemia, or prematurity.
2. Less commonly, hypoglycemia is caused by hypermetabolic states, usually a result of erythroblastosis or hyperinsulinism in infants of diabetic mothers. Rare causes also include congenital hyperthyroidism and genetic inborn errors, predominantly disorders of glycogen storage or release, amino acid metabolism, and mitochondrial enzymopathies. These last disorders are often associated with severe lactic acidosis.

Diagnostic Findings

1. Adrenergic: pallor, cool extremities, irritability
2. Central: jitteriness, poor feeding, seizures, apnea

NOTE: Hypoglycemia may not be accompanied by identifiable symptoms, particularly in the premature or asphyxiated newborn.

Management

Anticipatory management is important, particularly in premature and other high-risk infants.

1. In initial management, maintain a high suspicion for hypoglycemia in any infant with a history of maternal diabetes (discussed later), asphyxia, sepsis, or other risk factors.
2. In at-risk but stable infants of more than 34 weeks' gestation, begin enteral feedings with 15 to 30 ml of 5% or 10% dextrose in water (D5W or D10W), formula, or breast milk, and advance the diet as tolerated, with feedings every 2 to 3 hours. Perform serial determinations of serum glucose (Dextrostix or Chemstrip) until three normal readings (>45 mg/dl) are recorded. At least one confirmatory serum glucose level determination is indicated.
3. In unstable or premature infants of less than 34 weeks' gestation, begin D10W at

100 to 150 ml/kg/24 hr IV. Begin enteral feedings when stable.

4. In an infant who is symptomatic or has a serum glucose less than 35 mg/dl, administer D10W, 2 ml/kg IV over 5 minutes. Stable venous access is required. Follow with a constant infusion of D10W, 100 to 150 ml/kg/24 hr. Avoid higher concentrations of glucose in hyperinsulinemic or premature neonates because of the risks of rebound hypoglycemia and hypertonicity. It is sometimes necessary to administer more concentrated dextrose solutions via a central venous catheter, particularly when the sugar demands of the patient equate to excessive fluid intakes (e.g., >150 ml/kg/24 hr). In symptomatic infants the goal should be to administer sufficient substrate to keep blood glucose level above 60 mg/dl.
5. If neither IV glucose solution nor an infusion site is available, glucagon 0.1 to 0.2 mg/kg IM may be given in an emergency. Glucagon is ineffective in states of limited substrate availability, as in prematurity or growth restriction.

INFANT OF DIABETIC MOTHER

Births of infants of diabetic mothers (IDMs) are common because the mortality and fetal morbidity rates attributable to this disorder have fallen dramatically over the last 20 to 30 years. Common findings in infants of mothers with gestational or insulin-dependent diabetes include macrosomia and postnatal metabolic disorders such as hypoglycemia, hypocalcemia, polycythemia, and hyperbilirubinemia. Infants born to mothers with insulin-dependent diabetes have an increased risk of RDS and of anomalies of the heart (VSD, transposition of great vessels [TGV], coarctation), central nervous system (CNS) (holoprosencephaly, myelocele), skeleton (sacral dysgenesis), gastrointestinal (GI) system (anal atresia, small left colon), and renal system. Cardiac septal hypertrophy is commonly seen but is rarely symptomatic.

Diagnostic Findings

Excessive weight and length for gestational age and cushingoid or "cherubic" facies are common. Other findings relate to a particular anomaly, metabolic disorder, or concurrent problem. In addition, because of excessive fetal weight, birth trauma (clavicular fracture, axillary nerve injury) may occur during vaginal delivery. Cardiac septal hypertrophy is evidenced by cardiomegaly and occasionally heart failure or cyanosis.

Management

1. A comprehensive history of the mother's diabetes and complications is essential, as is a thorough newborn physical examination.
2. Observe the newborn closely for early hypoglycemia and hypocalcemia. Treat each disorder as previously described (p. 99). Hypomagnesemia may coexist with hypocalcemia. Hypomagnesemia may be treated with magnesium sulfate, 25 to 50 mg/kg dose q4-6hr for three or four doses.
3. Watch closely for development of hyperbilirubinemia, particularly on days 3 to 5. Office visits may be required after nursery discharge to assess severity of jaundice.
4. Even near-term and term IDMs may be hypotonic for several days postnatally. Poor feeding is also a transient problem.
5. If symptomatic cardiac septal hypertrophy is suspected, consultation with a pediatric cardiologist is necessary. Supportive therapy (sedation, oxygen supplementation) is usually all that is indicated. Avoid α and β agonists, such as dopamine and epinephrine.

HYPOCALCEMIA

Hypocalcemia is defined as a serum calcium level below 7 mg/dl or an ionized serum calcium level below 1 mmol/L. It is usually transient and in the neonate may be associated with maternal diabetes, prematurity, or perinatal asphyxia. After the first week of postnatal life, hypocalcemia may also be noted in infants with poor renal function. Rare causative disorders include isolated parathyroid hormone deficiency and DiGeorge syndrome (typical facial appearance, conotruncal cardiac anomalies, thymic and parathyroid dysfunction, and frequent association of deletion of a small portion of chromosome 22 [22q11del]).

Diagnostic Findings

Findings include jitteriness and irritability, occasional seizures in infants, low serum calcium level, and prolonged QT interval on ECG.

Management

1. Calcium gluconate, 100 mg/kg IV slowly. Watch for extravasation and bradycardia. Do not administer intraarterially.
2. Begin maintenance calcium gluconate, 200 to 300 mg/kg/24 hr q6-8hr IV or PO, until full feedings are tolerated. Adjust diet. (Occasionally, dosages as high as 600 mg/kg/24 hr are required.)
3. If the patient has little response to calcium gluconate, obtain serum magnesium measurement. If level is less than 1.5 mEq/L, treat with magnesium sulfate, 20 mg/kg/dose q12hr IV.
4. For patients with potential parathyroid hormone deficiency (hypocalcemia, hyperphosphatemia, normal renal function), consultation with a pediatric endocrinologist is encouraged if hypocalcemia is not transient.

HYPERKALEMIA (p. 832)

Hyperkalemia is defined as a serum potassium concentration above 6.5 mEq/L. Sampling site should be taken into account, particularly in the newborn, because of the effects of hemolysis in samples from a bruised heel (capillary blood samples). Hyperkalemia is common in babies with renal failure or severe renal anomalies, severe depression, and very low birth weight (BW) (<1 kg). Although rare, congenital adrenal hyperplasia (CAH) should be considered, particularly if the genitalia are ambiguous. Males with CAH have normal genitalia at birth.

Diagnostic Findings

Neonates often remain asymptomatic until the hyperkalemia is well advanced. Dysrhythmias are common. Earlier ECG findings include peaked T waves and widened QRS complex.

Management (see Chapter 85)

1. If the condition is stable, but potassium is 7.5 to 8.0 mEq/L or greater, give sodium polystyrene sulfonate (Kayexalate), 1 gm/kg/dose (25% sorbitol solution) q6hr rectally. Insulin and glucose have a more rapid onset of action and are also recommended. Infusion of human insulin in 5% albumin solution, 0.05 to 0.1 U insulin/kg/hr (1 unit of insulin per 10 ml of 5% albumin is given); piggyback into existing IV fluid such as D7.5W or D10W at 100 to 150 ml/kg/24 hr. Follow serum glucose and dipstick glucose levels closely.
2. If dysrhythmia is present, treat immediately with calcium gluconate, 100 to 200 mg/kg IV over 5 to 10 minutes and sodium bicarbonate, 1 to 3 mEq/kg IV over 10 to 20 minutes.
3. Determine and treat (if possible) the cause of the hyperkalemia.

OTHER DISORDERS

Hyponatremia (see Chapter 8)

Hypernatremia (see Chapter 8)

Gastrointestinal Disorders

Most significant GI diseases in neonates are caused by obstruction, which is usually evident shortly after birth or in the first few weeks of life (see Chapter 44).

ESOPHAGEAL ATRESIA AND TRACHEOESOPHAGEAL FISTULA

Symptoms of tracheoesophageal fistula (TEF) may or may not be present at birth. The incidence of premature delivery increases with TEF and polyhydramnios. Esophageal atresia is associated with fistula between the trachea and distal esophagus in 85% of patients with TEF.

Diagnostic Findings

Early respiratory distress, overabundant secretions, hoarse cry, and stridor are frequent presenting symptoms. Vomiting and aspiration occur when the infant is fed. A nasogastric (NG) tube will not pass. Associated anomalies, such as imperforate anus, limb defects, and vertebral or renal anomalies, may be present.

Complication. Aspiration pneumonia.

Ancillary Data

1. X-ray films: Anteroposterior (AP) chest film shows the tip of the NG tube in an air-filled upper esophageal pouch. It may also show an associated skeletal anomaly.
2. A contrast study should not be attempted without surgical consultation and is usually unnecessary.

Management

1. Administer oxygen, establish NPO status, and replace fluid deficits (see Chapter 7) as required.
2. Elevate patient's head 15 to 20 degrees.
3. Perform intermittent low suction with double-lumen nasoesophageal tube or equivalent (e.g., 8 F to 10 F catheter).
4. Arrange immediate pediatric surgery referral.

OBSTRUCTIVE LESIONS

Obstructive lesions are most commonly congenital in origin, with an overall rate of 1 in 2700 live births.

Etiology

1. Esophageal atresia: see previous section.
2. Pyloric stenosis (p. 668).
3. Intestinal atresia: proximal jejunum and distal ileum are the most common sites. Duodenal atresia is common with Down syndrome.
4. Meconium ileus: ileal obstruction is most commonly associated with cystic fibrosis.
5. Volvulus (p. 669).
6. Imperforate anus: if imperforate anus is associated with intestinal obstruction, perineal fistula is either absent or inadequate to permit elimination, particularly in boys. Incidence of associated malformations (vertebral, cardiovascular, and tracheoesophageal) is as high as 50%.
7. Hirschsprung's disease (p. 662).

Diagnostic Findings

1. High obstructions (midjejunum and above) are associated with less abdominal distension but persistent vomiting, which may be bilious if the obstruction is distal to the ampulla of Vater. Patients are often hungry after emesis. There may be a history of polyhydramnios.
2. Low obstructions (ileum and below) are associated with more abdominal distension, less vomiting, and only occasionally a history of polyhydramnios. Palpable and visible bowel loops may be prominent. Respiratory distress or apnea caused by elevated intraabdominal pressure and limited diaphragmatic excursion may be noted. High-pitched bowel sounds are often present.
3. Palpable mass, if present, is caused by volvulus or meconium ileus. Perforation may be accompanied by hypotension and sepsis.

Ancillary Data

1. X-ray films: AP abdominal films are often helpful, demonstrating distended bowel and occasionally air-fluid levels or mass effects. Free air may be noted in the presence of a perforation.
2. Electrolyte measurements and complete blood count (CBC).

Management

1. Oxygen and fluid deficit replacement as required (see Chapter 7); NPO status.
2. Insertion of a large-bore (e.g., 8 F to 10 F) NG tube for drainage at atmospheric pressure or intermittent low suction.
3. Immediate surgical and radiologic consultation as indicated by specific process.

ABDOMINAL WALL DEFECTS

Abdominal wall defects occur in 1 in 2500 live births.

1. Gastroschisis: abdominal wall defect lateral to umbilicus with herniation of abdominal viscera. Associated anomalies are rare, but associated intestinal atresias are not uncommon.
2. Omphalocele: herniation of abdominal viscera through omphalomesenteric duct into umbilical cord. Sac may rupture. Associated congenital anomalies are common (e.g., trisomy 13, trisomy 18, Beckwith-Wiedemann syndrome).

Diagnostic Findings

A mass is noted at birth either in the cord itself (omphalocele) or paraumbilically (gastroschisis). The physician may visualize bowel loops, stomach, and, occasionally, the liver within the herniated mass. With the advent of intrauterine ultrasound scanning, prenatal diagnosis of this disorder is relatively common. Green-tinged amniotic fluid may be mistaken for meconium but, when nonparticulate, probably represents in utero bilious reflux.

Management

1. Promptly curtail fluid loss from the defect: Enclose mass and lower portion of patient in a plastic wrap or aluminum foil. Support the mass in a midline position if possible, and avoid inadvertent twisting of the exposed bowel.
2. Prevent hypothermia with a heated incubator or radiant warmer.
3. Promptly administer IV fluids: D5W and lactated Ringer's solution (LR) or D5W 0.9% NS at 20 to 40 ml/kg over 2 to 6 hours. Maintain NPO status.
4. Insert large-bore (e.g., 8 F to 10 F) NG tube for drainage.
5. Monitor BP, urine output, and serum electrolyte levels.
6. Arrange immediate surgical consultation.

NECROTIZING ENTEROCOLITIS

Intestinal immaturity, ischemia, and secondary bacterial invasion are thought to be the most likely causes of necrotizing enterocolitis (NEC). Pneumatosis intestinalis and portal venous "air" are probably the results of bacterial fermentation with production of hydrogen gas and methane. This condition may quickly progress to intestinal necrosis and, occasionally, perforation. It may be accompanied by symptoms of gram-negative septicemia and shock. NEC is commonly found in the middle of the distal ileum; portions of the small and large intestines and even the stomach may be involved. Prematurity, high tonicity, frequent and high-volume feedings, umbilical catheterization, hypoxic stress, polycythemia, and *Klebsiella* nosocomial infection have all been implicated as risk factors. NEC occurs predominantly in preterm infants after the onset of feedings. A somewhat more benign entity has been observed in near-term or term newborns with only colonic involvement.

Diagnostic Findings

Insidious or rapid onset of abdominal distension, with significant gastric residual (or emesis) of feedings, which are commonly bile stained. Nonspecific but early signs also include lethargy, tachycardia, and temperature instability. These may progress rapidly to more worrisome findings such as hypotension, pallor, tachypnea (or apnea), bloody stools, and tenderness to palpation on abdominal examination.

Ancillary Data

1. X-ray films: early findings include intestinal dilatation with or without evidence

of bowel-wall edema. The presence of pneumatosis intestinalis, with bubbly or linear air shadows in the bowel wall, confirms the diagnosis. Portal venous gas, which is occasionally seen, is a poor prognostic sign. Free air (best seen on cross-table lateral or lateral decubitus views) suggests intestinal perforation.

2. White blood cell (WBC) count is markedly elevated or depressed, with a shift to the left and the presence of toxic granulations. Thrombocytopenia (platelet count <50,000 cells/mm^3) is present in 50% of patients.
3. Serum electrolyte and glucose concentrations may demonstrate hyperglycemia and hyponatremia.
4. ABG results often show a significant metabolic acidosis.
5. A specimen for blood culture should be obtained before antibiotic therapy is started.
6. Disseminated intravascular coagulation (DIC) may be demonstrated by coagulation studies.

Management

1. IV hydration, with an initial bolus of LR or 0.9% NS at 20 to 40 ml/kg over 2 to 3 hours if fluid deficit is present. In addition, colloid or blood may be required when peripheral perfusion is diminished and unresponsive to crystalloid bolus. Maintain NPO status and provide maintenance fluids.
2. Large-bore NG (e.g., 8 Fr to 10 Fr) tube placed for drainage. Suction is unnecessary, but the tube should be irrigated every 2 to 3 hours with 1 to 2 ml of 0.9% NS.
3. Antibiotics are initiated after culture results are obtained:
   - **a.** Ampicillin, 100 to 150 mg/kg/24 hr q12hr IV; *and*
   - **b.** Gentamicin, 2.5mg/kg q12hr IM or IV (infant <7 days old) or 2.5mg/kg q8hr IM or IV (infant 7 to 28 days old). Spacing of the doses may have to be adjusted if the infant is premature or renal function is compromised. Experience with alternative regimens of gentamicin dosage (higher loading dose followed by a once-daily maintenance dose) is still limited, although the approach is promising. An alternative approach is to use the third-generation cephalosporin cefotaxime, 100 mg/kg/24 hr q12hr IV or IM (infant ≤7 days old) or 150 mg/kg/24 hr q8hr IV or IM (infant >7 days old).
   - **c.** If symptoms and signs develop rapidly, *Clostridium* or other anaerobe species must be considered as etiologic agents. Initiation of clindamycin, 5 mg/kg q12hr IV (preterm infant), q8hr (full-term infant <7 days old), or q6hr (term infant >7 days old) is warranted. Metronidazole, 7.5 mg/kg q48hr (neonate with BW <1200 g), q24hr (infant <7 days old with BW 1200 to 2000 g), or q12hr (infant <7 days old with BW >2000 g) or 15 mg/kg q12hr (infant >7 days old with BW >2000 g), can also be used. Either one of these agents is also commonly administered if intestinal perforation has occurred or is deemed likely.
   - **d.** Antibiotic therapy should not be delayed if there are technical problems with collection of a blood culture specimen.
4. Surgical consultation, preferably as soon as concerns regarding NEC as a potential diagnosis are raised.

Hematologic Disorders

ANEMIA (see Chapter 26)

Normal Hct at birth is 45% to 65%.

Etiology

1. Hemorrhage

a. Prenatal or intrapartum hemorrhage or transfusion (e.g., abruptio placentae or fetomaternal transfusion)
b. Internal hemorrhage caused by trauma or bleeding dyscrasia
2. Hemolysis
3. Immune: erythroblastosis fetalis (EBF) caused by Rh, ABO, or minor blood group incompatibilities
4. Nonimmune: relatively uncommon; caused by red blood cell (RBC) membrane defect (e.g., glucose-6-phosphate dehydrogenase [G6PD] deficiency, spherocytosis) or intravascular coagulation

Diagnostic Findings

1. Pallor, tachypnea, weak pulse, hypotension (BP <30 to 40 mm Hg), and tachycardia if hemorrhage is recent and significant (10% blood volume or greater). Acidosis is a late sign.
2. Hemolysis, usually chronic, often associated with jaundice, hepatosplenomegaly, edema, and other signs of CHF.

Ancillary Data. Hct and hemoglobin (Hb) concentration are low (in normal term newborn, Hct is 45% to 65% and Hb is 14 to 21 g/dl) if blood loss is chronic but may still be in normal ranges if blood loss is acute. RBC morphology may show a significant hemolytic picture. Chronic blood loss or hemolysis is usually accompanied by reticulocytosis. Blood and cerebrospinal fluid (CSF) cultures should be performed if symptoms are vague and there is any suspicion of sepsis.

Management

1. Hemorrhagic, hypovolemic shock (see Chapter 5).
2. Without shock but with Hct less than 25%: 10 ml/kg of packed RBCs over 1 to 2 hours.
3. If caused by EBF (Rh incompatibility), see p. 108.
4. If immune hemolysis is a result of ABO or minor blood group incompatibility, follow serial serum bilirubin levels and Hct readings and maintain adequate hydration. Use phototherapy. Patient may need an exchange transfusion.

POLYCYTHEMIA

Screening for polycythemia is currently not recommended for all newborns, being reserved for infants who are at risk or symptomatic. A venous Hct above 65% may be associated with increased blood viscosity and vascular resistance. A higher incidence of polycythemia is noted in infants with IUGR or Down syndrome, in IDMs, and in the recipient in monozygotic twins with twin-to-twin transfusion syndrome. Polycythemia caused by intercurrent dehydration is less common and can be dealt with by simply rehydrating the patient.

Etiology

There is an absolute increase in fetal RBC mass with normal blood volume (chronic in utero hypoxemia) or an actual increase in blood volume (cord "milking" or transfusion syndrome).

Diagnostic Findings

Most commonly, symptoms are absent. If pronounced hyperviscosity is present, the infant may have plethora, tachypnea, respiratory distress, hypoglycemia, hypocalcemia, irritability, jitteriness, or seizures. Less common findings are frank CHF, oliguria, cyanosis, gangrene, and NEC.

Ancillary Data. Venous blood Hct above 65%. Capillary blood Hct is usually 4% to 7% above the value obtained from a peripheral or central vein specimen.

Management

Guidelines for management of polycythemia are controversial because later neurologic outcome appears not to be affected by whether a partial exchange transfusion is performed for neonatal polycythemia. One protocol that has been found useful follows:

1. With Hct 65% to 70%, observation is warranted if the patient is asymptomatic (usually). However, if significant CNS, cardiopulmonary, or renal signs develop, partial exchange transfusion via the umbilical vein may be indicated. Because this procedure is less commonly performed than in previous decades, risk of the procedure versus risk of the disease (e.g., minor symptoms such as mild respiratory distress or irritability) must be considered. Exchange transfusion should use the umbilical venous approach with 0.9% NS as the replacement solution. The volume (milliliters) to be exchanged is calculated as follows:

$$\frac{\text{Weight (kg)} \times 90 \times (\text{initial Hct} - \text{Hct desired})}{\text{Initial Hct}}$$

2. With peripheral venous Hct above 70%, partial exchange transfusion is often indicated; symptoms (particularly oliguria, respiratory distress, CNS symptoms, and hypoglycemia) are more common.
3. Monitor for hypoglycemia and treat if present.
4. NPO status for 6 to 12 hours after exchange transfusion is a conservative but reasonable measure.
5. Watch for hyperbilirubinemia.

THROMBOCYTOPENIA (p. 709)

Thrombocytopenia may be a nonspecific finding in conditions such as sepsis, anoxia, prematurity, and DIC. It may be featured in rare genetic syndromes (e.g., thrombocytopenia with absence of the radius [TAR], Wiskott-Aldrich syndrome). Maternal factors include toxemia of pregnancy, collagen vascular disease, idiopathic thrombocytopenic purpura (ITP), and platelet group incompatibilities.

Diagnostic Findings

Findings reflect the underlying cause and potential sequelae of bleeding.

Management

1. Treat the underlying process, including sepsis, hypoxemia, and DIC if present.
2. Administer platelet transfusion if platelet count is less than 25,000 cells/mm^3 (<50,000 cells/mm^3 if the infant is premature) or the infant is bleeding: 10 ml/kg/dose over 1 to 2 hours. Half-life of random donor platelets should be 2 to 4 days in peripheral blood.
3. In isoimmune thrombocytopenia, half-life of transfused platelets is greatly reduced if they were collected from random donors. Treat with maternal platelet concentrates, 10 ml/kg over 1 to 2 hours. Consider infusion of IV gamma globulin, 0.4 to 0.5 g/kg/24 hr given over 4 to 6 hours IV.
4. Avoid intramuscular injections and other trauma.

DISSEMINATED INTRAVASCULAR COAGULATION (p. 694)

Etiology

Common initiating events (triggers) for DIC in the neonate include the following:

1. Maternal factors: acute hemorrhage, amniotic fluid embolism, and dead fetal twin
2. Neonatal factors: hypoxemia, bacterial or viral sepsis, erythroblastosis, NEC, and severe HMD

Diagnostic Findings

Findings include petechiae, purpura, and evidence of underlying disease. In the neonate DIC can range from extremely mild to severe in presentation. Results of clotting studies, presence of fibrin degradation products, and hemolysis noted on RBC smear are diagnostic.

Management

1. Treatment of trigger with oxygen, ventilation, antibiotics, etc.

2. Transfusion of fresh frozen plasma, 10 ml/kg over 1 to 2 hours.
3. Infusion of blood platelet concentrate if platelet count is less than 25,000/mm^3 (<50,000 cells/mm^3 if the infant is premature).
4. Vitamin K, 1 mg IV slowly.
5. If DIC continues, further therapy may be indicated:
   a. If fibrinogen concentration is low (<100 mg/dl) and partial thromboplastin time (PTT) remains very prolonged (>75 to 80 seconds), give cryoprecipitate, 1 bag (about 20 ml) per 3 kg IV.
   b. Two-volume (neonatal blood volume is 80 to 90 ml/kg) exchange transfusion with fresh heparinized blood or citrate-phosphate-dextrose (CPD) blood in infants less than 72 hours old via umbilical vein in 5- to 10-ml increments. Alternatively, packed RBCs reconstituted in fresh frozen plasma to an Hct of 50% to 55% is acceptable. For exchange transfusion in neonates, in particular premature neonates, use of cytomegalovirus (CMV)-negative, irradiated product is warranted because of the risk of graft-versus-host reaction and transfusion-acquired CMV infection.
6. Consideration of heparin infusion, 100 U/kg/dose every 4 hours IV, although it is rarely required.

UNCONJUGATED HYPERBILIRUBINEMIA (NEWBORN JAUNDICE)

Physiologic jaundice in the term newborn is common, self-limited, and generally without sequelae. However, more severe jaundice in the first week of life may be caused by an occult disease process and may require intervention. "Physiologic" unconjugated hyperbilirubinemia with peak bilirubin concentration below 12 mg/dl occurs by day 3 to 4 in the term neonate (mean concentration is 6 to 7 mg/dl on day 3). In preterm infants peak bilirubin concentrations occur later and are more severe if untreated.

Severe unconjugated hyperbilirubinemia in babies with EBF has been related to kernicterus with irreversible deafness, choreoathetosis, and mental retardation. Risk factors for kernicterus include not only elevation of bilirubin concentration (probably above 25 mg/dl in the term neonate) but also level of maturity, intactness of blood-brain barrier (influenced by recent neurologic insult or prematurity), acidosis, hypoxia, hypoalbuminemia, and perinatal depression. Significant uncertainty remains regarding a direct cause-and-effect relationship between the factors just listed and the development of kernicterus.

Etiology

The most common disorders associated with nonphysiologic unconjugated (indirect) hyperbilirubinemia in the first week of life are Rh or ABO incompatibility, prematurity, polycythemia, intestinal obstruction, sepsis, and asphyxia or dehydration (infants are more vulnerable to inadequate fluid intake and excessive water losses). IDMs also constitute a high-risk group. Hypothyroidism must also be considered but is a rare cause of early hyperbilirubinemia. Breast milk jaundice rarely occurs before 10 days of life, and the bilirubin level usually does not peak above 15 mg/dl. Conjugated (direct) hyperbilirubinemia must be excluded. For hyperbilirubinemia occurring after the first week of life, diagnostic considerations must include sepsis, biliary atresia, hepatitis, rubella, galactosemia, and hypothyroidism.

Diagnostic Findings

1. Serial bilirubin determination. Clinically apparent jaundice usually indicates a serum bilirubin concentration above 4 to 5 mg/dl.
2. Conjugated bilirubin level is normally less than 10% of total bilirubin (maximum normal concentration 2.0 to 2.5 mg/dl).
3. Blood typing and Coombs' test, CBC, and RBC morphology.

4. Hepatomegaly may indicate extramedullary hematopoiesis in response to chronic hemolysis (unconjugated hyperbilirubinemia) or hepatitis (conjugated hyperbilirubinemia).

Management

1. Adequate hydration. Treat sepsis, asphyxia, intestinal obstruction, or erythroblastosis as indicated. In cases of hyperbilirubinemia related to dehydration and inadequate milk intake in the first several days after birth, hydration (oral and IV) plus phototherapy often produces a marked fall in serum bilirubin concentration within 4 to 6 hours. No current evidence exists that excessive fluid administration in an otherwise normally hydrated infant will alter serum bilirubin concentrations.
2. Treat acidosis because bilirubin precipitates in acid media (CNS).
3. Phototherapy. Table 11-2 lists recommendations for phototherapy and other treatment of hyperbilirubinemia. Phototherapy is indicated at given indirect bilirubin levels as follows:
   a. Higher than 15 to 18 mg/dl in a term neonate.
   b. Higher than 7 to 15 mg/dl in a premature neonate, depending on degree of immaturity and associated illness.
   c. Cord blood bilirubin concentration higher than 5 mg/dl in an infant with evidence of hemolytic disease.
   d. In-home phototherapy, prescribed on the basis of preestablished guidelines related to specific risk factors, is now possible but, in general, requires strict criteria for recommendation and follow-up.
4. Exchange transfusion may be indicated on the basis of unconjugated bilirubin levels as follows:
   a. Higher than 25 mg/dl in a full-term neonate. Clinical judgment must still play a major role here, particularly in vigorous babies. Findings such as lethargy, hypotonia, and poor feeding are all worrisome, even in patients with lower serum bilirubin values, and may indicate early bilirubin encephalopathy.
   b. Higher than 12 to 15 mg/dl in a premature neonate (see Table 11-2).
   c. Higher than 10 to 12 mg/dl in first 24 hours of life in an infant with significant hemolysis with or without a falling Hct.
   d. At present, risk of kernicterus from hyperbilirubinemia in a specific neonate cannot be assessed with accuracy. The guidelines provided should be tempered by risk factors such as prematurity and acidosis. The risk of intervention (specifically, exchange transfusion) must also be considered.
5. Late anemia (4 to 6 weeks) is common sequelae of neonatal ABO or Rh incompatibility.
6. Hearing screening is indicated as follow-up for babies with severe postnatal unconjugated hyperbilirubinemia.

ERYTHROBLASTOSIS FETALIS

Erythroblastosis fetalis produced by Rh disease is now relatively unusual because of maternal prophylaxis with Rh immune globulin (RhoGAM). However, minor blood group incompatibility and Rh disease itself continue to occur with high enough frequency to warrant some discussion.

Etiology

Maternal-fetal passage of maternal antibodies to fetal RBC antigens.

Diagnostic Findings

1. As in unconjugated hyperbilirubinemia, evidence of hemolysis may be indicated by RBC morphology, anemia, or a positive Coombs' test result.
2. Hepatomegaly caused by a long-standing hematopoietic response to anemia.

TABLE 11-2 Suggested Phototherapy Guidelines: Premature (<37 wk) and Sick Term Infants

	SERUM BILIRUBIN LEVEL (mg/dl)						
	DAYS OF AGE						
Birth Weight (g)	**1**	**2**	**3**	**4**	**5**	**6**	**7**
<1000	3	3	3	5	5	7	7
1000-1249	5	5	5	7	8	10	12
1250-1499	8	8	8	10	12	12	12
1500-1749	10	10	10	12	12	13	13
1750-1999	10	10	12	13	13	13	13
2000-2499	10	12	12	15	15	15	15
>2500	10	12	13	15	17	17	17

Suggested Treatment Guidelines Term, Well* Newborns (Term ≥37 wk and/or ≥2500 g)

	TOTAL SERUM BILIRUBIN LEVEL (TSB) (mg/dl)			
Age (hr)	**Consider Phototherapy**	**Institute Phototherapy**	**Exchange Transfusion if Phototherapy Fails**	**Exchange Transfusion and Phototherapy**
≤24	Require further evaluation and treatment			
25-48	≥12	≥15	≥20	≥25
49-72	≥15	≥18	≥25	≥30
≥72	≥17	≥20	≥25	≥30

Modified from AAP Practice Parameter, Provisional Committee on Quality Improvement, October 1994. Used with permission of the American Academy of Pediatrics.

* No hemolysis, sepsis, or shock.

3. In severe disease, pronounced anemia (cord Hct <30%), edema (hydrops), CHF, pleural effusions, and ascites.

Management

The severely affected neonate who has EBF should be transferred to a tertiary care center as soon as possible. However, certain emergency measures may be required before or during transportation. Much depends on the degree of hemolysis apparent at birth.

Nonhydropic State

1. If cord blood bilirubin is below 5 mg/dl and/or Hct is above 30%, neonate may be observed in the nursery for increasing serum bilirubin concentration. High reticulocyte count (>10% to 15%) and hepatomegaly are useful indicators of severe prenatal hemolytic disease. Phototherapy should be started early. Many sensitized fetuses (particularly if several in utero transfusions were received) have clinically insignificant hemolysis postnatally.
2. If cord blood bilirubin is above 5 mg/dl and/or Hct is below 30%, administer immediate partial exchange transfusion via umbilical venous catheter. Exchange 20 to 25 ml/kg of patient's blood with O-negative packed RBCs with an Hct of 70% to 80%. This exchange should be done in the first hour of life, in 5- to 10-ml increments. Follow serial serum bilirubin determinations and Hct values. Give phototherapy. Neonatology consultation is indicated because once the patient is deemed stable, subsequent double-volume exchange transfusion is often performed to remove sensitized RBCs and to treat severe hyperbilirubinemia.
3. Subsequent exchange transfusions for hyperbilirubinemia may be performed

according to the guidelines just given in the unconjugated hyperbilirubinemia discussion. For exchange transfusions in neonates, particularly premature neonates, use of CMV-negative, irradiated product is warranted because of the risk of graft-versus-host reaction and of transfusion-acquired CMV infection. In emergent situations, however, this may not be practical, such as for the immediate partial exchange transfusion procedure recommended previously.

4. Late anemia (4 to 6 weeks) is common. Follow-up observation and serial Hct determinations are indicated.

Hydropic State. The hydropic state signifies advanced anemia and CHF.

1. Support airway; patients very often require mechanical ventilation. Abdominal tension from ascites, which may compromise respirations, must be relieved by paracentesis.
2. Chest x-ray film to diagnose pleural effusions (although these may be present, they are rarely large enough to cause major pulmonary dysfunction).
3. Obtain umbilical venous access and begin partial exchange transfusion, using the guidelines for nonhydropic states for immediate treatment of anemia as noted previously.
4. Metabolic acidosis, as evidenced by a serum bicarbonate concentration of 18 to 20 mEq/L or less, is worrisome and may indicate tissue hypoxia caused by anemia.
5. Neonatology and cardiology consultations are indicated.

NONIMMUNE HYDROPS

Hydrops is the term used to describe generalized edema in an infant. When severe, this disorder presents the practitioner with diagnostic and therapeutic challenges among the most difficult in newborn medicine.

Etiology

Since the advent of effective preventive measures for maternal Rh sensitization, nonimmune causes of hydrops fetalis predominate. A large number and variety of conditions may be responsible. Cardiac anomalies and arrhythmias, vascular, lung, or renal malformations, congenital infections, tumors, twin-to-twin transfusion, fetomaternal hemorrhage, and chromosomal anomalies are among the more common.

Diagnostic Findings

1. The condition is commonly recognized in utero from the presence of polyhydramnios or the discovery on ultrasound scan of cutaneous edema or body cavity effusions. Level II and III ultrasound examination of the fetus and analysis of a fetal blood sample, when feasible, may provide diagnostic clues. Serial assessments of the biophysical profile via ultrasound help guide the obstetrical practitioner in the appropriate management and timing of early delivery, which is often needed.
2. In the newborn the clinical findings in nonimmune hydrops are indistinguishable from those in immune hydrops (see section on erythroblastosis fetalis). However, anemia is not always present.

Management

Given the complexity of diagnosis and management of fetal hydrops, mothers recognized to carry fetuses with hydrops should be evaluated in a tertiary care center. Despite progress made in our preparedness for and the techniques used for resuscitation of such infants, mortality remains high, especially when prematurity is a complicating factor.

Immediate control of the airway is indicated in most cases. Thoracocentesis and paracentesis are often necessary to establishing gas exchange, which is already compromised by the presence of pulmonary edema. Umbilical vessel catheterization for vascular access and hemodynamic monitoring is recommended. Partial exchange transfusion with packed RBCs may help improve oncotic pressure and oxygen delivery to the tissues.

Infectious Disorders

CONGENITAL AND PERINATALLY ACQUIRED INFECTIONS

Congenital infectious disorders are commonly associated with TORCHS agents (*Toxoplasma gondii,* other viruses, rubella, cytomegalovirus, herpes, and syphilis). "Other viruses" of growing importance are human immunodeficiency virus (HIV) and hepatitis B or C (HBV, HCV). Overall, such infections may be associated with growth retardation, lethargy, thrombocytopenia, anemia, rash, hepatosplenomegaly, and seizures. Several "classic" congenital infections, such as those caused by toxoplasmosis or rubella, are now relatively rare (for rubella, in part because of enhanced efforts to screen for antibody during pregnancy). However, the incidences of sexually transmitted diseases that affect the newborn, such as HIV, HBV, and herpes simplex virus (HSV), are on the rise.

Acquired immunodeficiency syndrome (AIDS) is of major concern as a disease transmissible to the fetus or newborn. Predominant modes of transmission are sexual contact (heterosexual and homosexual), skin breakage (e.g., needles), and for the newborn, perinatal transmission. Postnatal transmission may occur via breast milk. The increase in infection rate in women of childbearing age has been alarming, with concern raised about a subsequent rise in the rate of maternal–infant transmission. Cord blood and postnatal HIV antibody screening may be helpful, but the legal status of maternal consent for performing such studies is still in question. Routine testing with consent of pregnant women for HIV has been discussed. Diagnosis of neonatal infection may be difficult in the neonatal period because of transplacental passage of maternal antibodies, which survive as long as 18 months after birth. Preferred testing of the newborn includes sampling blood for polymerase chain reaction (PCR) evidence of HIV RNA or direct culture for HIV itself.

Because of the proven risk of maternal–infant transmission of HBV or HCV, and the current data indicating a link between chronic hepatitis and liver carcinoma, stronger efforts to diagnose hepatitis during pregnancy and eradicate its passage to the newborn have been undertaken. Immunization against HBV in infancy is now recommended but no effective vaccine is yet available for HCV.

Perinatal acquisition of HSV type 2 (HSV-2) by the neonate is a growing concern because of rising rates of apparent and inapparent maternal genital infection as well as high neonatal mortality and morbidity rates associated with neonatal infection. Infection by HSV-1 (10% to 15% of neonatal HSV infections) may also occur and is related to contact with infected oral lesions or secretions. It is important to identify those children at risk early in life by obtaining an adequate history. The risk of neonatal acquisition of HSV-2 infection is far greater if the mother has primary genital infection and the baby is delivered vaginally. Although neonatal HSV infection has occurred after recurrent or occult HSV genital infection, the risk is much lower.

Diagnostic Findings

The signs and symptoms indicating a risk of infection warrant a physical and laboratory investigation to detect the etiologic agent. Findings of adjunct examinations include:

1. Radiographic findings:
   a. Syphilis: periostitis, epiphyseal bands, or osteochondritis in long bones
   b. CMV: osteitis in long bones, intracerebral calcifications
   c. Rubella: osteitis in long bones
2. Ophthalmologic findings:
   a. Rubella: cataract

b. Toxoplasmosis, CMV, and rubella: chorioretinitis

Ancillary Data

1. Toxoplasmosis: Specific immunoglobulin IgM and IgG antibody tests are available.
2. Other viruses:
   a. HIV: Viral DNA PCR has become the test of choice to diagnose HIV infection in infants. Antibody testing results are confounded by the presence of maternal antibodies in the infant serum. Viral cultures are slow to grow, are not readily available, and are expensive.
   b. HBV: Prenatal testing of all pregnant women is recommended to identify newborns at risk. The presence of hepatitis B surface antigen (HBsAg) in serum indicates acute or chronic infection; presence of antibody to surface antigen (anti-HBs) indicates past infection or response to vaccine.
   c. HCV: Anti-HCV antibodies can be detected in the serum of infected infants by enzyme immunoassay. Positive results must be confirmed by immunoblot. These tests do not distinguish between the infant's own antibodies and those acquired from the mother, however. An alternative approach for early diagnosis of infection is the PCR detection of the viral RNA, which obviates waiting for the disappearance of maternally transmitted antibodies.
3. Rubella: Diagnosis of congenital infection is based mainly on historical and clinical data. It can be confirmed by measurement of rubella-specific IgM in the serum of affected infants.
4. CMV: Positive results of urine culture for CMV obtained within 3 weeks of birth are diagnostic of congenital CMV infection. Maternal and newborn convalescent titers (CMV-specific IgM) may also be helpful.
5. HSV: Direct culture for HSV (e.g., conjunctiva, mouth, nasopharynx, vesicle scraping, blood, stool) remains the easiest technique for diagnosis. Other techniques such as direct immunofluorescence antibody staining and enzyme immunoassay are available. PCR detection of HSV DNA is especially valuable in identifying patients with CNS infection.
6. Syphilis: The Venereal Disease Research Laboratory (VDRL) and rapid plasmin reagin (RPR) tests remain the gold standard nontreponemal tests for screening. Positive results must be confirmed by treponemal tests: fluorescent treponemal antibody absorption (FTA-ABS) or microhemagglutination test for *Treponema pallidum* (MHA-TP).

Isolation of patients for infection with most agents listed here appears no longer indicated as long as "universal precautions" are taken. Pregnant hospital staff, however, should be particularly fastidious about precautions. Isolation for proven HSV infection (see later) is recommended.

Management

Treatment is usually supportive, supplemented by specific therapy:

1. Congenital toxoplasmosis: Pyrimethamine combined with sulfadiazine has been recommended for symptomatic newborns with proven disease after the risk of neonatal jaundice has passed. Optimal dosage and duration of treatment have not been determined. Treated patients should be given folinic acid supplementation.
2. Other viruses:
   a. HIV: Zidovudine (ZDV) is now routinely given to pregnant HIV-positive women and their newborns. Prenatal ZDV treatment has been shown to significantly decrease the transmission of HIV. Since 1993, perinatal AIDS has declined by 66% in the U.S. The protocol recommended by the Centers for

Disease Control and Prevention (CDC) for neonates born to HIV-positive women consists of ZDV syrup, 2 mg/kg/dose q6hr PO for 6 weeks, starting 8 to 12 hours after birth. This therapy is also recommended for babies of HIV-positive women who did not receive prenatal ZDV. Last, if practical, HIV-positive women should be discouraged from breastfeeding because of the known risk of transmission of HIV through infected milk.

b. HBV: Immunization against HBV in infancy is now recommended. Additional treatment with hepatitis B immune globulin (HBIG) is indicated if the mother proves to be antigen positive (see Chapter 76).

c. HCV: No specific therapy currently exists for HCV infection or its prevention. Routine serologic testing of pregnant women for HCV is not recommended and should be reserved for those at increased risk.

3. HSV: Although treatment is controversial, the following guidelines may be helpful:

a. With active maternal genital infection, contact precautions should be taken. Isolation of neonates with proven HSV infection is recommended. Specimens for HSV culture should be obtained 24 to 48 hours after birth. Use of fetal scalp monitors during labor should be avoided in women whose infants are at risk for neonatal herpes.

b. Infants born vaginally to mothers with presumed or proven primary HSV infection should be treated with empiric acyclovir (30 mg/kg/24 hr q8hr, continued until culture results show absence of the disease). Some experts recommend starting therapy immediately after sampling for culture, and others advocate waiting for results of the cultures or clinical evidence of infection. Currently no data exist in support of the benefits or risks of either approach.

c. Infants born vaginally to mothers with known recurrent and active infection should be evaluated for possible infection. Cultures should be performed, and CSF tested for the presence of viral DNA by PCR. Chemotherapy is initiated if lesions become apparent in the newborn, results of culture or PCR are positive, or suspicion of infection remains strong.

d. Infants born by cesarean section to women with active herpetic lesions should be observed closely, and cultures are recommended. Chemotherapy should be initiated if an infant becomes symptomatic or culture results are positive.

e. Infants with proven infection should be treated with acyclovir for 14 days if the disease is limited to mucocutaneous membranes, and 21 days if it is disseminated or involves the CNS.

4. Syphilis: Current recommendations are as follows:

a. For infants with proven or probable congenital syphilis (because of physical or x-ray evidence of syphilis, serum VDRL or RPR titer more than four times the mother's, positive CSF VDRL result or abnormal CSF protein or cell count, positive IgM test result, or histologic evidence of treponemes in placenta or cord):

(1) Aqueous crystalline penicillin G, 50,000 U/kg/dose IV q12hr for the first 7 days of life and q8hr thereafter for a total of 10 days; *or*

(2) Aqueous procaine penicillin G, 50,000 U/kg IM qd for 10 days; adequate CSF levels are not always achieved with this latter regimen, however.

In all cases, missing more than 1 day of therapy warrants restarting the entire course. Because accelerated progression to early neurosyphilis has been reported in babies with coexistent HIV infection, HIV testing in patients with congenital syphilis is strongly recommended.

   b. Asymptomatic infants born to mothers who received adequate therapy more than 4 weeks before delivery should be examined carefully and regularly until results of nontreponemal serologic tests are negative. Some practitioners advocate administering a single injection of benzathine penicillin (50,000 U/kg IM), especially if regular follow-up is not likely.

   c. Asymptomatic infants born to mothers whose therapy was deemed inadequate (inadequate or unknown dosage, nonpenicillin regimen, treatment given less than 4 weeks before birth, lack of a response of maternal serum titers) should be fully evaluated, including CSF examination. Under these circumstances, a full 10-day course of penicillin G or a single IM injection of benzathine penicillin has been advocated.

   d. All patients with congenital syphilis should also be tested for other sexually transmitted diseases, including HIV.

5. For gonococcal ophthalmia: 0.5% erythromycin ointment, 1% tetracycline ointment and topical 1% silver nitrate solution (causes more chemical conjunctivitis) are considered equally effective for the prophylaxis of ocular gonorrheal infection.

ACQUIRED NEONATAL BACTERIAL SEPSIS

Acquired neonatal bacterial sepsis occurs in 3 to 5 newborns per 1000 live births. Its incidence increases with prematurity, prolonged (>24 hours) rupture of membranes, recent fever in the mother, chorioamnionitis, urinary tract infection (UTI), foul lochia, intrapartum asphyxia, and use of intravascular catheters in the neonate.

Etiology

Acquired neonatal bacterial sepsis is commonly caused by organisms present in maternal perineal flora, including *Escherichia coli*, group B or D β-hemolytic streptococci, *Listeria monocytogenes*, *Haemophilus* spp., and *Staphylococcus aureus*. Nosocomial infection with *Staphylococcus epidermidis* is of increasing concern in premature infants, particularly those given IV fluids via indwelling venous catheters.

Diagnostic Findings

1. Often subtle, diagnostic findings include irritability, vomiting, poor feeding, temperature instability (usually hypothermia), and lethargy. They may progress to more overt (but nonspecific) symptoms, including respiratory distress, apnea, poor peripheral perfusion, abdominal distension, jaundice, and excessive bleeding or bruising.
2. Group B streptococci and *L. monocytogenes* commonly have an early form (up to 3 days), with sepsis predominating, and a late form (4 to 14 days) with meningitis as the primary presentation.

Ancillary Data

1. Severe neutropenia (<2000 polymorphonuclear leukocytes [PMNs] per mm^3) or neutrophilia (>16,000 PMNs/mm^3), immature band forms, toxic granulations, thrombocytopenia, and coagulopathy may be present. Erythrocyte sedimentation rate (ESR) and C-reactive protein concentrations may be elevated.
2. Cultures of blood, CSF, and urine should be obtained once the diagnosis is suspected.
3. Chest x-ray films should be taken to exclude pneumonia.

Management

1. Treat under the following circumstances:
   a. If there are any of the overt signs discussed previously, unless other obvious causes (e.g., jaundice caused by incompatibility) exist.
   b. In the presence of any symptoms noted previously and with an abnormal WBC count, particularly neutropenia.
   c. If the delivery is premature, with any overt symptoms, or if risk factors (maternal fever, asphyxia, amnionitis) are present.
   d. For babies who are at increased risk of invasive group B streptococcal (GBS) disease, see later.
2. Perform cultures, particularly of blood, urine, and CSF.
   a. Collect specimens before initiating antibiotics. If venipuncture is unsuccessful, heelstick specimen for blood culture (0.2 ml) is acceptable if the skin is properly cleansed with antiseptic (povidone-iodine) and alcohol.
   b. If conditions of hemodynamic or respiratory instability warrant, lumbar puncture may be delayed 6 to 12 hours; blood cultures should be obtained. However, treatment should not be delayed, nor should prolonged attempts at lumbar puncture be allowed to compromise the patient's clinical status.
3. Administer antibiotics:
   a. Ampicillin, 100 mg/kg/24 hr q12hr IV or IM, *and*
   b. Gentamicin, 5 mg/kg/24 hr q12hr IV or IM (infant ≤7 days old) or 7.5 mg/kg/24 hr q8hr IV or IM (infant 7 to 28 days old). Intervals between doses may have to be lengthened in sick premature infants (see #5 also).
   c. Clindamycin should not be used for neonatal sepsis unless specifically indicated by culture and sensitivity data and then only if serum concentrations can be assessed. The dosage is 15 mg/kg/24 hr q8hr IV.
   d. Specific therapy for resistant organisms should await full culture reports. However, if conditions or suspicions warrant or the patient's condition continues to deteriorate, oxacillin (or equivalent) may be added, 75 mg/kg/24 hr q12hr IV or IM. For penicillin-resistant *S. epidermidis* septicemia, give vancomycin, 15 mg/kg/dose IV q12hr (infant ≤7 days old) or q8hr (infant >7 days old).
4. The decision whether to continue antibiotic therapy should be made only after the cultures are 48 hours old. Treat for 10 days if the blood culture findings are positive or if the patient is clinically precarious or showed great improvement upon initiation of antibiotic therapy, making sepsis likely. The last two situations may be associated with negative blood culture results. If meningitis is present, treatment should be lengthened to 14 days or more, guided by the condition of the patient, the nature of the infection, and the time to sterility of the CSF.
5. In cases in which potential toxicity of aminoglycosides is a concern, cefotaxime may be substituted for gentamicin (see #3b), at a dosage of 100 mg/kg/24 hr q12hr IM or IV (infant ≤7 days old) or 150 mg/kg/24 hr q8hr (infant >7 days old).
6. Crystalloid or blood (10 ml/kg over 2 to 3 hours) for shock or decreased peripheral perfusion.
7. IV gamma globulin, 0.75 g/kg, has been advocated by some, but its efficacy remains clinically in question. Similarly, the efficacy and safety of leukocyte transfusions are in large part unproven, if such transfusions are even available. Usage of recombinant human granulocyte colony-stimulating factor (rhG-CSF)

and granulocyte-macrophage colony-stimulating factor (rhGM-CSF), although promising, has not been studied enough to be recommended routinely.

Strategies for Group B Streptococcal Disease

GBS invasive disease in the newborn remains a significant cause of morbidity and mortality. The organism is relatively ubiquitous and the colonization rate in pregnant women may be as high as 10% to 30%. Specific strategies (Center for Disease Control and Prevention) have been suggested to deal with treatment and prevention of this deadly disease and are summarized here.

For the Mother

1. It is recommended that all pregnant women be screened at 35 to 37 weeks' gestation for vaginal and rectal colonization by GBS.
2. Women at risk (positive culture results) should receive intrapartum penicillin prophylaxis.
3. If culture results are unavailable or cultures have not been obtained, it is recommended to give intrapartum penicillin prophylaxis to a pregnant woman who:
   - **a.** Had a previous baby with invasive GBS disease, *or*
   - **b.** Had GBS bacteriuria during the current pregnancy, *or*
   - **c.** Has one of the following risk factors:
     - **(1)** gestation less than 37 weeks
     - **(2)** rupture of membranes for more than 18 hours
     - **(3)** a temperature greater than 38° C
4. Women in whom GBS culture result was negative within 5 weeks of delivery need not receive prophylaxis, even if one of these risk factors develops or if a planned cesarean delivery is to occur before labor begins or membranes rupture.
5. Women with threatening preterm delivery should receive prophylactic penicillin unless culture has shown them to be GBS negative in the previous 4 weeks. It is therefore recommended to perform GBS cultures in these women if delivery does not appear imminent.

For the Delivered Newborn. If the mother received intrapartum penicillin prophylaxis for GBS, current recommendations for the neonate are:

1. For asymptomatic newborns of less than 35 weeks' gestation, a limited diagnostic evaluation consisting of CBC and blood culture is indicated. Such infants should then be observed for at least 48 hours, but no specific antibiotic treatment is necessary.
2. For asymptomatic newborns of 35 weeks' gestation or more, the duration of maternal prophylaxis determines the course of action:
   - **a.** If intrapartum prophylaxis was administered at least 4 hours before delivery, no specific antibiotic treatment or evaluation is necessary, but observation for at least 48 hours is recommended.
   - **b.** If intrapartum prophylaxis was administered less than 4 hours before delivery, a limited diagnostic evaluation consisting of CBC and blood culture is indicated. Observation as in #1 is then indicated.
3. Symptomatic newborns should be treated as in the guidelines listed previously for newborn sepsis in general.

No single strategy is recommended for the management of infants born to mothers who did not receive intrapartum penicillin prophylaxis. Evaluation and intervention must be timely and individualized, reflecting the newborn's risk.

BACTERIAL MENINGITIS (p. 741)

The organism most commonly responsible for bacterial meningitis is the group B streptococcus *(S. agalactiae)*. Less commonly, *E. coli*, group D streptococcus, *Haemophilus* spp., and *Klebsiella* organisms are noted. High rates of significant neurologic sequelae and mortality (20% to 40%) make early diagnosis of paramount importance.

Intoxication

NEONATAL NARCOTIC ABSTINENCE

The neonatal narcotic abstinence symptom complex is caused by withdrawal from passive addiction caused by maternal use of a narcotic such as heroin, morphine, codeine, or methadone.

Diagnostic Findings

Symptoms are voracious appetite, vomiting, sneezing, hypertonicity, diarrhea, jitteriness, and irritability. Seizures are uncommon. Symptoms usually begin within 48 hours of delivery. Later manifestations (2 to 3 weeks) may occur in some patients, particularly with methadone withdrawal.

Cocaine use in pregnancy appears to be associated with an increased incidence of fetal loss and neonatal depression but not with classic symptoms of withdrawal. Although irritability and tremulousness may be prominent, they more likely represent toxicity rather than withdrawal from cocaine.

Management

1. Oral morphine is now commonly used to treat symptomatic opiate withdrawal in the newborn. In general, opiates are preferred over other agents (see later) if irritability is accompanied by GI symptoms such as diarrhea or vomiting. Morphine dosage is 0.08 mg/kg/dose PO q3-4hr; it may be increased by 0.02 mg/kg/dose to a maximum of 0.2 mg/kg/dose. Tincture of opium has been used previously, but the solution is not well standardized and may no longer be available in many hospital pharmacies. (Dose: tincture of opium = 2 mg/5 ml or 0.4 mg morphine/ml; give 0.2-0.3 ml/dose q3-4hr PO; maximum dosage 1-2 ml/kg/24 hr). The use of paregoric is discouraged because of the potential toxicity of the vehicle components (e.g., alcohol, camphor, benzoate).
2. Other agents occasionally used are chlorpromazine (Thorazine), 0.5 mg/kg/dose q6-8hr IV, IM, or PO, and phenobarbital, 5 mg/kg/24 hr q8-12hr IV, IM, or PO. Diazepam (1.0-2.0 mg q8hr) may be useful as an adjunct.
3. Treat for 1 to 3 weeks while gradually tapering dosage.
4. Monitor for apnea and bradycardia until the patient's condition is stable.
5. Testing for syphilis (VDRL), hepatitis B antigen, and HIV may be warranted.
6. As noted in Chapter 10, use of naloxone is contraindicated in babies exposed in utero to opiates because it may induce convulsions. In the event of seizures after administration of naloxone to a depressed newborn in the context of unsuspected maternal narcotic abuse, parenteral morphine, 0.1 mg/kg IV, may be the most efficacious therapy.

Neurologic Disorders

SEIZURES (p. 754)

Etiology

1. Seizures result from widely divergent CNS insults. Time of appearance after birth and history of pregnancy, delivery, drugs, and nutrition may be helpful in determining cause.
2. Intrapartum complications: symptoms apparent at less than 24 hours of age:
   a. Hypoxia and cerebral ischemia during labor: increased incidence in IUGR, large-for-gestational-age infants, multifetal gestations, and premature infants and after prolonged labor.
   b. Hemorrhage: subarachnoid and subdural hemorrhages are more common in term infants with breech birth, forceps extraction, or asphyxia. Intraventricular or intracerebral bleeding occurs in premature infants of less than 34 weeks' gestation, with

increased risk if asphyxia or respiratory distress is present. In term infants with intracerebral or intraventricular hemorrhage, arteriovenous malformation should be considered.

3. Infection:
   a. Bacterial meningitis (group B streptococci [*S. agalactiae*] and *E. coli* are most common), accounting for two thirds of cases. Increased incidence with prolonged rupture of membranes (PROM), chorioamnionitis, prematurity, and maternal UTI.
   b. Viral and other infections: Seizures caused by congenital herpes, CMV, and toxoplasmosis infection usually appear shortly after birth. Echovirus and coxsackievirus B infections are seasonal and rarely seen in the first few days of life.
4. Metabolic disorders:
   a. Hypoglycemia (see Chapter 38 and previous section in this chapter): blood glucose concentration less than 35 mg/dl. Prematurity, postdate delivery, maternal diabetes, polycythemia, and IUGR are all common causes of hypoglycemia.
   b. Hypocalcemia (serum calcium level <7 mg/dl). Peak incidence at less than 3 days after birth is related to prematurity or neonatal asphyxia; peak incidence at 4 to 10 days after birth is due to elevated intake of phosphorus, dehydration, or renal failure.
   c. Hyponatremia or hypernatremia, amino or organic acid abnormalities, severe hyperbilirubinemia, and pyridoxine dependency are all rare causes of neonatal seizures.
5. Drug abuse in the mother, including use of cocaine and amphetamines.

Diagnostic Findings

1. Subtle evidence of seizures, including eye deviation, drooling, repetitive movements of mouth, and writhing movements of hips and shoulders, are more common than classic tonic-clonic seizures seen in older patients.
2. Focal seizures are most commonly found during infections such as herpes; generalized disturbances are caused by asphyxia and metabolic problems.
3. Color change (flushing, cyanosis), bradycardia, and apnea or hypoventilation may accompany motor manifestations but are rarely found alone.
4. Associated asphyxia, hemorrhage, or infection, with bulging fontanelle, lethargy, pallor, or apnea may be present.

Ancillary Data

1. Serum glucose and calcium concentrations and lumbar puncture (cell count, protein and glucose concentrations, culture, and Gram staining). Urine toxicology screen may be indicated.
2. For an infant who is unstable or of less than 34 weeks' gestation, ultrasound to rule out intracerebral or intraventricular hemorrhage or midline shift. For stable neonate of more than 34 weeks' gestation, computed tomography (CT) is preferred. Magnetic resonance imaging (MRI), with or without flow studies, may better help identify arteriovenous malformation but is usually not indicated as an initial step in seizure evaluation.
3. Electroencephalogram (EEG) may be useful if appropriate staff is available to interpret newborn study results.

Management (see Chapter 21 and p. 754)

1. Metabolic abnormalities (hypoglycemia, hypocalcemia) require immediate correction.
2. Anticonvulsant alternatives:
   a. Phenobarbital is the drug of choice. Loading dose: 20 mg/kg IV; may be repeated at 5 to 10 mg/kg until seizures stop or a total of 40 mg/kg

has been administered; maintenance: 5 mg/kg/24 hr q12hr PO or IV. Monitor blood drug levels; 20 to 40 μg/ml is adequate.

b. Phenytoin (Dilantin) is a useful adjunct to phenobarbital in the asphyxiated newborn with persistent seizures. Its enteral absorption is poor in the newborn. Loading dose: 20 mg/ kg IV; maintenance: 5 mg/kg/24 hr q12hr IV. Monitor blood drug levels; maintain at 10 to 20 μg/ml; avoid IV extravasation.

c. Lorazepam (Ativan), 0.05 to 0.1 mg/kg/dose q6-8hr IV, for acute control.

3. Supportive care, including maintenance of IV fluids, oxygen, incubator, and monitoring of electrolyte, glucose, and calcium levels.
4. Consultation with neurologist for ongoing seizures.
5. Serial head circumference measurements and ultrasound evaluations to exclude posthemorrhagic and postinfectious hydrocephalus.
6. Long-term follow-up observation is essential; many children need maintenance anticonvulsants and supervision to monitor for potential developmental delays. Hearing screening is advisable if bacterial meningitis is the cause of the seizures.

MYELOMENINGOCELE

Myelomeningocele occurs in 1 in 500 live births. The posterior neuropore fails to close, leaving a spinal defect containing both neural and meningeal components. Distal limb and sphincter disturbances reflect the level of defect. Associated disorders include hydrocephalus (90% of patients with repaired myelomeningocele eventually require placement of ventriculoperitoneal shunts), Arnold-Chiari malformation, and talipes equinovarus.

Diagnostic Findings

A posterior midline deficit (with or without dural or epidermal covering) reflects the level of the vertebral defect. The infant may have an enlarged head circumference or full fontanelle. A sacral dimple alone (unless draining or infected) is usually benign.

Management

1. Keep the patient prone.
2. Cover the defect with sterile saline–soaked gauze pads, and wrap the lower trunk in plastic to prevent drying. Avoid the use of latex gloves in the handling of the infant.
3. Consult a neurosurgeon. Although some controversy still clouds the issues of survival and quality of life (if associated hydrocephalus or other major malformations exist), supportive care and early closure of defects are recommended in most cases.
4. Other manifestations of neurologic deficit (e.g., neurogenic bladder or vocal cord paralysis) should be watched for closely.

Pulmonary Disorders

APNEA (see Chapter 13)

Apnea (cessation of respiratory activity) is considered significant when it lasts more than 20 seconds or is associated with bradycardia (<100 beats/min). Shorter periods of apnea interspersed with normal respiratory activity (periodic breathing) are considered a normal developmental feature of the newborn.

Etiology

1. Apnea in infants may be symptomatic of a variety of conditions:
   a. Metabolic disorders: hypoglycemia, hypothermia.
   b. Infection: sepsis, pneumonia, meningitis.
   c. CNS damage: hemorrhage, hypoxic injury, seizures.
   d. Pulmonary disorders: respiratory distress caused by HMD, pneumonia, airway obstruction.

   e. Gastrointestinal disorders: Gastrointestinal reflux (GER) may exacerbate apnea, although the temporal relationship has yet to be established.
2. Apnea is also commonly observed in the premature (apnea of prematurity). Apnea of prematurity is most often mixed: the central component is due to immaturity of breathing control, and the obstructive component to softness of the chest wall, airway, and pharyngeal soft tissues and possibly to occult reflux.

Diagnostic Findings

Examination is indicated for rales, rhonchi, stridor, quality of air exchange, abnormal neurologic status, anterior fontanelle tension, temperature, and gestational age.

Ancillary Data

1. Chest x-ray films, pulse oximeter saturation, ABG analysis, electrolyte and glucose measurements, WBC count. Blood culture and lumbar puncture, as indicated.
2. Barium swallow or esophageal pH probe may be necessary to diagnose GER.
3. Standard monitors utilize thoracic impedance as an indicator of respirations and therefore detect only central apnea.

Management

1. Resuscitation, support, and treatment of any defined underlying disease.
2. Ongoing cardiac and apnea monitoring.
3. Apnea of prematurity is a diagnosis based on exclusion of other causes. Normally transient and developmentally regulated, this disorder in any patient with significant manifestations requires inpatient cardiac and apnea monitoring.
   a. Mild spells require gentle stimulation. Rocking water beds are recommended by some clinicians but are of indeterminate value. Use of supplemental oxygen in infants who have not demonstrated a baseline need for it is considered dangerous and should be avoided.
   b. Frequent or severe spells may require ventilation or continuous positive airway pressure (CPAP), applied using a nasal CPAP device, without placement of an ET tube. Pharmacologic approaches include the use of caffeine citrate, 20 mg/kg IV or PO initially followed by maintenance of 2.5 to 5 mg/kg/24hr q24hr PO, or theophylline, loading dose of 5 mg/kg IV followed by 1 to 2 mg/kg/dose q8hr IV or PO. Whereas therapy with theophylline requires monitoring of drug levels (therapeutic: 7-13 μg/ml), it is rarely necessary to follow serum levels with caffeine therapy (therapeutic: 5-25 μg/ml).
4. Neonatal and pulmonary consultations.
5. Proven or suspected GER may be partially dealt with as follows:
   a. Thickening of feedings with rice cereal.
   b. Smaller, more frequent feeding schedule.
   c. Bed or crib elevation, prone positioning, upright positioning ("Danny" sling).
   d. Metoclopramide, 0.1 mg/kg/dose qid IV or PO (maximum dosage: 0.5 mg/kg/24 hr), remains of questionable efficacy. The prokinetic agent cisapride has been shown to help relieve symptoms of GER but concerns about its proarrhythmic toxicity argue against its routine use.

RESPIRATORY DISTRESS SYNDROME (OR HYALINE MEMBRANE DISEASE)

Risk of respiratory distress syndrome (RDS, HMD) increases in premature infants (<36 weeks' gestation), particularly boys, IDMs, and infants with intrapartum asphyxia.

Etiology

This respiratory disorder is caused by developmental deficiency of surfactant (surface active lipoprotein) with subsequent generalized microatelectasis and pulmonary edema.

Diagnostic Findings

Tachypnea, nasal flaring, grunting and chest wall retractions, and an oxygen requirement characterize the usual presentation of infants with RDS. Auscultation may reveal decreased air entry and fine rales within 2 to 4 hours after delivery. Peak of disease occurs at 36 to 48 hours of age.

Ancillary Data

1. Chest x-ray films: diffuse fine reticulogranular densities, outlining air bronchograms; loss of volume may be bilateral, especially in smaller infants.
2. CBC, blood cultures to exclude sepsis, serial ABG determinations.

Management

1. Administer oxygen by hood with ongoing monitoring of arterial pulse oximetry and ABG levels. Umbilical artery catheter is recommended if Pao_2 is less than 50 mm Hg in 40% to 50% O_2. CPAP may be administered by nasal prongs or by nasal or ET tubes. Normally, CPAP is begun at 4 to 6 cm H_2O. Ventilator support may be needed if patient is unable to maintain Pao_2 above 50 mm Hg (oximeter saturation 90%-95%) or if $Paco_2$ is more than 55 to 60 mm Hg. Ventilator support (or ventilation using a resuscitation bag attached to an ET tube, if a mechanical ventilator is unavailable) should also be considered on purely clinical grounds if severe respiratory distress and cyanosis are present and blood gas analyses are unavailable.
2. Increase ambient temperature (via an incubator or other device) to achieve a core temperature of 37° C.
3. With significant distress, establish NPO status, and begin D10W at 60 to 80 ml/kg/24 hr IV. Salt is usually not needed during the first 24 hours because of a postnatal physiologic contraction of the extracellular fluid compartment. Withhold potassium supplementation until urine output is well established and patient is more than 24 hours old.
4. Consult neonatal specialists, with consideration of transfer to tertiary care nursery.
5. Studies have demonstrated the efficacy of surfactant administration via ET tube in the first 24 to 48 hours of postnatal life. FDA-approved preparations of exogenous surfactant consist of animal extracts of either porcine or bovine origin. Great caution should be used during administration of surfactant because of rapid changes that occur in neonatal lung compliance and occasional airway obstruction. In general, surfactant should be administered in an intensive care setting by professionals experienced in its use. Dose is 3 to 5 ml/kg by ET tube and may be repeated.

MECONIUM ASPIRATION SYNDROME

(see Chapter 10)

Prenatal aspiration of meconium-stained amniotic fluid below the glottis causes MAS. After delivery, meconium progresses into bronchi and, with postnatal respiratory activity, moves distally. Meconium causes intense tissue reaction and chemical pneumonitis as well as mechanical obstruction.

Diagnostic Findings

Early asphyxial syndrome (low Apgar score, apnea, flaccidity), meconium staining of the skin, umbilicus, and nails, and the presence of meconium at the level of the vocal cords are usual findings. Respiratory distress, with chest wall retractions, dyspnea, and cyanosis, is present, often within 1 to 2 hours of birth, and peaks in severity at 24 to 48 hours. Coarse rales and rhonchi are heard on auscultation.

Complication. Pneumothorax and pneumomediastinum occur in 15% to 30% of cases.

Ancillary Data

1. X-ray films: patchy asymmetric infiltrates, often perihilar in nature, with greater involvement of right middle and lower lobes. Hyperinflation is common.
2. CBC and glucose and electrolyte measurements: values usually normal. Blood cultures should be performed to exclude sepsis.

Management

1. For delivery room management of the newborn with meconium-stained amniotic fluid, see Chapter 10.
2. After delivery room resuscitation, if respiratory symptoms develop, treat as with RDS. Give humidified oxygen by hood, keeping pulse oximeter saturations above 95%. Serial blood gas determinations via umbilical artery catheterization or transcutaneous Po_2/Pco_2 monitors are recommended. As in RDS, NPO status should be established for patients with significant respiratory distress and D10W at 60 to 70 ml/kg/24 hr should be initiated. Monitor glucose concentration.
3. Neonatology consultation is advisable, with probable transfer to a neonatal intensive care unit if a patient has any of the following characteristics:
   a. More than 40% O_2 required to maintain Pao_2 above 50 mm Hg
   b. Severe respiratory distress in the first 24 hours of life
   c. $Paco_2$ above 50 mm Hg (exclude pneumothorax); intubation may be required
   d. Recurrent apnea
   e. Evidence of pneumothorax or pneumomediastinum
4. Patients with meconium aspiration pneumonia often have pulmonary hypertension (PPHN, see earlier discussion). Pulmonary vasodilation may be achieved through hyperoxia, alkalinization (sodium bicarbonate, 2-4 mEq/kg IV over 2-4 hours), sedation, and inhaled nitric oxide. Pressor support may also be of assistance (dopamine and/or dobutamine).
5. Surfactant administration via ET tube has been found efficacious in selected patients with MAS. As noted for RDS, surfactant should be administered in an intensive care setting by professionals experienced in its use.

BACTERIAL PNEUMONIA (p. 811)

Bacterial pneumonia is generally associated with prematurity and in infants with prolonged rupture of membranes (>24 hours) or other signs of chorioamnionitis.

Etiology

Most common causes of bacterial pneumonia are β-hemolytic streptococci (particularly group B), *S. aureus*, *E. coli*, and other gram-negative organisms.

Diagnostic Findings

As in HMD, tachypnea, expiratory grunting, and chest wall retractions are the usual presenting symptoms. Fine rales and asymmetrically decreased breath sounds are often noted. Peripheral vasoconstriction with decreased pulses and hypothermia indicate shock and suggest sepsis.

Ancillary Data

1. X-ray films: asymmetric patchy infiltrates, often unilateral; a minority of patients have pleural effusion. X-ray findings in the infant with GBS pneumonia may mimic those noted with HMD.
2. WBC may be increased or greatly decreased with a shift to the left and a decrease in platelets. Serial ABG determinations may show hypoxemia and metabolic acidosis. PMNs and bacteria may be noted in tracheal effluent and gastric aspirate if samples are obtained within 6 hours of delivery. Cultures of blood, CSF, and urine should be performed.

Management

1. Oxygen, support of ventilation, and serial ABG analyses as outlined for HMD. Umbilical artery catheterization may be useful.
2. Antibiotics: Administer after appropriate specimens (blood, CSF, and urine) are obtained for culture:
   a. Ampicillin, 100 mg/kg/24 hr q12hr IV; if culture results are positive for GBS, treatment may be changed to penicillin G, 100,000 U/kg/24 hr q12hr IV.
   b. Gentamicin, 2.5 mg/kg/dose q8-12hr IM or IV. When aminoglycosides are contraindicated, cefotaxime may be substituted for gentamicin at a dosage of 100 mg/kg/24 hr q12hr IM or IV (infant ≤7 days old) or 150 mg/kg/24 hr q8hr (infant >7 days old).
   c. If *S. aureus* is a concern, add oxacillin, 75 mg/kg/24 hr q12hr IV.
3. Neonatology consultation is suggested, particularly for a patient with severe respiratory distress or vascular instability.

TRANSIENT TACHYPNEA OF THE NEWBORN

The symptoms of transient tachypnea of the newborn (TTN) likely are due to excessive fetal lung fluid, both intravascular and extravascular. TTN is usually a self-limited disorder of term or near-term infants and is often evident 2 to 4 hours postnatally. It is somewhat more common after cesarean section or heavy maternal narcotic administration. A severe variant with associated pulmonary hypertension is seen in less than 10% of cases.

Diagnostic Findings

Tachypnea with a respiratory rate often at 80 to 100 breaths/min. Dyspnea is common but less prominent than in MAS or RDS. There are mild to moderate chest wall retractions with coarse rales and rhonchi; increased AP diameter of the chest is possible. Maximum severity of distress occurs within 24 to 48 hours, followed by gradual resolution.

Ancillary Data

1. X-ray films: nonspecific increase in perihilar markings with fluid in the right minor fissure; mild to moderate hyperinflation may be present, best seen in lateral views.
2. CBC and blood cultures to exclude sepsis. Pulse oximeter saturation readings should be monitored to guide adjustments in oxygen delivery, and regular ABG determinations are recommended, although umbilical arterial catheterization is usually unnecessary.

Management

1. Administer oxygen by hood with FiO_2 adjustment based on serial ABG determinations. More than 40% O_2 is rarely required to maintain oximeter saturation at 90% to 95%.
2. If respiratory rate is above 60 breaths/min, establish NPO status and give D10W, 60 to 70 ml/kg/24 hr IV.
3. Consider neonatology consultation if:
   a. There is respiratory distress with PaO_2 less than 50 mm Hg in 40% O_2 or $PaCO_2$ more than 55 mm Hg.
   b. Apnea develops or distress increases.

PNEUMOTHORAX

Pneumothorax is usually associated with sudden deterioration of the patient with preexisting respiratory distress, particularly MAS or RDS. "Spontaneous" pneumothorax may be present at birth.

Diagnostic Findings

Worsening of the respiratory symptoms is the norm and signs of tamponade may be present if the pneumothorax under tension. Breath sounds are decreased on the affected side and heart sounds are often displaced to the side without the air collection.

Ancillary Data

1. X-ray films: AP and lateral decubitus views are best for diagnosis, displaying a clear shadow lateral to the lung field with no lung markings. Shift in mediastinal structures or depression of ipsilateral hemidiaphragm indicates tension pneumothorax. In pneumomediastinum (seldom is life threatening or requires therapy), the air is noted lateral to the heart borders, with lung markings seen peripherally.
2. Asymmetric fiberoptic transillumination.

Management

1. If distress is not severe, there is no evidence of tension pneumothorax, and the infant is not premature, an increase of the ambient oxygen to 100% may be all that is needed, especially if the pneumothorax is small (<10% to 20%) and little underlying lung disease is present. In all cases, close monitoring for worsening condition (including x-ray films and ABG analysis) is paramount.
2. If large or tension pneumothorax is present, insert a 14- or 16-gauge intravenous cannula (over-the-needle type) at the anterior axillary line, at the fourth to fifth interspace, with the tip angled anteromedially. Take care to introduce the needle only far enough to enter the pleural space. Remove the needle and advance the cannula 1 cm. Attach the cannula to IV extension tubing; connect tubing to a three-way stopcock and a 30-ml syringe. An alternative insertion location is the second rib interspace on the midclavicular line. Tape the cannula in place and evacuate the air collection as needed until a chest tube is inserted, preferably by a person experienced in newborn care. Attach the chest tube, once in place, to a neonatal water seal and suction device (see Appendix A-9).
3. Repeat chest x-ray film to ensure adequate air evacuation.
4. Obtain neonatal or surgical consultation.

Renal and Genitourinary Disorders

ACUTE RENAL FAILURE (p. 828)

Most neonates (95%) void their bladders before 36 hours of age. Failure to void should initiate a diagnostic evaluation, particularly if certain risk factors are present, including hypotension, sepsis, polycythemia, dehydration, perinatal asphyxia, and drug toxicity.

RENAL DISORDERS

Renal disorders may manifest as functional disturbances (oliguria or anuria, uremia, acidosis, failure to thrive) or abnormal physical findings (abdominal mass) or may be clinically silent. When severe, they may lead to early death in infancy.

Etiology

1. Renal agenesis: may be unilateral, may involve only segments of the kidneys, or may be partial (renal hypoplasia). Bilateral renal agenesis leads to Potter's syndrome and is lethal.
2. Renal ectopy, horseshoe kidney: These disorders are often familial and functionally well tolerated.
3. Cystic diseases:
   a. Solitary, unilateral cysts are usually well tolerated and are rare.
   b. Multiple cysts may be part of various entities, such as polycystic kidney disease, either autosomal recessive or dominant. The dominant form of the disease is normally a condition of the adult but may be diagnosed in infancy, usually from the family history. Recessive polycystic kidney disease is often severe and may involve the liver as well. Multicystic dysplastic

kidney(s) is often the result of long-standing urinary obstruction.

4. Renal tumors: Congenital mesoblastic lymphoma, Wilms' tumor, and neuroblastoma are the most common renal tumors encountered in infancy.
5. Renal disturbances are part of the presentation in a number of genetic conditions (e.g., Fanconi's syndrome, Bartter's syndrome, Zellweger's syndrome) and vascular disorders (thrombosis of the renal vein).

Diagnostic Findings

1. Unilateral or bilateral flank mass. Palpable bladder may indicate a urinary obstruction. Poor feeding and emesis are common.
2. Ultrasound findings are usually diagnostic.
3. Blood urea nitrogen (BUN) and serum creatinine levels at least should be determined before more specialized tests (e.g., radionuclide scans, kidney biopsy) are considered.

Management

Renal disorders require referral to a nephrologist for complete evaluation. Although some need only dietary adjustment, other conditions evolve to end-stage renal disease, for which dialysis or transplantation is required.

OBSTRUCTIVE UROPATHY

Obstructive uropathy must be considered if there is an early history of oliguria with maternal history of oligohydramnios or abnormal in utero ultrasound findings and the presence of abdominal mass or spontaneous pneumothorax.

Etiology

1. Ureteropelvic or ureterovesical obstruction, megaloureter (may be present in the context of duplication of ureters), or urethral obstruction (posterior urethral valves being the more common form of obstruction in males).
2. Neurogenic bladder resulting from myelomeningocele or severe CNS insult.

Diagnostic Findings

1. Unilateral or bilateral flank mass (hydronephrosis), often cystic in nature. Palpable bladder may indicate urethral obstruction or neurogenic bladder. Poor feeding and emesis are common.
2. Ultrasound findings may be diagnostic.
3. Voiding cystourethrogram is most often part of the evaluation to assess bladder function and check for vesicoureteral reflux.

Management

1. Gentle bladder catheterization with 3.5 Fr to 5 Fr feeding tube should be considered only when the anatomy of the urinary tract has been established, to avoid injury to the urethra.
2. Urologic consultation is advisable, if not necessary, in most cases.

AMBIGUOUS GENITALIA ("INTERSEX")

Many patients with ambiguous genitalia are identified at birth. More minor degrees of ambiguity, such as hypospadias, would not generally qualify as a disorder requiring emergency management. In these minor cases, request for circumcision should be deferred until a pediatric urologist has been consulted. Similarly, cryptorchidism may need to be addressed only in later infancy, if the infant is otherwise well.

However, more serious anomalies of the genital area should be addressed by qualified professionals, urologists, pediatric surgeons, geneticists, endocrinologists, pediatricians, and neonatologists working as a team. Virilization of a genotypic female (e.g., adrenogenital syndrome, maternal androgens) and absence (e.g., penile agenesis, cloacal exstrophy) or incompleteness (hypopituitarism, septo-optic dysplasia) of virilization in a genotypic male are examples of ambiguous genitalia disorders that carry a high risk of early metabolic disturbances (e.g., adrenal failure, hypothyroidism). These disorders should be considered in any patient with a potential intersex anomaly. Qualified medical professionals, as previously listed, should be consulted immediately. In addition, although the issue is difficult because of parental concerns and anxiety, the assignment of male or female sex to a patient with more serious genital ambiguity disorders should be deferred until definitive diagnostic testing can be accomplished.

BIBLIOGRAPHY

AIDS Clinical Trials Group Protocol (Centers for Disease Control and Prevention): Recommendations for the use of zidovudine to reduce perinatal transmission of human immunodeficiency virus, *MMWR* 43(RR-11):1, 1994.

American Academy of Pediatrics and American College of Obstetrics and Gynecology: *Guidelines for perinatal care,* ed 4, Evanston, Ill, 1997, American Academy of Pediatrics, American College of Obstetrics and Gynecology.

American Academy of Pediatrics Committee on Infectious Diseases and Committee on Fetus and Newborn: Revised guidelines for prevention of early-onset group B streptococcal infection, *Pediatrics* 99:489, 1997.

American Academy of Pediatrics Policy Statement: Drugs for pediatric emergencies (Committee on Drugs), *Pediatrics* 101:e13, 1998.

American Academy of Pediatrics Policy Statement: Hepatitis C virus infection (RE9733), *Pediatrics* 101:481, 1998.

American Academy of Pediatrics Policy Statement: Neonatal drug withdrawal (RE9746), *Pediatrics* 101:1079, 1998.

American Academy of Pediatrics Provisional Committee for Quality Improvement, Subcommittee on Hyperbilirubinemia: Practice parameter: management of hyperbilirubinemia in the healthy term newborn, *Pediatrics* 94:558-565, 1994.

American Heart Association: Guidelines for cardiopulmonary resuscitation and emergency cardiac care, *JAMA* 268:2276, 1992.

American Heart Association and American Academy of Pediatrics: *Textbook of neonatal resuscitation,* ed 4, Dallas, 2000, American Heart Association, American Academy of Pediatrics.

Centers for Disease Control and Prevention (CDC): Prevention of perinatal group B streptococcal disease: revised guidelines, *MMWR* 51(RR11):1-22, 2002.

Committee on Infectious Diseases, American Academy of Pediatrics: *Report of the Committee on Infectious Diseases,* ed 25, Elk Grove, Ill, 2000.

Cornblath M, Hawdon JM, Williams AF et al: Controversies regarding definition of neonatal hypoglycemia: suggested operational thresholds, *Pediatrics* 105:1141, 2000.

Manroe BL, Weinberg AG, Rosenfeld CR et al: The neonatal blood count in health and disease. I. Reference values for neutrophilic cells, *J Pediatr* 95:89, 1979.

Rudolph CD, Mazur LJ, Liptak GS et al: Pediatric GE reflux clinical practice guidelines, *J Pediatr Gastroenterol Nutr* 32:S1, 2001.

Saugstad OD, Rootwelt T, Aalen O: Resuscitation of asphyxiated newborn infants with room air or oxygen: an international controlled trial: the Resair 2 Study, *Pediatrics* 102:e1, 1998.

Wiswell TE et al. Meconium in the Delivery Room Trial Group: delivery room management of the apparently vigorous meconium-stained neonate: results of the multicenter collaborative trial, *Pediatrics* 105:1, 2000.

Wolcoff LI, Davis J: Delivery room resuscitation of the newborn, *Clin Perinatol* 26:641-658, 1999.

V

Emergent Complaints

12 Anaphylaxis

Also See Chapter 20 (Respiratory Distress)

ALERT Acute respiratory distress caused by upper airway obstruction or lower airway bronchospasm requires prompt intervention.

Anaphylaxis is a multisystem allergic reaction elicited in a hypersensitive subject on reexposure to a sensitizing antigen. The syndrome is caused by antibodies, usually immunoglobulin E (IgE), which release chemical mediators, including histamine, leukotrienes, and other vasoactive substances.

ETIOLOGY

Antigens that produce a systemic reaction may be ingested, inhaled, or administered by injection. Although parenteral exposures have the highest risk, anaphylaxis may occur with oral ingestion.

Common agents responsible for anaphylaxis include the following:

1. Antigen extracts used for desensitization of skin testing
2. Antibiotics, particularly penicillin
3. Insect stings, including Hymenoptera order (bee, wasp, yellow jacket, hornet, certain ants) (p. 312)
4. Foods, ranging from shellfish to nuts, eggs, milk, and legumes
5. Insulin and adrenocorticotropic hormone (ACTH)
6. Biologic agents, including foreign serum (usually horse), gamma globulin, and vaccines
7. Latex, especially in health care workers and children with spina bifida or urogenital anomalies
8. Inhaled allergens such as dust, animal danders, and pollens
9. Diagnostic agents (e.g., radiologic contrast media); low-osmolarity contrast media reduce the risk
10. Local anesthetics
11. Aspirin
12. Narcotics such as morphine and codeine

NOTE: Reactions to agents listed in 9 through 12 are not IgE mediated and are called *anaphylactoid*.

DIAGNOSTIC FINDINGS

There is a wide range of reaction to antigenic exposures, from mild distress with a sense of anxiety to true anaphylaxis with respiratory distress and cardiovascular collapse. Patients often note a sense of "impending doom."

There may be upper and lower airway involvement of the respiratory tract. Patients may have rhinorrhea and initial sneezing that do not progress. Patients with significant distress have dyspnea, tachypnea with retractions, respiratory compromise, and cyanosis:

1. Upper airway problems may cause stridor, laryngeal and epiglottic edema, and obstruction.
2. Lower airway bronchospasm may cause coughing, wheezing, and marked distress.

Circulatory collapse may develop. Patients have mild hypotension or true vascular collapse and shock:

1. Initially, chest pain may be noted, sometimes secondary to myocardial ischemia.
2. Dysrhythmias and syncope are common.

Other findings are:

1. Urticaria, pruritus, and erythema.
2. Nausea, vomiting, abdominal cramping, and diarrhea.

Complications

The major life-threatening complications include the following:

1. Upper airway obstruction
2. Bronchospasm
3. Dysrhythmias and cardiac ischemia
4. Circulatory collapse and shock

Ancillary Data

1. Arterial blood gas (ABG) determinations are obtained for all patients with moderate or severe respiratory distress. Oximetry is performed in all patients. Severity of airway obstruction is reflected in ABG results.
2. Electrocardiogram (ECG) is obtained to assess for dysrhythmias, conduction abnormalities, and ischemic changes.

DIFFERENTIAL DIAGNOSIS

The differential diagnosis is usually distinctly established by the clear temporal relationship between the reaction and exposure to an antigenic agent. Special diagnostic considerations include the following:

1. Asthma
2. Infection—septic shock (see Chapter 5)
3. Vasovagal reaction
4. Procaine reaction from inadvertent intravascular injection of penicillin (may cause confusion, syncope, or seizures)

MANAGEMENT

The management of the patient must reflect the severity of the illness and must focus on stabilization.

1. Patients with *mild* disease and no evidence of respiratory distress or cardiovascular compromise may be easily treated with antihistamines (diphenhydramine [Benadryl], 5 mg/kg/24 hr q4-6hr PO), and epinephrine given subcutaneously if indicated.
2. The patient with *moderate* or *severe* distress represents a potentially life-threatening emergency for which immediate stabilization and intervention are required (see Chapter 4).
3. Attention must be directed to the airway, ventilation (assisted ventilation is rarely needed), and circulation:
   a. Oxygen administered at 3 to 6 L/min by mask or cannula
   b. Intubation if there is airway obstruction or respiratory failure
   c. With significant bronchospasm, administration of bronchodilators:
      (1) Albuterol can be given by inhalation (p. 790) as a supplement to epinephrine.
      (2) *Epinephrine*: Administer 0.01 ml/kg subcutaneously (maximum 0.35 ml of 1:1000 dilution). With absence of or partial response, repeat twice at 20-minute intervals. Do not give until heart rate is 180 beats/min or less.

   Epinephrine may also be injected directly into the site of administration of the offending agent, if appropriate, in cases of insect or allergen injections. After a tourniquet is applied (in case of parenteral drugs), inject 0.05 to 0.2 ml of 1:1000 solution.
4. Antihistamines may be helpful. Administer diphenhydramine (Benadryl) at a dosage of 2 mg/kg/dose IV, IM, or PO, and repeat every 4 to 6 hours to treat urticaria, itching, and angioedema.

5. Histamine (H_2) blockers have been found useful in cases of refractory anaphylaxis:
   a. Mild: Give cimetidine, 5 to 10 mg/kg/dose PO (adult: 300 mg/dose), or ranitidine, 1 to 2 mg/kg/dose PO (adult: 150 mg/dose).
   b. Moderate (angioedema, decreased blood pressure): Give cimetidine, 5 to 10 mg/kg/dose IM or IV q6hr (adult: 300 mg/dose), or ranitidine, 0.5 to 1 mg/kg/dose q8hr IV (adult: 50 mg).
6. Steroids are usually indicated, although their benefit is delayed: hydrocortisone (Solu-Cortef), 4 to 5 mg/kg/dose q6hr IV.
7. For hypotension, several maneuvers are indicated:
   a. Keep the patient with legs raised in Trendelenburg's position.
   b. Initiate appropriate fluids, initially infusing 20 ml/kg IV of 0.9% normal saline (NS) or lactated Ringer's (LR) solution over 10 to 20 minutes. May repeat infusion.
   c. If the patient is in shock, epinephrine should be administered IV. For severe disease, many prefer administration by continuous infusion:
      (1) Start in a child with 0.1 μg/kg/min, titrating to response with increasing dosage up to 1.5 μg/kg/min to maintain pressure (prepared by adding 1 mg or 1 ml of 1:1000 solution to 250 ml of 5% dextrose in water [D5W] to make a concentration of 4 μg/ml).
      (2) In an adult, administer bolus with 0.1 mg (0.1 ml of 1:1000 solution mixed in 10 ml D5W to make a dilution of 1:100,000), followed by infusion of 1 μg/min, which may be increased to 4 μg/min if needed (prepared by adding 1 mg or 1 ml of 1:1000 epinephrine to 250 ml D5W to make a solution of 4 μg/ml).

      The risk of dysrhythmias increases when epinephrine is infused at a rate greater than 5 μg/kg/min.

      NOTE: 0.1 ml of 1:1000 solution contains 100 μg, whereas 0.1 ml of 1:10,000 solution contains 10 μg.
   d. If hypotension continues, initiate dopamine, to be administered as a continuous IV infusion at a rate of 5 to 20 μg/kg/min.
8. A tourniquet placed proximal to the site of injection of antibiotics, insulin, antigen extract, or insect sting may be useful.

DISPOSITION

1. Patients with only mild reactions may be observed for 4 to 6 hours and discharged to continue antihistamine therapy at home.
2. All patients with moderate or severe disease must be admitted to an intensive care unit.
3. Prevention of anaphylaxis is an important aspect of its management:
   a. Patients should be aware of allergies and avoid exposure. They should also wear Medic-Alert bracelets or tags.
   b. Parenteral medications should be used only when appropriate. Patients should be observed at least 20 to 30 minutes after administration of such medications.

      NOTE: Prophylaxis with steroids and antihistamines may be indicated before use of radiocontrast media in patients with previous reactions.
   c. In settings where parenteral medications are administered, personnel should have access to emergency supplies, including epinephrine, oxygen and airway support, diphenhydramine (Benadryl), and aminophylline.

d. The patient with a history of anaphylaxis, particularly to insect bites, should carry an emergency kit, including syringes, epinephrine, and diphenhydramine. Epinephrine is available as autoinjectable premeasured kits:

Kit	Amount Delivered
EpiPen	0.3 ml (1:1000)
EpiPen Jr.	0.3 ml (1:2000)
Ana-Kit	0.6 ml (1:1000) (0.3 ml at one time)

Such patients should be considered for desensitization.

BIBLIOGRAPHY

Atkinson TP, Kaliner MA: Anaphylaxis, *Med Clin North Am* 76:841, 1992.

Bochner BS, Lichtenstein LM: Anaphylaxis, *N Engl J Med* 324:1785, 1991.

Edwards KH, Johnston C: Allergic and immunologic anaphylaxis. In Barkin RM, editor: *Pediatric emergency medicine: concepts and clinical practice*, ed 2, St Louis, 1997, Mosby.

Reisman RE: Staging insect bites, *Med Clin North Am* 76:889, 1992.

13 Apnea

Also See Chapters 20 (Respiratory Distress) and 22 (Sudden Infant Death Syndrome)

ALERT Apnea may be a nonspecific sign of a systemic illness or the prelude to other life-threatening events.

Apnea occurs with the cessation of airflow for more than 20 seconds or for less than 20 seconds if accompanied by bradycardia, cyanosis, pallor, or limpness. It must be distinguished from normal periodic breathing irregularities during sleep, which may consist of alternating periods of regular breathing and respiratory pauses of 10 seconds without color change during up to 3% of sleep time. If this latter pattern occurs in a premature infant, it is considered apnea of prematurity and generally resolves by 37 weeks of age. Those older than 37 weeks of age who experience an apneic episode have apnea of infancy.

An episode characterized by a combination of apnea, color change (usually cyanosis but occasionally erythema or plethora), marked change in muscle tone (usually limpness), and choking or gagging is referred to as an *apparent life-threatening event* (ALTE), previously termed "near-miss SIDS" (sudden infant death syndrome) (see Chapter 22).

DIAGNOSTIC FINDINGS AND ETIOLOGY

Central apnea is marked by an absence of respiratory efforts caused by a lack of activation of the musculature that produces flow. It is particularly common in newborn infants. The incidence in the preterm infant is inversely proportional to the gestational age and decreases with maturation. Other conditions that exacerbate the condition are infection, metabolic derangements, anemia, and hypoxic or vascular cerebral damage. Some premature infants have periodic breathing, and rarely, some fail to maintain central ventilation during sleep (*Ondine's* curse) (see Chapter 11).

Obstructive apnea occurs when airflow ceases even though the movements of chest and abdominal breathing continue—that is, respiratory efforts continue. Airway patency is a reflection of both airway constricting and dilating forces and the size of the upper airway lumen. Apnea caused by mixed mechanisms also occurs.

Infants may experience apnea from a wide variety of clinical conditions, often reflecting a mixed pathophysiologic mechanism with components of central and obstructive mechanisms. Although ALTE is the most common and widely recognized, seizures, trauma, breath-holding, and problems with gastroesophageal reflux or feeding are also seen.

Children may experience obstructive apnea, often related to sleep. They demonstrate restless sleep patterns and apnea. Tonsillar and adenoidal hypertrophy resulting in a relative upper airway obstruction is the most common cause. Pulmonary hypertension may be a secondary complication.

TABLE 13-1 Apnea: Diagnostic Considerations

	Apnea in Infancy	Obstructive Apnea
HISTORY	Intercurrent illness Relationship to sleep, feeding, position (reflux) Prenatal, neonatal history Appearance (color, tone) Duration, sequelae Response to stimuli History of seizures	Sleeping: snoring, fitful, restless, hypersomnolence Irritability Obesity Mouth breathing Pattern of progression Response to stimuli
ETIOLOGY		
Infection	Viral: respiratory syncytial virus (RSV), enterovirus, parainfluenza Bacterial: pertussis (p. 731)	**Tonsillitis, pharyngitis** (p. 613)
CNS	**Seizure** (p. 754) **Trauma** (p. 401) **Meningitis/encephalitis** (p. 741) Encephalopathy	Muscular dystrophy Cerebral hypotonia
Endocrine/metabolic	Hyponatremia Hypoglycemia Hypocalcemia	Hypothyroidism (p. 631) Cushing's disease Obese: Prader-Willi, pickwickian syndromes Mucopolysaccharides
Congenital		Pierre Robin syndrome

DIAGNOSTIC FINDINGS

A history is essential in evaluating the child with apnea. Ultimately, the issue is to determine the significance of the episode.

1. Nature of the episode, including appearance of the child with respect to color, tone (increased with seizures, choking, and aspiration; decreased with prolonged seizures or hypoxia), activity, respirations, precipitating events, duration, sequelae, response to intervention, and pattern of progression.
2. Nature of sleep, presence or absence of feeding reflux and chalasia. Sleep pattern should be defined with respect to snoring, fitfulness, restlessness, and hypersomnolence.
3. Intercurrent illnesses, including viral and bacterial diseases. Recurrent episodes of tonsillitis.
4. Medical history, including prenatal and neonatal history, seizures, and metabolic or congenital abnormalities.
5. Family history of apnea, SIDS, ALTE, and respiratory or cardiac problems.

The physical findings are commonly normal, revealing no specific entity to account for the episode. The clinician should ensure that the child is stable without evidence of cardiac, neurologic, or respiratory disease and should search for underlying organic conditions.

A variety of assessment tools are available to evaluate the child for the significance of apneic spells and potential causes.

MANAGEMENT

Evaluation, as outlined in Table 13-1, must focus on the suspected pathophysiologic mechanism and the underlying condition. Treatment after stabilization must account for contributing

TABLE 13-1 Apnea: Diagnostic Considerations—cont'd

	Apnea in Infancy	Obstructive Apnea
ETIOLOGY—cont'd		
Vascular	Vascular ring Congenital heart disease: atrial septal defect (ASD), patent ductus arteriosus (PDA), ventricular septal defect (VSD) Dysrhythmia (Chapter 6)	
Miscellaneous	**Near–sudden infant death syndrome (near-SIDS) or apparent life-threatening event (ALTE)** (Chapter 22) Anemia (Chapter 26) **Gastroesophageal reflux** **Feeding problems** **Breath holding** (p. 740) **Overdose or ingestion** (Chapter 54)	**Tonsillar/adenoidal hypertrophy** **Laryngomalacia** Anemia (Chapter 26) Tumors
ANCILLARY DATA (selectively indicated)	CBC, electrolytes, glucose, Ca^{++}, ABG Chest x-ray films Cerebrospinal fluid (CSF) Cultures: bacterial, viral ECG (consider Holter monitoring) EEG CT scan Barium swallow, manometry, nuclear scanning or esophageal pH studies as appropriate Oximetry monitoring and pneumogram (sleep study)	Lateral neck x-ray film ECG Chest x-ray film Laryngoscopy Formal sleep study
MANAGEMENT	Admit if episode occurred within 2 days of contact or is life threatening, or if follow-up is difficult Treat underlying cause Reflux precautions Consider CPAP or pharmacologic approach (p. 119) Close home monitoring	Admit as indicated Treat underlying problem Consider supplemental O_2, continuous positive airway pressure (CPAP) by nasal prongs Consider nasopharyngeal tube Consider tonsillectomy and adenoidectomy (nasal beclomethasone may provide temporary aid) Tracheostomy only as last resort

abnormalities while being supportive. Patients normally must be admitted for observation and evaluation if the episode occurred within 2 days of contact, if it was clinically significant or potentially fatal, or if follow-up observation and evaluation would otherwise be difficult.

Consultation, monitoring, support, or pharmacologic intervention (p. 119) may be appropriate. Evaluation should be specific for the individual child, often including a barium swallow study to exclude reflux, pulse oximetry, and electrolyte measurements.

BIBLIOGRAPHY

Brouillette RT, Morielli A, Leimonis A et al: Nocturnal pulse oximetry as an abbreviated testing modality for pediatric obstructive sleep apnea, *Pediatrics* 105:405, 2000.

Demain JG, Goetz DW: Pediatric adenoidal hypertrophy and nasal airway obstruction: reduction with aqueous nasal beclomethasone, *Pediatrics* 95:355, 1995.

Gray C, Davies F, Molyneux E: Apparent life-threatening events presenting to a pediatric emergency department, *Pediatr Emerg Care* 15:105, 1999.

Kattwinkel J, Brooks J, Myerberg D: Positioning and SIDS: AAP Task Force on Infant Positioning and SIDS, *Pediatrics* 89:1120, 1992.

National Institutes of Health: Consensus development conference on infantile apnea and home monitoring—986, *Pediatrics* 79:292, 1987.

Stradling JR, Thomas G, Warley ARH et al: Effect of adenotonsillectomy on nocturnal hypoxemia, sleep disturbance and symptoms in snoring children, *Lancet* 335:249, 1990.

Weese-Mayer DE, Morrow AS, Conway LP et al: Assessing clinical significance of apnea exceeding fifteen seconds with event reading, *J Pediatr* 117:568, 1990.

14 Chest Pain

ALERT Potentially life-threatening conditions must be excluded by history, physical examination, and ancillary data.

Chest pain in children is usually not an ominous symptom and rarely suggests a serious underlying condition. In 65% of patients who have the problem for less than 6 months, there is a definable cause (Table 14-1). More than one fifth of children who experience chest pain have no defined cause, 15% have a musculoskeletal origin, 10% a cough, 9% costochondritis, 9% a psychogenic basis, and 7% asthma. Up to 15% of children who receive medical attention have cardiac disease. In 47% of the children ill enough to require admission, the chest pain is secondary to heart disease (dysrhythmia, pericarditis, cardiomyopathy, myocarditis, and coronary ischemia [Kawasaki disease]) (see Box 14-1 and Table 14-1).

Somatic and visceral structures share sensory pathways. Visceral abnormalities may have somatic manifestations at the level of T1 to T6. Abdominal disorders may cause chest pain because the posterior and lateral portions of the diaphragm are innervated by intercostal nerves and may be referred to the lower thorax and abdomen. The central and anterior portions are referred to the shoulder and neck regions.

The focus of the history is on past medical problems of the heart and lungs, family history of heart disease, and the presence of trauma, medications (particularly cocaine or oral birth control pills), coagulopathies, sickle cell disease, and other predisposing factors. The pain should be characterized with respect to onset and progression, character, intensity, location, radiation, relationship to position, breathing, activity, reproducibility, ameliorating factors, and associated signs and symptoms. The presence of other somatic complaints, sleep disturbances, syncope, shortness of breath, and exercise intolerance requires specific questioning.

During the physical examination, attention to vital signs is crucial, as are careful auscultation, percussion, and palpation of the lungs, heart, and abdomen. Trauma should be excluded.

A minimal evaluation should include a chest x-ray film. Other ancillary studies, such as electrocardiography (ECG), arterial blood gas (ABG) determinations, echocardiography, cardiac enzyme evaluation, ventilation-perfusion scanning, and abdominal evaluation, are appropriate for specific indications, detected with the history or physical examination, of underlying cardiac or systemic disease. An exercise stress test or Holter cardiac monitoring may be helpful in unique circumstances.

If the patient appears symptomatic on arrival or if the pain is not obviously functional or musculoskeletal, oxygen and cardiac monitoring are appropriate until the diagnosis is clarified and no significant disease is defined. Treatment of the underlying abnormality and reassurance are indicated. An empiric trial of nonsteroidal antiinflammatory agents may be useful after trauma once a significant abnormality is excluded.

BOX 14-1

CAUSES OF MYOCARDIAL INFARCTION IN CHILDREN

CATEGORY	SPECIFIC CONDITIONS
Congenital cardiac disease	Stenosis or atresia of any of the valves, supravalvular aortic stenosis, atrioventricular canal, truncus arteriosus, patent ductus arteriosus, transposition of the great vessels, tetralogy of Fallot, coarctation of the aorta
Coronary artery anomalies	Anomalous origin of coronary arteries, single right or left coronary artery, aneurysm of the coronary arteries (Kawasaki disease)
Primary endocardial or myocardial disease	Endocardial fibroelastosis, cardiomyopathy
Collagen disorders	Rheumatic fever, systemic lupus erythematosus, mucocutaneous lymph node syndrome, rheumatoid arthritis
Hematologic/oncologic	Polycythemia, hemoglobinopathy (S-C, SS, H types), anemia, leukemia
Neuromuscular disease	Friedrich's ataxia, muscular dystrophy
Primary cardiac tumors	Myxoma, rhabdomyosarcoma, teratoma, fibroma, lipoma, hamartoma
Miscellaneous	Cocaine use

Causes of myocardial infarction in pediatric patients. In Perry LW: *Contemp Pediatr* 27: Nov-Dec, 1985.

TABLE 14-1 Chest Pain: Diagnostic Considerations

Condition	Diagnostic Findings
TRAUMA (Chapter 62)	
Muscle strain	Point tenderness; pain reproducible with pressure or activity; often associated with new activity, particularly weightlifting; also may be secondary to prolonged coughing
Direct trauma to chest wall	
Fractured rib Contusion	History of trauma or hard, paroxysmal coughing; localized, point tenderness; may be associated with pneumothorax
Costochondritis (Tietze's syndrome)	Firm, painful, tender swelling over one or more costochondral or chondrosternal junctions; localized, superficial, nonexertional; may be painful with deep inspiration or direct palpation
Pneumothorax	Acute onset of pain, often associated with shortness of breath, respiratory distress, and cyanosis; decreased breath sounds with hyperresonance; often no history of trauma
Abdominal trauma (Chapter 63) Splenic or liver laceration/bleeding Diaphragmatic injury	Acute onset of abdominal or referred chest pain (often shoulder pain as well); abdominal examination and vital signs variable; possible anemia

TABLE 14-1 Chest Pain: Diagnostic Considerations—cont'd

Condition	Diagnostic Findings
INFECTION/INFLAMMATION	
Pneumonia (p. 811)	Cough, fever, tachypnea, variable respiratory distress, systemic illness; abnormal lung findings; possible shoulder pain
Pleurisy	Superficial, localized, sharp pain, and tenderness; accentuated with deep breathing, cough, and movement of arms
Pleurodynia	Sharp pain, tenderness; unilateral or bilateral; accentuated by movement, breathing, cough; may have fever and abdominal pain; cause: coxsackievirus B
Pericarditis/myocarditis (p. 574) Viral Bacterial Tuberculosis Rheumatic fever Uremic	Sudden onset, sharp pain, substernal over precordium, epigastrium, or entire thorax; friction rub; pulsus paradoxus; accentuated by deep breathing, cough, swallowing, twisting; may have associated myocarditis (p. 572)
Herpes zoster (Chapter 42)	May be prodrome before development of vesicles
Abdomen (Chapter 24) Esophagitis/gastritis Peritonitis Appendicitis Hepatitis Pancreatitis Cholecystitis	Referred pain; symptoms specific for disorder; empiric trial of antacids may be useful
VASCULAR	
Angina, ischemia, and infarct (see Table 14-2) Sickle cell disease (p. 714) Pulmonary stenosis Aortic stenosis and left ventricular outflow obstruction Dysrhythmia (Chapter 6) Anomalous coronary artery	Crushing, sharp pain over left chest with radiation to left arm, neck, or jaw; associated shortness of breath, anxiety, and other signs of cardiac decompensation, including tachycardia, tachypnea, gallop, rales, edema, associated signs and symptoms; ECG indicated
Pulmonary embolism and infarct (p. 578)	Acute onset of dyspnea, tachypnea, tachycardia, hemoptysis, and chest pain; $\dot{V}/\dot{Q}$ scan indicated; exclude hyperventilation, rare without predisposing condition
Dissecting aortic aneurysm	Acute onset of sharp pain in chest, abdomen, or back; pulsating mass; asymmetric lower extremity blood pressures; murmur or bruit; rare in children; Marfan's syndrome predisposes
Mitral valve prolapse	Usually asymptomatic but may have chest pain, palpitations, syncope; midsystolic click with late systolic murmur; most likely seen in young adults
INTRAPSYCHIC	
Functional (p. 774)	Acute stress, attention getting; story inconsistent; no effect on sleep or desired activity
Hyperventilation	Rapid and deep respirations; weakness, tingling; dyspnea; response to rebreathing; may mimic pulmonary embolism

Continued

TABLE 14-1 Chest Pain: Diagnostic Considerations—cont'd

Condition	Diagnostic Findings
CONGENITAL	
Hiatal hernia/esophagitis/reflux (Chapter 44)	Acute or chronic substernal pain and discomfort, vomiting, fullness after eating, and evidence of reflux; influenced by position and food; response to antacids
NEOPLASM	
Thoracic Mediastinal Spinal	May have organ involvement, pressure, or cord compression
MISCELLANEOUS	
Idiopathic	Most common category
Pneumothorax/pneumomediastinum, (Chapters 20 and 62)	Acute onset of pain, often associated with tachypnea, respiratory distress, and cyanosis; may be spontaneous, traumatic, or associated with pulmonary disease (asthma, pneumonia, cystic fibrosis) or with forced inspiration (marijuana)
Asthma	Exercise-induced asthma; usually midsternal sharp pain

BIBLIOGRAPHY

Hirsch P, Landt Y, Porter S et al: Cardiac troponin I in pediatrics: normal values and potential use in the assessment of cardiac injury, *J Pediatr* 130:872, 1997.

Hoffman JI, Lister G: The implication of a relationship between prolonged QT interval and the sudden infant death syndrome, *Pediatrics* 103:815, 1999.

Reynolds JL: Precordial catch syndrome in children, *South Med J* 82:1228, 1989.

Rowe BH, Dulberg CS, Peterson RG et al: Characteristics of children presenting with chest pain to a pediatric emergency department, *Can Med Assoc J* 143:388, 1990.

Selbst SM, Ruddy RM, Clark BJ et al: Pediatric chest pain: a prospective study, *Pediatrics* 82:319, 1988.

Wiens L, Sabath R, Ewing L et al: Chest pain in otherwise healthy children and adolescents is frequently caused by exercise-induced asthma, *Pediatrics* 90:350, 1992.

Zavaras-Angelidou KA, Weinhouse E, Nelson DB: Review of 180 episodes of chest pain in 134 children, *Pediatr Emerg Care* 8:189, 1992

15 Coma

Also See Chapter 81 (Neurologic Disorders)

ALERT The child with an altered level of consciousness requires evaluation of airway, breathing, and circulation and administration of oxygen, dextrose, and naloxone (Narcan). Diagnostic considerations need rapid evaluation.

ETIOLOGY

Coma in children is caused by a wide variety of pathologic processes. Physiologically, hypoxia, hypoglycemia, or direct tissue injury is usually present. Most patients have meningitis, encephalitis, head trauma, or poisoning. Metabolic and endocrine abnormalities, prolonged seizures, and vascular accidents must also be considered. Tables 15-1 and 15-2 outline the common causes of coma, focusing primarily on signs and symptoms noted with the deterioration of mental status from lethargy to stupor to coma. Common treatable causes of coma include infection (meningitis, empyema, abscess, encephalitis), trauma (subdural or epidural hematoma), intoxications (alcohol, barbiturates, opiates, carbon monoxide, lead), endocrine or metabolic disorders (hypoglycemia, uremia), vascular disorders (shock, hypertension), and epilepsy. Intussusception does not cause coma but does produce lethargy, with decreased response to environmental stimuli (p. 664).

A useful diagnostic mnemonic is I SPOUT A VEIN: *i*nsulin (too much, too little), *s*hock, *p*sychogenic, *o*piates and other drugs, *u*remia and other metabolic abnormalities, *t*rauma, *a*lcohol, *v*ascular, *e*ncephalopathy, *i*nfection, and *n*eoplasm. Another mnemonic is AEIOU TIPS: *a*lcohol, *e*ncephalopathy/endocrinopathy/electrolytes, *i*nsulin/intussusception, *o*piates, *u*remia, *t*rauma, *i*nfection, *p*sychiatric, and *s*eizure.

DIAGNOSTIC FINDINGS

A thorough history should be obtained from friends or relatives and should focus on the progression of changes in mental status, medical history, associated signs and symptoms, and localized findings. A history of head trauma, medications, or possible ingestions (see Table 54-3) is imperative in the assessment.

Physical examination is crucial, not only in determining the patient's status, but also in providing diagnostic information to ascertain the level of injury. A complete neurologic examination is imperative. Useful diagnostic clues are outlined in Box 15-1. The Glasgow Coma Scale (p. 49) provides a means of serially monitoring patient responsiveness after trauma.

The location of the lesion may be further delineated by findings, as follows:

Supratentorial lesions have findings suggestive of focal hemispheric disease that progress from a rostral to a caudal direction. Pupillary reflexes are usually depressed, and motor signs are asymmetric.

Infratentorial lesions cause brainstem findings and are not rostral to caudal in evolution. Respiratory patterns may be abnormal, and cranial nerve palsies are common.

Toxic or metabolic lesions are associated with changes in mental status that occur before changes in motor signs develop; the latter are symmetric. Pupillary reactions are preserved,

TABLE 15-1 Coma: Diagnostic Considerations

Condition	Diagnostic Findings	Ancillary Data	Comments
INFECTION (p. 741)			
Meningitis	Fever, headache, nuchal rigidity, seizures, lethargy, irritability, usually no focal findings; may have otitis media or concurrent infection	CSF: ↑ WBC, ↑ protein, ↓ glucose, ↑ pressure, culture result positive	Viral or bacterial; consider in febrile patient with mental status change; antibiotics
Encephalitis	Fever, headache, variable nuchal rigidity, tremor, ataxia, hemiplegia, cranial nerve VI palsy, irritability, lethargy, or focal findings; may have only minimal symptoms	CSF: ↑ WBC (mononuclear), ↑ protein, ↑ pressure, culture result negative	Viral: measles, mumps, rubella, chickenpox, Epstein-Barr virus (infectious mononucleosis); bacterial: pertussis; immunization: pertussis, mumps
Intracranial abscess	Fever, headache, focal neurologic signs, increased ICP	CT scan; CSF: ↑ WBC, ↑ protein, culture negative	Extension otitis media, mastoiditis; predisposing risks: congenital heart disease and polycythemia
Subdural empyema	Toxic, fever, focal neurologic signs, increased ICP	CT scan; subdural tap; CSF: ↑ WBC, ↑ protein, ↑ pressure, culture result negative	Follows trauma or complication of meningitis
TRAUMA (Chapter 57)			
Cerebral concussion	Dizziness, nausea, vomiting, headache, lethargy, amnesia, ataxia, transient blindness, no focal findings	Variable CT scan, depending on course	Rule out mass lesions
Subdural hematoma	After trauma, immediate onset of altered mentation, headache, focal neurologic findings, increased ICP	CT scan immediately	Symptoms usually progress immediately after injury; rarely, findings may be delayed days to weeks
Epidural hematoma	Patient often awakens from concussion and, after a brief period of lucidity, lapses into coma; focal findings, headache, increased ICP	CT scan immediately	Delayed onset unless injury is very severe
Drowning (Chapter 47)	No focal findings, variable increased ICP	CSF WNL; CT WNL or edema	Injury reflects hypoxia
Heat stroke (Chapter 50)	Febrile (>40° C), headache, anorexia, confusion, posturing, acidosis	CSF WNL; ABG, electrolytes variable	Complications can be life threatening

ABG, Arterial blood gas; *CSF*, cerebrospinal fluid; *CT*, computed tomography; *ICP*, intracranial pressure; *WBC*, white blood cell; *WNL*, within normal limits.

TABLE 15-1 Coma: Diagnostic Considerations—cont'd

Condition	Diagnostic Findings	Ancillary Data	Comments
INTOXICATION (Chapter 54 and 55; Table 54-2)			
Sedatives/ hypnotics	Lethargy, stupor, possibly dilated pupils, no focal findings	Toxicology screen	Support; forced alkaline diuresis
Narcotics	Miotic, pinpoint pupils, depressed respiratory, GI, and GU activity, findings	Narcotic screen	Support; Narcan 0.1 mg/kg/dose (0.4-2.0 mg/dose) IV, repeated prn
Ethanol	Lethargy, ataxia, slurred speech, visual hallucinations, poor coordination, seizures; no focal findings	Levels >100 mg/dl (depending on chronicity)	Support; metabolized at about 30 mg/dl/hr; glucose, K^+
Salicylates	Tachypnea, hyperthermia, vomiting, tinnitus, excitability; lethargy, seizures; no focal findings	Level >90 mg/dl at 6 hr, ABG, electrolytes, ↓ glucose	Chronic ingestion—levels not helpful; metabolic acidosis with anion gap
Carbon monoxide	Throbbing headache, dizziness, nausea, vomiting, collapse, therapy; progressing with diminished brainstem function; no focal findings	Carboxyhemoglobin level	Emergency oxygen hyperbaric chamber
Lead	Weakness, irritability, weight loss, vomiting, personality change, ataxia, increased ICP, seizures; no focal findings	Urine lead levels; glycosuria, proteinuria, acidosis; CSF: ↑ WBC, ↑ pressure	Dimercaprol, EDTA
EPILEPSY (p. 754)			
	Following prolonged seizures, postictal period; may have focal findings (Todd's paralysis)	Anticonvulsant levels; evaluation of cause	Support, oxygen; need to evaluate cause of seizures
ENDOCRINE/METABOLIC			
Hypoglycemia (Chapter 38)	Sweating, weakness, tachycardia, tachypnea, tremor, anxiety; no focal findings; seizures	Hypoglycemia; CSF WNL	Administer 0.5-1.0 gm/kg/dose IV of D25W—rapid improvement; maintain glucose
Diabetic ketoacidosis (p. 624)	Kussmaul breathing, orthostatic BP changes, polydipsia, polyphagia, weight loss; no focal findings	Hyperglycemia, ketonemia, acidosis; CSF WNL	Fluids, insulin; variable bicarbonate therapy
Hyponatremia/ hypernatremia (Chapter 8)	Dehydration, edema, seizures, intracranial bleeding; no focal findings	Electrolytes abnormal; CSF WNL	Treat multiple causes in addition to sodium imbalance

EDTA, Ethylenediamine tetraacetic acid; *D25W*, 25% dextrose in water; *GI*, gastrointestinal; *GU*, genitourinary; *IV*, intravenous.

Continued

TABLE 15-1 Coma: Diagnostic Considerations—cont'd

Condition	Diagnostic Findings	Ancillary Data	Comments
ENDOCRINE/METABOLIC—cont'd			
Renal failure (p. 828)	Decreased urine output, edema, lethargy, dysrhythmia (secondary to ↑ K^+), CHF, tachypnea, hypertension; no focal findings	Electrolytes, BUN, creatinine levels abnormal; CSF WNL	Support; multiple causes; dialysis may be needed
Reye syndrome (p. 655)	URI with vomiting followed by lethargy, stupor, hepatic dysfunction, delirium, increased intracranial pressure; no focal findings	Liver function test results abnormal, elevated ammonia, bilirubin WNL; CSF WNL	Multiple causes; support; intracranial monitor
Addison's disease (p. 623)	Muscle weakness, pigmentation of skin, lethargy, anorexia, hypotension, weight loss; no focal findings	Electrolytes: ↓ Na^+, ↑ K^+, ↓ glucose; CSF WNL	May follow stress (trauma, infection); IV glucose, hydrocortisone (Solu-Cortef) 5 mg/kg/dose IV q6hr IV
Amino/organic acid abnormality	Deteriorating growth and development; mental status change; no new focal findings	Acidosis, hypoglycemia; CSF WNL	Evaluation of inborn errors; infection often precipitates problem
VASCULAR			
Subarachnoid hemorrhage	Acute onset of severe headache, nuchal rigidity, listlessness; usually no focal findings	CT scan; CSF bloody	May be caused by trauma, AV malformation
Hypertensive encephalopathy (Chapter 18)	Rapid rise in BP, headache, vomiting, seizures, hemiparesis, lethargy	CSF WNL; evaluate potential causes	Responds rapidly to reducing diastolic BP to 100 mm Hg
Cerebral vascular accident	Usually focal findings; seizures, hemiplegia after dehydration (cerebral vein or sagittal sinus thrombosis); papilledema, proptosis, conjunctival hemorrhage, ophthalmoplegia (cavernous sinus thrombosis)	CT scan; CSF variable	Support, anticoagulation; causes include cyanotic heart disease, endocarditis, sickle cell disease, thrombocytopenia, hemophilia, trauma, birth control pills, and anticoagulants
INTRAPSYCHIC (Chapter 83)			
Hysterical	Inconsistent findings, often focal; if arm is held up, when dropped it does not hit patient; history of depression, anxiety	CSF WNL	Usually history of mental illness
NEOPLASM			
Multiple cell types	Variable presentation	CT scan	Neurosurgical consultation

AV, Arteriovenous; *BP*, blood pressure; *BUN*, blood urea nitrogen; *CHF*, congestive heart failure; *URI*, upper respiratory infection.

TABLE 15-2 Differential Diagnosis of Coma

Focal Signs?	Normal Cerebrospinal Fluid*	Abnormal Cerebrospinal Fluid*

None present	Postictal
	Intoxication
	Concussion
	Metabolic/endocrine disorder
	Hypertensive encephalopathy
	Hysteria
	Hydrocephalus
		Infection
		  Meningitis
		  Encephalitis
		Subdural hematoma
		Epidural hematoma
		Subarachnoid hemorrhage
		Cerebral vein thrombosis
		Lead poisoning
		Midline tumor

Present	Subdural hematoma
	Epidural hematoma
	Todd's paralysis
	Hypertensive encephalopathy
		Subdural hematoma
		Epidural hematoma
		Infection
		  Brain abscess
		  Subdural empyema
		  Encephalitis
		Arteriovenous malformation
		Neoplasm

* Check for cells, protein, glucose, Gram stain response, culture, and pressure, if lumbar puncture is done. Perform lumbar puncture after computed tomography and obtain consultation for clinical suspicion of elevated pressure.

seizures are common, and abnormal motor movement is seen.

Acid-base imbalance may suggest the underlying cause. A *metabolic acidosis* with increased anion gap may be due to lactic acidosis (hypoxia or inadequate perfusion), diabetic ketoacidosis, renal failure, or ingestion (methanol, ethylene glycol, salicylates [late]). *Respiratory acidosis* associated with apnea or hypoventilation may be secondary to supratentorial or infratentorial lesions, ingestion (sedative, narcotics), respiratory muscle fatigue, neuromuscular disease, metabolic encephalopathy, and generalized seizures. *Respiratory alkalosis* caused by an increased respiratory rate is associated with intracranial hypertension, septic shock, hepatic failure, salicylate ingestion, Reye's syndrome, and brainstem dysfunction.

Laboratory evaluation should focus on potential causes. Chemical evaluations should always include glucose and electrolyte concentrations, liver function tests, and ammonia and blood urea nitrogen (BUN) levels. Specific tests should be performed as indicated. Complete blood count (CBC) and cultures are appropriate for evaluation of an infectious origin. Oximetry should be continuous. A lumbar puncture is particularly helpful once increased intracranial pressure is excluded (see Table 15-2). Urine and blood toxicologic screens may be done. Radiologically, computed tomography (CT), often with contrast medium if a nontraumatic condition is suspected, should take place early in the assessment.

A number of concurrent conditions may interfere with the assessment of the child's responsiveness, potentially leading to an incorrect diagnosis of brain death. Findings that may be associated with brain death and their other possible causes are:

1. Pupils fixed: anticholinergic drugs (systemic or topical), neuromuscular blockade, and preexisting eye disease
2. No oculovestibular reflex: ototoxic agent, vestibular suppressant, and preexisting disease
3. No respirations: post-hyperventilation apnea and neuromuscular blockade

Box 15-1
DIAGNOSTIC SIGNS IN COMA

RESPIRATORY PATTERN

Cheyne-Stokes (alternating apnea and hypernoia)
1. Bilateral cerebral or diencephalic lesion
2. Metabolic abnormality
3. Incipient temporal lobe herniation

Hyperventilation
1. Lesion between low midbrain and midpons
2. Metabolic acidosis
   a. Diabetic ketoacidosis
   b. Uremia
   c. Intoxication—ethanol, salicylates
   d. Fluid or electrolyte abnormalities
3. Hypoxia

Ataxic Breathing (irregular rate and depth): lesion of medulla

POSITION

Decorticate (arms flexed and abducted, legs extended): corticospinal tract lesion within or near the cerebral hemisphere

Decerebrate (arms extended and internally rotated against the chest, legs extended)
1. Midbrain—midpons lesion
2. Metabolic abnormality (hypoxia, hypoglycemia)
3. Bilateral hemispheric lesion

PUPILS

Pinpoint (1-2 mm), Fixed
1. Pontine lesions
2. Metabolic abnormality
3. Intoxication—opiates, barbiturates (not fixed)

Small (2-3 mm), Reactive
1. Medullary lesion
2. Metabolic abnormality

Midsize (4-5 mm), Fixed: midbrain lesion

Dilated, fixed
1. Bilateral
   a. Irreversible brain damage (shock, massive hemorrhage, encephalitis)
   b. Anticholinergic (atropine-like) drugs
   c. Barbiturates (late, secondary to hypoxia)
   d. Hypothermia
   e. Seizures
2. Unilateral
   a. Rapidly expanding lesion on ipsilateral side (subdural hemorrhage, tumor)
   b. Tentorial herniation
   c. Cranial nerve (CN) III nucleus lesion
   d. Anticholinergic eyedrops
   e. Seizures

Dilated, reactive
1. Postictal
2. Anticholinergic drugs

Box 15-1
DIAGNOSTIC SIGNS IN COMA—cont'd

BLOOD PRESSURE

Hypertension

1. Increased intracranial pressure
2. Subarachnoid hemorrhage
3. Intoxication

Hypotension

1. Associated injury with hypovolemia, spinal shock, or hypoxemia
2. Adrenal failure

NUCHAL RIGIDITY

1. Meningitis/encephalitis
2. Subarachnoid hemorrhage
3. Posterior fossa tumor

EYE MOVEMENT

Oculocephalic Reflex (Doll's eye): with the eyes held open, the head is turned quickly from side to side. Clear cervical spine first.

1. Comatose patient with an intact brainstem responds with eye movement in the direction opposite to the direction in which the head is turned, as if still gazing ahead in initial position.
2. Comatose patient with midbrain or pons lesions has random eye movement.

Oculovestibular Reflex with Caloric Stimulation: with head elevated 30 degrees, ice water is injected through a small catheter lying in the ear canal (up to 200 ml is used in an adult)

1. Comatose patient with an intact brainstem responds by conjugate deviation of the eyes toward the irrigated ear.
2. Comatose patient with brainstem lesions demonstrates no response.

Conjugate Deviation

1. Cerebral lesion
   a. Toward destructive lesion
   b. Away from irritative lesion
2. Brainstem lesion: away from destructive lesion

CN IV Palsy—eye(s) cannot move laterally

1. Increased intracranial pressure
2. Meningeal infection
3. Pontine lesion
4. Injury (e.g., trauma, neoplasm)

CN III Palsy—eyes point down and out

1. Tentorial herniation
2. CN III nerve entrapment (skull fracture)
3. Intrinsic CN III lesion (e.g., diabetes)
4. Compression (aneurysm, tumor)

4. No motor activity: neuromuscular blockade and sedative drugs
5. Isoelectric electroencephalogram (EEG): sedative drugs, hypoxia, trauma, hypothermia, and encephalitis

MANAGEMENT

Management must initially focus on administering fluids and stabilizing the airway and providing oxygen to support cardiac and respiratory status. Active intervention may be required. Thereafter all patients should receive oxygen, glucose (0.5-1.0 g/kg/dose IV), and naloxone (Narcan), 0.1 mg/kg/dose IV initially, up to 2.0 mg/dose IV. A urinary catheter should be inserted, and urine should be evaluated for toxic substances as well as output. A blood specimen is sent for measurements of glucose, electrolytes, BUN, arterial blood gases (ABGs), toxicology screening, and other specific studies, as indicated. After stabilization, a rapid approach to delineating etiologic conditions is imperative to initiating specific therapy. Obviously, a parallel approach is indicated in patients with altered mental status.

BIBLIOGRAPHY

American Academy of Pediatrics: Guidelines for the determination of brain death in children, *Pediatrics* 80:298, 1987.

Fields AI, Coble DH, Pollack MM et al: Outcomes of children in a persistent vegetative state, *Crit Care Med* 21:1890, 1993.

Plum F, Posner JB: *The diagnosis of stupor and coma*, ed 3, Philadelphia, 1980, FA Davis.

Seshia S, Johnston B, Kasia G: Non-traumatic coma in childhood: clinical variables in prediction of outcome, *Dev Med Child Neurol* 25:493, 1983.

Yager JY, Johnston B, Seshia SS: Coma scales in pediatric practice, *Am J Dis Child* 144:1088, 1990.

16 Congestive Heart Failure

Also See Chapters 19 (Pulmonary Edema) and 71 (

ALERT Infants with congestive heart failure may have feeding di... weight gain, irritability, and labored respirations without rale. O... often have fatigue and anorexia accompanied by tachycardia, cardiomegaly, tachypnea with rales, rhonchi, and wheezing, cyanosis, ... evidence of venous congestion.

Congestive heart failure (CHF) is caused by the inability of the heart to pump adequate blood volume to meet circulatory and metabolic needs. Heart failure may result from volume overload (increased preload), pressure overload (increased afterload), myocardial dysfunction, and dysrhythmias.

Ninety percent of children in whom CHF develops experience it during the first year of life because of congenital heart disease. The younger the infant with initial signs and symptoms of heart failure, generally, the worse the prognosis if the condition remains untreated. Although older children may have CHF caused by congenital heart disease, they more commonly have CHF caused by acquired disease, such as cardiomyopathy, bacterial endocarditis, or rheumatic carditis. About 25% of children with congenital heart disease have associated extracardiac anomalies.

ETIOLOGY

See Box 16-1 and Table 16-1.

DIAGNOSTIC FINDINGS

Symptoms reflect cardiac decompensation and the underlying disorder. The acuteness of the process and the nature of any anatomic lesions determine the pattern of progression. Patients may have right-sided, left-sided, or combined heart failure, and the clinical findings reflect the chamber(s) involved.

A careful history is essential. It should focus on preexisting cardiac disease or surgery, hematologic conditions (sickle cell anemia or thalassemia), pulmonary problems, decreased exercise tolerance or associated orthopnea, altered behavior, and weight loss and eating habits.

The cardiac examination demonstrates evidence of dysfunction, reflecting a physiologic response to the inadequate cardiac output and underlying abnormality:

1. Tachycardia secondary to increased adrenergic tone and catecholamine release.
2. Cardiomegaly on examination and x-ray study. The point of maximal impulse is usually lateral to the midclavicular line in the fifth or sixth intercostal space. Hypertrophy occurs first with pressure overload, but dilation is initially more common with volume overload.
3. Gallop rhythm with prominent third sound, reflecting impaired ventricular compliance and increased resistance to filling.
4. Tachypnea, often with rales, rhonchi, wheezing, retractions, and symptoms of orthopnea and dyspnea. Pulmonary edema (see Chapter 19) is commonly present.

Box 16-1

CAUSES OF CONGESTIVE HEART FAILURE

VOLUME OVERLOAD (increased preload)

1. Vascular-congenital heart disease (Table 16-1)
   - Left-to-right shunt: ventricular septal defect (VSD)
   - Anomalous pulmonary venous return
   - Valvular regurgitation (aortic insufficiency)
   - Patent ductus arteriosus (PDA)
   - Arteriovenous fistula
2. Anemia
3. Hypervolemia (malnutrition, iatrogenic)

PRESSURE OVERLOAD (increased afterload)

1. Vascular-congenital heart disease (Table 16-1)
   - Ventricular outflow obstruction (aortic stenosis, coarctation of aorta)
   - Left ventricular inflow obstruction (cor triatriatum)
2. Hypertension (Chapter 18)

DYSRHYTHMIA (Chapter 6)

1. Vascular
   - Atrial or ventricular: ectopic pacemaker or reentry pathway
   - Conduction defect
2. Metabolic: electrolyte, Ca^{++}, Mg^{++} abnormalities
3. Intoxication: digitalis, cyclic antidepressants, etc.

MYOCARDIAL DYSFUNCTION

1. Vascular
   - Pulmonary embolism (p. 578)
   - Endocardial fibroelastosis (endocardial fibrosis)
   - Anomalous coronary artery
   - Pulmonary hypertension (obesity, pickwickian)
2. Infection/inflammation
   - Cardiomyopathy
     - Viral: coxsackie, influenza
     - Bacterial: diphtheria, meningococcemia, sepsis, toxic shock syndrome
     - Miscellaneous: toxoplasmosis, spirochetes, parasites
     - Bacterial endocarditis (p. 567)
     - Pericarditis: viral, bacterial, mycobacterial
     - Pulmonary disease: chronic infection, aspiration, cystic fibrosis
3. Endocrine/metabolic
   - Newborn: infant of diabetic mother, hypocalcemia, hypomagnesemia
   - Hypothyroidism or hyperthyroidism
   - Hypoglycemia: glycogen storage disease, etc.
   - Pheochromocytoma
   - α_1-Antitrypsin deficiency
4. Trauma/environment (Chapter 62)
   - Cardiac tamponade, contusion or rupture secondary to blunt or penetrating trauma (p. 480)
   - Hyperthermia (Chapter 50)
5. Autoimmune/allergic
   - Asthma
   - Acute rheumatic fever (ARF) (p. 575)
   - Systemic lupus erythematosus (SLE)
6. Deficiency/degeneration
   - Anemia
   - Central nervous system disease: progressive or degenerative
   - Malnutrition: kwashiorkor, beri beri (thiamine), etc.
7. Intoxication: alcohol abuse, heavy metals, cardiac toxins (digitalis, β blockers)
8. Neoplasm: metastatic or infiltration, atrial myxoma
9. Postsurgical condition

5. Venous congestion associated with hepatomegaly, jugular venous distension, and peripheral edema, especially with right-sided failure.
6. Peripheral pulses often are weak with impaired perfusion. Extremities are cool. Peripheral edema may develop on the dorsum of the hands and feet, over the sacrum, and in the periorbital region if right-sided failure is present.
7. Cyanosis resulting from pulmonary or cardiac causes. Primary cardiac cyanosis caused by significant shunting (see Table 16-1) does not respond to 100% oxygen

TABLE 16-1 Congenital Heart Disease: Differentiation by Chest X-Ray Film and ECG

CYANOTIC				
	DECREASED PULMONARY BLOOD FLOW (RIGHT-TO-LEFT SHUNT)		INCREASED PULMONARY BLOOD FLOW (RIGHT-TO-LEFT OR LEFT-TO-RIGHT SHUNT)	
RVH	**LVH**	**LVH, RVH, CVH**	**RVH**	**LVH, RVH, CVH**
Pulmonary stenosis with variable VSD: CHF Tetralogy of Fallot: CHF Pulmonary atresia with variable VSD Ebstein: CHF	Tricuspid atresia Pulmonary atresia with hypoplastic right ventricle: CHF	Transposition of great vessels with pulmonary stenosis: CHF Truncus arteriosus with hypoplastic pulmonary artery: CHF	Total anomalous pulmonary venous return: CHF Hypoplastic left heart: CHF	Transposition and VSD: CHF Single ventricle Truncus arteriosus: CHF Tricuspid atresia with transposition: CHF

ACYANOTIC			
NORMAL PULMONARY BLOOD FLOW (NO SHUNTS)		INCREASED PULMONARY BLOOD FLOW (LEFT-TO-RIGHT SHUNT)	
RVH	**LVH**	**RVH**	**LVH or CVH**
Pulmonary stenosis (severe): CHF Mitral stenosis: CHF	Coarctation: CHF Mitral regurgitation Aortic stenosis Anomalous left coronary artery: CHF	Atrial septal defect: CHF Left-to-right shunt (increased pulmonary pressure) (PDA, VSD, ASD): CHF	Patent ductus arteriosus: CHF Ventricular septal defect: CHF Arteriovenous fistula: CHF

ASD, Atrial septal defect; *CHF*, lesion is often associated with congestive heart failure; *CVH*, combined ventricular hypertrophy; *LVH*, left ventricular hypertrophy; *PDA*, patent ductus arteriosus; *RVH*, right ventricular hypertrophy; *VSD*, ventricular septal defects.

administration. In contrast, pulmonary disease (see Chapter 17) shows no significant improvement of the cyanosis with administration of oxygen.

8. Growth failure, undernutrition, and feeding difficulties are common in infants. Older children may experience fatigue and anorexia.
9. Altered mental status may result from decreased cerebral perfusion. Infants are typically irritable.
10. Pulsus paradoxus may accompany pericardial tamponade, pneumothorax, or severe asthma. The clinician may determine its presence by having the patient breathe quietly and by lowering the pressure on the blood pressure cuff toward the systolic level, noting the value at which the first sound is heard. The pressure is further dropped until sounds can be heard throughout the respiratory cycle. A difference of 15 mm Hg or more indicates the presence of a paradoxic pulse.
11. Pulsus alternans is evidence of left-sided failure. When it is present, the systolic pressure rhythmically alternates between high and low values.

Complications

1. Pulmonary edema (see Chapter 19)
2. Dysrhythmias (see Chapter 6)
3. Shock (see Chapter 5)
4. Superimposed pulmonary infection (p. 811)
5. Renal failure secondary to decreased renal perfusion (p. 828)
6. Cardiac arrest and death (see Chapter 4)

Ancillary Data

Specific studies clarify cardiac and pulmonary status. Additional studies may be indicated to further evaluate the underlying cause of CHF.

1. Chest x-ray films: posteroanterior (PA) and lateral views. An anteroposterior (AP) view may be sufficient for initial evaluation of the critically ill patient.
   a. Cardiac silhouette demonstrates cardiomegaly. Other findings reflect the nature of any anatomic or functional lesion and may be diagnostic of a specific congenital defect.
   b. Pulmonary edema causes fluffy infiltrates with perihilar haziness, Kerley B lines, and, periodically, pleural effusion. Pneumonia, if present, must be distinguished from pulmonary edema.
   c. Noncardiac causes may be partially excluded: aortic aneurysm (widened mediastinum on PA film), signs of trauma (e.g., broken ribs), and chronic pulmonary disease.
2. Electrocardiogram (ECG), which is useful in the evaluation of a number of entities:
   a. Congenital heart disease (ventricular enlargement; axis deviation; abnormalities of P, QRS, or T waves) (see Table 16-1)
   b. Cardiac ischemia, infarction, or contusion
   c. Cardiomyopathy or pericardial disease
   d. Metabolic abnormalities (e.g., hypokalemia, hypocalcemia) (see Chapter 8)
   e. Dysrhythmias (see Chapter 6)
3. Arterial blood gas (ABG) measurements to determine acid-base abnormalities on the basis of respiratory, circulatory (perfusion), or metabolic inadequacies. The response to oxygen may assist in distinguishing primary cardiac disease from pulmonary disease. Ongoing monitoring is essential.
4. Chemical evaluation: measurements of electrolyte, glucose, blood urea nitrogen (BUN), creatinine, calcium, and magnesium levels. This is particularly important for patients with dysrhythmias and for those receiving diuretic therapy as well as to evaluate renal status and exclude prerenal azotemia.
5. Hematologic evaluation: complete blood count (CBC) to evaluate for anemia or infection. Erythrocyte sedimentation rate (ESR) is often decreased in active CHF.
6. Measuring pulmonary artery end-diastolic pressure or mean pulmonary capillary wedge pressure (PCWP) with a Swan-Ganz catheter is often essential in monitoring the patient. These parameters must be measured carefully in patients with moderate or severe disease to assess cardiac function and fluid balance. The common inadequacy of central venous pressure (CVP) becomes particularly important to attempts to balance inotropic agents with volume administration. Consultation should be sought.
7. Cardiac enzymes: creatine phosphokinase (CPK-MB), serum glutamic-oxaloacetic transaminase (SGOT), and lactate dehydrogenase (LDH) if a perfusion abnormality, ischemia, or inflammatory response is suspected.
8. Thoracentesis (see Appendix A-8).
9. Pericardiocentesis (see Appendix A-5).
10. Ultrasonography: echocardiography is a safe, noninvasive technique that may be performed at the bedside with portable equipment. It is particularly useful in assessing cardiac function, pericardial thickening or effusion, cardiac valve vegetations, and atrial myxoma. Echocardiography is essential in monitoring the response of the failing heart to inotropic drugs. In the fetus, heart disease may be associated

with scalp edema, ascites, and pericardial effusion.

11. Nuclear scanning: useful in the assessment of ventricular contractility, myocardial perfusion, and cellular viability. The ejection fraction as a measure of function represents the percentage of end-diastolic volume that is ejected per stroke using technetiumTc 99m scanning. Experience with small infants is still limited.

DIFFERENTIAL DIAGNOSIS

1. Vascular.
   a. Noncardiogenic pulmonary edema. Evaluation of heart determines level of dysfunction, if any. History may be helpful in focusing on other causes (see Chapter 19).
   b. Intrapulmonary hemorrhage.
   c. Pulmonary embolism (p. 578).
2. Infection: pneumonia (p. 811).
3. Allergy: asthma (p. 781).

MANAGEMENT

Initial cardiac and respiratory stabilization must be achieved during evaluation and treatment of the underlying condition. General management focuses on improving cardiac contractility and reducing the workload. It is important to distinguish between pump and muscle function, because abnormal loads imposed on the heart may result in failure of the heart as a pump in the absence of depression of intrinsic myocardial contractility. Myocardial contractility may be depressed, but favorable loading conditions may reduce the impact of this impairment on the contractile quality of the myocardial fibers as reflected in the Frank-Starling curve. Often this interaction requires careful titration in dosages of inotropic and unloading agents in relation to volume status.

Therapeutic goals must focus on improving cardiac performance, augmenting peripheral perfusion, and decreasing systemic and pulmonary venous congestion.

The airway, breathing, and circulation need immediate attention. Oxygen should be administered. When the condition is stabilized, the patient should be kept in a semirecumbent position with ongoing cardiac monitoring and oxygen administration. Temperature should be normalized.

Inotropic Agents: Digoxin (Table 16-2)

Digoxin is the drug of choice for improving the inotropic action of the heart. The inotropic response is determined by pharmacokinetic variables, including bioavailability, absorption, volume of distribution, metabolism, and plasma protein binding. End-organ response is affected by the sensitivity of the myocardium and by myocardial uptake. Infants often require a larger dose than adults because of the infant's higher body clearance and larger volume of distribution; children need doses similar to or lower than adult doses. Digoxin is contraindicated in idiopathic hypertropic subaortic stenosis (IHSS) and tetralogy of Fallot and should be used with caution in patients with myocarditis or electrolyte abnormalities.

Characteristics

1. Onset of action: 5 to 30 minutes when administered IV (IM absorption is erratic)
2. IV dose: usually about 75% of oral dose
3. Renal excretion: 48 to 72 hours
4. Oral absorption: 66% to 75%

TABLE 16-2 Digoxin: Total Digitalizing Dose (TDD)

Age	IV	PO
Premature	0.01-0.02 mg/kg	0.02-0.03 mg/kg
Newborn-2 wk	0.03-0.04 mg/kg	0.03-0.05 mg/kg
2 wk-2 yr	0.03-0.05 mg/kg	0.04-0.06 mg/kg
>2 yr	0.04 mg/kg	0.05 mg/kg
Adult	0.5-1.0 mg	1.0-1.5 mg

1000 μg = 1 mg. IV dose is generally 75% of PO dose.
NOTE: Oral maintenance daily dose is usually one fourth to one third of total digitalizing dose (TDD).

5. Preparations:
   a. Vials: 0.1 mg (100 μg)/ml and 0.25 mg (250 μg)/ml
   b. Elixir: 0.05 mg/ml
   c. Tablets: 0.125, 0.25, and 0.50 mg

Dosage

1. Give half of total digitalizing dose (TDD) initially, then one fourth of TDD in 6 to 8 hours, then one fourth of TDD 6 to 12 hours later, depending on severity of CHF.
2. The condition of relatively stable patients may be digitalized slowly by beginning the maintenance dose of digoxin. Therapeutic levels are reached in 5 to 7 days.
3. Maintenance daily dose is one fourth to one third of TDD divided into morning and evening doses (mg/kg/24 hr in one or two daily doses): premature babies, 0.005 mg/kg/24 hr; newborns, 0.005-0.010 mg/kg/24 hr; infants (younger than 2 years), 0.010-0.012 mg/kg/24 hr; children older than 2 years, 0.008-0.010 mg/kg/24 hr; and adults, 0.125-0.375 mg/24 hr.
4. Therapeutic level: 1 to 2.0 ng/ml
   a. Infants and children may not show toxicity until levels of 4 ng/ml are reached; some require this level for therapeutic effect.
   b. Measure serum drug levels 4 hours after IV dose and 8 hours after PO dose.
   c. Variability exists among laboratories and the individual toxic level in a specific patient.

Other Considerations

1. The dose of digoxin should be reduced in the patient with myocarditis, pulmonary hypertension, decreased renal function, electrolyte abnormalities, hypoxia, or acidosis. Digoxin is contraindicated in IHSS and tetralogy of Fallot.
2. Pulse and rhythm strips should be obtained before each parenteral dose until therapeutic levels are achieved. Normal ECG findings associated with therapeutic digoxin include T wave depression, ST segment depression (scooped), and prolonged PR interval.

Toxicity

The range between the optimal therapeutic dose and toxicity is relatively narrow. Factors that predispose to toxicity caused by *high serum digoxin levels* include decreased renal excretion (premature infant, renal disease), hypothyroidism, high dosage, and drug interaction (quinidine, verapamil). *Increased sensitivity of the myocardium* results from an altered myocardium (ischemia, myocarditis), hypokalemia, hypercalcemia, hypoxemia, alkalosis, sympathomimetic drugs, and a postoperative state.

The *signs of toxicity* are diverse:

1. Dysrhythmias (see Chapter 6):
   a. Bradycardia: infant, <80-90 beats/min; child, <60-70 beats/min; and older child and adult, <50-60 beats/min
   b. Atrioventricular (AV) dissociation with second- and third-degree block
   c. Premature ventricular complex (PVC)
   d. Ventricular bigeminy
   e. Paroxysmal atrial tachycardia (PAT) with block
2. Vomiting, nausea, and decreased intake
3. Blurring of vision (rare in children)

Treatment of toxicity is as follows:

1. Discontinue the drug, which has a half-life of 24 to 36 hours.
2. Give an infusion of 5% dextrose in water (D5W) with KCl, 40 to 80 mEq/L, at a rate of 0.3 mEq KCl/kg/hr IV with close monitoring. Do not use if second- or third-degree block is present.
3. Give atropine, 0.01 to 0.02 mg/kg/dose (minimum: 0.1 mg/dose; maximum: 0.6 mg/dose) IV, for severe bradycardia.
4. For dysrhythmias (see Chapter 6):
   a. Give phenytoin, 1 mg/kg/dose IV over 1 to 2 minutes, which may be

repeated every 5 minutes up to a total dose of 5 mg/kg. Hypocontractility may develop.

b. Lidocaine and propranolol are sometimes helpful.

NOTE: These drugs depress the myocardium and aggravate failure and must be used carefully.

c. Digoxin-specific Fab antibody fragments are useful in life-threatening situations. Cardiology consultation is advised.

Inotropic Agents: Shock (see Chapter 5)

CHF is often accompanied by cardiogenic shock and low-output states requiring aggressive management. Fluid status must be evaluated before therapy is initiated.

1. A *fluid* push may improve cardiac output by increasing filling pressure, particularly if the PCWP is 15 to 20 mm Hg or less; 0.9% NS (normal saline) solution at 5 ml/kg over 30 minutes may be administered with careful monitoring of response.
2. *Pressor* agents are usually necessary when the response to fluid challenge is inadequate once normovolemia has been achieved. The agents of choice (see Table 5-2) are the following:
   a. Dopamine administered by continuous IV infusion at a rate of 5 to 20 μg/kg/min up to 40 μg/kg/min (the higher infusion), the latter only if an α-blocking agent is used simultaneously; *or*
   b. Dobutamine administered by continuous IV infusion at a rate of 2 to 20 μg/kg/min (usually 10 to 15 μg/kg/min). Patients may respond to a low dosage, 0.5 μg/kg/min, but others require 40 μg/kg/min. Dobutamine is more effective in children older than 12 months of age; *or*
   c. Low dosage of dopamine (2 to 5 μg/kg/min) to maintain renal flow combined with inotropic dosage of dobutamine.

Pulmonary Edema (see Chapter 19)

1. Airway and ventilation require immediate attention:
   a. Administer oxygen at 3 to 6 L/min by mask or nasal cannula.
   b. Determine the need for intubation and mechanical ventilation. Intubation is indicated for the patient receiving supplemental oxygen with FiO_2 of 50% if PaO_2 is less than 50 mm Hg (sea level) and known cyanotic heart disease is not present. Other indications for intubation with ventilation are a $PaCO_2$ greater than 50 mm Hg (without preexisting disease), decreasing vital capacity, severe acidosis, and progressive disease or fatigue.
   c. If intubation is indicated, initiate positive end-expiratory pressure (PEEP) at 4 to 6 cm H_2O if severe pulmonary edema is present. Titrate upward as necessary, monitoring ABGs to maximize PaO_2 without decreasing cardiac output.
2. Fluid resuscitation: Fluids (D5W) should be used to maintain urine output, administered at 0.5 ml/kg/hr after stabilization of intravascular volume. Although fluids can usually be kept at about 60% of normal maintenance, this issue must be individualized for each patient. Observe for renal failure (p. 828) and fluid overload.
3. Diuretics (Table 16-3). In the acute situation, use furosemide (Lasix), 1 mg/kg/dose up to 6 mg/kg/dose q8-12hr IV. May be repeated q2hr if indicated. Do not use if anuria is present.
   a. Morphine sulfate lowers the PCWP and relieves anxiety.
   b. In severe pulmonary edema with CHF, 0.1 to 0.2 mg/kg IV should be administered slowly.

TABLE 16-3 Diuretics

				DOSAGE			
Drug	**Availability**	**Route**	**Frequency**	**Initial**	**Maximum**	**Onset of Action**	**Comments/ Site of Action**
Chlorothiazide (Diuril)	Solution: 50 mg/ml Tablet: 250, 500 mg	PO	q8-12hr	10 mg/kg/ 24 hr	20 mg/kg/24 hr (2 g/24 hr)	1-2 hr	$\downarrow K^+$, $\downarrow Na^+$, alkalosis, hyperglycemia; distal tubule
Hydrochlorothiazide (HydroDiuril)	Tablet: 25, 50, 100 mg	PO	q8-12hr	1 mg/kg/ 24 hr	2 mg/kg/24 hr (200 mg/24 hr)	1-2 hr	$\downarrow K^+$, $\downarrow Na^+$, alkalosis, hyperglycemia; distal tubule
Furosemide (Lasix)	Ampule: 10 mg/ml	IV, IM	q6-12hr	1 mg/kg/ dose	6 mg/kg/dose	5-15 min	$\downarrow K^+$, $\downarrow Na^+$, alkalosis, deafness; may give more often; ascending loop of Henle
	Solution: 10 mg/ml Tablet: 20, 40 mg	PO	q6-12hr	1-3 mg/kg/ dose	6 mg/kg/dose	30-60 min	
Spironolactone (Aldactone)	Tablet: 25 mg	PO	q8-12hr	1 mg/kg/ 24 hr	3 mg/kg/24 hr (200 mg/24 hr)	3-5 days	$\uparrow K^+$, $\downarrow Na^+$; useful as adjunct, not alone; aldosterone antagonist; collecting tubule
Mannitol	Vial: (250 mg/ml) 25%	IV (slow)		0.5 g/kg/ dose	2 g/kg/ dose	10-30 min	Reduced intracranial pressure
Acetazolamide (Diamox)	Vial: 500 mg Tablet: 125, 250 mg	IV PO	q6-24hr	5 mg/kg/ 24 hr	8 mg/kg/24 hr	1-6 hr	Carbonic anhydrase inhibitor; hyperchloremic acidosis
Metolazone (Zaroxolyn)	Tablet: 2.5, 5, 10 mg	PO	q24hr	0.2 mg/kg/ 24 hr	0.4 mg/kg/24 hr (adult: 10 mg/ 24 hr)	1-2 hr	Useful when marked $\downarrow$ glomerular filtration rate; no experience in children; renal tubule
Bumetanide (Bumex)	Tablet: 0.5, 1, 2 mg	PO	q12-24hr	0.015-0.1 mg/kg/ dose	0.5-2 mg/dose (max: 10 mg/ 24 hr)		Limited experience in children; side effects: cramps, dizziness, $\downarrow K^+$, $\downarrow Ca^{++}$, $\downarrow Na^+$, encephalopathy; 40 mg furosemide comparable to 1 mg bumetanide; cross-allergenicity to sulfonamides
	Vial: 0.25 mg/kg	IV	q8-12hr	0.1 mg/kg dose	0.5-1 mg/dose over 1-2 min (max: 10 mg/ 24 hr)		

c. Respirations may be depressed. Do not give in the presence of unstable vital signs, intracranial hemorrhage, chronic pulmonary disease, asthma, or narcotic withdrawal.

d. Bronchodilators are indicated if there is wheezing or evidence of bronchoconstriction (p. 781).

VOLUME OVERLOAD

Reducing the volume and cardiac preload may be beneficial if the PCWP and CVP can be maintained. Fluids and diuretics, as outlined in the previous section, must be cautiously monitored to provide the best balance between volume status and cardiac function. In patients with volume overload and renal failure, peritoneal dialysis has been used successfully.

PRESSURE OVERLOAD (see Table 18-2)

Afterload reduction may be useful if the response to digoxin, diuretics, pressors, and fluid management is inadequate. Agents that diminish afterload by decreasing peripheral resistance may improve cardiac output. Pharmacologic reduction of afterload should be used only with indwelling arterial monitoring and a Swan-Ganz catheter in place; it usually is deferred until the patient is admitted to the intensive care unit (ICU).

1. Sodium nitroprusside (Nipride) dilates systemic veins.
   - **a.** Dosage: 0.5 to 10 μg/kg/min IV by infusion. Begin with an infusion rate of 0.1 μg/kg/min and increase until the desired response is achieved. The average therapeutic dosage is about 3 μg/kg/min.
   - **b.** The clinical response is noted in 1 to 2 minutes and lasts 5 to 10 minutes after the infusion is stopped. Do not use in the presence of renal failure.
2. Nitroglycerin dilates the systemic veins and is occasionally useful for patients taking digoxin and diuretics who have severe CHF and pulmonary edema, particularly if these conditions are secondary to aortic or mitral regurgitation.
   - **a.** Dosage for sublingual administration has not been established for children (nor is there adequate experience); administration must be adjusted according to clinical response. The adult dosage is 0.15 to 0.6 mg q5min sublingually up to a maximum of three doses in a 15-minute period. May be routinely repeated in 1 to 2 hours. Onset of action is 1 to 2 minutes, lasting 30 minutes.
   - **b.** IV nitroglycerin (Nitrostat) has been used effectively in adults. In adults the infusion is usually begun at 5 μg/min with increments of 5 μg/min q3-5min until a therapeutic response is noted. Suggested pediatric dosage is not defined.
3. Other pharmacologic options are captopril (Capoten), hydralazine (Apresoline), and prazosin (Minipress) (see Table 18-2).

DYSRHYTHMIAS (see Chapter 6)

Dysrhythmias require urgent attention. Bradyrhythmias are primarily secondary to slowing of the intrinsic pacemaker or a conduction defect; tachyrhythmias result from ectopic pacemakers or reentrant pathways.

Other Considerations

1. *Sedation* may be essential in the anxious patient. If morphine sulfate is not used because of concern for depression of respiration, chloral hydrate, 20 mg/kg/dose PO up to 50 mg/kg/24 hr, or phenobarbital, 2 to 3 mg/kg/dose PO, IV, or IM up to q8hr, may be used.
2. *Anemia* should be treated if significant (hematocrit [Hct] <20%) to improve oxygenation. Give 5 to 10 ml/kg of packed red blood cells (RBCs) over 4 to 8 hours with careful monitoring. An exchange transfusion may have to be considered.

3. CHF secondary to large patent ductus arteriosus (PDA) in *premature* infants may respond to indomethacin, 0.1 to 0.2 mg/kg administered q12hr up to a maximum dose of 0.6 mg/kg IV, after consultation with a cardiologist to exclude a ductal-dependent lesion.

   Closure of the PDA in coarctation of the aorta or other ductal-dependent lesion may produce severe CHF, requiring immediate intervention. Dilation of the PDA to maintain patency may be achieved by prostaglandin E_1, 0.05 to 0.1 µg/kg/min IV infusion, administered in consultation with a cardiologist.
4. *Surgery* may occasionally be required on an emergent basis if medical management is unsuccessful and the lesion is amenable to surgical correction, such as PDA, total anomalous pulmonary venous return, transposition of the great vessels, pulmonic stenosis, aortic stenosis, ventricular septal defect, atrioventricular canal, and coarctation of the aorta.
5. For unresponsive cases, cardiology and cardiac surgery (if appropriate) consultations should be sought immediately. Other entities that must be considered are:
   a. Reactivation of rheumatic heart disease or concurrent infection (endocarditis, pericarditis, pneumonia, urinary tract infection)
   b. Electrolyte abnormality: hypochloremic alkalosis, hypokalemia, hyponatremia
   c. Digitalis toxicity (pp. 154 and 380)
   d. Dysrhythmias (see Chapter 6)
   e. Pulmonary embolism (p. 578)

DISPOSITION

Patients with CHF should be admitted to the hospital for immediate therapy. Those with moderate or severe disease must be monitored in an ICU with appropriate expertise and equipment. Rarely, patients with mild, slowly progressive or chronic CHF and pulmonary edema of known cause may be relatively asymptomatic and may show response to an oral digitalizing regimen over 5 to 7 days as outpatients, if compliance can be ensured and appropriate follow-up observation can be arranged.

A cardiologist should be involved in the management of all patients to ensure follow-up attention. Most patients need digoxin and diuretic therapy on a long-term basis.

BIBLIOGRAPHY

O'Laughlin MP: Congestive heart failure in children, *Pediatr Clin North Am* 46:263, 1999.

Park MK: Use of digoxin in infants and children with specific emphasis on dosage, *J Pediatr* 108:871, 1986.

Steinberg C, Notterman DA: Pharmacokinetics of cardiovascular drugs in children: inotropes and vasopressors, *Clin Pharmacol* 27:345, 1994.

Talner NS: Heart failure. In Emmanouilides AC, Riemenschneider TA, Allen HD et al, editors: *Heart disease in infants, children, and adolescents,* ed 5, Baltimore, 1995, Lippincott Williams & Wilkins.

17 Cyanosis

ALERT Impairment of ventilation or perfusion caused by cardiac or pulmonary abnormality is very common. Pending evaluation, oxygen should be administered and airway and ventilation evaluated and stabilized.

Cyanosis results from decreased oxygenation of the blood. For it to be clinically apparent, there must be at least 5 g of reduced hemoglobin (Hb) per deciliter of blood. Because of the increased affinity of fetal hemoglobin for oxygen, the infant may have hypoxia without cyanosis. Cyanosis is most evident where the epidermis is relatively thin, pigmentation is minimal, and capillaries are abundant (tips of finger and toes, under the nail beds, and in buccal mucosa).

Central Cyanosis

Central cyanosis involves cyanosis of the tongue, mucosal membranes, and peripheral skin. It may be caused by the following:

1. Decreased pulmonary and alveolar ventilation with impaired oxygen intake.
2. Decreased pulmonary perfusion.
3. An abnormal Hb content. Methemoglobin produces cyanosis when it represents more than 15% of the total Hb. It should be considered when there is a history of exposure or of central cyanosis that does not respond to oxygen and congenital heart disease is not suspected.

The history should focus on potential contributing conditions. Congenital heart, lung, or gastrointestinal (GI) disease should be excluded in the patient and family. The pattern of onset of cyanosis and respiratory distress may be distinct, as may the factors that exacerbate the finding. Recent fever, infection, shortness of breath, trauma, foreign body ingestion, and neurologic changes should be sought.

The physical examination must assess cardiovascular stability as well as seek clues to the cause.

Evaluation for central cyanosis should consist of oximetry, arterial blood gas (ABG) analysis, chest x-ray film, complete blood count (CBC), and electrocardiogram (ECG) as well as other studies related to the differential possibilities (see Chapter 13). In addition, the response to 100% oxygen should be measured by comparing ABG values in blood collected while the patient was breathing room air and during the administration of high-flow oxygen (see Table 17-1). This maneuver assists in

TABLE 17-1 Response to Oxygen: Differentiating Pulmonary and Heart Disease

	PULMONARY DISEASE (VENTILATION)		**HEART DISEASE (PERFUSION)**	
	Room Air	**100% O_2**	**Room Air**	**100% O_2**
Color	Blue	Pinker	Blue	Blue
Pao_2 (mm Hg)	35	120 (range: 60-250)	35 or less	Little change
Saturation	60%	99%	60%	62%

TABLE 17-2 Central Cyanosis: Diagnostic Considerations

Condition	Mechanism	Respiratory Pattern	Response to 100% O_2	Ancillary Data	Comments
VASCULAR: CARDIAC (Chapter 16)					
Congenital heart disease*					
↓ *PBF* Pulmonary vascular obstruction Pulmonary atresia Pulmonary stenosis Tetralogy of Fallot Tricuspid atresia Transposition with pulmonary stenosis	↓ perfusion	RR 20-50 breaths/min	Little	ABG: ↓ Pao_2, ↓ ↑ pH CXR: ↓ PBF, ↑ heart ECG: Variable Hypoglycemia	R → L shunt; prostaglandin E may be helpful
↑ *PBF* Transposition of great vessels Total anomalous venous return Truncus arteriosus Hypoplastic L heart		RR 30-60 breaths/min	Little	ABG: ↓ Pao_2, ↑↓ pH CXR: ↑ PBF, ↑ heart ECG: Variable Hypoglycemia	R → L shunt
Congestive heart failure	↓ alveolar ventilation, perfusion	RR 40-120 breaths/min	Moderate	ABG: ↓ Pao_2, ↓ pH ↓↑ $Paco_2$ CXR: ↑ PBF, variable pulmonary edema, ↑ heart ECG: Variable	
Pulmonary edema (Chapter 19)	↓ alveolar ventilation	RR 40-120 breaths/min	Moderate	ABG: ↓ Pao_2, ↓ ↑ pH, ↑ $Paco_2$ CXR: Interstitial infiltrate ECG: Variable	Variable associated CHF
Shock (Chapter 5)	↓ perfusion	RR 20-80 breaths/min	Good	ABG: ↓ Pao_2, ↓ pH, ↑ ↓ $Paco_2$ CXR: Variable	Associated conditions
VASCULAR: PULMONARY					
Pulmonary hemorrhage	↓ alveolar perfusion	RR 30-60 breaths/min	Moderate	ABG: ↓ Pao_2, ↑↓ pH, ↑↓ $Paco_2$ CXR: Abnormal	May have shunt

				ECG: WNL or RVH	
Pulmonary embolism (p. 578) Persistent fetal circulation (newborn) (Chapter 11)				ABG: ↓ Pao_2, ↑↓ pH, ↑ $Paco_2$	R → L shunt
Pulmonary AV fistula Pulmonary hypertension	↓ perfusion	RR 30-60 breaths/min	None	CXR: Variable ECG: Variable	
Vascular ring	↓ ventilation	Stridor, retraction	Good	ABG: ↓ Pao_2, ↑ $Paco_2$ CXR: Hyperexpansion ECG: WNL or RVH	Barium swallow or bronchoscopy may be useful Catheterization
VASCULAR: CNS HEMORRHAGE (Chapters 18 and 57)					
Subdural Intracranial	↓ ventilation	RR <20 breaths/min, apnea, seizures	Moderate	ABG: ↓ Pao_2, ↑ $Paco_2$ CXR, ECG: WNL	Associated CNS findings
INTOXICATION (Chapter 54)					
Nitrates } Well water, Nitrites } vegetables	Methemoglobinemia	Little distress unless >50%	None	ABG, CXR, ECG: WNL Methemoglobin high in blood; chocolate color when exposed to air	Rx: Methylene blue 1-2 mg (0.1-0.2 ml)/kg/dose IV over 5-15 min
Aniline dyes Sulfonamides					
Carbon monoxide (p. 376)	Displacement of O_2 by CO	RR 30-60 breaths/min	Good	Carboxyhemoglobin level	May have CNS symptoms, pulmonary edema
INFECTION/INFLAMMATION					
Lower airway disease (Chapter 20)	↓ alveolar ventilation, perfusion	RR 30-120 breaths/min, flaring, grunting, wheezing	Moderate	ABG: ↓ Pao_2, ↓ pH, ↑↓ $Paco_2$ CXR: Abnormal ECG: WNL or RVH	Some shunting; also see asthma below Rx: 100% O_2

ABG, Arterial blood gas; *AV*, arteriovenous; *CHF*, congestive heart failure; *CNS*, central nervous system; *CXR*, chest x-ray, *ECG*, electrocardiogram; *L*, left; *PBF*, pulmonary blood flow; *R*, right; *RR*, respiratory rate; RVH, right ventricular hypertrophy; *RX*, therapy; *WNL*, within normal limits.
* Complex heart lesions may have variable blood flow.

Continued

TABLE 17-2 Central Cyanosis: Diagnostic Considerations—cont'd

Condition	Mechanism	Respiratory Pattern	Response to 100% O_2	Ancillary Data	Comments
INFECTION/INFLAMMATION—cont'd					
Pneumonia (p. 811)					
Bronchiolitis					
Emphysema					
Hyaline membrane disease (Chapter 11)					
Bronchopulmonary dysplasia (Chapter 11)					
Atelectasis					
Aspiration					
Cystic fibrosis					
Upper airway disease (Chapter 20)	↓ ventilation	Stridor, retraction	Good	ABG: ↓ Pa_{O_2}, ↑↓ pH, ↑↓ Pa_{CO_2}	
Croup (p. 800)					
Epiglottitis					
Retropharyngeal abscess (p. 617)					
Meningitis (p. 741)	↓ perfusion ↓ ventilation	RR 10-80 breaths/min	Good	ABG: ↓ Pa_{O_2}, ↓ pH, ↑↓ Pa_{CO_2}	
DEGENERATIVE					
CNS: Seizures	↓ ventilation	RR 10-30 breaths/min, apnea, seizures	Good	ABG: ↓ Pa_{O_2}, ↓ pH, ↑ Pa_{CO_2}	Associated CNS findings
Progressive disease					
ALLERGIC					
Asthma (p. 781)	↓ ventilation	RR 40-80 breaths/min, flaring, wheezing, coughing	Good	ABG: ↓ Pa_{O_2}, ↑↓ pH, ↑↓ Pa_{CO_2} CXR: Variable	Also see infection/inflammation, lower airway disease, above
Anaphylaxis (Chapter 12)	↓ alveolar ventilation				
TRAUMA (Chapter 62)					
Upper airway foreign body (p. 808)	↓ ventilation	Stridor, retraction	Good	ABG: ↓ Pa_{O_2}, ↑↓ pH, ↑↓ Pa_{CO_2} CXR: Lateral neck positive result	

Lower airway Pneumothorax Drowning (Chapter 47) Contusion	↓ ventilation ↓ alveolar ventilation	RR 30-120 breaths/min, flaring	Good	ABG: ↓ Pao_2, ↑ $Paco_2$ CXR: Abnormal	
Cardiac	↓ perfusion	RR 20-80 breaths/min	Good	ABG: ↓ Pao_2, ↓ pH CXR: Variable ECG: Variable	
INTRAPSYCHIC					
Breath holding (p. 740)	↓ ventilation	RR 0-10 breaths/min	Moderate	ABG: ↓ Pao_2, ↑ $Paco_2$	Self-limited
CONGENITAL (Chapters 11 and 20)					
Hereditary hemoglobinemia	Methemoglobinemia	Little distress unless >50%	None	ABG, CXR, ECG: WNL Methemoglobin high in blood: chocolate color when exposed to air	Rx: Methylene blue 1-2 mg (0.1-0.2 ml)/kg/dose IV over 5-15 min
Diaphragmatic hernia Atresia nasal choanal Macroglossia Hypoplastic mandible Tracheolaryngomalacia	↓ ventilation	RR 30-80 breaths/min	Good	ABG: ↓ Pao_2, ↑↓ pH, ↑ $Paco_2$ CXR: Abnormal ECG: WNL or RVH	Requires surgery

differentiating primarily cardiac disease resulting from major shunting and decreased perfusion from pulmonary disease, which has primarily ventilation deficits (Table 17-2).

The hypoxemic spells seen in tetralogy of Fallot may cause sudden onset or deepening of cyanosis, dyspnea, alterations in consciousness, and decreased intensity of the systolic murmur. These episodes usually begin in the neonatal period. Treatment consists of providing oxygen, attending to the airway, breathing, and circulation (ABCs), and placing the child in the knee-chest position. Acidosis should be corrected. Sedation with morphine sulfate, 0.1 mg/kg/dose IV, is helpful, as well as causing beneficial hemodynamic changes. Pharmacologic agents that should be considered include the following:

1. Propranolol: 0.05 to 0.1 mg/kg/dose IV (maximum: 0.1 mg/kg/dose not to exceed 1 mg/dose).
2. Esmolol (ultrashort-acting β-blocker): initial bolus 0.5 to 1.0 mg/kg IV followed by infusion of 100 to 300 μg/kg/min.
3. Phenylephrine: initial bolus 10 to 20 μg/kg/min. Bolus may be repeated and may be doubled to a maximum total bolus of 50 μg/kg/min. Follow by continuous infusion of 0.1 to 0.5 μg/kg/min. Avoid digitalis preparations.

Peripheral Cyanosis

Peripheral cyanosis is accompanied by a bluish discoloration of the skin, which is caused by increased arterial-venous oxygen differences, with normal arterial saturation. It has a vascular origin:

1. Vasomotor instability:
   a. Common in newborns, particularly with temperature changes, sepsis, or metabolic abnormalities
   b. May be related to sepsis in older children
2. Capillary stasis or venous pooling.
3. Raynaud's phenomenon.
4. Hematologic disorder:
   a. Polycythemia
      (1) Congenital heart disease or chronic hypoxia
      (2) Maternofetal transfusion or twin-to-twin transfusion
   b. Hyperviscosity
5. Harlequin color changes: Half of body becomes pale or acutely reddened. This lasts only a few minutes and is not physiologically significant.

BIBLIOGRAPHY

Driscoll DJ: Evaluation of the cyanotic newborn, *Pediatr Clin North Am* 37:1, 1990.

Martin L, Khalil H: How much reduced hemoglobin is necessary to generate central cyanosis? *Chest* 97:182, 1990.

18 Hypertension

The definition of *high blood pressure* in children is relative to the age and size of the patient. In adults diastolic blood pressure (BP) of 90 to 104 mm Hg is regarded as mild elevations, 105 to 114 mm Hg as moderate, above 115 to 128 mm Hg as severe, and 129 mm Hg or higher as malignant. Children are considered hypertensive if their BP is at or above the 95th percentile for their age, unless they have excessive height or lean body mass for that age. Two classes of hypertension are further defined: significant, pressure between the 95th and 99th percentiles, and severe, pressure at or above the 99th percentile. BP measurements should be obtained on at least three occasions before such diagnoses are considered.

Hypertensive crisis occurs with a severe sudden increase in BP without end-organ damage. The diastolic BP may rise to 140 mm Hg or more, with a corresponding rise in systolic pressure to 250 mm Hg or more (values for an adolescent or adult). These potentially life-threatening episodes may result from acute glomerulonephritis, head injury, drug reaction, pheochromocytoma, toxemia, or pregnancy. Commonly the result is an accelerated phase of poorly controlled chronic hypertension.

Hypertensive emergencies have associated symptoms affecting the central nervous system (CNS) (confusion, visual problems, seizures), heart (congestive heart failure [CHF]), or kidneys. *Malignant and accelerated hypertension* implies severe hypertension with progressive end-organ damage.

Assessment of a child's BP requires the use of a cuff of appropriate size, based on the size of the inner inflatable bladder. The cuff should be long enough to encircle the arm completely (with or without overlap) and wide enough to cover about 75% of the upper arm between the top of the shoulder and the olecranon. A cuff that is too narrow shows a false elevation of BP; a cuff that is too wide gives a falsely low reading. Commonly available BP cuffs include the following:

Cuff	Age	Bladder Width (cm)	Bladder Length (cm)
Newborn	Newborn	2.5-4.0	5.0-9.0
Infant	6 mo	4.0-9.0	11.5-18.0
Child	1-10 yr	7.5-9.0	17.0-19.0
Adult	>10 yr	11.5-13.0	22.0-26.0

Measurement of BP by auscultation, palpation, flush, and Doppler methods is useful, the last being particularly important for the young infant. Normal values for diastolic and systolic BP values vary with age (see Appendix B-2).

ETIOLOGY

Hypertension in children younger than 12 years is usually associated with anatomic abnormality; older children more commonly have essential hypertension. Conditions suggesting a greater risk for hypertension in infants include abdominal bruit or mass, coarctation of the aorta, congenital adrenal hyperplasia, neurofibromatosis, failure to thrive, history of indwelling umbilical artery catheter, unexplained heart failure or seizure, and renal disease.

Hypertension in *neonates* is most commonly caused by coarctation of the aorta, renal artery thrombosis, renal artery stenosis, congenital renal malformations, bronchopulmonary dysplasia, and intracranial hemorrhage. Underlying conditions causing hypertension in children

Box 18-1

COMMON CAUSES OF HYPERTENSION IN CHILDREN

RENAL PARENCHYMAL DISEASE

1. Glomerulonephritis
2. Pyelonephritis
3. Henoch-Schönlein purpura (nephritis)
4. Hemolytic-uremic syndrome
5. Polycystic kidney disease
6. Dysplastic kidney
7. Obstructive uropathy
8. Autoimmune process: systemic lupus erythematosus, other vasculitides

RENAL VASCULAR DISEASE

1. Arterial anomalies or thrombosis, especially in newborns
2. Venous anomalies or thrombosis

VASCULAR DISEASE

1. Coarctation of the aorta
2. Renal artery stenosis
3. Vasculitis
4. Aortic or mitral insufficiency

NEUROLOGIC DISEASE

1. Encephalitis
2. Brain tumor
3. Dysautonomia
4. Guillain-Barré syndrome
5. Stress, including major burns

ENDOCRINE DISEASE

1. Pheochromocytoma
2. Steroid therapy—Cushing's disease, congenital adrenal hyperplasia, birth control pills
3. Hyperthyroidism
4. Neuroblastoma

INTOXICATION

Lead, mercury, amphetamine, cocaine, LSD, licorice, steroids

ESSENTIAL HYPERTENSION

younger than 6 years include renal parenchymal disease (cystic, hydronephrosis, pyelonephritis, and Wilms' tumor), renal artery stenosis, and coarctation of the aorta. Children *6 to 10 years old* with hypertension most commonly have renal artery stenosis, renal parenchymal disease (cystic, pyelonephritis), or primary hypertension. Causes in *older* children are renal parenchymal disease (cystic, pyelonephritis, glomerulonephritis, and collagen) and essential, primary hypertension.

A systematic approach is required to determine the cause and achieve control. Many entities that cause mild hypertension on a chronic or transient basis are outlined in Box 18-1.

DIAGNOSTIC FINDINGS

It is often difficult to define juvenile hypertension and to distinguish children with this disorder from normotensive children. When a BP measurement is stipulated, the average of at least two measurements should be used. Appendix B-2 may be used as a guide in evaluating children with hypertension.

In the medical history, it is essential to focus on any family history of hypertension, preeclampsia, toxemia, renal disease, tumor, complicated neonatal history, headaches, dizziness, epistaxis, joint pain, edema, weight loss, weakness, abnormal menses, or drug ingestion.

The physical examination may indicate underlying renal, endocrine, or genetic disease as well as cardiovascular, abdominal, retinal, or neurologic abnormalities (Box 18-2).

Ancillary Data

1. Hematologic: complete blood count (CBC) (hemolytic anemia, thrombocytopenia), elevated erythrocyte sedimentation rate (ESR)
2. Chemical evaluation: elevated blood urea nitrogen (BUN) and creatinine levels; electrolytes and PO_4^{--} (consistent with renal function; uric acid; fasting

Box 18-2

SIGNS AND SYMPTOMS OF HYPERTENSIVE PATIENT

CAUSE	SIGNS AND SYMPTOMS
Pheochromocytoma	Flushing, palpitations, diarrhea, tachycardia
Renal	Poor growth, fever, UTI, edema, hematuria, proteinuria, trauma, family history
Congenital adrenal hyperplasia	Virilization
Cushing's syndrome	Striae, moon facies, truncal obesity
Coarctation of the aorta	Heart murmur, decreased femoral pulse or leg BP, abdominal bruit
Chronic hypertension	Funduscopic changes, Bell's palsy, stroke, CHF, cardiomegaly

cholesterol, triglycerides, high-density lipoprotein cholesterol, and calculated low-density lipoprotein cholesterol)

3. Urinalysis: microscopic hematuria, proteinuria, and red blood cell (RBC) casts (see Chapter 85)
4. Chest x-ray film: cardiomegaly and left ventricular hypertrophy; possibly pulmonary edema
5. Electrocardiogram (ECG): left ventricular hypertrophy
6. Studies indicated to evaluate specific diagnostic considerations, including radiologic and radioisotope (intravenous pyelography, ultrasonography, angiography, computed tomography) and hormonal studies (e.g., quantitation of urine or plasma catecholamines and metabolites, urinary aldosterone, and electrolytes)

Malignant Hypertension

Malignant or accelerated hypertension is a subacute, accelerated phase of BP elevation accompanied by retinopathy. Common underlying disorders include acute glomerulonephritis, hemolytic-uremic syndrome, obstructive uropathy, pyelonephritis, and other causes of hypertension.

BP should be brought under control in hours to days to prevent complications, including encephalopathy, intracranial hemorrhage, acute left ventricular failure, and renal failure.

Diagnostic Findings

Headaches are common, classically described as constant, occipital, and most severe in the morning. Blurred vision, dizziness, anorexia, nausea, vomiting, and weight loss are common. Retinal hemorrhages, exudate, and papilledema are often present. Cardiomegaly is common. Patients are neurologically normal but persistent focal deficits may develop.

Ancillary data, obtained as indicated, may be useful.

Hypertensive Cerebrovascular Syndromes

Hypertension associated with changes in mental status may be caused by a number of cerebrovascular events that have a pathognomonic presentation and require rapid control of BP. The decision to lower BP must be individualized and may be accomplished by a variety of modalities.

1. Hypertensive encephalopathy:
   a. Associated with rapid increase in BP
   b. Gradual onset over 24 to 48 hours
   c. Variable neurologic findings: confusion, apprehension, and lethargy,

progressing to stupor and coma, seizures, and hemiparesis

d. Headache, nausea, vomiting, and anorexia concomitant with progression of mental status deterioration; visual blurring with transient blindness may be accompanied by retinal hemorrhages, exudates, and papilledema

NOTE: Patients show dramatic response to a decrease in diastolic BP to less than 100 mm Hg (adolescent or adult values).

2. Intracerebral hemorrhage:
   a. Rapid onset with loss of consciousness, hemiplegia, and sensory loss
   b. Often accompanied by headache, nausea, and vomiting
   c. Focal neurologic findings usually fixed
3. Subarachnoid hemorrhage:
   a. Rapid onset of a violent headache, with initial pain localized. Most patients have a stiff neck and progress to loss of consciousness; often have unequal pupils and variable, transient focal neurologic findings.
   b. Spinal fluid is usually bloody.
4. Trauma: head or neck (see Chapter 57)
5. Neoplasm

Other Presentations

1. Left ventricular failure with pulmonary edema (see Chapters 16 and 19).
2. Dissection of leaking aortic aneurysm.
3. Pheochromocytoma.
4. Monoamine oxidase (MAO) inhibitors. Patients taking MAO inhibitors should not use alcoholic beverages or eat ripened cheeses (Brie, cheddar, Camembert, and Stilton), because these contain tyramine, which might produce an acute catecholamine release.
5. Emergency surgery on individuals with uncontrolled hypertension may exacerbate hypertension. Anesthesia and postoperative care must be individualized for these patients.
6. Intoxication (see Table 54-1): sympathomimetics (amphetamine), hallucinogens (PCP, LSD), heavy metals.
7. Toxemia of pregnancy with maternal convulsions, left ventricular failure, or fetal distress.

MANAGEMENT

All patients must be evaluated rapidly to assess the acuteness of the rise in BP, preexisting medical problems, potential etiologic factors, clinical factors related to the BP, and compliance with medications.

The patient's hemodynamic status must be evaluated by measuring orthostatic BP changes and the potential effect on cardiac, cerebral, and renal perfusion.

Mild Hypertension

For the patient with only mild hypertension without evidence of crisis, a slow, sequential, *stepped-care* approach is appropriate.

Nonpharmacologic therapy consists of:

1. Weight reduction if the patient is obese
2. Exercise and conditioning
3. Dietary modification (sodium intake 1.5-2.0 mEq/kg/24 hr)

Pharmacologic therapy is indicated when the BP is between the 90th and 95th percentiles for age and sex, when there is evidence of target organ injury, or when symptoms or signs related to elevated BP are present. The goals of the stepped-care approach to therapy are as follows:

1. Reduce diastolic BP to below the 90th percentile
2. Minimize side effects
3. Minimize drugs used to maximize patient compliance

Ultimately, the choice of agents depends on urgency of treatment, knowledge of agents, availability of monitoring equipment, and source of long-term follow-up. Pharmacologic therapy should follow these steps:

1. Initiate a thiazide-type diuretic at a low dosage, which may be increased to full dosage. In adolescents and young adults

with hyperkinetic hypertension (rapid pulse), a β-blocker may be preferable if the patient is neither diabetic nor asthmatic. Loop diuretics (furosemide) should be reserved for patients with impaired renal function (<50%).

a. Hydrochlorothiazide (HydroDIURIL), 1 mg/kg/24 hr q12hr PO; *or*

b. Chlorothiazide (Diuril), 10 mg/kg/24 hr q12hr PO.

c. Spironolactone (Aldactone), 1 to 3 mg/kg/24 hr q6-12hr PO, if potassium losses are not compensated by supplements and diet and if additional diuresis is needed.

2. If the BP is still not controlled, add a β-adrenergic inhibitor at a small dose and slowly increase to maximal dose. Do not use if CHF or asthma is present.

a. Propranolol (Inderal), 0.5 to 3 mg/kg/dose q6hr PO. Another increasingly used alternative is labetalol, 0.4 to 1.0 mg/kg IV slow push, which may be repeated up to three times (up to 3 mg/kg) in the first hour of management. Nifedipine, 0.25 to 0.5 mg/kg, may also be used; it is often given sublingually or by having patient bite into a capsule (see p. 172).

b. Another β-blocker that is used extensively in *adults* and more recently in children is atenolol (Tenormin), 1 mg/kg/24 hr PO q12-24hr (adult dose: 50-100 mg/24 hr).

3. If BP is still uncontrolled, add a third agent, such as a vasodilator, after consultation. Hydralazine (Apresoline), 0.75 to 3.0 mg/kg/24 hr q6-12hr PO, is the common dose. Availability of hydralazine may be limited because it is being reformulated.

When several drugs are required, consultation is appropriate for immediate management and follow-up.

Hypertensive Crisis

Hypertensive crisis requires more rapid control, reflecting the clinical presentation and the

TABLE 18-1 Agent of Choice in Hypertensive Crisis

Hypertensive Crisis	Agent of Choice	Contraindicated Agents
Malignant (accelerated) hypertension	Nitroprusside, diazoxide	Reserpine (causes sedation)
Primary renal disease	Nitroprusside, labetalol, diazoxide	Trimethaphan (decreases renal flow), β agonists
Encephalopathy	Nitroprusside, labetalol, diazoxide	Trimethaphan (dilates pupils), β agonist Reserpine/methyldopa (causes sedation)
Head injury	Nitroprusside	Reserpine/methyldopa (causes sedation) Trimethaphan (dilates pupils) Diazoxide (causes hypotension), β agonists
Acute left ventricular failure with pulmonary edema	Nitroprusside, labetalol, nitroglycerin	Diazoxide/hydralazine (increases cardiac output), minoxidil
Aortic dissection	Propranolol and nitroprusside*	Diazoxide/hydralazine (increases cardiac output), minoxidil
Pheochromocytoma/monoamine oxidase inhibitor	Phentolamine, nitroprusside	All others
Eclampsia	Hydralazine, nitroprusside, labetalol, diazoxide, magnesium sulfate	Trimethaphan (decreases uterine flow), diuretics, β agonists

* Initiate propranolol first.

TABLE 18-2 Useful Drugs in Management of Hypertensive Emergencies

Drug	Availability	ACTION: Onset	ACTION: Duration	Dose
DIURETICS		See Table 16-3		
PERIPHERAL VASODILATOR				
Sodium nitroprusside (Nipride) (arterioles and veins)	50 mg/vial for reconstitution	1-2 min	1-5 min	0.5-10 μg/kg/min IV; average: 3 μg/kg/min; initial 0.25 μg/kg/min for eclampsia and renal insufficiency
Diazoxide (Hyperstat) (arterioles)	15 mg/ml (20 ml)	3-5 min	½-12 hr	1-3 mg/kg/dose rapid push
Hydralazine (Apresoline) (arterioles)	20 mg/ml (1 ml)	10-30 min (IV)	3-6 hr	0.1-0.4 mg/kg/dose q6hr (1.7-3.5 mg/kg/24 hr) (use with propranolol)
	10, 25, 50, 100 mg			0.5-7.0 mg/kg/24 hr
Minoxidil (Loniten)	2.5, 10 mg	1 hr	4-8 hr	0.1-1.0 mg/kg/24 hr
CALCIUM CHANNEL BLOCKER				
Nifedipine (Procardia)	10, 20, 30, 60, 90 mg	5-15 min	3-5 hr	0.25-0.5 mg/kg
GANGLIONIC BLOCKER				
Trimethaphan (Arfonad)	50 mg/ml (10 ml)	5-10 min	5-10 min	50-150 μg/kg/min
CENTRALLY ACTING AGENTS				
Clonidine (Catapres)	0.1, 0.2, 0.3 mg	½-2 hr	6-8 hr	5-10 μg/kg/24 hr initial dose up to 5-25 μg/kg/24 hr q6hr PO (maximum: 0.9 mg/24 hr)
Methyldopa (Aldomet)	50 mg/ml (5 ml)	2-3 hr	4-8 hr	2.5-5 mg/kg/dose (maximum: 20-40 mg/kg/24 hr)
	125, 250, 500 mg			10 mg/kg/24 hr (maximum: 40 mg/kg/24 hr)
Reserpine	0.1, 0.25 mg	2-4 hr	4-8 hr	0.01-0.02 mg/kg/dose

Frequency/Route	Adult dose (>12 yr)	Advantages	Disadvantages
Continuous light-shielded IV infusion	0.5-10 μg/kg/min	Precise control; protects myocardial perfusion	Constant monitoring; light sensitive; cyanide poisoning; fatigue, nausea, disorientation
q4-24hr IV (if first dose ineffective, repeat in 30 min)	75-150 mg/dose	Prompt; no reduction of renal or coronary perfusion	↑ HR, ↑ cardiac output, variable hypotension, hyperglycemia, sodium retention; requires close monitoring
q4-6hr IV	10-20 mg/dose (maximum: 300 mg/24 hr)	Prompt; maintains cerebral, renal, coronary perfusion	↑ HR, ↑ cardiac output; tachyphylaxis, systemic lupus erythematosus (SLE) reactions; if sole agent, higher dose needed; limited availability
q6-12hr PO	10-75 mg (maximum: 300 mg/24 hr)		
q12hr PO	10-40 mg/24 hr	Gradual decrease	Limited experience in children; fluid retention, tachycardia; often used in conjunction with propranolol and furosemide
Titrate q15-30min PO, sublingual, buccal	10-20 mg	Rapid onset	Negative inotropic effect; contraindicated in intracranial hemorrhage; variable response
Continuous IV infusion	0.5-1 mg/min	Precise control	Constant monitoring; use with dissecting aortic aneurysm; tachyphylaxis; autonomic blockage—paralysis, pupils, bladder, bowel
q12hr PO	Initial: 0.1-0.2 mg/dose Maintenance: 0.2-0.8 mg/24 hr	Rapid onset; oral	Little experience in children; sedation; central sympatholytic agent
q6-8hr IV	500-1000 mg/dose	Gradual decrease	Variably effective; somnolence; ulcerogenic; orthostatic hypotension; bradycardia
q6-12hr PO	250-750 mg/dose		
q12hr PO	0.1-0.25 mg/24 hr	Gradual decrease	Somnolence, depression, ulcerogenic; rarely used, often combined with other agents

Continued

TABLE 18-2 Useful Drugs in Management of Hypertensive Emergencies—cont'd

Drug	Availability	ACTION		Dose
		Onset	Duration	
α-β-ADRENERGIC BLOCKERS				
Propranolol (Inderal)	10, 20, 40, 80 mg	1-2 min	12 hr	0.5-3 mg/kg/dose and increase (maximum: 320 mg/24 hr)
Labetalol	5 mg/ml	5-10 min	3-6 hr	0.4-1.0 mg/kg IV slow push; repeat up to 3 mg/kg in 1 hour
Esmolol (Brevibloc)	250 mg/10 ml	2-10 min	10-30 min	0.5-0.6 mg/kg/dose IV over 1-2 min; then 0.3-1.0 mg/kg/min beginning at 0.2 mg/kg/min and titrate by 0.05 μg/kg/min q5min
Atenolol (Tenormin)	25, 50, 100 mg	2-4 hr	4-6 hr	1 mg/kg/24 hr PO
Prazosin (Minipress)	1, 2, 5 mg	3 hr	8 hr	First dose 5 μg/kg PO up to 25 μg/kg/dose
Phentolamine (Regitine)	5 mg/ml (1 ml)	1-2 min	5-20 min	0.05-0.1 mg/kg/dose (repeat q5min until control)
ANGIOTENSIN-CONVERTING ENZYME INHIBITOR				
Captopril (Capoten)	25, 50, 100 mg	15 min	4-6 hr	0.5-6 mg/kg/24 hr (newborn; 0.1-0.4 mg/kg/dose q6-12hr PO)

urgency of signs and symptoms. The level of control must reflect the hemodynamic status of the patient. *Usually only a moderate reduction in pressure is needed in the acute situation, often to the range of 100 mm Hg diastolic pressure:*

1. Furosemide (Lasix), 1 to 3 mg/kg/dose q6-12hr IV. May be repeated every 2 hours. In most cases, the physician cannot wait for significant diuretic effect but must use specific antihypertensive drugs.
2. Antihypertensive drugs:
   a. Agents are summarized in Tables 18-1 and 18-2.
   b. Parenteral therapy (usually vasodilators such as nitroprusside, diazoxide, and hydralazine) is indicated with severe acute hypertension (greater than the 95th percentile) associated with acute glomerulonephritis, hemolytic-uremic syndrome, or head injuries.

Frequency/Route	Adult dose (>12 yr)	Advantages	Disadvantages
Titrate IV	2 mg/min or 20 mg/dose initially; then 20-80 mg q10min	Can be followed by some drug orally	Hypotension; first dose evaluates effect
q6-12hr IV	10-40 mg/dose (maximum: 320 mg/ 24 hr)		Dysrhythmia (monitor); fatigue; hypoglycemia; β blocker; contraindicated: CHF, asthma
Titrate IV	0.5 mg/kg/min over 1 min; then 0.1-0.3 mg/kg/min beginning at 0.05 mg/kg/min and titrate q5min		Hypotension, dysrhythmia
q12-24hr	50-100 mg/24 hr	β selective	Limited experience in children; headache, nausea, hypotension, bradycardia, exacerbates CHF
q6hr PO	0.5-7 mg/dose		
q1-4hr IV	2.5-5 mg/dose	Rapid onset; specific for pheochromocytoma and MAO inhibitor	Hypotension, dysrhythmia
q6-12 hr PO	25-150 mg/dose	Rapid onset; oral; useful when other drug combinations fail, esp. if high plasma renin level	Variable response, hypotension; proteinuria, neutropenia, azotemia; absorption falls if taken with food

c. In general, nitroprusside is an excellent agent for initial control in most conditions that cause a hypertensive crisis.

d. Oral antihypertensive therapy lowers BP less rapidly than parenteral medications and has been used extensively in hypertensive emergencies without encephalopathy or cardiac decompensation. Many prefer this approach. Medications for this purpose include the following:

(1) Clonidine (Catapres): Adult dose is 0.2 mg PO initially, then 0.1 mg/hr PO up to a maximum dose of 0.8 mg/24 hr. Onset of action: 2 hours; duration: 6 to 8 hours. Disadvantages: sedation, hypertension. Mechanism: central sympatholytic.

(2) Nifedipine (Procardia): 0.25 to 0.5 mg/kg/dose PO or sublingually may be useful in severe hypertension. May be repeated in 30 minutes but usually q6-8hr (average: 0.33 mg/kg total dose [adult: 10 to 20 mg/dose PO or sublingually]). Onset of action: 5 to 15 minutes; duration: 3 to 5 hours. To give sublingually, draw contents of a 10-mg capsule (0.34 ml) into a 1-ml syringe. Disadvantages: may cause tachycardia (β-blocker may be given concurrently); variable response. Mechanism: calcium channel blocker.

DISPOSITION

A patient with only *mild* hypertension may be observed closely as an outpatient if compliance with therapy can be ensured.

A *hypertensive crisis* requires immediate hospitalization in an intensive care unit.

BIBLIOGRAPHY

Beronson GS: Combined low-dose medication and primary intervention over a 30-month period for sustained high blood pressure in childhood, *Am J Med Sci* 299:79, 1990.

Blassak RT, Savage JA, Ellis EN: The use of short-acting nifedipine in pediatric patients with hypertension, *J Pediatr* 139:34, 2001.

Bunchman TE, Lynch RE, Wood EG: Intravenously administered labetalol for treatment of hypertension in children, *J Pediatr* 120:140, 1992.

Calhoun DA, Oparil S: Treatment of hypertension crisis, *N Engl J Med* 323:1177, 1990.

Harshfield GA, Alpert BS, Pulliam DA et al: Ambulatory blood pressure recordings in children and adolescents, *Pediatrics* 94:180, 1994.

Hulman S, Edwards R, Chen YQ et al: Blood pressure patterns in the first three days of life, *J Perinatol* 11:231, 1991.

Ingelfinger JR: Pediatric hypertension, *Curr Opin Pediatr* 6:198, 1994.

National Institute of Health: Update on the task force report on high blood pressure in children and adolescents: NIH Publication No. 96.3790, 1996.

Sinaiko AR: Treatment of hypertension in children, *Pediatr Nephrol* 8:603, 1994.

19 Pulmonary Edema

Also See Chapters 16 (Congestive Heart Failure) and 71 (Cardiovascular Disorders)

ALERT Cardiac causes of pulmonary edema often are accompanied by congestive heart failure; noncardiogenic causes result from a wide variety of clinical entities. The chest x-ray film is particularly helpful in making this differentiation. All patients need oxygen and respiratory support.

Pulmonary edema may occur secondary to diverse mechanisms, including increased pulmonary capillary pressure (cardiac or noncardiac), decreased colloid osmotic pressure (renal or hepatic dysfunction, malnutrition), altered membrane permeability (pneumonia, drowning, adult respiratory distress syndrome [ARDS], drugs, toxins), changes in transpulmonary pressure (upper airway obstruction and relief), decreased lymphatic drainage, and mixed mechanisms (high-altitude pulmonary edema [HAPE], head trauma, seizures).

Most patients have cardiogenic pulmonary edema resulting from an elevated left atrial pressure with increased pulmonary hydrostatic pressure.

ETIOLOGY

1. Vascular:
   - **a.** Congestive heart failure (see Chapter 16)
   - **b.** Pulmonary embolism (p. 578)
   - **c.** Cerebrovascular accident
   - **d.** Fat embolism
2. Trauma or physical agent:
   - **a.** Central nervous system (CNS): cerebral anoxia, embolism, head trauma (see Chapter 57)
   - **b.** Near-drowning (see Chapter 47)
   - **c.** HAPE (see Chapter 49)
   - **d.** Radiation exposure
   - **e.** Upper airway foreign body or after removal of obstruction
3. Intoxication:
   - **a.** Inhaled toxins: smoke, CO, phosgene, ozone, etc.
   - **b.** Circulating toxins: snake venom, endotoxin
   - **c.** Drugs: sulfonamides, narcotics (methadone, heroin), naloxone, propoxyphene, salicylates, hydrocarbon, phenytoin, organophosphates, amphetamines, thiazides
4. Infection or inflammation:
   - **a.** Pneumonia or other pulmonary infection (p. 811)
   - **b.** Pulmonary aspiration
   - **c.** Pancreatitis (p. 654) or peritonitis
   - **d.** Upper airway obstruction (croup, epiglottitis, markedly enlarged tonsils and adenoids) or after relief of obstruction
   - **e.** Disseminated intravascular coagulation (DIC): infection, eclampsia (p. 694)
5. Iatrogenic:
   - **a.** Fluid overload
   - **b.** Decompression of pneumothorax

6. Metabolic: decreased oncotic pressure from hypoalbuminemia, as in liver failure.
7. Seizures.
8. Allergic or autoimmune:
   a. Asthma (p. 781)
   b. Systemic lupus erythematosus
9. Neoplasm: CNS, pulmonary.

DIAGNOSTIC FINDINGS

Although there are specific findings with pulmonary edema, most presenting signs and symptoms are related to the underlying cause and must be evaluated systematically. Historically, patients report progressive dyspnea with orthopnea, cough, and pink, frothy sputum.

Vital signs are variable. Blood pressure is often elevated with cardiac decompensation. It may be increased in noncardiogenic pulmonary edema secondary to anxiety and catecholamine release. Tachycardia is present. Patients have pale, clammy skin.

Tachypnea is uniformly apparent (unless decreased by narcotics). Cyanosis results from ventilation-perfusion abnormalities. Patients demonstrate rale, wheezing, and occasionally, pleural effusions. Unilateral effusions, when present, are usually on the right.

Cardiac findings reflect the underlying disorder associated with congestive heart failure, demonstrating gallop rhythm, increased heart sounds, and elevated jugular venous pressure (see Chapter 16).

Mental status may be decreased, with associated anorexia, listlessness, and headache, and occasionally, the patient may progress to coma, Cheyne-Stokes respirations, or apnea, which occurs with cerebral hypoxia.

Complications

1. Cardiac failure with left or right ventricular failure (see Chapter 16)
2. Superimposed pulmonary infection (p. 811)
3. Acute respiratory failure with $Pa{O_2}$ less than 50 mm Hg and $Pa{CO_2}$ greater than 50 mm Hg with room air, at sea level, with progressive disease or fatigue, and with respiratory acidosis
4. DIC (p. 694)
5. Cardiopulmonary arrest and death

Ancillary Data

Studies must reflect the primary cause, in addition to those directly related to pulmonary status:

1. Chest x-ray findings
   a. Fluffy alveolar infiltrates, with diffuse perihilar haziness, Kerley B lines, cardiomegaly, and possibly pleural effusions.
   b. If edema is cardiac in origin, findings are usually associated with underlying cardiac lesion(s). Cardiomegaly is usually present.
2. Arterial blood gas (ABG) analysis: hypoxia with respiratory acidosis or alkalosis; continuous oximetry
3. Electrocardiogram (ECG): reflects underlying heart disease, strain, or ischemia
4. Electrolyte values: abnormalities particularly with diuretics (hypokalemia, blood urea nitrogen [BUN], creatinine)
5. Thoracentesis: if patient has pleural fluid leading to respiratory decompensation (see Appendix A-8)

   NOTE: Analysis should include cell counts, measurements of protein, glucose, and lactic dehydrogenase (LDH), culture, and Gram stain.
6. Other studies, as indicated:
   a. Placement of Swan-Ganz catheter to measure pulmonary wedge pressure when cardiac failure is severe. The catheter is usually inserted in the intensive care unit (ICU).
   b. Echocardiogram to evaluate pulmonary hypertension and cardiac function and to determine whether effusion is present.

DIFFERENTIAL DIAGNOSIS

1. Infection: pneumonia (p. 811)
2. Vascular:

a. Intrapulmonary hemorrhage, accompanied by hemoptysis, chest pain, and infiltrate on chest x-ray film
b. Pulmonary embolism (p. 578) with hemoptysis, pleuritic chest pain, and dyspnea
3. Allergy: asthma (p. 781)

MANAGEMENT

The pulmonary status initially may be stabilized during the treatment of the underlying condition. For treatment of specific entities, see appropriate chapter.

The patient should be kept in a semirecumbent position with cardiac monitoring.

1. Airway and breathing:
   a. Oxygenation is a necessity. Administer humidified oxygen at 3 to 6 L/min by mask or nasal cannula (or 50%).
   b. Intubate and initiate positive end-expiratory pressure if the Pao_2 less than 50 mm Hg at an Fio_2 of 50%, beginning at 5 cm H_2O and increasing with close monitoring in ICU.
   c. Perform mechanical ventilation after intubation for respiratory failure (Pao_2 <50 mm Hg and $Paco_2$ >50 mm Hg at room air, sea level) to protect airway, to avoid rapid progression of disease or fatigue, or to treat unresponsive metabolic acidosis.
   d. Bronchodilator therapy including albuterol may be useful (p. 790).
2. Fluid resuscitation:
   a. Fluid therapy must be a balance between expanding the intravascular volume necessary to improve cardiac output and controlling the subsequent increased pulmonary flow and edema. This goal may require the insertion of a Swan-Ganz catheter and observation of the patient for renal failure.
   b. Crystalloid solution is used to maintain urine output at 0.5 ml/kg/hr in cardiogenic pulmonary edema but must be individualized in noncardiogenic pulmonary edema. Patients in general are maintained with fluids at a rate well below maintenance, and urine output is monitored.
   c. Albumin (25% salt poor administered 1 g/kg/dose over 2-4 hours) is indicated if pulmonary edema is secondary to hypoalbuminemia.
   d. Fluid management for patients with cardiac tamponade requires pushing of fluids and pericardiocentesis (see Appendix A-5).
3. Diuretics to reduce volume overload (see Table 16-3):
   a. Administer diuretics for pulmonary edema that is cardiogenic in origin. For noncardiogenic edema, use diuretics only if the underlying pathophysiologic condition is associated with fluid overload.
   b. Furosemide (Lasix): 1 mg/kg/dose up to 6 mg/kg/dose q6hr. May be repeated every 2 hours if indicated. Not to be used if patient is anuric.
4. Morphine sulfate: lowers pulmonary wedge pressure and relieves anxiety:
   a. In severe pulmonary edema, slowly administer 0.1 to 0.2 mg/kg IV.
   b. Do not give morphine if patient has unstable vital signs, asthma, or signs of intracranial hemorrhage, chronic pulmonary disease, or narcotic withdrawal.
   c. Use with caution in patients with respiratory depression or progressive disease. Close monitoring is essential.
   d. Nalbuphine (Nubain) is a useful substitute for morphine. The experience with this agent in children is still-limited.
5. Shock: cardiogenic shock or low-output state may accompany pulmonary edema and must be treated aggressively. The adrenergic agents of choice (see Chapter 5) are as follows:
   a. Dopamine administered by continuous IV infusion at a rate of 5 to

20 μg/kg/min. May be used at a higher dosage if α-blocking agents are used. Experience with this drug in children is extensive.

b. An alternative is dobutamine administered by continuous IV infusion at a rate of 2 to 20 μg/kg/min. Some patients may respond to a low dosage of 0.5 μg/kg/min; others may require 40 μg/kg/min. This agent may be used with low-dose dopamine (0.5-3 μg/kg/min).

6. Afterload reduction to diminish pressure overload. If response to these measures is inadequate, agents that diminish afterload by decreasing peripheral resistance may improve cardiac output. These drugs should be used only with indwelling arterial monitoring and a Swan-Ganz catheter in place (see Appendix A-3):
   a. Sodium nitroprusside (Nipride). Dosage: 0.5 to 8 μg/kg/min IV by infusion. Begin with rate of infusion of 0.1 μg/kg/min, and increase until the desired response is achieved. Average therapeutic dose is about 3 μg/kg/min. The clinical response is noted in 1 to 2 minutes and lasts for 5 to 10 minutes after the infusion is stopped. Do not use if renal failure is present.
   b. Nitroglycerin has no established dosage in children. Sublingual administration in adults (0.15-0.6 mg q5min up to a maximum of three doses in a 15-minute period) may be useful for acute treatment, particularly in the prehospital setting in the patient with obvious cardiac decompensation. IV nitroglycerin (Nitrostat) has similarly been used in adults (5 μg/min with increments of 5 μg/min q3-5min titrated to response) in the hospital environment.
7. Other considerations:
   a. Dysrhythmias require urgent treatment (see Chapter 6).
   b. Steroids are not useful unless they have efficacy for the underlying condition.
   c. Bronchodilators are indicated if there is wheezing and evidence of bronchoconstriction (p. 790).

DISPOSITION

Patients must be admitted to an ICU for appropriate intervention, immediate treatment and monitoring of the pulmonary edema, and management of the underlying condition.

The rare patient with mild, slowly progressive pulmonary edema of known cause may be managed on an ambulatory basis, if compliance with therapy and follow-up care can be ensured.

A cardiologist should be involved immediately.

BIBLIOGRAPHY

Feinberg AN, Shabino CL: Acute pulmonary edema complicating tonsillectomy and adenoidectomy, *Pediatrics* 75:112, 1985.

Kanter RK, Watchko JF: Pulmonary edema associated with upper airway obstruction, *Am J Dis Child* 138:356, 1984.

20 Respiratory Distress (Dyspnea)

ALERT Note any of the following findings: acuteness of onset; accompanying fever; voice changes; trauma; underlying heart, liver, or kidney disease; metabolic abnormalities; abnormal upper airway findings; asymmetric findings; stridor; or wheezing. These assist in rapidly evaluating potential causes. Oximetry is essential in assessing oxygenation. Airway and ventilation must be stabilized immediately. Never leave the patient with dyspnea unattended.

Dyspnea or labored, rapid respirations usually reflect an impairment of ventilation, perfusion, or a metabolic or central nervous system (CNS) drive. Upper airway problems produce primarily ventilatory abnormalities associated with stridor; lower airway disease may impair both ventilation and perfusion.

Respiratory failure is commonly associated with altered consciousness, increases in work of breathing and respiratory rate, poor color, sweating, grunting and flaring, decreased air movement, and abnormal arterial blood gas (ABG) or oximetry values.

ETIOLOGY

Stridor is the major complaint with significant upper airway disease. A variety of entities may commonly produce stridor (Table 20-1):

1. Infection: croup, epiglottitis, tracheitis
2. Allergic: anaphylaxis, angioneurotic edema
3. Congenital or anatomic: laryngeal edema, web
4. Neurologic
5. Psychogenic

Inspiratory stridor is usually supraglottic, whereas expiratory stridor emanates from the trachea. Patients with both inspiratory and expiratory stridor or expiratory stridor alone usually have more significant obstructions, demanding urgent intervention.

Supraglottic stridor is usually quiet and wet, and it is associated with a muffled voice, dysphagia, and a preference to sit; a patient with subglottic lesions producing a loud stridor often has a hoarse voice, barky cough, and possibly, facial edema.

Lower airway disease consists of a more diverse group of entities that inhibit the ability of oxygen to diffuse into the capillaries. The most common are pneumonia and asthma. Pulmonary disease is often associated with exertional dyspnea; cardiac disease, on the other hand, causes orthopnea and paroxysmal nocturnal dyspnea.

Most upper and lower airway disease result from one of several entities:

Upper Airway Disease	Lower Airway Disease
Stridor present	**Stridor absent**
Croup	Pneumonia
Epiglottitis	Asthma
Foreign body	Bronchiolitis
Tracheitis	Foreign body

Common causes of respiratory distress in children younger than 2 years are pneumonia, asthma, croup, congenital heart disease, foreign body inhalation, congenital anomalies of the

Text continued on p. 184

TABLE 20-1 Respiratory Distress: Diagnostic Considerations

Disease	Etiology	Signs and Symptoms	Ancillary Data	Comments/Management
		UPPER AIRWAY OBSTRUCTION		
INFECTION				
Epiglottitis (p. 800)	*Haemophilus influenzae*	Toxic, febrile, inspiratory stridor, cyanosis, muffled voice, drooling, labored respirations, cherry-red epiglottis	↑ WBC (shift left), positive lateral neck x-ray	Visualization and intubation, optimally in operating room; antibiotics; incidence down with routine immunization
Croup (laryngotracheal bronchitis) (p. 800)	Virus: parainfluenza, respiratory syncytial virus	Inspiratory stridor, hoarse voice, croupy cough, variably labored respirations, epiglottis WNL	Variable WBC, negative lateral neck x-ray	Cool mist; nebulized racemic epinephrine if needed; steroids
Peritonsillar abscess (p. 612)	Group A streptococci	Fever, severe throat pain, late inspiratory stridor, drooling, dysphagia, tonsil displaced, posterior pharyngeal mass	↑ WBC	Nafcillin (or equivalent), surgical incision and drainage; usually child <3 yr old
Retropharyngeal/ esophageal abscess (p. 617)	*Staphylococcus aureus*, group A streptococci		↑ WBC, positive lateral neck x-ray	
Bacterial tracheitis	*S. aureus*	High temperature, toxic, inspiratory stridor, brassy cough, no response to croup therapy	↑ WBC (shift to left)	Nafcillin (or equivalent); may require intubation to remove thick secretions
Diphtheria (p. 724)	*Corynebacterium diphtheriae*	Toxic, slight fever, membrane, hoarse	Culture	History of exposure, no immunization; antitoxin and penicillin
TRAUMA				
Foreign body (p. 808) Pharynx, larynx, trachea, esophagus	Aspiration of vegetable or inanimate matter	History reflects level of obstruction, inspiratory or expiratory stridor, cyanosis, labored respirations, wheezing, variable respiratory arrest	Chest (inspiratory and expiratory) and lateral neck x-ray; foreign body, wide mediastinum; findings vary with location	Back blow, chest/abdominal thrust, mechanical removal, surgical airway
Neck injury (Chapter 61)		History and findings of trauma, instability or disruption of neck, larynx, variable stridor	Clear cervical spine, look for signs of laryngeal injury	Stabilization of airway and neck
Cord paralysis	Congenital, traumatic, iatrogenic	Acute or chronic, voice change, inspiratory stridor, respiratory distress	Direct laryngoscopy	If acute, intubation or surgical airway

Subglottic stenosis	Trauma to glottis such as intubation; rarely congenital	Respiratory distress, usually insidious; may be exacerbated by respiratory infection	Direct laryngoscopy	Surgical airway may be needed
CONGENITAL (Chapters 10 and 11)				
Vascular ring Laryngeal web or polyp Small mandible (Pierre Robin) Large tongue (hypothyroid)	Congenital or acquired	Chronic inspiratory or expiratory stridor, variable respiratory distress (or both), wheezing	Laryngoscopy/bronchoscopy	Surgical or medical approach to underlying problem
Choanal atresia	Congenital	Nasal obstruction, discharge; variable respiratory distress	Catheter passage, visualization	Oral airway; surgical correction may be required if significant
Tracheomalacia	Abnormal collapse of supraglottic area	Expiratory stridor		Need oxygen until stable; usually resolves spontaneously; may have feeding problem
Laryngomalacia	Floppiness of trachea	Inspiratory stridor		
ALLERGIC				
Spasmodic croup (p. 800)	Exposure to irritant or sensitizing agent	Rapid onset inspiratory stridor, croupy cough, variable labored respirations		Cool mist; nebulized racemic epinephrine
Anaphylaxis (Chapter 12)	Allergic response	Rapid onset stridor, respiratory distress, wheezing		Removal of sensitizing agent; β agonists, antihistamines, steroids
Angioneurotic edema	Allergic response, hereditary	Rapid onset after eating, bee sting, environmental exposure		Airway support, epinephrine, etc. (Chapter 12)
NEOPLASM				
Tracheal, laryngeal, esophageal, neck	Carcinoma, teratoma, hemangioma, polyp	Insidious progression of stridor, dysphagia, labored respirations		Radiologic and surgical evaluation

Continued

TABLE 20-1 Respiratory Distress: Diagnostic Considerations—cont'd

Disease	Etiology	Signs and Symptoms	Ancillary Data	Comments/Management
		LOWER AIRWAY DISEASE		
INFECTION				
Pneumonia (p. 811)	Viral Bacterial: *Streptococcus pneumoniae, H. influenzae* Other	Febrile, recent onset tachypnea, cough, unequal breath sounds or rhonchi, variable chest pain	Variable WBC count; chest x-ray: infiltrate; blood culture (if toxic)	Antibiotics as indicated
Bronchiolitis (p. 797)	Viral: parainfluenza, respiratory syncytial virus	Variable fever, very tachypneic, nontoxic, wheezing, variable cyanosis	Chest x-ray: hyperexpanded, infiltrate variable; oximetry	Support: hydration, oxygen; nebulized β agonists (albuterol); ribavirin in selected children
Pleural effusion	Infections (viral or bacterial), CHF, nephrosis, liver failure	No fever, tachypneic with unequal breath sounds, variable chest pain	Chest x-ray (include lateral decubitus)	May need to aspirate; exudate (LDH >200 U, LDH fluid/blood ratio >0.6, or protein fluid/blood ratio >0.5)
Empyema	*S. aureus*	Fever, toxic, tachypneic, cough, variable pain, unequal breath sounds	Chest x-ray, fluid culture, blood culture	Thoracentesis for diagnosis, then closed chest tube drainage and antibiotics
VASCULAR				
Congestive heart failure (Chapter 16)	Congenital or acquired heart disease	Fatigue, anorexia, cough, orthopnea, basilar rale, edema	Chest x-ray, ECG, ABG	Diuretics, oxygen, digitalis, morphine, nitrates
Congenital heart disease	R → L shunt, pulmonary edema	Cyanosis	Chest x-ray, ECG, ABG	Cardiology consultation
Pulmonary edema (Chapter 19)	Heart, liver, renal vascular disease	Tachypnea, basilar rales, fatigue, cough, orthopnea, wheezing	Chest x-ray, serum protein, BUN, SGOT, electrolytes, UA	Evaluate systems involved; diuretics
Pulmonary embolism (p. 578)	Abnormal clotting, trauma, birth control pills	Tachypnea, hemoptysis, chest pain, variable fever	Chest x-ray, ABG, ventilation-perfusion scan	Immediate anticoagulation
Polycythemia	Heart, pulmonary, renal disease, abnormal Hb	Plethoric	CBC with indexes	Hematology consultation; may require partial exchange
Anemia (Chapter 26)	↓ production or ↑ loss; high output failure	Pale, fatigue, poor exercise tolerance	CBC with indexes, reticulocyte count	Hematology consultation; transfusion

ALLERGIC				
Asthma (p. 781)	Exposure to irritant or sensitizing agent; infection; emotional stress	Insidious or rapid onset of tachypnea, wheezing, cough		Oxygen, nebulized β agonists, bronchodilators, and steroids
Anaphylaxis (Chapter 12)	Exposure to sensitizing agent	Rapid onset wheezing, tachypnea	Chest x-ray, ABG	
TRAUMA				
Foreign body				
Bronchial (p. 808)	Vegetable or inanimate material	History, cough, wheezing, asymmetric breath sounds	Chest x-ray; inspiratory and expiratory fluoroscopy	Bronchoscopy
Pneumothorax (Chapter 62)	Chest wound, spontaneous	Tachypnea, chest pain, asymmetric breath sounds	Chest x-ray	Needle aspiration, chest tube
CONGENITAL				
Cystic fibrosis	Autosomal recessive, Caucasians	Progressive pulmonary disease (hemoptysis, atelectasis, pneumothorax, obstructive pulmonary disease, concurrent infection); poor growth; GI (steatorrhea, pancreatitis, rectal prolapse); hyponatremia	Chest x-ray, sweat test	Pulmonary consultation
NEOPLASM		Progressive pulmonary disease	Chest x-ray	Oncology consultation
DEGENERATIVE				
Kyphoscoliosis, progressive CNS disease	Multiple	Progressive pulmonary disease, secondary hypoventilation	Chest x-ray, ABG, pulmonary function	Neurology, pulmonary, orthopedic consultation

airway (tracheal web, cysts, lobar emphysema), and nasopharyngeal obstruction (large tonsils and adenoids). The underlying disorder in older children is more often asthma, pneumonia, foreign bodies, poisoning, drowning, trauma, cystic fibrosis, peripheral neuritis, or encephalitis.

In addition to the conditions listed in Table 20-1, oxygen demand may be increased (increased activity, fever, hyperthyroidism), oxygen transport may be deficient (anemia, methemoglobinemia, or shock), the respiratory system may be stimulated as a compensatory mechanism in metabolic acidosis (diabetes mellitus, uremia, drug ingestions), the ambient oxygen may be low, or there may be a central neurogenic stimulation.

Adult respiratory distress syndrome (ARDS) may result from a variety of conditions that cause pulmonary damage (p. 41).

DIAGNOSTIC FINDINGS (Fig. 20-1)

The initial focus must be on the assessment of the airway and ventilatory status with intervention on an emergent basis as required. This often must occur before definitive diagnostic evaluation has been completed. Oximetry is a more reliable indicator of hypoxemia than a solely clinical evaluation.

Airway integrity and ventilatory status can be rapidly assessed initially by evaluation for the presence of stridor and auscultation to determine the adequacy of air movement and to check for wheezing, rales, and rhonchi.

The history must focus on the presenting problems. The characterization of the current episode should include the nature of progression, associated signs and symptoms, cough (productive versus unproductive), fever, chest pain, trauma, and foreign body ingestion. Evidence of retractions, tachypnea, wheezing, stridor, and relationship to eating should be defined. Past medical problems related to respiratory distress; recurrent problems with shortness of breath, cough, pneumonia, retractions, fever; and exposure to chemical or environmental irritants should be noted. Pulmonary or cardiac disease, infectious exposures, tuberculosis, and early death in other family members may be important.

On physical examination, after stability has been ensured, respiratory status, including air entry, type of breathing, color (and oximetric findings), retractions, and breath sounds, should be evaluated. Stridor, adequacy of air movement, wheezing, rale, and rhonchi must be excluded.

Respiratory rates suggestive of pneumonia by age group: less than 6 months, >59 breaths/min; 6 to 11 months, >52 breaths/min; and 1 to 2 years, >42 breaths/min.

Ancillary Data

1. *Upper airway obstruction.* Laboratory evaluation is usually ancillary to direct visualization, particularly in patients with respiratory distress. Visualization must be performed with great caution and anticipation of problems. Specific measures are indicated for patients with potential foreign bodies (p. 808).
2. *Lower airway disease.* Chest x-ray films and ABG analysis (or oximetry) provide initial data. Specific tests for the suspected causes must be obtained (see Table 20-1).

MANAGEMENT

Stabilization of the airway is central to any management plan and must not be delayed by the search for excessive confirmatory data before definitive therapy is instituted. All patients with respiratory distress must be evaluated for airway and ventilatory status, and intervention must be performed as needed, often on an empiric basis. Oxygen and cardiac monitoring should be initiated on the patient's arrival in the emergency department.

It is important to remember that upsetting the child should be prevented when possible. The degree of distress should never be underestimated, and the child should never be left unattended in the emergency department, x-ray department, or any other area of the hospital.

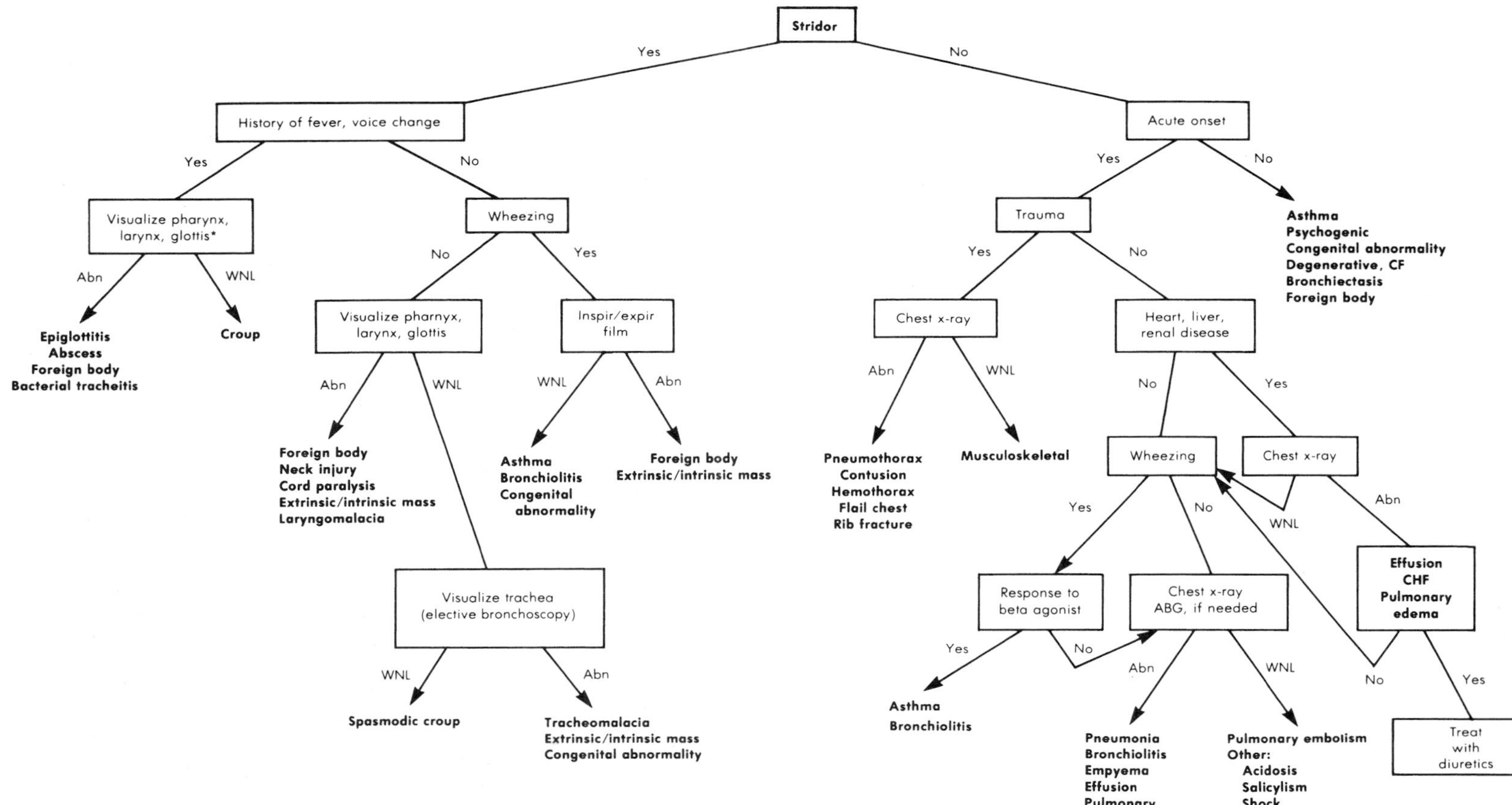

Fig. 20-1 Respiratory distress. *Do not visualize without immediate capability of airway intervention. If epiglottitis is suspected, procedure should be performed under controlled conditions, often in the operating room.

Specific intervention must reflect the severity of respiratory distress and the potential causative conditions.

BIBLIOGRAPHY

Meneker AJ, Petrack EM, Krug SE: Contribution of routine pulse oximetry to evaluation and management of patients with respiratory illness in a pediatric emergency department, *Ann Emerg Med* 25:36, 1995.

Ruddy RM: Respiratory distress in a child in the office, *Pediatr Emerg Care* 6:314, 1990.

Santamaria JD, Schafermeyer R: Stridor: a review, *Pediatr Emerg Care* 8:229, 1992.

Taylor J, DelBeccaro M, Done S et al: Establishing clinically relevant standards for tachypnea in febrile children younger than 2 years, *Arch Pediatr Adolesc Med* 149:283, 1995.

21 Status Epilepticus

Also See Chapter 81 (Neurologic Disorders)

ALERT Maintain airway; administer oxygen, dextrose, and naloxone (Narcan) (if appropriate) and then anticonvulsants. Consider diagnostic entities.

Patients are considered to be in status epilepticus when they experience continuous seizures for 20 to 30 minutes or have two or more seizures without a lucid period.

Poor compliance with antiseizure therapy is the most common explanation, although some patients may have lowered thresholds for seizure because of fever and infection, head trauma, hypoglycemia and metabolic abnormalities, ingestions, drug interactions, hypertension, or an exacerbation of the underlying condition. Status epilepticus may be the first seizure in a child who goes on to have epilepsy (p. 754). Animal studies have shown that cellular ischemic changes begin within 10 to 15 minutes of onset of continuous seizures.

The morbidity rate of aggressively treated status epilepticus in the absence of an acute neurologic result or progressive neurologic disorder is low. Status epilepticus is the initial seizure in most children with epilepsy. Seventy-five percent of episodes in children younger than 1 year, and 47% of episodes in children younger than 3 years, have an acute cause.

DIAGNOSTIC FINDINGS

Grand mal seizures are most common, although other categories of seizure are seen. Several patterns may occur:

1. Recurrent generalized seizures with persistent cortical depression between them
2. Nonconvulsive seizures producing continuous or fluctuating alteration in mental status
3. Recurrent partial seizure producing focal motor convulsions, focal sensory symptoms, or focal impairment of function (i.e., aphasia) not associated with alteration in consciousness

Patients experience seizure activity, loss of consciousness, and cyanosis. Temperature may be increased because of meningitis or other infection or secondary to the increased muscle activity related to the seizure. Tachycardia and elevated blood pressure are common.

Mydriasis and upward deviation of the eyes are present. The corneal reflex is decreased, and Babinski's reflex is present. Fecal and urinary incontinence occur.

Complications

1. Death resulting from anoxia, aspiration, or trauma associated with the loss of consciousness
2. Encephalopathy from hypoxia
3. Acute renal failure associated with myoglobinuria and rhabdomyolysis
4. Respiratory arrest caused by medications

Ancillary Data

Appropriate studies should be performed:

1. Sample obtained for serum glucose determination before infusion of 25%

dextrose in water (D25W); also, rapid serum glucose approximation (Dextrostix or Chemstrip)

2. Arterial blood gas (ABG) analysis for acidosis and hypoxia
3. Anticonvulsant drug level measurement, if patient has been taking medications
4. If the cause is unknown: measurements of electrolytes, Ca^{++}, Mg^{++}, and PO_4^{--}, complete blood count (CBC), and toxicologic screen; consider lumbar puncture and computed tomography (CT) scanning as appropriate

MANAGEMENT

Initial management must be supportive, with particular attention to the airway and ventilation and administration of supplemental oxygen.

1. Intubation may be required to oxygenate the patient and minimize the risk of aspiration. Prophylactic intubation is rarely indicated unless seizures are unresponsive or the airway or ventilation is compromised.
2. Traumatic injuries should be prevented by protecting the patient against self-injury. Trauma to the tongue rarely causes significant problems. Putting a soft cloth in the mouth to keep the teeth from closing may prevent dental damage. Attempting to force an airway into the mouth can cause obstruction.

Glucose has an immediate metabolic effect and should be considered. A blood specimen for glucose measurement should be drawn before administration of glucose, for later confirmation, if possible.

- Glucose (D25W), 0.5 to 1.0 g (2-4 ml)/kg/dose IV slowly; for preterm infant, use D10W.

The following measures should be considered:

1. Naloxone (Narcan), 0.1 mg/kg/dose up to 2 mg IV. If no response and with suspicion of opiates, give 2 mg IV. Available in vials of 0.4 mg/ml and 1.0 mg/ml. Very large doses may be required for propoxyphene (Darvon) and pentazocine (Talwin) overdoses.
2. Consider thiamine, 100 mg/dose IV or IM initially and then bid PO for maintenance. Administer if alcoholism or malnutrition is suspected.
3. All metabolic abnormalities must be corrected. Rarely are anticonvulsants totally effective in the presence of a significant metabolic abnormality.
   a. Hypoglycemia: D25W, 0.5 to 1.0 g (2-4 ml)/kg/dose IV; then use extra glucose in maintenance fluids (at least D10W).
   b. Hyponatremia: 3% saline solution (0.5 mEq Na^+ per ml) given at a rate of 4 ml/kg over 10 minutes; then correct deficit over 16 hours.
   c. Hypernatremia: correct over 48 hours.
   d. Hypocalcemia: 20 to 30 mg/kg/dose IV (max: 500 mg/dose) of 10% calcium chloride slowly over 5 min.
   e. Hypomagnesemia: $MgSO_4$, 25 to 50 mg/kg/dose q4-6hr for three to four doses IM or IV slowly (adult: 1 g 10% solution IV slowly).

Anticonvulsants (see Table 81-6) should be considered, although the appropriate drug and the order of administration are controversial. Diazepam (Valium), lorazepam (Ativan), phenobarbital, or phenytoin (Dilantin) may be used. Diazepam or lorazepam are usually preferred for immediate termination of seizures; both require initiation of a second drug for long-term management. The risk of respiratory depression is thereby increased.

1. Diazepam (Valium):
   a. Dosage: 0.2 to 0.3 mg/kg/dose IV over 2 to 3 minutes at a rate of 1 mg/min. May need to be repeated in 5 to 10 minutes if seizures continue. Maximum total dose: child, 10 mg; adult, 30 mg.
   b. Although it is not preferred, rectal administration has been successfully used. Undiluted commercial IV

preparation is administered directly into the rectum through a plastic tube or angiocatheter.
   - An initial dosage of 0.5 mg/kg/dose PR is recommended

c. Intramuscular administration is unreliable, largely being dependent on site and method of administration. In adults there have been good results when diazepam is administered intramuscularly into the deltoid. Endotracheal administration may cause pneumonitis.

d. Peak effect: 1 to 2 minutes, with an anticonvulsant effect for 20 to 30 minutes.

e. Toxicity: respiratory depressive effect synergistic with that of barbiturates. Flumazenil (Romazicon) (0.1 mg/ml) may be used to reverse suspected benzodiazepine overdose. Pediatric dosage is 10 μg/kg/dose IV, which may be repeated. Adult dose is 0.2 to 0.3 mg IV, which may be repeated up to 3 mg; if only partial responses, total dose may be increased to 5 mg.

   NOTE: Intramuscular (and possibly intranasal) midazolam (Versed), 0.2 mg/kg, may be an alternative if venous access is unavailable. Further studies are necessary.

2. Lorazepam (Ativan):
   a. Dosage: 0.05 to 0.15 mg/kg/dose IV over 1 to 3 minutes at a rate of 2 mg/min. Repeated doses have decreasing effectiveness but may be considered. Maximum total dose in child, 0.15 mg/kg up to a total dose of 4 mg; adult, 2.5 to 10 mg.
   b. Intramuscular injection is somewhat erratic in absorption. Sublingual (0.05 mg/kg) administration has been used.
   c. Onset: 5 minutes (peak level: 45 to 60 minutes).
   d. Half-life: 16 hours.
   e. Toxicity: respiratory depressive effect synergistic with that of barbiturates. See flumazenil dosage given for diazepam.
3. Midazolam:
   a. Dosage: 0.15 to 0.30 mg/kg IM, resulting in cessation of seizures within 10 minutes.
   b. Buccally administered midazolam has been found, in one study, to be equivalent to rectally administered diazepam.
   c. Further studies are indicated.
4. Phenobarbital:
   a. Loading dosage: 15 to 20 mg/kg/dose IV; infusion not to exceed 1 mg/kg/min. Adult: 100 mg/dose IV q20min prn at a rate of 30 mg/min but not to exceed three doses. If more is given as a loading dose, clinician must be prepared to support blood pressure and ventilation. Although not preferred, phenobarbital may be given as a deep IM injection, but there is a somewhat erratic absorption. If status epilepticus does not respond, additional dose may be given.
   b. Maintenance dosage: 3 to 5 mg/kg/24 hr IV, IM, or PO.
   c. Therapeutic serum level: 10 to 25 μg/ml.
   d. Toxicity: respiratory depressive effect synergistic with that of diazepam or lorazepam.
5. Phenytoin (Dilantin):
   a. Loading dosage: 10 to 20 mg/kg/dose IV infusion (concentration of 6.7 mg/ml or less in saline solution, not water; not to exceed 40 mg/min or 0.5 mg/kg/min). Maximum: 1250 mg total dose. Fosphenytoin (Cerebyx), 50 mg/ml, is available for IV or IM administration with less toxicity and local reaction.
   b. Maintenance dosage: 5 mg/kg/24 hr IV or PO.
   c. Peak effect in 15 to 20 minutes.

   d. Therapeutic serum level: 10 to 20 μg/ml.
   e. Toxicity: cardiac conduction block.
6. Paraldehyde:
   a. Dosage: 0.3 ml/kg (maximum: patient <10 years old, 5 ml; adult, 10 ml) mixed 1:2 in mineral or vegetable oil (1:3 in neonate) and given rectally.
   b. Useful for intractable seizures. Contraindicated in presence of hepatic, pulmonary, or renal disease.

If seizure control is difficult, a neurologist should be involved in the pharmacologic management of the patient. A common practice is to use drugs in a sequential fashion until control is achieved. Although there is no agreement, many clinicians start with diazepam (Valium) or lorazepam (Ativan) and concurrently administer phenytoin (Dilantin) or phenobarbital. Another option is to omit diazepam or lorazepam and proceed directly to phenytoin or phenobarbital to avoid the marked respiratory depression noted in young children given diazepam or lorazepam, particularly in combination with phenobarbital. In children who have received diazepam or lorazepam, phenytoin has the advantage as the second drug because there is no synergistic respiratory depressive effect.

Patients with seizures that are still resistant after loading with phenobarbital and phenytoin may receive paraldehyde or other agents. Another modality for resistant seizures after administration of appropriate drugs is general anesthesia (e.g., pentobarbital, 5 mg/kg IV slowly, followed by 1-3 mg/kg/hr infusion). Respiratory support is required along with continuous blood pressure monitoring in conjunction with neurologic consultation. The barbiturate coma is followed with electroencephalogram (EEG), with dosage titrated to achieve a burst suppression pattern.

If the patient previously had taken an anticonvulsant and the levels are subtherapeutic, the maintenance dosage should be increased. If poor compliance is the basis for low serum drug levels, the patient should be given another loading dose (in full or part, depending on the level) and then educated about the importance of taking the medication. Close follow-up observation with measurements of drug levels is necessary.

Concurrently with the attempt to treat seizure activity with anticonvulsants, a therapeutic and diagnostic evaluation must be performed to determine the potential cause. For seizures with metabolic causes, correction of the underlying abnormalities, rather than additional anticonvulsants, is required. Mass lesions and cerebral edema, for example, need specific therapeutic intervention. Infections should be treated expeditiously.

DISPOSITION

All patients with status epilepticus should be admitted to the hospital to ensure ongoing control of seizure activity. When poor compliance with therapy is the causative factor, a period of observation (4 hours) after reloading may substitute for admission if intervention is possible in the home environment. Careful follow-up observation is required.

If seizures are refractory to normal medications, a neurologist should immediately be involved, and the patient admitted to an intensive care unit.

BIBLIOGRAPHY

Chamberlain J, Altieri M, Futterman C et al: A prospective, randomized study comparing intramuscular midazolam with intravenous diazepam for the treatment of seizures in children, *Pediatr Emerg Care* 13:92, 1997.

Dieckman RA: Rectal diazepam for prehospital pediatric status epilepticus, *Ann Emerg Med* 23:216, 1994.

Epilepsy Foundation of America Working Group on Status Epilepticus: Treatment of convulsive status epilepticus, *JAMA* 270:854, 1993.

Haafiz A, Kissoon N: Status epilepticus: current concepts, *Pediatr Emerg Care* 15:119, 1999.

Lowenstein DH, Alldrege BK: Status epilepticus, *New Engl J Med* 338:970, 1998.

Phillips SA, Shanahan RJ: Etiology and mortality of status epilepticus in children, *Arch Neurol* 48:74, 1989.

Scott RC, Besag FM, Neville BG: Buccal midazolam and rectal diazepam for treatment of prolonged seizures in childhood and adolescence: a randomized trial, *Lancet* 353:623, 1998.

Selbst SM: Office management of status epilepticus, *Pediatr Emerg Care* 7:106, 1991.

Towne AR, DeLorenzo DJ: Use of intramuscular midazolam for status epilepticus. *J Emerg Med* 17:323, 1998.

22 Sudden Infant Death Syndrome

Also See Chapter 13 (Apnea)

ALERT The child who suffers near-sudden infant death syndrome (SIDS) or an apparent life-threatening event (ALTE) requires aggressive resuscitation and support. Families who have lost a child through SIDS or ALTE should receive immediate and ongoing support.

Sudden infant death syndrome (SIDS) is the sudden death of a young child between 1 month and 1 year of age that is not predicted by history and in which a thorough postmortem examination fails to define an adequate cause of death. The peak incidence of SIDS is in infants 2 to 4 months of age; 88% of deaths occur in those younger than 5.5 months. SIDS commonly occurs in the fall and winter months; many children who die in this manner have experienced a recent respiratory infection. The overall incidence of SIDS in the United States has decreased with the onset of the "Back to Sleep" campaign, which has emphasized the benefits of infants sleeping on the back rather than on the side or prone. Supine sleeping results in a less quiet sleep and greater heart rate variability during the first sleep after a feeding.

As discussed in Chapter 13, near-SIDS is commonly referred to as an *apparent life-threatening event* (ALTE), which is characterized by a combination of apnea, color change (usually cyanosis but occasionally erythema or plethora), marked change in muscle tone (usually limpness), and choking or gagging.

ETIOLOGY

Multiple contributing factors (e.g., infection, sleep, poor growth, aspiration, maternal smoking or multiparity, absence of prenatal care, low birth weight, genetics) lead to respiratory obstruction and central apnea with associated hypoxia and death. Infants born to mothers who smoke have a reduced drive to breathe and a blunted ventilatory response to hypoxia, contributing to a higher risk of SIDS. Siblings of prior victims of SIDS or ALTE are also at increased risk. Although infantile apnea (see Chapter 13) may precede SIDS, no evidence suggests that it does so in most cases of SIDS.

Well infants who are born at term and have no medical complications should be optimally placed down for sleep on their back to reduce the incidence of SIDS.

DIAGNOSTIC FINDINGS

The child with SIDS has experienced irreversible cardiac and respiratory arrest. The child who has experienced near-SIDS or ALTE has variable vital signs, depending on the duration of cardiac and respiratory arrest before intervention.

Complications of Near-SIDS or ALTE

1. Pulmonary edema (see Chapter 19)
2. Aspiration pneumonia
3. Neurologic sequelae secondary to hypoxia, including seizures

Ancillary Data

1. An autopsy should be performed by a competent and experienced pathologist on all children with SIDS.

2. Supportive data should be obtained in accordance with procedures for resuscitation (see Chapter 4).
3. In the child with near-SIDS or ALTE, an evaluation for causes of apnea (see Chapter 13) must be conducted, including oximetry, electrolyte and calcium measurements, complete blood count (CBC), chest x-ray, and electrocardiogram (ECG). Infection and other metabolic abnormalities should be excluded. Evaluations may also include pneumography, polysomnography, continuous ECG recording, electroencephalography (EEG), and computed tomography (CT) of the head. Because gastroesophageal reflux is a common associated finding, a barium swallow study is usually indicated.

DIFFERENTIAL DIAGNOSIS

1. Trauma: Head trauma or child abuse may be difficult to distinguish in the absence of a reliable history.
2. Infection:
   a. Overwhelming and acute infection may occur; preceding signs and symptoms should be consistent with an infectious process.
   b. Central nervous system (CNS) infection (encephalopathy or meningitis) may have a similar presentation.
3. Congenital: Metabolic derangements, particularly those producing hypoglycemia (e.g., glycogen storage disease or severe acidosis) may result in apnea and seizures. Hypoadrenalism.
4. Gastroesophageal reflux or aspiration may contribute to ALTE.
5. Vascular:
   a. Subarachnoid bleeding may occur, with acute loss of consciousness and cardiac arrest.
   b. Cardiac dysrhythmias rarely occur in children.
6. Intoxication: Accidental or intentional poisoning can produce coma, with subsequent hypoventilation, arrest, hypoxia, and death.
7. Infantile apnea (see Chapter 13).

MANAGEMENT

The child with near-SIDS or ALTE needs rapid evaluation and resuscitation efforts (as described in Chapter 4). Admission to the hospital for ongoing management is indicated, usually in the intensive care unit. Eventually a pneumogram is required.

Intense psychologic support for families and friends is required, both immediately and on a long-term basis. Parents of children who die of SIDS normally demonstrate denial, anger, and then self-reproach and guilt. Verbalization of feelings, with reunion and ultimate separation from the child, are important. Assistance in arranging the funeral may be helpful.

Ongoing support must be ensured. Many communities have parents' groups. Where they are not available, contacting the Sudden Infant Death Syndrome Alliance, 1314 Bedford Avenue, Suite 210, Baltimore, MD 21208 (800-221-7437), may be helpful.

DISPOSITION

After stabilization in the hospital, the child with near-SIDS (ALTE) may be discharged. Counseling must be provided. Many of these patients should be started on chalasia regimens with slow, careful feedings and an upright position for 30 to 60 minutes after meals.

When appropriate, apnea monitors are available for home use. Although no evidence documents its effectiveness, sleeping on the back is also beneficial. Encourage "tummy time" for the awake child, for development and to prevent flat spots on the occiput. Children with gastroesophageal reflux or upper airway problems are managed individually. Long-term follow-up care provided by supportive health personnel is mandatory.

Well infants who are born at term and have no medical complications should optimally be placed down for sleep on their back to reduce the incidence of SIDS.

BIBLIOGRAPHY

AAP Task Force on Infant Positioning and SIDS: Positioning and SIDS, *Pediatrics* 89:1120, 1992.

Goto K, Mirmiran M, Adams MM et al: More awakenings and heart rate variability during supine sleep in preterm infants, *Pediatrics* 103:603, 1999.

Haglund B, Cnattingius S: Cigarette smoking as a risk factor for sudden infant death syndrome: a population based study, *Am J Public Health* 80:29, 1990.

Hunt CE: Sudden infant death syndrome, *Pediatrics* 95:431, 1995.

Paris CA, Remler R, Daling JR: Risk factors for sudden infant death syndrome: changes associated with sleep position recommendation, *J Pediatr* 139:771, 2001.

Ueda Y, Stick SM, Hall G et al: Control of breathing in infants born to smoking mothers, *J Pediatr* 135:226, 1999.

Willinger M, Hoffman HJ, Hartford RB: Infant sleep position and risk of sudden infant death syndrome, *Pediatrics* 93:814, 1994.

23 Syncope (Fainting)

ALERT Unless syncope is obviously self-limited, patients should be connected to a cardiac monitor and should be given glucose and oxygen. The history is essential to determining potential causes.

Syncope is a transient, acute loss of consciousness. It is generally caused by relative cerebral hypoxia or hypoglycemia. Although it most commonly results from benign conditions, cardiac, vascular, and infectious causes should be excluded.

The history must focus on recent medications, past medical problems, intercurrent illness, metabolic abnormalities, social interactions, and family history. The episodes of syncope must be carefully described in regard to the precipitating factors and accompanying signs and symptoms (Table 23-1). A history of syncope during exercise points toward cardiac disease such as aortic stenosis. Syncope should be characterized with regard to suddenness of onset and progression, duration, sequelae, and accompanying problems, such as seizures.

Syncope may be a prelude to a number of cardiac conditions, including prolonged QT syndrome and other dysrhythmias, hypertropic cardiomyopathy, and coronary artery anomalies. Significant problems may occur during exercise. Patients with such a history should generally be screened for the prior occurrence of exertional chest pain; syncope or near syncope, a history of unexpected or unexplained shortness of breath, a family history of premature death or significant cardiovascular disability in a close relative younger than 50 years, hypertrophic cardiomyopathy, dilated cardiomyopathy, long QT syndrome, Marfan syndrome, or dysrhythmia should be noted.

The physician should focus on cardiac and pulmonary status and should perform a careful neurologic examination. A head-up tilt test may be useful in reproducing syncope if associated with vasovagal reactions, neurocardiogenic syncope, or hyperventilation. Vital signs should include orthostatic measurements.

The patient with positional syncope has venous pooling with decreases in venous return, stroke volume, and cardiac output. This combination produces baroreceptor inhibition, increased adrenergic tone, myocardial contraction, and parasympathetic tone. Syncope may be blocked acutely in older children with metoprolol, 0.2 mg/kg IV. If there is a response, the patient may be treated with 1 to 2 mg/kg/24 hr PO given in two doses (morning and early afternoon). The dosage should be rounded to the nearest 25 mg/24 hr.

Ancillary data may include a chest x-ray study, two-dimensional (2D) or Doppler echocardiogram; electrolyte, Ca^{++}, Ma^{++}, and glucose concentrations; complete blood count (CBC); and drug screening. An electrocardiogram (ECG) (Holter monitoring as indicated) should be obtained if there was a significant episode of syncope, especially if accompanied by any associated signs and symptoms. Measurement of arterial blood gases (ABGs) (or oximetry) is sometimes helpful, but procedures such as electroencephalogram (EEG) and computed tomography (CT) are not routinely needed unless indicated by the history or

TABLE 23-1 Syncope: Diagnostic Considerations

Condition	Diagnostic Findings	Comments
INTRAPSYCHIC (Chapter 83)		
Hyperventilation	Rapid and deep respirations; secondary weakness, tingling, numbness of hands; feeling of dyspnea	Response to anxiety; common in adolescents; responds to rebreathing
Breath holding (p. 740)	Cyanosis and frequent unconsciousness after vigorous crying	Usually self-limited; triggers usually easily defined (e.g., crying, anger)
Hysteria	No preceding nausea, vomiting, or somatic symptoms; no anxiety; avoids injury (falls while sitting)	Responds to environmental stimulus, unconscious; adolescents (females)
VASCULAR (decreased cardiac output)		
Vasomotor (vasovagal)	Rapid drop in blood pressure (BP), bradycardia; accompanying nausea, vomiting, sweating, pallor, numbness, blurred vision, weakness	Precipitated by fear, pain, anxiety, noxious stimuli; usually in hot, humid, closed space; common in adolescents; vasodilation and decreased vascular resistance
Postural hypotension (orthostatic)	Episode follows prolonged standing or upon rising from a recumbent position; orthostatic changes variably present on examination	Poor cerebral perfusion initially; avoid rapid position changes; check hematocrit (Hct), BP standing and supine
Neurocardiogenic	Episode follows standing	Overlap with vasomotor and postural hypotension
Congenital or acquired heart disease (Chapter 16) Pulmonary stenosis Aortic stenosis Tetralogy of Fallot	Cardiac murmur, low output with poor perfusion, pallor, variable large pulse pressure	Poor cerebral perfusion
Congestive heart failure (Chapter 16)	Tachypnea, dyspnea, rales, wheezing, tachycardia, cardiomegaly, diaphoresis, cyanosis	Poor cerebral perfusion
Dysrhythmia (Chapter 6) Heart block Others Prolonged QT syndrome	Bradycardia, irregular rhythm	Stokes-Adams attack: ECG required; if finding normal, Holter monitor and exercise evaluation; Ca^{++}, Mg^{++}, echocardiogram; antidysrhythmics
Supraventricular tachycardia Ventricular tachycardia WPW	Abnormal rhythm, rate, poor perfusion; vital signs variable	
Hypertension, malignant (Chapter 18)	Headache, dizziness, visual change, nausea, vomiting; variable change in mental status and focal neurologic signs	May require treatment for encephalopathy
Posttussive cough	Episode after coughing	Caused by decreased venous return; may require cough suppressant

VI

Urgent Complaints

24 Acute Abdominal Pain

Also See Chapter 76 (Gastrointestinal Disorders)

ALERT Severe abdominal pain lasting more than 6 hours in a previously well patient usually requires surgery; evaluation and support are always indicated.

Acute abdominal pain in the child presents a diagnostic dilemma. The most common medical problem is acute gastroenteritis, although more serious causes must be excluded. Beyond this, the clinician must synthesize historical and physical data with anatomic and physiologic considerations.

ETIOLOGY

Diffuse abdominal pain results from one of several processes. A ruptured viscus produces peritonitis with rebound, guarding, and tenderness, commonly accompanied by sepsis and shock. Abdominal distension with high-pitched sounds and minimal rebound results from intestinal obstruction. Systemic disease may produce a diffuse pattern.

Pain that is sudden in onset may be related to a perforation, intussusception, ectopic pregnancy, or torsion, whereas a more insidious pattern is associated with appendicitis, pancreatitis, or cholecystitis. Colicky pain is usually related to intestinal abnormality as well as the biliary tree, pancreatic duct, uterus, or fallopian tube.

Pain is commonly referred. Diaphragmatic involvement from such entities as basilar pneumonia, subphrenic abscess, pleurisy, pancreatitis, peritonitis, or disease of the spleen, gallbladder, or liver may produce shoulder pain, which may be bilateral if the median segment of the diaphragm is irritated. Testicular pain may represent renal or appendiceal abnormality. Complaints of back pain may be referred from a retroperitoneal hematoma, pancreatitis, or uterine or rectal disease. Pelvic abscesses may not produce diffuse peritonitis because of the relative absence of sensory innervation in that region.

Common diagnostic considerations vary with the age of the child. In the *infant* acute gastroenteritis is most common, but it is essential to exclude intussusception, volvulus, perforated viscus, incarcerated hernia, colic, and Hirschsprung's disease. In *preschool* children the most common underlying causes of acute abdominal pain are acute gastroenteritis, urinary tract infections, trauma, appendicitis, pneumonia, viral syndromes, and constipation. The *school-age* child often has acute gastroenteritis, urinary tract infection, trauma, appendicitis, gynecologic entities such as pelvic inflammatory disease (PID) or ectopic pregnancy, inflammatory bowel disease, functional pain, constipation, or a viral syndrome associated with the pain.

DIAGNOSTIC FINDINGS

The history must define the acuteness and progression of the pain and its timing, quality, location, radiation, severity, and effect on activity.

Factors that worsen or lessen the pain may provide clues. The potential for referred pain must be considered. If the pain is recurrent, events surrounding the initial episode and the nature of the subsequent pain should be defined. The response to therapeutic trials such

TABLE 24-1 Acute Abdominal Pain: Diagnostic Considerations

	Infection/Inflammation	Congenital	Trauma	Endocrine/Metabolic	Other
SYSTEMIC	**Influenza** Acute rheumatic fever	Sickle cell disease	Black widow spider bite	Diabetic ketoacidosis Porphyria Uremia Hyperparathyroidism Hypothyroidism	**Constipation, functional** Henoch-Schönlein purpura Neoplasm: leukemia, lymphoma, neuroblastoma Lead, heavy metal poisoning
SKIN	Herpes zoster Cellulitis		Contusion		
ABDOMINAL WALL		Hernia—inguinal, umbilical	Retroperitoneal hematoma		
PULMONARY	Pneumonia Pleurodynia				
GASTRO-INTESTINAL	**Acute gastroenteritis** (virus, bacteria, parasite) **Mesenteric adenitis** **Appendicitis** Gastritis Hepatitis Cholecystitis, cholelithiasis Pancreatitis Esophagitis Diverticulitis Peptic ulcer Peritonitis	Meckel's diverticulum Volvulus Intussusception Hiatal hernia Hirschsprung's disease	Laceration: spleen, liver Perforation Intramural hematoma Pancreatic pseudocyst		**Colic** Mesenteric infarct Ulcerative colitis Regional enteritis Neoplasm
URINARY	**Pyelonephritis** **Cystitis**	Hydronephrosis	Renal contusion	Renal stone	Wilms' tumor
GENITAL	**Pelvic inflammatory disease** Salpingitis Tuboovarian abscess Epididymitis/oophoritis	Testicular torsion		**Mittelschmerz** **Dysmenorrhea** Hematocolpos Ovarian cyst Threatened abortion Ectopic pregnancy	
OTHER	Osteomyelitis Pelvic abscess		Pelvic or vertebral fracture Herniated disk		Lactose intolerance Dissecting aortic aneurysm Abdominal epilepsy

as antacids often focuses on specific disease processes.

Associated vomiting, diarrhea, nausea, dysuria, frequency, vaginal discharge, and other systemic signs and symptoms must be carefully delineated. Menstrual history should be defined. Concurrent events such as toilet training, stress at home or school, and trauma may be contributory. Secondary gain from the abdominal pain may require attention.

Physical examination must include vital signs (including orthostatic responses), temperature, and an overall assessment of the appearance and hydration status of the patient. The chest must be examined. The abdomen should be auscultated to assess bowel sounds and then palpated for masses and evidence of rebound, guarding, tenderness, and psoas or obturator sign. Hyperesthesia indicates parietal peritoneum inflammation. Rectal examination, with specimen testing for occult blood and polymorphonuclear leukocytes, is indicated in most patients. A pelvic examination should be performed in all pubescent female patients with lower abdominal pain or any signs of pelvic disease.

Laboratory evaluation should include a urinalysis in all patients and, in those with severe pain, a complete blood count (CBC) and measurements of electrolytes and blood glucose. Gonorrhea cultures and a Pap smear should be done if a pelvic examination is performed. Abdominal (supine and upright) and posteroanterior and lateral chest x-ray films may be helpful. Abdominal radiographs are particularly helpful in patients with prior abdominal surgery, foreign body ingestion, abdominal distension, peritoneal signs, or abnormal bowel sounds. If there is a significant abnormality and further diagnostic evaluation is indicated, other useful studies that may be considered are erythrocyte sedimentation rate (ESR), amylase concentration, liver function tests (LFTs), pregnancy test, peritoneal lavage, ultrasound, computed tomography (CT), esophagoscopy, and contrast studies, including intravenous pyelogram (IVP), upper gastrointestinal (GI) series, barium enema study, and cholecystogram. See Table 24-1 for diagnostic considerations.

MANAGEMENT

The management of the patient with abdominal pain must reflect the severity, acuteness, and likely causes. Patients who must be seen immediately include those with prolonged, severe pain, high temperatures (>39° C), crying and doubling over with pain, associated trauma, potential dehydration, tachypnea or grunting; patients with more prolonged fever (>2 days) in whom progression of pain is made more comfortable by lying down should be seen on an urgent basis. Observation may be an important option.

Many patients with prolonged pain, particularly those with nausea, vomiting, or diarrhea, have fluid deficits and benefit from intravenous hydration during the evaluation process (see Chapter 7). Gastric decompression (nasogastric tube) also may be useful. Surgical consultation should be sought for all patients with severe pain and a significant abdominal examination finding. Pain relief may be administered after consultation.

A therapeutic trial of antacids may be useful if gastritis or esophagitis is suspected.

BIBLIOGRAPHY

Attard AR, Corlett MJ, Kidner NJ et al: Safety of early pain relief for acute abdominal pain, *BMJ* 305:554, 1997.

Miltenburg DM, Schaffer R, Breslin T et al: Changing indications for pediatric cholecystectomy, *Pediatrics* 105:1250, 2000.

Reef S, Sloven DG, Lebenthal E: Gallstones in children, *Am J Dis Child* 145:105, 1991.

Rothrock SG, Green SM, Hummel CB: Plain abdominal radiography in the detection of major disease in children: a prospective analysis, *Ann Emerg Med* 21:1423, 1992.

25 Abuse

Also See Chapters 56 (Evaluation and Stabilization of the Multiply Traumatized Patient) and 78 (Gynecologic Disorders)

SUZANNE Z. BARKIN

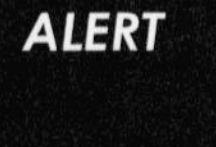

Suspicion is the key to recognition of abuse, particularly when the history and findings are inconsistent or a pathognomonic finding is present. All suspected or proven cases must be reported. Children must be medically stabilized when indicated.

Child Abuse: Nonaccidental Trauma

Children younger than 18 years who have a nonaccidental trauma (NAT) or physical injury that threatens their health or welfare are abused. Abuse may take any one of several forms, including physical or emotional abuse, neglect (physical, emotional, medical, or educational), and sexual assault. Consideration of abuse is mandatory in the evaluation of children who have suspicious injuries, particularly in emergency departments in which patients who are transient and whose care lacks continuity are seen.

DIAGNOSTIC FINDINGS

Unique interpersonal dynamics form the basis for potential abuse and identify children who are at greatest risk.

1. The abused child has the following characteristics:
   - **a.** Usually younger than 4 years
   - **b.** Often handicapped, retarded, hyperactive, or temperamental
   - **c.** History of premature birth or neonatal separation from parent(s)
   - **d.** Part of a multiple birth
2. The abusive parent has the following characteristics:
   - **a.** Low self-esteem, depression, substance abuse
   - **b.** Often abused as a child
   - **c.** History of mental illness or criminal activity
   - **d.** Violent temper outbursts aimed at the child
   - **e.** Rigid and unrealistic expectations of the child
   - **f.** Young parental age
3. The family in which child abuse occurs has the following features:
   - **a.** Monetary problems, often with unemployment
   - **b.** Isolation and high mobility
   - **c.** Marital problems
   - **d.** Pattern of husband or wife abuse
   - **e.** Poor parent-child relationships
   - **f.** History of unwanted pregnancies, illegitimate children, or youthful marriage

The introduction of one of the following triggers exacerbates the individual and family stresses, possibly resulting in child abuse: a family argument, a discipline problem, substance abuse, loss of a job, eviction, illness, and other environmental stresses. The child is often brought for care with a complaint other than the one associated with abuse or neglect ("somatic complaint").

Characteristics of History

1. Injury is inconsistent with the history
2. Parents are reluctant to give information or deny knowledge of how trauma might have occurred
3. Child is developmentally incapable of specified self-injury (e.g., 9-month-old falling off tricycle)
4. Response to severity of the injury is inappropriate
5. There was a delay in seeking health care

Physical Examination (Table 25-1)

Bruises on the skin go through a typical evolutionary pattern that is useful in relating the objective findings to the history. The age of the bruise should be only one criterion in a child's evaluation because the accuracy of timing is limited. Factors to consider include the following:

1. Bruise with any yellow is older than 18 hours
2. Red, blue and purple, or black coloring may occur at any time from 1 hour after injury to resolution
3. Red may be present in any bruise, irrespective of age
4. Bruises of identical age and cause on the same person may look different

The mechanism of a *burn* may be distinguished by physical findings. Accidental burns have an irregular pattern, often a splash configuration, and varying degrees of damage. Inflicted burns often have a clear line of demarcation without splash marks and with a uniform degree of burn throughout. Palm and sole burns suggest prolonged immersion in hot water.

Specific patterns include the dunking burn, in which the buttocks and genitalia are involved. Stocking or glove burns or doughnut-shaped burns may be noted after immersion injuries. Cigarette burns are usually second degree.

Retinal hemorrhage, although commonly associated with child abuse, has also been reported secondary to cardiopulmonary resuscitation, usually in children younger than 2 years (because of elevated intrathoracic pressures), as well as to accidental trauma, blood dyscrasias (leukemia, sickle cell disease), infections (Rocky Mountain spotted fever, tick fever), general anesthesia, intraocular surgery, and intracranial disease (aneurysm, subarachnoid hemorrhage, subdural hemorrhage).

Behavioral signs that may either provoke or result from abuse or neglect include the following:

1. Anger, social isolation, or destructive patterns, with evidence of negativism
2. Difficulty in developing relationships
3. Evidence of developmental delays
4. Depression or suicidal signals
5. Repeated ingestions
6. Poor school attendance and poor performance
7. Poor self-esteem
8. Regressive behavior

Ancillary Data (see Table 25-1)

1. *X-ray studies* are indicated for all children younger than 5 years to rule out unsuspected injuries in cases of physical abuse. For those older than 5 years, x-ray films are taken of areas of tenderness, deformity, etc.

   Skeletal injuries with high specificity for child abuse in infants are metaphyseal lesions and fractures of the rib (especially posterior), scapula, spinous process, and sternum. Injuries with moderate specificity are multiple fractures (especially bilateral), fractures of different ages, epiphyseal separation, vertebral body fractures and subluxations, digital fractures, and complex skull fractures. Common but nonspecific findings are subperiosteal bone formation, clavicular fractures, long

TABLE 25-1 Differential Diagnosis of Child Abuse

DIAGNOSTIC FINDINGS		
Physical Examination	**Ancillary Data**	**Differential Diagnosis**
CUTANEOUS LESIONS		
Bruising (rope, tie, bite, cigarette burns)	History	Trauma, accidental
	Bleeding screen	Hemophilia, von Willebrand
	Sepsis workup	Henoch-Schönlein purpura
	Sepsis workup	Purpura fulminans/meningococcemia
	CBC, bone marrow	Malignancy—leukemia
	History	Mongolian spot
Local erythema or bullae	History	Burn, accidental
(abrasion or burns)	Culture, Gram stain	Impetigo, cellulitis
(shape delineated)	History, sensitizing agent	Contact dermatitis or photodermatitis
SKELETAL PROBLEMS (Chapters 66–70)		
Fractures (multiple, unexplained, various stages of healing, metaphyseal or epiphyseal, subperiosteal ossification)	History	Trauma, accidental
	Radiograph, blue sclera	Osteogenesis imperfecta
	Nutritional history, levels	Nutritional deficiency, copper, rickets, scurvy
	History	Birth trauma
	Complete blood count, bone marrow	Malignancy—leukemia, neuroblastoma
	History	Neurogenic sensory deficit
	Serology	Syphilis
	History	Drugs—prostaglandin, methotrexate, vitamin A toxicity
ACUTE ABDOMEN (Chapters 24 and 63)		
Lacerated/contused liver, spleen, kidney, intramural hematoma, retroperitoneal hematoma	History	Trauma, accidental
	Radiographs, stool tests, etc.	GI disease (obstruction, peritonitis, inflammatory bowel disease)
	Urinalysis, culture	Urinary tract infection, anomaly
	Ultrasound, IVP	Other (e.g., genital problem, mesenteric adenitis, hernia)
	Specific studies	
MENTAL STATUS CHANGE (Chapter 15, 54, and 57)		
	CT scan	Trauma, accidental (subdural, epidural, intracranial)
	Drug screen	Intoxication
	Lumbar puncture	Meningitis
	Specific studies	Hypoglycemia, methylmalonic acidemia
OCULAR FINDINGS (Chapter 59 and p. 635)		
Retinal hemorrhage	History	Trauma, accidental or resuscitation
	Bleeding screen	Bleeding disorder
Conjunctival hemorrhage	History	Trauma, accidental or coughing
	History	Conjunctivitis
Hyphema	History	Trauma, accidental
SUDDEN INFANT DEATH (Chapter 22)		
	Sepsis workup	Infection
	History, autopsy	Trauma, accidental, SIDS

bone shaft fractures, and linear skull fractures.

The standard skeletal survey using high-resolution, high-contrast techniques may include:

a. *Appendicular skeleton*: humeri (AP), forearms (AP), hands (oblique PA), femurs (AP), lower legs (AP), feet (AP).
b. *Axial skeleton*: thorax (AP and lateral), pelvis (AP, including middle and lower lumbar spine), lumbar spine (lateral), cervical spine (lateral), skull (frontal and lateral).

2. A bleeding screen (see Chapter 29) is appropriate if there is a history of recurrent bruising and bruising is the predominant manifestation of abuse. Is usually performed as an elective procedure.
3. Specific studies as indicated. For example, methylmalonic acidemia is a genetic disorder leading to an accumulation of propionic acid; the condition may be seen with lethargy caused by central nervous system (CNS) hemorrhage.

DIFFERENTIAL DIAGNOSIS

See Table 25-1 for differential diagnosis.

MANAGEMENT (Fig. 25-1)

The key to management of child abuse is early recognition of actual and potential abuse situations. Of course, the immediate medical problems must receive attention.

1. Evaluate the family and the child's environment in a nonjudgmental and supportive fashion. A social worker should be involved in this phase of the evaluation.
2. Determine the extent of ongoing risk to the child.
3. Contact the appropriate protective services worker immediately. *There is a legal obligation to report suspected abuse.* A representative of the agency will discuss the case and arrange for involvement of a staff member. A full written report is required within 24 to 48 hours (depending on the state). Each hospital should have its own routine for expediting this process. Usually a special form is completed and forwarded with the encounter form.

DISPOSITION

Hospitalization is indicated when it is medically appropriate, in the absence of an alternative placement facility, or if the child cannot return home because of ongoing danger. The child should not be discharged until the medical problems are receiving appropriate treatment, social and protective services have agreed on a temporary disposition, and the case has been fully evaluated.

Optimally, a temporary crisis center is utilized if the patient is medically stable. If there is no ongoing risk, the patient may be discharged and sent home, with close monitoring and continuing evaluation. Attention should also be focused on the potential of ongoing domestic violence. Follow-up observation for medical problems should be arranged before the patient is discharged.

Social services and protective services must arrange for continuing evaluation and management of psychosocial problems.

BIBLIOGRAPHY

American Academy of Pediatrics, Section of Radiology: Diagnostic imaging of child abuse, *Pediatrics* 105:1345, 2000.

Dumaine AC, Christian CW, Rorke LB et al: Nonaccidental head injury in infants: the "shaken baby syndrome," *New Engl J Med* 338:1822, 1998.

Gayle MO, Kissoon N, Hered RW et al: Retinal hemorrhage in the young child: a review of etiology, predisposed conditions and clinical implications, *J Emerg Med* 13:233, 1995.

Hartley LM, Khwaja OS, Verity CM: Glutaric aciduria type 1 and nonaccidental head injury, *Pediarics* 107:174, 2001.

Hymel KP, Abshire TC, Luckey DW et al: Coagulopathy in pediatric abusive head trauma, *Pediatrics* 99:371, 1977.

Johnson DC, Braum D, Friendly D: Accidental head trauma and retinal hemorrhage, *Neurosurgery* 33:231, 1993.

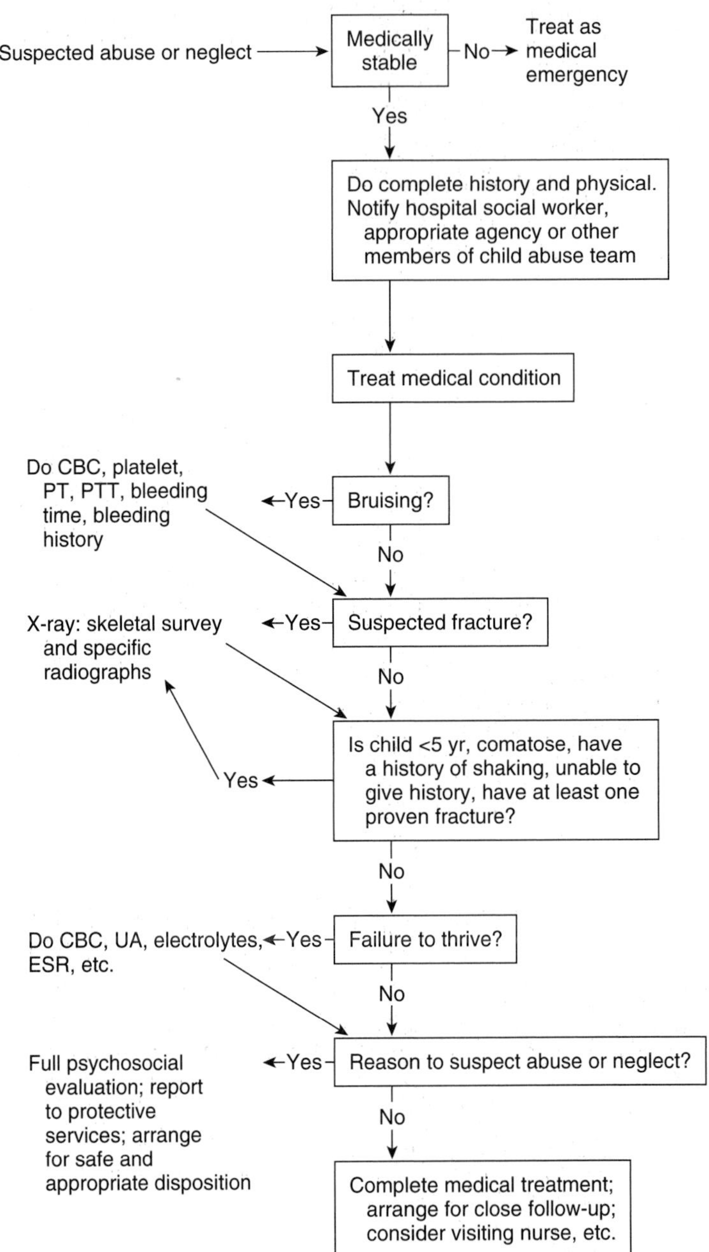

Fig. 25-1 Management of suspected child abuse.

Kleinman PK: *Diagnostic imaging of child abuse,* ed 2, St Louis, 1998, Mosby.

Schwartz AJ, Ricci LR: How accurately can bruises be aged in abused children? literature review and synthesis, *Pediatrics* 97:254, 1996.

Stewart GM, Rosenberg NM: Conditions mistaken for child abuse, part I and II, *Pediatr Emerg Care* 12:116, 217, 1996.

Wright RJ, Wright RO, Isaac NE: Response to battered mothers in the pediatric emergency department: a call for an interdisciplinary approach to family violence, *Pediatrics* 99:186, 1997.

Sexual Abuse

Sexual assault—rape, molestation, or incest—may occur at any age. Evaluation and management require considerable suspicion and sensitivity. Young boys as well as girls may be victims. Appropriate authorities should be notified, and the assessment must reflect local guidelines.

DIAGNOSTIC FINDINGS

Initially, confidence and rapport must be established with the patient. When a young child has been sexually assaulted, it is often the parent who is most upset. A detailed history of the incident must be documented. In addition, information about the medical history, menstrual and pregnancy history, contraceptive status, recent intercourse, and bathing or douching since the assault should be obtained.

The examination should be individualized, and with younger children, the mother should usually be present. Time, patience, and gentleness are needed. Patients who experienced severe assault may be angry and withdrawn.

The child's general appearance must be assessed, and signs of external trauma, abrasions, lacerations, contusions, bites, and child abuse noted. An internal examination is often not required in infants and young children. Younger girls often can be examined in the froglike position; older ones may require the lithotomy position (p. 676).

The patient with acute trauma has perineal contusions or lacerations and hymenal tears with bleeding, fissures, erythema, and discharge. The uterus and adnexa may be tender. Signs of chronic molestation are residual findings of hymenal remnants, healed lacerations, a large introitus, and discharge (p. 682). A hymenal diameter of 4 mm may be associated with sexual abuse. Less than 1 mm of hymenal tissue at the 6 o'clock position is generally found only in victims of abuse. However, there is tremendous natural variation in the shape and location of the opening of the hymen, and the assessment should be regarded as only one component of the evaluation.

Beyond the neonatal period, nonsexual transmission of sexually transmitted diseases is uncommon in prepubescent females. In general, sexual abuse should be considered in infants and prepubertal children with any of the following:

1. Genital or rectal *Chlamydia trachomatis* or herpes simplex virus
2. Genital or pharyngeal *Neisseria gonorrhoeae*
3. Anogenital warts in children older than 2 years
4. Human immunodeficiency virus (HIV) infection or syphilis in an infant or child whose mother is seronegative for the disease
5. Vaginal *Trichomonas vaginalis*
6. *Phthirus pubis* (crab louse) infestations of the eyelashes

Complications

Emotional trauma varies with the age of the victim and the circumstances of the assault.

Ancillary Data

1. Specimens and data are used to assist in documenting the circumstances and appropriately treating the patient. Many centers have kits for collecting specimens. Their use should be individualized. However, their value is minimal if more than 48 hours have elapsed or if the patient has bathed since the assault.
2. Culture specimens are taken from the cervix for *N. gonorrhoeae* and *C. trachomatis* as well as of the rectum and pharynx, if appropriate; further specimens are collected for culture 2 weeks after the assault. Antigen or nucleic acid amplification methods such as polymerase chain reaction (PCR) may be considered, given their enhanced sensitivity. Wet preparations are used to evaluate for trichomoniasis. A urethral swab may be useful in boys.

3. A wet mount preparation of vaginal discharge is made for *Gardnerella vaginalis* and *T. vaginalis* testing.
4. The Venereal Disease Research Laboratory (VDRL) (syphilis) test, a specimen for which is taken at the first visit, is also repeated in 2 weeks on a second specimen.
5. A pregnancy test (if appropriate) is used to determine status at the time of assault.
6. Vaginal fluid is collected to test for spermatozoa (wet and dried preparations) and the prostatic acid phosphatase concentration is studied.
7. Saliva for ABO-antigen typing determines whether the victim is a "secretor."
8. Hair specimens are obtained by combing the pubic area of the victim.
9. Clothing and other items are submitted for forensic examination when appropriate.

NOTE: To maintain the chain of custody, all specimens must be handled carefully and must remain in the physician's possession at all times until sealed. To ensure that the specimens are not altered before the introduction of the data in the courtroom, the "chain of evidence" must not be violated.

MANAGEMENT

The initial management of the patient must be supportive and understanding. The examination should proceed only after appropriate support services have assisted the patient and parents in dealing with the episode. Many institutions have specially trained individuals (often volunteers) to participate in this process. The examination must be individualized, reflecting the age of the child and the circumstances of the assault. If more than 48 hours have elapsed since the assault, specimens will be of little value. The episode must be reported to the appropriate child protective services agency.

Pregnancy may be prevented; a number of options exist for this purpose:

1. Yutzpe method: 100 mg ethinyl estradiol and 0.5 mg of levonorgestrel q12hr PO. Failure rate (rate at which the agent does not prevent pregnancy) is 2.5% if these drugs are taken within 72 hours of the event.
2. Progestin only: 0.75 mg levonorgestrel q12hr PO. Failure rate is 2.4% if the drug is taken within 48 hours of the event.
3. Do nothing, and await next menses.
4. Recheck result of monoclonal antibody agglutination to the beta subunit of human chorionic gonadotropin (hCG) test in urine or radioimmunoassay against the beta subunit of hCG in blood 7 days after the incident. If the result is negative, likelihood of pregnancy is low; if the result is positive, consider therapeutic alternatives.

Prophylactic antibiotic regimens for sexual abuse include the following:

1. Tetracycline, 500 mg QID PO for 7 days, or doxycycline, 100 mg BID for 7 days (*N. gonorrhoeae, C. trachomatis,* incubating syphilis). Tetracycline-resistant *N. gonorrhoeae* may be present. Do not use in children 9 years or younger.
2. For pregnant patient, 3 g amoxicillin plus 1 g probenecid, as single dose (*N. gonorrhoeae,* syphilis).
3. Erythromycin base, 500 mg QID PO for 7 days *(C. trachomatis)*.
4. Ceftriaxone, 125 to 250 mg IM (*N. gonorrhoeae,* syphilis).

Follow-up observation with appropriate support groups and health care professionals is crucial. The patient should be seen in 2 weeks to assess the reaction and collect specimens for second cervical culture and VDRL test. If follow-up care will be difficult, treatment for gonorrhea should be considered at the initial encounter (p. 683).

Presumptive antibiotic treatment of prepubertal children is not widely recommended because of the lower risk of ascending infection in this group.

Ongoing support may be necessary because of persistent problems.

BIBLIOGRAPHY

American Academy of Pediatrics: Guidelines for the evaluation of sexual abuse in children, *Pediatrics* 87:254, 1991.

Bays J, Jenny C: Genital and anal conditions confused with child sexual abuse trauma, *Am J Dis Child* 144:1319, 1990.

Berenson AB, Chacko MR, Wiemann CM et al: Use of hymenal measurements in the diagnosis of previous penetration, *Pediatrics* 109:228, 2002.

Dubowitz H, Black M, Starrington D: The diagnosis of child sexual abuse, *Am J Dis Child* 146:688, 1992.

Gardner JJ: Descriptive study of genital variation in healthy, nonabused premenarchal girls, *J Pediatr* 120:251, 1992.

Golden NH, Seigel WM, Fisher M et al: Emergency contraception: a pediatricians' knowledge, attitudes and opinions, *Pediatrics* 107:287, 2001.

Hermann-Giddens ME, Frothingham TE: Prepubertal female genitalia: examination for evidence of sexual abuse, *Pediatrics* 80:203, 1987.

McCann J, Voris J, Simon M: General injuries resulting from sexual abuse: a longitudinal study, *Pediatrics* 89:307, 1992.

Ricci LR: Photographing the physically abused child, *Am J Dis Child* 145:275, 1991.

Swanson HY, Tebbutt JS, O'Toole BI et al: Sexually abused children 5 years after presentation: a case-controlled study, *Pediatrics* 100:600, 1997.

26 Anemia

Also See Chapter 79 (Hematologic Disorders)

THOMAS J. SMITH and JULIE D. ZIMBELMAN

ALERT Anemia requires a systematic evaluation of hematologic parameters including hemoglobin (Hb), white blood cell count, and platelet count.

Anemia can be a manifestation of a primary disease, secondary to a systemic disease, or caused by nutritional deficiency. Because the hemoglobin (Hb) and hematocrit (Hct) values vary with age, anemia in children and adolescents is defined as an Hb concentration below the third percentile for the patient's age group (Fig. 26-1).

ETIOLOGY (Fig. 26-2)

Nutritional iron deficiency is the most common cause of anemia in children between 6 months and 2 years of age. It typically results from excessive intake of cow's milk (>24 to 30 ounces/day) and inadequate consumption of iron-rich foods as the child outgrows inborn iron stores. Iron deficiency in infants younger than 6 months is rare unless associated with prematurity or blood loss. Iron deficiency anemia in those older than 2 years should prompt an investigation for causes of chronic blood loss. Iron deficiency anemia may adversely influence performance on developmental testing; this effect may persist beyond correction of the anemia.

Anemias unrelated to iron deficiency can be divided into two major categories:

1. Anemias caused by impairment of red blood cell (RBC) production, maturation, or release from the bone marrow:

Disease	Mechanism
Malignancy: storage disease	Marrow infiltration
Fanconi's anemia, drugs, Blackfan-Diamond anemia, transient erythroblastopenia of childhood (TEC), aplastic anemia	Marrow aplasia or hypoplasia
Infection	Marrow hypoplasia or hemolysis
Folate, vitamin B_{12}, or copper deficiency	Impaired maturation of RBC precursors in bone marrow
Thalassemia syndrome, iron deficiency, lead poisoning, sideroblastic anemia, pyridoxine deficiency	Impaired Hb production, intramedullary hemolysis (thalassemias)
Chronic disease, inflammation, renal disease, hypothyroidism	Impaired erythropoiesis

2. Destruction, sequestration, or acute loss of circulating RBCs:

Disease	Mechanism
Sickle cell disease and other hemoglobinopathies, ABO or Rh incompatibility (in newborn), vitamin E deficiency, autoimmune hemolytic anemia, RBC enzyme deficiency, RBC membrane defect, hemolytic-uremic syndrome (HUS), disseminated intravascular coagulation (DIC), hemangioma, cardiac defect, prosthetic heart valve	Hemolysis

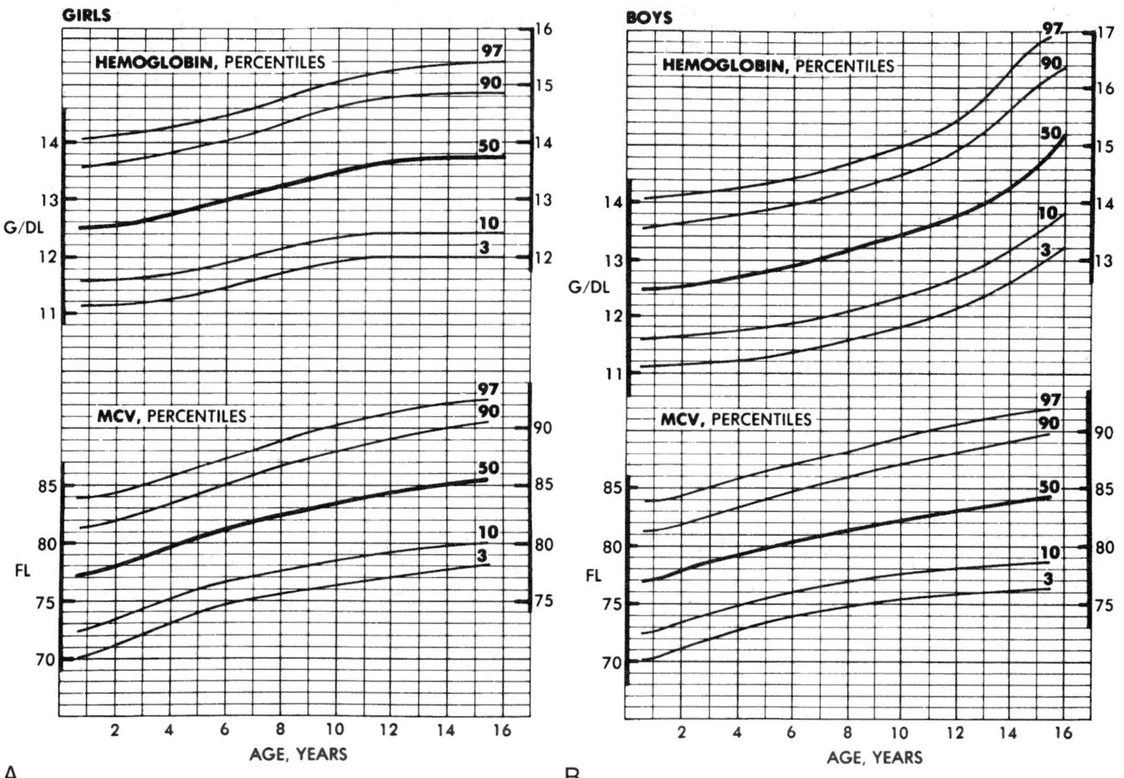

Fig. 26-1 Normal hemoglobin value by age. **A,** Hemoglobin and MCV percentile curves for girls. **B,** Hemoglobin and MCV percentile curves for boys. MCV, Mean corpuscular volume.

(From Dallman PR, Siimes MA: *J Pediatr* 94:26, 1979.)

Portal hypertension, sickle cell disease	Splenic sequestration
Trauma, surgery, bleeding disorder, peptic ulcer disease	Hemorrhage

The physiologic nadir of Hb level occurs at 6 to 12 weeks of age. In normal term infants the Hb level can drop to 9 g/dl, and in normal preterm infants, to 7.5 g/dl (see Chapter 11).

DIAGNOSTIC FINDINGS

Historically, it is important to consider age, sex, ethnic background, blood type (in infants), and dietary history (especially intake of cow's milk); to determine the duration of symptoms; and to inquire about chronic illness or infection, bleeding, and pica. Family history must be reviewed in regard to history of anemia, jaundice, gallbladder disease, splenomegaly, and splenectomy.

The presenting signs and symptoms reflect the severity of the anemia, the rapidity of onset, and the underlying cause.

1. With rapid onset of anemia (e.g., blood loss, sudden hemolysis), headache, dizziness, postural hypotension, tachycardia, hypovolemia, or high-output cardiac failure may be present (see Chapters 5 and 16). Intravascular hemolysis may manifest as these symptoms and tea-colored urine.
2. Insidious onset (e.g., nutritional deficiency, leukemia) is typically associated with pallor and decreased exercise tolerance.

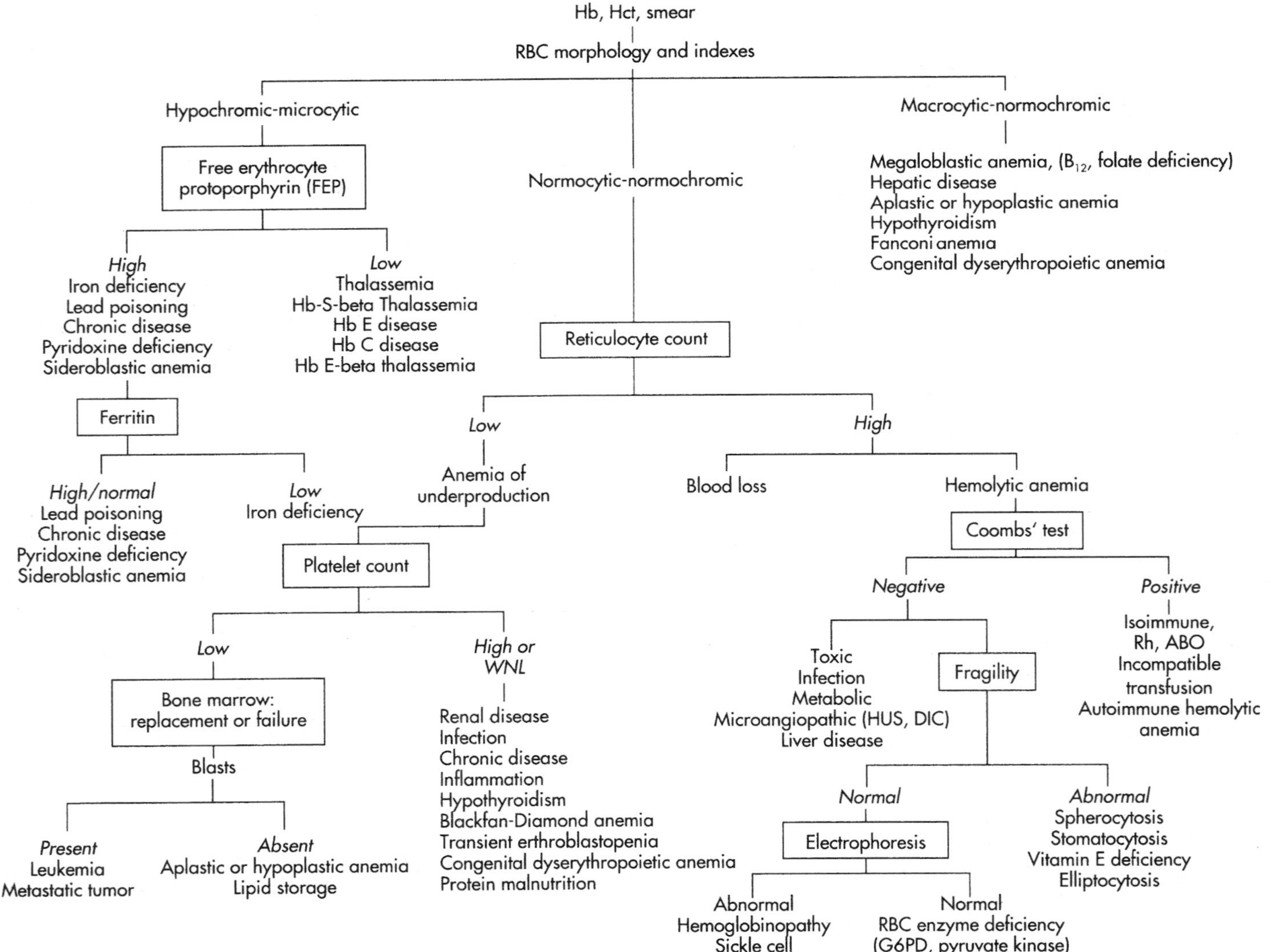

Fig. 26-2 Evaluation of anemia.

3. Children with iron deficiency anemia may display behavioral disturbances, learning problems, and delayed motor development. Severe iron deficiency disrupts the integrity of the gastrointestinal (GI) mucosa and may lead to a protein-losing enteropathy with blood in the stools, along with decreased iron absorption.
4. Hemolytic anemia typically causes jaundice and splenomegaly. If it is chronic, symptomatic cholelithiasis may develop during the teenage years. Underlying autoimmune disease (e.g., systemic lupus erythematosus) may be present.

Complications

Diminished oxygen-carrying capacity is generally well compensated for by an increased cardiac output. However, severe tissue hypoxia can occur if the anemia is rapid in onset or there is concomitant high-output cardiac failure.

Ancillary Data

1. Initial laboratory evaluation includes complete blood count (CBC) with measurements of Hb and Hct, RBC indexes, white blood cell (WBC) count, platelet count, peripheral smear, and reticulocyte count.
2. Anemia in association with microcytosis strongly suggests iron deficiency. For further confirmation, the free-erythrocyte protoporphyrin (FEP), iron saturation, or serum ferritin level should be determined. An FEP level greater than 3 μg/gm of Hb and a serum ferritin level of less than 12 ng/ml are typical of iron deficiency. Fasting iron saturation (serum iron/total iron-binding capacity × 100) of less than 20% also indicates iron deficiency but is subject to greater error because of diurnal and acute diet-related fluctuations in serum iron level. Serum ferritin is an acute-phase reactant and can be elevated in inflammatory states. An FEP level greater than 18 μg/gm of Hb strongly suggests lead poisoning.
3. Check stool for occult blood.
4. Perform other studies, as indicated in Fig. 26-2.

Samples for diagnostic studies to determine the cause of anemia are best collected before transfusion therapy, if such therapy is required.

MANAGEMENT

In children 6 months to 2 years of age with no history of blood loss or prematurity, a hypochromic, microcytic anemia is most likely caused by dietary iron deficiency anemia. It is appropriate to forgo iron studies and initiate a therapeutic trial with careful follow-up observation. Many authorities recommend that iron supplementation be started in breast-fed children at 9 months of age. However, in children older than 2 years, among whom nutritional deficiency is less common, a more extensive evaluation to confirm iron deficiency and exclude chronic blood loss is indicated.

For initial treatment of suspected iron deficiency anemia:

1. Prescribe elemental iron, 5 to 6 mg/kg/24 hr q8hr PO. Ferrous sulfate (Fer-In-Sol), 75 mg (15 mg elemental iron)/0.6-ml dropper, is a useful formulation. To replenish iron stores, the iron supplement should be continued for 2 months after anemia is corrected.

   NOTE: With good compliance, normal absorption, and no ongoing iron losses, the reticulocyte count should increase in 3 to 5 days, and the Hb level should begin to rise during the first week of treatment.
2. Encourage iron-rich foods.
3. Limit intake of cow's milk to 24 oz/day or less.
4. Blood transfusions should be reserved for patients with evidence of cardiovascular compromise.

Rapid-onset or profound anemia may produce life-threatening cardiovascular instability, requiring emergency intervention with blood products and fluids (see Chapters 5 and 16). Other forms of anemia requiring specialized evaluation and treatment should be handled on an individual basis in consultation with a hematologist.

DISPOSITION

Most children may be monitored as outpatients. Admission is indicated if the Hct is below 20% (Hb <7 mg/dl) or if there is evidence of cardiac decompensation, hypoxia, rapid ongoing blood loss, or hemolysis.

Parental education for iron deficiency anemia:

1. Give an iron supplement three times a day, preferably between meals to enhance absorption.

   If there is any nausea, the iron may be given with foods. Keep the medication in a safe place because accidental ingestion of a large amount can be dangerous.
2. Increase your child's intake of iron-rich foods such as meat, eggs, green vegetables, and enriched cereals and breads. Limit milk intake to 24 oz/day.
3. Take your child back for a recheck of blood counts in 1 to 2 weeks and at 1 and 2 months to be certain he or she is no longer anemic.
4. Vitamin C (200 mg Vit C/30 mg iron) may enhance absorption.

BIBLIOGRAPHY

Beutler E: The common anemias, *JAMA* 259:2433, 1988.

Eden AN, Mir MA: Iron deficiency in 1- to 3-year-old children, *Arch Pediatr Adolesc Med* 151:986, 1997.

Lozoff B, Jimenez E, Wolf AW: Long-term developmental outcome of infants with iron deficiency, *N Engl J Med* 325:687, 1991.

Walter T, De Andraea I, Chadud P et al: Iron deficiency anemia: adverse effects on infant psychomotor development, *Pediatrics* 84:7, 1989.

27 Arthralgia and Joint Pain

Also See Chapter 82 (Orthopedic Disorders)

ALERT Septic arthritis must be excluded in all patients.

Pain, swelling, and joint discomfort accompany arthralgia. If the joint is inflamed with accompanying redness, warmth, swelling, and pain, the patient has arthritis.

The patient or parents must be questioned regarding the nature of the joint discomfort or pain with specific reference to the progression of signs and symptoms: severity, duration, and type of pain, ameliorating factors, and family history. Any relationship to trauma and infection or systemic, vascular, or degenerative disease must be defined. Associated signs and symptoms, especially gastrointestinal, renal, and neurologic, should be sought. Knowledge of previous medical problems and exposures and consideration of the patient's age may be helpful.

The patient must undergo a careful examination of the joint, with particular attention to the severity of involvement—defining objective parameters, including warmth, tenderness, pain, presence of fluid, and limitation of motion. Hip pain may be referred to the knee.

Ancillary data are often essential. If a fever or an elevated erythrocyte sedimentation rate (ESR) (>30 mm/hr) is present, an infectious or autoimmune process is eight times more likely than if both are absent. Only 7% of patients with joint pain and both fever and elevated ESR have neither an infectious nor an autoimmune process. Radiographs should be obtained. Follow-up plain films are often useful, given that callus or periosteal reaction may not be present for 7 to 10 days in patients with hairline fractures or osteomyelitis. Complete blood count (CBC), blood culture, bone scan, antinuclear antibody (ANA) tests, and rheumatoid factor and immunoglobulin measurements may be selectively obtained.

If there is any question of the diagnosis and joint fluid is present, a joint aspirate should be obtained, usually after consultation with an orthopedist (see Appendix A-2). The procedure is usually contraindicated, however, if there is any overlying infection of the joint or if only small joints are involved. Typical findings are outlined in Tables 27-1 and 82-1.

A therapeutic trial of nonsteroidal antiinflammatory agents or aspirin may be useful in inflammatory diseases.

BIBLIOGRAPHY

Ilowite NT: Current treatment of juvenile rheumatoid arthritis, *Pediatrics* 109:109, 2002.

Kunnamo I, Kallio P, Pelkonen P et al: Clinical signs and laboratory tests in the differential diagnosis of arthritis in children, *Am J Dis Child* 141:34, 1987.

TABLE 27-1 Arthralgia and Joint Pain: Diagnostic Considerations and Management

Condition	Diagnostic Findings	Joints	Ancillary Data	Comments/Management
TRAUMA (Chapter 66)				
Sprain **Fracture**	History of trauma; joint tenderness, swelling; fracture may be occult	Usually monoarticular	X-ray study findings variable	Orthopedic consult; consider child abuse (NAT)
"Little League elbow"	Swelling, tenderness; pitcher's elbow	Elbow on dominant arm	X-ray study findings WNL	Restrict pitching
INFECTION				
Toxic synovitis of the hip (Chapter 69)	Preceding viral illness; nontoxic; often accompanied by limp; rarely warm, tender, limited range of motion	Hip	CBC, ESR: WNL; x-ray study findings—variable effusion; aspirate if question of septic arthritis	Self-limited; common in children 1½ to 7 years old
Arthritis, septic (p. 767)	Acute onset, febrile; local swelling, warmth, tenderness	Monoarticular, large weight-bearing: knee, hip, wrist, elbow, shoulder; rarely polyarticular (gonococcal)	↑ WBC, ↑ ESR; x-ray study findings; joint aspirate; may need bone scan	Requires urgent drainage and antibiotics
Arthritis, viral Rubella Rubella vaccine Hepatitis Epstein-Barr virus Chickenpox	Local swelling, warmth, tenderness; associated symptoms	Polyarticular; often large joints (knee)	CBC, viral titers, liver functions; x-ray study findings—effusion; joint aspirate	Usually self-limited
Arthritis, uncommon Mycobacteria Fungi Syphilis	Often indolent with subacute progression; joint swelling, tenderness	Usually monoarticular, large joints	Joint aspirate; CBC, syphilis serologic test, PPD, as indicated	
Osteomyelitis	Fever, variable systemic toxicity, local swelling, tenderness, warmth	Monoarticular long bones (femur, tibia)	↑ CBC, ↑ ESR; x-ray study; bone scan; joint and bone aspirate	Arthritis and osteomyelitis may be concurrent; antibiotics

AUTOIMMUNE				
Juvenile rheumatoid arthritis				
Acute febrile systemic (Still's) disease (30% JRA patients)	Irritable, listless, anorexic; hyperpyrexia (may precede arthritis); 90% have light salmon-colored maculopapular rash; organomegaly; lymphadenopathy; extraarticulor manifestations	Minimal or widespread; often only arthralgia; 25% severe arthritis	↑ CBC, ↑ ESR (70%); negative ANA, negative rheumatoid factor results	Peak onset: 1-3 yr; NSAIDs; if fails methotrexate, sulfasalazine; average age: 7½ yr
Polyarticular (25% JRA patients)	Listless, anorexic; low-grade fevers, daily spike; rare macu-lopapular rash; rare iridocyclitis	≥5 joints during first 6 months of illness (knee, ankle, wrist, elbow, hand); abrupt or insidious onset; swollen, red, tender; morning stiffness	↑ CBC, ↑ ESR (70%); positive ANA result (25%); positive rheumatoid factor result (10%-15%)	Trial of NSAIDs
Pauciarticular (45% JRA patients)	Low-grade to no fever; rare rash; iridocyclitis (25%)	<5 joints—knee most common during first 6 months of illness (others: ankle, elbow, wrist, fingers, sacroiliac); swollen, red, tender; morning stiffness	CBC, ESR: WNL; positive ANA result (25%), positive rheumatoid factor result rare; bone x-ray study finding: acclimated maturation, periosteal proliferation; synovial fluid aspiration	Average age: 7½ yr; trial of NSAIDs
Rheumatic fever (p. 575)	Carditis, chorea, rheumatoid nodule, erythema marginatum, fever	Migratory, polyarticular, involving knee, ankle, wrist, elbow, shoulder; joints swollen, red, tender, hot, and painful	Variable CBC, ↑ ESR; ↑ streptozyme, throat culture result variably positive	ASA trial; consider steroids; penicillin
Henoch-Schönlein purpura (anaphy-lactoid purpura) (p. 822)	Purpuric rash on ankles, buttock, elbow, beginning on lower extremity on extensor surface; abdominal pain, diarrhea, bleeding, intussusception; nephritis	Migratory polyarthritis of large joints	CBC, platelets: WNL; hematest stool, urine; ↑ streptozyme, throat culture	Monitor for renal failure

Continued

TABLE 27-1 Arthralgia and Joint Pain: Diagnostic Considerations and Management—cont'd

Condition	Diagnostic Findings	Joints	Ancillary Data	Comments/Management
AUTOIMMUNE—cont'd				
Kawasaki's disease (p. 726)	Persistent fever (<5 days), conjunctivitis, rash, mucosal membrane changes, migratory polyarthritis, erythema and induration of hand and feet		CBC, platelets: elevated; ↑ ESR, ↑ CRP	Specific diagnostic criteria; IV gamma globulin, aspirin
Systemic lupus erythematosus	Multisystem disease: weakness, fever, butterfly cheek eruption, hepatosplenomegaly, lymphadenopathy, nephritis; CNS: seizures, psychosis	Migratory; transient with arthralgia or redness, swelling, stiffness	↓ WBC, ↑ Hct, ↑ platelets; positive ANA result; variable hematuria and proteinuria	Prednisone, 1 mg/kg/24 hr PO; involve nephrologist
Serum sickness	Fever, rash, lymphadenopathy	Polyarthritis with redness, swelling, pain, stiffness, and large-joint effusion	↑↓ WBC; variable hematuria and proteinuria; reduced complement	Prevent exposure; antihistamine; consider NSAIDs or steroids
Inflammatory bowel disease Ulcerative colitis Regional ileitis	Diarrhea, variable rectal bleeding, abdominal pain	Polyarthritis, large joints	Sigmoidoscopy, barium swallow study	Antiinflammatory agents, possibly surgery
Reiter syndrome	Insidious onset; conjunctivitis, urethritis	Polyarticular, small joints	CBC, ESR: WNL, UA: WNL	Rare in children
CONGENITAL				
Hemophilia (p. 696)	Healthy male, variable history of trauma; history of hemophilia	Monoarticular; joint swollen, tender with hemarthrosis	X-ray study result; abnormal bleeding screen result	Factor replacement
Sickle cell disease (p. 714)	Systemic disease	Usually polyarticular; often insidious onset joint and bone pain	X-ray study finding: Hct; positive result of rapid sickle cell test (Sickledex); bone scan findings variable	May have concurrent infection; may be crisis or infarct
Developmental hip dislocation	Normal newborn except for instability of joint; presence of Ortolani's sign (abduction)	Abnormal placement and range of motion of hip	X-ray study result abnormal	Orthopedic consultation; splint hip in flexion and abduction

VASCULAR				
Legg-Calvé-Perthes (avascular necrosis of proximal femoral head)		Insidious onset; pain of hip with limp or limitation of movement; pain may be referred to knee	X-ray study result: bulging capsule, widening joint space, decreased bone density around joint	Peak: boys, 4-10 yr; orthopedic consultation; treat hip in abduction and internal rotation
DEGENERATIVE				
Slipped capital femoral epiphysis	Usually obese child or tall, thin child with rapid growth	Unilateral or bilateral; knee pain (referred) on medial aspect thigh above knee; hip or knee pain made worse by activity; limp; limitation abduction and internal rotation	X-ray study result: widening of epiphyseal growth plate	Peak: 12-15 yr; orthopedic consultation, surgical immobilization
OSTEOCHONDROSIS				
Osteochondritis dissecans	No systemic signs	Knee is painful, stiff with effusion	X-ray, tunnel view shows demineralization of medial femoral condyle	Teenagers; decreased activity; muscle stengthening
NEOPLASM				
Ewing's sarcoma Osteogenic sarcoma Leukemia Neuroblastoma	Systemic signs often present	Local pain, effusion, with warmth and tenderness	CBC; x-ray study; biopsy	Orthopedic consultation

28 Ataxia

ALERT Ataxia in children requires attention to the diagnostic alternatives that permit early initiation of therapy when appropriate.

Ataxia is a disorder that causes impaired balance and incoordination of intentional movement. Infectious and inflammatory processes and intoxication cause most incidents of acute ataxia in children. Hysteria, trauma, ear problems, sinusitis, migraines, and cerebellar and spinal cord tumors may also be causative (Table 28-1). Insidious onset of ataxia is a component of presentation in a host of congenital conditions (Friedreich's ataxia, ataxia

TABLE 28-1 Acute Ataxia: Diagnostic Considerations

Condition	Diagnostic Findings	Ancillary Data	Comments
INFECTION/INFLAMMATION			
Acute cerebellar ataxia	Prodrome of fever, respiratory or GI illness; abrupt onset; cerebellar ataxia; no evidence of intracranial pressure increase; normal mental function	CSF: WNL or slight lymphocytosis	Affects primarily 2- to 6-year-olds; resolves in 2-3 mo; usually viral (consider varicella)
Postinfectious encephalitis	Preceding headache, exanthem, stiff neck, fever; changed mental status; cerebellar ataxia	CSF: ↑ protein, lymphocytosis	Usually viral; usually resolves
Bacterial: meningitis/ encephalitis (p. 741)	Fever, toxic, stiff neck, changed mental status; cerebellar ataxia may be early symptom or postinfectious sequela	CSF: ↑ protein, ↑ WBC, ↓ glucose	Usually resolves after treatment
Cerebellar abscess	Fever, headache, cerebellar ataxia; may be signs of increased intracranial pressure	CT scan	Neurosurgical consultation
Acute labyrinthitis/ sinusitis	Cerebellar ataxia, vertigo, nystagmus, tinnitus, hearing loss, headache, nausea, vomiting; may accompany otitis media		May also be traumatic
Multiple sclerosis	Cerebellar ataxia; spastic weakness; optic neuritis, diplopia; multiple neurologic deficits; relapsing	CSF: ↑ cells, ↑ protein, ↑ gamma globulin	Steroids (ACTH); physiotherapy

telangiectasia) and metabolic disorders (Hartnup disease, maple syrup urine disease).

Neurologic findings should be defined historically. Progression, acuteness, and recurrence of ataxia and other neurologic findings should be assessed. Preceding events such as trauma, ingestion of drugs, infection, and respiratory symptoms should be delineated. A family history may be useful.

Cerebellar ataxia is associated with a wide-based, unsteady, and staggering gait, with difficulty in turning. The patient cannot stand with the feet together whether the eyes are open or closed (absence of Romberg's sign). *Sensory* ataxia from injury of the peripheral nerve or posterior column of the spinal cord also appears as a wide-based gait. However, the patient can stand with the feet together when the eyes are open but not when closed (presence of Romberg's sign). This often is associated with lethargy, stupor, and altered mental functioning, although ataxia may be the predominant finding.

Examination of the younger child must rely heavily on observation and cerebellar function demonstrated through play activities.

Ancillary data should usually include a spinal tap and serum drug levels, if indicated. A computed tomography (CT) or magnetic resonance imaging (MRI) scan may exclude mass lesions and increased intracranial pressure. Other tests must focus on potential causes.

BIBLIOGRAPHY

Chutorian AM, Pavlaxis SG: Acute ataxia. In Pellock JM, Meyer EC, editors: *Neurologic emergencies in infancy and childhood*, ed 2, Boston, 1993, Butterworth-Heinemann.

Peters ACB, Versteeg J, Lindeman J et al: Varicella and acute cerebellar ataxia, *Arch Neurol* 35:769, 1978.

TABLE 28-1 Acute Ataxia: Diagnostic Considerations—cont'd

Condition	Diagnostic Findings	Ancillary Data	Comments
INTOXICATION (Chapter 54)			
Phenytoin	Cerebellar ataxia, nystagmus	Level >30 μg/ml	
Phenobarbital	Cerebellar ataxia, lethargy	Level >50 μg/ml	Tranquilizers also
Alcohol	Cerebellar ataxia, slurred speech, visual impairment, progressing to stupor and coma	Level depends on whether use is acute or chronic	
Carbon monoxide	Headache, confusion, cerebellar ataxia, seizures, stupor to coma	CO elevated	Oxygen therapy, hyperbaric oxygen
Lead (also mercury and thallium)	Anorexia, vomiting, lethargy, cerebellar ataxia, increased intracranial pressure, papilledema, anemia; history of pica		Dimercaprol, EDTA
TRAUMA			
Head injury (Chapter 57)	Head trauma; headache; concussion; cerebellar ataxia	CT scan	Close monitoring
Heat stroke/exhaustion (Chapter 50)	Fatigue, weakness, headache, cerebellar ataxia, seizures, psychosis, coma	Electrolytes; variable ABG and ECG	Treatment varies with condition
INTRAPSYCHIC (Chapter 83)			
Hysteria	Anxious; inconsistent findings		Psychiatric consultation

CSF, Cerebrospinal fluid; *GI*, gastrointestinal; *WNL*, within normal limit.

29 Bleeding

Also See Chapter 79 (Hematologic Disorders)

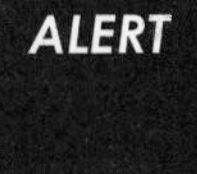

Patients with abnormal bleeding should be evaluated by an initial assessment that includes complete blood count (CBC), platelet count, and bleeding (BT), prothrombin (PT), and partial thromboplastin (PTT) times. Hemorrhage should be controlled when significant, usually by application of direct pressure. Resuscitation may be required with severe hemorrhage.

The evaluation of the patient with bleeding requires careful attention to the pattern of bleeding, its location, and whether it is spontaneous or a response to minor or major trauma. A history of bleeding problems should be pursued by asking about prior experience with procedures, such as circumcision, lacerations, tooth extraction, and menstruation, which typically cause transient bleeding. A family history may indicate a hereditary basis for the bleeding disorder.

The physical examination should classify the nature of the bleeding and ascertain its severity and any potential hemodynamic complications. Orthostatic vital signs may be helpful. If bruises or bleeding is unexplained or is inconsistent with the history, additional evaluation for child abuse should be considered (Table 29-1).

Ancillary data that should be obtained for all patients with excessive or abnormal bleeding include the following:

1. CBC, peripheral blood smear, and platelet count
2. Bleeding time (BT)
3. (PTT)
4. (PT) and international normalized ratio (INR)
5. Thrombin time (TT)
6. Fibrinogen level

TABLE 29-1 Patterns of Bleeding

Diagnostic Findings	Small-Vessel Hemostasis Defect (Platelet or Capillary)	Intravascular Defect (Coagulation)
Preceding injury		
None (spontaneous)	Small, superficial, diffuse bleeding involving mucous membranes (epistaxis, gastrointestinal, menorrhagia)	Major bleeding (musculoskeletal, central nervous system)
Superficial cut or abrasion	Profuse, prolonged	Minimal
Deep cut or tooth extraction	Immediate; good response to pressure	Delayed; poor response to pressure
Joint trauma	Hemarthrosis uncommon	Hemarthrosis common
Petechiae	Common	Rare
Ancillary data	Prolonged bleeding time Abnormal platelets	Prolonged partial thromboplastin time, prothrombin time

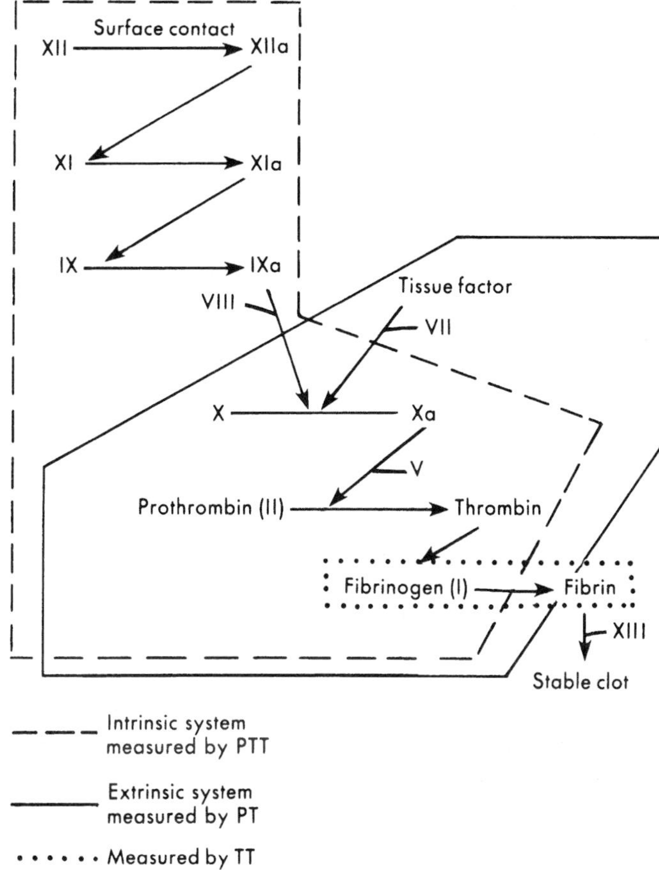

Fig. 29-1 Blood coagulation scheme.

These tests assess various components of hemostasis (Fig. 29-1) and, in combination with factor assays and platelet-function studies, define most common bleeding abnormalities (Table 29-2).

Once the disorder has been classified, specific management can be initiated in consultation with a hematologist.

BIBLIOGRAPHY

Bennett JS: Blood coagulation and coagulation tests, *Med Clin North Am* 68:557, 1985.

Clouse LH, Comp PC: The regulation of hemostasis: the protein C system, *N Engl J Med* 314:1298, 1986.

TABLE 29-2 Screening of the Bleeding Patient

Condition	SCREENING TESTS					Comments
	Platelet Count	BT	PTT	PT	TT	
NORMAL (WNL) (varies with lab)	150,000-400,000/ml	4-9 min	25-35 sec	12-13 sec	8-10 sec	Fibrinogen level 190-400 mg/dl
HEREDITARY DISORDERS						
Hemophilia						
Factor VIII (Classic: A)	WNL	WNL	↑	WNL	WNL	Factor assay
Factor IX (Christmas: B)	WNL	WNL	↑	WNL	WNL	Factor assay
Factor XI	WNL	WNL	↑	WNL	WNL	Factor assay
Factor XII	WNL	WNL	↑	WNL	WNL	Factor assay
Factor II, V, X	WNL	WNL	↑	↑	WNL	Factor assay
Factor VII	WNL	WNL	WNL	↑	WNL	Factor assay
vWF* (many variants)	WNL	↑	↑	WNL	WNL	vWF antigen, vWF activity, ristocetin cofactor
Platelet dysfunction	WNL/↓	↑	WNL	WNL	WNL	Platelet aggregation studies
ACQUIRED DISORDERS						
Disseminated intravascular coagulation (p. 694)	↓	↑	↑	↑	↑	↓ Fibrinogen level, ↑ fibrin split products, ↑ D-dimer, microangiopathy
Idiopathic thrombocytopenic purpura (p. 709)	↓	↑	WNL	WNL	WNL	Increased destruction of platelets—immune
Henoch-Schönlein purpura (p. 822)	WNL	WNL	WNL	WNL	WNL	
Liver failure (severe)	WNL/↓	WNL/↑	↑	↑	WNL/↑	↓ Fibrinogen level, ↑ fibrin split products
Uremia (p. 828)	WNL/↓	↑	WNL	WNL	WNL/↑	Secondary to hepatic dysfunction or protein loss
Anticoagulants						
Heparin	WNL	WNL	↑	WNL/↑	↑↑	Also lupus-like and inactivating anticoagulant
Warfarin	WNL	WNL	WNL/↑	↑	WNL	
Aspirin, other NSAID	WNL	↑	WNL	WNL	WNL	
Hemolytic-uremic syndrome (p. 819), thrombotic thrombocytopenic purpura	↓	Varies with platelet count	WNL	WNL	WNL	Platelet activation, microangiopathic hemolytic anemia, renal failure

* von Willebrand.

30 Constipation

ALERT Constipation is commonly functional, although organic conditions must be excluded.

Constipation is present when children have difficulty with bowel movements for longer than 2 weeks because of an abnormality in the character of the stool rather than solely frequency.

Guidelines to the frequency of normal stooling may be useful:

- 5 to 40 stools/week in breast-fed infants until 3 months of age (mean/day: 2.9)
- 5 to 28 stools/week in formula-fed infants until 3 months of age (mean/day: 2.0)
- 5 to 28 stools/week in children 6 to 12 months of age (mean/day: 1.8)
- 4 to 21 stools/week in children 1 to 3 years of age (mean/day: 1.4)
- 3 to 14 stools/week in healthy children >3 years of age (mean/day: 1.0)

With persistent pain and discomfort, frequency decreases. Elimination patterns reflect familial, cultural, and social factors. It is essential to determine whether the stool pattern being described is actually normal. Constipation in the newborn is often associated with an anatomic problem, but in older children it is usually functional (caused by voluntary withholding of feces to avoid unpleasant defecation) or dietary in origin.

ETIOLOGY

1. Dietary:
   a. Lack of fecal bulk, causing an inadequate peristaltic stimulus; inadequate intake of roughage
   b. Excessive intake of cow's milk and early introduction of solids such as cereals and yellow vegetables
2. Intrapsychic:
   a. Abnormal or difficult toilet training, voluntary retention, or habit; possible history of prolonged, difficult toilet training; or constipation may begin with an anal fissure and then be perpetuated
   b. Psychogenic; associated with parent-child and environmental problems and stresses; commonly fecal impaction, with secondary liquid stools soiling around the fecal mass (encopresis)
3. Trauma: Anal fissures appear as small tears at the anus, often accompanied by blood streaking of the stools and pain
4. Intoxication:
   a. Excessive use of suppositories and enemas, causing the bowel to be insensitive to normal physiologic peristalsis
   b. Excessive use of antihistamines, diuretics, calcium channel blockers, diphenoxylate (Lomotil), or codeine-containing substances
5. Congenital (see Chapter 11):
   a. Atresia or stenosis of the colon or rectum
   b. Meconium plug syndrome in newborns, associated with cystic fibrosis and Hirschsprung's disease

   c. Hirschsprung's disease (p. 662)
   d. Myelomeningocele and other neurologic problems
   e. Cystic fibrosis
6. Ileus secondary to infection or inflammatory bowel disease
7. Neurologic:
   a. Degenerative central nervous system (CNS) diseases
   b. Spinal cord abnormality or trauma, neurofibromatosis
8. Metabolic or endocrine:
   a. Hypothyroidism
   b. Hypercalcemia
   c. Hypokalemia
   d. Gluten enteropathy
9. Abnormal abdominal musculature:
   a. Prune belly
   b. Gastroschisis
   c. Down syndrome
10. Drugs:
    a. Phenobarbital
    b. Antacids
    c. Anticholinergics
    d. Sympathomimetics
    e. Antidepressants
    f. Opiates

DIAGNOSTIC FINDINGS

It is imperative to determine whether the stool pattern is abnormal and whether the constipation is an isolated finding or is associated with systemic signs and symptoms. The characteristics of the stool must be assessed with respect to frequency, consistency, color, odor, and previous patterns. Weight loss (or failure to thrive), fecal soiling, and the relationship to toilet training should be pursued. Common complaints are anorexia, tenesmus, and abdominal pain. The pain may be crampy or constant and is usually recurrent. Occasionally, it may be severe enough to mimic a surgical abdomen. Urinary incontinence and recurrent urinary tract infections may develop but generally resolve with relief of constipation. Personal and family stresses, behavioral issues, and maternal-paternal interactions should be evaluated.

Previous dietary manipulation and therapeutic trials should be determined with special attention to these changes, recent medications, and behavioral therapy.

Physical examination may demonstrate a palpable, cylindric abdominal mass. Bowel sounds are variable. Distension and minimal diffuse tenderness are often present. Look for perianal fissures, dermatitis, abscess, fistulas. The rectum is usually full of stool.

Ancillary Data

If the diagnosis is in doubt, abdominal x-ray films may demonstrate retained stool that is granular or rocklike in appearance. Stool should be assessed for blood. Ultimately, rectal manometry is diagnostic of aganglionic megacolon. Rectal biopsy or barium enema study may be useful.

MANAGEMENT

Simple Constipation

Usually, the elimination pattern is normal, and reassurance is all that is necessary after the determination that there is no organic cause. Generally, dietary manipulation is sufficient, depending on the patient's age, the severity of symptoms, and the level of parental anxiety. If constipation develops during bowel training, the pressure on training must be reduced.

1. For babies, add 1 to 2 tsp of corn syrup (Karo) to each bottle. If the child is older than 4 months, strained apricots, peaches, pears, and other fruits may be introduced. Avoid rectal stimulation with suppositories.
2. Older children should be encouraged to increase their intake of fruits and vegetables. These include prunes, figs, raisins, beans, celery, and lettuce. Prune juice is excellent and may be diluted with soda to improve the taste. Bran should be given in cereals, muffins, crackers, and other sources. Milk products may be

constipating in some children. Other fluids should be pushed temporarily.

3. Maltsupex (proprietary preparation of nondiastatic barley malt extract), increasing up to 2 tbsp/day BID PO, may be helpful. Docusate (Colace), 5 to 10 mg/kg/24 hr q6-12hr PO, may be initiated for 5 to 7 days.
4. Stool softeners may also be helpful in the child *without* impaction. Mineral oil (1-2 ml/kg/dose BID PO; adolescent: 60 ml/dose) may be used; emulsified forms have a better taste. This may occasionally be supplemented by laxatives to stimulate the bowel. Such agents include milk of magnesia (1 ml/kg/dose BID PO), senna concentrate (Senokot) (child <5 years, 1-2 tsp syrup; child >5 years, 2-3 tsp syrup), and Castoria (child <5 years, 1-2 tsp; child >5 years, 2-3 tsp).
5. Enemas and suppositories should not be given routinely.

Anal fissures usually disappear once the bowel movement pattern has improved. Very rarely, chronic fissures require surgical excision.

Long-Standing Constipation

Severe constipation in the older child, often with fecal impaction, requires a more aggressive approach after organic causes have been excluded. Cleanout may be accomplished "from above and below."

1. Perform fecal disimpaction by manual removal or by administering hypertonic phosphate enema (Fleet pediatric, 30 to 60 ml/10 kg/dose; adolescent: 120 ml/dose) the day after a dose of mineral oil has been administered. Add 100 mg docusate (Colace) to each enema. Enemas must usually be repeated once or twice.
2. Begin mineral oil at 1 to 2 ml/kg/dose up to 120 ml/dose BID PO for 2 to 7 days until the rectal effluent contains no fecal material. The dose may gradually be increased to 300 ml BID PO as a maximum. Senna concentrate may be used as an alternative.
3. Referral for complete psychologic evaluation, support, and follow-up observation may be indicated.

BIBLIOGRAPHY

Baker SS, Liptak GS, Collectti RN et al: Constipation in infants and children: evaluation and treatment: a medical position statement of the North American Society of Pediatric Gastroenterology and Nutrition, *J Pediatr Gastroenterol Nutr* 29:612, 1999.

Bulloch B, Tenenbein M: Constipation: diagnosis and management in the pediatric emergency department, *Pediatr Emerg Care* 18:254, 2002.

Dohil R, Roberts E, Verries Jones K et al: Constipation and reversible urinary tract abnormalities, *Arch Dis Child* 70:56, 1994.

Gleghorn EE, Heyman MB, Rudolph CD: No-enema therapy for idiopathic constipation and encopresis, *Clin Pediatr* 30:669, 1990.

Hoew AC, Walker CE: Behavioral management of toilet training, enuresis and encopresis, *Pediatr Clin North Am* 39:413, 1992.

Leoning-Baucke V: Urinary incontinence and urinary tract infection and their resolution with treatment of chronic constipation of childhood, *Pediatrics* 100:228, 1997.

Leoning-Baucke V, Cruickshank B, Savage C: Defecation dynamics and behavioral profiles in encopretic children, *Pediatrics* 80:672, 1987.

31 Cough

Also See Chapters 20 (Respiratory Distress) and 84 (Pulmonary Disorders)

ALERT Upper and lower airway disease may produce coughing. Patients should be evaluated for respiratory distress (see Chapter 20).

Coughing follows forceful expiration and opening of a closed glottis. An initial inspiration is followed by closure of the glottis. The intrathoracic pressure increases with sudden opening of the glottis and release of intrathoracic air and contraction of the diaphragm, chest, abdominal wall, and pelvic floor musculature. The cough reflex, which is controlled in the medulla, receives vagal stimuli from the pharynx, larynx, trachea, and other large airways, as well as the ear. A number of different stimuli trigger the reflex, including mechanical, chemical, thermal, and psychogenic factors.

ETIOLOGY AND DIAGNOSTIC FINDINGS

The predominant cause of coughing is upper respiratory tract infection (Table 31-1). Other significant causes vary by age group. In *infants*, structural abnormalities of the airway, gastroesophageal reflux, tracheoesophageal fistula, vascular rings, and physiologic mechanisms must be considered. *Toddlers* may have a foreign body, irritation of the airway (especially passive smoking), or asthma. *School-age* children often have asthma, sinusitis, or chronic rhinitis. *Adolescents* commonly have a cough caused by smoking or psychogenic factors. A chronic cough may be the only clinical presentation of reactive airway disease, but other entities to be considered with a prolonged cough include foreign body, unusual infection, and congenital anomaly.

The type of cough may be useful in considering specific differential diagnoses. Staccato, paroxysmal coughs accompany pertussis or chlamydia infections, but productive coughs imply a lower airway or parenchymal infection. Purulent sputum is associated with bacterial pneumonia, lung abscess, bronchiectasis, and cystic fibrosis. Coughs that worsen at night are usually caused by posterior nasal drips from allergy or infection, and coughs that improve during sleep often are psychogenic in origin.

Historically, it is imperative to determine the duration, frequency, quality, timing, and productivity of the cough. Inciting and ameliorating conditions should be defined as well as associated signs and symptoms such as fever, shortness of breath, wheezing, allergies, and growth pattern. A family history should be obtained, with particular focus on asthma, cystic fibrosis, tuberculosis, and any chronic pulmonary disease.

The physical examination must assess the patient's clinical condition, primarily in terms of a careful evaluation of the airway, lungs, and heart. Color, oximetry, respiratory rate, pattern, effort, retractions, and flaring should be noted. The level of respiratory tract involvement may be defined by the presence of stridor, wheezing, rhonchi, rales, altered breath sounds, and symmetry. Evidence of acute infection may be supported by the presence of fever, adenopathy, productive cough, rhinorrhea, or rash. Allergic disease usually has accompanying eczema,

TABLE 31-1 Cough: Diagnostic Considerations

Condition	Diagnostic Findings	Ancillary Data	Comments
INFECTION/INFLAMMATION			
Upper respiratory infection (p. 618)	Acute onset, prolonged course; rhinorrhea, congestion, fever, pharyngitis, laryngitis, nonproductive cough	Throat cultures, if indicated	Self-limited; vagal stimulation; also croup (p. 800)
Pneumonia (p. 811)	Variable onset; fever, tachypnea, anorexia, irritability, productive cough, pleuritic pain; hemoptysis (group A streptococcus, TB)	Chest x-ray study; CBC; oximetry, ABG as needed	Viral, bacterial, mycoplasma, tuberculosis, chlamydial, pneumocystis; antibiotics, if needed
Bronchiolitis (p. 797)	Wheezing, tachypnea, nonproductive cough, fever, relatively little respiratory distress early but may develop with cyanosis	Chest x-ray study; oximetry, ABG, if needed	Viral; children <1 yr; support, hydrate, bronchodilator (albuterol)
Aspiration pneumonia	History of incident or patient with reduced level of consciousness; fever, productive cough; respiratory distress may be delayed 12-24 hr	Chest x-ray study; serial ABG	May follow aspiration of gastric contents, bacteria, hydrocarbons; may be recurrent
Pulmonary abscess	Insidious; fever, malaise, anorexia, hemoptysis, productive cough; chest pain	Chest x-ray study; culture of abscessed material	Aspiration of infected material or complication of pneumonia; drainage, antibiotics
Pertussis (whooping cough) (p. 731)	Catarrhal phase followed by paroxysmal cough with cyanosis and vomiting; prolonged cough	Chest x-ray study; ↑ CBC (lymphocytes); fluorescent antibody	Hospitalize, support; erythromycin with catarrhal phase
Measles (Chapter 42)	Coryza, conjunctivitis, and productive cough, with generalized morbilliform rash, fever	Chest x-ray study if significant and prolonged	Self-limited; complications of secondary infection
Pleurisy	Sharp, intense pain, worsens with inspiration; irritative, dry cough	Chest x-ray study to exclude pneumonia, effusion	Self-limited; analgesia
Retropharyngeal abscess (p. 617)	Fever, difficulty swallowing, drooling, sore throat; irritative, dry cough	Lateral neck x-ray study, CBC, culture material	Incision and drainage, antibiotics, analgesia

Continued

TABLE 31-1 Cough: Diagnostic Considerations—cont'd

Condition	Diagnostic Findings	Ancillary Data	Comments
ALLERGIC			
Asthma (p. 781)	Wheezing, tachypnea, mild to moderate respiratory distress; nonproductive cough may be only symptom, unaccompanied by wheezing (may be induced by exercise); may be worse at night	Chest x-ray study; oximetry, ABG, pulmonary functions, as indicated	Responds to bronchodilator, steroids, oxygen
Posterior nasal drip (p. 618)	Prolonged, productive cough, often after respiratory infection; worse when lying down; rhinorrhea, bronchorrhea, congestion		Empiric treatment with decongestant before bedtime
TRAUMA			
Foreign body (p. 808)	If tracheal: partial or total obstruction of airway; bronchial: nonproductive cough, without accompanying illness; asymmetric wheezing	Chest x-ray study; inspiration and expiration; direct visualization	Remove by bronchoscopy; bronchial and <24 hr, consider postural drainage
Atelectasis	Fever, productive cough, hemoptysis; may have splinting; may be caused by trauma	Chest x-ray study	Postural drainage; IPPB
VASCULAR			
Congestive heart failure (Chapter 16)	Tachypnea, tachycardia, murmur, rales, wheezing, cyanosis, cardiomegaly, productive cough	Chest x-ray study; ABG; ECG	Diuretics, digitalis; evaluate underlying cause
Mitral stenosis	Dyspnea, cyanosis, pulmonary edema, CHF, hemoptysis	Chest x-ray study; ABG; ECG	Congenital or rheumatic; cardiology consultation
INTOXICATION			
Hydrocarbon ingestion aspiration (p. 385)	Initially asymptomatic, then in 12-24 hr tachypnea, fever; prolonged productive cough	Baseline and follow-up chest x-ray studies	Postural drainage; treat complications of secondary infection, central nervous system toxicity

CONGENITAL (Chapter 11)			
Cystic fibrosis	Chronic productive cough, recurrent pulmonary infection; frequent illness, poor weight gain; abnormal stools	Chest x-ray study; ABG, pulmonary functions; positive sweat test result	Postural drainage; antibiotics for acute exacerbations; dietary supplement
Tracheoesophageal fistula	Variable cough with feedings; poor weight gain, vomiting	Barium swallow study	Surgery
Diaphragmatic hernia	As newborn, acute-onset cyanosis, poor feeding, vomiting, nonproductive cough, respiratory distress	Chest x-ray study, barium swallow study	Surgery
NEOPLASM			
Pulmonary or mediastinal	Insidious onset, variable cough, hemoptysis, weight loss, chronically ill	Chest x-ray study; nuclear scan, biopsy	Refer to oncologist

boggy nasal mucosa, clear rhinorrhea, hypertrophic lymphoid follicles, or allergic "shiners."

Ancillary data must be individualized and may include a complete blood count (CBC), chest x-ray study (inspiratory and expiratory films if a foreign body is suspected), examination of sputum, pulmonary function tests, and specific studies, such as a sweat chloride analysis, sinus or neck x-ray studies, and barium swallow study, to explore diagnostic considerations. Arterial blood gas (ABG) analysis or oximetry may be useful in selected conditions.

Hemoptysis, or coughing up of blood often mixed with sputum (appearing red and frothy), is an unusual pediatric condition that may occur with a number of clinical entities.

1. Infection or inflammation
   a. Pneumonia: group A streptococci, tuberculosis
   b. Pertussis
   c. Pulmonary abscess
   d. Bronchiectasis, especially cystic fibrosis
   e. Viral infections: most common
2. Trauma: foreign body
3. Vascular: pulmonary hypertension, mitral stenosis, pulmonary embolism
4. Neoplasm: mediastinal or pulmonary
5. Bleeding diathesis
6. Idiopathic pulmonary hemosiderosis
7. After an acute asthmatic attack
8. Cystic fibrosis
9. *Pseudohemoptysis*: Munchausen syndrome or an upper airway lesion such as epistaxis, gingival bleeding, or gastrointestinal bleeding

Most patients with coughing have only minimal signs and symptoms and may be discharged with an appropriate therapeutic regimen. Those with respiratory distress or significant hemoptysis should be hospitalized to allow identification of the underlying disease and facilitate treatment.

MANAGEMENT

The focus of management must be on determining the cause of the cough and instituting specific therapy for that condition. Beyond these specific steps, cough suppression may be necessary in older children if the cough interferes significantly with activities, sleep, or eating or causes significant vomiting.

Therapeutic options for cough suppression, if desired, include mixtures of equal parts of honey (corn syrup in children younger than 1 year), lemon concentrate, and an alcoholic drink (for older children), medicines with dextromethorphan (DM), or antitussives with 10 mg codeine per 5 ml, administered in a dosage of 1 mg codeine/kg /24 hr q4-6hr PO (adult, 10-20 mg codeine/dose PO). However, antitussive medications have limited use in pediatrics because a specific therapy (i.e., bronchodilator for asthma, sputum production) may be more important to minimize lower airway disease; furthermore, narcotics are sedating and reduce mucokinesis.

Parental Education

The following instructions apply to the child discharged with a cough, commonly after an upper respiratory tract infection.

Sucking on cough drops or hard candy may be useful for the older child. A good cough medicine can be made at home by mixing equal amounts of honey (corn syrup for children younger than 1 year), lemon concentrate, and an alcoholic drink such as Scotch or bourbon. You may omit the liquor for younger children.

1. Cough syrups are rarely useful. Stronger cough medicines containing DM or codeine must be prescribed by a physician, but they have the danger of reducing the cough reflex that protects the lungs.
2. Humidifiers and pushing warm fluids may be helpful.
3. Call your physician if any of the following occurs:
   a. Difficulty in breathing or shortness of breath develops.
   b. Cough lasts more than 2 weeks.
   c. Cough changes to croup ("barking-seal cough") or wheezing develops.

d. Child develops fever that lasts more than 72 hours.
e. Cough spasms occur that cause choking, passing out, a bluish color of lips, or persistent vomiting.
f. There is blood in the mucus.
g. Chest pain develops.

BIBLIOGRAPHY

Braman SS, Corrao WM: Cough: differential diagnosis and treatment, *Clin Chest Med* 8:177, 1987.

Hannaway PJ, Hopper DK: Cough variant asthma in children, *JAMA* 247:206, 1982.

Reisman J, Canny GJ, Levinson H: The approach to chronic cough in childhood, *Ann Allergic* 61:163, 1988.

32 Acute Diarrhea

Also See Chapters 44 (Vomiting) and 76 (Gastrointestinal Disorders)

ALERT Initial evaluation of the child with diarrhea must include assessment of the hydration status. If there is evidence of dehydration, fluids should be administered to correct deficits. Therapy for specific pathogens may be indicated.

ETIOLOGY

Acute diarrheal disease in childhood is primarily infectious in origin, resulting from a host of viral and bacterial agents delineated in Chapter 76. Acute gastroenteritis commonly leads to postinfectious malabsorption, secondary to lactose intolerance. Rarely do patients with peritoneal irritation, pneumonia, otitis media, or urinary tract infections have associated diarrhea. Antibiotics (e.g., ampicillin) are commonly associated with diarrhea (Table 32-1). When other obvious causes are ruled out, infectious diarrhea is the probable diagnosis if the patient has unformed bowel movements at twice the normal rate associated with one or more of the following: fever, nausea, vomiting, abdominal pain, cramps, bloody or mucoid stools, and tenesmus.

Evaluation of more chronic diarrhea should account for inflammatory bowel disease, irritable bowel syndrome, malabsorption, secretory disorders, anatomic abnormality (especially Hirschsprung's disease), parasites, systemic disease, overfeeding, antibiotics, toxins, and secondary lactase deficiency (Box 32-1).

DIAGNOSTIC FINDINGS

The onset of symptoms and the characteristics of bowel movements (consistency, mucus, blood, frequency) are important, with particular attention to factors that increase (e.g., time, diet) or decrease (e.g., dietary elimination, withdrawal of drugs) elimination. Related signs and symptoms, including fever, rash, and arthralgia, must be assessed. Recurrence and exposures may be important clues. Urine output should be evaluated.

Bacterial gastroenteritis is more likely in children with a history of blood in the stool in combination with a fever greater than 38° C or at least 10 stools in 14 hours.

The physical examination should focus on the state of hydration, hemodynamic stability, and associated findings. Abdominal and rectal examinations may be useful. Serial monitoring is essential.

Ancillary Data

Hydration status may require evaluation, including measurements of electrolytes, blood urea nitrogen (BUN), and urine specific gravity. Complete blood count (CBC) is variably helpful. Methylene blue smears for stool polyps are particularly useful in excluding a number of bacterial causes; for example, bacterial gastroenteritis is commonly associated with the presence of polymorphonuclear cells in the smear. Rapid tests for rotavirus may be diagnostic. On rare occasions, stool samples for culture and ova and parasite examination are appropriate.

TABLE 32-1 Acute Diarrhea: Diagnostic Considerations

Condition	Character of Stool	Associated Symptoms	Evaluation	Comments
INFECTION				
Acute gastroenteritis (p. 640)				
Virus	Loose; rare blood; rare WBC	Respiratory symptoms, vomiting	ELISA for rotavirus; electron microscopy	Acute onset
Bacteria	Loose/watery; variable blood; PMNs common	Vomiting; fever; seizure (*Shigella*); crampy abdominal pain	Culture; methylene blue for PMNs	Acute onset; toxic; may be related to food poisoning
Parasite	Variable	Multisystem involvement; weight loss	Ova and parasite	May be insidious
Postinfectious malabsorption	Watery	Recovering from acute gastroenteritis	Reducing substance in stool (≥0.5%); pH <5.0	Usually patient is lactose intolerant; may be primary
Food poisoning	Profuse	Abdominal pain, cramping, vomiting	Epidemiologic	Usually temporally related to food ingestion
Acute appendicitis (p. 658) **or peritonitis**	Loose	Reflects associated problems	Abdominal x-ray study; CBC	Surgical exploration
Extraintestinal				
Respiratory infection (p. 618)	Variable	Fever, rhinorrhea	Chest x-ray study, if needed	Antibiotics
Urinary tract infection (p. 833)	Variable	Dysuria, frequency, burning	Urinalysis, urine culture	Antibiotics
INTOXICATION				
Antibiotics Iron (p. 386) Antimetabolites	Loose; fat (variable)	Vomiting, anorexia; adverse reactions of medication	Withdrawal of drug	Clindamycin causes pseudomembranous enterocolitis
AUTOIMMUNE/ALLERGIC				
Ulcerative colitis	Mucus; pus; blood; nocturnal	Urgency; tenesmus, abdominal pain, fever, weight loss; systemic signs (e.g., arthritis)	Sigmoidoscopy; barium enema study	Insidious; age: 10-19 yr; treatment: sulfasalazine, steroids
Regional enteritis (Crohn's disease)	Loose; blood (variable); nocturnal	Abdominal pain; weight loss, fever; perianal disease	Sigmoidoscopy; barium enema study	Insidious; teenagers; treatment; surgery, sulfasalazine, steroids
Milk allergy	Watery; blood (occult or gross)	Vomiting, anemia	Dietary elimination	May also be caused by soy formula

Continued

TABLE 32-1 Acute Diarrhea: Diagnostic Considerations—cont'd

Condition	Character of Stool	Associated Symptoms	Evaluation	Comments
AUTOIMMUNE/ALLERGIC—cont'd				
Gluten sensitivity (celiac disease)	Profuse; bulky; pale; frothy	Failure to thrive, anemia, vomiting, abdominal pain	Peroral intestinal biopsy, stool fat	Onset reflects age of introduction of gluten (wheat, rye, oats); eliminate gluten foods
IRRITABLE BOWEL SYNDROME	Watery; mucus	None; normal growth	Therapeutic response	Treatment: bland diet; reduce snacks; peak: 6-36 mo; multiple inciting causes
INTRAPSYCHIC				
Fear/anxiety	Loose	Anxiety	History helpful	Stress-reducing activities; needs long-term therapy
Fecal impaction (encopresis) (Chapter 30)	Watery	Variable abdominal pain	History; rectal examination; x-ray study	Chronic constipation
CONGENITAL				
Cystic fibrosis	Fatty; bulky; foul smelling	Respiratory infections; poor growth	Sweat test	Needs enzyme replacement; long-term follow-up
Hirschsprung's disease (p. 662)	Green, watery; foul-smelling	Abdominal distension; vomiting; fever; lethargy; poor growth	Barium enema study; rectal biopsy	Surgical intervention
ENDOCRINE				
Hyperthyroid (p. 631)	Watery	Systemic signs	Thyroid studies	
NEOPLASM				
Lymphoma Carcinoma Neuroblastoma Zollinger-Ellison syndrome	Watery, variably severe	Associated problems	Variable	Important cause to exclude

Box 32-1

PRESENTATION AS DIAGNOSTIC CONSIDERATION FOR DIARRHEA

ACUTE ONSET

Fever common, ± vomiting/dehydration

Acute infectious gastroenteritis
- Viral (rotavirus, calicivirus, enteric adenovirus)
- Bacteria or toxin (*Campylobacter, Shigella, Salmonella, Staphylococcus* toxin)

"Parenteral" diarrhea (secondary to otitis, UTI)
Medication related
- Antibiotic-associated diarrhea
- Pseudomembranous colitis

Usually afebrile, hydrated

Transient malabsorption
- High fat intake
- Food intolerance/adverse reaction to food

Protozoal gastroenteritis (*Giardia, Entamoeba, Cryptosporidium*)
Psychogenic—anxiety/stress

CHRONIC COURSE

Failing to thrive, ± dehydration

Postinfectious diarrhea
- Starvation stools (prolonged liquid diet)
- Lactose intolerance postenteritis
- Inflammatory bowel disease

Hirschsprung's disease
Chronic malabsorption
- Protein (celiac disease)
- Fat (cystic fibrosis, pancreatic diseases)
- Carbohydrates (acquired lactase deficiency)

Protozoal diarrhea (also cause of acute process)

Thriving, afebrile, hydrated

Age-specific variant of normal
- Breast-feeding stools (0-2 mo old infant)
- Chronic nonspecific diarrhea of infancy/childhood (up to age 3)

Medication related
- Laxative abuse in adolescents
- Sorbitol content of cough syrups/bronchodilators

Encopresis—overflow incontinence

From Boenning DA: Diarrhea. In Barkin RM, editor: *Pediatric emergency medicine: concepts and clinical practice*, ed 2, St Louis, 1997, Mosby.

More exhaustive evaluations are rarely indicated unless the diarrhea has been prolonged. Sigmoidoscopy, barium enema, rectal biopsy, and other studies are performed for severe disease in the absence of an infectious cause.

MANAGEMENT

Management must focus on correcting any fluid deficits (see Chapter 7) and treating the specific condition. Hospitalization should be considered when there is dehydration, intractable vomiting, young age (especially less than 2 to 3 months), underlying disease, systemic toxicity, and disrupted social or physical environment. Patients with severe abdominal pain associated with bloody stools require immediate evaluation and surgical consultation.

The patient whose clinical status is stable can usually be monitored at home. Clear liquids should be given until there is some resolution of the diarrhea or specific therapy can be instituted.

Parental Education

1. Give only clear liquids; give as much as your child wants. The following may be used during the first 24 hours:
   a. Rehydralyte during initial rehydration followed by Pedialyte or Lytren is ideal
   b. Defizzed, room-temperature soda for older children (>2 years) if diarrhea is only mild
2. If your child is vomiting, give clear liquids slowly. In younger children, start

with 1 teaspoonful and slowly increase the amount. If vomiting occurs, let your child rest for a while and then try again. About 8 hours after vomiting has stopped, the child can gradually return to a normal diet.

3. After 24 hours your child's diet may be advanced if the diarrhea has improved. If your child is taking only formula, mix the formula with twice as much water to make up half-strength formula, which should be given over the next 24 hours. Applesauce, bananas, rice, and toast may be given if your child is eating solids. If these foods are tolerated, your child may be advanced to a regular diet over the next 2 to 3 days.
4. If your child has had a prolonged course of diarrhea, it may be helpful in the young child to advance from clear liquids to a soy formula (Isomil, ProSobee, or Soyalac) for 1 to 2 weeks.
5. Do not use boiled milk. Kool-Aid and soda are not ideal liquids, particularly in younger infants, because they contain few electrolytes.
6. Call your physician if any of the following occurs:
   - **a.** The diarrhea or vomiting is increasing in frequency or amount.
   - **b.** The diarrhea does not improve after 24 hours of clear liquids or resolve entirely after 3 to 4 days.
   - **c.** Vomiting continues for more than 24 hours.
   - **d.** The stool has blood, or the vomited material contains blood or turns green.
   - **e.** Signs of dehydration develop, including decreased urination, less moisture in diapers, dry mouth, no tears, weight loss, lethargy, and irritability.

33 Dysphagia

ALERT After correcting hydration, diagnostic considerations should be evaluated before initiating definitive therapy.

Patients with dysphagia have difficulty swallowing because of pharyngeal, laryngeal, or esophageal lesions. Clinically, patients experience associated choking, regurgitation, pain and discomfort, and a sense of food sticking. When such symptoms are caused by esophageal lesions, the patient commonly has a subjective sensation of a bolus of food failing to pass, with accompanying pain and discomfort.

Dysphagia results from either anatomic obstruction or compression or a physiologic dysfunction of the neuromuscular process of swallowing; that is, swallowing requires coordination with sucking and breathing (Table 33-1). *Obstructive* or compressive lesions can usually be evaluated by careful physical examination and radiologic studies, including lateral neck film, barium swallow study, and fluoroscopy. Patients with obstructive or compression lesions usually have difficulty only in swallowing solids. *Physiologic* dysfunction, often associated with systemic disease, is rarely isolated to the alimentary tract. Patients commonly have difficulty with both solids and liquids.

The assessment of patients with dysphagia must delineate the mechanism and degree of dysfunction. The rapidity of onset and recurrence and the nature of any progression are important diagnostic clues. Accompanying pain, discomfort, vomiting, and a preceding history of trauma should be noted. Systemic findings should be evaluated.

Laboratory studies may include cultures and measurement of serum drug levels and electrolytes. Manometry to measure the upper and lower esophageal pressures and peristaltic wave may provide physiologic information. Radiologic studies, including a barium swallow study to exclude narrowing, stricture, and presence of a foreign body, are essential, as is examining the swallowing mechanism. A lateral neck radiograph to look for masses and a computed tomography (CT) scan of the neck or head may be diagnostic.

A therapeutic trial of edrophonium (Tensilon) may be warranted.

Management of the patient must focus on stabilization by ensuring adequate vital signs and hydration, followed by diagnostic testing.

TABLE 33-1 Dysphagia: Diagnostic Considerations

	PRIMARY MECHANISM		
Condition	**Obstruction/ Compression (Mechanical)**	**Physiologic Dysfunction (Motor)**	**Comments**
INFECTION/INFLAMMATION			
Tonsillitis (p. 613)	Yes		Group A streptococci, diphtheria, mononucleosis, etc.
Stomatitis (p. 621)	Yes		Herpes, apthous
Peritonsillar abscess (p. 612)	Yes		Direct visualization required to define
Retropharyngeal abscess (p. 617)	Yes		Lateral neck
Epiglottitis, croup (p. 800)	Yes	Yes	Direct visualization imperative
Botulism, rabies, polio (Chapter 80)		Yes	Cranial nerves affected; also after polio
Guillain-Barré syndrome (Chapter 41)		Yes	Ascending paralysis
Esophagitis		Yes	Retrosternal discomfort (e.g., hiatal hernia, reflux)
Chalasia/gastroesophageal reflux	Yes	Yes	May be physiologic in infants
Pericarditis	Yes		Associated symptoms present
INTOXICATION			
Caustic ingestion (p. 372)	Yes	Yes	Requires immediate intervention to minimize injury
Phenothiazine overdose (p. 392)		Yes	Associated with dystonia
CONGENITAL (Chapter 11)			
Cleft palate	Yes	Yes	
Macroglossia	Yes		Consider hypothyroidism, Beckwith's syndrome
Esophageal web, atresia, stenosis	Yes		May be associated with trachea anomaly (trachoesophageal fistula)
Riley-Day syndrome		Yes	
DEGENERATIVE			
Central nervous system disease		Yes	
Hypotonia		Yes	
Myasthenia gravis		Yes	Trial of Edrophonium (Tensilon)
INTRAPSYCHIC			
Globus hystericus		Yes	Psychiatry consultation
TRAUMA			
Foreign body (p. 647)	Yes		History crucial
ENDOCRINE (p. 631)			
Goiter	Yes		Thyroid studies required
Hashimoto's thyroiditis	Yes		Thyroid studies required
NEOPLASM			
Carcinoma, Hodgkin's disease	Yes		Usually associated nodes, weight loss

TABLE 33-1 Dysphagia: Diagnostic Considerations—cont'd

Condition	PRIMARY MECHANISM Obstruction/ Compression (Mechanical)	PRIMARY MECHANISM Physiologic Dysfunction (Motor)	Comments
VASCULAR			
Vascular ring	Yes		Chest x-ray study, ECG, catheterization
Heart disease	Yes		Chest x-ray study, ECG, echocardiogram, catheterization
Aortic aneurysm	Yes		Chest x-ray study, ECG, ultrasound, catheterization
AUTOIMMUNE			
Various collagen-vascular diseases (dermatomyositis)	Yes	Yes	Evaluate in detail

BIBLIOGRAPHY

Sonies BC, Dalakas MC: Dysphagia in patients with post-polio syndrome, *N Engl J Med* 324:1162, 1991.

Weiss MH: Dysphagia in infants and children, *Otolaryngol Clin North Am* 21:4, 1988.

34 Fever in Children

ALERT A systematic approach to the acutely ill, febrile child is required to exclude serious systemic disease. Evaluation and management must reflect the child's age, medical history, physical findings, toxicity, environment, and family compliance.

Fever is an important symptom of illness and is a common complaint in children, accounting for up to 20% of emergency department (ED) visits. Most children seeking medical care for evaluation of a fever can be easily diagnosed and have minor illnesses. The clinical challenge is to identify those with significant underlying infections.

Physiologic mechanisms to control body temperature include sweating and hyperventilation to lower temperature and vasoconstriction and shivering to raise temperature. Circulating interleukins, prostaglandins, and prostacyclins mediate the febrile response.

MEASUREMENTS

A child is generally considered febrile when the rectal temperature is 38.0° C (100.4° F) or higher. The reliability of other methods of temperature measurement is variable. There is a normal diurnal variation in children of up to 1.1° C; the variation is less pronounced in younger children. Seriously ill infants may be euthermic or hypothermic. The absence of fever is not a reliable basis on which to eliminate the possibility of serious disease.

The *site* for temperature measurement must reflect proximity to major arteries, absence of inflammation, degree of precision required, safety, and insulation from external factors (e.g., drinking). *Rectal* temperatures provide precision and should be the technique in infants, especially those younger than 90 days. Care should be exercised to avoid rectal perforation and emotional trauma. *Axillary* temperatures are appropriate in thermostable environments or when absolute precision is not mandatory; neither of these conditions is present in the ED setting. The *oral or sublingual* site is useful in a cooperative older child who does not have a rapid respiratory rate. The *tympanic membrane* has been used with great reproducibility but appears to be less accurate in infants younger than 6 months, yielding falsely low values. It measures the infrared radiation emitted by the tympanic membrane. Speed of measurement must be balanced by the relative inaccuracy of the method. With the tympanic membrane approach, pulling posteriorly and superiorly on the external ear at the midpoint between the apex of the helix and the inferior border of the lobule may improve accuracy. Temperature in children younger than 90 days should be measured rectally. Bundling has little impact on rectal temperature.

Although most underlying illness is infectious, the obligation is to ensure that children with significant and potentially life-threatening conditions are distinguished from those with self-limited problems. The nonspecific presentation in neonates and infants and their impaired immunocompetency require aggressive evaluation and treatment in children younger than 90 days, although new patterns of management have introduced greater support for individualizing treatment in children older than 30 days.

DIAGNOSTIC FINDINGS

1. History usually reflects nonspecific observations related to behavior and associated signs and symptoms rather than data that permit an early focus on the involved system. The history is important in defining the nature of the illness, the height and duration of fever, dosage of, frequency of, and response to antipyretics, and past medical problems. A measured elevated temperature within the previous 6 hours is usually considered significant. Associated symptoms and behavioral patterns should be reviewed, with particular attention to irritability, response to the environment, respiratory or gastrointestinal abnormalities, limpness, and other localizing findings. Information about exposures to other ill children or adults, immunizations, travel, and source of water may be useful. Preexisting medical conditions (e.g., sickle cell disease, immunodeficiency, respiratory, cardiac, or renal disease) should be delineated. Prematurity and associated problems may affect the assessment and blur specific age parameters, especially during the first 6 months of life.
2. Physical examination should be systematic and thorough. While the child is distracted with play objects, obvious physical abnormalities such as limitations of limb movement, rashes, and points of tenderness should be defined. Examination of the chest, heart, and abdomen require a gentle hand and patience. Tachypnea disproportionate to fever (>59 breaths/min in a child <6 months old, >52/min in those 6 to 11 months old, and >42/min in children 1 to 2 years old) may suggest underlying pneumonia. Once these areas have been assessed, a full examination of the eyes, ears, throat, neck, extremities, and skin is required to look for specific findings.
3. Behavioral observation of the child at play while encouraging the youngster to follow lights, bring objects to parents, and so forth may be helpful in defining mental status:
   - Child looks at and focuses on the clinician and spontaneously explores the room.
   - Child spontaneously makes sounds or talks in a playful manner.
   - Child plays and reaches for objects.
   - Child smiles and interacts with parent or practitioner.
   - Child quiets easily when held by parents.
4. Antipyretic therapy is imperative in facilitating observation. Many children who are irritable and uninterested in their environment improve markedly with antipyretic management. Acetaminophen, 15 mg/kg/dose q4-6hr PO or PR, should be administered to children with temperatures greater than 38.5° to 39° C on arrival in the ED to ensure optimal observation by reducing temperature and permitting a more accurate assessment of the child. Studies have demonstrated that a *one-time loading dose* of acetaminophen, 30 mg/kg PO, produces a larger temperature decrease over a longer duration. Ibuprofen, 5 to 10 mg/kg/dose q6-8hr PO, may be useful as an ancillary agent. Children who are particularly uncomfortable may also benefit from a lukewarm-water sponge bath. Studies have documented that the clinical response to antipyretics is not predictive of whether a child has a serious bacterial infection; the response may facilitate evaluation.
5. Studies have suggested that in the first few months of life, febrile children are far more likely to have serious illness. Fever may be the only early symptom; few signs and symptoms may exist. Children with serious disease, as mentioned, may be

normothermic. The absence of specific findings mandates complete laboratory evaluation, admission, and antibiotics in this age group.

The older the patient, the more reliable are the findings. Meningitis in youngsters may merely manifest as irritability or lethargy, whereas in the teenager, meningismus, pain on extension of the knee with the leg positioned in flexion at the hip (Kernig's sign), and reflex flexion at the knee and hip when the neck is flexed (Brudzinksi's sign) are noted.

Ancillary Data

1. No laboratory or historical factors definitively exclude serious underlying bacterial disease. A peripheral white blood cell (WBC) count above 15,000 cells/mm^3 or below 5000 cells/mm^3 may indicate a serious infection. Meningococcemia, disseminated intravascular coagulation (DIC), and septic shock classically cause low WBC counts. Studies have suggested that a ratio of bands to neutrophil of 0.2 is associated with bacterial infections.
2. Blood cultures for aerobic and anaerobic organisms should be obtained in patients in whom bacteremia is suspected.
3. Urinalysis in children with fever and no source. Urinalysis results may be unremarkable in up to 80% of neonates with a documented positive culture result. Twenty percent of older children with urinary tract infections have a normal urinalysis result with negative leukocyte esterase or nitrite result. If nitrite or leukocyte esterase are both positive, the specificity is 96%. A Gram stain of the spun urine sediment increases the sensitivity screening test. Gram stain and dipstick analysis for nitrite and leukocyte esterase have similar sensitivity and both are superior to microscopic analysis for pyura.

   The only reliable methods to obtain a urine sample are straight catheterization or suprapubic bladder aspiration. Table 85-2 provides an interpretation of culture results. Bagged urine is useful to screen for dehydration, hematuria, proteinuria, or glucosuria. Urine cultures should be processed promptly.
4. Lumbar puncture (LP) is appropriate to exclude meningitis when this diagnosis is considered. Febrile children with seizures deserve special consideration, especially those 12 months or younger in whom a spinal tap is generally done. The fluid should be cultured and studies should include cell count, Gram stain, measurements of protein and glucose (with concurrent blood glucose level) (see Table 81-3). Performing an LP in a bacteremic child does not significantly increase the risk of development of meningitis.
5. Erythrocyte sedimentation rate (ESR) is a nonspecific test for infection, inflammatory bowel disease, and collagen-vascular disease. Its usefulness is limited by the length of time required for the study.
6. Stool smear examination for polymorphonuclear leukocytes (PMNs) is useful in children with diarrhea because 90% of infections with *Salmonella* or *Shigella* are associated with the presence of PMNs; infections with *Campylobacter*, toxigenic *Escherichia coli*, and *Yersinia* species may also cause PMNs in stool.
7. Chest x-ray studies are recommended in young febrile children with evidence of lower respiratory tract disease, such as coughing, wheezing, tachypnea, dyspnea, retractions, grunting, nasal flaring, and focally decreased breath sounds. Tachypnea disproportionate to the child's age, as noted previously, may be an additional risk factor. In febrile child (>39° C), children older than 3 months with no clinical evidence of lower respiratory tract infection and a WBC >20,000 cells/mm^3, a chest x-ray should be considered to exclude radiographic evidence of pneumonia.

An abnormal radiographic result in the absence of cough, rales, or wheezing is unusual in children younger than 8 weeks.

8. Coagulation studies, cultures, and radiographs as indicated.

SPECIFIC ENTITIES

Occult Bacteremia

Although bacteremia occurs in association with a host of clinical entities, including meningitis, septic arthritis, epiglottitis, cellulitis, pneumonia, and kidney infection, about 6% of febrile patients without a defined focus have positive blood culture results. The most common pathogen is *Streptococcus pneumoniae*, accounting for 85% of positive cultures. With the availability of the pneumococcal vaccine, the incidence of invasive pneumococcal disease caused by vaccine serotypes has dropped by more than 50%. *Haemophilus influenzae* type B infections are less common, particularly following the remarkable impact of immunization in decreasing incidence. *Neisseria meningitidis, Salmonella* species, and other pathogens may also be found.

The group at highest risk for occult bacteremia are those 24 months or younger with a fever 39.4° C or higher and a WBC count of 15,000 cell/mm^3 or greater. The differential blood cell count does not increase predictive value. An ESR greater than 30 mm/hr may also be suggestive.

Each degree elevation above 39° C increases the risk; children with a temperature of 39.5° to 39.9° C have about a 3% incidence of bacteremia, those with a temperature of 40° to 40.9° C have a 4% risk, and those with a temperature higher than 41° C have a 10% risk. The risk of a serious bacterial infection developing in a bacteremic child is probably less than 1%.

It is essential to evaluate such children carefully to be certain no underlying disease exists. If pneumococcal bacteremia is suspected, consideration should be given to initiating prophylactic antibiotics, but the benefit is controversial. Retrospective review of *H. influenzae* and *N. meningitidis* bacteremia suggested that children sent home with oral antibiotic therapy may do better compared with those sent home without therapy; parenteral administration of antibiotics may have further benefit. Another study demonstrated that starting oral amoxicillin therapy enhanced defervescence but questionably prevented major morbid events. A meta-analysis of studies involving *S. pneumoniae* bacteremia had similar findings; oral antibiotics decrease the incidence of serious bacterial infections but did not reduce the risk of meningitis. In general, children younger than 60 to 90 days old with suspected occult bacteremia in whom empiric antibiotics are initiated should undergo a full sepsis evaluation, including an LP.

Hyperpyrexia

True hyperpyrexia, defined as a temperature greater than 41° C (105.8° F), is rare but is more commonly associated with serious infections. About 20% of children with temperatures higher than 41° C have convulsions. Ten percent of children younger than 2 years with temperatures higher than 41.1° C have bacterial meningitis; an additional 7% have bacteremia without meningitis. Another study has noted that 8 of 15 (53%) children with temperatures over 41.1° C had serious disease (2 bacterial meningitis, 2 with bacteremia, 2 pneumonia, 1 pericarditis, and 1 Kawasaki disease).

Temperatures greater than 42° C often have noninfectious causes, such as hyperthermia, head injury, ingestion of psychotropic drugs, and malignant hyperthermia during anesthesia.

Antipyretic management is appropriate, and patients should receive a minimum of a complete blood count (CBC), urinalysis, and blood culture. LP should be considered and a chest x-ray obtained if there is any suggestion of respiratory findings.

Immunocompromise

Children with a history of recurrent serious bacterial infection should be evaluated for immunodeficiency. Children who are undergoing cancer chemotherapy or have a history of asplenia (e.g., congenital, traumatic) are obviously at risk. Those with sickle cell disease have a 400-fold greater risk of pneumococcal septicemia if they are younger than 5 years old, and a fourfold risk of *H. influenzae* septicemia if younger than 9 years.

Fever and Petechiae

Children with fever and petechiae may have a viral illness, Rocky Mountain spotted fever, or invasive bacterial disease. Rapid intervention is required. In one study of 90 patients with fever and petechiae, 15 had bacterial disease, half of which was meningitis. The most common pathogen was *N. meningitidis*, accounting for 13 of the 15 patients with invasive disease; group A streptococcus and respiratory syncytial virus were the most common causes of noninvasive bacterial disease. Most well-appearing children do not have serious bacterial invasive infections.

Children with fever and petechiae who have a normal LP, a WBC count that is neither elevated nor decreased, normal absolute neutrophil and band counts, and a temperature less than 40° C are less likely to have a bacterial infection.

Fever of Unknown Origin

Fever of unknown origin (FUO) is commonly used to refer to a febrile illness without identified cause that lasts 14 days or more. Most children have actually had two or more febrile illnesses within a short period. When the prolonged fever is continuous, numerous causes need to be considered (Box 34-1). In a study of 100 children, 52 had an infectious origin, 20 had collagen inflammatory disease, 6 had

Box 34-1

ETIOLOGY OF PEDIATRIC PROLONGED FEVER OF UNKNOWN ORIGIN

INFECTION

Bacterial
- Sinusitis
- Pyelonephritis
- Mastoiditis
- Endocarditis
- Adenitis

Viral
- Infectious mononucleosis
- Hepatitis A, B, or C
- Cytomegalovirus

Chlamydial

Mycoplasma

Fungal
- Cysticercosis, blastomycosis, histoplasmosis

Rickettsial
- Q fever
- Rocky Mountain spotted fever

Parasitic
- Malaria
- Toxoplasmosis

COLLAGEN-VASCULAR

Juvenile rheumatoid arthritis
Lupus erythematosus
Vasculitis, postinfectious
Acute rheumatic fever
Ulcerative colitis/regional enteritis

MALIGNANCY

Leukemia, lymphoma, neuroblastoma, Wilms' tumor

DRUG-INDUCED

Antineoplastic, anticonvulsants, antituberculosis agents
Quinidine, procainamide
Serum sickness

OTHER

Kawasaki disease
AIDS
Hypothalamic dysfunction
Factitious

From Fetter RA, Bower JR: Infectious diseases. In Barkin RM, editor: *Pediatric emergency medicine: concepts and clinical practice*, ed 2, St Louis, 1997, Mosby.

malignancy, and 12 were undiagnosed. A systematic approach to evaluation and referral for ongoing management are appropriate.

MANAGEMENT

A conservative yet responsible approach appears mandatory for the febrile child, with the recognition that assessment and care must be individualized. Antibiotic sensitivity patterns constantly evolve, with resistance to *H. influenzae* and *S. pneumoniae* being increasingly prevalent.

Infants Younger Than 90 Days

A rational and conservative approach is essential in young infants. The history is rarely more specific than the triad of fever, irritability, and poor feeding. The physical examination may fail to yield specific focal findings, despite the presence of systemic infections, which may be enteric as well as the more common organisms infecting older children. Children younger than 3 months with a temperature above 38.5° C have more than a 20-fold higher risk of having a serious infection than older children with similar temperatures. High fever has some correlation with serious illness, but the absence of this finding does not exclude bacterial infections. Prematurity makes such age cutoffs less distinct.

Prospective studies have demonstrated that clinical judgment alone is not adequate in the assessment of febrile infants. No clear factors are sensitive or specific enough to be relied on in decision-making. However, factors that have been most consistently associated with bacterial disease are age less than 1 month, breastfeeding, history of lethargy, no contact with an ill person, polymorphonuclear neutrophil count above 10,000 cells/mm^3, and band count greater than 500 cells/mm^3. *No laboratory or historical factors should be used to exclude underlying bacterial infection.*

1. During the first 30 days of life, infants undergo tremendous developmental and immunologic changes and are difficult to assess. In one study, one in nine neonates with serious bacterial infection appeared clinically well. Furthermore, the etiologic agents evolve from vaginal flora (*E. coli*, group B streptococcus, *Listeria monocytogenes*, herpes, and chlamydia) to more traditional community-acquired diseases. Febrile children in this age group require admission, after a full sepsis work-up, for administration of parenteral antibiotics and monitoring until culture results are negative at 48 to 72 hours. Blood, urine, and cerebrospinal fluid (CSF) cultures should be performed, and other studies as indicated. Antibiotics should be initiated, including ampicillin, 100 to 200 mg/kg/24 hr q4-6hr IV, and cefotaxime, 50 to 100 mg/kg/24 hr q8hr IV. Gentamicin, 5 to 7.5 mg/kg/24 hr q8hr IV, or ceftriaxone, 50 to 100 mg/kg/24 hr q12hr IV, may substitute for cefotaxime, the latter in children older than 30 days.
2. In children 30 to 60 days old, the assessment has greater validity because of the enhanced developmental skills of the child and maturing of the immune system. Blood and urine cultures, CBC, and LP should generally be performed in febrile children in this age group. An LP is indicated in children with abnormal physical or laboratory findings or in whom antibiotics are to be prescribed. Admission is indicated in children with systemic findings, toxic appearance, or any abnormal laboratory findings and those who do not meet the low-risk for serious bacterial infection Rochester criteria delineated in Box 34-2. These criteria are *not* reliable in children younger than 30 days.

   Children 30 to 60 days old who need treatment may be given the antibiotics described above.
3. In children 60 to 90 days of age, a CBC, urinalysis, and urine culture should be considered. If results of any of these evaluations are abnormal, a blood culture should be done. An LP is appropriate

Box 34-2

LOW-RISK ROCHESTER CRITERIA

Well-appearing infant; normal vital signs; good hydration and perfusion
Healthy infant
- Term (≥37 weeks' gestation)
- No antibiotic therapy—antenatal or postnatal
- No unexplained hyperbilirubinemia
- No underlying illness
- No previous hospitalizations; discharged with mother as newborn

No focal infection (skin, soft tissue, bone/joint)
Good social situation
Laboratory criteria
- WBC count 5000 to 15,000/mm^3
- Band form count ≤1500/mm^3
- Normal urinalysis (<5 WBC/HPF)
- Normal stool (<5 WBC/HPF, if done)

WBC, White blood cell(s); *HPF*, high-power field.

if indicated by the examination of the child or if antibiotics are to be started. Admission is appropriate if the child is not at low risk or appears toxic, or if the physical or laboratory findings are abnormal in any respect. Additional studies should be considered.

Children 90 Days to 36 Months

In children 90 days to 36 months old, the evaluation is more specific, and the examination may provide information about a specific diagnostic direction. Studies have shown that most children with serious infections can be identified by the initial evaluation. Furthermore, beyond the greater reliability of the examination, the mature immune status provides reassurance regarding the nature of infection. Clearly, toxic-appearing children need extensive evaluations, whereas children without specific findings who appear nontoxic can generally be managed by ambulatory observation. When the temperature is greater than 39.4° C or 103° F, a CBC is indicated; when the WBC is greater than 15,000 cells/mm^3, a blood culture to exclude occult bacteremia is appropriate, particularly if the child has not received immunizations to *H. influenzae* and *S. pneumoniae*. Those who are to receive antibiotics, males younger than 6 months, and girls should have a urinalysis and urine culture obtained.

If blood cultures are obtained, empiric treatment with antibiotics during the wait for results may be considered; controversy exists about whether the incidence of significant complications is reduced. *Follow-up observation is essential*, usually in 12 to 24 hours, depending on clinical and logistical constraints; this is particularly important in children at high risk for bacteremia.

If the elevated temperature has been present for less than 24 hours and the child looks well without any high-risk factors, follow-up observation for 4 to 12 hours may substitute for laboratory evaluation at the time of the first encounter, particularly if the child is fully immunized. Close follow-up is essential.

Children Older Than 3 Years

Children older than 3 years need a careful evaluation focused on specific findings. Although viral illness predominates in this age group, such organisms as group A streptococcus, *Mycoplasma*, and Epstein-Barr virus are more common etiologic agents than in younger children.

DISPOSITION

Obviously, close follow-up is essential in every child discharged with a febrile illness, usually within 24 hours; follow-up may be accomplished either by phone or return visit to the ED or visit to the primary care physician. Children younger than 30 days are routinely admitted, whereas those 30 to 60 days old are often hospitalized. Changing clinical status, evolving foci, or other parameters should be evaluated as well as the cultures obtained initially checked for results.

If the blood culture result is negative, follow-up on an outpatient basis is appropriate if the patient remains well without any focal findings. Antibiotic therapy, if started, should be stopped after 48 hours, and the patient monitored until the illness resolves.

If the blood culture result is positive, thereby documenting bacteremia, reexamination of the patient is essential. If the patient is totally normal and the culture yields a gram-positive organism, close follow-up and antibiotic therapy may be continued for a total 10-day course. If the child is febrile or toxic or has an evolving focus, or the organism is gram negative, admission and intravenous antibiotics are indicated.

Parental Education

Parental education is important in the management of the febrile infant. Obviously, instructions are indicated in the management of the specific diagnostic entity, but additional information about fever control must be provided. Fever control is of utmost importance for the initial assessment of the child and may also make the child more comfortable throughout the duration of the illness. Fever is a means of fighting infection, and the level of fever does not always reflect the severity of the illness.

1. *Fever* is a temperature over 99.7° F (37.6° C) when measured orally or 100.4° F (38.0° C) when measured rectally (Fig. 34-1). If the fever is between 100° F and 101° F when measured orally or rectally, the temperature should be taken again in 1 hour. Temperatures may be temporarily elevated from too much clothing or exercise. Oral temperatures can be raised by recently eaten warm food. Teething does not cause marked elevations of temperature. Bundling has little impact on rectal temperature.

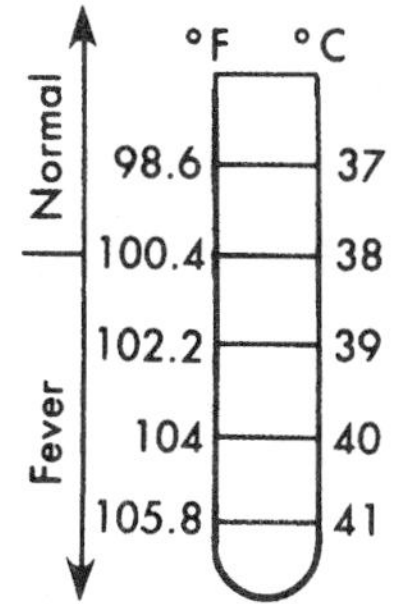

Fig. 34-1 Conversion scale.

2. Take the rectal temperature:
   a. Shake the thermometer down to below 97° F (36° C).
   b. Lubricate the thermometer with petroleum jelly (Vaseline), cold cream, or cold water.
   c. Gently insert the thermometer ½ inch into the rectum. Often, holding the child stomach down on your lap is helpful.
   d. Leave the thermometer in 3 minutes or until the silver line stops rising.
   e. Do not leave the child unattended. Hold the child still.
   f. Remove the thermometer, and read the temperature by turning the sharp edge of the triangle toward you. Turn it slightly in each direction until you can see the end of the silver column.
   g. On the centigrade (Celsius) thermometer, each line is 0.1° C; on the Fahrenheit thermometer, each line is 0.2° F.

      NOTE: In unusual circumstances, axillary temperatures may be taken as a screen, holding the tip of the thermometer under the dry armpit for 4 minutes. The elbow should be held against the chest. If the axial temperature is above 99° F (37.2° C), recheck by taking a rectal temperature.
3. Fever medicines should be used if the temperature is above 101.5° F (38.6° C) and your child is very uncomfortable, or if any fever is present at bedtime (see Table 34-1). If your child is acting normally, fever medicines may be delayed until the temperature is 102.2° F (39.0° C).

TABLE 34-1 Dosage of Fever Medicine According to Age

Agent	0-3 mo	4-11 mo	12-23 mo	2-3 yr	4-5 yr	6-8 yr	9-10 yr	11-12 yr
Acetaminophen drops (80 mg/0.8 ml)	0.4 ml	0.8 ml	1.2 ml	1.6 ml	2.4 ml			
Acetaminophen elixir (160 mg/tsp)		½ tsp	¾ tsp	1 tsp	1½ tsp	2 tsp	2½ tsp	
Chewable tablet acetaminophen or aspirin (80 mg)			1½	2	3	4	5	6
Junior swallowable tablet (160 mg)				1	1½	2	2½	3
Adult tablet acetaminophen or aspirin (325 mg)						1	1	1½
Ibuprofen suspension (100 mg/5 ml)	½ tsp	¾ tsp	1 tsp	1¼ tsp	1¾ tsp	2 tsp		
Ibuprofen capsule (200 mg)						1	1½	2

a. If your child is older than 3 months, give fever medicine if the temperature is above 101.5° F (38.6° C). Acetaminophen (Tylenol or equivalent) is recommended every 4 to 6 hours in the dosage indicated in Table 34-1. Many clinicians use 10 to 15 mg/kg/dose. Younger febrile children should be evaluated immediately.

b. Ibuprofen is a useful addition or single-agent antipyretic, usually given at a dosage of 10 mg/kg/dose PO QID. It is available over the counter in tablets of 200 mg or as a prescription suspension with 100 mg/5 ml.

c. Do not use aspirin if your child has chickenpox or an influenza-like illness because of the association between Reye's syndrome and aspirin.

4. Sponging is rarely needed but may be useful if the temperature remains over 104° F (40° C) after antipyretic medicines and your child remains uncomfortable or irritable. Sponge or partially submerge your undressed child in lukewarm water (96° to 100° F). This can be done for 15 to 30 minutes as often as necessary. Some parents prefer laying the undressed child on a towel; another towel or washcloth soaked in lukewarm water is placed over the child, being resoaked and replaced every 1 to 2 minutes for 15 to 30 minutes.
5. Dress your child lightly. Push fluids.
6. Call your physician if any of the following occurs:
   a. The fever goes above 105° F (40.5° C).
   b. The fever lasts beyond 48 to 72 hours.
   c. Your child is younger than 3 months and has a rectal temperature over 100.4° F (38° C).
   d. Your child has a seizure (convulsion) or abnormal movements of face, arms, or legs, stiff neck, purple spots, or fullness of the soft spot; looks sicker than expected; or has difficulty breathing, burning on urination, decreased urination, abdominal pain, marked change in behavior, or level of consciousness or activity.

BIBLIOGRAPHY

Baker D, Avner J, Bell J: Failure of infant observation scales in detecting serious illness in febrile four to eight-week-old infants, *Pediatrics* 85:1040-1043, 1990.

Baker MD, Bell LM, Avner JR: Outpatient management without antibiotics of fever in selected infants, *N Engl J Med* 329:1437-1441, 1993.

Baker RC, Sequin JH, Leslie N et al: Fever and petechiae in children, *Pediatrics* 84:1051, 1989.

Baker RC, Tiller T, Bausher JC et al: Severity of disease correlated with fever reduction in febrile infants, *Pediatrics* 83:1016-1019, 1989.

Baraff LJ: Management of fever without source in infants and children, *Ann Emerg Med* 36:602, 2000.

Baraff U, Bass JW, Fleisher GR et al: Practice guidelines for the management of infants and children 0 to 36 months of age with fever without source, *Ann Emerg Med* 22:1198-1210, 1993.

Baraff U, Oslund SA, Schriger DL et al: Probability of bacterial infections in febrile infants less than three months of age: a meta analysis, *Pediatr Infect Dis J* 11:257, 1992.

Black S, Shinefield H, Hansen J et al: Postlicensure evaluation of the effectiveness of seven valent pneumococcal conjugate vaccine, *Pediatr Infect Dis* 20:1105, 2001.

Bonadio WA, Webster H, Wolfe A et al: Correlating infectious outcome with clinical parameters of 1130 consecutive febrile infants aged zero to eight weeks, *Pediatr Emerg Care* 9:84, 1993.

Brannan DF, Falk JL, Rothrock SG et al: Reliability of infrared tympanum thermometry in the determination of rectal temperature in children, *Ann Emerg Med* 25:21, 1995.

Crain EF, Bulas D, Bijur PE et al: Is a chest radiograph necessary in the evaluation of every febrile infant less than 8 weeks of age? *Pediatrics* 8:821, 1991.

Cram E, Gershel J: Urinary tract infections in febrile infants younger than 8 weeks of age, *Pediatrics* 86:363, 1990.

Goldsmith B, Campo J: Comparison of urine dipstick, microscopy and culture for the detection of bacteriuria in children, *Clin Pediatr* 29:214, 1990.

Graneto JW, Soglin DF: Maternal screening of childhood fever by palpation, *Pediatr Emerg Care* 12:183, 1996.

Grover G: The effects of bundling on infant temperatures, *Pediatrics* 94:669, 1994.

Jaskiewicz JA, McCarthy CA, Richardson AC et al: Febrile infants at low risk for serious bacterial infection: an appraisal of the Rochester criteria and implications for management, *Pediatrics* 94:390, 1994.

Klassen TP, Rowe PC: Selecting diagnostic tests to identify febrile infants less than 3 months of age as being at low risk for serious bacterial infection: a scientific overview, *J Pediatr* 121:671, 1992.

Kramer MS, Shapiro ED: Management of the young febrile children: a commentary on recent practice guidelines, *Pediatrics* 100:128, 1997.

Mandl KD, Stack AM, Fleisher GR: Incidence of bacteremia in infants and children with fever and petechiae, *J Pediatr* 131:398, 1997.

Muma BK, Treloar DJ, Wurmlinger K et al: Comparison of rectal, axillary and tympanic membrane temperatures in infants and young children, *Ann Emerg Med* 20:41, 1991.

Pikis A, Akram S, Donkerscoot JA et al: Penicillin resistant pneumococci from pediatric patients in the Washington DC area, *Ann Pediatr Adolesc Med* 149:30, 1995.

Pizzo PA, Rubin M, Freifeld A et al: The child with cancer and infection. I: empiric therapy for fever and neutropenia and preventive strategies, *J Pediatr* 119:679, 1991.

Pollack CV, Pollack ES, Andrew ME: Suprapubic bladder aspiration versus urethral catheterization in ill infants: success, efficiency, and complication rates, *Ann Emerg Med* 23:225, 1994.

Rothrock SG, Harpee MB, Green SM et al: Do oral antibiotics prevent meningitis and serious bacterial infections in children with *Streptococcus pneumoniae* occult bacteremia? a meta-analysis, *Pediatrics* 99:438, 1997.

Walson PD, Galletta G, Chomilo F et al: Comparison of multidose ibuprofen and acetaminophen therapy in febrile children, *Am J Dis Child* 146:626, 1992.

35 Gastrointestinal Hemorrhage: Hematemesis and Rectal Bleeding

Also See Chapter 76 (Gastrointestinal Disorders)

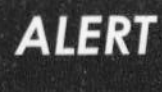

The initial focus must be on assessing the severity of bleeding, initiating necessary stabilization measures, and determining diagnostic considerations.

Gastrointestinal (GI) hemorrhage, whether it be manifested by vomiting (hematemesis) or rectal bleeding (melena), reflects an infectious, inflammatory, or anatomic abnormality (Tables 35-1 and 35-2). It must be differentiated from hemoptysis (p. 234), which is indicated by red, frothy material mixed with sputum.

ETIOLOGY

In the newborn, swallowed blood,* bleeding diathesis, and stress ulcers are the most common causes of GI bleeding. Necrotizing enterocolitis (NEC) is occasionally noted in the nursery. During the first year of life, anal fissures and intussusception account for 70% of noninfectious gastrointestinal hemorrhage, with gangrenous bowel, peptic ulcers, and Meckel's diverticulum less common. Lesions in older children include colonic polyps (50%), anal fissures (13%), peptic ulcers (13%), intussusception (9%), and esophageal varices (9%). Infectious diarrhea is a frequent cause.

*Apt test for maternal blood: Mix 1 part bright red stool or vomitus with 5 to 10 parts water and centrifuge. Add 1 ml 0.2N NaOH to supernatant fluid. Pink color that develops in 2 to 5 minutes indicates fetal hemoglobin; brown color indicates adult hemoglobin.

DIAGNOSTIC FINDINGS

Initially, the urgency of intervention must reflect hemodynamic instability, which is assessed by history and physical examination. The history should determine the onset, progression, character, frequency, and quality of bleeding. Associated vomiting, diarrhea, and abdominal pain should be noted. A history of drug ingestion, especially aspirin, alcohol, caustic agents, and gastric irritants, should be delineated, as should previous episodes of bleeding or family history of problems.

The physical examination should determine vital signs and assess for abdominal tenderness, sounds, and rebound, guarding, and rectal disease.

The diagnostic evaluation focuses on defining the site of hemorrhage, with particular reference to whether it is proximal or distal to the ligament of Treitz, after baseline laboratory data—including complete blood count (CBC), platelets, type and cross-match, and coagulation studies (platelets, prothrombin time [PT], partial thromboplastin time [PTT])—have been obtained (Fig. 35-1). The approach must be individualized.

1. Lesions proximal to the ligament of Treitz usually result in nasogastric (NG) aspirates positive for blood (see Fig. 56-1).

TABLE 35-1 Gastrointestinal Hemorrhage: Diagnostic Considerations by Age

Infant (<3 mo)	Toddler (<2 yr)	Preschooler (<5 yr)	School-Age Child (>5 yr)
UPPER GASTROINTESTINAL BLEEDING			
Swallowed maternal blood	Esophagitis	Esophagitis	Esophagitis
Gastritis	Gastritis	Gastritis	Gastritis
Ulcer, stress	Ulcer	Ulcer	Ulcer
Bleeding diathesis	Pyloric stenosis	Esophageal varices	Esophageal varices
Foreign body (NG tube)	Mallory-Weiss syndrome	Foreign body	Mallory-Weiss syndrome
Vascular malformation	Vascular malformation	Mallory-Weiss syndrome	Inflammatory bowel disease*
Duplication	Duplication	Hemophilia	Hemophilia
		Vascular malformation	Vascular malformation
LOWER GASTROINTESTINAL BLEEDING			
Swallowed maternal blood	Anal fissure	Infectious colitis*	Infectious colitis*
Infectious colitis*	Infectious colitis*	Anal fissure	Inflammatory bowel disease*
Milk allergy	Milk allergy	Polyp	Pseudomembranous enterocolitis*
Bleeding diathesis*	Colitis	Intussusception*	Polyp
Intussusception*	Intussusception*	Meckel's diverticulum	Hemolytic-uremic syndrome*
Midgut volvulus*	Meckel's diverticulum	Henoch-Schönlein purpura	Hemorrhoid
Meckel's diverticulum	Polyp	Hemolytic-uremic syndrome*	
Necrotizing enterocolitis (NEC)*	Duplication	Inflammatory bowel disease*	
	Hemolytic-uremic syndrome*	Pseudomembranous enterocolitis*	
	Inflammatory bowel disease*		
	Pseudomembranous enterocolitis*		

* Commonly associated with systemic illness involving multiple organ systems either primarily or secondarily.

a. Bright red hematemesis indicates that there is little or no contact with gastric juices; it results from an active bleeding site at or above the cardia. In children it is usually caused by varices, esophagitis, or, rarely, Mallory-Weiss syndrome. Occasionally, duodenal or gastric bleeding may be so brisk that it is bright red.

b. A "coffee grounds" appearance to the aspirate indicates that it has been altered by the gastric juices.

c. Melena may be present, indicating a blood loss in excess of 50 to 100 ml/24 hr.

d. Evaluation should involve endoscopy and an upper GI series, depending on the stability of the patient and the likely cause.

2. If rectal bleeding is the primary presentation, the stool should be examined for stool leukocytes and a culture obtained. The color of the blood in the stool reflects the amount and site of bleeding.

a. Hemorrhage proximal to the ileocecal valve produces tarry stools, but lower GI bleeding is red.

b. Streaks of blood on the outside of the stool indicate a lesion in the rectal ampulla or anal canal, most commonly fissures.

c. Depending on the suspected cause and clinical status, other evaluations can include anal inspection, sigmoidoscopy, colonoscopy, technetium scan, and double-contrast barium enema.

TABLE 35-2 Hematemesis and Rectal Bleeding: Diagnostic Considerations

		CHARACTER OF BLEEDING	
Condition	**Age**	**Gastric Aspirate**	**Stool**
INFECTION/INFLAMMATION			
Acute diarrhea (p. 640) Bacteria, virus, parasites	Any	—	Small (variable)
Gastritis (Chapter 44)	Any	Mild-moderate, coffee grounds	Tarry
Ulcer			
Peptic	>6 yr	Small/large; red/coffee grounds	Small/large; tarry
Duodenal	>6 yr	Small/large; red/coffee grounds	Small/large; tarry
Stress	Any	Small/large; red/coffee grounds	Small/large; tarry
Esophagitis	Any	Small	
Ulcerative colitis	Any	—	Small/large
Crohn's disease (regional enteritis)	10-19 yr	—	Variable, red
ANATOMIC			
Intussusception (p. 664)	<2 yr (5-12 mo)	—	"Currant jelly"
Volvulus (p. 669)	Neonate	—	Red/tarry
Rectal fissure (Chapter 30)	Infant	—	Blood-streaked stool
Polyps	2-10 yr	—	Small/moderate; red, intermittent
Meckel's diverticulum (p. 666)	4 mo-4 yr	—	Large; red and tarry
VASCULAR			
Esophageal varices	>2 yr (3-5 yr)	Large; red	Large, tarry
Hemangioma/hematoma/ telangiectasia	Any	—	Occult blood/large
TRAUMA			
Foreign body (p. 647)	2-6 yr	—	Variable, red
Mallory-Weiss syndrome		Large; red	
AUTOIMMUNE/ALLERGIC			
Henoch-Schönlein purpura (p. 822)	3-10 yr		Small/large; red/tarry
Idiopathic thrombocytopenia purpura (p. 709)	Any		
Milk allergy (cow or soy)	<12 mo	—	Occult blood/small; red

Signs and Symptoms	Evaluation	Comments
Fever, diarrhea, polymorphonuclear cells (bacterial)	Stool leukocytes, culture, CBC, ova and parasites	Dietary manipulation useful
Vomiting		Acute gastroenteritis, ASA, alcohol, *Helicobacter pylori*
Vomiting, pain, anemia	Endoscopy with biopsy/culture; upper GI series; exclude Zollinger-Ellison syndrome; determine diet, family history	May be life threatening; peptic ulcer often associated with *H. pylori* and treated with bismuth, amoxicillin, metronidazole, cimetidine/ranitidine for 14-28 days; cimetidine, ranitidine, or antacids (30 ml 1 and 3 hr after meals and before bed)
Vomiting, retrosternal pain	Upper GI, esophagoscopy	May be caused by hiatal hernia, chalasia; cimetidine
Insidious weight loss and pain	Proctoscopy, barium enema	Multiple complications
Insidious weight loss and pain	Protoscopy, barium enema	
Acute onset, crampy, abdominal pain	Hydrostatic barium enema	Life threatening, requires immediate surgery
Bile-stained vomit, shock, abdominal distension	Barium enema	
Well child	Inspection of anus	Stool softener
Well child, variable anemia	Proctoscopy, barium enema	Severe if Peutz-Jeghers syndrome; may be inflammatory, adenoma or hemartoma
Well child with acute, massive bleeding	Pertechnetate scan	
Painless, cirrhosis, portal vein thrombosis	Esophagoscopy, barium swallow	
Painless, mucocutaneous lesions	Angiography, laparotomy	Familial (Peutz-Jeghers syndrome)
History, rectal pain	Digital examination, proctoscopy	
History, vomiting	Esophagoscopy	
Abdominal pain, arthritis, hematuria, purpura	Physical examination, CBC, platelet count	Risk of intussusception
Recurrent vomiting, diarrhea, colic, failure to thrive; rarely, fulminant enterocolitis	Dietary change	

Continued

TABLE 35-2 Hematemesis and Rectal Bleeding: Diagnostic Considerations—cont'd

		CHARACTER OF BLEEDING	
Condition	**Age**	**Gastric Aspirate**	**Stool**
CONGENITAL			
Hemophilia (p. 696)	Any (male)	Occult blood/large; red/coffee grounds	Occult blood/large; red/tarry
DEGENERATIVE			
Vitamin K deficiency	1-2 days	Mild/large; red	Mild/large; red/tarry
ENDOCRINE			
Zollinger-Ellison syndrome	>7 yr	Small/large; coffee grounds	Tarry
NEOPLASM			
Esophageal/gastric carcinoma		Occult blood/large	Tarry; occult blood/large
MISCELLANEOUS			
Iron deficiency anemia (Chapter 26)	<18 mo	—	Occult blood/small
Swallowed blood	Any	Small/large; coffee grounds	Occult blood/small

Occult blood may be identified by the guaiac test (most conveniently supplied as Hemoccult packets), which produces a blue discoloration for a positive result. Stools may appear black from ingestion of iron, large numbers of chocolate sandwich cookies, bismuth, Pepto-Bismol, lead, licorice, charcoal, or coal, or they may be red from ingestion of gelatin. False-positive findings may result from ingestion of iron, red fruit, and meats; false-negative findings occur when the fecal specimen is stored and dried or the patient has recently ingested ascorbic acid. The guaiac test for detecting occult blood in stool is not useful for detecting gastric bleeding. A test specifically for use with gastric juice (e.g., Gastroccult) should be used instead.

There is an inconsistent correlation between esophageal pH and findings.

Helicobacter pylori associated with peptic ulcer may be diagnosed by the carbon 13-labeled urea breath test in older children, although upper endoscopy is still more commonly used in younger children.

MANAGEMENT

Management of significant GI bleeding involves stabilization of the patient, initially with crystalloid, followed by whole blood or packed red blood cells. Coagulopathies must be treated. Patients should be given oxygen, an intravenous line or lines should be started, and patients should be monitored closely from the time they enter the emergency department (ED). A hematocrit evaluation should be done immediately and blood specimens sent for typing and cross matching. If upper GI bleeding is present, a large-caliber NG tube should be passed and the stomach lavaged with cooled saline solution to decrease mucosal blood flow while monitoring blood in the returned aspirate. Lavage is continued until the aspirate is clear. Consultation with a gastroenterologist should usually be obtained, and if bleeding stops within 30 to 45 minutes, gastroduodenoscopy is often performed to provide direct visualization. If the bleeding is massive or ongoing,

Signs and Symptoms	Evaluation	Comments
History of bleeding diasthesis	Coagulation screening	Factor replacement
Well child or bleeding	PT	Vitamin K, 1-2 mg (infant), 5-10 mg (child, adult)
Vomiting, pain, anemia	Endoscopy, upper GI series, gastric acid	Recurrent ulcers
Variable with location and histology	Endoscopy, barium contrast study	Rare in infants
Well child, pale	CBC	Iron supplementation
Usually obvious source	CBC, Apt test (newborn)	Newborn—maternal blood, epistaxis, etc.

endoscopy may not be useful, and scanning or arteriography may be required.

Vasopressin (Pitressin) may rarely be required for intractable variceal bleeding. After consultation, an initial bolus of 20 units/1.73 m^2 IV diluted in 2 ml/kg of 5% dextrose in water (D5W) is given over 20 minutes followed by a continuous infusion of 0.2 to 0.4 units/1.73 m^2/min. If bleeding ceases, infusion is maintained at the initial dosage for 12 hours and then is tapered over 24 to 36 hours. If it fails, sclerosing agents or a Sengstaken-Blakemore tube may be needed.

Surgical intervention is required for life-threatening hemorrhage, intussusception (if not reducible), volvulus, Meckel's diverticulum, ulcer (if perforated), or a neoplasm.

All patients must be hospitalized for evaluation, monitoring, and intervention. After stabilization and diagnostic evaluation, a long-term management plan must be developed. Mucosal lesions may be treated with antacids containing magnesium hydroxide and aluminum hydroxide (e.g., Maalox, Mylanta). During an acute episode, patients are given the antacids at a dose of 0.5 ml/kg (maximum: 30 ml/dose) q1-2hr PO to keep gastric pH at 5 or above. On a maintenance basis, the same dose is given at 1 and 3 hours after meals and before bedtime.

Pharmacologic agents (histamine [H_2] receptor antagonist) that are equally effective include cimetidine (Tagamet), 20 to 30 mg/kg/24 hr q6hr PO (adult 600-1800 mg/24 hr PO) or 20 to 30 mg/kg/24 hr q4hr IV slowly as 15-minute infusion; ranitidine (Zantac), at either 4 to 5 mg/kg/24 hr [max: 300mg/24 hr] q8-12hr PO or 2 to 4 mg/kg/24 hr q6-8hr IV; and famotidine (Pepcid), 0.5 mg/kg/dose q8-12hr PO, IV (adult: 40 mg q24hr PO or 20 mg q12hr IV).

In patients with peptic ulcer associated with *H. pylori*, triple therapy should be considered; it consists of omeprazole, 10 or 20 mg/dose PO BID; amoxicillin, 25 mg/kg/dose PO BID; and clarithromycin, 7.5 mg/kg/dose PO BID.

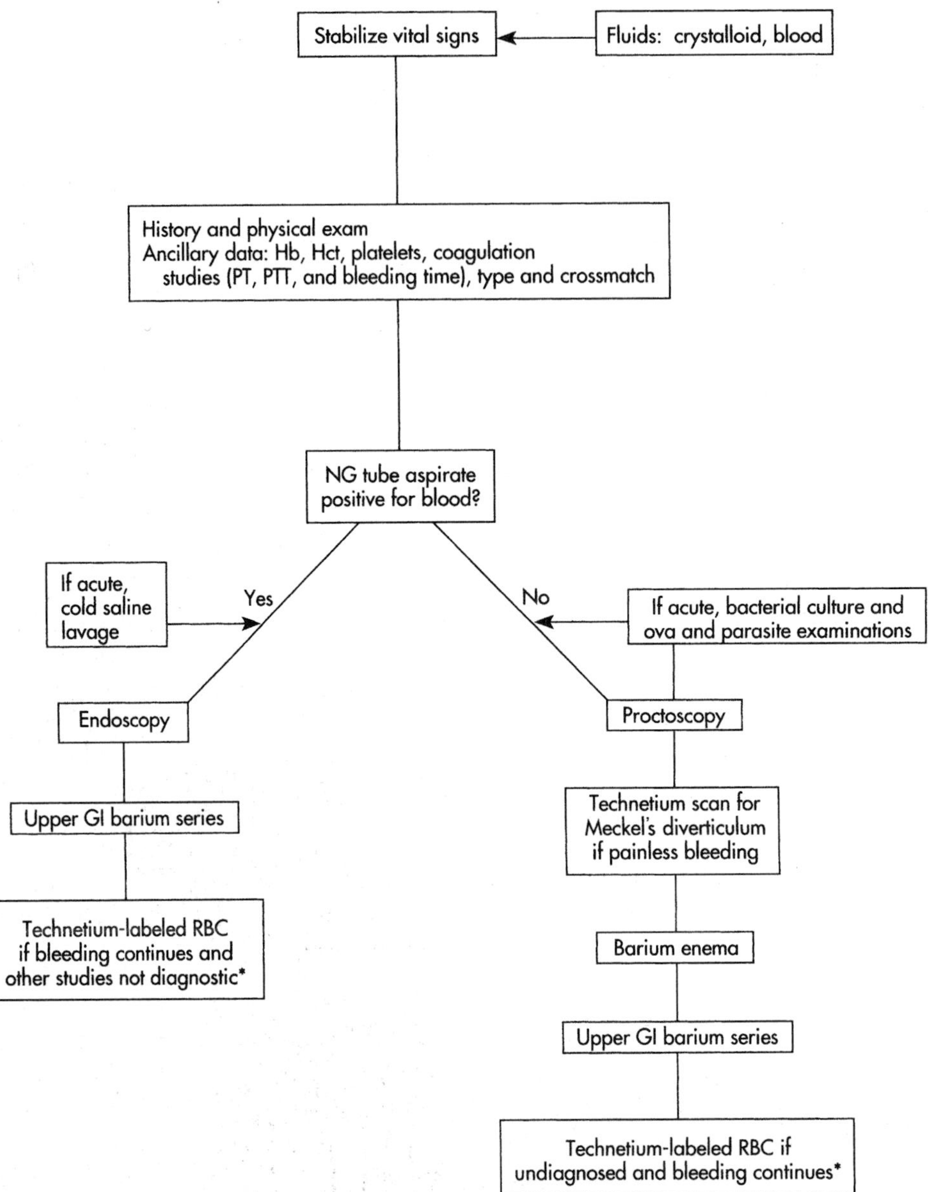

Fig. 35-1 Diagnostic options for gastrointestinal (GI) hemorrhage. *Study may be useful in detecting and localizing sites of active bleeding. Assumes history, physical examination, and ancillary data do not indicate a cause. Consultation is generally indicated. If study is nondiagnostic and bleeding continues, arteriogram may be indicated.

BIBLIOGRAPHY

Jenkins HR, Pincott JR, Soothill JF et al: Food allergy: the major cause of infantile colitis, *Arch Dis Child* 59:326, 1984.

36 Headache

Also See Chapter 84 (Neurologic Disorders)

ALERT Children younger than 5 years rarely have headaches and must be evaluated for an organic cause. Progressive, recurrent, or severe headaches need evaluation. Life-threatening conditions must be excluded.

Because the brain has no pain-sensitive structures, headaches secondary to intracranial disease arise from irritating pain fibers that innervate the dura or vessels of the pia-arachnoid. Headaches may also be extracranial, involving muscles, blood vessels, epithelial tissue of the sinuses, orbit, and eye. Nearly two thirds of headaches in children are associated with extracranial infections (viral syndrome, sinusitis, pharyngitis). The pain associated with headaches has several mechanisms:

1. Muscle contraction: tension
2. Vascular: migraine, cluster, hypertension
3. Traction: subarachnoid hemorrhage, mass lesion, postconcussion
4. Inflammatory: meningitis, sinusitis, arteritis
5. Secondary to extracranial structures: refractive error, sinusitis
6. Psychogenic: depression, conversion

DIAGNOSTIC FINDINGS

The initial evaluation of the patient with a headache who is otherwise stable must determine the characteristics with regard to location, nature of pain, age of onset, frequency, duration and progression, precipitating and ameliorating factors, pica, ingestions, exposures, associated signs and symptoms, medications, medical history (especially hypertension, sinusitis, heart disease, ear infections, and seizures), and family history. The temporal pattern is particularly important for determining whether the headache is acute (single event with no previous episodes), acute and recurrent, chronic and progressive (suggesting potential raised intracranial pressure with increasing severity and frequency), or chronic and nonprogressive (several times per day or week, with no change in severity or signs and symptoms). Recent stresses and emotional stability should be delineated. A careful physical examination must be performed with a complete neurologic evaluation, including visual acuity and fields, cerebellar signs, and auscultation for bruits.

Because children younger than 5 years rarely have headaches, an organic cause is highly likely. Increased intracranial pressure is suggested by a headache that awakens the patient from sleep, occurs in the morning, is associated with vomiting without nausea, or is related to a change in position from prone to supine or erect. Occipital pain is often associated with an anatomic abnormality. Presenting signs and symptoms are helpful in differentiating cause of the headache (Tables 36-1 and 36-2).

Ancillary Data

Ancillary data should reflect positive findings. Studies that may be useful under specific circumstances are computed tomography (CT),

TABLE 36-1 Differentiation of Headache Type By Signs and Symptoms

Clues	Type of Headache
ASSOCIATED EVENTS	
Abrupt onset	Convulsive, subarachnoid hemorrhage
Afternoon	Muscle contraction
Present on arising	Convulsive (following nocturnal seizure), emotional depression, traction (tumor), vascular
Preceded by aura	Convulsive, vascular (migraine)
Exacerbated by coughing	Paranasal sinus, traction (tumor, increased intracranial pressure), vascular
Followed by lethargy	Convulsive, vascular
Followed by focal central nervous system deficit	Convulsive (Todd's paresis), traction (tumor), vascular (hemiplegic migraine)
Fever, neck stiffness	Meningitis
Related to posture	Posttraumatic, traction (tumor and after lumbar puncture)
Related to stress	Muscle contraction, vascular (migraine)
Nausea and vomiting	Migraine, convulsive, traction (tumor)
Elevated diastolic pressure	Hypertensive encephalopathy
CHARACTER OF PAIN	
Steady	Emotional depression, muscle contraction, sinus, traction (tumor, increased intracranial pressure)
Throbbing	Convulsive, posttraumatic, traction (tumor, increased intracranial pressure), vascular (migraine, vasculitis, inflammatory)
LOCATION	
Frontal	Traction (supratentorial tumor), vascular
Occipital and neck	Muscle, contraction, sinus (ethmoid), traction (posterior fossa tumor)
Unilateral	Traction (lateralized supratentorial tumor), vascular (migraine), intracranial hemorrhage

Modified from Kriel RL: Headache. In Swaiman KF, Wright FS, editors: *The practice of pediatric neurology*, ed 2, vol 1, St Louis, 1982, Mosby.

TABLE 36-2 Headache: Diagnostic Considerations

Condition	Diagnostic Findings	Comments
INTRAPSYCHIC		
Tension	Common; anxiety, stress, recurrent headache; pain—occipital, neck, or generalized, although it can be bifrontal or frontotemporal; sense of pressure or constriction; no prodrome, aura; spasm of muscles of neck and shoulder	Attempt to reduce anxiety; analgesia, stress control
Conversion reaction (p. 774)	Inconsistent physical findings	
Depression	Inciting event; history of behavioral disturbance; difficulty sleeping	

TABLE 36-2 Headache: Diagnostic Considerations—cont'd

Condition	Diagnostic Findings	Comments
INFECTION		
Meningitis/encephalitis (p. 741)	Acute onset, infectious prodrome, and associated findings; pain on movement; diffuse headache; lumbar puncture diagnostic	Hospitalize; antibiotics; support
Abscess, cerebral	Low-grade fever; focal neurologic findings; localized headache; meningism; lumbar puncture: variable WBC, negative culture results; CT scan	Neurosurgical referral
Sinusitis (p. 619)	Unilateral or bilateral frontal headache; pain on percussion of sinus; if sphenoid, may be occipital; purulent rhinorrhea; sinus x-ray studies	Antibiotics; rare drainage and referral; other ear, nose, and throat infections can cause headache including otitis media, mastoiditis, and retropharyngeal abscess
Dental abscess (p. 599)	Insidious onset; local pain; dental x-ray studies	Dental referral
VASCULAR		
Migraine (p. 750)	Unilateral recurrent headache (young children—generalized); throbbing; associated visual, sensory, motor deficit; abdominal pain, nausea, vomiting, positive family history; 25%–50% of chronic headaches	Supportive; analgesia, steroids, ergotamine (Cafergot); prophylaxis if frequent (atenolol, propranolol, calcium channel blocker, serotonin antagonist, cyclic antidepressant); sumatriptan useful in older children
Cluster	Paroxysmal, unilateral, explosive retroorbital, periorbital, or frontal headache; unilateral autonomic symptoms—nasal stuffiness, lacrimation, Horner syndrome; cluster in short period separated by long pain-free interval; rare in children; lasts 30–120 min but extremely severe; may occur several times in 24-hr period	Oxygen; DHE (IV or IM) plus antiemetic or sumatriptan; intranasal lidocaine (4%); trial of prophylactic verapamil and tapering steroids
Subarachnoid or cerebral bleeding; AV malformation (Chapter 18)	Acute onset; intense headache; focal neurologic examination; obtundation; meningism; CT scan; lumbar puncture bloody	Predisposing factors: trauma, bleeding diathesis
Hypertensive encephalopathy	Diffuse headache, nausea, vomiting, confusion, seizure, focal neurologic finding; high blood pressure	Associated illness: acute glomerulonephritis, etc.
TRAUMA (Chapter 57)		
Postconcussive	Diffuse headache, often occipital, neck, or generalized bifrontal; vertigo, dizziness, confusion, sensitivity to noise, movement, heat, light; emotional instability; normal neurologic finding	Observation; frequent examinations; analgesia, muscle relaxants

Continued

TABLE 36-2 Headache: Diagnostic Considerations—cont'd

Condition	Diagnostic Findings	Comments
TRAUMA (Chapter 57)—cont'd		
Subdural	Acute or insidious onset headache; CT	Neurosurgical intervention, observation; frequent examination
Fracture	Local tenderness and swelling; skull x-ray study	Neurosurgical consultation
INTOXICATION		
Carbon monoxide (p. 376)	Headache, weakness; dizziness; respiratory arrest, coma; carboxyhemoglobin level	Oxygen; hyperbaric chamber
Lead	Diffuse headache; weakness; irritability, personality change; ataxia; seizures, coma; pica; red cell δ-amino-levulinic acid dehydratase	Dimercaprol and EDTA; penicillamine
NEOPLASM		
Cerebral	Frontal unrelenting headache, unilateral or bilateral; usually worse on rising; papilledema; increased intracranial pressure	Neurosurgical consultation
Cerebellar	Occipital unrelenting headache; vomiting; ataxia	Neurosurgical consultation
Pseudotumor cerebri (p. 753)	Nausea, vomiting, diplopia, acute or insidious generalized headache; full fontanelle, variable papilledema, ↑ CSF pressure	Predisposing factors: viral illness, intoxication, head trauma, steroids, etc.
AUTOIMMUNE		
Temporal arteritis	Local headache with tenderness and pain over temporal artery	Steroids; rare; increased ESR
Trigeminal neuralgia	Unilateral, recurrent headache and pain over distribution of second branch, trigeminal nerve	Carbamazepine, phenytoin
MISCELLANEOUS		
Eye		
Glaucoma	Generalized headache; blurred vision, dilated pupil; tonometry	Miotic, osmotic, diuretic
Refractive error	Generalized headache	Glasses
Epilepsy (p. 754)	Paroxysmal onset of headache and abrupt termination; brief duration; loss of contact with environment; variable abdominal pain	Rare cause of headaches
High altitude (Chapter 49)	Diffuse headache; weakness	
Temporomandibular joint (TMJ) disease	Frontotemporal or temporal pain; bilateral or unilateral severe, steady ache; limited mandibular movement, tenderness in muscles of jaw and neck	Refer to dentist
Status postlumbar puncture	Diffuse headache after procedure; unusual in young children	Bed rest, supine; occasional patch

often with special views to evaluate sinuses (elevated intracranial pressure, progressive or new neurologic signs, behavioral change, growth drop-off, reduced visual acuity, increasing frequency or severity of headaches, or increasing pain on awakening, coughing, straining, or changing position, focal electroencephalogram [EEG], meningismus, focal headache, seizures), electroencephalography, and lumbar puncture.

MANAGEMENT

Management should focus on suitable analgesia and treatment of the underlying condition, excluding life-threatening conditions. An empiric trial is sometimes indicated. Hospitalization is indicated if there is any evidence of increased intracranial pressure, progressive or new neurologic signs, or intractable pain.

BIBLIOGRAPHY

Burton LJ, Quinn B, Pratt-Cheney JL et al: Headache etiology in a pediatric emergency department, *Pediatr Emerg Care* 13:1, 1997.

Singer HS, Rowe S: Chronic recurrent headache in children, *Pediatr Ann* 21:369, 1992.

Stafstrom CE, Rostasy K, Minster A: The usefulness of children's drawings in the diagnosis of headache, *Pediatrics* 109:460, 2002.

Stratton SJ: Sumatriptan: a clinical standard, *Ann Emerg Med* 25:538, 1995.

Svenson J, Cowen D, Rogers A: Headache in the emergency department: importance of history in identifying secondary etiologies, *J Emerg Med* 15:617, 1997.

37 Hematuria and Proteinuria

Also See Chapter 85 (Renal Disorders)

ALERT Hematuria and proteinuria require a systematic evaluation to exclude glomerular or extraglomerular disease on the basis of the history and physical and laboratory findings.

*H*ematuria is present when there are 5 or more red blood cells per high-power field (RBCs/HPF) in a sediment of 10 ml of centrifuged urine (also see Chapter 85). It can result from nonrenal as well as glomerular and extraglomerular abnormality, which can often be clinically distinguished by urinalysis as follows:

	Glomerular	Extraglomerular or Nonrenal
Urine color	Brown, smoky "cola color"	Red, pink, or bright red blood
RBC casts	May be present	Absent
Blood clots	Absent	May be present

Hematuria in newborns results primarily from vascular disorders such as hypoxia, thrombosis, and circulatory compromise; in older children, urinary tract infections account for most cases, followed by glomerulonephritis and trauma. Hypercalciuria and nephrolithiasis also can cause hematuria.

Hemoglobinuria or myoglobinuria can cause false-positive test results, as can iodine. Obviously, a microscopic examination for RBCs should be done. With myoglobinuria, the hematocrit is normal and the serum is clear (not pink). Common causes of hemoglobinuria are hemolytic anemia, incompatible blood transfusions, disseminated intravascular coagulation (DIC), hemolytic-uremic syndrome, infection (sepsis, malaria), burns, exertion, cold, nocturnal and exertional hemoglobinurias, and drugs (carbon monoxide, sulfonamides, snake venom). Myoglobinuria may be caused by muscle injury (crush, burn), myositis, or rhabdomyolysis.

Drugs and other agents that turn the urine red or dark include aniline dyes, blackberries, phenolphthalein, phenazopyridine (Pyridium), rifampin, and urates (p. 365).

Proteinuria is present when more than 200 mg/m^2/24 hr of protein is excreted in the urine. It is usually transient, occurring with fever, exercise, seizures, pneumonia, congestive heart failure (CHF), or environmental stress. *Orthostatic proteinuria* occurs when an individual is in an upright position; resolution is seen in 50% of patients by early adulthood. Evaluation of orthostatic proteinuria requires careful collection and comparison of standing and recumbent urine samples. During a 24-hour collection, the voids during the night and upon awakening (recumbent position) must be separated from the remainder of the urine collected during the day. Ideally this is done by having the patient fast (NPO) after 9 pm and void before bed. Urine specimens are then collected at midnight and 5 AM while the patient remains recumbent, again at 7 AM, and then while the patient is active through the day until bedtime.

Urine dipstick tests for hematuria change color with the oxidation of orthotoluidine to cumene hyproperoxide with the catalysis of hemoglobin or myoglobin. Oxidizing agents

TABLE 37-1 Hematuria and Proteinuria: Diagnostic Considerations*

Condition	Site of Involvement	Diagnostic Findings	URINALYSIS Hematuria	URINALYSIS Proteinuria	Comments
INFECTION					
Urinary tract infection (p. 833)	Nonrenal/extraglomerular	Acute onset fever, dysuria, frequency, burning; if pyelonephritis, may appear toxic, with CVA tenderness, WBC casts	Gross/microscopic	Positive	Cystitis or pyelonephritis; bacterial, viral, tuberculosis, other; culture
AUTOIMMUNE					
Glomerulonephritis, acute (p. 817)	Glomerular	Malaise, headache, vomiting, fever, abdominal pain; oliguria, edema, high BP	Gross/microscopic	Positive	Poststreptoccal; high ASO titer; low complement
Membranoproliferative glomerulonephritis (p. 817)	Glomerular	Often insidious; malaise, headache, vomiting, edema, high BP	Gross/microscopic	Positive	Low complement; biopsy
Henoch-Schönlein purpura (p. 822)	Glomerular	Purpuric rash, arthritis, GI involvement	Microscopic	Variable	Variable involvement; may have elevated IgA level
Lupus nephritis	Glomerular	Associated signs and symptoms	Microscopic	Positive	Variable involvement; positive ANA result, low complement; biopsy
Nephritis Bacterial endocarditis (p. 567) Shunt	Glomerular	Acute illness, fever, toxicity, signs and symptoms of related disease	Microscopic	Positive	Low complement
Nephrotic syndrome (p. 824)	Glomerular	Periorbital swelling and oliguria followed by edema, malaise, abdominal pain	Rare (25%)	Positive	Low albumin, high lipid levels; cause unknown
TRAUMA (Chapter 64)					
Renal calculi	Nonrenal	Asymptomatic to severe back and abdominal pain, nausea, vomiting	Gross/microscopic	Negative	Idiopathic, UTI, ↑ Ca^{++}, cystinosis, hyperuricemia VP; IVP indicated
Foreign body	Nonrenal	Frequency, urgency, pain	Microscopic	Negative	Usually experimenting or masturbating

Continued

TABLE 37-1 Hematuria and Proteinuria: Diagnostic Considerations*

Condition	Site of Involvement	Diagnostic Findings	URINALYSIS Hematuria	Proteinuria	Comments
TRAUMA (Chapter 64)—cont'd					
Direct trauma (Chapter 64)	Variable	History of trauma with variable complaints	Gross/microscopic	Negative	Usually renal contusion; if gross, laceration or rupture; IVP
Exercise	Nonrenal	Follows heavy exercise	Microscopic	Variable	
Meatal excoriation (p. 671)	Nonrenal	Local lesion	Gross/microscopic	Negative	Local treatment
CONGENITAL					
Hydronephrosis	Extraglomerular	Abdominal mass	Microscopic	Positive	Most common ureteropelvic junction
Polycystic kidney	Extraglomerular	Large kidney, other cystic anomalies	Microscopic	Positive	Infant, adult types
Hemangioma/ telangiectasis	Extraglomerular	Hemangioma, telangiectasia	Microscopic	Negative	Rendu-Osler-Weber disease
Hemoglobinopathy/ hemophilia Sickle cell trait, SC (p. 714)	Extraglomerular	Associated signs and symptoms	Microscopic	Negative	Difficulty concentrating urine; factor levels
Coagulopathy thrombocytopenia (p. 709)	Extraglomerular	Bleeding problems elsewhere	Gross/microscopic	Negative	Bleeding screen, platelets
Hereditary nephritis	Glomerular	Hearing deficit	Microscopic	Negative	Alport syndrome
Benign familial hematuria	Glomerular	Intermittent or persistent	Microscopic	Negative	Benign
INTOXICATION					
Anticoagulants Aspirin Methicillin Sulfonamides	Extraglomerular	Nephritis or crystalluria	Gross/microscopic	Variable	Temporally related to drug use
NEOPLASM					
Wilms' tumor	Extraglomerular	Abdominal mass	Gross/microscopic	Negative	Surgical consultation
Leukemia	Extraglomerular	Systemic disease	Microscopic	Variable	Oncology consultation
OTHER					
Renal vein thrombosis	Extraglomerular		Gross/microscopic	Variable	Occurs in acutely ill children
Congestive heart failure (Chapter 16)	Extraglomerular	Dyspnea, tachycardia, tachypnea	Microscopic	Negative	Accompanies cardiac disease

such as povidone-iodine, hexachlorophene, and hypochlorite may cause false-positive results, as can markedly alkaline urine. False-negative findings can result from ascorbic acid.

Proteinuria results may be expressed as follows: 0, trace (15 mg/dl), 1+ (30 mg/dl), 2+ (100 mg/dl), 3+ (300 mg/dl), and 4+ (2000 mg/dl). Fifty percent of patients with "trace" proteinuria have normal quantitation results. False-positive results occur with highly alkaline urine (pH >6.5) or contamination with benzalkonium.

A ratio may allow use of a single specimen. Semiquantitative protein excretion may be estimated by determining, on a spot urine, the ratio of mg protein divided by mg creatinine, preferably with use of the first morning urine. A ratio above 0.2 in children older than 2 years or more than 0.5 in children 6 to 24 old is abnormal.

The evaluation of a child with hematuria or proteinuria is outlined in Figs. 37-1 and 37-2 and Table 37-1.

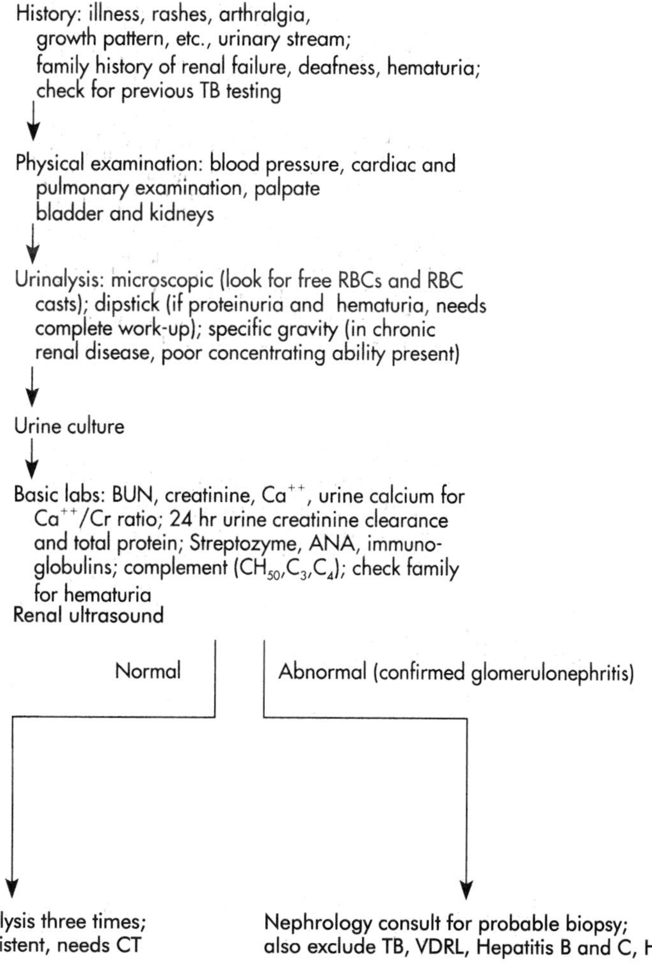

Fig. 37-1 Evaluation for hematuria. Evaluation of hematuria after trauma is discussed in Chapter 64.

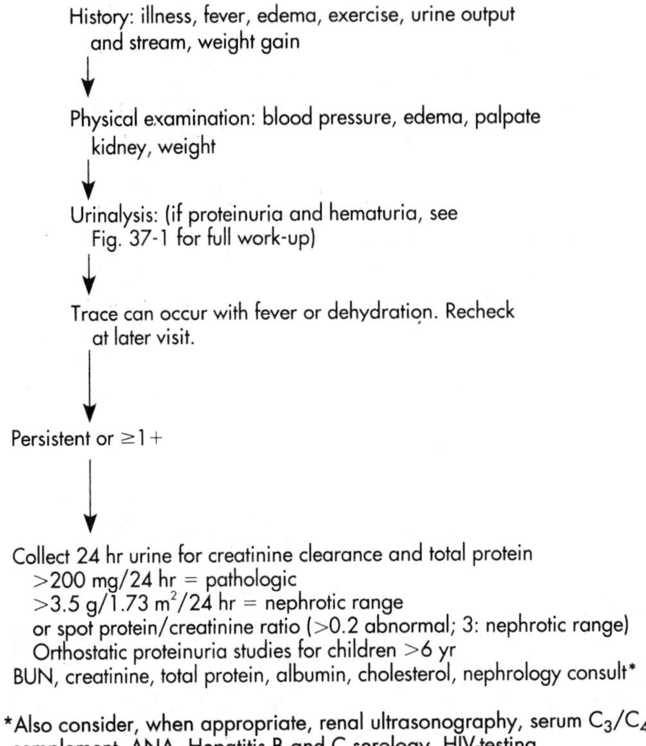

History: illness, fever, edema, exercise, urine output and stream, weight gain
Physical examination: blood pressure, edema, palpate kidney, weight
Urinalysis: (if proteinuria and hematuria, see Fig. 37-1 for full work-up)
Trace can occur with fever or dehydration. Recheck at later visit.
Persistent or ≥1+
Collect 24 hr urine for creatinine clearance and total protein
>200 mg/24 hr = pathologic
>3.5 g/1.73 m²/24 hr = nephrotic range
or spot protein/creatinine ratio (>0.2 abnormal; 3: nephrotic range)
Orthostatic proteinuria studies for children >6 yr
BUN, creatinine, total protein, albumin, cholesterol, nephrology consult*
*Also consider, when appropriate, renal ultrasonography, serum C3/C4 complement, ANA, Hepatitis B and C serology, HIV-testing

Fig. 37-2 Evaluation for proteinuria.

BIBLIOGRAPHY

Abitol C, Zilleruelo G et al: Quantitation of proteinuria with urinary protein/creatinine ratios and random testing with dipstick in nephrotic children, *J Pediatr* 116:243, 1990.

Fitzwater DS, Wyatt RJ: Hematuria, *Pediatr Rev* 15:102, 1994.

Hogg RJ, Portman RJ, Milliner D et al: Evaluation and management of proteinuria and nephrotic syndrome in children: recommendations from a pediatric nephrology panel established at the National Kidney Foundation Conference on Proteinuria, Albuminuria, Risk, Assessment, Detection and Elimination (PARADE), *Pediatrics* 105:1242, 2000.

White RHR: The investigation of hematuria, *Arch Dis Child* 64:259, 1989.

Yadin O: Hematuria in children, *Pediatr Ann* 23:474, 1994.

38 Hypoglycemia

Also see Chapter 74 (Endocrine Disorders)

ALERT If signs and symptoms are consistent, an emergent therapeutic trial of glucose administration should be attempted after specimens for glucose determination have been obtained.

Hypoglycemia is generally considered to be associated with a blood glucose level of less than 40 mg/dl in the child. The blood glucose level in most newborns exceeds 50 mg/dl by 48 hours of life. The currently recommended operational threshold for intervention is 45 mg/dl in symptomatic neonates. In the absence of symptoms in a neonate, hypoglycemia is a serum glucose value less than 35 mg/dl (p. 99). Initial use of Dextrostix or Chemstrips is helpful for emergency approximations before confirmation by clinical analysis in the laboratory. Obviously, clinical signs and symptoms must be correlated with laboratory measurements.

Fasting hypoglycemia, which is related to an imbalance between glucose production and use, is most common in thin male children between 18 months and 5 years. Reactive hypoglycemia produces a low glucose level within 5 hours after eating; it accompanies increased insulin and is usually severe. Drugs also can cause hypoglycemia.

ETIOLOGY (Table 38-1)

Newborns experience transient hypoglycemia, often in association with perinatal complications caused by excessive insulin secretion, including maternal diabetes or erythroblastosis. After the first day of life, and often in association with hypoxia and intrauterine growth retardation, a more prolonged hypoglycemia produced by inadequate glycogen stores may develop. Congenital abnormalities of the central nervous system (CNS) or heart may cause hypoglycemia; sepsis and hypocalcemia may develop.

Inborn errors of carbohydrate and glycogen storage, amino acid and organic acid metabolism, and endocrine abnormalities may cause hypoglycemia during *infancy*. Hypoglycemia occurs shortly after the ingestion of protein in patients with idiopathic leucine sensitivity and defects in amino acid and organic acid metabolism. Ingestion of lactose may stimulate hypoglycemia associated with galactosemia; sucrose ingestion may produce hypoglycemia in the presence of hereditary fructose intolerance. Patients with medium-chain acyl-CoA dehydrogenase deficiency (MCADD) typically are seen between 3 months and 2 years of age with minor illnesses or when a baby first sleeps through the night. This disorder of fatty acid oxidation impairs ketogenesis.

In *childhood*, fasting hypoglycemia may result from ketotic hypoglycemia as well as hormonal deficiencies, hyperinsulinism, glycogen storage disease, or fructose 1,6-diphosphatase deficiency. *Preschool* children may be symptomatic after prolonged fasting, which exacerbates the physiologic response to starvation. Poisons and toxins may be contributory in other patients.

TABLE 38-1 Hypoglycemia: Diagnostic Considerations

Condition	Type	Hepatomegaly (Variably Abnormal Liver Function-test)	Ketonuria/ Ketonemia
NEONATAL (TRANSIENT) (Chapter 11)			
Small-for-gestational age infant	Fasting	No	No
Hyperinsulinism	Fasting	No	No
Infant of diabetic mother			
Erythroblastosis			
Perinatal insult	Fasting	No	No
Asphyxia, infection			
HEPATIC ENZYME DEFICIENCY			
Glycogen storage disease (I, III, VI)	Fasting	Yes	Variable
Disorder of gluconeogenesis	Fasting	Yes	No
LIMITED SUBSTRATE			
Ketotic hypoglycemia (onset 1½-5 yr; resolves by 9-10 yr)	Fasting	No	Yes
Endocrine (Chapter 74)			
Panhypopituitarism	Fasting	No	Yes
Growth hormone deficiency			
ACTH deficiency			
Addison's disease			
Hypothyroidism			
HYPERINSULINEMIA			
Beta-cell tumor, adenoma, hyperplasia	Fasting	No	No
Leucine sensitivity	Reactive	No	No
Extrapancreatic tumor	Fasting	No	No
Prediabetes	Fasting	No	No
INTOXICATION (Chapter 54)			
Salicylates		No	Yes
Ethanol		No	Variable
Propranolol		No	No
Insulin		No	No
MISCELLANEOUS			
Malnutrition	Fasting	Yes	Yes
Hepatic damage	Fasting	Variable	Variable
Reye syndrome (p. 655)			
Hepatitis (p. 649)			
Fructose intolerance, galactosemia	Reactive	Yes	No
Amino acid abnormalities	Fasting	No	No
Gastroenteritis	Fasting	No	No

Idiopathic ketotic hypoglycemia accounts for more than one fourth of significant hypoglycemia unrelated to diabetes in children older than 6 months. It generally manifests in children 7 months to 5 years with symptomatic hypoglycemia in the morning hours after a moderate fast and with ketonuria. They respond to administration of glucose.

DIAGNOSTIC FINDINGS

The patient's history may be helpful in focusing on the appropriate cause. Onset; frequency;

relationship to food (fruits and fructose intolerance, high-protein diet intolerance, or leucine sensitivity), drugs, or fasting; family history; and concurrent medical problems must be explored. Evidence of abnormalities in growth and development must be sought (Table 38-2).

The systemic response primarily reflects excessive catecholamine release. Clinically, patients have sweating, weakness, tachycardia, tachypnea, variable elevations of blood pressure and temperature, anxiety, tremulousness, and hunger. Neonates may be asymptomatic.

If the hypoglycemia is not treated, cerebral dysfunction may progress, the presentation and complications paralleling those seen with hypoxia. Patients may have headaches; disturbed mental status with confusion, irritability, and psychotic behavior; ataxia; seizures; and coma. The signs and symptoms of the underlying cause may also be present.

A ***complication*** of hypoglycemia is permanent brain damage from frequent or prolonged hypoglycemia.

Ancillary Data

1. Serum insulin, serum, and urine glucose and ketone, lactate, and phosphate levels and liver function test results.
2. Specific tolerance tests, response to ketogenic diet, enzymes in urine, liver biopsy, and so on, may all have to be considered, depending on the differential diagnosis.

DIFFERENTIAL DIAGNOSIS

See Chapters 15 and 54.

MANAGEMENT

Concurrently with stabilization, the hypoglycemia must be treated. Patients with clinical

TABLE 38-2 Hypoglycemia: Etiologic Differentiation

	Inborn Error of Metabolism (Carbohydrate/Amino Acid)	Hormonal Deficiency	Hyperinsulinism
HISTORY			
Hypoglycemia			
Fasting (time after fasting)	Common* (many hours)	Common (few hours)	Common (few hours)
After lactose	Galactosemia	No	No
After sucrose	Hereditary fructose intolerance	No	No
After protein	Amino acid, organic acid	No	No
Family history	Common	Variable	Variable
PHYSICAL			
Hepatomegaly	Common	No	No
Failure to thrive	Common	Variable	Variable
LABORATORY			
Ketosis	Common†	Variable	No
Acidosis	Common	No	No
Nonglucose urine reducing substance	Galactosemia, hereditary fructose intolerance		
Hyperammonemia	Amino acid, organic acid		
Liver function abnormality	Common	No	No

* Glycogen storage disease. Fructose 1,6-diphosphatase deficiency.

† If no ketosis, consider 3-hydroxy-3-methylglutaric aciduria, glutaric aciduria type II, systemic carnitine deficiency, and carnitine palmitoyl transferase deficiency.

components of hypoglycemia require emergency intervention.

1. In the newborn, early, frequent feedings with very close monitoring are often adequate. If the glucose remains low, intravenous administration may be indicated.
2. In the older child, if there are no vital sign or central nervous system abnormalities, oral glucose may be given, with frequent feedings.
3. If the patient is unstable with altered mental status, glucose should be administered parenterally:
   a. Give 0.5 to 1 g/kg/dose IV, usually administered as 25% dextrose in water (D25W) (2-4 ml/kg/dose) slowly; a rapid response is to be expected if hypoglycemia is the prominent cause. D10W should be used for preterm infants; D10W has 10 g of glucose per dl.
   b. Thereafter, maintain adequate glucose homeostasis and fluid balance: 10% glucose in 0.2% normal saline (NS) solution at a rate of about 7 mg of dextrose/kg/min.
4. If glucose is unavailable, glucagon, 0.03 to 0.1 mg/kg/dose IM, IV (1 mg may be given at any age), will provide transient elevation of glucose level in a patient whose liver stores are adequate. The dose may be repeated in 20 minutes.
5. Sources of 20 g of glucose commonly available include Kool-Aid with sugar (13.4 oz), Coca-Cola (13.3 oz), orange soda (10 oz), ginger ale (15.5 oz), Hershey's milk chocolate bar (2.5 oz bar), orange juice (12 oz), and apple juice (12 oz). Obviously, the glucose levels may change with variations in products or mixing technique.
6. In severe hyperinsulinemia, diazoxide, 6 to 12 mg/kg/24 hr q12hr PO, is usually required on an ongoing basis. Frequent feedings alone are often successful in preventing fasting types of hypoglycemia. Underlying diseases must receive prompt treatment.

DISPOSITION

Most patients with suspected hyperinsulinemia or any vital sign abnormalities or cerebral dysfunction should be admitted to the hospital until the cause is clear and future episodes can be prevented. Patients with only minimal symptoms and a known cause can, with adequate follow-up observation, often be monitored as outpatients. The ultimate disposition and management must reflect the cause.

BIBLIOGRAPHY

Bonham JR: Investigation of hypoglycaemia during childhood, *Ann Clin Biochem* 30:238, 1993.

Haymond M: Hypoglycemia in infants and children, *Endocrinol Metab Clin North Am* 18:211, 1989.

Pershad J, Monroe K, Atchison J: Childhood hypoglycemia in an urban emergency department: epidemiology and a diagnostic approach to the problem, *Pediatr Emerg Care* 14:268, 1998.

39 Irritability

ALERT Irritability may be the presenting complaint for a potentially life-threatening systemic disease. It is essential to consider such conditions in determining management.

Children tend to be irritable with acute infections, particularly those associated with fever. The febrile child needs careful evaluation to ensure that no underlying significant disorder is associated with the behavioral change. Chronic illnesses, such as juvenile rheumatoid arthritis, may cause a child to be irritable.

Most children tend to be most irritable during a particular period of the day, usually toward the evening. When this irritability becomes marked, it is known as *colic*, a disorder that occurs in as many as 10% of children. Irritability from teething usually begins at 6 months of age with the appearance of the first teeth. Because medications commonly cause irritability, this factor should be considered in the prescription of drugs. Unrecognized trauma must also be excluded (Table 39-1).

The history and physical examination should focus on the pattern of irritability and contributing findings. Time and duration, frequency, and factors that reduce or exacerbate the behavior should be defined. The child's response to being consoled, fed, and rocked should be noted. Factors such as loud noises, hunger, wet diapers, and search for attention may affect behavior. Potential contributing conditions, including trauma, medication, infection, congenital anomalies, and metabolic abnormalities, should be excluded. The parent-child interaction should be evaluated. Tooth eruption should be noted.

In children with suspected esophagitis, it is essential to realize there is an inconsistent correlation between esophageal pH monitoring and disease.

Attempts must be made to ensure the child's comfort while ascertaining that there is no significant disorder and that the parents are dealing with the child's irritability from an appropriate perspective. In addition to specific therapeutic interventions, support, empathy, and frequent follow-up observation are essential. If infantile colic is suspected, dietary manipulation (avoidance of milk and fruit juices containing sorbitol) should be attempted.

TABLE 39-1 Irritability: Diagnostic Considerations

Condition	Diagnostic Findings	Comments
INFECTIONS		
Minor acute infections		
Upper respiratory infections (p. 618)	Rhinorrhea, cough, variable fever, decreased activity, nontoxic	Irritability decreases with antipyretic therapy; must rule out other abnormality
Otitis media (p. 605)	Rhinorrhea, fever, ear pain	Irritability usually decreases with antipyretic therapy and local therapy (eardrops) if needed
Urinary tract infection (p. 833)	Fever, dysuria, frequency, burning	Irritability decreases in 24 hr with appropriate antibiotics
Other	Associated signs and symptoms	
Meningitis (p. 741)/ encephalitis	Fever, anorexia, changed mental status, lethargy, variable stiff neck, headache	Important infection to consider in irritable child; may exist even in presence of other infection such as otitis media
Osteomyelitis (p. 769)	Bone pain, redness	Orthopedic consultation
COLIC	Episodic, intense, persistent crying in an otherwise healthy child; usually occurs in late afternoon or evening	Usually begins at 2-3 wk and continues until 10-12 wk; must be certain no abnormality exists; advise soothing rhythmic activities (rocking, wind-up swing), avoiding stimulants (coffee, tea, cola) if breast-feeding, and minimizing daytime sleeping; soy or hydrolyzed casein formula may be transiently beneficial; make sure that mother gets adequate sleep and is handling stress; colic may have long-term impact on family; diagnosis of exclusion
TEETHING	Irritated, swollen gum; does *not* cause high fevers, significant diarrhea, or diaper rash	Advise teething ring, wet washcloth to chew on; rubbing gums with small amount of Scotch (or other liquor) or proprietary products; avoiding salty foods
INTRAPSYCHIC		
Parental anxiety	Insecure, anxious parents; overly responsive, irritable well child	Unstable or changing home environment, inconsistent parenting; attempt to support parents
INTOXICATION (Chapter 54)		
Phenobarbital Aminophylline Amphetamines Ephedrine	In therapeutic or high dosage may cause irritability as either a primary or paradoxical effect	May try different form of drug or substitute
Lead	Weakness, weight loss, vomiting, headache, abdominal pain, seizures, increased intracranial pressure	Dimercaprol, EDTA
Narcotics withdrawal in newborn (Chapter 11)	Yawning, sneezing, jitteriness, tremor, constant movement, seizures, vomiting, dehydration, collapse	Symptoms begin in first 48 hr but may be delayed; support child: phenobarbital, 5 mg/kg/24 hr q8hr IM or PO with slow tapering over 1-3 wk

TABLE 39-1 Irritability: Diagnostic Considerations—cont'd

Condition	Diagnostic Findings	Comments
TRAUMA		
Foreign body, fracture, tourniquet (hair around digit) (Chapter 66)	Local tenderness, swelling, often following injury; thread or cloth around digit or penis	Splinter or other foreign body, hairline fracture; contusion; tourniquet around digit or penis
Subdural hematoma (Chapter 57) Epidural hematoma	History of head trauma; progressively impaired mental status; vomiting, headache, seizures	May be acute or chronic; requires recognition, computed tomography scan; neurosurgical consultation
Corneal abrasion (p. 443)	May not have history; patch; fluorescein positive	Value of patching is not proven
DEFICIENCY		
Iron deficiency anemia (Chapter 26)	Pallor, learning deficit, anorexic, poor diet, microcytic, hypochromic anemia	Peaks at 9 and 18 mo of age; diet insufficient; elemental iron 5 mg/kg/24 hr q8hr PO
Malnutrition	Wasted, distended abdomen	May be caused by neglect or poverty
ENDOCRINE/METABOLIC		
Hyponatremia/ hypernatremia (Chapter 8)	Dehydration, edema, seizures, intracranial bleeding	Multiple causes
Hypocalcemia	Tetany, seizure, diarrhea	Multiple causes
Hypercalcemia	Abdominal pain, polyuria, nephrocalcinosis, constipation, pancreatitis	Multiple causes
Hypoglycemia (Chapter 38)	Sweating, tachycardia, weakness, tachypnea, anxiety, tremor; cerebral dysfunction	Multiple causes; dextrose 0.5-1.0 g/kg/dose IV
Diabetes insipidus	Polydipsia, thirst, constipation, dehydration, collapse	May be hyponatremic; urine specific gravity <1.006; inability to concentrate urine on fluid restriction
VASCULAR		
Congenital heart disease	Cyanosis, other cardiac findings	Usually cyanotic
Congestive heart failure (Chapter 16)	Tachypnea, tachycardia, rales, pulmonary edema	Cardiac and noncardiogenic
Paroxysmal atrial tachycardia (Chapter 6)	Heart rate >180 beats/min, restless, variably cyanotic, variable congestive heart failure	Irritability if prolonged
MISCELLANEOUS		
Incarcerated hernia Intussusception	Specific abdominal findings	Surgical consultation; may be more common cause than expected
Diphtheria-pertussis-tetanus reaction	Immunization within 48 hr	Analgesia

BIBLIOGRAPHY

Barr RG: Colic and crying syndromes in infants, *Pediatrics* 102: 1282, 1998.

Duro D, Rising R, Cedillo M et al: Association between infantile colic and carbohydrate malabsorption from fruit juices in infancy, *Pediatrics* 109:797, 2002.

Forsythe BWC: Colic and the effect of changing formula: a double-blind multiple crossover study, *J Pediatr* 115:521, 1989.

Harkness MJ: Corneal abrasion in infancy as a cause of inconsolable crying, *Pediatr Emerg Care* 5:242, 1989.

Hawley TL: New developments: cocaine-exposed children, *Curr Probl Pediatr* 24:259, 1994.

Heine RG, Cameron DJS, Chow CW et al: Esophagitis in distressed infants: poor diagnostic agreement between esophageal pH monitoring and histopathologic findings, *J Pediatr* 140:14, 2002.

Rautava P, Lehtonen L, Helenius H et al: Infantile colic: child and family three years later, *Pediatrics* 96:43, 1995.

Ruiz-Contreras J, Urquia L, Bastero R: Persistent crying as the predominant manifestation of sepsis in infants and newborns, *Pediatr Emerg Care* 15:113, 1999.

Trocinski DR, Pearigen PD: The crying infant, *Emerg Med Clin North Am* 16:895, 1998.

Zuckerman B, Stevenson J, Bailey V: Sleep problems in early childhood: continuities, predictive factors, and behavior correlates, *Pediatrics* 80:664, 1987.

40 Limp

Also See Chapter 27 (Arthralgia and Joint Pain)

ALERT Septic arthritis, osteomyelitis, and fracture must be considered early in the evaluation. Hip abnormality may appear as knee pain.

The child with a limp requires a systematic assessment of gait to determine the functional problem and cause. In children it is often difficult to isolate the abnormality on clinical grounds alone because of the difficulty in eliciting specific signs and symptoms.

ETIOLOGY

By age group, the following conditions are most commonly associated with limping (Table 40-1):

1-5 years	5-10 years
Toxic synovitis	Toxic synovitis
Occult fracture	Legg-Calvé-Perthes disease
Osteomyelitis	
Septic arthritis	**10-15 years**
Juvenile rheumatoid arthritis	Slipped capital femoral epiphysis
	Osgood-Schlatter disease
	Osteochondroses

Limping may be associated with *back* pain, and the differential diagnostic considerations should encompass additional conditions, including trauma resulting in musculoskeletal soft tissue injury (most common), fractures, and osteomyelitis. The diagnosis of low back pain in the adolescent should also consider the following:

1. Lumbar strain
2. Spondylolysis
3. Spondylolisthesis
4. Disk syndrome
5. Spinal cord tumor
6. Diskitis
7. Scheuermann's disease
8. Ankylosing spondylitis

DIAGNOSTIC FINDINGS

The history is particularly important in helping localize the exact site of abnormality. The progression of signs and symptoms, precipitating factors, relationship to trauma, and infection and systemic disease are crucial in the initial evaluation. Previous medical problems, exposures, family history, and patient's age are helpful in considering diagnostic entities.

In physically evaluating the child, the clinician must watch the child walk, focusing on the components of gait. First, the hips, knees, and ankles should be examined for pain, warmth, effusion, asymmetry, and limitation of motion, and then the femur, tibia, fibula, and foot and ankle bones. Length of legs from the anterior iliac crest to the medial malleolus should be compared. Circumference should also be measured. A complete neurologic examination of the lower extremities (motor strength, sensory, reflexes) and examination of the abdomen, rectum, and genitalia are required. Hip pain is often referred to the knee.

If the results of the physical examination and history are inconclusive, complete blood count (CBC), measurement of the erythrocyte sedimentation rate (ESR), and blood cultures may be useful in evaluating a potential infectious cause.

TABLE 40-1 Limp: Diagnostic Considerations

Condition	Diagnostic Findings	Ancillary Data	Comments/Management
TRAUMA (Chapters 66-70)			
Sprain/contusion	History of trauma; local pain, tenderness, swelling, ecchymosis; variably unstable	X-ray study result negative	Support, restrict weight-bearing
Fracture	Variable history of trauma; local pain, tenderness, swelling; may be occult	X-ray study result may be positive; if negative, do serial studies, looking for buckle fracture in the cortex of tibia, fibula, or femur; be certain x-ray study includes all potentially involved areas; technetium bone scan rarely needed	Orthopedic consultation; stress fracture may occur after repeated indirect trivial injuries; consider child abuse
Periostitis	Minor trauma to tibia, femur; local tenderness, fullness	X-ray study for subperiosteal hemorrhage (may be delayed)	Periosteum is loosely attached, with minor trauma; may have periosteal hemorrhage
Foreign body/ splinter in foot	Acute onset pain, local tenderness, variable erythema	X-ray study rarely needed, but foreign body may localize if radiopaque	Remove; location will dictate need for consult
Poorly fitting shoe	Limp disappears when shoe is removed		
Vertebral disk injury	Motor defect—weakness, asymmetric reflexes; sensory defect	X-ray study may show injury	Orthopedic and neurosurgical consultation
INFECTION/INFLAMMATION			
Toxic synovitis of hip (Chapter 69)	Preceding viral illness, nontoxic; hip rarely warm, tender, or limited range of motion	CBC, ESR: WNL; x-ray study: variable effusion; aspirate if question of septic arthritis	Self-limited; common in children 1½ to 7 yr old
Osteomyelitis (p. 769)	Fever, variable systemic toxicity; local swelling, tenderness, warmth; monoarticular, long bones (femur, tibia)	↑ CBC, ↑ ESR; x-ray study; technetium bone scan; joint and bone aspirate	May have arthritis and osteomyelitis concurrently; antibiotics
Arthritis, septic (p. 767)	Febrile, monoarticular, large weight-bearing (knee, hip) joints; local swelling, warmth, tenderness	↑ WBC, ↑ ESR; x-ray study; bone scan; joint aspirate	Requires urgent drainage and antibiotics
Arthritis, viral Rubella Rubella vaccine Hepatitis Chickenpox	Local swelling, warmth, tenderness; polyarticular, particularly large joints (knee); associated symptoms	CBC, viral titers, liver functions; x-ray study: effusion; joint aspirate	Usually self-limited

Arthritis, uncommon *Mycobacterium* Fungal	Insidious, commonly hip with progression; leg is flexed, well abducted	Joint aspirate; CBC; variable syphilis serologic findings; tuberculin skin test	
Appendicitis (p. 658)	RLQ pain, psoas/obturator sign, limited hip movement	↑ WBC, variable pyuria	Important to consider in differential as well as other abdominal problems
Polio (Chapter 41)	Systemic disease with asymmetric flaccid paralysis, bulbar involvement	CSF pleocytosis; ↑ WBC; positive viral culture finding	Decreased incidence
Guillain-Barré syndrome (Chapter 41)	Ascending symmetric paralysis with pain, paresthesias, and paralysis; may involve cranial nerves; preceding viral illness	CSF: high protein	Danger of respiratory insufficiency; associated with viral infection; supportive care with IV gamma globulin (? plasma exchange)
VASCULAR			
Legg-Calvé-Perthes disease (Chapter 69)	Insidious onset pain of hip with limp or limitation of motion	X-ray study: bulging capsule with widened joint space; technetium scan: ↓ uptake	Peak: 4:1 males, 4-10 yr; orthopedic consultation—treat hip in abduction and internal rotation
Discitis	Gait problem (<3 yr); local back, abdominal pain with limp (>3 yr); irritable, no systemic illness	X-ray study result normal for 4-8 wk; disc space may narrow by 3-4 wk; result of technetium scan abnormal after 7 days	Vascular disruption of epiphyseal end-plate of vertebrae; prognosis good; treatment: support, antibiotics controversial
DEGENERATIVE			
Slipped capital femoral epiphysis (Chapter 69)	Unilateral or bilateral pain in knee (referred) or in medial aspect of thigh; hip or knee made worse by activity; limitation of abduction and internal rotation	X-ray study: widening epiphyseal growth plate	Peak: 12-15 yr; orthopedic consultation; surgical immobilization; child obese or tall and thin, with rapid growth spurt
Osgood-Schlatter disease (Chapter 69)	Pain in knee caused by patellar tendonitis at insertion into tibial tubercle	X-ray study result: fragmentation of tibial tuberosity	Peak: 11-15 yr; symptomatic treatment, rest, avoid activities that cause pain
Osteochondroses			
Chrondomalacia patellae	Irregularity of patella, pain on compression of patellar at intercondylar notch with contraction of quadriceps	X-ray study result: WNL	Teenagers, female > males; symptomatic; treatment: quadriceps strengthening
Osteochondritis dissecans	Pain, stiffness, swelling, clicking of knee	X-ray study result: tunnel view shows demineralization of medial femoral condyle	Teenagers; decreased activity, muscle strengthening
Neuromuscular disease	Associated motor and sensory findings		Often progressive

Continued

TABLE 40-1 Limp: Diagnostic Considerations—cont'd

Condition	Diagnostic Findings	Ancillary Data	Comments/Management
CONGENITAL			
Hemophilia (p. 696)	Variable history of trauma; muscle bleeding; monoarticular joint swollen, tender with hemarthrosis	X-ray study result: variable bleeding screen	Factor replacement
Sickle cell disease (p. 714)	Systemic disease; bone pain; polyarticular joint involvement	X-ray study result; Hct; positive sickle preparation; variable technetium bone scan	Concurrent infection may be present; may be crisis or infarct
Dislocated hip	Normal newborn except for instability and range of motion of joint; positive hip click (abduction)	X-ray study	Orthopedic consultation, splint hip in flexion and abduction
Unequal leg length	Unequal length from anterior iliac crest to medial malleolus		Orthopedic consultation
Testicular torsion (p. 673)	Acute onset of scrotal or groin pain; mass, tender swollen		Surgical emergency
Incarcerated hernia (p. 672)			
AUTOIMMUNE (Table 27-1)			
NEOPLASM			
Osteochondroma	Local pain with exostosis		
Leukemia	Systemic disease with associated symptoms		
Neuroblastoma			
Ewing			
Spinal cord tumor			
INTRAPSYCHIC			
Attention getting	Inconsistent signs and symptoms		May be functional habit after resolution of physical problem, particularly in children <5 yr old

RLQ, Right lower quadrant.

X-ray studies for infection, trauma, neoplasm, congenital abnormalities, and degenerative problems are often diagnostic. A technetium bone scan may be obtained for further clarification. When infectious arthritis or osteomyelitis is suspected, collecting a joint aspirate may be useful, with appropriate stains and cultures (pp. 767 and 769). If the initial evaluation is unrevealing, serial examinations with close follow-up may be required because an occult or stress fracture, osteomyelitis, infectious arthritis, or other condition may be delayed in manifesting objective signs and symptoms.

BIBLIOGRAPHY

Barkin RM, Barkin SZ, Barkin AZ: The limping child, *J Emerg Med* 18:331, 2000.

Blatt SD, Rosenthal BM, Barnhart DC: Diagnostic utility of lower extremity radiographs of young children with gait disturbances, *Pediatrics* 87:138, 1991.

Olson TL, Anderson RL, Dearwater SR et al: The epidemiology of low back pain in an adolescent population, *Am J Public Health* 82:606, 1992.

Sills EM: What's causing the back pain? *Contemp Pediatr* 5:85, 1988.

41 Paralysis and Hemiplegia

ALERT After assessment of respiratory and circulatory status, the diagnostic evaluation must quickly establish the underlying process to provide guidelines for support and therapy.

The acute onset of paralysis in children may be indicated by a youngster's not wanting to walk. Infectious and inflammatory causes are most common (Table 41-1). In addition, spinal cord or central nervous system (CNS) injury resulting from trauma can cause transient or permanent deficits. Heavy metal intoxications can induce paralysis. Hysterical conversion reactions may mimic paralysis, but usually the physical findings are inconsistent.

CNS lesions are generally accompanied by a flaccid paralysis and loss of tone and deep tendon reflexes (DTRs). After about a week the patient may become spastic with hyperactive reflexes. The evaluation should include a careful neurologic examination as well as a check for associated symptoms. Spinal fluid should normally be examined.

The major complications encountered by patients with CNS lesions are respiratory failure (rarely requiring ventilatory support) and secondary bacterial infections. Treatment is generally supportive.

Rarely, patients have *acute hemiplegia*, secondary to emboli, thromboses, or intracerebral hemorrhage. Emboli produce a rapidly evolving clinical picture, but thromboses often evolve over hours to days. Predisposing factors include the following:

1. Infection:
   a. Viral: herpes or coxsackievirus encephalitis
   b. Bacterial meningitis
2. Vascular-embolic:
   a. Congenital heart disease
   b. Endocarditis
   c. Dysrhythmias: atrial fibrillation
   d. Arteriovenous malformations
   e. Acute infantile hemiplegia: seizure followed by coma, hemiplegia, and fever caused by occlusion of the middle cerebral artery
3. Vascular:
   a. Hemiplegic migraine
   b. Vasculitis
4. Trauma:
   a. Blunt trauma to the neck (or intraoral trauma): may produce delayed onset of symptoms in 24 to 48 hours
   b. Penetrating trauma: may produce immediate loss or vascular foreign body emboli
5. Congenital:
   a. Sickle cell disease (thrombosis, spasm)
   b. Hemophilia (hemorrhage)
6. Todd's paralysis: transient paralysis after seizures that resolve without therapy

Fig. 41-1 provides a summary of the anatomic and functional correlations in upper and lower motor neuron disease; Table 41-2 helps differentiate the site of injury. Treatment must focus on the underlying disorder as well as complicating conditions.

TABLE 41-1 Paralysis: Diagnostic Considerations

	Guillain-Barré Syndrome	Secondary Polyneuropathy	Poliomyelitis	Tick-Bite Paralysis	Transverse Myelitis/ Neuromyelitis Optica
Etiology	Unknown; role of viral, mycoplasm infections unknown	Infectious or inflammatory: viral, bacterial (diphtheria, botulism), immunizations; autoimmune; intoxication	Poliovirus	Toxin release by tick	Unknown but may be inflammatory and related to multiple sclerosis
Prodrome	Nonspecific respiratory or gastrointestinal symptoms 5-14 days before onset	Low-grade fever and other signs and symptoms reflecting the underlying disease	Fever, respiratory or gastrointestinal symptoms; may have meningism	1 wk after tick bites and remains attached; fatigue, irritability	
Neurologic findings	Symmetric flaccid ascending paralysis; greater involvement of lower extremities, greater proximally; facial diplegia, cranial nerve, bulbar involved; muscle tenderness; sensory-distal hyperesthesia with impaired position, vibration	Variable involvement; flaccid paralysis with loss of DTRs and position and vibration senses; ataxia; cranial nerve involvement with dysphagia; generalized weakness	Flaccid, asymmetric paralysis with maximum deficit 3-5 days after onset; lower extremities more involved than upper; bulbar involvement may occur very early; sensory examination normal; marked muscle tenderness, pain, fasciculations, and twitching	Rapid progression of muscle pain with ascending flaccid symmetric paralysis; pain and paresthesias	Rapid progression; may have ataxia, weakness, multiple neurologic deficits; optic neuritis; paralysis develops with sensory loss below lesion and hyperesthesia above; bowel and bladder problems
Ancillary data	CSF: few WBCs, high protein after 10 days	CSF: few monocytes with high protein; tests to determine underlying disease; nerve conduction velocity	CSF: pleocytosis (initially PMNs, then monocytes), elevated protein level	CSF: normal	CSF (not done routinely): pleocytosis, increased protein level; myelogram if indicated
Comments	Peaks in 5- to 9-yr-old children; usual recovery in 1-3 wk; supportive care and IV gamma globulin	Major systemic illness reflects nature of underlying disease	May be asymptomatic or nonparalytic; summer epidemic; unimmunized individuals	Tick usually attached to head or neck; rapid improvement with removal of tick (Table 45-1)	Steroids (ACTH) may be useful in treatment

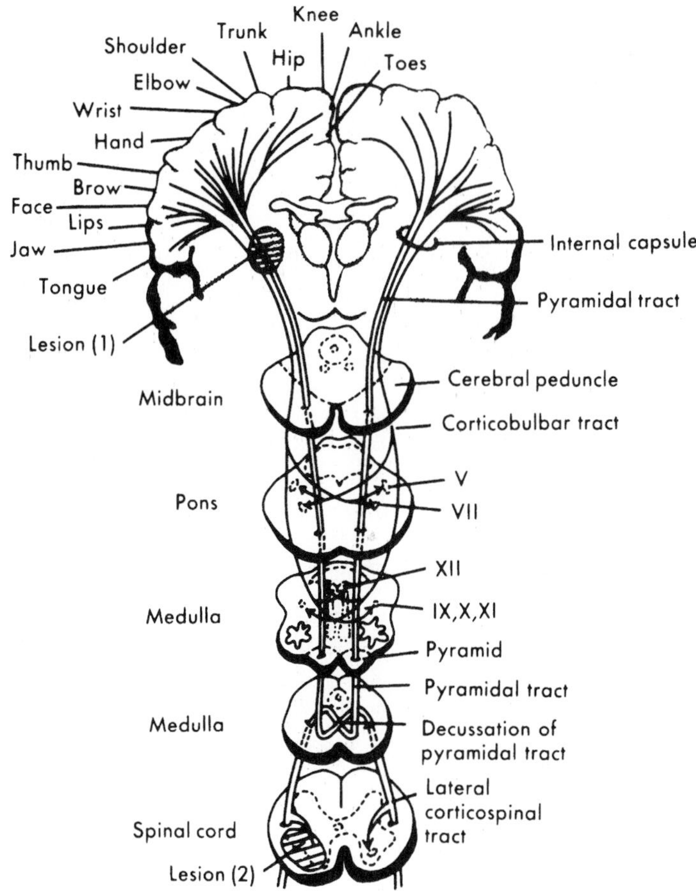

Lesion (1)

Upper motor neuron lesion

Contralateral hemiparesis
Postural flexion of arm, extension of leg
Muscles hypertonic
Tendon reflexes hyperactive
Atrophy not prominent
No muscle fasciculations
Pathologic reflexes present

Lesion (2)

Lower motor neuron lesion

Paresis limited to specific muscle groups
Gait depends on muscles affected; flail-like movements common
Muscles flaccid
Tendon reflexes absent or hypoactive
Atrophy prominent
Muscle fasciculations present
Contractures and skeletal deformities may develop

Fig. 41-1 The pyramidal system.

(From Gilman S, Newman SW, editors: *Essentials of clinical neuroanatomy and neurophysiology,* Philadelphia, 1987, FA Davis.)

TABLE 41-2 Differentiating Findings Noted by Level of Injury

	Motor Neuron	Muscle	Neuromuscular Junction	Nerve
Reflexes	–	–	–	–
Muscle bulk	↓	↓	↓	↓
Fasciculations	+	+	–	–
Tone	↓	↓	↓	↓
Strength	↓	↓	↓	↓
Sensation	WNL	↓	Variable	↓

–, Absent; +, present; ↓, decreased.

Bell's palsy is a seventh cranial nerve paralysis of sudden onset and unknown cause. The patient has a flattened nasolabial fold on the affected side and is unable to close the eyelids, pucker the lips, or wrinkle the brow. Recovery usually occurs over 3 to 6 weeks. Therapy should include protection of the cornea with artificial tears. Steroids may be useful if initiated within 2 days of onset of symptoms. Prednisone can be initiated at 1 mg/kg/24 hr PO, and then the dosage tapered over 7 to 10 days.

BIBLIOGRAPHY

Birse GS, Strauss RW: Acute childhood hemiplegia, *Ann Emerg Med* 14:74, 1985.

Freeman JM: Diagnosis and evaluation of acute paraplegia, *Pediatr Rev* 4:327, 1983.

42 Rash

Also See Chapter 72 (Dermatologic Disorders)

ALERT	Lesions requiring emergency evaluation include petechiae, purpura, burns, cellulitis, and those with other evidence of systemic infection or child abuse.

Although rash is a common presenting complaint, the term requires careful definition. The identification of a rash disease requires examination of the lesions, focusing on whether there are blisters, or if solid, whether the lesions are red or scaling (Table 42-1). It is important to define the configuration and distribution of findings and relate the chronology of the evolution with the development of systemic signs and symptoms.

Most urgent encounters related to rashes have an infectious origin. Tables 42-2, 42-3, and 42-4 divide the common exanthems into categories on the basis of structure: maculopapular, vesicular, and petechial or purpuric.

TABLE 42-1 Rash: Evaluation

Appearance	Diagnostic Considerations
BLISTER (FLUID-FILLED)	
Clear	*Vesicular* (Tables 42-2 and 42-4): herpes simplex, varicella-zoster, scabies *Bullous:* bullous impetigo, erythema multiforme, burn, contact dermatitis, friction blister
Pustular	Acne, folliculitis (bacterial, fungal), candidiasis, bacteremia (gonococcemia, meningococcemia)
SOLID (NONRED)	
Skin-colored	*Keratotic* (rough-surfaced lesion): wart, corn, callus *Nonkeratotic* (smooth lesion): wart, molluscum contagiosum, epidermoid (sebaceous) cyst, basal and squamous cell carcinoma, nevi
White	Pityriasis alba, vitiligo, pityriasis versicolor, postinflammatory hypopigmentation, milia, molluscum contagiosum
Brown	Café-au-lait patch, nevi, freckle, melanoma, hypopigmentation secondary to systemic disease, medication, or postinflammatory condition
Yellow	Jaundice, nevi sebaceous
SOLID (RED, NONSCALING)	
Inflammatory papule/nodule	*Papule (maculopapular):* (Tables 42-2 and 42-3): viral exanthem, erythema multiforme, insect bite, scarlet fever, angioma *Nodule:* furuncle, erythema nodosum
Vascular (flat-topped)	*Nonpurpuric:* toxic erythema (viral exanthem, medication, photosensitivity), urticaria (infection, medication), erythema multiforme, cellulitis (erysipelas) *Purpuric* (Table 42-2): vasculitis, petechiae, ecchymosis

TABLE 42-1 Rash: Evaluation—cont'd

Appearance	Diagnostic Considerations
SOLID (RED, SCALING)	
Papulosquamous disease	No epithelial disruption: pityriasis rosea; tinea corporis, capitis, pedis or cruris; lupus erythematosus; syphilis
Eczematous disease	Epithelial disruption: atopic (eczema); seborrheic, diaper, contact, or stasis dermatitis; tinea cruris; capitis or pedis; nummular eczema, impetigo, candidiasis

Modified from Lynch PJ, Edminister SC: *Ann Emerg Med* 13:603, 1984; and Weston WL: *Primary Care* 11:469, 1984.

TABLE 42-2 Acute Exanthems

	Maculopapular	Vesicular	Petechial or Purpuric
Infection	Viral Measles, Rubella, Roseola, Enterovirus (Table 42-3) Infectious mononucleosis (p. 730) Pityriasis rosea (p. 593)	Viral Chickenpox (Table 42-4) Herpes zoster (Table 42-4) Herpes simplex Enterovirus (Table 42-2) Hand, foot, and mouth Herpangina Molluscum contagiosum (p. 597) Historical: smallpox	Viral Enterovirus Hemorrhagic measles Rubeola (atypical) Chickenpox
	Other Scarlet fever (Table 42-3) Staphylococcal scalded skin (p. 595) Toxic shock syndrome (p. 736) Kawasaki's disease (p. 726) Meningococcemia (p. 729) *Mycoplasma pneumoniae* Tick diseases (Table 45-1) Rocky Mountain spotted fever Typhus	Other Impetigo (p. 591) Rickettsialpox Candidiasis Staphylococcal scalded skin syndrome (p. 595) Erythema multiforme (p. 589)	Other Meningococcemia (p. 729) *Haemophilus influenzae* Pneumococcemia Rocky Mountain spotted fever Sepsis (with thrombocytopenia or DIC) Gonococcemia (p. 679) Endocarditis (p. 567) Plague
Intoxication	Ampicillin Penicillin Barbiturates Anticonvulsants Sulfonamides		
Other	Sunburn Juvenile rheumatoid arthritis Serum sickness	Insect bites (p. 310)	Henoch-Schönlein purpura (p. 822) Idiopathic thrombocytopenic purpura (p. 709) Coagulation disorder Trauma Tourniquet (distal) Coughing (head and neck) Leukemia Aplastic anemia

TABLE 42-3 Common Maculopapular Exanthems

	Measles (Rubeola)	Rubella (German, 3-Day Measles)	Roseola (Exanthema Subitum)
Incubation	10-14 days	14-21 days	10-14 days
Prodrome	3 days high fever, cough, conjunctivitis, and coryza; child appears toxic, lethargic	May be none; lymphadenopathy (especially postauricular, suboccipital), malaise, variable low-grade fever	3-4 days of high fever in otherwise well child, preceding rash
Exanthem	Reddish brown; begins on face and progresses downward; generalized by third day; confluent on face, neck, upper trunk; lasts 7-10 days; desquamates; atypical measles; maculopapular, purpuric, petechial, or vesicular rash	Pink; begins on face and progresses rapidly downward; generalized by second day; discrete; lasts 2-3 days; fades in order of appearance	Appears after defervescence; rose, discrete; initially on chest, spreads to involve face and extremities; fades quickly
Enanthem	Koplik's spots (2 days before rash, on buccal mucosa opposite molars)	None	None
Complications	Pneumonia Encephalitis Otitis media Thrombocytopenia Hemorrhagic measles Pneumothorax Hepatitis Exacerbation of TB	Arthritis (common in women) beginning after 2-3 days of illness; knee, wrist, finger Congenital rubella syndrome Encephalitis Thrombocytopenia	Febrile seizures Meningoencephalitis Pseudotumor cerebri
Management	Supportive; may require hospitalization; active immunization of contacts within 72 hr of exposure; immune serum globulin (0.25 ml/kg) for children <1 yr and pregnant women within 6 hr of exposure; reportable	Supportive; isolate from pregnant women; active immunization of contacts; reportable	Supportive; good fever control
Comments	Rare with immunization	Rare with immunization; serologic diagnosis	Usually in 1-to 4-yr-old children Probably caused by human herpesvirus-6 (HHV-6)

Fifth Disease (Erythema Infectiosum)	Enterovirus	Scarlet Fever
7-14 days	Variable (short)	2-4 days
None	Variable; fever, malaise, vomiting, sore throat, rhinorrhea	1-2 days of fever, vomiting, sore throat; often toxic
Erupts in 3 stages: (1) red-flushed cheeks with circumoral pallor (slapped cheek), (2) maculopapular eruption on extremities (lacelike), (3) may recur secondary to heat, sunlight, trauma	Maculopapular, discrete, nonpruritic, generalized; rubella-like; hand, foot, and mouth distribution	Erythematous, punctate, sandpaper texture; appears first in flexion areas, then generalized; most intense on neck, axilla, inguinal, popliteal skin fold; circumoral pallor; lasts 7 days, then desquamates
Variable	Variable	Red pharynx, tonsils; palatal petechiae; strawberry tongue
Transient arthritis	Aseptic meningitis Myocarditis Hepatitis	Rheumatic fever Acute glomerulonephritis
Rarely needs care	Supportive	Penicillin
Caused by human parvovirus B19 associated with hypoplastic anemia, arthropathy, myocarditis, vasculitis, multiple organ failure; may be role for IVIG	Concurrent family illness, gastroenteritis, herpangina	Group A streptococci (p. 613)

TABLE 42-4 Vesicular Exanthems

	Varicella (Chickenpox)	Herpes Zoster (Shingles)	Herpes Simplex
Diagnostic findings	Rapid progression of erythematous macules, developing into papules and vesicles; vesicles are thin-walled and superficial, surrounded by an erythematous area; pruritic; distribution is central with relative sparing distally; marked variability in severity of exanthem—may only be a few lesions; usually febrile; enanthem—shallow mucosal ulcers; different ages of lesions; may initially resemble insect bites	Erythema followed by red papules that become vesicular in 12-24 hr, pustular in 72 hr, and crusts in 10-12 days; distribution is unilateral after peripheral dermatome or cranial nerve; preeruptive pain with hyperesthesia over involved skin	Multiple presentations **Gingivostomatitis:** fever, irritability, pain in mouth, throat, and with swallowing; shallow ulcers on mucosa (buccal, tonsillar, and pharyngeal); crusts on lips; cervical lymphoadenopathy; lasts 1-14 days **Vulvovaginitis:** similar shallow ulcers on vagina and vulva; pain on urination **Keratoconjunctivitis:** corneal ulceration
Complications	Pneumonia Secondary bacterial infections: cellulitis, bacterial pneumonia, especially group A streptococcus Encephalitis, myelitis Hepatitis Reye syndrome	Ophthalmic: neuralgia, corneal dendrites, iritis Postherpetic neuralgia and death	Ophthalmic: corneal ulceration Encephalitis Neonatal viremia with encephalitis
Management	Antipruritic agents Topical: calamine lotion; cold baths with small amount of baking soda (⅓ tsp) in water Systemic: diphenhydramine Antipyretics—*Do not* use aspirin Treatment of complications: Acyclovir, 80 mg/kg/24 hr (maximum: 3200 mg/24 hr) PO QID for 5 days; begin within 24 hr of rash in high-risk patients* Zoster-immune globulin (VZIG) for exposure in high-risk patient; 125 units/10 kg (maximum: 625 units)	Support, analgesia Eye involvement requires ophthalmology consultation Famciclovir, 500-750 mg/dose TID for 7 days; decreases duration, accelerates lesion healing, and decreases duration of viral shedding Acyclovir may have a role in specific circumstances Steroids or amitriptyline may reduce postherpetic neuralgia	General support Gingival: topical analgesia—antacid or mixture of viscous lidocaine (Xylocaine), diphenhydramine, Kaopectate; acyclovir (Zovirax): topical, IV, PO for initial and recurrent lesions
Comment	Incubation: 14-21 days Vaccine Particularly dangerous in newborns, pregnant females, immunosuppressed or immunodeficient individuals	Common history of chickenpox	Sexual spread of vulvovaginitis Potentially life-threatening to newborn, immunodeficient, or immunosuppressed; consider systemic acyclovir (p. 686)

* Nonpregnant patients ≥13 yr, children >12 mo with chronic cutaneous or pulmonary disorder, and children receiving long-term salicylate therapy. Children receiving short-term, intermittent, or aerosolyed corticosteroid therapy are probably not immunocompromised, and the risk is unknown. If patient is taking high-dose corticosteroids, acyclovir IV is probably indicated.

The condition must be treated as an emergency if the lesions are purple or look like blood (purpura); do not blanch (petechiae); are burnlike (scalded skin); are red, blue, or tender to the touch (cellulitis); have red streaking; or are pustular. Lesions that are pruritic, are associated with fever of more than 24 hours' duration, may be related to a medication, or are pustular and associated with a red or cola-colored urine should also be seen.

Chapter 72 provides a more detailed summary of the common dermatologic problems that require evaluation and treatment.

BIBLIOGRAPHY

American Academy of Pediatrics Committee on Infectious Diseases: Use of oral acyclovir in otherwise healthy children with varicella, *Pediatrics* 91:674, 1993.

American Academy of Pediatrics: *Report of the committee on infectious diseases*, Elk Grove Village, Ill, 2000, American Academy of Pediatrics.

Balfour HF, Rotbart HA, Feldman S et al: Acyclovir treatment of varicella in otherwise healthy adolescents, *J Pediatr* 120:627, 1992.

Doctor A, Harper MB, Fleisher GR: Group A beta-hemolytic streptococcal bacteremia: historical overview, changing incidence, and recent association with varicella, *Pediatrics* 96:428, 1995.

Peterson CL, Mascola L, Chao SM et al: Children hospitalized with varicella: a prevaccine review, *J Pediatr* 129: 529, 1996.

Tyring S, Barbarash RA, Nahlik JE: Famciclovir for the treatment of acute herpes zoster: effects on acute disease and post herpetic neuralgia, *Ann Intern Med* 123:89, 1995.

Vugia DJ, Peterson CL, Meyers HB et al: Invasive group A streptococcal infections in children with varicella in Southern California, *Pediatr Infect Dis J* 15:146, 1996.

43 Vaginal Bleeding

Also See Chapter 78 (Gynecologic Disorders)

ALERT Third-trimester bleeding requires immediate obstetric consultation. Dysfunctional uterine bleeding is most common in pubescent females, but ectopic pregnancy should be excluded; in younger girls the cause is commonly trauma or foreign bodies. Hypotension may develop.

In the pubescent female, vaginal bleeding is most commonly related to menstruation. The most common problem associated with vaginal bleeding is dysfunctional uterine bleeding because of anovulatory cycles in which the bleeding is scanty, watery, and irregular. Most young girls begin their cycles with anovulatory ones, and it may be several years before ovulation occurs. Other causes, including complications of pregnancy, trauma, vulvovaginitis, and pelvic inflammatory disease, must be considered (Table 43-1).

After ensuring that there is no vascular instability, the clinician must perform a thorough pelvic examination, including an evaluation of both the internal and external genitalia (p. 679). Appropriate cultures (*Neisseria gonorrhoeae* and *Chlamydia trachomatis*) and microscopic examination (potassium hydroxide and saline solution) are usually indicated if the bleeding is not caused by obvious trauma. If there is any question of potential pregnancy (and often even if there is no question), a serum pregnancy test should be performed. Ultrasound examination may confirm an intrauterine pregnancy and identify pelvic abnormality. A hematocrit determination is usually indicated in the assessment if bleeding is significant. A bleeding screen may be helpful.

Pregnant women with third-trimester bleeding should be examined in the operating room, with preparations for a double setup whereby the baby can be delivered vaginally or by cesarean section. As appropriate, cultures of the cervical os and rectum (and pharynx), analysis of discharges, and a Papanicolaou smear should be done.

Bleeding in the prepubescent girl is commonly caused by foreign bodies or hymenal trauma. Vulvovaginitis may produce a bloody discharge. Tumors are uncommon unless the patient had an intrauterine exposure to diethylstilbestrol (DES). Vaginal bleeding may accompany endocrine and hematologic disorders.

TABLE 43-1 Vaginal Bleeding: Diagnostic Considerations*

Condition	Signs and Symptoms	Evaluation/Comments
ENDOCRINE		
Uterine dysfunction (p. 677)	Irregular menses; flow too frequent, heavy, or prolonged	Diagnosis of exclusion; anovulatory cycle
Pregnancy complications (p. 686)		
Abortion	First trimester; cervix variably dilated; various products of conception	Treatment depends on type of abortion
Placenta previa	Third trimester; painless; may have profuse bleeding	Ultrasound; avoid pelvic examination in ED; double setup; fetal monitor
Abruptio placentae	Third trimester; abdominal pain; tender uterus; bleeding may be concealed	Ultrasound; avoid pelvic examination in ED; double setup; fetal monitor; common in blunt trauma
Ectopic pregnancy	Missed menses, pelvic pain, rebound, adnexal mass; low Hct, hypotension	Culdocentesis or ultrasound; rapid pregnancy test; potentially life-threatening
Following delivery	Bleeding without pain	Pharmacologic curettage (rarely mechanical); consider endometriosis
Thyroid disease (p. 631)	Associated signs and symptoms	Thyroid functions
Physiologic	Newborn may have bleeding at 5-10 days	Caused by withdrawal from maternal estrogens
TRAUMA		
Foreign body	Foul-smelling discharge	Peak is 5-9 yr (may occur at any age); forgotten tampon common in adolescent; also IUD
Laceration	Signs of trauma	Secondary trauma, intercourse, heavy exercise, molestation
INFLAMMATION		
Vulvovaginitis (p. 682)	Characteristic discharge and inflamed introitus	Culture, wet and KOH preparation of discharge
Pelvic inflammatory disease (p. 679)	Abdominal, pelvic tenderness, fever, chills, nausea, vomiting	Elevated CBC and ESR; culture and Gram stain
INTOXICATION		
Birth control pills	Irregular intake or acute overdose	Adjust or control dosage
Anticoagulants	Bleeding sites elsewhere	Coagulation studies
DEFICIENCY		
Bleeding diathesis	Bleeding sites elsewhere	Coagulation studies
Idiopathic thrombocytopenic purpura (p. 709)	Bleeding elsewhere	Platelet count and coagulation studies
NEOPLASM		
Tumors, polyps, fibroid tumors	Physical examination reveals mass, spotty bleeding	Unusual; may occur in children with DES exposure; Pap smear

* See also Chapter 78.

BIBLIOGRAPHY

American College of Emergency Physicians, Clinical Policy Committee: Clinical policy in the initial approach to patients presenting with a chief complaint of vaginal bleeding, *Ann Emerg Med* 29:435, 1997.

Anderson M, Lewin CE, Sayder DL: Abnormal vaginal bleeding in adolescents, *Pediatr Ann* 15:696, 1986.

Baldwin DD, Landa HM: Common problems in pediatrics and gynecology, *Urol Clin North Am* 22:161, 1995.

44 Vomiting

Also See Chapters 32 (Diarrhea) and 76 (Gastrointestinal Disorders)

ALERT Assessment must initially determine the child's hydration status, and stabilization must be initiated. Cause must be determined.

Vomiting is the forceful ejection of the stomach contents into the esophagus and through the mouth. It may be caused by irritation of the peritoneum or mesentery, obstruction of the intestine, action of a toxin on the medulla, or primary central nervous system (CNS) disorder.*

ETIOLOGY

In children the most common cause of vomiting is acute gastroenteritis, followed by other infections, including otitis media, urinary tract infections, and meningitis. Infants often vomit as a result of faulty feeding techniques or chalasia. Other conditions that must be considered are congenital obstructions of the gastrointestinal tract, particularly pyloric stenosis; CNS lesions producing increased intracranial pressure; and a variety of endocrine, metabolic, and toxic problems. Newborns often have congenital obstructions.

Intestinal obstruction in the neonate should be suspected if there is more than 20 ml of fluid in the gastric aspirate (especially bile stained), he or she vomits and has abdominal distension in the first 24 to 36 hours of life, or meconium is not passed in the first 48 hours of life (Tables 44-1 and 44-2).

* See also Acute Gastroenteritis, p. 640, and Chapter 32.

DIAGNOSTIC FINDINGS

The history must determine precipitating factors, such as trauma, recent illness, medications, poor feeding techniques, and environmental instability leading to emotional upheaval. Associated symptoms and family history are important. The nature of the vomiting must be determined: its color, composition, relationship to eating and position, onset, progression, and whether it was projectile. The expelled material should be examined.

1. Undigested food suggests an esophageal lesion at or above the cardia.
2. Nonbilious vomitus may result from lesions proximal to the pylorus.
3. Bile-containing material indicates obstruction beyond the ampulla of Vater or an adynamic ileus, found in sepsis, significant other infections, or serious underlying disease. Bile turns green upon exposure to air.
4. A fecal odor is consistent with peritonitis or a lower obstruction.
5. A bloody vomitus usually signifies a lesion proximal to the ligament of Treitz. If it is bright red, there has been little contact with gastric juices and the site is at or above the cardia. A "coffee grounds" appearance to vomitus results from alteration by gastric juices.

The physical examination should include inspection of the abdomen for trauma,

TABLE 44-1 Vomiting: Diagnostic Considerations

Condition	Diagnostic Findings	Evaluation	Comments/Management
INFECTION/INFLAMMATION			
Acute gastroenteritis (p. 640)	Acute onset with nausea, fever, diarrhea, and evidence of systemic illness	Fluid status, stool culture if needed	NPO, if indicated; clear liquids, advance slowly
Posttussive/posterior nasal drip	Follows vigorous coughing; may be greatest at night when recumbent; associated cough, rhinorrhea	Chest x-ray study if needed	Therapeutic trial: cough suppressant or decongestant
Otitis media (p. 605)	Fever, irritability, painful ear		Antibiotics; topical therapy for extreme pain
Esophagitis/gastritis (Chapter 35)	Variably "coffee grounds," bloody; epigastric or substernal pain, discomfort; reflux	Endoscopy; upper GI series	Associated reflux, hiatal hernia; drugs; trial of antacids
Ulcer, peptic/duodenal (Chapter 35)	Usually "coffee grounds" appearance; epigastric, abdominal pain; may be chronic or acute; possible anemia	Endoscopy; upper GI series	May be life-threatening
Hepatitis (p. 649)	Associated liver tenderness; icterus	Liver function tests	Usually infectious; viral, EB virus
Peritonitis Appendicitis (p. 658) Cholecystitis Pancreatitis	Generalized or localized tenderness, guarding, rebound	WBC, x-ray studies, UA	Surgical exploration usually needed
Cystitis Pyelonephritis (p. 833)	Associated fever, dysuria, frequency, burning, variable CVA tenderness	UA, urine culture	Initiate antibiotics during wait for culture results
Meningitis (p. 741) CNS abscess Subdural effusion/empyema	Fever, systemic toxicity; changed mental status; local neurologic signs, variable signs of increased ICP	Lumbar puncture; CT if needed	Antibiotics; neurosurgical consultation if indicated
CONGENITAL			
Pyloric stenosis (p. 668)	Regurgitation progressing to projectile vomiting; palpable olive-sized tumor in RUQ; vigorous gastric peristalsis present; variable dehydration, poor weight gain	Upper GI series—delayed gastric emptying, narrow pyloric channel ("string sign"), ultrasound may substitute; electrolytes to assess hydration	Usually male, 4-6 wk of age; treat fluid deficits, then surgery (pyloromyotomy)

GI obstruction (Chapter 11) Intestinal obstruction/stenosis/bands Imperforate anus Malrotation	Obstructive pattern beginning in newborn period, >20 ml in gastric aspirate; if proximal to ampulla of Vater, distension epigastrium or LUQ and gastric peristaltic wave; if distal to ampulla of Vater, vomitus contains bile, distension is generalized	Abdominal x-ray study with contrast studies if needed; electrolytes to assess fluid status	Immediate decompression; correction of fluid deficits; surgical consultation
Meconium ileus/plug			Associated with cystic fibrosis
Volvulus, sigmoid/midgut (p. 669)			Life-threatening
Intussusception			Life-threatening
Hydrocephalus	Excessive growth of head circumference; irritability, lethargy, headache, bulging of fontanelle	CT	May involve blockage of ventricular shunt; neurosurgical consultation; urgent care
TRAUMA			
Concussion (Chapter 57)	Trauma; headache, minimally changed mental status; often, projectile vomiting	Skull x-ray study, CT	Support; monitoring
Subdural hematoma (Chapter 57)	Marked change in mental status, signs of increased intracranial pressure: headache, ataxia, sixth nerve palsy, seizures; focal neurologic signs	CT	Immediate neurosurgical consultation; support: intubation, hyperventilation, diuretics, etc.
Foreign body (p. 647)	History: patient may have dysphagia or total obstruction; may have respiratory distress	X-ray study; esophagoscopy	If in esophagus, attempt to remove by use of Foley catheter under fluoroscopy; if elsewhere, endoscopy or surgery, depending on foreign body
Intramural duodenal hematoma (Chapter 63)	After even minimal blunt trauma: nausea, bilious vomiting, pain, tenderness, ileus; may have abdominal mass	Upper GI series	May be delay in symptom presentation
Ruptured viscus (Chapter 63)	Trauma followed by abdominal tenderness, rebound, guarding	Peritoneal lavage; x-ray study for free air	Immediate surgical intervention; fluids, antibiotics
Subarachnoid hemorrhage (Chapter 18)	Headache, stiff neck, progressive loss of consciousness; focal neurologic signs	CT; bloody spinal fluid	Neurosurgical consultation; supportive care
Cerebral edema	Signs of increased ICP: headache, ataxia, sixth nerve palsy; altered mental status	CT	Diuretics, steroids, hyperventilation, elevation

Continued

TABLE 44-1 Vomiting: Diagnostic Considerations—cont'd

Condition	Diagnostic Findings	Evaluation	Comments/Management
INTOXICATION (Chapter 54)			
Alkali burns	Associated mouth burns, difficulty swallowing	Endoscopy	Lye, bleaches most common; surgery consultation
Salicylates	Nausea, vomiting, tinnitus	Salicylate level	Stop medication; antacids, fluids
Iron	Hematemesis, shock, acidosis	Iron level, ABG, CBC	Urgent treatment with deferoxamine
Lead	Usually chronic exposure; signs of increased intracranial pressure	Lead level	Dimercaprol, EDTA
Digitalis	Underlying heart disease; nausea, dysrhythmias	Digitalis level; ECG	Stop digitalis; institute active treatment of dysrhythmia, etc.
VASCULAR			
Migraine (p. 750)	Unilateral, throbbing headache, aura; family history	Evaulation to exclude other causes	Consider therapeutic trial of ergotamine; analgesia, steroids
Hypertensive encephalopathy (Chapter 18)	Rapid increase in BP; changed mental status; headache, nausea, anorexia	Evaluation of underlying disease	Rapid response when diastolic BP brought below 100 mm Hg
ENDOCRINE/METABOLIC			
Acidosis (Chapter 8)	Underlying cause; rapid, deep breathing	ABG	Correction
Diabetic ketoacidosis (p. 624)	Kussmaul's breathing; history of diabetes; nausea, abdominal pain; ketones on breath	Electrolytes; ABG; glucose; ketone levels	Hydration, insulin, K^+
Uremia (p. 575)	Oliguria, often predisposing cause	BUN, creatinine levels; tests for underlying conditions	Evaluate and treat underlying cause
Inborn errors of metabolism Amino/organic acids	Associated acute-onset vomiting and acidosis, progressive deterioration, or poor growth and development	Urine and blood for amino and organic acids; electrolytes, ABG: acidosis	Exacerbation precipitated by acute illness
Fructose intolerance	Associated with ingestion of sugar or fruits	Challenge test under controlled conditions	
Addison disease (p. 623)	Dehydration, circulatory collapse; if chronic: weakness, fatigue, pallor, diarrhea, increased pigmentation	Serum Na^+, K^+ urine adrenocorticoids low	Adrenal genital syndrome in newborns
Reye syndrome (p. 655)	Associated liver failure, with marked change in mental status (often combative)	Liver function test results and ammonia level elevated	

INTRAPSYCHIC			
Attention getting	Inconsistent history; times usually related to seeking attention	Psychiatric evaluation	Organic causes must be ruled out
Hysteria/hyperventilation	Anxiety, nausea, and other psychosomatic symptoms; may hyperventilate	Psychiatric evaluation	Exclude organic causes
NEOPLASM			
GI	Related to location, type, and extent of neoplasm; insidious onset of symptoms	Specific for tissue considerations	Rare in children
Intracerebral			
MISCELLANEOUS			
Improper feeding techniques	Often regurgitation; bad nipple on bottle; improper position; usually occurs shortly after feeding; usually vomited material is undigested	Rarely upper GI series needed to rule out abnormality	Implement support system; make sure child not overfed
Chalasia	May be small amounts; associated with feeding, usually within 30–45 min of feeding; child well, good growth	Upper GI series if needed	Trial of slow, careful, prone, upright feedings; child usually <6 mo old; avoid overfeeding
Pregnancy	Increased intraabdominal pressure; usually first trimester		
Epilepsy (p. 754)	Aura or seizure may involve vomiting	EEG	Requires good neurologic follow-up evaluation
Ascites	Increased intraabdominal pressure	As related to cause; total serum protein, albumin levels	
Environmental heat illness (hyperthermia) (Chapter 50)	Abnormal mental status; variably febrile, leg cramps, dehydrated	Electrolytes	Fluids, cooling
Superior mesenteric artery syndrome	Compression of duodenum in child (adolescent female) leading to obstruction; usually recent marked weight loss	Upper GI series	Usually requires psychiatric therapy for underlying problems; support

TABLE 44-2 Vomiting: Gastrointestinal Causes According to Age

Newborn (0-28 days)	Infant	Child (>2 yr)
OBSTRUCTIVE		
Intestinal atresia/stenosis	Pyloric stenosis	Foreign body
Malrotation of bowel	Foreign body	Duodenal hematoma
Volvulus	Malrotation/volvulus	Intussusception
Meconium ileus/plug	Intussusception	Meckel's diverticulum
Hirschsprung's disease	Meckel's diverticulum	Hirschsprung's disease
Imperforate anus	Hirschsprung's disease	Incarcerated hernia
Incarcerated hernia	Incarcerated hernia	Adhesions
INFECTIOUS/INFLAMMATORY		
Necrotizing enterocolitis	Gastroenteritis	Gastroenteritis
Gastroesophageal reflux	Gastroesophageal reflux	Peptic ulcer disease
	Peritonitis	Appendicitis
	Milk allergy	Pancreatitis
		Paralytic ileus
		Peritonitis

Adapted from Fuchs S, Jaffe D: Vomiting, *Pediatr Emerg Care* 6:664, 1990.

distension, hyperactivity of the bowel, and congenital abnormalities as well as systemic illness.

MANAGEMENT

Management should focus on correction of fluid deficits (see Chapter 7) as well as definitive treatment of underlying abnormality. The well-hydrated patient with a self-limited problem can usually be discharged and sent home to follow a clear-liquid regimen. Antiemetics are usually unnecessary for children. A good balance of efficacy and sedation is achieved by promethazine (Phenergan), 0.25 to 0.5 mg/kg/dose q4-6hr PO, PR, or IM prn (adult, 12.5-25 mg/dose). Ondansetron [Zofran] may be given as 2 ml (1.6 mg) q6hr PO in children 1 to 3 years old or 5 ml (4 mg) q6hr PO in those 4 to 12 years old. Hospitalization is indicated for the child who is dehydrated or cannot tolerate oral intake.

Parental Education

Give only clear liquids slowly: Pedialyte, Lytren, Gatorade, defizzed soda pop (cola, ginger ale), and so on. With younger children, start with a teaspoon and slowly enlarge the amount. If vomiting occurs, let your child rest for a while and then try again.

1. About 8 hours after vomiting has stopped, your child can gradually return to a normal diet. With older infants and children, give bland items (toast, crackers, clear soup) slowly.
2. Call your physician if any of the following occurs:
   a. Vomiting continues for more than 24 hours or increases in frequency or amount.
   b. Signs of dehydration develop, including decreased urine level, less moisture in diapers, dry mouth, no tears, or weight loss.
   c. Child becomes sleepy, difficult to awaken, or irritable.
   d. Vomited material contains blood or turns green.

Many children will spit up *(regurgitate)* food, particularly during the first few months of life. This is normal in most children but may be exaggerated by faulty feeding techniques or gastroesophageal reflux **(chalasia)**. If the child is well and growing normally, the problem may be reduced by careful attention to feeding techniques. Suggestions for parents that may be useful include the following:

1. Keep your child in an upright position during feeding and prone for 30 to 45 minutes after feeding.
2. Feed your baby smaller amounts more often.
3. Burp your baby frequently.
4. Thickened liquids may be helpful.

BIBLIOGRAPHY

Edstrom CS: Hereditary fructose intolerance in the vomiting infant, *Pediatrics* 85:600, 1990.

Ramsook C, Sahagun-Carreon I, Kozinetz CA et al: A randomized clinical trial comparing oral ondansetron with placebo in children with vomiting from acute gastroenteritis, *Ann Emerg Med* 39:397, 2002.

Reeves J, Shannon W, Fleisher G: Ondansetron decreases vomiting associated with acute gastroenteritis: a randomized, controlled study, *Pediatrics* 109:e62, 2002.

Squires RH: Intracranial tumors: vomiting as a presenting sign, *Clin Pediatr* 28:351, 1989.

VII

Environmental Emergencies

45 Bites

ALERT Bites must be evaluated to determine the extent of local tissue injury and potential immediate and long-term systemic or local infectious reactions.

Animal and Human Bites

Children commonly experience animal bites, as many as 20% of which are dog bites. The peak age range is 5 to 14 years, with the highest incidence in boys during the spring and summer. Management involves minimizing skin and soft tissue injury to achieve a good cosmetic and functional result, and providing prophylaxis against infection in the initial encounter and adequate follow-up observation to ensure prompt treatment of delayed infection.

DOG AND CAT BITES

Large dogs are responsible for most animal bites, although smaller dogs and cats may bite and scratch. It is estimated that 0.5 to 2 million dog bites occur each year, representing about 1% of emergency department visits. Up to 5% of dog bites and 20% to 50% of cat bites become infected. In most cases, the dog belongs to the family or a neighbor.

Etiology

1. *Pasteurella multocida* infection is often involved in children with early evolving cellulitis; *Staphylococcus aureus*, usually a common secondary infection beginning at 2 to 4 days, is grown from culture of as many as 50% of infected wounds. Mixed infections are common. Anaerobic bacteria are present in approximately one third of infected wounds.
2. Rabies virus is an unusual pathogen but must be considered. Rodents (e.g., rats, mice, gerbils, hamsters, squirrels) do not carry rabies virus (p. 733).

Diagnostic Findings

Patients commonly have soft tissue injuries, which are usually a combination of crush injury and lacerations. Injuries to the face, head, and neck are most common.

Complications

Cellulitis may develop, with the onset of erythema, swelling, or tenderness. Lymphadenitis may also develop. If no signs of infection are present within 3 days of trauma, infection is unlikely to occur. Puncture wounds have a higher rate of infection than lacerations because the bacterial inoculum in a puncture wound is deeper, and the wound more difficult to cleanse.

Cat-scratch disease may occur after a cat bite, producing regional lymphadenitis of an extremity 14 days (range: 3 to 50 days) after the scratch. Cats younger than 1 year are more likely to be involved; 80% of cat-scratch disease occurs in people younger than 21 years. *Bartonella henselae* (formerly *Rochalimaea henselae*) most commonly causes the disease.

All patients have adenopathy, which is the only clinical feature in half the cases. The most common site is the axilla. Parinaud's oculoglandular syndrome (POGS), associated with cat scratches in 97% of cases, consists of neuroretinitis, encephalopathy (headache, lethargy, transient hemiplegia, aphasia, hearing loss), thrombocytopenic purpura, angiomatous papules, hepatomegaly, and splenomegaly. Atypical cases in about 5% of patients with cat-scratch disease may involve prolonged fever, malaise, fatigue, myalgia, arthralgia, or POGS.

The immunofluorescent antibody (IFA) assay is 98% to 100% sensitive for diagnosis of cat-scratch disease; the antibody titer peak occurs at 6 to 8 weeks after the onset of illness. The skin test is not generally recommended. Biopsy of the lymph nodes may be useful in atypical disease.

Complications

Complications of animal bites include the following:

1. Crush injuries
2. Osteomyelitis (p. 769)
3. Septic arthritis (p. 767)
4. Tenosynovitis

Ancillary Data

Cultures and Gram staining are unnecessary with routine animal bites. However, if a wound becomes infected, cultures should be performed, particularly if the infection has been unresponsive to previous therapy, or if the patient either is taking prophylactic antibiotics or is immunosuppressed. IFA assay should be performed for cat-scratch disease.

Management (see Chapter 65)

1. Mechanical irrigation and debridement are crucial to the treatment of animal bites:
   a. Adequate cleansing may require local or regional anesthesia.
   b. The wound should be irrigated extensively with 1% povidone-iodine solution (Betadine), not scrub. Some prefer to use sterile saline solution, but the iodine solution is preferable. Peroxide and isopropyl alcohol may cause tissue damage. Using pressure for the irrigation is ideal. A 19-gauge needle attached to a 35-ml syringe can generate 7 pounds per square inch (PSI), whereas a standard bulb syringe creates only 0.05 PSI. Irrigation is best done at 7 PSI or higher through a 19-gauge or larger needle syringe system. The fluid is directed at various angles so that all surfaces are cleansed.
   c. Debridement of wound edges and devitalized tissues is essential to reduce nonvital tissue and facilitate a good plastic closure.
   d. Scrubbing (except for wounds with rabies potential) is usually harmful to tissues.
   e. Particular attention must be given to irrigation and debridement of wounds with extensive damage.
2. Suturing is indicated for cosmetic and functional reasons:
   a. It should be done only after thorough irrigation and debridement.
   b. Hand injuries, injuries involving extensive soft tissue injury or damage to deep tissues, puncture wounds, and injuries older than 24 hours should not be sutured if any question exists about the extent of the wound, the adequacy of irrigation and debridement, or the completeness of follow-up. Sterile bandaging (Steri-strips) may be useful.
   c. One study of dog bites to the hand showed a small difference in infection rate between sutured (5.5%) and unsutured (4.5%) wounds. Human bites of the hand are not usually sutured.
3. Wounds that have a high risk of becoming infected include the following:
   a. Bites of the hand, wrist, or foot. On infants, the scalp and face are problematic.
   b. Extensive wounds in which devitalized tissue cannot be entirely debrided.
   c. Wounds older than 12 hours.
   d. Wounds involving tendons, joints, or bone.

e. Sutured wounds.
f. Puncture wounds.
g. Crush injuries that cannot be debrided.
h. Wounds in patients with peripheral vascular insufficiency (e.g., diabetes), asplenia, or immunocompromise, and in patients older than 50 years. Generally, the risk of infection is highest for cat bites.

4. Antibiotics may be considered prophylactically with high-risk injuries (as defined previously). About 14 patients are treated with antibiotics for every patient in whom an infection is thus prevented. The estimated relative risk for development of an infection is 0.56% for patients who are treated with antibiotics, and 16% for those who are not.
   a. Penicillin VK, 25 to 50 mg/kg/24 hr q6hr PO, and cephalexin (Keflex) or cephradine (Velosef), 25 to 50 mg/kg/24 hr q6hr PO; *or* amoxicillin–clavulanic acid (Augmentin), 30 to 50 mg amoxicillin/kg/24 hr q8hr PO.
   b. Wounds that become infected, particularly those in high-risk locations, generally require parenteral therapy:
      - Penicillin G, 100,000 U/kg/24 hr q4hr IV, and nafcillin (or equivalent), 100 mg/kg/24 hr q4hr IV; or less ideally, a cephalosporin such as cefazolin (Ancef), 50 to 100 mg/kg/24 hr q6-8hr IV.
      - Infections in low-risk areas may be initially treated orally if the child is nontoxic and follow-up observation is good.
5. Although antibiotics are generally not recommended for cat-scratch disease, they may be indicated if systemic disease is present. Recommended agents, in decreasing order of effectiveness, are oral rifampin, ciprofloxacin, and trimethoprim-sulfamethoxazole; parenteral gentamicin may also be used.
6. Other considerations include the following:
   a. Tetanus toxoid should be administered as indicated (p. 734).
   b. Wounds with great soft tissue injury should be immobilized and, if on an extremity, elevated.
   c. If an abscess forms, surgical drainage is required.
   d. Suture material should be removed from a sutured wound that becomes infected.
   e. Rabies should be considered in some geographic areas, depending on the animal inflicting the scratch or bite, the location of the injury, and other factors outlined on p. 733.

Disposition

Patients with uncomplicated animal bites may be discharged, with careful instructions to monitor for infection. Those with high-risk bites should receive antibiotic therapy. Careful follow-up observation is essential. If a bite is sutured, it should be reexamined within 24 hours. Patients with high-risk bites that become infected must be hospitalized for parenteral therapy.

Parental Education

1. Instruct children about not playing with unfamiliar animals. Do not allow a child to place the face near a dog's face; do not leave children unattended with dogs. Dogs may misinterpret human gestures as threatening. Obey leash laws and be particularly careful with large dogs. Dogs must be treated with respect, which includes never hurting or teasing them or taking things from them.
2. Call your physician if any of the following occurs:
   a. The wound gets red, tender, or swollen or develops a discharge.
   b. Child has a fever.

BIBLIOGRAPHY

Bass JW, Vincent JM, Person DA: The expanding spectrum of *Bartonella* infections. II: cat-scratch disease, *Pediatr Infect Dis* 16:163, 1997.

Brogan TV, Bratton SL, Dowd MD et al: Severe dog bites in children, *Pediatrics* 96:5, 1995.

Cummings P: Antibiotics to prevent infections in patients with dog bite wounds: a meta-analysis of randomized trials, *Ann Emerg Med* 23:535, 1994.

Dire DJ, Hogan DE, Walker JS: Prophylactic oral antibiotics for low risk dog bite wounds, *Pediatr Emerg Care* 8:194, 1992.

Goldstein EJ: Bite wounds and infection, *Clin Infect Dis* 14:633, 1992.

Margileth AM: Antibiotic therapy for cat-scratch disease: clinical study of therapeutic outcome in 268 patients and a review of the literature, *Pediatr Infect Dis J* 11:474, 1992.

Midani S, Ayoub EM, Anderson B: Cat-scratch disease, *Adv Pediatr* 43:397, 1996.

Rosenkrans JA: Animal and human bites. In Barkin RM, editor: *Pediatric emergency medicine: concepts and clinical practice*, ed 2, St. Louis, 1997, Mosby.

HUMAN BITES

Human bites have a greater risk of tissue damage and infection than bites inflicted by dogs and cats.

Etiology

More than 40 organisms have been identified as human mouth flora and may be potential pathogens.

Diagnostic Findings

The most common bite injury involves a clenched fist striking an opponent's mouth, with potentially great tissue damage from the teeth. Examination of damage to soft tissues and tendons must include repositioning of the hand in the clenched and neutral positions. Other tissues may be involved.

Infection produces cellulitis, with potential closed-space infections and abscess formation, as well as osteomyelitis and septic arthritis.

Management

Irrigation and debridement are performed as described for animal bites (p. 308) and must be done with meticulous care. These wounds should never be sutured because of the high rate of infection.

1. Antibiotics should be administered as noted for animal bites (p. 305). Tetanus toxoid should be administered as indicated (p. 718).
2. Patients who have infections associated with human bites are usually admitted to the hospital for parenteral therapy. Medications should provide coverage for *S. aureus*, streptococci, anaerobes, and *Eikenella corrodens* (often resistant to first-generation cephalosporins, clindamycin, and aminoglycosides). The response should be monitored closely.
   - Ampicillin, 100 mg/kg/24 hr q4hr IV, and nafcillin (or equivalent), 100 mg/kg/24 hr q4hr IV; *or* a cephalosporin such as cefazolin (Ancef), 50 to 100 mg/kg/24 hr q6-8hr IV.

Disposition

Patients with uncomplicated human bites may be discharged with antibiotic therapy and good follow-up monitoring. Patients with infected bites should be admitted to the hospital.

BIBLIOGRAPHY

Leung AKC, Robson WLM: Human bites in children, *Pediatr Emerg Care* 8:225, 1992.

Arthropod (Insect) Bites

BROWN RECLUSE SPIDER

The brown recluse spider *(Loxosceles reclusa)* is 1 inch long and is distinguished by violin-like markings on the dorsum of its thorax. The spider introduces a venom containing necrotizing, hemolytic, and spreading factors in the skin. It seeks out dry, warm habitats, spinning the webs in protected places, such as under stones and cliffs; in rarely disturbed areas such as attics, closets, and garages; and in corners and crevices of houses. It is not aggressive toward humans and generally attacks only when trapped or crushed against the skin.

Diagnostic Findings

Local pain and erythema at the site develop 2 to 8 hours after the bite, followed by formation of a bleb or blister, with a surrounding area of pallor. The pain is out of proportion to the size of the lesion. Over the ensuing 48 to 72 hours, central induration occurs, and a dark violet color develops, surrounded by a larger area of reactive erythema. This "red, white, and blue" sign is typical of severe bites. The area then ulcerates, and a black eschar forms within a week, which heals over 6 to 8 weeks. If these changes have not occurred by 58 to 96 hours, the patient usually does not have any significant necrosis. Necrosis develops from bites in the fatty areas such as the abdomen, buttocks, and thighs with greater frequency than from bites elsewhere.

Systemic signs appear in the initial 24 to 48 hours, including headache, fever, nausea, vomiting, joint pains, and, very rarely, cyanosis, hypotension, and seizures. The variability of the response reflects the immune status of the patient, the amount of venom injected, and the location of the bite.

Complications

1. Hemolysis with hemoglobinemia, hemoglobinuria, and renal failure. Bites less than 1 cm in diameter rarely cause hemolysis. If the bite has enlarged on serial examinations, monitoring of the urine should continue. If the bite is larger than 1 cm, the patient's urine must be monitored closely. If hemolysis occurs, hydrate the patient and consider steroid therapy.
2. Disseminated intravascular coagulation (DIC) (p. 694).
3. Seizures (see Chapter 21).
4. Rarely, death.

Ancillary Data

A complete blood count (CBC), prothrombin time (PT), partial thromboplastin time (PTT), platelet count, and urinalysis should be obtained.

Management

1. Assess airway and ventilation. Manage anaphylaxis (see Chapter 12).
2. Local care of the site of bite. Rest the bitten site, put ice compresses on the area, and elevate it.
3. Give parenteral steroids. Hydrocortisone (Solu-Cortef), 5mg/kg/dose q6hr IV, should be administered for a minimum of 24 hours if any systemic signs develop.
4. Give analgesia for pain.
5. Excise if the ulceration and necrotic area exceed 1 cm (rarely needed).
6. Provide specific treatment for complications.
7. Studies suggest the efficacy of dapsone, 1 to 4 mg/kg/24 hr q12hr PO (adult, 50-100 mg/24 hr PO) for 3 days, in reducing ulceration because of its leukocyte-inhibiting properties, but no randomized data are available for confirmation. Potential adverse effects include hemolysis, agranulocytosis, aplastic anemia, methemoglobinemia, rashes, and toxic epidermal necrolysis.
8. Hyperbaric oxygen has been studied but no clear benefit has been shown.

Disposition

Patients with systemic signs and symptoms should be admitted to the hospital; others may be monitored closely as outpatients.

BIBLIOGRAPHY

Eitzen EM, Seward PN: Arthropod envenomations in children, *Pediatr Emerg Care* 4:266, 1988.

Phillips S, Kohn M, Baker D et al: Therapy of brown spider envenomation: a controlled trial of hyperbaric oxygen, dapsone, and cyproheptadine, *Ann Emerg Med* 25:363, 1995.

Wright SW, Wrenn KD, Murray L et al: Clinical presentation and outcome of brown recluse spider bite, *Ann Emerg Med* 30:28, 1997.

Wilson DC, King LE Jr: Spiders and spider bites, *Dermatol Clin* 8:2, 1990.

BLACK WIDOW SPIDER

The black widow spider *(Latrodectus mactans)* is identified from a shiny, black button-shaped body with a red hourglass marking on the underside. The venom is a neurotoxin.

Diagnostic Findings

At the site of the bite, there is immediate pain with burning, swelling, and erythema. Double fang markings can be seen. Other local features are piloerection, mild edema, perspiration, and lymphangitis.

The severity of systemic signs and symptoms reflects the number of bites, the amount of venom injected, and the toxicity of the spider's venom. Within 30 minutes of the bite, crampy abdominal pain occurs, accompanied by dizziness, nausea, vomiting, headache, and sweating. The abdomen is characteristically boardlike, mimicking an acute abdomen. Other findings are salivation, lacrimation, tremors, tachycardia or bradycardia, and anxiety. The patient's condition usually resolves in 24 hours, but the bite is associated with hypertension rather than hypotension.

In one study 79% of patients had pain at the bite site, 71% had abdominal pain, and 57% had lower extremity weakness.

Complications

1. Ascending motor paralysis (see Chapter 41)
2. Seizures (see Chapter 21)
3. Shock (see Chapter 5)
4. Coma, respiratory arrest, death

Management

Supportive therapy should be instituted at the first sign of systemic symptoms. Options include the following:

1. Muscle relaxant: diazepam (Valium), 0.1 to 0.3 mg/kg/dose IV; *and*
2. Analgesics: meperidine (Demerol), 1 to 2 mg/kg/dose q4-6hr IM, IV. Morphine, 0.1 to 0.2 mg/kg/dose q2hr IV, may be an alternative.
3. Calcium gluconate (10%), 50 to 100 mg (0.5-1 ml)/kg/dose (up to a maximum dose of 10 ml) IV slowly, has been reported to have a variable and transient efficacy. Dose may have to be repeated. The use of this agent is controversial.

An equine antivenin, ethacrynate (Lyovac)—in a vial containing 2.5 ml—is administered, according to package directions, after negative skin test results for horse serum sensitivity have been obtained. This agent has a limited role, given the efficacy of the preceding therapy, but may be important for young children and individuals with hypertension and cardiac disease. Some authorities have suggested that antivenin is indicated if all of the following conditions are present or if three have been present for more than 12 hours: abdominal pain, hypertension, muscular pain, and agitation or irritability.

Disposition

All patients with known black widow spider bite must be admitted for observation and potential treatment.

BIBLIOGRAPHY

Clark RF, Wethern-Kestner S, Vance NV et al: Clinical presentation and treatment of black widow spider envenomation: a review of 163 cases, *Ann Emerg Med* 21:782, 1992.

Moss HS, Binder LS: A retrospective review of black widow spider envenomation, *Ann Emerg Med* 16:188, 1987.

HYMENOPTERA

Hymenoptera (honey bees, wasps, yellow jackets, and hornets) produce a variety of systemic effects, reflecting individual sensitivity and the number of bites or stings inflicted by the offending insect.

Diagnostic Findings

1. Local reactions commonly produce edema and pain.
2. Toxic reactions occur with multiple stings (10 or more): vomiting, diarrhea, dizziness, muscle spasms, and, rarely, convulsions.

3. Anaphylactic reactions, such as wheezing and urticaria (see Chapter 12), occur in sensitive individuals.
4. Delayed serum-sickness reaction occurs 10 to 14 days after the sting, with morbilliform rash, urticaria, myalgia, arthralgia, and fever.

Management

1. Local attention to the point of sting—cleansing, removing the stinger with a scraping motion, and cold compresses—may provide symptomatic relief. Local application of papain, found in meat tenderizer, is believed by some to relieve pain.
2. Diphenhydramine (Benadryl), 5 mg/kg/24 hr q6-8hr PO, IM, or IV, may reduce local as well as systemic signs and symptoms.
3. Systemic signs of anaphylaxis are treated with epinephrine, nebulized β-agonist agents, and steroids (see Chapter 12).

Disposition

1. Patients with only local reactions can usually be discharged with symptomatic treatment.
2. Those with severe reactions should be admitted for continuation of emergent care.
3. After resolution of severe systemic and anaphylactic reactions, the patient should be referred to an allergist for hyposensitization.
4. People who have experienced severe local or systemic reactions should carry bee sting kits containing epinephrine and syringes (see Chapter 12). Children should be warned to avoid clothing with bright colors and flowery patterns as well as perfumes, hair sprays, and colognes, all of which attract insects.

TICKS

Most tick bites are benign and simply require removal of the tick. However, a number of diseases may be transmitted by ticks, with specific types serving as the vectors (Table 45-1).

As indicated in Table 45-1, *Lyme disease* has three clinical phases. The first stage occurs within a few days up to weeks after the tick inoculation. Erythema chronicum migrans (ECM) begins as a red papule or macule at the site and expands to an annular lesion with central clearing. Viral-like syndromes may be present. Stage 2, associated with spirochete dissemination, has neurologic, cardiac (atrioventricular nodal block), and ophthalmologic findings. Stage 3 involves ongoing neurologic findings and synovitis. Long-term sequelae include neuropathy, encephalopathy, fibromyalgia, chronic fatigue syndrome, and recurrent arthralgia. An antibody response does not protect against subsequent infection. A vaccine is being developed.

Tick-bite paralysis presenting as an ascending paralysis is discussed on page 285.

An embedded tick can usually be withdrawn by covering it with alcohol, mineral oil, nail polish, or an ointment. Another suggested protocol for tick removal is the following:

1. Using a blunt, curved forceps or tweezer, grasp the tick close to the surface and pull upward in a steady motion.
2. If steady traction is unsuccessful, the tick and superficial attached skin can easily be cut away. Brief pressure on the wound will stop the bleeding.
3. Do not squeeze, squash, or puncture the body of the tick because its fluids (saliva, hemolymph) may contain infective agents.
4. Do not touch the tick with bare hands.

The wearing of protective clothing when in tick-infested areas should reduce potential exposure.

NOTE: A small study has suggested that antimicrobial prophylaxis with a single 200-mg dose of doxycycline given within 72 hours of a bite from an *Ixodes scapularis* tick in a patient older than 8 years may prevent the development of Lyme disease.

TABLE 45-1 Tick-Transmitted Diseases

	Etiology	Tick Vector	Incubation (days)	Diagnostic Findings	Antibiotics
Tularemia	*Francisella tularensis*	*Dermacentor*	1-14	Headache, persistent fever, malaise, anorexia, lymphadenopathy	Streptomycin, tetracycline,* chloramphenicol
Relapsing fever	*Borrelia recurrentis*	*Ornithodoros*	5-9	Relapsing fever, occipital headache, malaise, myalgia, cough, meningismus, lymphadenopathy, conjunctivitis leukocytosis	Tetracycline,* penicillin, chloramphenicol
Rocky Mountain spotted fever	*Rickettsia rickettsii*	*Dermacentor*	2-14	Resistant fever, headache, malaise, arthralgia, periorbital edema, conjunctivitis, meningismus, coma, centrifugal hemorrhagic rash, petechiae; history of tick bite in 60%–70% of patients	Tetracycline,* doxycycline,* chloramphenicol
Colorado tick fever	Colorado tick fever virus	*Dermacentor*	3-6	Sudden onset of fever, retroorbital headache, myalgia, anorexia, meningismus, rash, conjunctivitis, leukopenia	None (support)
Ehrlichiosis	*Ehrlichia chaffeensis*	*Amblyomma americanum*	7-20	Fever, headache, malaise, arthralgia, myalgia, nausea, rash (30% of cases); low platelet count and WBC	Tetracycline,* doxycycline,* chloramphenicol (less effective)
Lyme disease	*Borrelia burgdorferi*	*Ixodes scapularis/ pacificus*	3-32	ECM (macular/papular becoming annular), flulike symptoms (headache, anorexia, chills) during stage 1; 15% of patients progress to stage 2, with neurologic complications (encephalopathy, cranial neuropathy, peripheral radiculoneuropathy), joint complications; 50%–60% have pericarditis; stage 3 may occur with persistent CNS findings and arthritis (arthralgia); pericarditis; remissions; ELISA	Tetracycline,* doxycycline,* cefuroxime, or amoxicillin for 10-30 days; late-stage or toxic child needs additional therapy (ceftriaxone)

ECM, Erythema cronicum migrans.
* Do not use in children <9 yr.

BIBLIOGRAPHY

Committee on Infectious Diseases, American Academy of Pediatrics: Treatment of Lyme borreliosis, *Pediatrics* 88:176, 1991.

Feder HM, Hunt MS: Pitfalls in the diagnosis and treatment of Lyme disease in children, *JAMA* 274:66, 1995.

Gerber MA, Shapiro ED: Prognosis of Lyme disease in children, *J Pediatr* 121:157, 1992.

Gerber MA, Shapiro ED, Burke GS et al: Lyme disease in children in southeastern Connecticut, *N Engl J Med* 335:1270, 1996.

Jacobs RF, Schutze GE: Ehrlichiosis in children, *J Pediatr* 131:184, 1997.

Nadelman RB: Prophylaxis with single-dose doxycycline for the prevention of Lyme disease after an *Ixodes scapularis* tick bite, *N Engl J Med* 345:79, 2001.

Shadick NA, Phillips CB, Logigian EL et al: The long-term clinical outcome of Lyme disease: a population based retrospective cohort study, *Ann Intern Med* 121:560, 1994.

Williams CL, Strabino B, Lee A et al: Lyme disease in childhood: clinical and epidemiologic features of ninety cases, *Pediatr Infect Dis* 9:10, 1990.

Snake Bites

ALERT It is crucial to determine rapidly whether a snake is potentially poisonous. If it is, urgent local treatment, support, and administration of antivenin are required.

Of the known species of snakes, only 5% are venomous. In the United States, the most commonly encountered venomous snakes are Crotalidae (pit vipers, water moccasins, and copperheads) and Elapidae (coral snakes). Their venom consists of multiple poisonous proteins and enzymes that are absorbed through the lymphatic system after envenomation. Most snake bites occur in the summer during the afternoon or evening.

The severity of injury from a poisonous snake bite reflects, among other factors, the amount of venom released and the size of the victim. The following factors should be considered:

1. Age, size, and health of the patient.
2. The size of the snake; larger snakes produce more venom. Juvenile snakes may produce a more lethal venom to compensate for the diminished venom volume. Not all strikes result in envenomation; thus the biting and the envenomation can be distinct processes.
3. The location of the injury. Peripheral injuries account for more than 90% of bites and are usually less severe. Bites to the distal aspect of a digit may be associated with less severe clinical manifestations.

Distinguishing venomous from nonvenomous snakes is sometimes difficult. Venomous snakes usually have vertically elliptic pupils, a facial pit between the eye and the nostril, a rattle, fangs, and subcaudal plates behind oval plates, which in pit vipers are arranged in a single row. Nonvenomous snakes have round pupils; no pit, rattle, or fangs; and a double row of subcaudal plates.

DIAGNOSTIC FINDINGS

1. The site of the poisonous snake bite may display fang marks, with subsequent burning, pain or numbness, swelling, and erythema. These symptoms may progress rapidly to hemorrhage and necrosis. A compartment syndrome may develop, which is difficult to distinguish from the local effects of the venom.
2. Regional effects of extremity bites include edema of the arm or leg, ecchymoses, and lymphadenopathy.
3. Systemic signs and symptoms may develop within 15 minutes, depending on the severity of the injury:
   a. Nausea, vomiting, sweating, chills, numbness, and paresthesias of the tongue and perioral region may occur.
   b. Fasciculations, dysphagia, bleeding, and hypotension are common.
4. Nonpoisonous snake bites often leave the patient with major psychologic trauma, which may result in mild nonspecific symptoms similar to those of actual envenomation.

Complications

1. DIC and hemolysis (p. 694)
2. Respiratory failure caused by noncardiogenic pulmonary edema
3. Renal failure (p. 828)
4. Seizures (see Chapter 21)
5. Shock and death

Ancillary Data

1. CBC, platelet count, coagulation studies (PT, PTT, fibrinogen, fibrin split products [FSPs]).
2. Urinalysis and measurements of blood urea nitrogen (BUN), serial electrolyte, creatinine levels.
3. Blood typing and cross-match; should be performed initially because it may be difficult to accomplish once hemolysis occurs.
4. In moderate to severe cases, consider a chest radiograph, electrocardiogram (ECG), and arterial blood gas analysis.

MANAGEMENT

1. If possible, the snake should be killed and identified, with careful handling of the head because it can still deliver venom for as long as 1 hour after death.
2. Initially, a broad, firm, constrictive bandage should be applied proximal to the bitten area and around the limb. It should be tight enough to reduce superficial lymphatic drainage.
3. The extremity should be splinted to reduce motion.
4. Activity of the patient should be minimized, and cooling, which can cause further tissue damage, should be avoided.
5. Surgical excision of the wound site or fasciotomy is probably unnecessary because the muscle necrosis is probably due to proteolytic enzymes rather than increased compartmental pressure. Incision and suction have not proven efficacious. Fasciotomy is indicated in rare circumstances of documented true compartment syndrome.
6. Hyperbaric oxygen may be an adjunctive treatment if severe envenomation occurs with a large open wound and a significant volume of necrotic muscle.

Antivenin Therapy

Transport to the hospital should be expedited for support and administration of antivenin. Indications for the use of antivenin after a venomous bite by a Crotalidae is the presence of progressive injury associated with a worsening local injury (i.e. swelling, ecchymoses), a clinically important coagulation abnormality, or systemic effects (hypotension, altered mental status). Recurrent coagulopathy may require ongoing therapy beyond the first doses.

1. Antivenin of purified, mixed, monospecific crotalid polyvalent immune (ovine) antigen-binding fragment (Fab) (CroFab or FabAV). Initial control dose of 3 to 12 vials with subsequent scheduled therapy of 2 vials at 6, 12, and 18 hours.
2. Antivenin (Crotalidae) polyvalent; horse serum requiring reconstitution. The exact dose is difficult to determine; for information call Wyeth Laboratories 215-688-4400:
   - 2 to 4 vials for *minimal* reaction (local swelling without systemic symptoms)
   - 5 to 9 vials for *moderate* reactions (progressive symptoms with marked swelling and systemic signs, including metallic taste, and paresthesias or laboratory abnormalities)
   - 10 to 15 vials for *severe* reactions (rapid swelling, severe systemic symptoms [muscle fasciculations, hypotension, oliguria] and abnormal laboratory findings)

If horse serum is to be used, skin tests for hypersensitivity must be done. Reactions can be managed by slowing down or temporarily stopping infusions and pretreating with diphenhydramine (Benadryl) and a histamine (H_2) blocker (cimetidine). The antivenin infusion should begin slowly at a dilution of 1:10, and the dilution should be increased gradually if no reaction is noted. If anaphylactic reactions are noted despite pretreatment, it is possible to titrate response with an epinephrine infusion after consultation (see Chapter 12). Monitoring is mandatory.

Information, consultation, and antivenin for rare species may be obtained from Oklahoma Poison Control Center: 405-271-5454.

Complications of horse serum administration include anaphylactic shock, DIC, and serum sickness. Serum sickness may develop 7 to 14 days after antivenin administration. Treatment of complications is essential to the ultimate outcome. Tetanus toxoids should also be given if indicated.

DISPOSITION

All patients with poisonous snake bite should be admitted to the hospital for supportive care. Patients with unidentified snake bites may be discharged if no signs and symptoms develop during 4 hours of observation. Reassurance may be necessary.

BIBLIOGRAPHY

Burgess JL, Dart RC, Egan NB et al: Effects of constriction bands on rattlesnake venom absorption: a pharmacokinetic study, *Ann Emerg Med* 21:1086, 1992.

Dart RC, McNally J: Efficacy, safety and care of snake antivenoms in the US, *Ann Emerg Med* 37:181, 2001.

Dart RC, Seifert SA, Carroll L et al: Affinity-purified mixed monospecific crotalid antivenom ovine Fab for the treatment of crotalid venom poisoning, *Ann Emerg Med* 30:33, 1997.

Hall EL: Role of surgical intervention in the management of Crotalidae snake envenomation, *Ann Emerg Med* 37:175, 2001.

McKinney PE: Out-of-hospital and interhospital management of crotaline snakebite, *Ann Emerg Med* 37:168, 2001.

Moss ST, Bogen G, Dart RC: Association of rattlesnakes bite location with severity of clinical manifestations, *Ann Emerg Med* 30:58, 1997.

Tully SA, Wingert WA: Venomous animal bites and stings. In Barkin RM, editor: *Pediatric emergency medicine: concepts and clinical practice*, ed 2, St Louis, 1997, Mosby.

46 Burns, Thermal

Also See Chapters 53 (Smoke Inhalation) and 55 (Specific Ingestions)

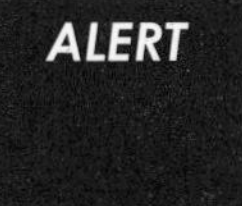

Rapid assessment of the depth, location, and extent of a burn should determine the severity of the injury. Airway and pulmonary status and associated trauma must be treated, and volume deficits corrected. Specific burn therapy should be initiated immediately after stabilization.

ETIOLOGY

The mechanism of heat transfer and injury influences the type of burn.

Scald burns result from contact with a hot object or hot liquid. They are most commonly seen in children younger than 3 years and may be sharply demarcated and of partial thickness, except in young infants, in whom full-thickness injury may be noted.

Flame burns occur with direct-flame exposure resulting from ignition of clothing. They are commonly seen in children older than 2 years, who often play with matches, fire, and flammable materials. The borders are irregular and may be of full thickness.

Flash burns, caused by exposure to an explosion, are uniform and of partial thickness.

Electrical burns are discussed in Chapter 48.

DIAGNOSTIC FINDINGS

Initial evaluation must include information about the mechanism of injury, time since the burn, patient's age and weight, underlying disease, past medical problems, and associated injuries.

Body surface area (BSA) in children may be estimated to determine the extent of burns (Fig. 46-1). In adults, the *rule of 9's* is easily used for estimating involved body surface: head and neck (9%), anterior trunk (18%), posterior trunk (18%), each leg (18%), each arm (9%), and anorectal area (1%).

The patient should be thoroughly examined for other associated traumatic injuries as well as signs of smoke inhalation, including hoarseness, cough, singed nasal hairs, oral burns, carbonaceous sputum, wheezing, rhonchi, and cyanosis (see Chapter 53).

Depth of burn is an important determinant of severity and potential complications:

1. Superficial partial-thickness (first-degree) burns involve only the epidermis and are characterized by erythema and local pain.
2. Partial-thickness (second-degree) burns involve the epidermis and corium:
   a. Partial-thickness burns produce erythema and blisters.
   b. Deep partial-thickness burns are white and dry and have reduced sensitivity to touch and pain. They blanch with pressure.
3. Full-thickness (third-degree) burns are numb, with a tough, brownish surface and a hard eschar. Spontaneous healing will not occur.

Severity of burns is determined by the depth of the burn, BSA affected, location of the injury, age and health of the patient, and associated injuries, as follows:

1. *Major* burn:
   a. Partial-thickness burn of more than 25% BSA in adults or more than 15% to 20% BSA in children or full-thickness burn of more than 10% BSA

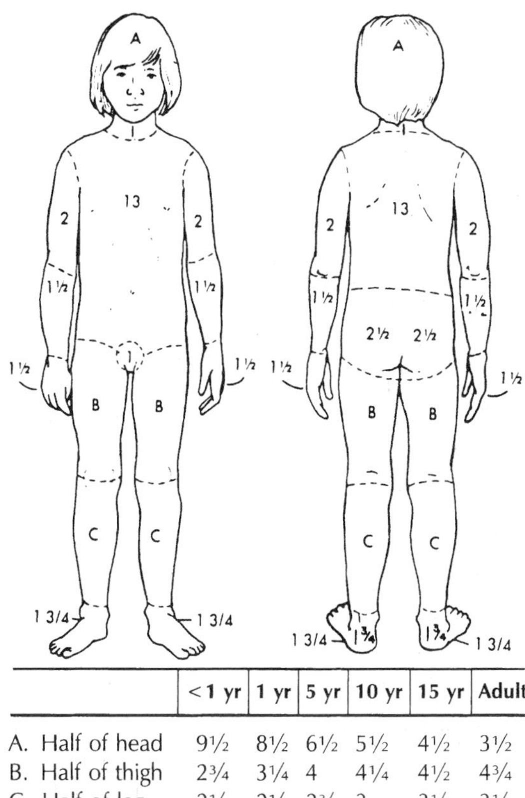

	<1 yr	1 yr	5 yr	10 yr	15 yr	Adult
A. Half of head	9½	8½	6½	5½	4½	3½
B. Half of thigh	2¾	3¼	4	4¼	4½	4¾
C. Half of leg	2½	2½	2¾	3	3¼	3½

Fig. 46-1 Calculation of burn surface area.
(After Lund and Browder.)

   b. Burns of the hands, face, eyes, ears, feet, or perineum
   c. Patients with inhalation injury, electrical burns, burns complicated by fractures or other major trauma
   d. Burns that encircle a limb, neck, or chest
   e. Poor-risk patients, including those with underlying disease, associated major injuries, or suspicion of child abuse
2. *Moderate* uncomplicated burn: partial-thickness burn of 15% to 25% BSA in adults or 10% to 15% BSA in children or full-thickness burn of 2% to 10% BSA
3. *Minor* burn: partial-thickness burn of less than 15% BSA in adults or less than 10% BSA in children or full-thickness burn of less than 2% BSA

Complications

1. Smoke inhalation. Direct inhalation of toxic particles or exposure to hot smoke and air may produce respiratory distress on the basis of upper or lower respiratory abnormality (see Chapter 53).
2. Carbon monoxide poisoning (p. 376).
3. Circumferential third-degree burns may produce an eschar (dead, coagulated skin). This may cause vascular or respiratory compromise depending on the location of the burn.
4. Dehydration and shock from fluid losses and inadequate fluid therapy.
5. Renal failure secondary to myoglobinuria or dehydration.
6. Sepsis and death. Very young children (0 to 4 years) who die in house fires account for 47% of deaths. Survival has improved markedly during the last decade. One study demonstrated no mortality in children with burns of less than 60% BSA and a 14% mortality in those with 60% to 100% BSA involvement.

Ancillary Data

1. Blood tests for moderate or major burns should include, when appropriate, complete blood count (CBC), measurement of electrolytes, blood urea nitrogen (BUN), and serum creatinine levels; arterial blood gas (ABG) analysis; determination of carbon monoxide level; blood type and cross-match; and measurement of carboxyhemoglobin level.
2. A chest x-ray film is useful for all patients with major burns and for those with any question of smoke inhalation. The initial film is useful for comparison with later x-ray studies. Abnormal findings are often delayed for up to 24 hours.
3. Urinalysis should be performed for specific gravity, sugar, protein, myoglobin,

and hemoglobin. Urine output is useful in assessing fluid status.

MANAGEMENT OF MINOR AND SOME MODERATE BURNS

1. Burn wounds should initially be covered by a cloth cooled with saline solution. Minimize contact with nonsterile objects.
2. Intact blisters should be left unbroken unless they are at flexion creases. Ruptured vesicles should be debrided, and the area cleansed gently.
3. Superficial partial-thickness burns require no topical therapy except for symptomatic relief. Aloe vera gel facilitates healing.
4. Partial-thickness injuries may be treated with 1% silver sulfadiazine or by application of a fine-mesh gauze impregnated with a petroleum jelly (Xeroform, Adaptic, Vaseline). Very small burns, particularly those in difficult areas, may be left exposed. Sulfadiazine may cause transient leukopenia and should be avoided in patients with sulfa allergies; in vitro studies demonstrate some retardation in healing.
5. Alternative approaches to burns exist. Second-degree burns may be covered with a biologic or synthetic dressing (Polyurethane film [Tegaderm, OpSite] or hydrocolloid semi-open dressing [Biobrane]) without topical application of an antibiotic. This approach speeds wound healing but has no clear advantage over topical antimicrobial therapy. Fluid may have to be aspirated from under such a dressing on occasion.
6. If a bulky dressing is used as reviewed in #4, the dressing should be changed in 24 hours and then every 2 to 3 days or sooner if an odor develops or if the area becomes painful.
7. Tetanus immunization should be given, if necessary.
8. Pain medication is rarely needed. Nonsteroidal antiinflammatory agents may be useful in reducing pain.
9. If the patient has evidence of group A streptococcal disease, penicillin (50,000 U/kg/24 hr q6hr PO or IV) should be given to prevent colonization of the burn.
10. Exclude child abuse in cases of inconsistent or suspicious injury.

Disposition

Patients with minor burns can routinely be sent home unless other medical problems, associated injuries, or suspicion of child abuse or lack of compliance precludes such management. Infants with burns that involve more than 10% to 15% BSA and adults with burns that involve more than 25% BSA or with major burns should be admitted.

Parental Education

1. Keep the wound clean and dry.
2. Change the dressing in 24 hours and then twice daily. Wash burn gently, apply cream, and dress as directed.
3. Call your physician if any of the following occurs:
   a. Increasing redness or discolorations of the normal tissue around the burn site develop or the area becomes odorous or painful.
   b. Red streaks develop around the area.
   c. Fever and chills are present.
   d. Swelling or progressive inability to use fingers or toes (if extremities are involved) is noted.
   e. Pain increases.
   f. Shortness of breath, increased cough, or difficulty in swallowing is present.
   g. Blurred vision develops if face is involved.
4. Sunblock should be used for up to 6 months and on the burn area once healing has occurred.

MANAGEMENT OF MAJOR AND MOST MODERATE BURNS

Assessment of airway and ventilation is crucial to seek evidence of respiratory distress or smoke inhalation injury. Oxygen should be administered to all patients, and if respiratory distress or abnormal ABG values are present, the patient should be intubated. Pulmonary disease may have a delayed onset of up to 24 hours, secondary to smoke inhalation or CO intoxication (see Chapter 53 and p. 376).

Intravenous fluid resuscitation must be initiated immediately with one to two large-bore catheters. Initial stabilization should include infusion of 20 ml/kg 0.9% normal saline (NS) or lactated Ringer's (LR) solution over 20 to 30 minutes. Although controversial, the following is then suggested as an initial guideline for fluid therapy:

Day 1: 4 ml LR solution with 5% dextrose × body weight in kg × [BSA of burn as number, (e.g., 70% = 70)], given over the first 24 hours, in addition to normal maintenance fluids (see Chapter 8). Half of the total volume of fluids should be given during the first 8 hours after the burn, and the remainder over 16 hours.

For instance, a 10-kg child with 20% BSA burn would require the following fluid management, with adjustments as necessitated by urine output:

- Maintenance: 1000 ml H_2O with 30 mEq NaCl and 20 mEq KCl—approximately 5% dextrose in water (D5W) 0.2% NS with 20 mEq KCl/L.
- Replacement: 800 ml of D5WLR = 4 ml D5WLR × 10 (kg) × 20 (% BSA)

One half of replacement dose and one third of maintenance dose to be given during first 8 hours

Day 2: Crystalloid solution infused at about one half to three fourths of the previous day's needs. In addition, colloid is useful at this time when administered as a 5% albumin solution at 0.5 gm/kg/% BSA.

The following considerations should be kept in mind:

1. Potassium should generally not be added to the fluid.
2. If fluid management is difficult, a central venous pressure line should be inserted.
3. Urine output and vital signs are the most sensitive indicators of the adequacy of therapy. A Foley catheter should be inserted to monitor urine flow. Optimal flow output should be 2 to 3 ml/kg/hr, but a minimal level of 1 ml/kg/hr is acceptable.
4. A nasogastric tube should be inserted.

Wound Management

1. Initially, cover the wound with a cloth cooled in saline. Place the patient on a sterile sheet, and make sure anyone touching the patient wears sterile gloves, gowns, and a cap.
2. Gently scrub the wound, using povidone-iodine soap (Betadine) diluted in saline followed by irrigation. Cool saline or water may reduce pain.
3. Obtain surgical consultation.
4. Debride all dead material. Intact blisters should be left unbroken unless they are at flexion creases. Ruptured vesicles should be debrided.
5. Dress wounds with a liberal application of a 1% silver sulfadiazine cream. Apply an absorbent dressing of fine (36 × 44) mesh gauze or 4 × 4 fluffs, using several layers and a role of gauze to hold the dressing. Biobrane, a bilayer semisynthetic dressing, may decrease pain and total healing time in thermal partial-thickness fresh burns without contamination.
6. Leave the face and perineum open after applying antibiotic cream.
7. Escharotomy is indicated with full-thickness, circumferential burns of the extremities accompanied by impaired neurovascular function. Eschars of the chest may impair ventilation and thus require surgical intervention.

8. Depending on the depth and severity of the wounds, dressings may be left on for 24 hours. At each change, the wound can be cleansed with warm water and debrided; this process is often facilitated by a whirlpool. The burns may then be redressed after application of silver sulfadiazine and fine mesh gauze.
9. Skin grafting after early (within 3 to 5 days) burn excision is useful in some injuries with large deep burns. Early excision may reduce mortality risk and hospital stay. Biologic and synthetic dressings have an increasing role in treatment.
10. A burn should be epithelialized in 2 to 3 weeks. If healing is not occurring by 14 days, consider excision and grafting. Superficial partial-thickness injuries should be examined for up to 6 weeks for hypertrophic scarring.

Other Considerations

1. Pain medication may be used once vital signs have normalized. Optimally, drugs such as morphine and meperidine should be given intravenously.
2. Update tetanus immunization if appropriate.
3. Initiate peptic ulcer (Curling's ulcer) prophylaxis with antacid therapy—antacids, cimetidine (20-30 mg/kg/24 hr q6hr IV or PO), or famotidine (Pepcid) (adult: 20-40 mg q24hr PO or 20 mg q12hr IV)—in the first 6 hours after burn.
4. Antibiotics should be administered not prophylactically, but for specific signs and symptoms of infection after appropriate cultures. Give penicillin if there is evidence of a group A streptococcal infection.
5. Begin intravenous, tube, and oral nutrition after the stabilization period. An increased metabolic response is noted after a thermal injury.
6. Keep body temperature normal. Do not apply cold or ice dressings.
7. Provide psychologic support of the family when dealing with a major burn; this issue is imperative from the first encounter through the entire hospitalization. It also is often complicated by concerns about potential child abuse.
8. Initiate rehabilitation after stabilization.
9. Exclude child abuse if the cause of injury is suspicious.

Disposition

All patients with moderate or major burns should be admitted to the surgical service with appropriate consultation as necessary.

Major burns can often best be cared for in burn centers, where the burn team can deal with the patient's total needs on a more routine basis.

If transport is necessary, the initial stabilization should be achieved at the primary receiving hospital, often involving a surgical consultant at that time. The same level of care must be maintained throughout the transport process.

BIBLIOGRAPHY

Carvasal HF: Fluid resuscitation of pediatric burn victims: a critical approach, *Pediatr Nephrol* 8:357, 1994.

Goldstein AM, Weber JM, Sheridan RL: Femoral venous access is safe in burned children: an analysis of 224 catheters, *J Pediatr* 130:442, 1997.

McLoughlin E, McGuire A: The causes, cost and prevention of childhood burn injuries, *Am J Dis Child* 144:677, 1990.

Nagel RT, Schunk JE: Using the hand to estimate the surface area of a burn in children, *Pediatr Emerg Care* 13:254, 1997.

Parish RA: Thermal burns. In Barkin RM, editor: *Pediatric emergency medicine: concepts and clinical practice*, ed 2, St Louis, 1997, Mosby.

Sheridan RL, Remensnyder JP, Schnitzer JJ et al: Current expectations for survival in pediatric burns, *Arch Pediatr Adolesc Med* 154:245, 2000.

Singer AJ, Clark RAF: Cutaneous wound healing, *New Engl J Med* 341:738, 1999.

Yowler CJ, Fratianne RB: Current status of burn resuscitation, *Clin Plast Surg* 27:1, 2000.

47 Drowning, Near-Drowning, and Dysbarism

ALERT After initial resuscitation, evaluate for associated injuries. Monitor patient for evolving pulmonary or cerebral edema. Diving injuries require carefully controlled recompression.

Drowning and Near Drowning

The victim of a submersion episode may die immediately or within 24 hours of the hypoxic insult of complications (*drowning*) or may survive the incident but require intensive support (*near-drowning*). Most accidents occur in swimming pools, ponds, lakes, and bathtubs, with peak incidences in children younger than 4 years and 15 to 24 years old. Among boys 15 to 19 years old, 38% of drownings are alcohol related. Nearly two thirds of bathtub near-drownings have evidence of abuse or neglect.

Freshwater and saltwater drownings have distinct pathophysiologies leading to hypoxemia and similar clinical presentations. Freshwater drowning disrupts surfactant, causing atelectasis and ultimately pulmonary edema; saltwater drowning causes fluid movement along an osmotic gradient, producing flooding of alveoli with protein-rich plasma and pulmonary edema. Electrolyte and erythrocyte abnormalities may also develop in both cases; however, they rarely do because large amounts of water are usually not aspirated.

Prolonged immersion in cold water is associated with a better prognosis than prolonged immersion in warm water.

ETIOLOGY: PRECIPITATING FACTORS

1. Trauma:
   a. Head or neck (see Chapters 57 and 61)
   b. Barotrauma: scuba diving
   c. Hypothermia (see Chapter 51)
   d. Child abuse (see Chapter 25)
2. Seizures (see Chapter 21)
3. Intoxication: alcohol, sedatives, phencyclidine (PCP), lysergic acid diethylamide (LSD) (see Chapter 54)
4. Exhaustion, boating accident, poor swimmer

DIAGNOSTIC FINDINGS

The signs and symptoms reflect pulmonary and cerebral hypoxic injury. The spectrum of illness may range from minimal or negative findings initially, with a delayed onset in 2 to 6 hours, to complete cardiac and respiratory arrest. Vital signs and temperature must be determined. Hypothermia may be protective.

Pulmonary findings include cyanosis, pallor with pulmonary edema, and aspiration pneumonitis often associated with intrapulmonary shunting. Patients may demonstrate rales, frothy sputum, and rhonchi or wheezing and progress to respiratory failure or arrest. Seizures, change in mental status, and stupor or coma may be present with or without focal findings, reflecting hypoxia and cerebral edema.

The patient may be postictal if a seizure precipitated the episode. Cardiac dysrhythmias and asystole are possible.

Evidence of trauma must be evaluated as possible precipitating factors, particularly head and neck injuries. Other unexplained signs may indicate child abuse.

Several researchers have defined factors that are *unfavorable* prognosticators in cases of pediatric near-drowning. Outcome is usually a reflection of hypoxia, not the toxicity of the water. Patients who are conscious or have only blunted levels of consciousness on arrival in the emergency department (ED) usually do well. Such patients usually have pupillary light responses, even if the reaction is slightly blunted.

Clinical indicators suggestive of a poor outcome include the following:

1. Patient is younger than 3 years.
2. Maximum submersion time is more than 5 minutes.
3. Resuscitation efforts not attempted for at least 10 minutes after rescue.
4. Presence of seizures, fixed and dilated pupils, decerebrate posture, flaccid extremities, and coma.
5. Cardiopulmonary resuscitation required on admission in a patient who is not hypothermic. Of those arriving at the ED with asystole in the studies, 76% died and the remainder remained vegetative.
6. Glasgow Coma Scale (GCS) (see Table 57-1) score less than 5. In the studies, a GCS score less than 5 was associated with an 80% mortality rate; patients with GCS scores of 6 or greater had no sequelae.
7. Arterial pH 7.10 or less.
8. Initial blood glucose increase of more than 200 mg/dl.

Children with an intracranial pressure (ICP) of 20 mm Hg or less and a cerebral perfusion pressure (CPP) (difference between systemic arterial and intracranial pressure) of 50 mm Hg or more had the best prognosis, with only an 8% mortality rate. Sustained late intracranial hypertension is more likely a sign of profound neurologic insult than its cause.

Complications

1. Pulmonary edema, respiratory failure, adult respiratory distress syndrome (ARDS), and cardiorespiratory arrest (see Chapters 4 and 19)
2. Aspiration pneumonia
3. Hypoxic encephalopathy and seizures
4. Acute tubular necrosis and renal failure (p. 828)
5. Spinal cord injury
6. Disseminated intravascular coagulation (DIC) (see Chapter 79)
7. On-site resuscitation complications: pneumothorax, abdominal visceral tears, etc.

Ancillary Data

1. Electrolytes: levels are usually normal, but when drowning occurs in water with high concentrations of electrolytes (i.e., Dead Sea), marked elevations of calcium and magnesium levels, as well as the more common electrolytes, may be noted.
2. Complete blood count (CBC) and coagulation screen: usually normal.
3. Arterial blood gas (ABG) analysis.
4. Chest x-ray film: result may be normal initially with delayed appearance of evidence of aspiration or pulmonary edema.
5. Head, neck, and other x-ray studies as indicated by condition.
6. Other studies, as indicated by possible precipitating factors.

MANAGEMENT

In cases of significant near-drowning, initial management must focus on stabilization of the airway, removal of foreign material, maintenance of ventilation, and administration of oxygen and fluids. Vital signs must be meticulously monitored. A nasogastric (NG) tube and urinary catheter should be inserted. If the patient is febrile, antipyretics and a cooling mattress should be used. If the patient is hypothermic, body temperature should be normalized aggressively. Rapid prehospital intervention can improve outcome (p. 340). Furthermore, immediate resuscitation before arrival of prehospital personnel is associated with a better neurologic outcome.

Consideration must be directed toward precipitating conditions, with particular attention to head trauma, neck injury, hypothermia, and barotrauma. Trauma requires neck immobilization until the lateral neck x-ray film and, ultimately, the full cervical spine series have documented no problems. Patients should be rewarmed in accordance with the clinical protocol outlined in Chapter 51. Slow decompression is required if the injury was secondary to barotrauma.

1. Pulmonary management:
   a. Oxygenation is essential. Humidified oxygen at 3 to 6 L/min is given by mask or nasal cannula until stabilization and evaluation are completed. Continuous positive airway pressure (CPAP) should be considered if an Fio_2 greater than 40% is needed. In the awake, cooperative patient, a CPAP of 10 to 12 cm H_2O can be administered by a tightly fitting face mask or other device. Otherwise, intubation may be required.
   b. Intubation and initiation of positive end-expiratory pressure (PEEP) or CPAP are indicated if there is clear evidence of progressive pulmonary edema with an Fio_2 greater than 40% required, particularly if CPAP delivered by mask has been unsuccessful. PEEP should be initiated at 5 cm H_2O and increased slowly, with monitoring of oxygenation and cardiac output. If the cardiac output falls, increasing the intravascular volume may be useful.
   c. Intubation and mechanical ventilation are indicated if the patient is unable to handle secretions, if respiratory failure (Pao_2 less than 50 mm Hg and $Paco_2$ greater than 50 mm Hg in room air at sea level) is present, if there is a severe metabolic acidosis, or if the patient has shown evidence of cerebral edema.
   d. Monitor ABGs and oximetry.
   e. Bronchospasm may require specific β-adrenergic (albuterol) therapy (p. 790).
2. Cerebral edema secondary to hypoxic injury (or head trauma): ICP monitor may be useful in measuring the therapeutic effect (p. 424). Optimally, maintain ICP at less than or equal to 20 mm Hg and CPP at greater than or equal to 50 mm Hg. Measures to reduce ICP may include one or more of the following:
   a. Hyperventilate the patient to maintain a $Paco_2$ of 35 mm Hg.
   b. Elevate the head of bed 30 degrees if vital signs, cervical spine, and head injuries from trauma are stable.
   c. Give furosemide (Lasix), 1 mg/kg/dose up to 3 mg/kg/dose q6hr, which may be repeated q2hr if indicated.
   d. Give mannitol, 0.5 gm/kg/dose over 30 minutes q3-4hr prn IV. Effect lasts 2 to 3 hours, and there may be rebound. Use only when patient is symptomatic.
   e. Restrict fluids to 50% to 60% of maintenance rate while keeping central venous pressure (CVP) in the low to normal range (8 to 10 mm Hg) and urine output between 0.5 and 1 ml/kg/hr. Initial resuscitation may require a fluid bolus.
   f. Barbiturates are controversial. No evidence that they affect outcome independently of associated hyperthermia. Intracranial monitoring is necessary if these agents are used:
      - Pentobarbital (Nembutal): initial dose of 3 to 20 mg/kg IV slowly push while blood pressure (BP) is monitored. Maintain infusion of

1 to 2 mg/kg/hr. Blood drug level should be maintained between 25 and 40 μg/ml; levels above 30 μg/ml are associated with hypotension in as many as 60% of patients.

g. Muscle relaxants may be required if the patient is symptomatic and requires ventilation. Intubate. Pancuronium (Pavulon), 0.1 mg/kg/dose q1hr or prn IV.

3. Other considerations:
   a. Acidosis, if present, requires treatment. Sodium bicarbonate, 1 mEq/kg/dose IV, may be given. Subsequent doses may be required in response to changes in ABG values.
   b. Hypoxic seizures may be controlled by oxygen, ventilation, and diazepam (Valium), 0.2 to 0.3 mg/kg/dose IV, or lorazepam (Ativan), 0.05 to 0.15 mg/kg/dose IV over 1 to 3 minutes, until seizures stop. Control airway. Begin phenobarbital or phenytoin (Dilantin) therapy (see Chapter 21).
   c. Antibiotics are administered only for specific indications.
   d. Steroids have no proven value beyond their controversial role in the treatment of cerebral edema or aspiration pneumonia after near-drowning.
   e. Fever may indicate a secondary infection, such as pneumonitis. It should be treated aggressively with appropriate antibiotics and antipyretics.
   f. Maintain normal levels of electrolytes, glucose, etc.
   g. Avoid procedures that may be poorly tolerated.
   h. Emotional support for the family and friends is imperative.

DISPOSITION

All patients with significant episodes of near-drowning must be admitted to the hospital, particularly in view of the delayed onset of symptoms. Most require the monitoring available in an intensive care unit. Cessation of treatment may be guided by the prognostic factors that have been defined and the clinical response to support.

Parental Education

1. Teach swimming and water safety techniques at an early age but probably not before 3 years.
2. Define water areas that children cannot use. Fence them off.
3. Children require supervision near water and boats. Always have appropriate supervision. Keep rescue devices and first aid equipment near pools.
4. Children with seizure disorders may swim if they have been seizure free for 1 to 2 years but then only with supervision.

Dysbaric Diving Injuries

Divers are subject to barotrauma resulting from barometric pressure changes within body structures. Inadequate pressure adaptation between air-containing cavities and ambient atmosphere causes tissue damage, most commonly in the ear, paranasal sinuses, gastrointestinal (GI) tract and chest (Table 47-1). *Barotrauma of descent* is produced by compression of air that is trapped during descent, potentially occurring in water as shallow as 4.5 feet. Barotitis is common. *Barotrauma of ascent* develops from expansion of air that is trapped in bodily spaces during ascent. Conditions may involve the ear, sinuses, teeth, mediastinum (subcutaneous and interstitial emphysema), pneumothorax, and pulmonary air embolism. *Nitrogen narcosis* and *decompression sickness* result from the indirect effect of pressure changes in the body secondary to breathing gases at higher than normal atmospheric pressure. Problems may also be caused by breathing gases of elevated partial pressure (i.e., nitrogen narcosis and decompression sickness). As indicated for the specific

TABLE 47-1 Dysbarism Syndrome: Diagnostic Findings

	BAROTRAUMA				
	Otolaryngolic, Dental, Gastrointestinal	**Pulmonary Overpressurization Syndrome (POPS)**	**Dysbaric Air Embolism (DAE)**	**Nitrogen Narcosis**	**Decompression Sickness**
Ascent or descent	Both	Ascent	Ascent	Descent	Ascent
Onset	Variable	Before surfacing or at the surface	Within 10 min of surfacing	Variable depths	>10 min after surfacing
Diagnostic findings	Pain in the sinuses, ears, teeth, and abdomen; vertigo; flatulence; hearing impairment	Hoarseness, subcutaneous emphysema, dyspnea, cyanosis, neurologic deterioration, hemoptysis	Seizures, visual impairment, aphasia, altered mental status, multiplegia, hemoptysis, chest pain, cardiac arrest	Incoordination, altered mental status, obtundation	Pruritus, lymph node pain, joint pain, vertigo, deafness, paralysis, seizures, headache, respiratory failure, shock
Ancillary data	Electronystagmogram, audiogram	ABG, chest x-ray film	ABG, electrolytes, coagulation profile, chest x-ray film	None	ABG, electrolytes, coagulation profile, urinalysis, ECG, chest x-ray film
Differential diagnostic considerations	Otitis media, labyrinthitis, sinusitis, head trauma, gastroenteritis	Pulmonary contusion, head trauma, coagulopathy, pneumonitis, spontaneous pneumothorax	Cerebrovascular disease, coronary vascular disease, cerebral AVM or aneurysm, stroke due to cyanotic heart disease	Metabolic derangement drugs or ethanol intoxication, CNS hemorrhage or infection	Barotrauma, POPS, DAE, exhausion, dermatitis, muscle strain
Management:					
Admit	Variable	Yes	Yes	Immediate ascent	Yes
Oxygen	No	Yes	Yes	No	Yes
IV hydration	No		Yes	No	Yes
Recompression	No	Yes	Yes	No	Yes

From Smith KM: High altitude illness and dysbarism. In Barkin RM, editor: *Pediatric emergency medicine: concepts and clinical practice*, ed 2, St Louis, 1997, Mosby.

conditions listed in Table 47-1, decompression using a chamber may be required.*

Diving by pregnant women is associated with a higher incidence of low birth weight infants, prematurity, congenital malformations, stillbirths, and spontaneous abortions.

BIBLIOGRAPHY

American Academy of Pediatrics Council on Injury and Poison Prevention: Drowning in infants, children, and adolescents, *Pediatrics* 92:292, 1993.

Boltron M: Scuba diving and fetal well-being: a survey of 208 women, *Undersea Biomed Res* 7:183, 1989.

Graf WD, Cummings P, Quan L et al: Predicting outcome in pediatric submersion victims, *Ann Emerg Med* 26:312, 1995.

Habib DM, Tecklenburg FW, Webb SA et al: Prediction of childhood drowning and near drowning morbidity and mortality, *Pediatr Emerg Care* 12:255, 1996.

Harley JR, Ochsenschlager DW: Near drowning. In Barkin RM, editor: *Pediatric emergency medicine: concepts and clinical practice*, ed 2, St Louis, 1997, Mosby.

Kizer KW: Dysbaric cerebral air embolism in Hawaii, *Ann Emerg Med* 16:535, 1987.

Kyriacou DN, Arcinue EL, Peek C et al: Effect of immediate resuscitation of children with submersion injury, *Pediatrics* 94:133, 1994.

LaVelle JM, Shaw KN, Seidl T et al: Ten-year review of pediatric bathtub near-drownings: evaluation for child abuse and neglect, *Ann Emerg Med* 25:344, 1995.

Shupak A, Doweck I, Greenberg E et al: Diving-related inner ear injuries, *Laryngoscope* 101:173, 1991.

Spack L, Gebeit R, Splaingard M et al: Failure of aggressive therapy to alter outcome in pediatric near drowning, *Pediatr Emerg Care* 13:98, 1997.

Weinstein MD, Krieger BF: Near drowning: epidemiology, pathophysiology, and initial treatment, *J Emerg Med* 14:461, 1996.

Wintemute GJ: Childhood drowning and near-drowning in the United States, *Am J Dis Child* 144:663, 1990.

* Information about decompression chambers can be obtained from the Diver's Alert Network: telephone 919-684-8111.

48 Electrical and Lightning Injuries

ALERT Extent of burns does not reflect severity of injury.

Electrical injuries and lightning injuries have similar clinical presentations, both affecting the electrical charge of functional cells, particularly the conductive tissue of the nervous system and heart, and causing cell death by intense heat. The patient may have direct contact with electrical sources, such as high-tension wires or faulty wiring in a home, or may be struck by lightning. The injury reflects the resistance of the tissue, the path and type of current (alternating current [AC] is three times more dangerous than direct current [DC]), the voltage, and the duration of contact.

Lightning acts as a massive DC countershock, instantly depolarizing the myocardium and causing asystole, whereas ventricular fibrillation occurs with a high-voltage electrical current. Injury may be caused by a direct hit, by a charge jumping from object to object, or by ground current.

DIAGNOSTIC FINDINGS

The patient may have only minor burns or may undergo full cardiac respiratory arrest. Most patients have some evidence of burns. Electrical thermal burns, caused by energy transformation into heat as it passes through tissue, cause most of the damage. Tissues vary in electrical resistance, ranging from low to high as follows: nerves < vessels < muscles < skin < tendons < fat < bone.

1. Entry-exit burns: The entry wound is ischemic, with a well-circumscribed area of whitish yellow material and charred center. The exit wound is extensive, often with indistinct margins.
2. Arc burns, usually across joints: The current has struck the skin but not entered the body.
3. Flame burn, resulting in direct thermal injury, usually from ignition of clothing.
4. Lip burns: In children they may initially look innocuous but often involve the labial artery, possibly resulting in significant hemorrhage after some delay. Lip burn commonly results from a child's biting on an electrical cord.

Patterns of lightning injury are direct strike (flow of current internally to externally), contact (touching an object that is directly struck), side splash, ground and current, and blunt trauma.

The extent of the burns rarely reflects the potential severity of the injury.

Cardiac dysrhythmias and even infarction may occur. Lower voltages produce ventricular fibrillation; higher voltage may produce asystole.

Neurologic assessment in most patients shows impaired mental status, with associated paresthesias, headache, aphasia, and paralysis. Abnormalities of memory, mood, and affect may persist for months. There may be permanent damage.

Additional findings include the following:

1. Pulmonary contusion and chest pain
2. Retinal detachment and burns; cataracts (a delayed sequela)
3. Tinnitus, hearing loss, and perforated tympanic membranes
4. Rhabdomyolysis

5. Nonspecific abdominal pain, with nausea, vomiting, splenic rupture, intestinal perforation, stress ulcers, and pancreatitis (rarely noted)

Complications

Complications of electrical and lightning injuries include the following:

1. Cardiac respiratory arrest caused by central respiratory apnea, dysrhythmias, or cardiac ischemia leading to death. AC most commonly produces ventricular fibrillation.
2. Neurologic complications, such as amnesia, headache, sensorineural deafness, visual blurring, sensory complaints, confusion, motor findings (paraplegia or quadriplegia), cerebellar ataxia, and cerebral edema and intracranial hemorrhages with seizures. Some findings may be persistent.
3. Fractures, dislocations, cervical spine injury, and amputations secondary to falls, sustained muscle contraction, or direct cell death and neurovascular compromise.
4. Acute tubular necrosis resulting from crush injury and myoglobinuria or because of third spacing.
5. Complications related to extensive burns.
6. Vascular injury with thrombosis.
7. Adynamic ileus.
8. Trauma: AC causes muscle tetany, whereas DC produces a violent contraction, often throwing the patient.
9. Pregnancy: electrical and lightning injuries are associated with a 15% to 73% fetal mortality. Abruptio placentae is common.

Ancillary Data

1. Complete blood count (CBC) with elevated white blood cells (WBCs), platelet level.
2. Electrolytes to check on potassium level, which may be elevated.
3. Blood urea nitrogen (BUN) and creatinine levels.
4. Urinalysis (myoglobinuria or hemoglobinuria).
5. Cardiac enzymes. Peak creatine kinase (CK) reduces the amount of muscle injury and the extent of injury.
6. Arterial blood gas (ABG) analysis.
7. Electrocardiogram (ECG).
8. X-ray films:
   a. Chest, to check for pulmonary contusion, cardiac decompensation.
   b. Bones, cervical spine, and others as indicated.

MANAGEMENT

The key to outcome is the adequacy of prehospital care, which must involve the rapid removal of the individual from the source, the institution of appropriate resuscitation, and immobilization of the cervical spine.

Stabilization in the emergency department (ED) should focus on airway and cardiac status and ensure that the cervical spine is stable:

1. Oxygen, IV fluids, nasogastric (NG) tube, and urinary catheter as indicated.
2. ECG and cardiac monitoring. This should be prolonged if the patient has a dysrhythmia, loss of consciousness, significant injury, chest pain, or hypoxia. Cardiac monitoring is also indicated if the skin was wet at the time of injury or the current flowed across the heart region.
3. Fluid resuscitation must be given empirically on the basis of vital signs and urinary output. Patients with significant myoglobinuria require diuresis. Alkalinization (urine pH $\geq$7.45), achieved by using fluids with one ampule of $NaHCO_3$ per liter of infusate, increases the solubility of myoglobin in the urine.
4. Burn care should be initiated (see Chapter 46). Tetanus vaccine may be required.

Lip burns should not be debrided. Patients with lip burns should be observed for hemorrhage in the hospital for 3 to 4 days. Bleeding is controlled by pressure, with the area kept clean. Special feeding devices and splints may be needed to prevent microstomia. Patients are at risk for bleeding for 5 to 10 days after injury.

In cases of cerebral edema and seizures (p. 424), the following measures should be considered:

1. Hyperventilate to maintain $Paco_2$ at 35 mm Hg.
2. Elevate head of bed 30 degrees if possible.
3. Give furosemide (Lasix), 1 mg/kg/dose q4-6hr IV.
4. Give mannitol, 0.5 g/kg/dose q3-4hr prn IV, if patient has neurologic symptoms or seizures.
5. Control seizure initially with diazepam (Valium), 0.2 to 0.3 mg/kg/dose q2-5min prn IV. Initiate other anticonvulsants (see Chapter 21).

Other management techniques include the following:

1. Insertion of NG tube
2. Treatment of associated complications
3. Tetanus immunization, if indicated

DISPOSITION

All patients with a high-voltage injury (>1000 volts) or with any evidence of cardiac, pulmonary, gastrointestinal, or neurologic abnormalities should be hospitalized. Patients with lip burns or potential neurovascular compromise must be observed. Neurologic, ophthalmologic, otolaryngologic, and plastic surgery consultations may be useful in the management of the patient.

Asymptomatic patients may be discharged after they have been observed for a minimum of 4 hours and arrangements for follow-up have been made.

Pregnant patients should be referred for fetal monitoring.

Parental Education

1. Instruct your child about the dangers of electrical injury.
2. Eliminate your child's access to electrical plugs and wires.
3. In case of lightning, have your child stay indoors or seek shelter in a building away from windows and telephones. If there is no shelter, instruct your child to avoid the highest object in the area, hilltops, open spaces, metal clotheslines, and wire fences. Avoid contact with metal objects such as golf clubs. Remaining in a closed automobile may be protective. Lightning rods and streamer retardants may be useful.
4. If lightning does strike, initiate cardiopulmonary resuscitation (CPR) immediately, if necessary. If contact with an electrical source occurs, remove the patient from it without exposing yourself to potential injury.

BIBLIOGRAPHY

Bailey B, Guadreault P, Thirierge RL et al: Cardiac monitoring of children with household electrical injuries, *Ann Emerg Med* 25:612, 1995.

Baker MD, Chiaviello C: Household electrical injuries in children, *Am J Dis Child* 143:59, 1989.

Cherington M: Lightning injuries, *Ann Emerg Med* 25:516, 1995.

Epperly TD, Stewart JR: The physical effects of lightning injury, *J Fam Pract* 29:267, 1989.

Fish RM: Electrical injury, Part III: cardiac monitoring indications—the pregnant patient and lightning, *J Emerg Med* 18:181, 2000.

Hall ML, Sills RM: Electrical and lightning injuries. In Barkin RM, editor: *Pediatric emergency medicine: concepts and clinical practice*, ed 2, St Louis, 1997, Mosby.

49 High-Altitude Sickness

ADAM Z. BARKIN

ALERT Acute onset of fatigue, respiratory distress, headache, or confusion during adaptation to a high altitude requires intervention.

People often have difficulty making the physiologic adaptation to altitudes above 7500 ft (2500 m), particularly on the initial exposure to the low oxygen content of the air at that height. In up to 25% of cases, evidence of acute mountain sickness develops at 6000 ft, whereas 50% of nonacclimated people who ascend rapidly to 10,000 ft experience acute mountain sickness within 6 to 8 hours and respond well to conservative therapy. Most symptoms of hypoxia occur within 48 to 96 hours of arrival at high altitudes.

The adaptation to increasing altitude is inadequate when symptoms occur. People may have only self-limited fatigue and mild headaches. High-altitude illnesses are characterized by one of three typical clinical presentations (Table 49-1). The illness may be rapid in onset, may affect the young and healthy, and may be life threatening if not promptly recognized and treated.

Factors predisposing individuals to high-altitude sickness include the following:

1. Rapid ascent (airplane versus car versus walking)
2. Return of a high-altitude resident after a period of being at a lower altitude
3. Exercise
4. Preexisting infection
5. Preexisting pulmonary disease
6. Previous episodes

The underlying pathogenesis is a response to relative or absolute hypoxia.

High-altitude rétinal hemorrhage (HARH) is rare, occurring in 50% of climbers who ascend to 16,500 ft and 100% of those who ascend to 21,000 ft, usually within 2 to 3 days of arrival at these altitudes. HARH findings include increased dilation of the retinal veins and arteries, retinal hemorrhages, and papilledema without pain. The disease may be a warning sign of impending high-altitude pulmonary edema (HAPE). If visual changes occur, descent is recommended. Prevention is key, achieved by acclimatization.

Patients with sickle cell (SC) disease may be affected by the hypoxemia of altitudes above 5000 ft. Oxygen is recommended, even for air travelers who have SC disease.

Caution is usually advised for pregnant women from low altitudes who wish to travel above 13,000 ft and for pregnant women who reside at high altitudes for prolonged periods because of concerns of potential fetal growth retardation and hypoxemia.

Treatment for HAPE is descent to a lower altitude. Nifedipine may be useful, particularly when descent is not readily possible, because the agent reduces pulmonary artery pressure through its vasodilatory effect. The adult protocol that has been shown to be efficacious is 10 mg of nifedipine sublingually and 20 mg of slow-release nifedipine. If the systolic blood pressure does not drop more than 10 mm Hg within 10 minutes, the sub-

TABLE 49-1 High-Altitude Sickness

	Acute Mountain Sickness (AMS)	High-Altitude Pulmonary Edema (HAPE)	High-Altitude Cerebral Edema (HACE)
Diagnostic findings	Nausea, vomiting, headache, lethargy, sleep disturbance, tinnitus, vertigo	Shortness of breath, tachypnea, tachycardia, cough, variable cyanosis	Headache, mental confusion, delirium, ataxia, hallucination, seizure, focal neurologic signs, coma; long-term neurologic deficits
Onset	4-6 hr after reaching high altitude	24-96 hr	48-72 hr
Altitude	>8000 ft	8000-14,000 ft	Usually >12,000 ft
Ancillary data (in addition to those indicated for diagnostic evaluation)	ABG Chest x-ray study Electrolytes	ABG Chest x-ray study ECG Bleeding screen	ABG Electrolytes CT of head
Differential diagnostic considerations:			
Trauma	Concussion Gastroenteritis	Pulmonary confusion	Head Meningitis
Infection	Respiratory or CNS infection	Pneumonia	Encephalitis
Metabolic		Uremia	Diabetic ketoacidosis Uremia Encephalopathy ↑↓ Na^+, ↑ Ca^{++}
Intoxication	Salicylates	Multiple	Narcotics
Vascular		CHF	Subarachnoid hemorrhage
Management (all respond to descent):			
Admit	Variable	Yes	Yes
Oxygen	Yes	Yes	Yes
Acetazolamide	Prophylactic	Prophylactic	Prophylactic
Bronchodilator	No	Yes	No
Steroids	Controversial	Yes	Yes
Ventilation with PEEP	No	Yes, if severe	Hyperventilation

From Smith KM: High-altitude illness and dysbarism. In Barkin RM, editor: *Pediatric emergency medicine: concepts and clinical practice*, ed 2, St Louis, 1997, Mosby.

lingual dose is repeated after 15 minutes. Subsequently, 20 mg of slow-release nifedipine is administered every 6 hours for the period at high altitude. Furosemide is also beneficial but must be counterbalanced by the accompanying dehydration.

Dexamethasone has been demonstrated to prevent acute mountain sickness (AMS) as well as to decrease the symptoms of AMS once it is evolving. This agent is specifically recommended when descent is impossible or when it is necessary to facilitate cooperation in the evacuation process. Some patients have experienced a rapid onset of AMS after discontinuation of dexamethasone that was used for prophylactic purposes.

Prevention must be emphasized. Acclimatization is essential, with attention to the rate of ascent and initiation of a graded exercise program. Acetazolamide (Diamox) is useful in preventing high-altitude sickness (5-10 mg/kg/24 hr PO q12hr or in an adult either 250 mg q12hr PO or 500 mg in sustained-release form q24hr). It should be taken 1 to 2 days before ascent (it is not useful once illness has commenced) and should be continued during ascent. Dexamethasone (initially 8 mg PO followed by 4 mg q6hr PO for at least six doses) may reduce the incidence of AMS by 50% in those ascending to 10,000 ft or above. Prophylactic use of nebulized β-adrenergic agents may reduce the risk of pulmonary edema.

BIBLIOGRAPHY

Hackett PH, Roach RC: Medical therapy of altitude illness, *Ann Emerg Med* 16:980, 1987.

Levine BD, Yoshimura K, Kobayasizi J et al: Dexamethasone in the treatment of acute mountain sickness, *New Engl J Med* 321:1907, 1989.

Montgomery AB, Luce JM, Michael P et al: Effects of dexamethasone on the incidence of acute mountain sickness at two intermediate altitudes, *JAMA* 261:734, 1989.

Oelz O, Ritter M, Jenni R et al: Nifedipine for high altitude pulmonary edema, *Lancet* 867:1241, 1989.

Sartor C, Allemann Y, Duplain H et al: Salmeterol for prevention of high altitude pulmonary edema, *New Engl J Med* 346:1631, 2002.

Theis MK, Honigman B, Yip R et al: Acute mountain sickness in children at 2835 meters, *Am J Dis Child* 147:143, 1993.

Tso E: High-altitude illness, *Emerg Med Clin North Am* 10:231, 1992.

Yaron M, Waldman N, Neirmeyer S et al: The diagnosis of acute mountain sickness in pre-verbal children, *Arch Pediatr Adolesc Med* 152:683, 1998.

50 Hyperthermia

ALERT Prompt attention must be given to fluid management and cooling.

Exposure to environmental heat without appropriate acclimatization, equipment, or fluid replacement may lead to a variety of clinical presentations that are usually preventable. Particularly at risk are athletes, laborers, soldiers, the chronically ill, and the very young or old when the air temperature exceeds the skin temperature (Table 50-1).

Heat gain results from a combination of metabolic activity, environmental heat, and strenuous exercise. This is balanced by heat loss mechanisms: radiation, convection, conduction and evaporation.

Children acclimatize more slowly than adults to exercise in the heat. Youngsters have a greater surface area/mass ratio than adults and produce more metabolic heat per mass unit when walking or running. Sweating capacity is not as great in children as adults, nor is the ability to convey heat by blood from the body core to the periphery. Acclimatization is characterized by earlier onset of sweating as well as greater sweating volume accompanied by a decreased concentration of sodium in the sweat and urine.

HEAT CRAMPS

Etiology

Heat cramps are caused by sodium depletion from prolonged or excessive exercise, accompanied by profuse sweating, in an environment with high temperature and low humidity. Thirst is relieved by fluids that do not contain salt.

Diagnostic Findings

Patients are alert and oriented, with normal or slightly elevated temperatures. They experience severe cramps in those skeletal muscles subjected to intense exercise, most commonly the legs.

Ancillary Data. Low serum sodium level indicates heat cramps.

Differential Diagnosis

1. Intrapsychic: hyperventilation
2. Metabolic: hypokalemia
3. Trauma: black widow spider bite

Management

1. Hydration:
   a. If severe, 0.9% normal saline (NS) solution at 20 ml/kg/hr over 1 to 2 hours
   b. If mild, oral salt solution: 1 tsp NaCl (4 g) in 500 ml of water administered at same rate as in a
2. Rest

HEAT EXHAUSTION

Etiology

Heat exhaustion is caused by exposure to a high-temperature environment, with continuous sweating and lack of appropriate replenishment of water or salt.

Diagnostic Findings

Many individuals have a combination of the following:

1. *Water depletion:* inadequate water replacement (see Chapter 7 for hypernatremic

TABLE 50-1 Environmental Heat Illnesses: Clinical Presentation

Condition	Predisposing Cause	Central Nervous System	Skin	Muscle Cramps	Thirst	Rectal Temperature	Blood Pressure	Pulse	Management
Heat cramps	Muscle work, sodium depletion, drinking large quantities of water	WNL	Sweating	Severe	WNL	<40° C	WNL	WNL	Replace salt
Heat exhaustion	Heat exposure: (1) without access to water, (2) with replacement of sweat loss with water only	Fatigue, weakness, headache, anxiety	Sweating	Variable	Variable	<40° C	Tends to be low	Tends to be low	Replace salt or water
Heat stroke	Heat exposure, K^+-Na^+ depletion, impaired sweating, increased heat production	Headache, listlessness, confusion, seizure, psychosis, coma	Hot, dry	Variable	Abnormal	>40° C	Abnormal (high or low)	Elevated	Cooling and support

dehydration). Signs and symptoms of dehydration are thirst, irritability, fatigue, anxiety, and disorientation. Temperature is usually normal.

2. *Salt depletion:* inadequate salt replacement, the more common type of heat exhaustion. Signs and symptoms of salt depletion are fatigue, headache, nausea, vomiting, diarrhea, and muscle cramps. Temperature is normal or slightly increased. An acclimatized individual has a lower salt content of sweat.

Complications

1. Shock
2. Seizures and coma

Ancillary Data. Serum sodium level may be high (water depletion) or low (salt depletion).

Management

Necessary stabilization must be provided. Management must reflect the underlying cause. In patients with only modest elevations in body temperature, oral fluids and sprinkling water over the body to increase evaporative losses may be adequate. In severe disease with obtundation, intravenous administration of fluid should be initiated. If water depletion is accompanied by hypernatremic dehydration, fluid administration should be instituted slowly in accordance with the protocol in Chapter 7. In patients with salt depletion and isotonic or hypotonic dehydration:

- Initiate 20 ml/kg of 0.9% NS over 30 minutes; then follow protocol for dehydration (see Chapter 7).

Disposition

Patients with significant dehydration should be admitted for fluid management and monitoring. Those with no metabolic abnormalities and only mild symptoms may be discharged after initial fluid push.

Prevention requires the availability and intake of appropriate fluids.

HEAT STROKE

Etiology

In heat stroke, the body's heat dissipation system (sweating, radiation, and convection) has been overwhelmed by production and absorption of heat. Classic heat stroke occurs during periods of sustained high ambient temperatures and humidity, whereas exertional heat stroke accompanies strenuous exercise. Underlying conditions may contribute to this imbalance:

1. Trauma and physical:
   a. Environment: particularly in the newborn, who has immature thermoregulation and is more dependent on the environment
   b. Burns (see Chapter 46)
2. Congenital:
   a. Cystic fibrosis, from excessive sweating and salt loss
   b. Dermatologic: anhidrotic ectodermal dysplasia, ichthyosis
3. Intoxication (see Table 54-1):
   a. Decreased sweating: antihistamines, phenothiazines, anticholinergics, and cardiac β-blockers
   b. Increased heat production and impaired sweating: amphetamines, lysergic acid diethylamide (LSD), phencyclidine (PCP), and thyroid replacements
   c. Increased heat absorption: ethanol

Diagnostic Findings

Heat stroke may be caused by the following:

1. Exertion, which has a rapid course. Exertional heat stroke usually occurs in young, healthy patients.
2. A preexisting condition that has a slow onset (nonexertional).
3. Intoxication.

Symptoms include the following:

1. Anorexia, nausea, vomiting, headache, fatigue, and confusion or disorientation, possibly progressing to coma and posturing

2. Skin that is red, hot, and dry
3. High temperatures (>40°C), accompanied by tachycardia and hypotension

Complications

1. Coma with permanent neurologic sequelae
2. Acute tubular necrosis (p. 828)
3. Hypoglycemia, especially with exertional heat stroke
4. Acidosis
5. Dysrhythmias (see Chapter 6)
6. Rhabdomyolysis and myoglobinuria, particularly in patients with exertional heat stroke
7. Hepatic damage
8. Coagulopathy with disseminated intravascular coagulation (DIC) and thrombocytopenia (see Chapter 79); a mild coagulopathy is more common in classic heat stroke
9. Death

Ancillary Data

1. Arterial blood gas analysis. Changes in body temperature alter true values. For each degree greater than 37° C, the following physiologic changes are noted:

pH	↓0.015
$Pa{CO_2}$	↑4.4%
$Pa{O_2}$	↑7.2%

NOTE: The opposite adjustment is noted for each degree less than 37°C.

2. Electrolytes (hyperkalemia, hypokalemia, hyponatremia, hypernatremia), blood urea nitrogen (BUN) (increased), and glucose (hyperglycemia)
3. Complete blood count and platelet count
4. Electrocardiogram: ST depression, nonspecific T-wave changes, premature ventricular complex (PVC), supraventricular tachycardia
5. Bleeding and disseminated intravascular coagulation screen, if appropriate
6. Other studies to evaluate nature of underlying condition

Differential Diagnosis

1. Infection: meningitis or encephalitis; rickettsial disease: typhus, Rocky Mountain spotted fever; malaria
2. Endocrine: hypothalamic disorder

Management

Heat stroke is life threatening and requires rapid intervention. Initial stabilization in the field should include removing the patient from the heat and drenching or immersing the individual in cool water to enhance conductive heat loss. The airway should be stabilized, and oxygen administered. Circulatory status should be assessed, and intravenous fluids initiated. Patients require ongoing cardiac and rectal temperature probe monitoring.

Other management techniques include the following:

1. Iced water immersion (if unavailable, fan patient while sprinkling water or use ice packs to enhance evaporative cooling) until patient's body temperature reaches 38.5° C. Simultaneously massage extremities.
2. Intravenous fluids appropriate to the patient's electrolyte levels and fluid balance. Initially, give 0.9% NS at 20 ml/kg over 45 to 60 minutes. If cardiac status is unstable, insert a central venous line.
3. Foley catheter, with nasogastric tube to minimize aspiration.
4. Diazepam, 0.2 to 0.3 mg/kg/dose IV for treatment of shivering.

Disposition

All patients with heat stroke should be admitted to an intensive care unit (ICU).

Prevention includes ensuring adequate water and salt intake during heat exposure. The intensity of activities that last more than 30 minutes should be reduced when humidity and air temperature are relatively high. A warm-up period may be useful. Children should not be left unattended in automobiles.

Individuals with cystic fibrosis or a dermatologic problem should avoid prolonged exposure. Response to predisposing drugs should be monitored.

Runners in hot weather should drink 100 to 300 ml of water 10 to 15 minutes before a race and drink about 250 ml of water every 3 to 4 km. Fluid losses may exceed electrolyte abnormalities. Clothing should be lightweight; commercially available apparel is designed to facilitate activities in hot environments.

BIBLIOGRAPHY

Gentile DA, Kennedy BC: Wilderness medicine in children, *Pediatrics* 88:967, 1991.

Mellor MFA: Heat-induced illnesses. In Barkin RM, editor: *Pediatric emergency medicine: concepts and clinical practice,* ed 2, St Louis, 1997, Mosby.

Rek D, Olshaker JS: Heat illness, *Emerg Med Clin North Am* 10:299, 1992.

Robinson MD, Seward PN: Heat injury in children, *Pediatr Emerg Care* 3:114, 1987.

51 Hypothermia and Frostbite

ALERT Resuscitation must continue in the pulseless, apneic patient until the core temperature is at least 30° C.

Hypothermia exists when a patient's core temperature is 35° C or less. It results from prolonged exposure, conditions that secondarily contribute to hypothermia, or systemic diseases that interfere with thermoregulation.

Temperature control is a balance of heat loss and heat production. Loss is associated with heat flow from hot to cold by radiation or conduction, the latter including convection and evaporation. Heat dissipation results from blood flow, sweating, excretion of warm urine and feces, and exhalation of air. Voluntary muscle exercise, eating, and shivering produce heat.

Neonates are particularly at risk because of their relatively large surface area and small percentage of subcutaneous fat.

Progressive decrease in core temperature initially produces changes in basal metabolic rate, vasoconstriction, increased antidiuretic hormone (ADH), and impaired cerebral blood flow. Below 29° C, thermoregulation is lost; the loss is accompanied by vasodilation, impaired cardiac and central nervous system (CNS) function, slowed nerve conduction, and cardiac irritability. Eventually apnea and asystole become prominent.

ETIOLOGY (AND ASSOCIATED CONDITIONS)

1. Trauma/physical:
   - **a.** Exposure
   - **b.** Near-drowning (see Chapter 47)
   - **c.** Head or spinal cord injury (see Chapter 57)
   - **d.** Subdural hematoma (see Chapter 57)
2. Infection:
   - **a.** Bacterial meningitis (p. 741)
   - **b.** Encephalitis
   - **c.** Respiratory infection (p. 811)
   - **d.** Gram-negative septicemia
3. Endocrine and metabolic factors:
   - **a.** Hypoglycemia (see Chapter 38)
   - **b.** Diabetic ketoacidosis (p. 624)
   - **c.** Hypopituitarism
   - **d.** Myxedema (p. 631)
   - **e.** Addison's disease (see Chapter 74)
   - **f.** Uremia (p. 828)
4. Intoxication (see Table 54-1):
   - **a.** Alcohol
   - **b.** Barbiturates
   - **c.** Carbon monoxide
   - **d.** Narcotics
   - **e.** Phenothiazines
   - **f.** Anesthetics, general
   - **g.** Cyclic antidepressants
5. Degenerative or deficiencies:
   - **a.** CNS disease
   - **b.** Malnutrition and kwashiorkor
6. Vascular factors:
   - **a.** Shock (see Chapter 5)
   - **b.** Subarachnoid hemorrhage (see Chapter 18)
   - **c.** Pulmonary embolism (p. 578)
   - **d.** Cerebrovascular accident
7. Intrapsychic: anorexia nervosa
8. Neoplasm, intracranial

DIAGNOSTIC FINDINGS

The severity of the findings reflect the degree and duration of hypothermia and the nature of any underlying or predisposing condition. Special low-reading thermometers are required.

In general, the progression of signs and symptoms reflect the degree of hypothermia:

Core Temperature	Common Signs and Symptoms
35° C (95° F)	Slurred speech, lapse of memory, shivering maximum.
32° C (89° F)	Diminished mental status: drowsy, amnesic, confused, disoriented. Muscle rigidity, poor muscle coordination.
30° C (86° F)	Skin cyanotic, edematous. Stuporous, irritable. Progressive decline in basal metabolic state. Shivering stops. Myocardial irritability, bradycardia. J (or Osborne) waves on electrocardiogram (ECG), decreased cardiac output, and hypotension. Decreased minute ventilation.
28° C (82° F)	Dysrhythmias common. Bradycardia in up to 50% of cases, refractory to atropine with progression to ventricular fibrillation and asystole. This is the cardiac fibrillatory threshold at which ventricular fibrillation can be induced by cardiac stimulation.
26° C (79° F)	Loss of consciousness, areflexia.
25° C (77° F)	Respirations cease, dead appearance.

General Findings

1. Patients will initially have tachycardia, progressing to bradycardia associated with a decreased respiratory rate, tidal volume, and hypoxia at 30° C. Blood pressure declines with decreased cardiac output. On rewarming, patients may exhibit shock secondary to the initial vasodilation.
2. Myocardial irritability and impaired pacemaker function lead to atrial and ventricular dysrhythmias and bradycardia. Asystole and electromechanical dissociation (or pulseless electrical activity [PEA]) develop at 20° C.
3. Neurologic status progresses from slight ataxia, slurred speech, and hyperesthesias to frank coma. Recovery on warming may be slow. Progression is specific to the temperature level.
4. Body heat is partially maintained by shivering, which ceases somewhere between 30° and 33° C. Pallor and cyanosis are noted. Muscular rigidity develops.
5. Renal function is diminished with poor renal perfusion. Oliguria may be noted.
6. Pancreatitis appears and hepatic function decreases.
7. With profound hypothermia (often <25° C), the patient appears apneic, rigid, pulseless, areflexic, and unresponsive, with fixed, dilated pupils.
8. Infants with hypothermia have decreased feeding, lethargy, edema of the limbs, and cold, erythematous, and scleremic (hardened) skin. Bradycardia and abdominal distension may be observed. Metabolic acidosis, hypoglycemia, and hyperkalemia are usually present.

Complications

Frostbite

1. Ice crystallization in the cells is associated with vasoconstriction.
2. Fingers, hands, feet, toes, ears, and nose are the most common sites.
3. Severity of injury depends on temperature, duration of exposure, wind-chill factor, immobility, tightness of clothing, and dampness of environment.
4. Predisposing conditions include hypothermia, previous cold injury, dehydration, hypoxia, mechanical factors such as inadequate insulation, constricting or wet clothing, and immobility, environmental issues such as humidity, wind chill, low ambient temperature, and altitude, and

medical problems such as hypotension, sickle cell disease, and diabetes.

5. Classification:

Degree	Clinical Presentation
First	Skin is mottled, edematous, hyperemic, with burning and tingling. Peaks in 24 to 48 hours and may persist for 1 to 2 weeks.
Second	Blister formation with paresthesia and anesthesia.
Third (deep)	Necrosis of skin with ulceration and edema. Involves subcutaneous tissue.
Fourth (deep)	Necrosis with gangrene. Vesicle followed by eschar and ulceration. Progression over 24 to 36 hours. Demarcation may take several weeks.

6. The initial evaluation may be faulty because involvement is dynamic.

Other Complications

1. Metabolic abnormalities: metabolic acidosis, hypoglycemia, hyperkalemia
2. Gastrointestinal bleeding (see Chapter 35)
3. Acute renal failure (p. 828)
4. Pancreatitis (p. 654)
5. Hypovolemia secondary to shift of fluids into extracellular spaces
6. Sepsis
7. Dysrhythmias
8. Deep vein thrombosis (p. 578)
9. Coagulopathy, disseminated intravascular coagulation (DIC), thrombocytopenia, leukopenia (see Chapter 79)
10. Pulmonary edema (see Chapter 19)

Ancillary Data

1. Arterial blood gas analysis. Changes in body temperature alter values because cold blood buffers poorly. For each degree below 37° C, the following may be observed:

pH	↑0.015
P_{CO_2}(mm Hg)	↓4.4%
P_{O_2}(mm Hg)	↓7.2%

2. ECG: Dysrhythmias are noted with progression—for example, J (or Osborne) wave at about 30° C. It appears as a "camel-humped" deflection of the QRS-ST junction.
3. Chemical evaluation:
   a. Hyperkalemia secondary to metabolic acidosis, renal failure, or rhabdomyolysis. Hypokalemia may develop.
   b. Blood urea nitrogen (BUN) and creatinine levels increased.
   c. Increased amylase level.
   d. Glucose level increased when patient is cold and decreased during rewarming. Liver function test results elevated with hepatitis.
4. Hematologic evaluation:
   a. Hematocrit increases 2% for every 1° C fall in temperature.
   b. Possible coagulopathy with DIC.
   c. Thrombocytopenia and leukopenia secondary to sequestration; possible hemoconcentration.
5. Studies to assess status of underlying conditions.

MANAGEMENT

Initial management must stabilize the patient's condition and treat underlying conditions. In addition to standard resuscitation regimens, the patient should be moved to a warm environment and clothing should be removed. Handling of the patient should be minimized to avoid precipitating a dysrhythmia. Cardiac and rectal probe monitors are necessary. Hypoglycemia and hypoxia should be corrected with administration of oxygen, glucose, and warmed intravenous (IV) solutions. Underlying conditions need prompt attention. A low-reading thermometer is needed. Closed-chest compressions maintain neurologic viability in hypothermic patients hours longer than in normothermic patients. Prehospital misdiagnosis of cardiac arrest is a hazard.

Temperatures >32° C (Mild/Moderate Hypothermia)

1. Initiate passive external rewarming by warming the patient in blankets,

optimally in a warm room to maintain peripheral vasoconstrictors.

2. Attempt to raise the temperature 0.5° to 2° C/hr.
3. If no increase in temperature is seen in 2 hours, evaluate for underlying disease and initiate active rewarming.

Temperature <32° C (Moderate/Severe Hypothermia)

1. Begin active rewarming at 0.5° C/hr. Patient may experience rewarming shock during treatment (vasodilation may cause transient fall in blood pressure). Active rewarming is indicated in a number of specific circumstances:
   a. Cardiovascular instability
   b. Temperature less than 32° C
   c. Inadequate rate or failure of rewarming
   d. Endocrinologic insufficiency
   e. Hypothermia secondary to impaired thermoregulation
   f. Traumatic or toxicologic peripheral vasoconstriction
2. Monitor at all times. Handle patient carefully.
3. Avoid inserting intracardiac monitors and administering adrenergic drugs until the temperature is higher than 28° C, if possible. If necessary, preoxygenate patient before performing invasive procedures.
4. Administer oxygen, humidified and heated if possible. If intubation is required, preoxygenate well.

If the cardiovascular system is *stable,* active external rewarming is appropriate, with use of a radiant heater, warmed blankets, chemical hot packs, and heated objects (e.g., water bottle) applied primarily to the trunk. With temperature below 28° C, emergency intervention is needed.

If the cardiovascular system is *unstable,* the patient experiences diabetic ketoacidosis (insulin inactive at <30° C), endocrinologic insufficiency, peripheral vasodilation caused by trauma, ingestion, or spinal cord injury or external rewarming is ineffective, initiate active core rewarming, which may be used in conjunction with active external rewarming procedures. Techniques that may be used individually or in combination include the following:

1. Humidified oxygen delivered at about 40.5° C (105° F) to 42° C (107.6° F) by either mask or endotracheal tube.
2. Warmed (36° to 40° C) IV fluids: 5% dextrose in water (D5W) 0.9% normal saline (NS) without potassium is preferred.
3. Peritoneal dialysis using K^+-free dialysate heated to 40.5° to 42.5° C. Warmed lavage (gastric enema, bladder, pleural) fluid may be useful.
4. Hemodialysis and extracorporeal blood rewarming may be attempted if other approaches are unsuccessful. They are indicated in the unresponsive patient in cardiac arrest and in the stable patient without cardiac arrest who has concomitant significant drug overdose, infection, or trauma. The procedure should be continued until a core temperature of 30° to 32° C is achieved. It is logistically difficult and may produce complications, including bleeding.
5. To prevent overheating, active rewarming should generally be discontinued when the core temperature reaches 32° to 34° C.

Dysrhythmias

Lidocaine is effective in treatment of hypothermic ventricular dysrhythmias. Defibrillation is usually not effective at temperatures lower than 29.4° C (85° F). If ventricular fibrillation occurs at a temperature higher than 29.4° C, one attempt at defibrillation is warranted. If it fails, a single IV bolus of lidocaine may be useful. Bradycardia and atrial fibrillation usually revert with warming.

Frostbite

1. Primary attention must be directed at resuscitation.

2. Initial treatment in the field must include careful handling, with rewarming only if there is no chance of a second freezing during transport. Superficial first- and second-degree injuries of the hand may be treated in the field by holding the fingers in the armpits or blowing on them with hot air. Once warmed they should be covered with a dry, clean cloth. Stabilize core temperature.
3. Deep frostbite should be treated definitively by immersion of the extremity or part in tepid water (37° to 40° C that is monitored) for 20 minutes after core rewarming is well under way. A temperature higher than 42° C may cause additional injury. Protect the involved tissue from further damage. After warming, apply sterile gauze and elevate for 40 minutes. Elevate extremity after thawing.
4. Amputation of fourth-degree injuries must be delayed until there is good demarcation of necrotic tissue. Gentle debridement may be done.
5. Analgesics may be required. Handle involved area gently. Avoid friction massage.
6. Tetanus prophylaxis may be appropriate.

DISPOSITION

Patients with hypothermia require hospitalization, and those with core temperatures less than 32° C should be admitted to an intensive care unit (ICU). The best predictors of outcome are the underlying disease and the response to therapy. Patients with only superficial frostbite may be sent home.

Patients should be informed about the importance of appropriate clothing. Layering allows air trapping (air is an effective insulator), which reduces heat loss by conduction and convection. Wicking facilitates movement of sweat from the surface of the skin to outer layers of clothing. Garments should be nonconstricting and should provide special protection of hands, face, and feet.

BIBLIOGRAPHY

Cornelli HM: Accidental hypothermia, *J Pediatr* 120:671, 1992.

Danzl DF, Pozos RS: Accidental hypothermia, *N Engl J Med* 331:1756, 1994.

Dobson JAR, Burgess JJ: Resuscitation of severe hypothermia by extracorporeal rewarming in a child, *J Trauma* 40:483, 1996.

Heggers JP, Phillips LG, McCauley RL et al: Frostbite: experimental and clinical evolutions of treatment, *J Wilderness Med* 1:27, 1990.

Hofstrand HT: Accidental hypothermia and frostbite. In Barkin RM, editor: *Pediatric emergency medicine: concepts and clinical practice,* ed 2, St Louis, 1997, Mosby.

Jolly BT, Ghezzi KT: Accidental hypothermia, *Emerg Med Clin North Am* 10:311, 1992.

Lazar HL: The treatment of hypothermia, *N Engl J Med* 337:1545, 1997.

McAdams TR, Swenson DR, Miller AR: Frostbite: an orthopedic perspective, *Am J Orthop* 28:21, 1999.

Weinberg AD: Hypothermia, *Ann Emerg Med* 22:374, 1993.

52 Radiation Injuries

Radiation injuries most commonly result from transportation, nuclear facility, or industrial accidents. Enhanced concern exists with the potential utilization of weapons of mass destruction. Ionizing radiation may consist of alpha (noninjurious), beta (minimal surface injury), or gamma (penetrates deeply, causing acute radiation injury) exposure.

Radiation leads to ionization, release of free radicals from water, and breakage of DNA or RNA strands. Injury depends on the amount of body surface exposed, the duration of exposure, the distance from the source, the type of radiation, and shielding techniques. The dose of whole-body ionizing radiation that kills 50% of those exposed to it is 4.5 gray (Gy) (1 Gy is equivalent to 1 joule of radiation absorbed per kilogram of tissue).

The normal background annual radiation exposure is 110 mrem/year. A chest radiogram has about 10 mrem/study.

The clinical presentation is delineated in relation to dose in Table 52-1. It reflects the type and amount of radiation, length of exposure, distance of source to victim, amount and type of shields, and continuous nature of exposure. In general, the higher the dose of exposure, the earlier symptoms develop. Organs with higher cell division rates are more sensitive, so the hematopoietic and gastrointestinal systems are most affected; the central nervous system is most resistant.

The best predictor of survival is the absolute lymphocyte count at 48 hours after radiation exposure (>1200 cells/mm^3: good prognosis; 1200-300 cells/mm^3: moderate prognosis; <300 cells/mm^3: poor prognosis).

From the perspective of the receiving hospital, the following steps should be taken:

1. Advance notification of arrival should be received.
2. Treatment areas, with specific entrance, should be designated.

TABLE 52-1 Radiation Dose-Effect Relationship

Whole Body Radiation Dose (Gy)	Clinical Manifestations
<1.5	Asymptomatic or mild symptoms (anorexia, nausea, vomiting) Mild depression of white cells and platelets
4	Mild nausea and vomiting Hematologic change with lymphocyte depression within 48 hr
4–6	Serious symptoms: nausea, vomiting, diarrhea, bleeding, infection Hematologic depression of about 75% within 48 hr Mortality >50%
6–15	Severe nausea, vomiting, diarrhea, progressing to coma Severe hematologic changes Mortality up to 100%
>20	Fulminant course with GI, cardiovascular, and CNS complications Death within 48 hr

3. Personnel should wear operating room attire with gloves.
4. Life-saving measures should be performed first.
5. Contamination should be defined with radiation detectors.
6. Patient should be washed with washcloths, soap, and water.
7. After the patient's condition is medically stable, exposure should be evaluated:
   a. External contamination: Clothing should be removed with proper disposal. Swabs of orifices should be obtained for sampling and the patient washed with warm water and soap. Eyes and open wounds should be irrigated. All wastewater must be collected and placed in appropriate containers.
   b. Internal contamination: Prevent absorption and increase elimination. Gastric lavage is followed by administration of antacids to precipitate heavy metals. Chelation may be useful.
   c. Partial body exposure, whereby part of the body receives a large dose of radiation.
   d. Acute radiation syndrome (ARS).
8. Expert medical consultation is usually necessary to assist in management. Such resources are readily available from local, state, and federal agencies. Routine steps for symptomatic patients with significant exposure include isolation; fluids; bowel sterilization with antibiotics; infusions of red blood cells (RBCs), platelets, and granulocytes; and infection control and monitoring.

BIBLIOGRAPHY

Asch SM, Cosimi L: Radiation exposures. In Barkin RM, editor: *Pediatric emergency medicine: concepts and clinical practice*, ed 2, St Louis, 1997, Mosby.

Mettler FA, Voelz GZ: Major radiation exposure: what to expect and how to respond, *New Engl J Med* 346:1554, 2002.

Vyas DR, Dick RM, Crawford J: Management of radiation accident and exposure, *Pediatr Emerg Care* 10:232, 1994.

53 Smoke Inhalation

Also See Chapter 46 (Burns, thermal)

ALERT Airway stabilization is imperative.

Smoke inhalation most commonly accompanies major burns and is considered to be the major respiratory complication of thermal burns (see Chapter 46). Several factors affect toxicity:

1. Heat of gases. Inhalation of heated gas at 150° C may result in injuries to the face, nasal mucosa, oropharynx, and upper airway. Adding moisture to the air increases injury to the upper airway. Air is rapidly cooled after reaching the vocal cords.
2. Particulate matter. Particulate matter deposition with adsorbed toxins may lead to chemical injury, tracheobronchitis, and pulmonary edema.
3. Toxic gases. Most common is carbon monoxide (CO). Others are hydrogen cyanide, aldehydes, ammonia, chlorine, and hydrochloric acid.

ETIOLOGY

1. Direct thermal injury to respiratory tract, often associated with flame burns in a closed room:
   - **a.** Major burns
   - **b.** Nasopharyngeal—circumoral burns:
     - **(1)** Singed nasal hairs
     - **(2)** Singed eyelids and eyebrows
2. Inhalation of toxins, often secondary to noxious fumes that may be the products of combustion:
   - **a.** Acetic acid (petroleum products)
   - **b.** Formic acid or aldehydes (wood, cotton, paper, petroleum products)
   - **c.** Chlorine (polyvinyl chloride)
   - **d.** Hydrochloric acid or HCN (hydrocyanic acid) (plastics)
3. CO poisoning
4. Hypoxia, usually secondary to closed-space fire

DIAGNOSTIC FINDINGS

1. Patients usually demonstrate thermal burns (see Chapter 46) and may have evidence of CO poisoning (p. 376).
2. Patients demonstrate evidence of direct thermal damage to the upper respiratory tract (which may be delayed up to 24 hours), for example, stridor, hoarseness, and black or brown carbonaceous sputum.
3. Lower airway findings reflect the irritant effects of noxious gases and particulate matter, alveolar-capillary membrane damage, and, ultimately, pulmonary edema/infiltrates from impaired mucociliary transport, diminished surfactant production, and macrophage dysfunction.
4. Concurrently, patients may have CO poisoning, hypoxia, and upper airway obstruction. The relative hypoxia may cause confusion and agitation; rare cases progress to coma.

Complications

1. Upper airway obstruction, secondary to mucosal injury, similar to croup

2. Pulmonary edema (see Chapter 19), usually developing 1 to 4 days after injury: dyspnea, cough, wheezing, rales, and respiratory distress may be noted
3. Bacterial pneumonia about 1 week after injury

Ancillary Data

All patients require arterial blood gas (ABG) analysis, carboxyhemoglobin measurement, and chest x-ray film.

DIFFERENTIAL DIAGNOSIS

See Chapters 19 and 20.

MANAGEMENT

Humidified oxygen should be administered to all patients. This is appropriate treatment for CO poisoning (p. 376) and direct respiratory tract injury.

1. Manage airway:
   a. If the patient's airway is compromised, intubate and initiate active control. Positive end-expiratory pressure (PEEP) and constant positive airway pressure (CPAP) improve oxygen exchange in the lungs. Indications include the following:
      (1) Respiratory failure (Pao_2 <50 mm Hg and $Paco_2$ >50 mm Hg)
      (2) Severe acidosis
      (3) Laryngeal obstruction
      (4) Difficulty with secretions
2. If bronchospasm is present, useful bronchodilators include inhaled β agonists (see Chapter 84).
3. Early bronchoscopy is indicated for significant secretions or direct evaluation of injury when pulmonary lesion is suspected.
4. Consider hyperbaric oxygen if necessary for markedly elevated carboxyhemoglobin (p. 376). More aggressive approach is required in pregnant females because of potential risk to the fetus.
5. Manage associated burn, if present (see Chapter 46).
6. Corticosteroids, which increase the mortality rate, are not indicated.

DISPOSITION

All patients with the following findings should be hospitalized:

1. Respiratory failure
2. Carboxyhemoglobin level elevation requiring admission (p. 376)
3. High-risk category: major and most moderate burns, as well as facial or nasal burn
4. Upper airway signs of involvement (hoarseness, stridor)
5. Lower airway involvement (bronchospasm, dyspnea)

Patients with none of these factors may be discharged if follow-up care and observation can be ensured and there is no question of child abuse. Parents must watch for any changes in respiratory status.

Parental Education

1. Call your physician immediately if any of the following develops:
   a. Increasing difficulty in breathing
   b. Hoarseness, stridor, cough, or wheezing
   c. Lethargy, agitation, or other behavioral changes
   d. Fever
2. Read information about fire prevention.

BIBLIOGRAPHY

Baud FJ, Barriot P, Toffis V et al: Elevated blood cyanide concentrations in victims of smoke inhalation, *N Engl J Med* 325:1761, 1991.

Lee MJ, O'Connell DJ: The plain chest radiograph after acute smoke inhalation, *Clin Radiol* 39:33, 1988.

Parish RA: Smoke inhalation and carbon monoxide poisoning in children, *Pediatr Emerg Care* 2:36, 1986.

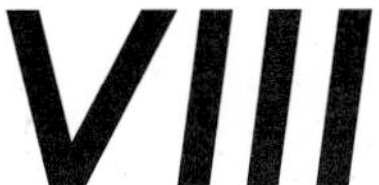

Poisoning and Overdose

KENNETH W. KULIG

54 Management Principles

Poisoning is a significant cause of morbidity and mortality in the United States; it is the fourth most common cause of death in children. Approximately 80% of accidental ingestions occur in children younger than 5 years, the peak incidence being between 1 and 3 years. In children younger than 1 year, poisoning usually results from therapeutic misuse of drugs. The preschooler is adventuresome and curious and ingests any accessible household product or medication. The adolescent may experiment with mind-altering drugs, often with peers; manipulative behavior and suicide become important motivators. Family turmoil is commonly present, and the poisoning tends to be recurrent.

Children younger than 6 years ingest a wide variety of substances, most commonly involving cosmetics, cleaning substances, analgesics, plants, cough and cold preparations, foreign bodies, topicals, pesticides, antimicrobials, vitamins, gastrointestinal (GI) preparations, arts, crafts, or office supplies, hydrocarbons, hormones, and food products. The most significant exposures commonly involve salicylates, alkaline corrosives, acetaminophen, iron, petroleum products, antihistamines, cardiac medications, street drugs, alcohols, cyclic antidepressants, benzodiazepines, barbiturates, pesticides, carbon monoxide, and opiates. Of childhood poisonings, 87% occur in the home. The volume of a normal swallow in an infant is about 0.21 ml/kg, 1 teaspoon (4.5 to 5 ml) in a child 18 to 36 months old, and 15 ml in an adult.

There is some controversy regarding the most effective means of gastric decontamination, and this is often patient specific. A number of distinguished toxicology organizations have issued joint position statements on these modalities:

1. Syrup of ipecac: There is insufficient data to support or exclude administration *immediately* after poisoning. Probably of no value in the emergency department (ED).
2. Gastric lavage: considered in patients with potentially life-threatening ingestions if undertaken within 60 minutes of ingestion. This is rarely additive to activated charcoal *alone* but might be useful in:
   - **a.** Significantly symptomatic patients presenting in the first hour after ingestion.
   - **b.** Symptomatic patients who have ingested agents that slow GI motility.
   - **c.** Patients ingesting sustained-release medications.
   - **d.** Patients taking massive or clearly life-threatening amounts of medication.
3. Activated charcoal alone: Most toxicologists would recommend charcoal alone if GI decontamination is thought to be of benefit. It is quicker to act, has less morbidity, and is more likely to be of benefit, than either syrup of ipecac or gastric lavage.

INITIAL CONTACT WITH THE POISONED PATIENT

1. Determine that the ABCs (airway, breathing, and circulation) are being maintained.
2. *Basic information* is essential. Obtain name, weight, and age. Address and

telephone number provide a means for later contact.

3. Determine the *type of ingestion.* Define the product name, exact ingredients, amount consumed, and any current symptoms. The amount taken relative to the patient's weight is often useful. If any question exists about the medication, ask for a prescription number, the dispensing pharmacy, or the prescribing physician. Always request that the product be brought to the ED if the patient gets there. The history is often inaccurate.
4. Determine *when ingestion occurred.*
5. Are there any other possible poisoning victims in the home?

INITIATION OF THERAPY AT HOME

Many accidental ingestions may be treated at home without an ED visit if the substance or the amount ingested is nontoxic (Box 54-1) or relatively so, or if the amount ingested is unlikely to cause symptoms.

1. Be certain to cover the areas of poison prevention. Dangerous substances that are often found in the household include medications, dishwasher soap and cleaning supplies, drain-cleaning crystals or

Box 54-1

LOW-TOXICITY INGESTIONS*

Abrasives
Adhesives
Antacids
Antibiotics
Baby product cosmetics
Ballpoint pen inks
Bathtub floating toys
Birth control pills
Calamine lotion
Candles (beeswax or paraffin)
Chalk (calcium carbonate)
Clay (modeling or Play Doh)
Corticosteroids
Cosmetics (most, except perfumes)
Crayons marked AP or CP
Dehumidifying packets (silica)
Deodorants and deodorizers
Etch-A-Sketch
Fabric softener
Fish bowl additives
Glues and pastes
Greases
Gums
Hair products (dyes, sprays, tonics)
Hand lotions and creams
Ink (black, blue, indelible, felt-tip markers)
Kaolin
Lanolin
Linoleic acid
Linseed oil
Lipstick
Lubricants and lubricating oils
Newspapers
Paint (indoor and latex)
Pencil (graphite)
Petroleum jelly (Vaseline)
Polaroid picture coating fluid
Putty (<2 oz)
Sachets (essential oils, powder)
Shampoos and soap (bubble baths, soap bar)
Shoe polish (not containing aniline dyes)
Spackle
Suntan preparations
Sweetening agents (saccharin, cyclamate)
Teething rings
Thermometers (mercury)
Toothpaste (without fluoride)
Vitamins without iron
Zinc oxide

* These materials generally do not produce significant toxicity except possibly in very large doses. Substances such as cologne, after-shave lotion, deodorant, fabric softeners, and oral contraceptives may be toxic in large amounts. Toxicity is altered if the patient is pregnant or has an underlying disease.

liquids, paints and thinners, automobile products, and garden sprays.

2. Regional poison control centers provide an effective means of disseminating information, providing medical consultation, and arranging for follow-up. Unnecessary hospital visits may therefore be eliminated.
3. If specific social problems are noted, referral is made to a public health nurse. Any child in whom nonaccidental ingestion or potential child abuse is suspected must be seen in a health care facility despite the seemingly benign nature of the exposure.

Prevention of Absorption

Techniques to prevent further absorption can and should be initiated before the patient arrives at the ED.

1. External:
   a. Skin exposed to insecticides (organophosphates or carbamates), hydrocarbons, medications designed to be well absorbed transdermally, or acidic or alkaline agents should be flooded with water and washed well with soap and a soft washcloth or sponge. Remove clothing.
   b. Eyes must be irrigated immediately, before any transport or other therapy is discussed. Have the patient hold head under the sink or shower, or pour water into the eye from a pitcher or glass. Irrigation should be continued for a steady 15 to 20 minutes.
2. Internal:
   a. Dilute any acidic or alkaline ingestions with milk or water; do not induce emesis.
   b. *Activated charcoal* has been used more extensively, usually in a dose of 15 to 50 g orally. This is usually done after consultation with a poison control center. Sixty percent of children between the ages of 8 months and 5 years in one study drank the entire recommended dose. Palatability is greater when the charcoal is mixed with a cola drink. This approach is probably more efficacious than inducing emesis.
   c. If advised by the regional poison control center, induce emesis with *syrup of ipecac* in children older than 6 months, particularly if it can be administered *immediately after the ingestion*. Do not use for children younger than 6 months. Give 10 ml (child younger than 1 year); 15 ml (child 1 to 12 years); or 30 ml (child older than 12 years), followed by 15 ml/kg of fluid (up to 250 ml or 8 oz of water). Do not use milk or heavily sugared liquids. Ambulate the patient and wait for vomiting, which usually occurs in the next 20 minutes. Pharyngeal stimulation may be useful. If the patient does not vomit, repeat dose in 20 minutes in children older than 12 months.

      The shelf life of syrup of ipecac is probably longer than indicated by the expiration date.

      NOTE: Induction of emesis is contraindicated in the home setting if any of the following conditions exists:

      (1) Patient is comatose, stuporous, or seizing, has no gag reflex, is younger than 6 months, or has a bleeding diathesis.
      (2) Ingestion involves acidic or alkaline substances (p. 372).
      (3) Ingestion involves hydrocarbons that contain *c*amphor, *h*alogenated or *a*romatic products, heavy *m*etals, or *p*esticides ("CHAMP") (p. 385).
      (4) Ingestion involves a rapid-acting central nervous system (CNS) depressant or convulsant.

Transport to Hospital

All patients who require evaluation or treatment should be transported. The ED to receive the patient should be notified and given information about the treatment plan initiated and the means of transport. The parent or patient should be reminded to bring the ingested material for identification.

Other Considerations

If a potentially toxic ingestion is treated at home, arrangements should be made for the patient to be contacted with a return phone call. Asking the older patient to make a follow-up phone call is risky because of the possibility of the patient's becoming obtunded or confused. Poison control centers can often facilitate this follow-up. All suicidal patients must be sent to a health care facility.

Records of all poison calls should be kept, including basic information, the type of ingestion, and therapy initiated.

Treatment information is available from multiple sources. *Poisindex* is a comprehensive information system available on microfiche or computer in many EDs. Poison control centers are a further source of data and management advice.

MANAGEMENT IN THE EMERGENCY DEPARTMENT

Stabilization and assessment are required of these potentially critically ill patients. Often an associated ingestion may change the clinical presentation and treatment plan. Dilution of acidic and alkaline ingestions with milk or water is of immediate priority, even before the patient arrives in the ED. Patients usually fast (NPO status) after the initial evaluation.

Cardiopulmonary Status

1. Ensure that airway, ventilation, and circulation are adequate.
2. Establish intravenous (IV) lines in potentially serious ingestions.
3. In any patient with altered mental status, seizures, or coma, simultaneously administer the following:
   - **a.** Oxygen at 4 to 6 L/min
   - **b.** Dextrose, 0.5 to 1 g (1-2 ml 50% dextrose in water [D50W]) per kg per dose IV, or STAT documentation of a normal blood glucose level
   - **c.** Naloxone (Narcan), 0.1 mg/kg/dose up to 2 mg IV

Other Considerations

1. Focus the physical examination on the cardiopulmonary and neurologic status. A specific toxic syndrome may be identified.
2. Start cardiac monitoring and perform an electrocardiogram (ECG) if the ingested drug or chemical might precipitate dysrhythmias.
3. Evaluate electrolyte levels and acid-base status.

Toxicologic Screen. Blood analysis provides quantitative levels of specific drugs. Urine toxicology screening can yield rapid qualitative information about the presence of certain drug classes but does not provide quantitation.

Agents requiring emergency quantitative laboratory analysis include acetaminophen, salicylates, alcohols (methanol, ethylene glycol), iron, theophylline, lithium, and carbon monoxide.

The timing of drug concentration determinations may be complicated by the ingestion of large amounts; absorption may be prolonged. Modified-release agents may also delay and prolong toxicity.

The toxicology laboratory alone should not be relied on to make the diagnosis. Patient history and physical examination are far more important and timely (Tables 54-1 and 54-2).

1. Always let the laboratory personnel know what drugs are suspected.
2. Because a negative toxicologic screen result does not exclude a drug overdose, knowing which drugs the laboratory has screened for in its analysis is a must.

Prevention of Absorption

1. External:
   - **a.** Skin—as described on p. 353.

TABLE 54-1 Clues to Diagnosis of Unknown Poison: Vital-Sign Changes

DYSRHYTHMIAS	**CYANOSIS** (secondary to methemoglobinemia; does not respond to oxygen)
Anticholinergics	Anesthetics, local
β-Blockers (e.g., propranolol)	Aniline dyes
Carbon monoxide	Chlorates
Cardiovascular drugs	Dapsone
Chloral hydrate	Hydrazines
Cyclic antidepressants (CADs)	Naphthalene
Digitalis	Nitrates
Halogenated solvents	Nitrites
Hypo/hyperkalemia	Nitroglycerine
Lithium	Nitroprusside
Phenothiazines	Phenacetin
Propoxyphene	Pyridium
Quinidine	Sulfonamides
Sympathomimetics (e.g., cocaine)	
Theophylline	
Thioridazine	

Increased	Decreased
BLOOD PRESSURE	
Amphetamines	Antidepressants
Anticholinergics (antihistamines, CADs)	Antihypertensives
Black widow envenomation	Antipsychotics
Sympathomimetics (phencyclidine, lysergic acid diethylamide, caffeine, cocaine, theophylline)	Cyanide
	Narcotics
	Sedatives/hypnotics (see Table 54-2, Coma)
HEART RATE	
Alcohol	Barbiturates
Anticholinergics	β-Blockers
Hallucinogens	Calcium channel blockers
Organophosphates	Cholinergics
Sympathomimetics (e.g., caffeine, amphetamines, cocaine)	Digitalis
Theophylline	Narcotics
	Organophosphates
	Sedatives/hypnotics
RESPIRATORY RATE	
Amphetamines	Alcohols (ethanol, isopropyl, methanol)
Anticholinergics	Barbiturates
Cocaine	Central nervous system depressants
Hydrocarbons	Narcotics
Nicotine	Sedatives/hypnotics
Organophosphates	
Secondary to metabolic acidosis ("MUDPILES") (p. 369)	

Continued

TABLE 54-1 Clues to Diagnosis of Unknown Poison: Vital-Sign Changes—cont'd

RESPIRATORY RATE—cont'd

Secondary to noncardiogenic pulmonary edema:

- Carbon monoxide
- Hydrocarbons
- Narcotics
- Organophosphates
- Salicylates
- Sedatives/hypnotics

TEMPERATURE

Anticholinergics	Alcohol (ethanol)
Atropine	Anesthetic, general
β-Blockers	Barbiturates
Calcium channel blockers	β-Blockers
Cyclic antidepressants	Carbon monoxide
Monoamine oxidase inhibitors	Clonidine
Pentachlorophenol	Cyclic antidepressants
Phencyclidine	Narcotics
Phenothiazines	Organophosphates
Salicylates	Phenothiazines
Selective serotonin reuptake inhibitors	Sedatives/hypnotics
Strychnine	
Sympathomimetics (e.g., cocaine, amphetamines)	

TABLE 54-2 Clues to Diagnosis of Unknown Poison: Neurologic Alterations

	FINDINGS ASSOCIATED WITH COMA		
	Seizures, Myoclonus, Hyperreflexia	**Hyporeflexia, Hypotension**	**Pulmonary Edema, Hypotension**
COMA			
Amphetamines	+		
Anticholinergics	+		
Barbiturates		+	+
Benzodiazepines		+	
Carbamazepine	+		
Carbon monoxide	+		
Chloral hydrate		+	
Cocaine	+		
Cyclic antidepressants	+		
Ethanol, isopropyl		+	+
Haloperidol	+		
Narcotics		+	+
Phencyclidine (PCP)	+		
Phenothiazines	+		
Phenytoin	+		
Salicylates			+
Sedatives/hypnotics			+

TABLE 54-2 Clues to Diagnosis of Unknown Poison: Neurologic Alterations—cont'd

SEIZURES ("CAP")

Camphor	Aminophylline	*Pesticides (organophosphates)*
Carbon monoxide	Amphetamines and sympathomimetics	*Phencyclidine (PCP)*
Cocaine	Anticholinergics	*Phenol*
Cyanide	Aspirin	*Propoxyphene*

Also lead, isoniazid, drug withdrawal, carbamazepine (Tegretol), lithium, strychnine, cyclic antidepressants, sympathomimetics, organophosphates, GHB, MOMA

BEHAVIOR DISORDERS

Toxic psychosis: hallucinogens (lysergic acid diethylamide [LSD], phencyclidine [PCP]), sympathomimetics (cocaine, amphetamines), anticholinergics, heavy metals, drug withdrawal, monoamine oxidase inhibitors, androgenic steroids

Paranoid, violent reactions: phencyclidine

Depression, paranoid hallucinations, emotional lability: sympathomimetics (cocaine, amphetamines)

Hallucinations, delirium, anxiety: anticholinergics, hallucinogens

MOVEMENT DISORDERS

Choreoathetosis, orofacial dyskinesis, nystagmus, ataxia: phenytoin

Extrapyramidal: anticholinergics, phenothiazines, haloperidol

Choreoathetoid movements: cyclic antidepressants, carbamazepine

Ataxia, choreiform movements: heavy metals

Ataxia, tremors: lithium

Nystagmus: "SALEMTIP" (*s*edative, *a*lcohol, *l*ithium, *e*thanol/ethylene glycol, *m*ethanol, *t*hiamine depletion/Tegretol, *i*sopropanol, *p*hencyclidine/phenytoin/primidone)

PUPILS

Pinpoint (miosis)	**Dilated** (mydriasis)
Barbiturates (late)	Alcohol
Cholinergics	Anticholinergics
Clonidine	Antihistamines
Narcotics (except meperidine)	Barbiturates
Organophosphates	Meperidine
	Phenytoin
	Sympathomimetics (e.g., amphetamines, cocaine, ephedrine, LSD, PCP)

b. Ocular exposures, particularly to caustic agents, require immediate irrigation before examination. Each eye should be washed with a minimum of 1 L of saline solution; eversion of the eyelids and cleaning of the fornices increases effectiveness.

2. Internal:

a. *Activated charcoal* can be given without a prior gastric emptying procedure (syrup of ipecac or lavage). Its palatability may be improved by mixing with a cola drink. As noted previously, there is little adjunctive value to gastric emptying except in specific circumstances. In patients who have undergone lavage, charcoal can be administered through the tube. A 12 to 16 Fr nasogastric tube may be inserted to facilitate administration if a patient is unable to take the charcoal orally. Clinical or radiographic verification of tube placement in the stomach is mandatory to prevent administration of charcoal in the lungs. Data would indicate that the administration of activated charcoal to intubated patients with overdose is associated with a low incidence of aspiration pneumonia.

Commonly, 1 g of activated charcoal per kg body weight is the dose. Adults usually receive 50 to 100 g, and children 15 to 50 g, orally. The agent can be mixed in 35% to 70% sorbitol for children older than 1 year to allow simultaneous administration of a cathartic.

The efficacy of activated charcoal is greatest when it is given early, usually within 1 hour of ingestion. Ingested substances that reduce gastric motility (i.e., anticholinergic agents) may continue to be absorbed up to 12 to 24 hours after ingestion and are usually treated with activated charcoal as well as more specific measures.

Most drugs are absorbed by activated charcoal:

(1) Analgesic/antiinflammatory agents: acetaminophen, salicylates, nonsteroidals, morphine, propoxyphene

(2) Anticonvulsants and sedatives: barbiturates, carbamazepine, chlordiazepoxide, diazepam, phenytoin, sodium valproate

(3) Other: amphetamines, atropine, chlorpheniramine, cocaine, digitalis, quinine, theophylline, cyclic antidepressants

Drugs that are NOT absorbed by activated charcoal include: caustics, corrosives, lithium, iron, ethanol, borates, bromide, potassium.

Multiple-dose activated charcoal (adult: 20-50 g q2-4hr PO; child: 1 g/kg/dose q2-4hr PO) increases the clearance of carbamazepine, meprobamate, phenobarbital, phenytoin, salicylates, theophylline, and other substances. Do not mix charcoal with a cathartic (including sorbitol) after the first dose in multiple-dose charcoal regimen.

b. *Lavage:*

(1) Indicated for patients who have ingested a potentially toxic substance, are seen within 1 to 2 hours of ingestion, and are seizing, comatose, or uncooperative or have lost their gag reflex. The procedure also facilitates later administration of activated charcoal and cathartics.

(2) Contraindicated for caustic or acid ingestions.

(3) A 24 to 36 Fr tube (36 to 40 Fr in adults) inserted orally with the patient tilted slightly to the left side in Trendelenburg's position, ideally in the left lateral decubitus position. Saline or half-normal saline solution at 200 to 300 ml per pass in adult (proportionately smaller in child) is administered, and the dosage is repeated until the return is clear. Often a funnel or other device attached to the tube facilitates the procedure.

If the patient is seen more than 1 to 2 hours after ingestion, administration of a single dose of activated charcoal may be the preferred approach to reducing absorption, rather than lavage or emesis performed first.

(4) In comatose patients or patients who lack protective reflexes (gag, cough, swallow), intubation is usually indicated before insertion of the lavage tube.

(5) The procedure is performed with the patient on the left side in the Trendelenburg's (head-down) position.

c. *Emesis with syrup of ipecac* is rarely if ever indicated in the ED. *Do not* give this agent if the patient is comatose, stuporous, or seizing, has no gag reflex, is younger than 6 months, has a bleeding diathesis, or has ingested an acidic, alkaline or hydrocarbon substance that does not contain camphor, halogenated or aromatic products, heavy metal, or pesticides. Ipecac also should not been given if the ingested substance can rapidly cause seizures or coma (i.e., a cyclic antidepressant) (p. 356).

Age	Amount of Ipecac Administered
6-12 mo	10 ml (do not repeat)
1-12 yr	15 ml
>12 yr	30 ml

If emesis does not occur in 20 minutes, repeat the dose if the child is older than 12 months.

d. *Catharsis*, with magnesium sulfate, 250 mg/kg/dose PO (adults 20 g PO), should be given to shorten transit time. It is contraindicated in patients with renal failure, severe diarrhea, adynamic ileus, or abdominal trauma. Do not use multiple doses. Sodium sulfate, sorbitol (2 ml/kg of 70% sorbitol [1-2 g/kg]), or magnesium citrate (4 to 8 ml/kg [maximum: 300 ml]) also may serve as a cathartic. Use one dose only.

e. *Whole-bowel irrigation*. Rapid administration of a specialized fluid solution (polyethylene glycol electrolyte or GoLYTELY) can be useful in cases in which iron, packets of street drugs, or large amounts of sustained-release drugs have been ingested. The patient must be alert and be able to protect the airway. Adults and adolescents receive 1 to 2 L/hr; toddlers and preschoolers may receive 250 to 500 ml/hr until the rectal effluent is similar in appearance to the infusate.

This approach is particularly useful with ingestions involving iron and other heavy metals, lithium, sustained-release or enteric-coated agents, body packers/stuffers, and foreign bodies (batteries, etc).

Enhancement of Excretion

1. *Diuresis* can hasten the excretion of a few substances, namely those with small volumes of distribution that are excreted by the kidneys. When a drug is ionizable, intracellular and CNS drug levels may be reduced and renal excretion increased by ion-trapping. Ionizable drugs cross lipid membranes (cell wall or blood barrier) only in a nonionized state. Alkaline pH favors dissociation (ion-trapping) of weakly acidic drugs (phenobarbital, salicylates). Potassium depletion may prevent excretion of salicylates. Substances whose excretion may be definitely enhanced by diuresis include phenobarbital (alkaline) and salicylates (alkaline). The goal of alkaline diuresis is to increase urinary pH to 7.5 or higher and to maintain brisk urine flow (2-5 ml/kg/hr). It is imperative to prevent fluid overload; hourly assessment of volume status is mandatory.
   a. Alkaline diuresis is achieved by giving $NaHCO_3$, 1 to 2 mEq/kg/dose IV over 1 hour, with K^+ supplement as necessary. Adding two to three adult ampules (44.5 mEq $NaHCO_3$ per ampule) to 1 L of D5W results in a solution that is not hypertonic and that facilitates alkalinization. Urine pH should be 7.5 or higher. Monitor electrolyte levels. Potassium usually must be given in concentrations of 30 to 50 mEq/L. Alkaline diuresis is contraindicated if pulmonary or

cerebral edema or renal failure is present.

b. Acid diuresis is not recommended.

2. *Dialysis,* usually considered after failure of conservative medical treatment, may be useful in only a few circumstances. It is indicated if life-threatening symptoms are present with markedly elevated serum levels. The following drugs are dialyzable:

Salicylates
Methanol
Lithium
Ethylene glycol

After methanol ingestion, immediate dialysis should be performed for unresponsive patients, significant acidosis, renal failure, visual symptoms, or peak levels (measured or extrapolated) greater than 50 mg/dl.

3. Hemoperfusion with charcoal or resin-filled devices is still controversial. Hemoperfusion appears particularly useful for significant theophylline overdoses, but because of the greater availability of hemodialysis, the latter is usually preferred.

Antidotes. (Table 54-3) Specific antidotes are useful when used appropriately. The antiquated "universal antidote" (burned toast, magnesium oxide, and tannic acid) has no place in modern therapy.

Disposition

1. The decision whether to discharge the patient from the ED must reflect the severity of the ingestion and potential life-threatening medical and psychiatric considerations.
2. Before the patient is discharged, specific attention must be focused on poison prevention, with emphasis on discarding old medications and placing needed drugs and toxic household substances in locked cabinets.
3. Children and their families should be cautioned about accident prevention. Families with 2- to 6-year-old children who have a possible poison exposure are at an increased risk of subsequent injury. Injury prevention education is essential.
4. Patients who take overdoses of substances as suicide gestures or environmental manipulation should receive *psychiatric evaluation* before discharge (p. 778).
5. Incidents of child abuse must be referred to the appropriate child welfare authorities (see Chapter 25).

TOXIC SYNDROMES

While a patient's history is being obtained and the physical examination is being performed, certain toxic syndromes may become evident. Such an occurrence can assist the physician by focusing on a class of toxins to which the patient may have been exposed.

Narcotics and Sedative-Hypnotics (p. 388)

Narcotic and sedative-hypnotic agents, which cause associated cardiorespiratory depression, can result in coma.

Diagnostic Findings

1. Narcotics (except meperidine) may produce miosis, noncardiogenic pulmonary edema, and seizures, especially with propoxyphene or meperidine.
   a. Anticholinergic findings—diphenoxylate (Lomotil) and atropine.
   b. Treatment: naloxone (Narcan), 0.4 to 2 mg IV. Ingestion of propoxyphene (Darvon) or pentazocine (Talwin) may require larger doses for reversal. The use of naloxone is both therapeutic and diagnostic. Occasionally, a continuous infusion may be required.
2. Sedative-hypnotics: benzodiazepines (e.g., diazepam), barbiturates, methaqualone (Quaalude), meprobamate (Miltown),

TABLE 54-3 Common Antidotes (See Chapter 55)

Drug	Diagnostic Findings Requiring Treatment	Antidote	Dosage
Acetaminophen	History of ingestion and toxic serum level	*N*-acetylcysteine	140 mg/kg/dose PO, then 70 mg/kg/dose q4hr PO × 17
Anticholinergics Antihistamines Atropine Phenothiazines Cyclic antidepressants	Supraventricular tachycardia (hemodynamic compromise) Unresponsive ventricular dysrhythmia, seizures, pronounced hallucinations or agitation	Physostigmine	Child: 0.02 mg/kg/dose up to 0.5 mg/dose IV slowly (over 3 min) q10min prn (maximum total dose: 2 mg) Adult: 1-2 mg IV slowly q10min prn (maximum: 4 mg in 30 min)
Benzodiazepines	Respiratory depression, coma	Flumazenil	10 μg/kg IV for 2 doses; adult: 0.2 mg, 0.3 mg, then 0.5 mg separated by 30 seconds, up to total of 3 mg
Cholinergics Physostigmine Insecticides	Cholinergic crisis: salivation, lacrimation, urination, defecation, convulsions, fasciculations	Atropine sulfate	0.05 mg/kg/dose (usual dose 1-5 mg; test dose for child 0.01 mg/kg) q4-6hr IV or more frequently prn Also pralidoxime (see below)
Carbon monoxide	Headache, seizure, coma, dysrhythmias	Oxygen, hyperbaric oxygen	100% oxygen (half-life 40 min); consider hyperbaric chamber
Cyanide	Cyanosis, seizures, cardiopulmonary arrest, coma	Amyl nitrite Sodium nitrite (3%) Sodium thiosulfate (25%) Also consider hyperbaric oxygen	Inhale perle q60-120 sec 0.27 ml (8.7 mg)/kg (adult: 10 ml [300 mg]) IV slowly (Hb 10 g) 1.35 ml (325 mg)/kg (adult: 12.5 g) IV slowly (Hb 10 g)
Ethylene glycol	Metabolic acidosis, urine Ca^{++} oxalate crystals	Ethanol (100% absolute, 1 ml-790 mg) Flumazenil	1 ml/kg in D5W IV over 15 min, then 0.15 ml (125 mg)/kg/hr IV; maintain ethanol level of 100 mg/dl 0.01 mg/kg (max: 0.2 mg) IV; may repeat × 2
Iron	Hypotension, shock, coma, serum iron level toxic	Deferoxamine	Shock or coma: 15 mg/kg/hr IV for 8 hr; if no shock or coma 90 mg/kg/dose IM q8hr
Isoniazid	Seizures	Pyridoxine	50-100 mg IV (adult)
Phenothiazines Chlorpromazine Thioridazine	Extrapyramidal dyskinesis, oculogyric crisis	Diphenhydramine (Benadryl)	1-2 mg/kg/dose (maximum: 50 mg/dose) q6hr IV, PO
Methanol	Metabolic acidosis, blurred vision; level >20 mg/dl	Ethanol (100% absolute) Flumazenil	1 ml/kg in D5W over 15 min, then 0.15 ml (125 mg)/kg/hr IV 0.01 mg/kg (max: 0.2 mg) IV; may repeat × 2

Continued

TABLE 54-3 Common Antidotes (See Chapter 55)—cont'd

Drug	Diagnostic Findings Requiring Treatment	Antidote	Dosage
Methemoglobin Nitrate Nitrite Sulfonamide	Cyanosis, methemoglobin level >30%, dyspnea	Methylene blue (1% solution)	1-2 mg (0.1-0.2 ml)/kg/dose IV: repeat in 4 hr if necessary
Narcotics Heroin Codeine Propoxyphene	Respiratory depression, hypotension, coma	Naloxone (Narcan)	0.4-2 mg/dose IV; repeat as necessary (nelmefene has longer half-life)
Organophosphates Malathion Parathion	Cholinergic crisis: salivation, lacrimation, urination, defecation, convulsions, fasciculations	Atropine sulfate	0.05 mg/kg/dose (usual dose 1-5 mg) IV prn or q4-6hr
		Pralidoxime	After atropine, 20-50 mg/kg/dose (maximum: 2000 mg) IV slowly or 500 mg/hr IV infusion

glutethimide (Doriden), ethchlorvynol (Placidyl):

a. Management: prevention of absorption and supportive care (alkaline diuresis for phenobarbital)

b. Benzodiazepine respiratory depression or coma reversed by flumazenil (Mazicon) in a dose of 0.01 mg/kg every 1 minute to a total of 1 mg. Adult: 0.2 mg/dose, 0.3 mg/dose, and then 0.5 mg/dose IV separated by 30 seconds between doses, up to a cumulative dose of 3.0 mg. Flumazenil should not be given if the patient has a seizure disorder or elevated intracranial pressure or has also overdosed on a cyclic antidepressant.

Anticholinergics (p. 374)

Classes of anticholinergic agents include the following:

1. Antihistamines
2. Antiparkinsonian—benztropine (Cogentin)
3. Belladonna alkaloids (atropine)
4. Butyrophenones (haloperidol)
5. GI and genitourinary (GU) antispasmodics
6. Over-the-counter (OTC) analgesics (Midol, Excedrin)
7. OTC cold remedies
8. OTC sleeping preparations
9. Phenothiazines
10. Cyclic antidepressants

Plants may also be sources, such as *Amanita muscaria*.

Diagnostic Findings. Peripheral signs include the following:

1. Tachycardia
2. Dry, flushed skin
3. Dry mucous membranes
4. Dilated pupils
5. Hyperpyrexia
6. Urinary retention
7. Decreased bowel sounds
8. Dysrhythmias
9. Hypertension
10. Hypotension (late)

Central anticholinergic syndrome causes:

1. Delirium—organic brain syndrome:
   a. Disorientation
   b. Agitation
   c. Hallucinations
   d. Psychosis
   e. Loss of memory
2. Extrapyramidal movements
3. Ataxia
4. Picking or grasping movements
5. Seizures
6. Coma
7. Respiratory failure
8. Cardiovascular collapse

A useful mnemonic for remembering the components of central anticholinergic syndrome is *Mad as a hatter, Hot as a hare, Blind as a bat, Dry as a bone, and Red as a beet.*

Phenothiazines may cause pronounced hypotension resulting from their α-blocking action (p. 393).

Treatment

1. Seizures: diazepam (Valium) or phenobarbital; for the unresponsive or psychotic patient, physostigmine
2. Dysrhythmias (cyclic antidepressants): alkalinization, phenytoin, lidocaine; for the psychotic patient, physostigmine (p. 381)
3. Pronounced hallucinations and agitation (in which patient may be in danger of harming self or others) may require physostigmine:
   - Physostigmine, 0.02 mg/kg/dose up to 0.5 mg/dose IV (children) or 1 to 2 mg IV (adults) slowly

Cholinergics

Cholinergics include organophosphates and carbamate pesticides (p. 391), physostigmine, neostigmine, pyridostigmine, and edrophonium (Tensilon).

Diagnostic Findings

1. "SLUDGE": *s*alivation, *l*acrimation, *u*rination, *d*efecation (diarrhea), GI cramping, and *e*mesis. Patients appear "wet."
2. CNS effects: headache, restlessness, and anxiety progressing to confusion, coma, and seizures.
3. Sweating, miosis, muscle fasciculations and weakness, bradycardia, bronchorrhea, and bronchospasm. Tachycardia is also common.

Treatment

1. Decontamination and support.
2. Atropine (blocks acetylcholine), 0.05 mg/kg/dose (usual dose 1-5 mg) q10min prn or q4-6hr IV. The end-point of atropinization should be drying of pulmonary secretions. Pupil size is unsatisfactory because the pupils may initially be dilated, and miosis is not the life-threatening condition.
3. Pralidoxime 2-PAM (cholinesterase reactivator), 20 to 50 mg/kg/dose IV slowly q8hr IV prn (three times), after atropine; may also be administered as an infusion at a rate of 500 ml/hr.

Sympathomimetics (p. 397)

Sympathomimetics include amphetamines, phenylpropanolamine, ephedrine, and cocaine.

Diagnostic Findings. Findings of sympathomimetic ingestion are similar to those in anticholinergic syndrome:

1. Psychoses, hallucinations, delirium
2. Nausea, vomiting, and abdominal pain
3. Possibly prominent piloerection
4. Tachycardia and cardiac dysrhythmias
5. Severe hypertension

Treatment

1. Supportive care after gastric emptying.
2. Diazepam (Valium), 0.1 to 0.2 mg/kg/dose q4-6hr IV or PO for sedation.
3. Haloperidol (Haldol), 0.05 to 0.15 mg/kg/24 hr q8-12hr PO; begin 0.5 mg/24 hr; dose not well established in children; adult: 0.05 to 2 mg (maximum: 5 mg) q8-12hr PO; may also be given parenterally if patient is extremity agitated. Adult emergent dose is 5 to 20 mg IV prn.

Drug-induced psychosis requires a reassuring attitude and maintaining verbal contact with the patient. Physical restraints should be avoided.

Classic Manifestations of Toxicity

See Tables 54-1 and 54-2 and Box 54-2.

Although tremendous variability exists in clinical presentations, certain manifestations of toxicity are commonly recognized and are particularly helpful in identifying unknown poisons.

BIBLIOGRAPHY

AACT/EAPCCT Position Statement on Gastric Lavage, *J Tox-Clin Tox* 35:711, 1997.

AACT/EAPCCT Position Statement on Ipecac Syrup, *J Tox-Clin Tox* 35:699, 1997.

AACT/EAPCCT Position Statement on Single-Dose Activated Charcoal, *J Tox-Clin Tox* 35:721, 1997.

Albertson TE, Derlet RW, Foulke GE et al: Superiority of activated charcoal alone compared with ipecac and activated charcoal in the treatment of acute toxic ingestions, *Ann Emerg Med* 18:56, 1989.

Baraff LF, Guterman JJ, Bayer MJ: The relationship of poison center contact and injury in children 2 to 6 years old, *Ann Emerg Med* 21:153, 1992.

Brent J, McMartin K, Phillips S et al: Fomepizole for the treatment of methanol poisoning, *New Engl J Med* 344:424, 2001.

Clark RF, Sage TA, Tunget C et al: Delayed onset lorazepam poisoning successfully reversed by flumazenil in a child, *Pediatr Emerg Care* 11:32, 1995.

Dagnone D, Matsu D, Rieder MJ: Assessment of the palatability of vehicles for activated charcoal in pediatric volunteers, *Pediatr Emerg Care* 18:19, 2002.

Hoffman JR, Schriger DL, Luo JS: The empiric use of naloxone in patients with altered mental status, *Ann Emerg Med* 20:246, 1991.

James LP, Nichols MH, King WD: A comparison of cathartics in pediatric ingestion, *Pediatrics* 96:235, 1995.

Kaczorowski JM, Wax PM: Five days of whole-bowel irrigation in a case of pediatric iron ingestion, *Ann Emerg Med* 27:258, 1996.

Keller RE, Schwab RS, Krenzelok EP: Contribution of sorbitol combined with activated charcoal in prevention of salicylate absorption, *Ann Emerg Med* 19:654, 1990.

Kornberg AE, Dolgin J: Pediatric ingestions: charcoal alone versus ipecac and charcoal, *Ann Emerg Med* 20:648, 1991.

Box 54-2

CLUES TO DIAGNOSIS OF UNKNOWN POISONS AND CONDITIONS: LABORATORY AND OTHER ALTERATIONS

TOXIC METABOLIC ACIDOSIS ("MUDPILES")*

Methanol
Uremia
Diabetes ketoacidosis
Paraldehyde
Isoniazid, iron, ibuprofen, inhalant (CO, cyanide)
Lactic acidosis
Ethanol, ethylene glycol
Salicylates, starvation, strychnine, solvent (benzene, toluene)

GLUCOSE

Increased

Salicylates
Isoniazid
Iron
Isopropyl alcohol

Decreased

Acetaminophen (if hepatic failure)
Isoniazid
Salicylates
Methanol
Insulin and oral hypoglycemics
Ethanol

URINE COLOR

Red: hematuria, hemoglobinuria, myoglobinuria, pyrvinium (Povan), phenytoin (Dilantin), phenothiazines, mercury, lead, iron, anthocyanins (food pigment in beets and blackberries)
Brown-black: hemoglobin pigments, melanin, methyldopa (Aldomet), cascara, rhubarb, methocarbamol (Robaxin)
Blue, blue-green, green: amitryptyline, methylene blue, indigo blue, triamterene (Dyazide), Clorets, *Pseudomonas*, propofol
Brown, red-brown: porphyria, urobilinogen, nitrofurantoin, furazolidone, metronidazole, aloe (seaweed)
Orange: dehydration, rifampin, phenazopyridine (Pyridium), sulfasalazine (Azulfidine, propofol)

X-RAY STUDY (radiopaque medications and chemicals: "CHIPE," i.e., heavy metals and enteric-coated tablets)†

Chloral hydrate, cocaine, "condos," calcium
Heavy metals (arsenic, lead)
Iron, iodides
Phenothiazines, psychotropics (cyclic antidepressants), potassium, Pepto-Bismol
Enteric coated tablets, slow-release capsules
Also, chlorinated hydrocarbon solvents

BREATH ODOR

Alcohol: ethanol, chloral hydrate, phenols
Acetone: acetone, salicylates, isopropyl alcohol, paraldehyde
Bitter almond: cyanide
Burned rope: marijuana
Fruity: ethanol, acetone, isopropyl alcohol, chlorinated hydrocarbon (i.e., chloroform)
Garlic: arsenic, phosphorus, organophosphates
Rotten eggs: disulfiram, *N*-acetylcystine
Wintergreen: methylsalicylates

---

* Metabolic acidosis may be caused by any drug, chemical, or condition that causes hypotension, seizures, or cellular metabolism dysfunction.

† Factors affecting radiopacity include the size of patient, the arrangement of the pills in the stomach, air-contrasting pills, and the composition of the enteric coating or pill matrix.

Kulig K: Initial management of ingestions of toxic substances, *N Engl J Med* 326:1677, 1992.

Lewander WJ, Lacouture PG: Office management of acute pediatric poisoning, *Pediatr Emerg Care* 5:262, 1989.

Litovitz T, Manoquerra A: Comparison of pediatric poisoning hazards: an analysis of 3.8 million exposure incidents, *Pediatrics* 89:999, 1992.

Litovitz TL, Smilkstein M, Felberg L et al: 1996 Annual Report of the American Association of Poison Control Centers Toxic Exposure Surveillance System, *Am J Emerg Med* 15:447, 1997.

Lovejoy FH, Robertson WO, Woolf AD: Poison centers, poison prevention, and the pediatrician, *Pediatrics* 94:220, 1994.

McDuffee AT, Tobias JD: Seizure after flumazenil administration in a pediatric patient, *Pediatr Emerg Care* 11:186, 1995.

McNamara RM, Aaron CK, Gemborys M et al: Efficacy of charcoal and cathartic versus ipecac in reducing serum acetaminophen in a stimulated overdose, *Ann Emerg Med* 18:934, 1989.

Merigian KS, Woodard M, Hedges JR et al: Prospective evaluation of gastric emptying in the self-poisoned patient, *Am J Emerg Med* 9:479, 1990.

Moll J, Kerns W, Tomaszewski C et al: Incidence of aspiration pneumonia in intubated patients receiving activated charcoal, *J Emerg Med* 17:279, 1999.

Mullins ME, Brands CL, Daya MR: Unintentional pediatric superwarfarin exposures: do we really need a prothrombin time? *Pediatrics* 105:402, 2000.

Osterloh JD: Utility and reliability of emergency toxicologic testing, *Emerg Med Clin North Am* 8:693, 1990.

Pond SM, Lewis-Driver DJ, Williams GM et al: Gastric emptying in acute overdose: a prospective randomised controlled trial, *Med J Aust* 163:345, 1995.

Rosenberg PJ, Livingston DJ, McLellan BA: Effect of whole bowel irrigation on the efficacy of oral activated charcoal, *Ann Emerg Med* 17:681, 1988.

Savitt DL, Hawkins HH, Roberts JR: The radiopacity of ingested medications, *Ann Emerg Med* 16:331, 1987.

Shannon M, Amitai Y, Lovejoy FH: Multiple dose activated charcoal for theophylline poisoning in young infants, *Pediatrics* 80:368, 1987.

Sugarman JM, Paul RI: Flumazenil: a review, *Pediatr Emerg Care* 10:37, 1994.

Sugarman JM, Rodgers GC, Paul RI: Utility of toxicity screening in a pediatric emergency department, *Pediatr Emerg Care* 13:194, 1997.

Tenenbein M: General management principles in poisoning. In Barkin RM, editor: *Pediatric emergency medicine: concepts and clinical practice,* ed 2, St Louis, 1997, Mosby.

Tenenbein M: Multiple doses of charcoal: time for reappraisal? *Ann Emerg Med* 20:529, 1991.

Tenenbein M, Cohen S, Sitar DS: Efficacy of ipecac induced emesis, orogastric lavage, and activated charcoal for acute drug overdose, *Ann Emerg Med* 16:838, 1987.

Tenenbein M, Cohen S, Sitar DS: Whole bowel irrigation as a decontamination procedure after acute drug overdose, *Arch Intern Med* 147:905, 1987.

55 Specific Ingestions

Acetaminophen

ALERT History and plasma level determine the need for therapy.

Acetaminophen is a widely used antipyretic and analgesic that is metabolized in the liver in part by conjugation with glutathione. After an acetaminophen overdose, the glutathione substrate can be overwhelmed, and a toxic metabolite is formed via an alternative pathway. The toxic metabolite may bind covalently to hepatic macromolecules, producing cellular necrosis.

In adults, 150 mg/kg is considered a toxic overdose, but the same dose may produce only minor changes in children younger than 10 years. Ingestion of 200 mg/kg or less is usually not associated with signs and symptoms of hepatic injury in children, who appear less susceptible to injury. Both children and adults, however, are susceptible to long-term overdose of acetaminophen, which causes hepatic damage. Chronic ingestion of alcohol, as well as malnutrition, appears to be a risk factor. Therapeutic levels are 10 to 20 μg/ml, whereas toxic levels are 150 μg/ml at 4 hours and 37.5 μg/ml at 12 hours.

DIAGNOSTIC FINDINGS

The history of ingestion is often inadequate and bears little correlation to the blood levels. Patients may experience hepatic failure secondary to necrosis of the centrilobular type. Encephalopathy, coma, and death may follow. Children are unlikely to have toxic levels if they experienced early, spontaneous emesis.

1. Gastrointestinal (GI) symptoms and diaphoresis may develop 6 to 12 hours after ingestion. Many patients remain asymptomatic.
2. An asymptomatic period follows for 12 to 48 hours after ingestion, although hepatic enzyme levels begin to rise.
3. After about 36 hours, evidence of liver injury becomes apparent, with marked elevations of hepatic enzymes, which usually then normalize over the ensuing 4 to 7 days.

Ancillary Data

1. Acetaminophen levels are obtained 4 hours after ingestion and plotted on a nomogram (Fig. 55-1)
2. Liver function tests, including serum glutamic oxaloacetic transaminase (SGOT), serum glutamic pyruvic transaminase (SGPT), and bilirubin measurements, and prothrombin time (PT)
3. Arterial blood gas (ABG) analysis and other evaluations as indicated by central nervous system (CNS) findings
4. Blood glucose level if hepatic damage occurs

DIFFERENTIAL DIAGNOSIS

1. Infection: acute gastroenteritis (see Chapter 76) and hepatitis (p. 649)
2. Encephalopathy (p. 141)
3. Chemical hepatitis from other drugs or chemicals (e.g., solvents, mushrooms)

MANAGEMENT

The decision regarding intervention is made on the basis of the presumed history of ingestion and, ideally, an acetaminophen level.

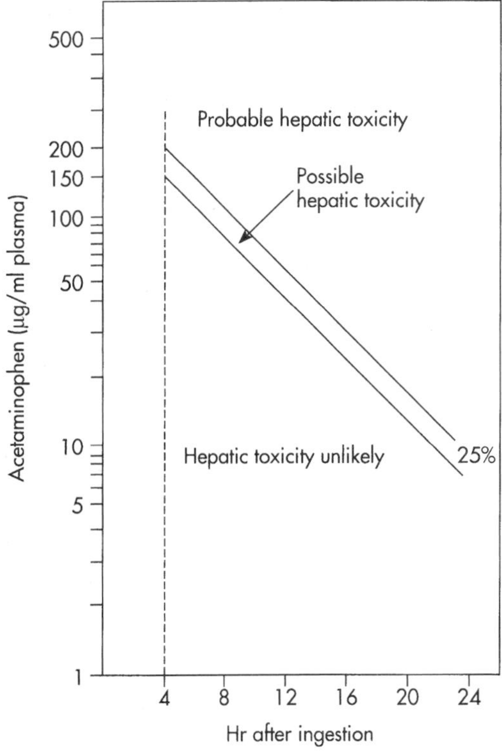

Fig. 55-1 Rumack-Matthew nomogram for acetaminophen poisoning.

(From Rumack BH, Matthew H: *Pediatrics* 55:871, 1975. Copyright American Academy of Pediatrics, 1975.)

1. Initial stabilization of the patient. Emesis or gastric lavage may be indicated if these procedures can be performed very soon after ingestion. Do not give syrup of ipecac to a patient who is already vomiting. Give activated charcoal as soon as possible, preferably without prior syrup of ipecac dose or gastric lavage. If given less than 4 hours after ingestion, charcoal may prevent development of a toxic acetaminophen level. Charcoal will not interfere with the absorption or efficacy of *N*-acetylcysteine 20% (NAC; Mucomyst).
2. NAC: diluted fourfold to a 5% solution in grapefruit juice, water, or cola. Can also be given IV. It is ideally indicated within 8 hours of ingestion but is still effective up to 24 hours after ingestion, or even after that in patients demonstrating hepatic failure.
   - **a.** Indicated if the serum acetaminophen level is in the toxic range and less than 24 hours has elapsed since ingestion. *Toxic levels* are considered to be those levels above the possible toxicity line on the nomogram. Levels obtained on blood collected less than 4 hours after ingestion may not be interpretable, because acetaminophen has a two-compartment kinetic pattern. Children appear to have more resistance to toxicity.
   - **b.** If no blood levels are immediately available and the ingestion is considered to be toxic (>150 mg/kg), therapy should be initiated; it may be stopped later if the blood level is determined to be in the nontoxic range. Whether ingestion of the new sustained-release form of acetaminophen should be managed differently from the regular form regarding use of the nomogram is unclear. A certified regional poison center should be contacted for the most current information.
   - **c.** Dosage. Load with 140 mg/kg/dose PO followed by 70 mg/kg/dose q4hr PO for 17 doses. Some toxicologists now recommend a shorter course of oral NAC, with treatment stopped at 24 hours if the acetaminophen blood level is nondetectable and hepatic transaminase values are normal. If the patient vomits within 1 hour of administration of the dose of NAC, repeat the dose. If vomiting persists, give by nasogastric (NG) or duodenal tube as slow drip or consider IV. Metoclopramide (Reglan), 1 mg/kg IV up to 10 mg, 30 minutes before NAC, or ondansetron (Zofran) may prevent vomiting.

DISPOSITION

All patients who need treatment with NAC should be admitted for treatment and monitoring. Long-term follow-up observation will be required.

BIBLIOGRAPHY

Anderson BJ, Hotford NHG, Armishaw JC et al: Predicting concentrations in children presenting with acetaminophen overdose, *J Pediatr* 135:290, 1999.

Bruno MK, Cohen SD, Khairallah EA: Antidotal effectiveness of *N*-acetylcysteine in reversing acetaminophen-induced hepatotoxicity, *Biochem Pharmacol* 37:4319, 1988.

Chamberlain JM, Gorman RL, Oderda GM et al: Use of activated charcoal in a simulated poisoning with acetaminophen: a new loading dose for *N*-acetylcysteine, *Ann Emerg Med* 22:1398, 1993.

Harrison PM, Keays R, Bray GP et al: Improved outcome of paracetamol-induced fulminant hepatic failure by late administration of acetylcysteine, *Lancet* 335:1572, 1990.

Heubi J: Therapeutic misadventures with acetaminophen: hepatotoxicity after multiple doses in children, *J Pediatr* 132:22, 1998.

Rivera-Penera T, Gugig R, Davis J et al: Outcome of acetaminophen overdose in pediatric patients and factors contributing to hepatotoxicity, *J Pediatr* 130:300, 1997.

Smilkstein MJ, Bronstein AC, Linden C et al: Acetaminophen overdose: a 48-hour intravenous *N*-acetylcysteine treatment protocol, *Ann Emerg Med* 20:1058, 1991.

Smilkstein MJ, Knapp GI, Kulig KW et al: Efficacy of oral *N*-acetylcysteine in the treatment of acetaminophen overdose, *N Engl J Med* 319:1557, 1988.

Alcohols: Ethanol, Isopropyl, Methanol, Ethylene Glycol

Ethanol is becoming an increasingly popular drug among adolescents. The immediate medical problems, as well as the long-term psychiatric ones, must be treated.

DIAGNOSTIC FINDINGS (see Table 55-1)

Classically, the progression of findings in nontolerant intoxicated individuals is related to the blood alcohol level (Table 55-2). A progressive change is seen in mental status and sensory impairment, ultimately leading to respiratory failure and death.

1. *Ethanol* equivalents: Approximately four drinks ingested quickly on an empty stomach will result in a peak blood level of about 100 mg/dl. If a comatose patient has a blood alcohol level less than 250 mg/dl, consider another cause for the coma.
2. *Isopropyl* alcohol is considered to be more of a CNS depressant and GI irritant than ethanol. There may be a smell of acetone on the breath after ingestion.
3. *Methanol* ingestion results in a nonintoxicated, acidotic patient with visual symptoms 3 to 24 hours after ingestion.
4. *Ethylene glycol* produces an intoxicated patient with severe acidosis, rapid progression of CNS signs, renal dysfunction commonly associated with calcium oxalate crystalluria, pulmonary edema, and shock.

Often, an associated ingestion of a drug or another alcohol is present, and there are many alcohol-drug interactions.

Ancillary Data

1. Ethanol, methanol, ethylene glycol, and isopropanol blood levels.
2. Blood glucose, electrolyte levels, osmolality (by freezing point depression), and ABG analysis. Osmolal gap, if high, may indicate high levels of methanol or ethylene glycol; if such levels are low or normal, however, methanol or ethylene glycol poisoning has not been ruled out. The laboratory specimen may have been drawn late in the course of the poisoning.

DIFFERENTIAL DIAGNOSIS

Differentiation of the alcohols may be made on the basis of blood levels, acid-base status, breath odor, and diagnostic findings.

A useful mnemonic for remembering the causes of metabolic acidosis is "MUDPILES":

TABLE 55-1 Alcohol Ingestion and Overdose

Alcohol (Uses)	"Toxic Dose" (Toxic Level)	CNS Depression	Acidosis	Ketonemia	Increased Osmolality at Level of 50 mg/dl
Ethanol (beverages, mouthwash, perfumes)	3-5 g/kg (>100 mg/dl)	+	±	±	11 mOsm/kg H_2O
Isopropyl (rubbing alcohol, solvent)	2-3 g/kg (>50 mg/dl)	+	+	++	8.5 mOsm/kg H_2O
Methanol (canned heat, antifreeze, solvent, denaturant)	1-2 ml/kg (>20 mg/dl)		+++	±	15.5 mOsm/kg H_2O
Ethylene glycol (antifreeze, deicer)	1-2 ml/kg (>20 mg/dl)	+	+++	–	8 mOsm/kg H_2O

Modified from Goldfrank LR, Starke CL: Metabolic acidosis in the alcoholic. In Goldfrank LR: *Toxicologic emergencies*, ed 6, New York, 1998, Appleton-Century-Crofts.

TABLE 55-2 Blood Ethanol Levels and Clinical Findings in the Nontolerant Adult

Blood Ethanol Level (mg/dl)	Clinical Findings
≤99	Changes in mood, personality, behavior Progressive muscular incoordination Impaired sensory function
100-199	Marked mental and sensory impairment Incoordination, ataxia Prolonged reaction time Grossly intoxicated
200-299	Nausea, vomiting, diplopia, marked ataxia
300-399	Amnesia, dysarthria, hypothermia
>400	Coma, respiratory failure, death possible

*m*ethanol, *u*remia, *d*iabetes mellitus, *p*araldehyde, *i*ron, *i*soniazid, *l*actic acidosis, *e*thanol, *e*thylene glycol, *s*alicylates, and *s*tarvation. Acidosis is caused by these agents as well as those that cause seizures, hypotension, and all cellular poisons (e.g., iron, cyanide, carbon monoxide).

MANAGEMENT

1. *Supportive care* with particular attention to the airway and fluids. Treatment of acidosis, hypoglycemia, hypocalcemia, respiratory and renal failure, or pulmonary edema.
2. *Gastric emptying* if it can be achieved soon after ingestion or if there is any question of an associated ingestion.
3. *Pharmaceutical therapy:*
   a. Ethanol, as outlined in Table 55-1, for methanol or ethylene glycol ingestions. Maintain blood ethanol level at 100 mg/dl or greater.

Diagnostic Findings	Odor on Breath	Treatment
Intoxication with nausea, vomiting, ataxia, uncoordination, slurred speech progressing to seizures, coma, hypothermia, respiratory failure, death	Ethanol	Gastric emptying, fluids, glucose support; blood level declines at 10-50 mg/dl/hr; consider dialysis if life threatening
Intoxication with significant CNS depression, hemorrhagic tracheobronchitis, gastritis; twice toxicity of ethanol	Acetone	Gastric emptying, fluid support; dialysis if life threatening
Not intoxicated; delayed onset; mild initial CNS depression may become severe; intractable acidosis; blurred vision with pink edema of optic disc in 12-24 hr; abdominal pain (pancreatitis)	None	Gastric emptying, fluid support; ethanol (100%) 1 ml/kg over 15 min, then 0.15 ml (125 mg)/kg/hr IV; flumazenil 0.01 mg/kg (max 0.2 mg) IV (may repeat × 2); dialysis if peak level >50 mg/dl, visual symptoms, or severe acidosis; prognosis associated to acidosis
Intoxicated; stupor, ataxia progressing to seizures, coma; severe acidosis; ocular nystagmus; CHF and pulmonary edema; shock; renal failure, calcium oxalate crystalluria, oliguria, hypocalcemia	None	Gastric emptying, fluid support; calcium prn; ethanol (100%) 1 ml/kg over 15 min, then 0.15 ml (125 mg)/kg/hr IV; flumazenil 0.01 mg/kg (max 0.2 mg) IV (may repeat × 2); dialysis if renal failure, severe acidosis, or peak level >50 mg/dl

b. Fomepizole, a competitive inhibitor of alcohol dehydrogenase, may also be useful to treat ethylene glycol ingestions. A loading dose of 15 mg/kg/dose IV (over 30 minutes) is followed by 10 mg/kg/dose q12hr IV for four doses; dosage is then increased to 15 mg/kg/dose q12hr until the ethylene glycol concentration is below 20 mg/dl. The agent is expensive, and there is only limited experience with its use in children Fomepizole is of value in patients after methanol poisoning as well.

4. *Dialysis* is indicated early in the treatment of methanol and ethylene glycol ingestions with peak levels that are or could have been greater than 50 mg/dl or for accompanying severe acidosis or visual symptoms, but only in life-threatening intoxication of ethanol and isopropyl alcohol.

Alcohol withdrawal and the hyperkinetic state associated with long-term use of ethanol may be partially controlled in adolescents and adults with clorazepate (Tranxene), 15 mg q6hr PO, lorazepam (Ativan), 0.5 to 1.0 mg q6hr PO, or chlordiazepoxide (Librium), 50 to 100 mg IM or IV in adult. Diazepam (Valium) also may be useful.

DISPOSITION

All pediatric patients with significant methanol or ethylene glycol ingestions should be admitted, as should those with toxic levels of ethanol and isopropyl alcohol.

Long-term psychiatric follow-up care is usually indicated.

BIBLIOGRAPHY

Brent J, Lucas M, Kulig K et al: Methanol poisoning in a 6-week old infant, *J Pediatr* 118:644, 1991.

Brent J, McMartin K, Phillips S et al: Fomepizole for the treatment of methanol poisoning, *New Engl J Med* 344:424, 2001.
Burkhart K, Kulig K: The other alcohols: methanol, ethylene glycol, and isopropanol. In Harwood-Nuss A, editor: *Emerg Med Clin North Am*, Philadelphia, 1990, WB Saunders.
Burns MJ, Graudins A, Aaron CK et al: Treatment of methanol poisoning with intravenous 4-methylpyrazole, *Ann Emerg Med* 30:829, 1997.
Casavant MJ: Fomepizole in the treatment of poisoning, *Pediatrics* 107:170, 2001.
Chabali R: Diagnostic use of anion and osmolal gaps in pediatric emergency medicine, *Pediatr Emerg Care* 13:204, 1997.
Jacobson D, McMartin KE: Antidotes for methanol and ethylene glycol poisoning, *Clin Toxicol* 35:127, 1997.
Shannon M: Fomepizole—a new antidote, *Pediatr Emerg Care* 14:170, 1998.

Alkalis and Acids

ALERT Immediate dilution with milk or water should be initiated.

A large number of household products contain alkali or acid and may be ingested by the curious child. Accidental ingestions usually occur in children younger than 4 years, whereas older individuals may be attempting suicide or self-mutilation.

ETIOLOGY

1. Common alkalis:
   a. Sodium or potassium hydroxide (lye), washing powders, paint removers, drain pipe and toilet bowl cleaners, Clinitest tablets
   b. Liquids: drain (Liquid Plumber, Drāno) and oven cleaners
   c. Solid: Drāno (granular), Clinitest (tablets)
   d. Other: sodium hypochlorite bleach (if >5%), some detergents, electric dishwashing agents
   e. Button (disk) batteries
2. Common acids:
   a. Hydrochloric acid (HCl): metal, swimming pool, and toilet bowl cleaners
   b. Sulfuric acid: battery acid, toilet bowl cleaners, industrial drain cleaners
   c. Other: slate cleaners, soldering flux

DIAGNOSTIC FINDINGS

The nature of the ingestion must be defined. Specific attention should be directed to the material ingested (solid or liquid, acid or alkali), to its volume, to the duration of contact (when? was there emesis? was diluent used?), to the volume of liquids or solids in the stomach at the time of ingestion, and to the presence of pain, dysphagia, drooling, or other symptoms.

Physical examination should include a check for drooling, respiratory distress, oral or pharyngeal burns, evidence of chest abnormality or mediastinitis, and abdominal pain, guarding, or tenderness.

1. Alkalis primarily produce liquefaction necrosis and thermal injury, with deep tissue penetration and a high risk of perforation. Skin burns and major ocular injury may occur (see Chapters 46 and 59). Esophageal burn is characterized initially by erythema, followed by shallow ulceration within 24 hours. Edema may lead to narrowing in 48 to 72 hours and to scar tissue and strictures 4 to 6 weeks after the initial injury.
   a. Oropharyngeal burns with associated drooling, dysphagia, vomiting, and chest pain are common. Crystalline caustics tend to attach to the oral mucosa and produce severe burns of the mouth rather than the esophagus. Gulping caustic liquids may spare the oral and pharyngeal mucosa but cause severe burns of the esophagus. Solid alkali, particularly lye, may lodge in the oropharynx or esophagus. Clinitest tablets cause a high incidence of esophageal burns with stricture, intestinal perforation, and laryngeal edema.
   b. The absence of oropharyngeal burns does not exclude esophageal injury.

Esophageal injury is most commonly present if two or more of the following are present: vomiting, drooling, or stridor. Esophageal perforation may result in mediastinitis and shock. Stricture may develop as a delayed complication.

   c. Soft tissue swelling of the upper airway caused by involvement of the larynx, epiglottis, or vocal cords or by tracheal aspiration may produce respiratory distress.

2. Acid substances cause coagulation necrosis and thermal injury. The skin may be burned by exposure, and a major ocular emergency may result from acid exposure (see Chapters 46 and 59). There may be associated soft tissue swelling, with potential respiratory obstruction. Specific effects may include the following:
   a. Oropharyngeal burns with significant ingestions; rare esophageal perforation
   b. Perforation of the stomach or small intestine, acute peritonitis, and shock
3. Bleach in combination with acids (HCl) may produce chlorine gas, resulting in pulmonary damage if inhaled. Ingestion of household bleach (about 3% concentration) rarely causes esophageal burns.

Ancillary Data

1. Complete blood count (CBC), blood type and cross-match, and oximetry or ABGs with significant exposure.
2. X-ray films. Lateral neck views may be useful in evaluating upper respiratory edema; chest and abdominal films are needed if there are extensive complications.

MANAGEMENT

The first priority must be to assess the airway and ensure that any obstruction, if present, is relieved. If extensive burns of the oropharynx are present, a cricothyrotomy may be indicated. Ventilation and circulatory insufficiency must be treated.

1. Administer oxygen, particularly if the exposure has been to chlorine gas.
2. Dilute ingested material with milk or water as soon as possible. This should optimally be initiated at home, before the patient is taken to the emergency department (ED). Do not use weak acids or alkalis for neutralization, because that combination can produce a tremendous amount of heat. If involved, the skin should be washed well; each eye, if exposed, is irrigated with 1 to 2 L saline solution for at least 20 minutes (see Chapter 59).

   NOTE: Dilution of ingested material is contraindicated if perforation, shock, or upper airway compromise is present.
3. Do not initiate emesis, lavage, or catharsis or give charcoal.

Other Considerations

1. Steroids may have a role in deep or circumferential esophageal burns, but their role is controversial. If used, they should be initiated as soon after injury as possible and continued for at least 3 weeks, usually in consultation with a surgeon:
   - Hydrocortisone (Solu-Cortef), 4 to 5 mg/kg/dose q6hr IV, or methylprednisolone (Solu-Medrol), 2 mg/kg/dose q6hr IV
2. Antibiotics are not indicated for prophylaxis but may be required if mediastinitis or perforation develops.
3. A surgeon should be involved early in the evaluation. Surgery is required immediately if perforation or mediastinitis develops.
4. Esophagoscopy should be performed in the first 24 to 48 hours after ingestion in all patients with oropharyngeal burns, symptoms, or history of significant ingestion.
   a. Should be performed only to the point of major burn and not beyond
   b. Contraindicated in patients with respiratory obstruction, perforation,

shock, or third-degree burns of the oropharynx

5. Button (disk) batteries require special considerations. For children with a history of ingesting such a battery, perform radiographs to localize the battery. If it is lodged in the esophagus, removal should be considered an emergency. Batteries smaller than 18 mm (penny size) are rarely stopped in the esophagus. When located beyond the esophagus, the battery must be retrieved if there are any signs or symptoms of GI injury. Batteries larger than 15 mm, although rarely, when ingested by children younger than 6 years may have a delayed transit time and are unlikely to pass in the stool if they have not done so within 48 hours of ingestion; camera batteries larger than 23 mm ingested by people of any age need similar management. Follow-up in 4 to 7 days is needed for all battery ingestions if the object has not been found in the stool. The National Button Battery Ingestion Hotline (202-625-3333) can provide chemical content of batteries when given the imprint code, and can update clinical management approaches.
6. The timing of esophageal dilation and bougienage is controversial; most authorities prefer to wait until several weeks after injury. Serial barium swallow studies may provide evidence of developing esophageal stricture; if stricture is present, discontinue steroids and begin dilation.
7. An intraluminal shunt may be indicated for patients with documented second- and third-degree esophageal burns.

DISPOSITION

All patients with oropharyngeal burns should be admitted for fluid management and observation of respiratory and GI complications, as well as for esophagoscopy. Nutrition must be maintained.

Long-term follow-up observation is essential to monitor for the development of esophageal or gastric stenosis, with esophagoscopy or barium studies. Dilation and bougienage may be necessary. In patients in whom complete obliteration of the esophagus develops from stricture or who have not responded to dilation, colon interposition may be considered.

Psychiatric involvement is required in self-inflicted injuries, and poison-prevention counseling is essential in all families.

BIBLIOGRAPHY

Anderson KD, Rouse TM, Randolph JG: A controlled trial of corticosteroids in children with corrosive injury of the esophagus, *N Engl J Med* 323:637, 1990.

Howell JM, Dalsey WC, Hartsell FW et al: Steroid for the treatment of corrosive esophageal injury: a statistical analysis of past studies, *Am J Emerg Med* 10:421, 1992.

Litovitz T, Schmitz BF: Ingestion of cylindrical and button batteries: an analysis of 2382 cases, *Pediatrics* 89:747, 1992.

Anticholinergics

ALERT Peripheral and central effects are prominent. Physostigmine is indicated for unresponsive seizures and dangerous psychoses.

A wide spectrum of drugs possesses anticholinergic properties. For most of these agents, there is good GI absorption with a peak effect at 1 to 2 hours.

PHARMACEUTICALS WITH ANTICHOLINERGIC PROPERTIES

1. Antihistamines: diphenhydramine (Benadryl), tripelennamine (Pyribenzamine)
2. Belladonna alkaloids and related synthetic compounds: atropine, scopolamine, glycopyrrolate
3. Phenothiazines: chlorpromazine (Thorazine), thioridazine (Mellaril), prochlorperazine (Compazine), trifluoperazine (Stelazine)
4. Butyrophenones: haloperidol (Haldol)
5. Thioxanthenes: thiothixene (Navane)
6. Cyclic antidepressants (CADs): amitriptyline (Elavil), nortriptyline (Pamelor),

imipramine (Tofranil), desipramine (Norpramin), doxepin (Sinequan)
7. GI and genitourinary (GU) antispasmodics: dicyclomine (Bentyl), propantheline bromide (Pro-Banthine)
8. Local mydriatics: tropicamide (Mydriacyl), cyclopentolate (Cyclogyl)
9. Over-the-counter (OTC) analgesics: pyrilamine (Excedrin P.M.), cinnamedrine (Midol)
10. OTC cold remedies
11. OTC sleep aids
12. Antiparkinsonian medications: benztropine (Cogentin), trihexyphenidyl (Artane)

PLANTS CONTAINING ANTICHOLINERGIC ALKALOIDS

1. *Amanita muscaria* (fly agaric)
2. *Amanita pantherina* (panther mushroom)
3. *Datura stramonium* (jimsonweed)
4. *Myristica fragrans* (nutmeg)
5. *Solanum carolinense* (wild tomato)
6. *Solanum dulcamara* (bittersweet)
7. *Solanum tuberosum* (potato)
8. *Lantana camara* (wild sage)

DIAGNOSTIC FINDINGS

Anticholinergics cause a consistent clinical picture, although some variability exists in findings with specific drugs. Initially patients with diphenoxylate and atropine (Lomotil) overdoses have primarily anticholinergic (atropine) findings, but many hours after ingestion, they may have cardiopulmonary depression, miosis, hypotension, and coma, consistent with a narcotic overdose.

1. Peripheral signs and symptoms of anticholinergic overdose result primarily from muscarinic blockage:
   a. Vital sign alterations: tachycardia, hyperpyrexia, hypertension. Hypotension may be a late finding (phenothiazines may cause hypotension because of their α-blocking action).
   b. Dry flushed skin and dry mucous membranes.
   c. Dilated pupils (mydriasis).
   d. Urinary retention and decreased bowel sounds.
   e. Dysrhythmias, primarily as a result of direct myocardial depressant effect. Only CADs predictably cause ventricular dysrhythmias. CADs also prolong atrioventricular (AV) conduction and prevent reuptake of norepinephrine, leading to ventricular dysrhythmias and heart block. Thioridazine (Mellaril) may have a similar effect.
2. Central anticholinergic syndrome: a delirium characteristic of an evolving organic brain syndrome. Signs are as follows:
   a. Disorientation, uncontrolled agitation, impaired long-term memory, and hallucinations. The patient is rarely violent or self-mutilating.
   b. Movement disorders:
      (1) Phenothiazines and CADs often cause extrapyramidal reactions, including myoclonus and choreoathetosis.
      (2) Picking and grasping movements are common with overdoses of most of the anticholinergics.
   c. Seizures, coma, respiratory failure, and cardiovascular collapse.

Ancillary Data

1. Urine toxicology screening may be useful, but the laboratory should be told which agents are suspected.
2. Glucose, electrocardiogram (ECG), and ABG as indicated.
3. X-ray films: Abdominal film taken before tablets dissolve may show phenothiazines.

MANAGEMENT

1. Supportive care (airway management and maintaining vital signs) is of highest priority. All comatose patients should

receive dextrose, 0.5 to 1 g/kg IV, and naloxone, 0.1 mg/kg up to 2 mg IV.

2. Physostigmine, a naturally occurring alkaloid, is a reversible cholinesterase inhibitor. Centrally, it crosses the blood-brain barrier and is capable of reversing coma, delirium, seizures, and extrapyramidal signs. Peripherally, it is effective in reversing the muscarinic blockage.
   a. Indications for physostigmine:
      (1) Supraventricular dysrhythmias resulting in hemodynamic instability.
      (2) Pronounced hallucinations and agitation in which patients may be a danger to themselves or others.
      (3) Coma caused by anticholinergic overdose. Physostigmine should be administered as a diagnostic test and not used just "to wake the patient up."

      NOTE: It is best to reserve physostigmine for life-threatening situations, because safer agents are available for treatment of seizures (phenytoin, phenobarbital, diazepam) and dysrhythmias (alkalinization, phenytoin, lidocaine).
   b. Dosage (administer slowly):
      (1) Children: 0.02 mg/kg/dose up to 0.5 mg/dose IV slowly over 3 minutes q10min up to a total dose of 2 mg.
      (2) Adults: 1 to 2 mg IV slowly over 3 minutes q10min until cessation of life-threatening condition or until it appears ineffective. Maximum dose: 4 mg in 30 minutes.
   c. Side effects include seizures, bradydysrhythmia, asystole, and cholinergic crisis (hypersalivation, bradycardia, and hypotension).
   d. Contraindications: asthma, gangrene, cardiovascular disease, or obstruction of the GI or GU tracts.
3. Initial treatment of seizures with diazepam (Valium), 0.2 to 0.3 mg/kg/dose IV, followed by phenobarbital (see Chapter 21).
4. Treatment of CAD overdoses. If the QRS is prolonged or ventricular dysrhythmias are present, treat with sodium bicarbonate, 1 to 2 mEq/kg/dose q10-20min IV, to achieve alkalinization (plasma pH >7.5), as well as phenytoin or lidocaine (p. 56).
5. Sedation: Can usually be achieved by treatment with diazepam (Valium).
6. Large amounts of naloxone (Narcan), 0.8 to 2.0 mg prn IV, for some cases of diphenoxylate (Lomotil) overdose.

DISPOSITION

All symptomatic patients need inpatient treatment and observation, usually in an intensive care unit (ICU) capable of cardiac and neurologic monitoring.

BIBLIOGRAPHY

Amitai Y, Singer R, Almog S et al: Atropine poisoning in children from automatic injectors during the Gulf Crisis, *Vet Hum Toxicol* 33:360, 1991.

Sennhauser FGH, Schwarz HP: Toxic psychosis from transdermal scopolamine in a child, *Lancet* 2:1033, 1986.

Carbon Monoxide

ALERT Several members of the same household with headache, nausea, or shortness of breath should be evaluated for carbon monoxide exposure.

Carbon monoxide (CO) is an odorless, colorless gas produced by internal combustion engines and by combustion of natural gas, charcoal, and coal gas. Fire victims often have high CO levels after exposure. Methylene chloride (a solvent used in paint strippers) is metabolized to carbon monoxide. Carbon monoxide binds to hemoglobin 210 times more avidly than does oxygen.

DIAGNOSTIC FINDINGS

All potential cases should be evaluated, especially if several members of the same household are experiencing similar symptoms.

Signs and symptoms progress with increased exposure, reflecting the levels of carboxyhemoglobin in the blood. The levels listed below are from data about adults. Children may have a greater susceptibility to CO toxicity. Children with CO levels higher than 25% carboxyhemoglobin (HgCO) consistently showed syncope and lethargy in one study. Symptoms in all patients may correlate more closely with the length of exposure than with the actual, measured carboxyhemoglobin levels. Furthermore, levels may be influenced by significant delays between exposure and presentation, particularly if oxygen therapy has been administered en route.

Complications

1. Cardiac:
   a. Dysrhythmias (see Chapter 6)
   b. Myocardial ischemia with ST-T wave changes (usually only in adults)
2. Pulmonary edema and hemorrhage either immediately or as delayed finding (see Chapter 19)
3. Renal failure secondary to myoglobinuria
4. CNS:
   a. Encephalopathy with associated agitation, seizures, and coma (see Chapters 15 and 21)
   b. Cerebral edema
   c. Long-term neuropsychiatric changes and memory defects if exposure is life threatening

Ancillary Data

1. HgCO level: Normal level is less than 1%, although it has been reported to be as high as 5% in persons who have driven on busy freeways. Heavy smokers may have levels of 15% or occasionally even higher. Fetal hemoglobin can contribute to a falsely elevated HgCO level in infants younger than 30 months.
2. ABG analysis with a measured, not calculated, oxygen saturation. Oximetry is not a reliable indicator of CO poisoning or lack thereof.
3. ECG for a patient with significant exposure or any evidence of myocardial ischemia, chest pain, or shortness of breath.
4. Chest x-ray film in patient with smoke inhalation. Findings often normal in first 24 hours (see Chapter 53).

MANAGEMENT

Although it is clear that hyperbaric oxygen is the treatment of choice for patients in coma from CO poisoning, in part because it produces a more rapid reduction in HgCO level, the level of HgCO requiring such treatment in a patient with no or minimal symptoms is a matter of controversy. Some factors that may be considered are transient loss of consciousness, ischemic changes on ECG, focal neurologic defects, and abnormal psychometric test results. Hyperbaric oxygen may theoretically decrease the long-term neurologic sequelae in patients with such findings. Some experts have suggested that patients with peak HgCO levels greater than 25%, a history of altered level of consciousness or persistent neurologic defect, cardiac abnormality, acidosis, or syncope should be treated in the hyperbaric chamber. The data regarding an absolute level indicating treatment are not available; symptoms may be more important than a specific HgCO level, and there is some inconsistency between the level of carboxyhemoglobin and clinical findings:

HgCO Level in Blood (%)	Common Clinical Findings
10-20	No apparent findings
20-30	Dyspnea (vigorous exertion), dizzy, mild headache, nausea
30-40	Dyspnea, worse headache
40-50	Severe headache, confusion, chest pain
50-60	Altered mentation, dyspnea, irritability, fatigue, dizziness, blurred vision
>60	Syncope, tachycardia, tachypnea, stupor, seizures, coma, cardiac dysrhythmias, death

1. Remove the patient from the source of combustion, and immediately administer high-flow oxygen while continuing resuscitation; 100% oxygen can be delivered through a mask or an endotracheal tube.

   NOTE: The half-life of HgCO at room air is approximately 4 hours; with 100% oxygen, it is approximately 40 minutes. With hyperbaric oxygen (2 atm), the half-life is reduced to less than 20 minutes.
2. Monitor for evolving complications and treat aggressively.

CO exposure in a pregnant woman places the fetus at great risk. The fetus is at relatively increased risk from elevated CO levels. Treatment of a pregnant woman should be continued for at least three times as long as the time recommended for the mother alone. Consultation should be obtained.

DISPOSITION

The following patients should be admitted for prolonged observation and treatment:

1. Those with HgCO levels greater than 20% to 25%. This decision must be individualized.
2. Those with abnormal neurologic findings, ECG findings, or acidosis.
3. Pregnant women with HgCO levels greater than 15%, who need longer oxygen therapy.

Before the patient is discharged, the source of CO must be eliminated. The clinician who suspects CO poisoning should evaluate all household residents if the incident was a household exposure. Long-term follow-up of patients who have been treated with hyperbaric oxygen is indicated to monitor for subtle but lasting memory deficits or personality changes.

BIBLIOGRAPHY

Bozeman WP, Myers RA, Barish RA: Confirmation of the pulse oximetry gap in carbon monoxide poisoning, *Ann Emerg Med* 30:608, 1997.

Buckley RG, Aks SE, Eshom JL et al: The pulse oximetry gap in carbon monoxide intoxication, *Ann Emerg Med* 24:252, 1994.

Hampson NB, Norkool DM: Carbon monoxide poisoning in children riding in the back of pickup trucks, *JAMA* 267:538, 1992.

Olson KR, Seger D: Hyperbaric oxygen from carbon monoxide poisoning: does it really work? *Ann Emerg Med* 25:535, 1995.

Seger D, Welch L: Carbon monoxide controversies: neuropsychologic testing, mechanisms and toxicity and hyperbaric oxygen, *Ann Emerg Med* 24:242, 1994.

Sloan EP, Murphy DG, Hart R et al: Complications and protocol considerations in carbon monoxide: poisoned patients require hyperbaric oxygen therapy: report from a 10-year experience, *Ann Emerg Med* 18:629, 1989.

Thom SR, Taver RL, Mendiguren IL et al: Delayed neuropsychologic sequelae after carbon monoxide poisoning prevention by treatment with hyperbaric oxygen, *Ann Emerg Med* 25:474, 1995.

Tibbles PM, Perrotta PL: Treatment of carbon monoxide poisoning: a critical review of human outcome studies comparing normobaric oxygen with hyperbaric oxygen, *Ann Emerg Med* 24:269, 1994.

Varon J, Marki PE, Fromm RE et al: Carbon monoxide poisoning: a review for clinicians, *J Emerg Med* 17:87, 1999.

Weaver LK, Hopkins RO, Larson-Lohr V: Neuropsychologic and functional recovery from severe carbon monoxide poisoning without hyperbaric oxygen therapy, *Ann Emerg Med* 27:736, 1996.

Cardiovascular Drugs

β-ADRENERGIC BLOCKING AGENTS

The primary indications for β-adrenergic blocking agents include angina, dysrhythmias, hypertension, migraines, glaucoma, and thyrotoxicosis. β-Adrenergic stimulation increases heart rate and cardiac inotropy (β_1) and relaxes bronchial and vascular smooth muscle (β_2). Blockade inhibits these effects and may have a direct myocardial depressant effect as well. Therapeutic doses vary with the individual drug but may include bradycardia, AV conduction defects, hypotension, congestive heart failure, bronchospasm, hypoglycemia, as well as fatigue, depression, and sexual dysfunction. Cardioselective agents (acebutolol, atenolol, metoprolol) cause little bronchospasm; pindolol is rarely associated with bradycardia and hypotension. After significant overdose, however, selectivity is lost, and the toxicities of nonselective and selective agents are similar.

Diagnostic Findings

Signs and symptoms occur with impaired cardiovascular function. Dizziness, syncope, and collapse may occur along with impaired mental status, lethargy, coma, and seizures. Bradycardia and hypotension may be present. Pulmonary edema may be noted.

The ECG may reveal sinus bradycardia and AV conduction defects. Asystole, disappearance of P waves, and widening of the QRS interval may be associated with massive overdose. Serum drug levels do not correlate with the severity of intoxication.

Management

1. Supportive care and monitoring are essential. Evaluate airway and breathing, and manage as appropriate. Gastric lavage may be performed initially. Administer charcoal as early as possible.
2. Treat symptomatic bradycardia initially with atropine, 0.02 mg/kg/dose IV.
3. Hypotension responds to fluids and dopamine, the latter often at very high dosages.
4. Seizures are best managed by diazepam, 0.2 to 0.3 mg/kg/dose IV, followed by standard management (p. 187).
5. Glucagon at high dosages and diluted is effective in a dose of 0.05 to 0.1 mg/kg IV (adult, 3 to 5 mg/dose IV q5min up to a total dose of 10 to 15 mg). Response is rapid but lasts only 10 to 20 minutes; a continuous infusion may be required, for which the initial successful dose is used as the determinant of the rate of infusion, usually in the range of 0.05 to 0.1 mg/kg/hr.

Disposition

Patients who are asymptomatic 6 hours after a trivial ingestion may be discharged. Those with any evidence of cardiovascular or CNS findings and those who have ingested a time-release formulation should usually be admitted.

CALCIUM CHANNEL BLOCKERS

Used increasingly in the management of angina, hypertension, and tachydysrhythmias, calcium channel blocking agents are available for ingestion. These calcium antagonists interfere with the entry of calcium into cells through the slow-calcium voltage-dependent channels. Toxicity is due to hypoperfusion associated with vasodilation, negative inotropism, and cardiac dysrhythmias.

Diagnostic Findings

Myocardial hypoperfusion may cause angina and evidence of ischemia. Mental status may be altered; focal neurologic findings (including hemiparesis) have been noted. Coma and seizures may occur.

ECG may demonstrate bradycardia, asystole, inverted P waves, tachycardia, conduction abnormalities, QRS prolongation, and nonspecific ST and T changes.

Management

1. Stabilize patient and begin gastric lavage if ingestion was very recent. Activated charcoal should be given as quickly as possible. Patients require constant monitoring.
2. Intravenous calcium chloride (10% solution), 25 mg/kg (maximum: 1 g) over 3 to 5 minutes followed by an infusion, may be used in unstable patients.
3. Vasodilation may respond to fluids and dopamine or other catecholamines.
4. There is preliminary evidence that insulin infusions with dextrose improve hemodynamics after calcium channel blocker overdose. This treatment should be considered in critically ill patients, but hypoglycemia must be avoided.

Disposition

Patients who are asymptomatic 8 hours after a trivial ingestion of a non–modified-release agent may be discharged. All others require ongoing monitoring.

CLONIDINE

Clonidine (Catapres) is the most common cardiovascular drug associated with pediatric ingestions. It is a central and peripheral α_2-adrenergic agonist used in the management of hypertension. The half-life is 9 hours.

Diagnostic Findings

Signs and symptoms that usually develop within 1 hour of ingestion include impaired level of consciousness, bradycardia, respiratory depression, miosis, hypotension, hypertension, and hypothermia. Hypotension may appear as a delayed finding. Symptoms and signs may mimic a narcotic overdose.

Laboratory studies are not useful except those obtained to maximize supportive care.

Management

Supportive care, gastric lavage (if performed very early), and charcoal therapy should be initiated. Hypotension may respond to fluids and dopamine; hypertension is transient and usually does not require therapy. In severe cases, it may be treated with a short-acting vasodilator such as nitroprusside, 0.5 to 10 μg/kg/min IV. Naloxone, 2 mg IV, supplemented by an IV infusion may have a beneficial role.

All children must be monitored for at least 4 hours. Symptomatic patients should be admitted.

DIGITALIS

Digoxin is widely used in the effort to improve cardiac inotropy, concurrently affecting electrical activity. Digitalis raises the level of intracellular calcium, promoting the initiation of muscle contraction. Excessive levels may result from dosing problems, decreased digoxin elimination (renal failure or drug interaction with quinidine, calcium channel blockers, or spironolactone), or decreased volume of distribution (starvation, muscle wasting). Toxicity can occur at therapeutic levels associated with hypokalemia, hypercalcemia, hypernatremia, alkalosis, hypoxia, hypomagnesemia, nodal disease, and primary cardiac diseases such as ischemia, cor pulmonale, and cardiac trauma or surgery.

Clinical presentation and management are discussed on p. 153. The dose of digoxin immune antibody fragment (ovine) (Digibind or DigiFab) is calculated on the basis of the body burden of digitalis.

BIBLIOGRAPHY

Heidemann SM, Sarnaik AP: Clonidine poisoning in children, *Crit Care Med* 18:618, 1990.

Love JN: Beta blocker toxicity: a clinical diagnosis, *Am J Emerg Med* 12:356, 1994.

Weiner DA: Calcium channel blockers, *Med Clin North Am* 72:83, 1988.

Wiley JF, Wiley CC, Torrey SB et al: Clonidine poisoning in young children, *J Pediatr* 116:654, 1990.

Woolf AD, Wendger T, Smith TW et al: The use of digoxin-specific Fab fragments for severe digitalis intoxication in children, *N Engl J Med* 326:1734, 1992.

Zaritsky AL, Horowitz M, Chernow B: Glucagon antagonism of calcium channel blocker-induced myocardial dysfunction, *Crit Care Med* 16:246, 1988.

Cocaine (p. 397)

ALERT Cardiovascular dysrhythmias and CNS stimulation must be monitored.

Cocaine may be used as an anesthetic, but it is often abused, causing sympathomimetic effects, CNS stimulation, and euphoria. Methods of administration are insufflation (30% to 60% absorption), intravenous use, smoking of the free base (onset of symptoms is in seconds), and oral ingestion. Cocaine may be teratogenic.

DIAGNOSTIC FINDINGS

The major findings in cocaine ingestion (Table 55-3) reflect sympathomimetic stimulation, which produces dilated pupils, tachycardia, dysphoric agitation, and respiratory stimulation. Chest pain, secondary to coronary

TABLE 55-3 Sympathomimetic Syndrome: Common Clinical Findings

Clinical Findings	Amphetamines	Cocaine (p. 397)	β-Adrenergic Agents
Central nervous system			
Stimulation	Yes	Yes	Yes
Hallucination	Yes	Yes	Yes
Seizures	Yes	Yes	
Coma	Yes	Yes	
Cardiovascular			
Tachycardia	Yes	Yes	
Dysrhythmias	Yes	Yes	Yes
Hypertension	Yes	Yes	Yes
Chest pain	Yes	Yes	
Nausea, vomiting, abdominal pain	Yes		Yes
Mydriasis	Yes	Yes	Yes
Hyperthermia	Yes	Yes	
Other	Intracranial hemorrhage, self-destructive behavior		

vasoconstriction and increased thrombogenesis, is reported.

Complications

1. Cardiovascular dysrhythmias, myocardial ischemia
2. Intestinal ischemia
3. Hypertensive emergency
4. Hyperthermia
5. Pneumomediastinum
6. Intracranial hemorrhage
7. Rhabdomyolysis
8. Seizures
9. Cardiovascular collapse

MANAGEMENT

After stabilization and initiation of monitoring, specific problems may also need to be treated:

1. Seizures (see Chapter 21): Use diazepam (Valium), lorazepam (Ativan), or phenytoin.
2. Dysrhythmias (see Chapter 6): Use phenytoin initially. Consider cardioversion. Tachydysrhythmic patients with hypertension may be treated with labetalol (0.25 mg/kg IV over 2 minutes and titrated). Esmolol may also be helpful. Benzodiazepines decrease myocardial oxygen consumption.
3. Hypertension is appropriately treated with phentolamine.
4. Decontamination:
   a. Nasal: Clean nasal passage with cotton applicator dipped in a non–water-soluble product such as petrolatum.
   b. GI: Give activated charcoal.

BIBLIOGRAPHY

Cravey RH: Cocaine deaths in infants, *J Anal Toxicol* 12:354, 1988.

Derlet RW, Albertson TE: Emergency department presentation of cocaine intoxication, *Ann Emerg Med* 18:182, 1989.

Garland JS, Smith DS, Rice TB et al: Accidental cocaine intoxication in a nine-month-old infant: presentation and treatment, *Pediatr Emerg Care* 5:245, 1989.

Hollander JE: Management of cocaine associated myocardial ischemia, *N Engl J Med* 333:1267, 1995.

Lyons Jones K: Developmental pathogenesis of defects associated with prenatal cocaine exposure: fetal vascular disruption, *Clin Perinatol* 18:139, 1991.

Cyclic Antidepressants

ALERT Anticholinergic effects and cardiotoxicity are prominent. Immediate intervention is necessary.

Cyclic antidepressants are a widely used class of medications. Beyond their use as antidepressants, they are popular in the treatment of enuresis (e.g., imipramine). Their major toxicity is from their anticholinergic and quinidine-like effects. Plasma CAD levels do not correlate with toxicity. Tricyclic antidepressants (TCAs), one type of this class of drugs, are lipophilic. TCAs may cross the placental barrier, although teratogenicity is not documented.

ETIOLOGY

Imipramine (Tofranil), amitriptyline (Elavil), desipramine (Norpramin), doxepin (Sinequan), and nortriptyline (Pamelor) are commonly used.

DIAGNOSTIC FINDINGS

Anticholinergic effects, both peripheral and central, may be prominent and usually develop within 6 hours (p. 374):

1. Peripheral findings include dry, flushed skin, dry mucous membranes, dilated pupils, and urinary retention, with decreased bowel sounds. Tachycardia, dysrhythmias, hyperpyrexia, and hypertension may be present.
2. Central effects: Patients have delirium with disorientation, agitation, hallucinations, and movement disorders. Seizures and coma are common.

Dysrhythmias result from the anticholinergic effects of TCAs and from direct cardiotoxicity, blockage of norepinephrine uptake, and a quinidine-like action (myocardial depression and AV conduction delay). Supraventricular tachydysrhythmias, conduction blocks, and ventricular dysrhythmias are common, although their onset may be delayed. The best correlate with risk of seizures is a QRS equal to or greater than 0.10 second, whereas ventricular dysrhythmias occur when it is 0.16 second or more.

TCA ingestion in a dose <5 mg/kg generally does not cause significant toxicity in children 6 years or younger, although each encounter must be individualized.

Hypotension is common, secondary to myocardial depression and alpha blockade. Patients with fatal ingestion may exhibit trivial signs and symptoms that may rapidly progress to coma, conduction defects, dysrhythmias, hypotension, and seizures.

Ancillary Data

1. CAD blood level. Although unreliable as an indicator of potential toxicity, documentation of the drug's presence with toxicology screens may be important. Toxicology screens are not of predictive value regarding complications.
2. ECG in all patients; oximetry, ABG analysis, and serum glucose measurements as indicated.

DIFFERENTIAL DIAGNOSIS

Intoxications must be differentiated from anticholinergic and quinidine reactions.

MANAGEMENT

1. Life support is crucial because of the potential for respiratory depression and hemodynamic compromise. Upon the patient's arrival, oxygen therapy and cardiac monitoring should be started, and IV access should be established. Administer dextrose and naloxone as indicated by mental status.
2. Perform gastric emptying (only by lavage, and only if performed very early); give charcoal as soon as possible.
3. Patients with prolongation of the QRS or ventricular dysrhythmias should receive alkalinization with $NaHCO_3$, 1 to 2 mEq/kg/dose IV q10-20min prn, to maintain a plasma pH of 7.5 or greater. The pH may be maintained in this range with an infusion of 150 mEq $NaHCO_3$ in one liter of 5% dextrose in water (D5W). This agent appears to be prophylactic in preventing progression of dysrhythmias.
   - Ventricular dysrhythmias or conduction delays (QRS >0.16 second) should be treated with phenytoin (Dilantin), 5 mg/kg as a loading dose IV and then with maintenance doses. This agent

also has the advantage of being an anticonvulsant. Lidocaine also may be used (see Chapter 6).

4. Physostigmine is effective as a treatment for the anticholinergic effects; its use should be reserved for situations in which other modalities have failed (p. 376).
   a. Dosage: children, 0.02 mg/kg/dose up to 0.5 mg/dose IV slowly over 3 minutes q10min up to a total dose of 2 mg; adult, 1 to 2 mg IV slowly over 3 minutes q10min until life-threatening condition ceases or the agent is ineffective. Maximum dose: 4 mg in 30 minutes.
   b. Indicated for hemodynamically unstable supraventricular dysrhythmias and also for behavior that is potentially harmful. It is best to reserve physostigmine for life-threatening situations because there are safer agents for treatment of seizures (phenytoin, phenobarbital, diazepam) and dysrhythmias (phenytoin, alkalinization, lidocaine).
5. Seizures should be treated initially with diazepam (Valium), 0.25 mg/kg/dose IV q10min prn (see Chapter 21).
6. Coma usually requires supportive care but is self-limited and is not an indication for physostigmine.
7. Hypotension may respond to fluid challenge. If the challenge is unsuccessful, use norepinephrine as the pressor agent (see Chapter 5).

DISPOSITION

All patients must be monitored for at least 6 hours after ingestion. Significant ingestions or symptomatic patients with CAD overdose must be admitted to an ICU for treatment and cardiac monitoring. Those with minimal ingestions who are asymptomatic after 6 hours may be discharged if they have bowel sounds and have been given cathartics and charcoal. Appropriate psychiatric evaluation should also be completed if the ingestion was deliberate. Follow-up observation is necessary.

BIBLIOGRAPHY

Boehnert MT, Lovejoy FH: Value of the QRS duration versus the serum drug level in predicting seizures and ventricular arrhythmias after an acute overdose of tricyclic antidepressants, *N Engl J Med* 313:474, 1985.

Ellison DR, Pentel PR: Clinical features and consequences of seizures due to cyclic antidepressant overdose, *Am J Emerg Med* 7:5, 1989.

Liebelt EL, Francis PD, Woolf AD: ECG lead a VR versus QRS interval in predicting seizures and arrhythmias in acute tricyclic antidepressant toxicity, *Ann Emerg Med* 26:195, 1995.

Niemann JT, Bessen HA, Rothstein RJ et al: Electrocardiographic criteria for tricyclic antidepressant cardiotoxicity, *Am J Cardiol* 57:1154, 1986.

Phillips S, Brent J, Kulig K et al: Fluoxetine versus tricyclic antidepressants: a prospective multicenter study of antidepressant drug overdoses, *J Emerg Med* 15:439, 1997.

Stremski ES, Brady WB, Prasad K et al: Pediatric carbamazepine, *Ann Emerg Med* 25:624, 1995.

Tokarski GF, Young MJ: Criteria for admitting patients with tricyclic antidepressant overdose, *J Emerg Med* 6:121, 1988.

Hallucinogens: Phencyclidine, LSD, Mescaline

ALERT Differentiate from other entities causing hallucinations

A wide variety of agents produce hallucinogenic states. Phencyclidine (PCP, angel dust), lysergic acid diethylamine (LSD, acid), and mescaline (buttons, peyote, cactus) produce similar behavioral changes, although their systemic effects are markedly different. Hallucinogens may be ingested along with other drugs, altering the presentation markedly.

DIAGNOSTIC FINDINGS

Phencyclidine (PCP)

Children younger than 5 years have symptoms different from those of older patients:

1. Bizarre behavior, including lethargy, staring spells, intermittent unresponsiveness, irritability, and poor feeding
2. CNS findings that may progress to coma—commonly ataxia, nystagmus, opisthotonos, and hyperreflexia

3. Tachypnea, tachycardia, and hypertension

Older patients have a progression of symptoms with increasing dosage:

1. Low doses (<5 mg) induce associated agitation, excitement, disorganized thought process, incoordination, nystagmus, blank-stare appearance, and intoxication with drowsiness and apathy.
2. Moderate doses (5 to 10 mg or 0.1 to 0.2 mg/kg) often induce stupor or coma, decreased peripheral sensation, muscular rigidity, myoclonus, nystagmus, flushing, hypersalivation, and vomiting.
3. Large doses (>10 mg) cause coma with seizures, decerebrate posturing, hypertension, nystagmus, opisthotonos, hypersalivation, and diaphoresis.

Lysergic Acid (LSD)

Effect lasts for 4 to 12 hours with an accompanying hallucinogenic state. The pupils are usually massively dilated. LSD may produce permanent psychosis in susceptible individuals and flashbacks months after the initial ingestion.

Ancillary Data

1. Order urine toxicology screen, analysis for PCP, and other studies indicated for support.
2. Let the laboratory know if phencyclidine is suspected because many urine screens do not specifically examine for it.

DIFFERENTIAL DIAGNOSIS

1. Intoxication:
   a. Sedative/hypnotics: do not generally cause hypertension or hyperreflexia. Respirations are usually decreased.
   b. Anticholinergics: There are prominent peripheral and central findings. May cause hallucinations.
   c. Stimulants: Tachycardia, hypertension, and piloerection are more prominent.
2. Encephalitis, meningitis, Reye syndrome, or high fever
3. Acute psychosis

MANAGEMENT

Supportive care is essential, and associated drug ingestion should be considered.

1. Administration of dextrose and naloxone as indicated.
2. Activated charcoal.
3. Diuresis: Acidifying the urine is not recommended because doing so may raise the risk of precipitating myoglobin crystals in the urine if rhabdomyolysis has occurred.

For agitated and hallucinating patients:

1. Avoid physical restraints, if possible.
2. With PCP, reduce stimuli.
3. Try to maintain verbal contact and reassure the patient.
4. Consult a psychiatrist for acute and long-term care.

If sedation is necessary, use diazepam (Valium) or midazolam (Versed). Hypertensive crisis may require treatment (see Chapter 18).

DISPOSITION

Most patients with significant findings need to be hospitalized for medical or psychiatric management.

BIBLIOGRAPHY

Farrar HC, Kearns GL: Cocaine: clinical pharmacology and toxicology, *J Pediatr* 115:665, 1989.

Kulig K: LSD, *Emerg Med Clin North Am* 8:551, 1990.

Tokarsk GF, Paganussi P, Urbanski R et al: An evaluation of cocaine-induced chest pain, *Ann Emerg Med* 19:1088, 1990.

Hydrocarbons

ALERT Pulmonary and CNS findings predominate, and specific guidelines for emesis or gastric lavage should be followed.

The ingestion of hydrocarbons is a common occurrence in children, but management remains controversial. The toxicity of hydrocarbons varies with the relative viscosity (expressed as SSU, the number of seconds for a quantity of liquid to pass through a standard aperture) and additives. The lower the viscosity, the higher the risk of pulmonary aspiration; certain additives have significant toxicity of their own.

ETIOLOGY

1. Viscosity (SSU):
   a. Less than 60 SSU: gasoline, turpentine, benzene, kerosene, mineral seal oil (furniture polish)
   b. Less than 100 SSU: lubricating grease, diesel oil, mothballs, paraffin
2. Toxic additives; "CHAMP" is a useful mnemonic:
   a. Camphor causes CNS excitement or depression.
   b. *H*alogenated hydrocarbons (i.e., carbon tetrachloride) produce hepatitis, nephritis, diarrhea, and CNS excitement or depression.
   c. *A*romatic (benzene) results in aplastic anemia, dysrhythmias, and CNS and respiratory depression.
   d. *M*etals (heavy metals such as mercury) result in GI bleeding, renal failure, and neurologic sequelae.
   e. *P*esticides, primarily organophosphates, also cause cholinergic signs and symptoms (p. 363).

DIAGNOSTIC FINDINGS

Diagnostic findings depend on the amount ingested (one swallow in a child is about 4 ml), the material ingested (container should be examined), and the time elapsed since the ingestion. Findings include the following:

1. Coughing, dyspnea, and choking accompany the initial ingestion.
2. Pulmonary symptoms may be delayed up to 6 hours; include tachypnea, wheezing, and respiratory distress. The pneumonitis produces a fever that does not necessarily reflect a bacterial infection.
3. CNS depression or excitement.
4. Nausea, vomiting, and abdominal pain.
5. Pulmonary edema and dysrhythmias (see Chapters 6 and 19).
6. Cyanosis developing shortly after ingestion. May be associated with a toxin that causes methemoglobinemia.
7. Toluene (glue or paint sniffing) produces psychiatric disturbances, CNS depression, abdominal pain, dysrhythmias, or renal tubular acidosis with associated hypokalemia and acidosis.

Ancillary Data

1. CBC. May demonstrate leukocytosis. Electrolyte measurements are indicated if toluene inhalation is suspected.
2. ABG analysis or pulse oximetry.
3. X-ray studies. Chest film findings are abnormal in 90% of symptomatic patients, usually with a multilobar fluffy infiltrate. These findings may be delayed. Pulmonary edema may be present.
4. Other studies as indicated, including red blood cell (RBC) cholinesterase measurement and ECG.

MANAGEMENT

Initial management should include stabilization, with administration of oxygen, and decontamination of the patient by removal of clothing and washing of the skin. Associated findings require treatment.

Indications for gastric emptying are controversial. At present they include the following: severe GI or CNS symptoms, and hydrocarbon that contains one of the "CHAMP" additives (Fig. 55-2). Intubation and protection of the airway should be considered before lavage.

Steroids and antibiotics are not indicated for prophylaxis.

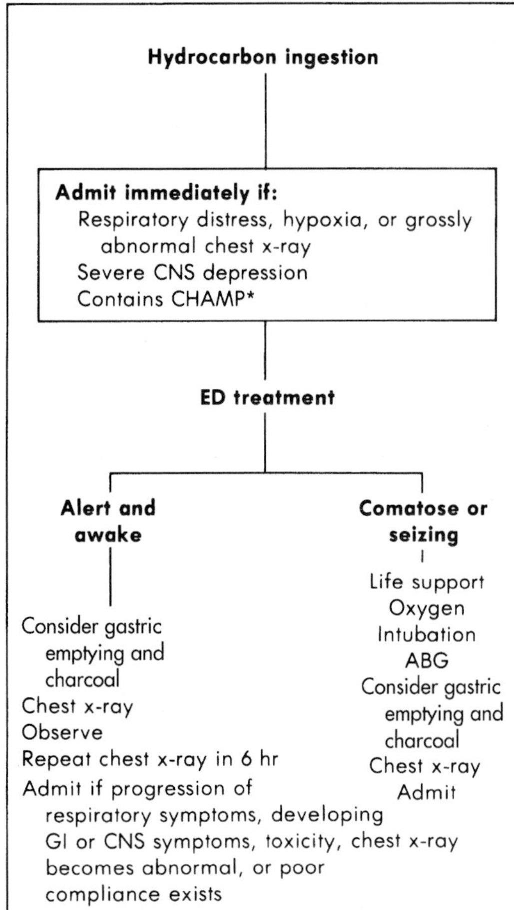

Hydrocarbon ingestion
Admit immediately if:
Respiratory distress, hypoxia, or grossly abnormal chest x-ray
Severe CNS depression
Contains CHAMP*
ED treatment
Alert and awake
Comatose or seizing
Consider gastric emptying and charcoal
Chest x-ray
Observe
Repeat chest x-ray in 6 hr
Admit if progression of respiratory symptoms, developing GI or CNS symptoms, toxicity, chest x-ray becomes abnormal, or poor compliance exists
Life support
Oxygen
Intubation
ABG
Consider gastric emptying and charcoal
Chest x-ray
Admit

Fig. 55-2 Management of hydrocarbon ingestion. *Camphor, halogenated, aromatic (benzene), metals (heavy), pesticides (organophosphates). Most of the common hydrocarbons ingested (e.g., gasoline, kerosene, oil) need not be removed regardless of the volume swallowed.

DISPOSITION

Patients must be admitted in accordance with the protocol outlined in Fig. 55-2. Before the patient is discharged, poison-prevention counseling is required, and long-term follow-up observation of pulmonary status should be arranged.

BIBLIOGRAPHY

Anene O, Costello FV: Myocardial dysfunction after hydrocarbon ingestion, *Crit Care Med* 22:529, 1994.

Zucker AR, Berger S, Wood LD: Management of kerosene induced pulmonary injury, *Crit Care Med* 14:303, 1986.

Iron

ALERT GI symptoms are followed by shock, acidosis, and liver failure. Rapid treatment is required.

Normal daily dietary iron intake is about 15 mg, of which 10% is absorbed. It is then transported in the plasma bound to ferritin. The elemental iron content of the ingested substance is a good measure of potential toxicity. Ferrous sulfate contains 20% elemental iron; ferrous gluconate, 12%; and ferrous fumarate, 33%. Normally the serum iron (SI) is 50 to 100 µg/dl, and the total iron-binding capacity (TIBC) of ferritin is 300 to 400 µg/dl. An ingestion of 60 mg/kg of elemental iron is considered dangerous. Ingestion of less than 20 mg/kg of elementary iron is rarely symptomatic.

DIAGNOSTIC FINDINGS

Toxicity from an iron ingestion has a fairly classic pattern of progression unless intervention is timely.

1. Stage 1: initial period (to 6 hours after ingestion). Vomiting, hematemesis, diarrhea, hematochezia, and abdominal pain occur.
2. Stage 2: latent period (2 to 12 hours). The patient improves.
3. Stage 3: systemic toxicity 4 to 24 hours after ingestion. Shock, metabolic acidosis, fever, hyperglycemia, bleeding, and death may occur.
4. Stage 4: hepatic failure beginning at 48 to 96 hours. This is associated with seizures and coma, and the patient has a poor prognosis.
5. Stage 5: late sequelae of pyloric stenosis may develop at 2 to 5 weeks.

Ancillary Data

1. Levels of SI and TIBC should be ascertained:
   a. Peak SI less than 350 μg/dl is rarely symptomatic.
   b. Peak levels greater than 500 μg/dl are considered toxic; most patients should undergo chelation.
   c. The presence of diarrhea, vomiting, leukocytosis, hyperglycemia, or a positive abdominal radiograph result is predictive of an SI greater than 300 μg/dl.
   d. Evidence now suggests that the relative relationship between the SI and the TIBC should not be used as the sole basis for deciding to use deferoxamine, because the TIBC is artificially increased in the presence of iron poisoning; nevertheless, patients in whom the SI is greater than the TIBC require careful evaluation for chelation.
2. Immediate release products peak at 2 to 4 hours; modified-release preparations may have a later peak.
3. If an SI level is not readily obtainable, the deferoxamine provocation test may be useful for asymptomatic patients. Either dose of 90 mg/kg IM or 1 hour of IV infusion at 15 mg/kg/hr IV is given. Rose coloration of the urine within 1 to 3 hours indicates the presence of free iron and feroxamine complex and is an indication for further treatment with deferoxamine.
4. Other data include the following:
   a. CBC, electrolyte and glucose levels, liver function tests, and ABG analysis with significant ingestion.
   b. X-ray film: abdominal flat plate. Should be obtained as soon as possible. The presence of intact tablets in the stomach mandates aggressive therapy for their removal.

DIFFERENTIAL DIAGNOSIS

1. Infection:
   a. Acute gastroenteritis (see Chapter 76)
   b. Hepatitis (p. 649)
2. Gastrointestinal bleeding (see Chapter 35)
3. Shock (see Chapter 5)

MANAGEMENT

Management should reflect the amount of iron ingested; the clinical status of the child in terms of problems with GI, CNS, or vital signs problems; and laboratory data.

Initial fluid and acid-base resuscitation is imperative when it is indicated. Shock, GI hemorrhage, and significant metabolic acidosis may be present. After initial measures are taken, the patient should undergo gastric lavage. Emesis or lavage to reduce or eliminate absorption is important. Some recommend adding some bicarbonate or deferoxamine to the lavage fluid. Radiographs should be taken as soon as possible to detect undissolved tablets (a second radiograph should be taken after lavage if tablets were present initially).

1. Patients with peak SI less than 350 μg/dl require no further treatment if TIBC is greater than 350 μg/dl.
2. Patients with SI greater than TIBC (see preceding note) or with SI greater than 350 μg/dl for whom TIBC is unavailable should be treated with IV or IM deferoxamine if symptomatic.
3. Patients with SI greater than or equal to 500 μg/dl should be treated immediately, with monitoring of electrolytes, hematocrit, and ABG analysis:
   a. For patients in shock or coma, give deferoxamine at 15 mg/kg/hr for 8 hours IV or as long as the urine remains rose colored. Start slowly and work up to this infusion rate over the first 15 to 30 minutes. In some cases, a higher dosage of IV deferoxamine may be used.

b. If patient is less seriously ill, give 90 mg/kg/dose IM q8hr.

Deferoxamine, 100 mg, can chelate 8.5 mg of elemental iron. It is contraindicated in renal failure and in patients shown to be sensitive to it.

1. Rapid IV administration of deferoxamine may cause hypotension, facial flushing, rash, urticaria, tachycardia, and shock. Give slowly.
2. If an SI value is unavailable or delayed and the patient is symptomatic, give deferoxamine, 90 mg/kg/dose IM, and repeat q8hr.
3. An exchange transfusion may be indicated in cases of life-threatening iron toxicity.

If the x-ray study demonstrates the presence of iron past the pylorus, whole-bowel irrigation can be useful with solutions such as polyethylene glycol electrolyte lavage solution. Surgical removal of the iron is rarely needed.

DISPOSITION

Asymptomatic patients with peak SI less than 350 μg/dl may be discharged after poison-prevention counseling.

All patients treated with deferoxamine should be admitted for observation and treatment. Such patients require follow-up observation after discharge to monitor long-term sequelae.

BIBLIOGRAPHY

Burkhart KK, Kulig KW, Hammond KB et al: The rise in the total iron binding capacity after iron overdose, *Ann Emerg Med* 20:532, 1991.

Gomez HF, McClafferty HH, Flory D et al: Prevention of gastrointestinal iron absorption by chelation from an orally administered premixed deferoxamine/charcoal slurry, *Ann Emerg Med* 30:587, 1997.

Schaubein JL, Augestein L, Cox J et al: Iron poisoning: report of three cases and a review of therapeutic intervention, *J Emerg Med* 8:309, 1990.

Tenenbein M: Whole bowel irrigation in iron poisoning, *J Pediatr* 111:142, 1987.

Tenenbein M, Yatschoff RW: The total iron binding capacity in iron poisoning, *Am J Dis Child* 145:437, 1991.

Narcotics and Sedative-Hypnotics

ALERT CNS and respiratory depression and hypotension are prominent.

Narcotics and sedative-hypnotics in overdoses consistently produce CNS and respiratory depression along with hypotension. Aggressive supportive care is the key to treatment.

ETIOLOGY

1. Narcotics:
   a. Heroin (skag, dope, horse)
   b. Morphine
   c. Codeine
   d. Meperidine (Demerol)
   e. Methadone
   f. Propoxyphene (Darvon)
   g. Diphenoxylate (Lomotil)
   h. Hydrocodone
   i. Oxycodone
2. Barbiturates:
   a. Long-acting (onset: 1 hour; peak: 6 hours; duration: days): phenobarbital
   b. Intermediate-acting (onset: 1 hour; peak: 3 to 6 hours; duration: 6 to 8 hours): amobarbital, butabarbital
   c. Short-acting (onset: minutes; peak: 3 hours; duration: 4 to 8 hours): pentobarbital, secobarbital
   d. Ultra–short-acting (onset: seconds; peak: seconds; duration: minutes): thiopental
3. Sedative-hypnotics:
   a. Benzodiazepines: chlordiazepoxide (Librium), diazepam (Valium)
   b. Cyclic ether: paraldehyde (Paral)
   c. Alcohols: chloral hydrate, ethchlorvynol (Placidyl)
   d. Propanediol carbamates: meprobamate (Miltown, Equanil)
   e. Piperidinediones: glutethimide (Doriden), methyprylon (Noludar)
   f. Quinazolines: methaqualone (Quaalude)

DIAGNOSTIC FINDINGS

Patients with overdoses of narcotics or sedative-narcotics demonstrate variable levels of CNS depression with associated respiratory impairment (Table 55-4). Other findings are outlined in Table 55-3. Associated ingestions may change the presentation.

Ancillary Data

1. Toxicologic measurements: Send urine and blood to analysis for all patients whose diagnosis is uncertain. Notify the laboratory as to which drugs are suspected.
2. Electrolyte and serum glucose measurements, CBC, and ABG analysis as indicated.
3. X-ray film: abdominal flat plate if chloral hydrate is suspected (radiopaque).
4. Other studies to exclude differential diagnostic considerations.

DIFFERENTIAL DIAGNOSIS

See Chapter 15.

MANAGEMENT

1. Good supportive care is of primary importance, with particular attention to the airway, ventilation, and circulation:
   a. For all patients with impaired mental status or respiratory function, oxygen,

TABLE 55-4 Narcotics and Sedative-Hypnotic Overdose: Clinical Findings and Treatment*

	Narcotics	Sedative-Hypnotics	Barbiturates
FINDINGS			
CNS			
Depressed/coma	Yes	Yes	Yes
Seizures (associated drugs)	Meperidine, propoxyphene	Methaqualone, meprobamate	Butabarbital, pentobarbital, secobarbital
Cardiovascular			
Hypotension/shock	Yes	Yes	Yes
Dysrhythmias	No	Chloral hydrate, haloperidol, meprobamate	No
Miosis	Yes (not meperidine)	Variable	Variable
Respiratory			
Depression	Yes	Yes	Yes
Pulmonary edema	Yes	Meprobamate, ethchlorvynol, paraldehyde	Yes
Anticholinergic	Lomotil (early)	Glutethimide, OTC sleep medications	No
Other	Analgesia (GI, GU motility; bronchoconstriction)	Paraldehyde—acute renal failure	Cutaneous bullae
MANAGEMENT			
Support	Yes	Yes	Yes
Charcoal	Yes	Yes	Yes
Antidote	Naloxone	No*	No
Diuresis	No	No	Phenobarbital (alkaline)
Dialysis	No	No	Phenobarbital

* Flumazenil for benzodiazepines.

cardiac monitor, and IV lines should be established.

   b. D50W, 0.5 to 1 g dextrose (1 to 2 ml)/kg/dose IV, often diluted; and naloxone, 0.1 mg/kg/dose up to 2 mg/dose. If no response, 2 mg (5 adult vials) IV should be given to all patients with altered mental status.

2. Gastric emptying, by lavage, may be indicated in patients with impaired mental status after very recent oral overdose. Give activated charcoal as early as possible.
3. For narcotic overdoses, administer naloxone (Narcan, 0.1 mg/kg/dose up to 2 mg) IV. Propoxyphene (Darvon) and pentazocine (Talwin) overdoses may require larger than usual amounts of naloxone for adequate reversal of effects. If a response to naloxone occurs, a continuous infusion may be indicated. Naloxone infusion should never replace careful observation and support. Use with caution after oral overdose; the effective half-life of naloxone is 30 to 60 minutes.
4. Benzodiazepine-induced respiratory depression and coma may be reversed by the antidote flumazenil (Romazicon) with an onset of effect of 1 to 2 minutes and an effective duration of 1 to 4 hours. The adult dose is 0.2 mg; dose may be repeated up to a total cumulative dose of 3 mg. The total dose may be repeated to 5 mg if there is only a partial response to 3 mg. The dose in children has not been well established, but 0.01mg/kg (max: 0.2 mg) for two doses has been suggested. Other authorities have recommended that this dose may be repeated every minute to a maximum total cumulative dose of 1 mg. Flumazenil should not be given if the patient has a seizure disorder or increased intracranial pressure, or has also overdosed on a TCA.
5. Alkaline diuresis may enhance excretion of phenobarbital. Urine flow should be established at 3 to 6 ml/kg/hr by giving an initial flush of 0.9% normal saline (NS) or lactated Ringer's solution (LR) at 20 ml/kg and then $NaHCO_3$, 1 to 2 mEq/kg/dose over 60 minutes with K^+ supplements as necessary. Fluids should be infused at twice the maintenance level. Urine pH should be 7.5 or greater. Dialysis or hemoperfusion is rarely required. Hourly intake and output should be measured.
6. Serial doses of activated charcoal (adults: 20 to 50 g q2-4hr PO) in 70% sorbitol increase the elimination of oral or intravenous phenobarbital, but the effect on the clinical course is unclear. Mixing every other dose with a cathartic may be beneficial.
7. Dialysis may be useful in severe phenobarbital ingestions.
8. Associated ingestions should be treated as necessary.

DISPOSITION

All patients with significant overdoses should be hospitalized, and after medical clearance, psychiatric consultation should be sought.

BIBLIOGRAPHY

Lewis JM, Klein-Schwartz W, Benson BE et al: Continuous naloxone infusion in pediatric narcotic overdose, *Am J Dis Child* 138:944, 1984.

Pond SM, Olson ICR, Osterloah JD et al: Randomized study of the treatment of phenobarbital overdose with repeated doses of activated charcoal, *JAMA* 251:3104, 1984.

Organophosphates and Carbamates

ALERT The classic cholinergic syndrome is recognized with the mnemonic "SLUDGE" (*s*alivation, *l*acrimation, *u*rination, *d*efecation, *G*I cramping, and *e*mesis).

Organophosphate pesticides are widely used and produce the classic cholinergic syndrome by the inhibition of acetylcholinesterase. There are many different organophosphates with widely varying toxicities, including chlorthion, parathion, diazinon, malathion, TEPP, OMPA, and systox. Parathion is 600 times more toxic than malathion, the latter being used for household purposes. Carbamates have similar uses as insecticides but are less toxic, partially because the carbamate-cholinesterase bond is reversible, and symptoms are of shorter duration (about 24 hours). Absorption is primarily through the skin and gastrointestinal tract.

DIAGNOSTIC FINDINGS

The symptoms of cholinergic syndrome are usually evident within hours of exposure (Table 55-5).

Specific findings reflect excessive acetylcholine:

1. Muscarinic (parasympathomimetic) findings:
   a. Sweat glands: increased sweating
   b. Lacrimal glands: increased lacrimation
   c. GU: urinary incontinence
   d. GI: anorexia, nausea, emesis, diarrhea, fecal incontinence
   e. Eye: miosis, blurred vision
   f. Bronchial: bronchoconstriction, pulmonary edema
   g. Cardiovascular: bradycardia, hypotension
2. Nicotinic (motor) findings:
   a. Striated muscle: fasciculations, cramping, weakness, hyperreflexia.
   b. Long-term peripheral neuropathy may be seen after serious exposure.
3. CNS: restlessness, ataxia, seizures, depression of respiratory and cardiovascular centers, emotional lability, impaired memory, confusion, coma

Ancillary Data

1. CBC, measurement of electrolytes, blood urea nitrogen (BUN), and glucose, liver function tests, PT, and ABG analysis.
2. Chest x-ray film if evidence of pulmonary edema, and ECG for dysrhythmias.
3. Serum cholinesterase level is a more sensitive but less specific indicator of organophosphate poisoning than is RBC cholinesterase level and will return to normal without treatment weeks after exposure. RBC cholinesterase regenerates at 1% or less per day and can require 3 to 4 months to regenerate.

   However, determination of these levels is only rarely available to the physician soon enough to make a difference in treatment and may not correlate directly with the clinical status of the patient. Such determinations are particularly useful in cases of chronic exposure, for which it is desirable to know whether

TABLE 55-5 Organophosphate Exposure: Clinical Manifestations and Management

Serum Cholinesterase Level*	Clinical Manifestations	Management
>50%	Usually none	Observe in hospital
20%-50%	Fatigue, headache, numbness, salivation, wheezing, abdominal pain	Atropinization Pralidoxime (2-PAM)
10%-20%	Weakness, dysarthria, muscle fasciculations, plus above	Atropinization Pralidoxime (2-PAM)
<10%	Miosis, loss of pupillary reflex, flaccid paralysis, pulmonary edema, plus above	Atropinization Pralidoxime (2-PAM) (multiple doses)

* Clinical manifestations rather than the serum cholinesterase level should be used in determining management in acute situations. Percentages best compared with baseline.

further protection from the organophosphate is needed.

DIFFERENTIAL DIAGNOSIS

1. Intoxication: physostigmine, neostigmine, pyridostigmine, edrophonium (Tensilon)
2. Noncardiogenic pulmonary edema

MANAGEMENT

Stabilization of the airway and resuscitation are imperative. Additional measures include decontamination by removal of clothing and washing of the skin for contact exposure and emesis or gastric lavage and administration of charcoal and cathartic for ingestion. Health care workers must be protected.

Organophosphate and carbamate insecticides are rapidly absorbed through the clothes and skin. Contaminated clothes must be removed, and the skin must be decontaminated; this treatment is optimally performed outside a medical facility by personnel wearing gloves, rubber aprons, and so on. Two separate water and detergent washes remove a total of 91% to 94% of organophosphates, even when performed up to 6 hours after exposure. Hospital personnel must be protected during and after decontamination.

Specific treatment involves administration of anticholinergic medications to the symptomatic patient:

1. Atropine binds at muscarinic receptors and is given first: 0.05 mg/kg/dose (maximum: 2 to 5 mg/dose) IV. A test dose (child: 0.01 mg/kg IV; adult: 2 mg IV) is usually given. This may be repeated every 5 minutes until atropinization is achieved, with drying of pulmonary secretions. Mydriasis is not an adequate endpoint. Some authorities advocate a continuous infusion of atropine at 0.02 to 0.05 mg/kg/hr IV.
   - Should be given for the first 24 hours as needed to maintain atropinization. Average adult dose is 40 mg/day. Adults may need 100 mg in the first 24 hours of therapy.
2. Pralidoxime (2-PAM) reactivates acetylcholinesterase and reverses cholinergic nicotinic stimulation. It is useful if given within 36 hours of exposure. It should be administered after adequate atropinization.
   a. Dosage: pralidoxime, 20 to 50 mg/kg/dose (maximum: 2 g/dose) IV slowly. In the adult, 1 g is mixed with 250 ml 0.9% NS and given over 30 to 60 minutes. If symptoms of weakness and fasciculations persist, it may be repeated in 1 hour and then every 8 hours for additional doses.
   b. No serious side effects noted from pralidoxime. Usually not required for carbamates, which have a lower toxicity of shorter duration.

DISPOSITION

All symptomatic patients with exposure or ingestion need admission and usually consultation with a poison control center for guidance in drug therapy.

BIBLIOGRAPHY

Tafuri J, Roberts J: Organophosphate poisoning, *Ann Emerg Med* 16:193, 1987.

Zwiener RJ, Ginsburg CM: Organophosphate and carbamate poisoning in infants and children, *Pediatrics* 81:121, 1988.

Phenothiazines

ALERT Symptoms include sedation and anticholinergic findings; occasionally there may be prominent dystonic reactions.

Phenothiazines are widely used antipsychotics as well as antinauseants. They have anticholinergic, antidopaminergic, and α-blocking actions.

ETIOLOGY

See Table 55-6.

DIAGNOSTIC FINDINGS

The major finding in phenothiazine overdoses reflects anticholinergic and antidopaminergic effects. An inverse relationship exists between the anticholinergic potency and extrapyramidal side effects (p. 374).

Extrapyramidal dystonic reactions may be divided into several categories, although clinically different patterns may appear simultaneously. Dystonia is not necessarily dose related.

1. Oculogyric: upward-gaze paralysis, bizarre tics
2. Torticollis: may involve one side, often with arm involvement
3. Buccolingual: facial grimacing with dysphagia, mutism, trismus
4. Opisthotonic
5. Tortipelvic: abdominal wall spasms, bizarre gait, lordosis, kyphosis

Other side effects include the following:

1. Reduced seizure threshold.
2. Anticholinergic findings.
3. Hypothermia may occur early, but the patient with sufficient thermal exposure may have hyperthermia.
4. Tachycardia and orthostatic hypotension are common.
5. Non–life-threatening side effects include hepatitis, photosensitivity, visual blurring, hirsutism, and gynecomastia. Thioridazine has been associated with retinal pigment degeneration.

Ancillary Data

1. Granulocytopenia, hyperglycemia, and acetonemia are reported.
2. Other studies should include toxicology screen (in seriously ill patients), ECG, and x-ray film.
3. A few drops of 10% ferric chloride added to 5 ml of urine will turn urine purple-brown. Urine turns purple in presence of salicylates.

MANAGEMENT

Initial focus must be given to stabilization, with particular attention to airway, ventilation, and circulation. Obtunded patients should receive oxygen, dextrose, and naloxone. Hypotension should be treated initially with IV fluids. Cardiac rhythm should be monitored, and dysrhythmias treated as appropriate.

TABLE 55-6 Phenothiazines and Antipsychotics: Related Side Effects*

	Sedation	Extrapyramidal	Hypotension
PHENOTHIAZINES			
Chlorpromazine (Thorazine)	+++	++	IM +++ PO ++
Triflupromazine (Vesprin)	++	+++	++
Thioridazine (Mellaril)	+++	+	++
Trifluoperazine (Stelazine)	+	+++	+
Prochlorperazine (Compazine)	++	+++	
OTHER ANTIPSYCHOTICS			
Thiothixene (Navane)	+ or ++	++	++
Haloperidol (Haldol)	+	+++	+
Quetiapine (Seroquel)	++	+	+
Risperidone (Risperdal)	++	+	+
Clozapine (Clozaril)	++	+	+
Olanzapine (Zyprexa)	+++	+	+

* *+, ++, +++,* Relative prominence.

Emesis in a child may remove some small amount of drug if performed within 30 minutes of ingestion. Gastric lavage may be necessary, followed by charcoal and catharsis.

Extrapyramidal dystonic reactions should be treated with diphenhydramine (Benadryl), 1 to 2 mg/kg/dose IV. Benztropine (Cogentin), 1 to 4 mg/dose (adult) IV, may have anticholinergic effects because of an atropine component. Patients are maintained with one of these drugs for 1 to 2 days.

DISPOSITION

Disposition must reflect the severity of symptoms. Patients with adequately treated extrapyramidal findings can usually be discharged with follow-up observation. Others often need hospitalization. Depending on the nature of the ingestion, psychiatric counseling or poison prevention should be stressed.

Salicylates (Aspirin)

ALERT Consider whether the patient has tachypnea, hyperthermia, or metabolic acidosis.

Ingestion of salicylates is common but has decreased with the widespread use of safety lids on medication bottles and the popularity of acetaminophen-containing products. A wide variety of products contain salicylates, and an acute, single ingestion of 250 mg/kg may produce toxicity. Signs and symptoms can be related to the salicylate levels diagrammed in the Done nomogram (Fig. 55-3). Therapeutic levels are 15 to 30 mg/dl in arthritic conditions. The Done nomogram cannot be used in cases in which chronic ingestion produces symptoms at levels lower than those normally considered to be toxic or for overdose of sustained-release aspirin products. Methyl salicylate (oil of wintergreen) is particularly toxic, containing 1365 mg of salicylate per ml.

DIAGNOSTIC FINDINGS

Patients with significant ingestions initially may have tachypnea and deep, labored respirations, hyperthermia, tinnitus, and vomiting. Mental status changes may develop with moderate ingestions, ranging from lethargy or excitability to seizures and coma. Slurred speech, hallucinations, vertigo, pulmonary edema, and cardiovascular collapse may develop.

Chronic salicylism is associated with accentuated CNS findings and less prominent acid-base abnormalities. Thus levels do not indicate the seriousness of ingestion.

Complications

1. Metabolic:
   - a. Hypoglycemia, sometimes preceded by an initial hyperglycemia.
   - b. Metabolic acidosis and respiratory alkalosis: In children younger than 4 years, metabolic acidosis develops more rapidly, without the concurrent respiratory alkalosis. This is often the predominant presentation.
   - c. Electrolyte abnormalities:
     - (1) Potassium deficit secondary to acidosis with urinary losses
     - (2) Hyponatremia because of inappropriate antidiuretic hormone (ADH)
2. Noncardiogenic pulmonary edema (see Chapter 19)
3. CNS findings in moderate to severe ingestions:
   - a. Seizures from hypoglycemia, hyponatremia, cerebral edema, or decreased ionized calcium caused by alkali therapy.
   - b. Coma: May occur in acute ingestions when the level is very high or the patient has ingested more than one agent. Coma is more common with chronic salicylism (see Chapter 15).
4. Bleeding from hypothrombinemia and platelet dysfunction
5. Chemical hepatitis

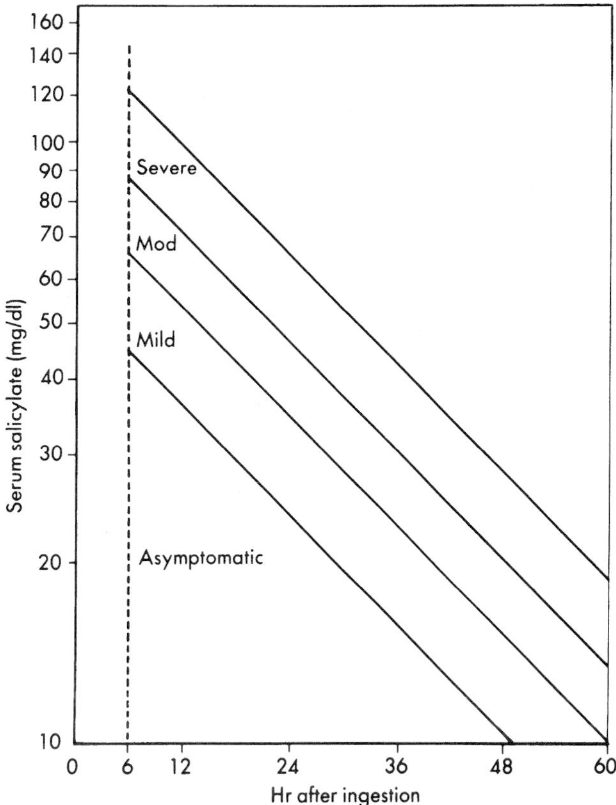

Fig. 55-3 Done nomogram for salicylate poisoning. Not to be used for anything other than a single acute aspirin overdose. Don't wait until 6 hours after overdose before drawing first level if patient is symptomatic. (From Done AK: *Pediatrics* 26:805, 1960. Copyright American Academy of Pediatrics, 1960.)

6. Allergic manifestations, particularly wheezing

Ancillary Data

A qualitative test for the presence of aspirin in urine may be performed by adding 5 ml of urine to a few drops of 10% ferric chloride. The urine turns purple and remains stable if salicylates are present, purple-brown with phenothiazines, purple-red (fades in minutes) with ketosis, and yellowish green with isoniazid. Normal urine turns brownish, whitish, or yellowish.

To provide a semiquantitative measure of salicylate level, one drop of serum may be applied to a urine test strip (Phenistix). A tan color is consistent with a level of less than 40 mg/dl, brown with a level of 40 to 90 mg/dl, and purple with a level higher than 90 mg/dl.

1. A quantitative salicylate level may be measured and interpreted with use of the Done nomogram (see Fig. 55-3). It is not useful in chronic ingestions. Therapeutic salicylate level is 15 to 30 mg/dl. The value of the Done nomogram is only a general reference. The clinical condition of the patient is far more important than where the salicylate level falls on the nomogram. It is unnecessary to wait until 6 hours after ingestion to obtain a salicylate level specimen in a symptomatic patient.

2. Electrolyte and glucose measurements and ABG analysis as indicated.
3. Coagulation studies if indicated. Prolonged PT and bleeding time.
4. ECG, if severe electrolyte problems are suspected.

DIFFERENTIAL DIAGNOSIS

1. Metabolic acidosis ("MUDPILES"):
   a. Ingestions: methanol, paraldehyde, iron, isoniazid, lactic acid, ethanol, ethylene glycol, salicylates, strychnine.
   b. Metabolic: uremia, diabetes mellitus, starvation.

      NOTE: In general, metabolic acidosis results from ingestions of the specific drugs listed previously as well as cellular poisons (e.g., iron, cyanide) and drugs that cause seizures. In addition, poor perfusion, ischemia, or cellular death produces metabolic acidosis.
2. Infection: meningitis, encephalitis, pneumonia, Reye syndrome.

MANAGEMENT

After stabilization, oral absorption should be reduced by emesis (syrup of ipecac) if within 30 minutes of ingestion or gastric lavage, activated charcoal, and catharsis. Mild ingestions require no additional therapy.

For moderate or severe ingestions, parenteral therapy with forced alkaline diuresis is required. Salicylates are weak acids (pKa = 3), and their elimination may be facilitated by alkalinization of the urine to pH of 7 to 8 and correction of potassium and acid-base abnormalities. Ancillary data should be monitored.

1. If the patient is initially dehydrated, expand the vascular volume with D5W 0.45% NS, adding 60 mEq/L $NaHCO_3$. Infuse at 10 to 20 ml/kg over 1 hour.
2. After the resuscitation and establishment of good urine flow (>2 ml/kg/hr), infuse D5W with $NaHCO_3$, 88 to 132 mEq (2-3 ampules)/L, and KCl, 30 to 40 mEq/L at a rate of 4 to 8 ml/kg/hr. May also use D5W 0.45% NS with $NaHCO_3$ at 40 to 60 mEq/L, and KCl at 30 mEq/L. Hypokalemia is very common.
   - If a severe metabolic acidosis is present, give additional $NaHCO_3$ at 1 to 2 mEq/kg IV slowly.
3. Multiple-dose activated charcoal may enhance elimination. Give 1 to 2 g/kg/dose (adult: 30 to 100 g/dose) q4hr PO.
4. Treat hyperpyrexia with a cooling blanket.
5. For seizures give diazepam (Valium), 0.2 to 0.3 mg/kg/dose IV q10min prn. Treat metabolic problems, if any.
6. For bleeding diathesis: vitamin K (infants: 1 to 2 mg/dose IV; children and adults: 5 to 10 mg/dose IV).
7. Dialysis is indicated for the following conditions; hemodialysis is more effective than peritoneal dialysis:
   a. Renal failure
   b. CNS deterioration or poor response, particularly with chronic salicylism
   c. Unchanging high or increasing salicylate level or level higher than 100 mg/dl at 6 hours
   d. Severe, unresolving metabolic acidosis
   e. Renal or hepatic failure
   f. Pulmonary edema

DISPOSITION

Patients with mild ingestions may be discharged with appropriate poison-prevention counseling. Hospitalization should be arranged for patients who are significantly symptomatic, who have serum levels equal to or greater than 60 mg/dl at 6 hours, who have ingested methyl salicylates, or who have a history of long-term ingestion or have ingested sustained-release preparations that are potentially toxic.

BIBLIOGRAPHY

Burton RT, Bayer MJ, Barron L et al: Comparison of activated charcoal and gastric lavage in the prevention of aspirin absorption, *J Emerg Med* 1:411, 1984.

Dugandzic RM, Tierney MG, Dickinson GE et al: Evaluation of the validity of the Done nomogram in the management of acute salicylate intoxication, *Ann Emerg Med* 18:1186, 1989.

Kulig K: Salicylate intoxication: is the Done nomogram reliable? *AACT Clin-Toxicol Update* 3:1, 1990.

McGuigan MA: A two-year review of salicylate deaths in Ontario, *Arch Intern Med* 147:510,1987.

Vertrees JE, McWilliams BC, Kelly HW: Repeated oral administration of activated charcoal for treating aspirin overdose in young children, *Pediatrics* 85:594, 1990.

Sympathomimetics

ALERT CNS and cardiovascular stimulants may produce ventricular dysrhythmias or sudden death.

The sympathomimetics are a diverse group of stimulant drugs with primarily CNS and cardiovascular toxicity.

TYPES

1. Amphetamines: methamphetamine, phenmetrazine (Preludin) (much greater toxicity with intravenous administration than oral ingestion).
2. Cocaine (street names: snow, gold dust, coke, speed ball—when combined with heroin) (p. 380).
3. β-Adrenergic agents: ephedrine (available alone or in combination with theophylline), pseudoephedrine, phenylpropanolamine, terbutaline, albuterol.

DIAGNOSTIC FINDINGS

See Table 55-3.

Ancillary data should include CBC, measurements of electrolytes, glucose, and BUN, oximetry or ABG analysis, ECG, and toxicology screens as indicated.

DIFFERENTIAL DIAGNOSIS

Sympathomimetics ingestions must be differentiated from intoxication caused by phencyclidine, hallucinogens, anticholinergics, sedative-hypnotics, alcohol, theophylline, caffeine, and camphor.

MANAGEMENT

1. Supportive care is important, being focused particularly on potential cardiovascular instability and altered mental status:
   a. Patients with altered mental status should receive oxygen, dextrose, and naloxone.
   b. Hyperthermia must be aggressively treated with cooling blankets.
   c. Hypoglycemia should be suspected and treated.
2. Gastric emptying should be achieved either by emesis or lavage (if performed very soon after ingestion) as well as by charcoal and catharsis as outlined previously.
3. A calming, reassuring approach to the patient with an acute psychosis or hallucinations is important, as is an attempt to reduce stimuli.
4. Sedation, if necessary, may be achieved with diazepam (Valium), 0.2 to 0.8 mg/kg/24 hr q6-8hr PO (adult: 5 to 10 mg/dose). Titrate dose according to response.
5. For behavioral changes caused by amphetamines and not responsive to benzodiazepine, haloperidol (Haldol), 2 to 10 mg IV, may be used.

BIBLIOGRAPHY

Spiler HA, Ramoska EA, Henretig FM et al: A two year retrospective study of accidental pediatric albuterol ingestions, *Pediatr Emerg Care* 9:338, 1993.

Wasserman D, Amitai Y: Hypoglycemia following albuterol overdose in a child, *Am J Emerg Med* 10:556, 1992.

Theophylline (p. 793)

ALERT Seizures and cardiac dysrhythmias may occur with toxicity.

Theophylline overdoses are uncommon in children with decreased use.

DIAGNOSTIC FINDINGS

Effects are primarily sympathomimetic in action, resulting in irritability and seizures as well as tachycardia, dysrhythmias (atrial fibrillation and ventricular tachycardia), and hypertension. Patients may be restless and agitated. Nausea, vomiting, diarrhea, and abdominal pain are seen frequently, even at nontoxic theophylline levels.

Overdoses with sustained-release preparations can produce severe and prolonged CNS and cardiovascular toxicity.

In one study, the mean theophylline level of patients who had seizures after long-term theophylline intoxication was 45 μg/dl.

Ancillary Data

Serum theophylline determinations are commonly available and should be obtained for all patients who are considered to have potentially toxic levels. Rapid office assays may also be used for measuring levels. An ECG should usually be performed.

MANAGEMENT

1. Supportive care is essential with ongoing cardiac monitoring. Gastric emptying by either emesis or lavage (reflecting level of consciousness, seizures, or absence of gag reflex), if performed very soon after ingestion and followed by charcoal and catharsis as outlined previously.
2. In the asymptomatic patient with minimal overdoses, withholding the drug and monitoring are usually adequate.
3. Significant theophylline overdoses may be treated initially with serial doses of activated charcoal (adult: 10 g q1hr or 20 g q2hr to total dose of 120 g; children: proportionately less). This approach markedly decreases the half-life of elimination. If the theophylline level is higher than 50 μg/dl, dialysis (and rarely, hemoperfusion) should be considered.
4. Whole-bowel irrigation may be useful, especially if long-acting medication is involved.
5. Seizures are treated initially with diazepam (Valium), 0.2 to 0.3 mg/kg/dose IV q2-5min prn (see Chapter 21), and dysrhythmias are treated with specific drugs (see Chapter 6).

DISPOSITION

Patients who are symptomatic or have drug levels higher than 30 μg/dl should generally be admitted for observation and treatment.

BIBLIOGRAPHY

Gal P, Miller A, McCue JD: Oral-activated charcoal to enhance theophylline elimination in an acute overdose, *JAMA* 251:3130, 1984.

Jain R, Tholl DA: Activated charcoal for theophylline toxicity in a premature infant on the second day of life, *Dev Pharmacol Ther* 19:106, 1992.

Paloucek FP, Rodvoid KA: Evaluation of theophylline overdoses and toxicities, *Ann Emerg Med* 17:135, 1988.

IX

Trauma

56 Evaluation and Stabilization of the Multiply Traumatized Patient

ALERT Aggressive, highly prioritized management must be implemented immediately, using a team approach to airway stabilization, ventilation, the spine, shock, and external hemorrhage. A multiply injured patient may be able to respond to only one major painful stimulus at a time. Thus a careful identification of all sites of injury is important.

The traumatized pediatric patient presents unique challenges to the physician, but the principles of establishing treatment priorities are identical to those for older patients. Beyond the principles of immediate stabilization, the psychologic impact on a child and family are immense and must be addressed with appropriate urgency through communication, support, and understanding. Anatomic and physiologic differences between adults and children affect the approach. The higher center of gravity in a child, which increases the risk of head injury; the shorter stature, which raises the risk of hypothermia; and the variability in the child's airway (p. 20) must all be considered. Furthermore, there are logistic problems in the care of the pediatric patient with respect to ensuring intravenous access, adjusting to limitations of equipment, monitoring and determining vital signs, and assessing fluid requirements.

Patterns of fatal childhood injury suggest that one third of deaths are due to homicides in an urban setting. House fires (34%), firearms (19%), drownings (11%), and motor vehicle accidents (7%) account for most fatal injuries.

It is important to recognize that infants depend on others for care, placing them in a uniquely vulnerable position. Of trauma victims younger than 3 months, 28% are injured in neglectful or abusive conditions. Peak incidence of trauma occurs from June to September. Many injuries are sustained in falls. Young infants are unable to roll; falls from a height less than 90 cm rarely result in fractures or serious injury. A fracture explained by a fall from a low height is suspicious for abuse, as are injuries with multiple or stellate skull fractures and spiral long bone extremity fractures.

There are three peak times for deaths after trauma:

- *Immediate death* occurs within seconds to minutes of injury, usually at the scene, and accounts for approximately 50% of trauma deaths. Usually, massive head injury, high cervical spine disruption, cardiac laceration, aortic rupture or laceration of great arteries, or airway obstruction is present.
- *Early death* occurs within minutes to a few hours (sometimes known as the "golden hour"). Death is due to subdural or epidural hematoma, ruptured spleen, lacerated liver, hypovolemic tamponade, massive hemothorax, or aortic rupture.
- *Delayed death* occurs days to weeks after the initial injury, usually as a result of multisystem organ failure or sepsis.

PRINCIPLES OF MANAGEMENT

Organization

For optimal treatment, trauma care requires organizational structure and coordination at several levels: the region and prehospital system, the hospital, and crucial health care professionals. This text focuses on the hospital-based physician-centered organization, but to be effective, the physician must understand the other components of the emergency medical services (EMS) system and must be able to communicate effectively with the prehospital system.

Triage

Triage often sends trauma patients to a trauma center, reflecting specific local guidelines and protocols. Familiarity with trauma and a multidisciplinary approach to managing traumatized patients are generally present in such settings. The triage criteria used by the American College of Surgeons Committee on Trauma purposely "over-triages" patients by 30%. The Florida Triage Study suggests that "under-triage" in the pediatric population occurs approximately 33% of the time, and triage criteria specific to the pediatric population must be developed. At present, a debate about the benefits of destination policies, including pediatric and general trauma centers, is ongoing, reflecting the substantive data that support the importance of personnel, resources, responsiveness, and system commitment.

Team Approach

Effective trauma resuscitation requires a trauma team led by a senior member designated as the trauma captain. Although the exact composition of the team varies with the institution and availability of personnel to include surgeons, emergency physicians, and pediatricians, some type of organized team approach is essential. Trauma injuries are complex, requiring the performance of multiple procedures and frequent reassessment in a timely fashion. Only through a team effort, orchestrated by a team captain, can optimal care be provided.

The team organization must reflect the resources and expertise of a specific institution, the clinical needs of the specific patient, and other resource demands at a specific moment. Prioritization of specific resources and manpower is always essential and must be individualized. The structure must be predetermined to enhance efficiency, define responsibilities, and ensure completeness of assessment and treatment. Criteria for activation of the trauma team should reflect the child's physiologic status, the injury, and the mechanism of the trauma. The Children's Hospital Medical Center in Cincinnati uses the following guidelines for trauma team activation:

- *Physiologic*: shock, respiratory distress/failure, cardiac arrest, Glasgow Coma Scale (GCS) score less than 8, or a low trauma score.
- *Injury*: penetrating wound of the head or thorax, potential airway compromise, inhalation airway burn, burn (>30% of body surface area [BSA] or 15% to 30% second- or third-degree burns), significant injuries below and above the diaphragm, two or more proximal long bone or pelvic fractures, traumatic amputation of a limb, crush injury of the torso, or spinal injury with paralysis.
- *Mechanism of injury*: ejection from a motor vehicle, extrication time longer than 20 minutes, at least one fatality from the event, intrusion into the passenger space of vehicle more than 20 inches, pedestrian struck at speed higher than 20 miles per hour (mph), unrestrained passenger in a motor vehicle crash occurring at a speed higher than 20 mph or restrained passenger in a crash at a speed higher than 40 mph, fall from more than 20 feet, passenger in a vehicle that has rolled over, struck by lightning.

Aggressive Management

Because the multiply injured child has a high potential for rapid deterioration, an aggressive approach must be the foundation for determining treatment priorities.

Treatment Based on Clinical Findings. Diagnosis need not always be confirmed by x-ray study or laboratory work before treatment is initiated. Such delays in treatment may prove detrimental to patient survival. For example, the treatment urgency of a tension pneumothorax, diagnosed from clinical findings of diminished breath sounds, subcutaneous emphysema, or hemodynamic compromise, necessitates immediate placement of a chest tube without x-ray study confirmation of the diagnosis.

Assuming the Most Serious Diagnosis. When a number of diagnostic possibilities explain a physical finding, the most serious of these possibilities should be assumed and appropriate treatment instituted, until that diagnosis can be excluded.

Consideration of the Nature of the Accident (i.e., the mechanism of injury). Victims of potentially serious accidents should be considered seriously injured until proven stable. For example, for the victim of a fall or an auto-pedestrian accident, IV lines should be started and careful monitoring performed despite an initially stable appearance and absence of complaints.

Assessment of Priorities. Evaluation of the trauma victim must be conducted in a prioritized and systematic fashion to guarantee that life-sustaining functions are addressed and maintained first.

Thorough Examination. The trauma team rapidly ensures that the airway, ventilation, and circulation are adequate; obtains a history; and then performs a more complete examination:

1. Remove all clothing to prevent overlooking an injury.
2. Perform a concise and systematic, yet thorough, examination to ensure detection of all injuries.
3. Do not stop looking for injuries after one serious injury has been detected.
4. Examine the patient's back. If there is potential cervical spine injury, obtain an x-ray film before examining the back if the patient's condition permits. Otherwise, the patient may be logrolled.

Frequent Reassessments. The clinical presentation of a trauma victim is dynamic and the patient is subject to sudden deterioration. Frequent assessment of vital signs and indicators of vital function (e.g., level of consciousness, pupils, ventilation) is essential. Vigilance in monitoring intake and output and its correlation with vital signs is imperative to determining additional fluid or blood requirements.

Technical Steps

Technical procedures should be accomplished early to facilitate monitoring and intervention in seriously ill patients:

1. *Intravenous (IV) lines* are placed and *oxygen* is administered.
2. *Urinary catheter* (6 months: 8 Fr; 2 to 3 years: 10 Fr; 6 to 8 years: 10 to 12 Fr; 8 to 10 years: 12 Fr) is inserted, and the urine is examined for blood and monitored for volume of output.
3. *Nasogastric (NG) tube* (6 months: 8 Fr; 2 to 3 years: 10 Fr; 6 to 8 years: 10 to 12 Fr; 8 to 10 years: 14 to 18 Fr) is inserted (after cervical spine is cleared). Fig. 56-1 provides guidelines for length of insertion of gastric tubes.

   NOTE: Insertion of the NG tube is usually delayed in patients with significant facial fractures.
4. *Cardiac monitoring* is started.
5. *Laboratory* and *x-ray studies* are ordered as discussed later.

Five tubes are virtually always required in a patient in whom major trauma is suspected: two IV tubes, an NG tube, a bladder tube, and tubes of blood for hematocrit (Hct) and type and cross-match determinations.

If prehospital IV cannulation is achieved, it is essential to ensure that it is clinically useful in the field by initiating adequate fluid resuscitation. On arrival in the emergency department (ED), the cannula should be

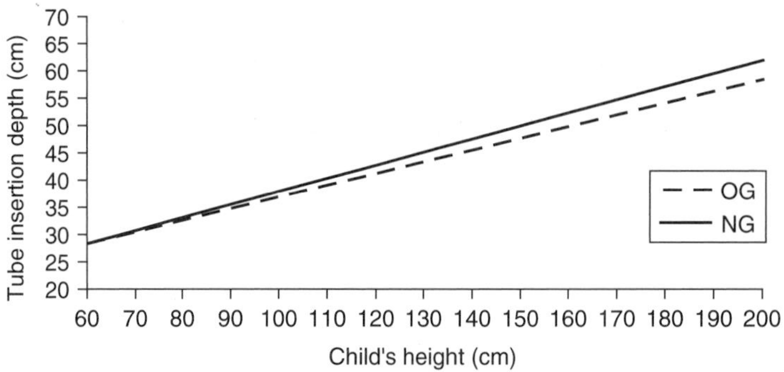

Fig. 56-1 Graphic representation of recommended tube insertion depths based on patient length. *NG*, Nasogastric tube; *OG*, orogastric tube.

(From Klasner AE, Luke DA, Scalzo AJ: *J Emerg Med* 34:268, 2002.)

reassessed and fluids continued with adequate monitoring of the rates and response.

The practice of typing and cross-matching the blood of every trauma patient has come under close scrutiny. Obtaining a type and screen is a cost-effective alternative that does not pull blood out of circulation in the blood bank and therefore saves resources. Cross-matching should take only an additional 5 minutes after the type and screen have been completed. Studies suggest that type and cross-match should be performed initially in patients with hypotension or obviously severely injured children with a Pediatric Trauma Score less than 7.

AGE AND SIZE CONSIDERATIONS

Age- and size-specific issues must be considered in management. The child's relatively large surface area increases the risk of heat loss, and abdominal distension may impede diaphragmatic breathing.

1. Vital signs, including respiratory rates, vary by age (see Appendix B-2). Systolic blood pressure (BP) may be estimated by adding twice the patient's age in years to 80. The heart rate varies with age (infant: 100 to 160 beats/min; child: 60 to 150 beats/min; adult: 59 to 90 beats/min).
2. Fluid replacement should be performed on the basis of the patient's blood volume (70 to 80 ml/kg), the vital signs, the nature of the injury, and the presence of ongoing hemorrhage. Unless the patient is in profound shock, the initial approach is to give a fourth of the patient's blood volume (20 ml/kg) as crystalloid (0.9% normal saline [NS] or lactated Ringer's [LR] solution). Direct further treatment toward the initial response and the other factors mentioned.
3. Venous access is somewhat more difficult in children, particularly if they are hypovolemic. If establishing a percutaneous line is impossible, establish a venous cutdown in the distal saphenous or external jugular vein. Intraosseous infusion during the initial fluid resuscitation may be particularly useful for transient venous access if access through traditional routes is difficult (see Appendix A-3). Central venous lines are rarely used in children because of the greater risk of pneumothorax and vascular injury, but they may be used, ideally with a Seldinger wire approach. If a central line is desired, the internal jugular or femoral vein may be cannulated by the customary approach.
4. Placement of tubes, including thoracostomy and endotracheal (ET) and NG tubes and urinary catheters, should be

accomplished with the largest tubes that the child can accommodate.

5. Administer medications on an age-specific basis. The Broselow tape may be useful in relating height to dose.

ASSESSMENT BY PRIORITIES

Preliminaries

1. Assemble the trauma team, the composition of which will vary according to the number and type of people available in the ED. A team captain must be identified who can orchestrate the resuscitation and task assignments on the basis of ambulance reports.
2. Take an updated report from ambulance personnel while the patient is being transferred from the ambulance stretcher. Attempt to acquire additional history, including the details of the accident, significant history, medications, and allergies.
3. Maintain any splinting and head and neck immobilization that has been instituted in the field.
4. Remove all clothing. Use overhead heating, lights, and warm blankets to maintain body temperature, especially in smaller children. Hypothermia may occur because of the relatively large body surface area of children.
5. Attach the patient to a cardiac monitor and oximeter, and administer oxygen. Initiate IV lines.
6. "AMPLE" history is essential: *a*llergy, *m*edications, *p*ast medical history, time of *l*ast meal, and *e*vents leading to injury.

Approach

Initial management can be divided into stabilization of immediate life-threatening conditions and a subsequent brief but systematic head-to-toe evaluation. Life-threatening conditions comprise five high-priority factors: airway, ventilation, the spine, shock, and level of consciousness; these five factors require rapid assessment and intervention to permit survival (see Chapter 4).

The second phase of management is a complete evaluation of other potentially injured systems. A reassessment of the high-priority factors and evaluation of neurologic status, abdomen, heart, musculoskeletal system, and soft tissue injuries is essential. Although of lower priority, these elements do have the potential for causing serious morbidity and mortality and must be addressed expeditiously.

Consistent patterns of injury should be sought. For instance, a child involved in a pedestrian–motor vehicle accident should be evaluated for injury to the head, abdomen, and lower extremities (Waddell's triad), although the actual incidence of this triad is low.

PRIMARY SURVEY AND RESUSCITATION

Airway

1. Check for patency. If there is any question, open the airway, suction secretions, remove foreign debris, and insert an oral or nasal airway. High-flow oxygen should be applied, often with a mask while monitoring is done with an oximeter.
2. Check for adequacy of air exchange; if insufficient, active intervention is necessary:
   a. If urgent airway management is needed before the cervical spine can be cleared, the decision to use oral or nasal intubation must be made. The comfort level and experience of the physician dictate the choice; both methods are safe and effective.
      (1) Nasotracheal intubation in a spontaneously breathing patient may be attempted unless there is a severe facial injury (which might allow the tube to pass into the cranium). Apnea is a contraindication to nasotracheal intubation because the breath sounds are used to guide tube placement.
      (2) In patients at risk for cervical spine injury and in whom nasal

intubation is contraindicated or unsuccessful, the preferred technique is oral intubation while in-line stabilization of the head and neck is maintained. Please note that in-line stabilization is not in-line traction. Most authorities prefer the in-line stabilization approach to a surgical airway, which is difficult in young children. In cases of significant head trauma, rapid-sequence induction with oral intubation is the preferred technique. Blind nasotracheal intubation is discouraged in these cases because it can increase intracranial pressure (ICP). The lower incidence of unstable neck fractures in children further supports this recommendation. If a surgical airway is established, cricothyroidotomy because of simpler anatomy is preferred over tracheostomy. However, size limitation precludes cricothyroidotomy in small children. Although recommendations vary, most suggest that children younger than 12 years undergo tracheostomy. Other options to consider are digital intubation, intubation guided by fiberoptic laryngoscopy, and transtracheal needle jet insufflation.

b. If no evidence of cervical spine injury is present (conscious patient with no nerve deficit or neck pain and normal cervical spine x-ray findings), standard oral intubation may be performed with caution while motion is minimized. Remember that normal cervical spine films do not rule out an unstable ligamentous injury.

Ventilation

1. Inspection: Look for signs of respiratory distress, including dyspnea, tachycardia, tachypnea, cyanosis, diaphoresis, retractions, flail segments, external evidence of trauma, and tracheal deviation.
2. Palpation: Feel for bony crepitus, subcutaneous emphysema, chest wall tenderness, and tracheal deviation.
3. Auscultation: Determine presence, character, and symmetry of breath sounds.
4. Management:
   - **a.** Evidence of inadequate ventilation indicates the need for active airway management or tube thoracostomy.
   - **b.** Airway management may be achieved as outlined previously. If necessary, *controlled intubation with paralysis (CIP)* or *rapid sequence induction (RSI)* may be used for specific patients to maintain adequate oxygenation, protect the airway, and reduce adverse cardiovascular or ICP responses to intubation (see Chapter 4).

     The patient's anatomy is initially evaluated, looking for oral or dental abnormalities, trauma to the neck or face, and systemic abnormalities. Equipment is checked.

     (1) The patient is preoxygenated. If the patient is hypoventilating, hyperventilate while the Sellick maneuver is performed. Position the head of an adolescent or adult on a towel to elevate the head about 10 cm off the bed.

     (2) Administer a nonparalyzing dose of nondepolarizing agent (i.e., vecuronium [Norcuron], 0.01 mg/kg IV [adult: 1 mg IV]), to reduce fasciculations. Allow 3 to 5 minutes before proceeding with succinylcholine. This step is *not* necessary in children younger than 5 years, and many believe it can be left out entirely unless fasciculations may cause injury. With extensive burns or crush injury more than 72 hours old, fasciculations may release potassium from damaged cells and cause a dangerous hyperkalemia; in those cases, a nondepolarizing agent should be used.

(3) Atropine, 0.01 to 0.02 mg/kg IV (minimum: 0.10 mg/dose), may be given to prevent bradycardia caused by vagal stimulation and to reduce secretions, particularly in children younger than 5 years. A minimum dose prevents paradoxic bradycardia. In the presence of significant head injury, administer lidocaine, 1 mg/kg IV, to blunt the rise in ICP caused by the stimulation of intubation, and allow 2 minutes before giving succinylcholine.

(4) Sedate the patient with thiopental, 3 to 5 mg/kg IV, if the patient is not hypotensive or in status asthmaticus.

Alternatives include:

- Normotensive: midazolam, etomidate, thiopental, propofol
- Hypotensive/hypovolemic; mild: etomidate, ketamine, midazolam; severe: etomidate, ketamine, none
- Head injury or status epilepticus; normotensive: etomidate, thiopental, propofol; hypotensive: etomidate, low-dose thiopental (1 to 2 mg/kg IV)

(5) Give succinylcholine, 1 to 1.5 mg/kg IV to adults and 2 mg/kg IV to children weighing less than 10 kg. Allow 45 to 60 seconds for muscle relaxation. Cricoid pressure should be maintained. Other choices of agents are vecuronium (0.1 mg/kg IV) and rocuronium (0.6 to 1.2 mg/kg IV)

(6) Perform oral intubation, verify tube position, and release cricoid pressure. When paralysis wears off, vecuronium, 0.1 mg/kg IV, may be used if needed.

(7) The use of CIP or RSI has been shown to reduce the complication rate of intubation. All facilities dealing with pediatric trauma should have protocols for its use in place, and the physicians should be comfortable with the use of these medications. Remember to continue to keep the patient sedated and comfortable after the initial medicines are given. Children are often undertreated with sedative and analgesic agents.

c. Insert a chest tube if there are any signs of pneumothorax or hemothorax (see Chapter 62). If the patient is relatively stable, tube thoracostomy may obviate active airway management.

Cervical Spine (see Chapter 61)

1. The cervical spine of every multiply traumatized patient beyond infancy should be considered fractured until proven otherwise. This principle has direct bearing on airway management. Fracture or dislocation is unusual in the patient younger than 3 years without neurologic defect.
2. In the awake, alert, and cooperative older child, palpation to detect misalignment or tenderness may be all that is needed to rule out injury. If any doubt exists, particularly in the younger, uncooperative child or in the patient with an impaired sensorium, a portable cross-table lateral x-ray film of the neck should be taken. This study, to be adequate, must include all seven cervical vertebrae and the top of the first thoracic vertebral body. One person should maintain axial traction while a second pulls the patient's arms caudad from the foot of the bed, thus lowering the shoulders enough to expose the lower cervical vertebrae (p. 461).

The criteria for obtaining a cervical spine x-ray series in the traumatized child are undefined. Factors that may be useful in defining high-risk patients include those with neck pain, tenderness, or limited mobility; involvement in a vehicular accident with head trauma; a history of trauma to the neck; and abnormalities of reflexes, strength, sensation, or mental status.

3. Management.
   a. Immobilize the head and neck with sandbags, tape, and a semirigid collar, if possible, until the entire cervical spine x-ray series is completed. Agitated or combative patients may also need to be immobilized manually by one of the trauma team members.
   b. If dislocation or fractures are detected or suspected, immobilize with a Philadelphia or 4-poster collar with tape and sandbags. Products such as the Stif Neck and Baby No-Neck (California Medical Products) are available. Request immediate neurosurgical consultation.

Thoracic and Lumbar Spine
(see Chapter 61)

1. Thoracic or lumbar fractures are easily overlooked in the child who is confused or obtunded or has other painful injuries.
2. Palpation of the spinal column often localizes tenderness and step-offs or, on logrolling, one may see ecchymoses.
3. Cross-table lateral x-ray films may not be easily obtainable anywhere but in the x-ray suite, but the anteroposterior (AP) view often shows thoracic or lumbar fractures. Moreover, the AP view is the one from which to assess stability if there is a fracture and also to obtain important information about other structures in the chest, abdomen, and pelvis.
4. Management:
   a. Keep the patient in a supine position on a hard stretcher. If it is necessary to move the patient, use a backboard or scoop stretcher rather than the logroll maneuver.
   b. Insert an NG tube and urinary catheter if the cervical spine is clear and no major facial trauma or meatal bleeding is present.

Shock (see Chapter 5)

1. Up to 25% to 30% of blood volume can be lost before a child exhibits hypotension in the supine position. More subtle findings, such as tachycardia, a narrowed pulse pressure, and poor perfusion should be sought and treated aggressively.
2. Normal age-specific values of pulse and blood pressure must be considered in the evaluation of the patient. Normal systolic blood pressure in individuals 1 to 18 years of age can be estimated by adding twice the age in years to 80. Diastolic blood pressure is usually two thirds of the systolic blood pressure (see Appendix B-2).
3. The initial hematocrit value obtained in the ED is usually normal in acute hemorrhages and is therefore a poor indicator of volume status. A low value may indicate preexisting anemia, chronic hemorrhage, or a massive acute hemorrhage.
4. The presence of shock demands a thorough, rapid evaluation to determine the source of bleeding. In the absence of external musculoskeletal hemorrhage, three cavity spaces must be evaluated: chest, abdomen, and retroperitoneum. Except in the small infant, isolated head trauma does not cause shock. Therefore another concurrent source of shock must be aggressively investigated in the presence of head trauma.
5. Management.
   a. Significant external hemorrhage should be controlled by direct pressure. If an isolated bleeding vessel can

be identified, it may be clamped, but blind clamping in the depths of a wound is never indicated.

b. Establish IV lines. Large-bore, peripherally placed, over-the-needle catheters are optimal for rapid fluid infusion. Larger catheters permit greater flow rates. Resistance is increased by longer catheters. The flow of whole blood (at 300 mm Hg pressure) through a 16-gauge subclavian line is 60 ml/min; when through a 16-gauge short catheter, it is 149 ml/min. In the case of shock, if intravenous access cannot be obtained within the first 5 minutes, the intraosseous route should be considered.

On occasion, central venous pressure (CVP) lines may be helpful, particularly if pericardial tamponade is suspected or if there is poor response to fluid administration.

c. Initially, administer a bolus of LR solution or 0.9% NS solution, 20 ml/kg IV, as rapidly as possible. Subsequent administration of crystalloid solution and blood should reflect the response to the initial infusion and ongoing hemorrhage. Once 40 to 50 ml/kg of crystalloid has been infused during the initial resuscitation, blood should be considered if evidence of hypovolemia persists.

d. Monitor urine output, and titrate crystalloid solution infusion to maintain output at 1 to 2 ml/kg/hr.

e. If completely cross-matched blood is not available, administer type-specific blood. It is usually available 10 to 15 minutes after delivery of a clot to the blood bank. O-negative blood should be reserved for those patients who are in profound shock or cardiac arrest. Warm, fresh blood is optimal when available.

f. If massive transfusions are necessary (equivalent to one total blood volume), use blood warmers and micropore filters and also consider administration of fresh-frozen plasma and platelets. One of the greatest risks of massive transfusions is hypothermia.

g. Medical antishock trousers (MAST) or suits are available for pediatric patients, but there is evidence that they may be detrimental in the patient with major trauma. A MAST may be useful in stabilizing large-bone fractures and in controlling hemorrhage caused by intraabdominal injury or pelvic fractures. The efficacy of this garment is controversial, and controlled data are not available to demonstrate an improved outcome.

The MAST suit is contraindicated in patients with pulmonary edema and cardiogenic shock. The abdominal compartment should not be inflated in pregnant patients or in patients with evisceration or abdominal impalement. Complications include compartment syndromes and metabolic acidosis.

h. Thoracotomy permits cross-clamping of the aorta and shunting of available blood to the cerebral and coronary circulations. It also permits immediate relief of pericardial tamponade and temporary control of certain cardiothoracic injuries.

ED thoracotomy should be selectively applied to patients with trauma arrest. The prognosis for survival is best among victims of penetrating trauma who show signs of life (palpable pulse, spontaneous respirations, reactive pupils) at the scene but who subsequently experience cardiac arrest and undergo thoracotomy within 10 minutes of initiation of cardiopulmonary resuscitation (CPR).

Conversely, patients with blunt trauma who present to the ED in pulseless cardiac arrest or with severe hypotension (systolic BP <50 mm Hg) have virtually a 100% mortality and should generally not undergo resuscitative thoracotomy. A 7-year study of pediatric patients with blunt trauma arrest yielded no functional survivors. The only survivor was neurologically devastated. Patients with blunt trauma who lose their vital signs and patients with penetrating trauma who show no signs of life at the scene have a dismal prognosis. Data in the adult population is similar, undermining the potential utility of this procedure except in unique circumstances.

Fortunately, the incidence of pediatric trauma arrest is low, and any extrapolation of data from the general population to pediatric patients should be made with caution. Furthermore, an initial full resuscitation may stabilize the patient enough for transport to and maintenance in the intensive care unit (ICU) for consideration as an organ transplant donor. It is doubtful that thoracotomy will improve outcome, and the risk to the physician performing the procedure, in the form of blood exposure, must be considered.

Loss of Consciousness and Pupillary Response

A detailed neurologic examination is not conducted at this point, but findings that need immediate intervention are investigated. Specifically, the level of consciousness, as indicated by response to verbal and painful stimuli, is determined. The patient's level of consciousness may be determined with the GCS (see Table 57-1) or the AVPU method, the latter providing a qualitative assessment. *"AVPU"* is an acronym for *a*lert, responds to *v*erbal stimuli, responds to *p*ainful stimuli, and *u*nresponsive.

Likewise, pupillary symmetry and reactivity to light are noted in an effort to identify an impending brain herniation. Patients with persisting coma and certainly those with evidence of herniation should receive prompt intubation and hyperventilation and should undergo neurologic evaluation. The use of furosemide (Lasix), 1 mg/kg/dose IV, and mannitol, 0.25 to 1.0 g/kg/dose IV, should be individualized, and if possible, these agents should be given in conjunction with neurosurgical consultation. Generally, these agents are reserved for patients who show signs of developing herniation during evaluation.

REASSESSMENT AND SECONDARY SURVEY

Once the high-priority factors listed on pages 405-410 have been evaluated and appropriate treatment has been administered, vital signs, urine output, perfusion, saturation, and overall status should be reassessed. If no further actions are necessary beyond those already initiated, a complete secondary survey, including a thorough examination and a more detailed history, should be initiated.

Neurologic Considerations
(see Chapter 57)

Level of consciousness is the most important indicator of prognosis. The GCS (see Table 57-1) is an objective, reproducible means of assessing level of consciousness. A numerical score is given on the basis of motor and verbal responses and eye movement. Because the head is relatively large in children in relation to the trunk, it is often the primary point of contact in an injury.

1. Head: Inspect and palpate the head for any hematomas, ecchymoses, lacerations, or bony instability. When possible, examine deep lacerations digitally using sterile gloves.
2. Eyes: Evaluation includes the size, shape, symmetry, and reactivity of pupils; the

fundus; the fullness of extraocular movements; and any evidence of obvious trauma.

3. Nose and ears: Hemotympanum, otorrhea, and rhinorrhea indicate a basilar skull fracture and often represent the only means of making that diagnosis.
4. Movement of extremities: Note spontaneous movement or movement of all extremities in response to pain. Is movement symmetric? Is there any evidence of posturing?
5. Rectal tone: The presence of rectal tone in a patient paralyzed from spinal cord injury may indicate a central cord syndrome, which has a good prognosis. Absence of rectal tone in a comatose patient may be the only discernible clue to spinal cord injury.
6. Reflexes: Absence of deep tendon reflexes is consistent with a cord injury; upward flexion of the toes (presence of Babinski's reflex) is consistent with upper motor neuron damage.

Management. Any alteration of consciousness or abnormal neurologic findings warrant close and repeated observation, neurosurgical consultation, and consideration of a computed tomography (CT) scan. Intubation is usually indicated for a GCS score of 8 or less.

Persistent loss of consciousness requires intubation and hyperventilation if there is evidence of cerebral herniation; also use furosemide (Lasix), 1 mg/kg/dose IV, or mannitol, 0.25 to 1.0 g/kg/dose IV, if the patient is hemodynamically stable. A neurosurgeon should be consulted.

Cardiac Considerations (see Chapter 62)

Although usually not very enlightening in trauma cases, a cardiac examination should be performed, and cardiac monitoring is imperative. A full 12-lead electrocardiogram (ECG) should be obtained in all patients with chest wall trauma and dysrhythmias, hypotension, or other signs of cardiac dysfunction.

1. Inspect for signs of anterior chest wall trauma that suggest the possibility of cardiac contusion. Persistent tachycardia may be the only sign of myocardial contusion.
2. Auscultate to determine the character of the heart sounds and the presence of rubs or murmurs.
3. In penetrating chest trauma, exclude cardiac tamponade. Inspect for evidence of hypotension, tachycardia, dilated (full) jugular veins (elevated CVP), and muffled heart sounds. A pericardiocentesis may be indicated.

Management

1. Cardiac tamponade requires immediate pericardiocentesis or thoracotomy, depending on the status of the vital signs.
2. Myocardial contusion requires ICU monitoring because of the potential for dysrhythmias and even of hemodynamic compromise in cases of severe contusion. Serial cardiac isoenzyme measurements should also be obtained.

The Abdomen (see Chapter 63)

The abdomen is difficult to examine. Older, cooperative children without evidence of injury or unexplained hemodynamic instability may require no further evaluation. Younger children and children with any alteration in mental status should undergo a diagnostic evaluation by CT if there is any indication of abdominal injury or unexplained vital sign abnormalities. The patient's stability is an important factor in choosing the diagnostic approach, with unstable patients more likely to undergo laparotomy or gastric lavage. Ultrasonography may become an increasingly important modality for evaluation and treatment, with laparoscopy as another option.

Examination of the Abdomen

1. Inspect for signs of trauma and distension, and for surgical scars.

2. Auscultate to determine the presence or absence of bowel sounds.
3. Palpate to elicit tenderness and rebound and to define any masses.
4. Examine the rectum to evaluate tone, the prostate, and the presence or absence of blood in stool.
5. Palpate, compress, and rock the pelvis over the iliac crest and pubis to detect movement, tenderness, or crepitus suggestive of pelvic fracture.
6. Examine the genitalia for obvious trauma. Blood at the urethral meatus precludes the insertion of a urinary catheter and requires investigation.
7. Perform a dipstick examination of urine for blood; if present, order a microscopic analysis. If there are more than 20 red blood cells per high-powered field (RBCs/HPF), further investigation should be considered, usually including a CT scan with a contrast agent (p. 497). With a pelvic fracture, a cystogram may be performed. In males, blood at the urethra indicates the need for a retrograde urethrogram after urologic consultation.

Management. Management of blunt abdominal trauma in children is controversial. Although persistent unexplained shock requires a laparotomy, the presence of hemoperitoneum is not uniformly managed. Some centers recommend laparotomy, whereas others favor a conservative, nonoperative approach in the hemodynamically stable child, consisting of ICU observation and hemodynamic support, including limited blood transfusion. A CT scan is usually indicated in this latter group to define the nature of the injury. Both approaches have merit; the point to stress is consistency and careful adherence to the protocol followed in a given institution. Laparoscopy may also have a role. Early consultation with a surgeon is imperative so that he or she can oversee and guide diagnostic and therapeutic interventions.

Musculoskeletal Injuries
(see Chapters 66 to 70)

Musculoskeletal injuries have relatively low priority. Obvious extremity injuries require splinting and referral for a more detailed examination. Nevertheless, major bone fractures can contribute significantly to hypovolemic shock.

Examination

1. Inspect and palpate all extremities for deformity, tenderness, bony crepitus, and joint laxity.
2. Assess distal pulses and neurovascular integrity distal to the injury.
3. Inspect and palpate the spine for deformity and tenderness.

Management. Management of musculoskeletal injuries involves appropriate x-ray studies, temporary splinting, and orthopedic consultation.

Facial and Soft Tissue Injuries
(see Chapters 58, 60, and 65)

Facial injuries, unless massive, are not life threatening and require little initial treatment, although they do affect airway management. Severe hemorrhage and distortion are indications for active intervention:

1. Define contusions and lacerations of the soft tissues, and apply pressure to control hemorrhage. Assess neurovascular function and, when time permits, place sutures as needed.
2. Carefully explore the depth and severity of penetrating or significant soft tissue injuries to the neck. A surgeon should be involved in evaluation and management if there is penetration of the platysma or extensive blunt soft tissue injury.

X-RAY AND LABORATORY EVALUATIONS

X-Ray Studies

1. Essential roentgenograms during the initial evaluation of any victim of multiple trauma include an AP chest view, an AP pelvis view, and a lateral cross-table view

of the cervical spine. The spine film is essential for diagnosis of fractures and dislocations, and the chest and pelvic films may identify serious abnormality requiring further assessment and treatment as well as define a source of blood loss. If an adequate examination can be performed, the trauma series radiographs can be ordered selectively on the basis of the clinical findings.

2. Obtain portable films. Do not transport unstable patients to the radiology department. After stabilization, additional films can be obtained while the patient is being appropriately monitored.
3. CT and angiography may be necessary. Exercise great care and judgment in obtaining these studies in the unstable patient. Other priorities of care, such as a laparotomy, must be carefully weighed before diagnostic x-ray studies are obtained. Careful monitoring must be maintained throughout the examination.
4. Ultrasonography has taken on a larger role in the ED, particularly with the growing use of this technology by emergency physicians. Focused ultrasonography performed by emergency physicians has been shown to be useful in the diagnosis of trauma (abdominal and thoracic), pulseless electrical activity (PEA), pericardial tamponade, suspected abdominal aortic aneurysm, gallbladder disease, ectopic pregnancy, and obstructive uropathy.

Laboratory Studies

1. Studies that should be performed in the ED include a spun hematocrit determination, urinalysis, and perhaps an oximetry or arterial blood gas (ABG) determination.
2. Blood typing and cross-match are essential in patients with all significant trauma cases but should be ordered selectively in other patients.
3. Routine studies include a complete blood count (CBC), platelet count, measurements of electrolytes, blood urea nitrogen (BUN), glucose, and amylase (with abdominal abnormality), and coagulation studies (prothrombin time [PT] and partial thromboplastin time [PTT]).

   Coagulation disorders are most common in patients with severe head trauma and less common in cases of gunshot wounds, blunt trauma, and stab wounds. Abnormalities are most commonly found in patients with a GCS score of 13 or less, low systolic blood pressure, open or multiple bone fractures, or major tissue injury. A rapid bedside screen may be accomplished by observing for clot formation in blood drawn into a clean tube. Normally, the blood clots and then retracts within 10 minutes. The absence of clotting indicates a major coagulopathy, whereas abnormal clot retraction suggests thrombocytopenia. If the blood clots and subsequently lyses, fibrinolysis is occurring.
4. Consider a urine drug screen (unfortunately, drug use is growing in every young population).
5. Perform an ECG if indicated by the nature of the injury.
6. Test for pregnancy in menstruating females.

SCORING PEDIATRIC TRAUMA

A number of scoring systems have been developed to facilitate consistency of evaluation of trauma in children. In one study using the Pediatric Trauma Score (PTS) (Table 56-1), 28% of patients with a score of 6 or lower died, whereas only 1% of those with a score of 7 or higher died. All children with a score lower than 2 died.

The Revised Trauma Score (RTS) (Table 56-2), which can be used in both adults and children, has been shown to be a valid predictor of

TABLE 56-1 Pediatric Trauma Score*

	SCORE FOR EACH VARIABLE*		
Component	**+2**	**+1**	**−1**
Weight	≥20 kg	10-20 kg	<10 kg
Airway patency	Normal	Maintainable	Unmaintainable
Systolic blood pressure	≥90 mm Hg	90-50 mm Hg	<50 mm Hg
CNS status	Awake	Obtunded/loss of consciousness	Coma/decerebrate
Open wound	None	Minor	Major/penetrating
Skeletal injury	None	Closed fracture	Open/multiple fractures

From Tepas JJ, Mollitt DL, Talbert JL et al: *J Pediatr Surg* 22:14, 1987.
* A score of +2, +1, or −1 is given to each variable and then added (range, −6 to 12). A score ≤8 indicates potentially important trauma.

TABLE 56-2 Revised Trauma Score*

Revised Trauma Score	Glasgow Coma Scale Score (Table 57-1)	Systolic Blood Pressure (mm Hg)	Respiratory Rate (breaths/min)
4	13-15	>89	10-29
3	9-12	76-89	>29
2	6-8	50-75	6-9
1	4-5	1-49	1-5
0	3	0	0

From Wesson DE, Spence LJ, Williams JL et al: *Can J Surg* 30:398, 1987.
* A score of 0-4 is given for each variable, then added (range, 1-12). A score ≤11 indicates potentially important trauma.

severity. It may define the severity of injury from the prehospital environment through the hospital stay.

The PTS predicts risk for severe injury or death but has performed less well in patients with isolated blunt abdominal injuries. The PTS and RTS are similar in their ability to identify severely injured children. However, the RTS has greater simplicity and is useful for adult and pediatric patients with trauma. The Trauma Score and Injury Severity Score (TRISS) and A Characterization of Trauma (ASCOT) are evolving as outcome analysis systems.

After motor vehicle crashes, predictive criteria for significant injury in children include a GCS score lower than 15, passenger space intrusion of 15 cm or more, and lack of use of passenger restraints.

After blunt trauma, patients who present to an ED with pulseless cardiac arrest have little chance of functional survival.

CONSULTATION

1. Notify a trauma surgeon as soon as the facility is alerted that a patient with serious trauma is en route to the hospital. Depending on the reliability of the prehospital care assessment, this initial surgical contact may await arrival and primary assessment if the surgeon is not in the hospital.
2. Notify a neurosurgeon if significant head injury is present.
3. Orthopedic, plastic surgery, and urology personnel may be notified after the patient has been stabilized. Premature consultation may add chaos and confusion to the initial resuscitation.

PSYCHOLOGIC CONCERNS

For many reasons, the child who is the victim of trauma may be terrified and crying hysterically on arrival in the ED. Pain is present from either the injuries or their treatment. The child is separated from parents, in a strange environment and surrounded by unfamiliar doctors and nurses.

Support is essential for the conscious child. Time must be taken to explain in a reassuring way that the youngster has been injured, is in the hospital, and is going to be all right. Touching the child in a soothing manner as well as speaking in a calm, controlled tone may be helpful in winning confidence and establishing rapport. Procedures should be explained if possible, and the child warned that there may be accompanying pain. The patient should not be surprised.

Parents should be allowed to stay with the child whenever possible. This may not be feasible when the youngster is critically ill, requiring major resuscitative efforts, or when the parents are so upset that they are actually contributing to the patient's hysteria. If parents are unavailable, a member of the resuscitation team should be designated to support the child as a surrogate parent in these circumstances; make sure that there is adequate communication and support for the family when contact is made.

Long-term follow-up is probably indicated to monitor for the evolution of poststress anxiety reactions. These may develop in children who have experienced a life-threatening event or have witnessed such an episode in a family member or friend.

DISPOSITION

Patients with multiple serious injuries should be admitted to the trauma service, with coordination of the appropriate consulting services.

Transfer of the patient to another institution is indicated only if definitive care cannot be provided at the initial facility. Lines of referral for specific types of injury (i.e., burns, amputation) should be established in advance to facilitate communication and transfer.

Before transfer, the patient's condition must be stabilized. During transfer, the levels of monitoring and treatment established in the ED should be maintained. All records, x-ray films, and laboratory data should accompany the patient (see Chapter 3).

COST OF TRAUMA

Trauma results in direct and indirect costs not just in terms of recovery after the initial injury but also in loss of future productivity of the child throughout his or her life, damage to parental marital relationships, and the financial affect on the family.

Studies of adults and children with severe head injuries found that more than 25% of families reported use of all or most of their fiscal resources after an injury. Nearly one third of families experienced marital difficulties, and more than half had new social and financial problems. Another study found that even for children who are only mildly injured, 60% of the families reported at least one financial or work-related problem at 1 month after discharge, and 40% reported at least one problem 6 months after discharge.

Families must be counseled about the impending stresses that they can expect in the recovery phase and must be made aware of any resources that they may have at their disposal.

BIBLIOGRAPHY

American College of Emergency Physicians: Clinical policy for the initial approach to patients presenting with acute blunt trauma, *Ann Emerg Med* 31:422, 1998.

American College of Emergency Physicians: Guidelines for trauma care systems, *Ann Emerg Med* 22:1079, 1993.

American College of Surgeons Committee on Trauma: *Advanced trauma life support program for physicians*, Chicago, 1993, American College of Surgeons.

Boulanger BR, McLellan BA, Brenneman FD et al: Emergent abdominal sonography as a screening test in a new diagnostic algorithm for blunt trauma, *J Trauma* 40:867, 1996.

Durham LA, Richardson RJ, Wall JM et al: Emergency center thoracotomy: impact of prehospital resuscitation, *Trauma* 32:775, 1992.

Esposito TJ, Jurkovich GJ, Rice CL et al: Reappraisal of emergency room thoracotomy in a changing environment, *J Trauma* 31:881, 1991.

Ferrera PC, Colucciello SA, Marx JA et al, editors: *Trauma management: an emergency medicine approach*, St Louis, 2001, Mosby.

Fitzmaurice LS: Approach to multiple trauma. In Barkin RM, editor: *Pediatric emergency medicine: concepts and clinical practice*, ed 2, St Louis, 1997, Mosby.

Furnival RA, Schunk JE: ABCs of scoring systems for pediatric trauma, *Pediatr Emerg Care* 15:215, 1999.

Gerardi MI, Sacchetti AD, Kantor RM et al: Rapid sequence intubation of the pediatric patient, *Ann Emerg Med* 28:55, 1996.

Gin-Shaw SL, Jorden RC: Multiple trauma. In Marx JA, Hockberger RS, Walls RM et al: *Rosen's Emergency medicine, concepts and clinical practice*, ed 5, St Louis, 2002, Mosby.

Gnauck K, Lungo JB, Scalzo A et al: Emergency intubation of the pediatric medical patient: use of anesthetic agents in the emergency department, *Ann Emerg Med* 23:1242, 1994.

Green SM, Rothrock SG: Is pediatric trauma really a surgical disease? *Ann Emerg Med* 39:537, 2002.

Grupp-Phelan J, Tanz RR: How rational is the crossmatching of blood in a pediatric emergency department? *Arch Pediatr Adolesc Med* 150:1140, 1996.

Hazinski MF, Chahine AA, Holcomb GW et al: Outcome of cardiovascular collapse in pediatric blunt trauma, *Ann Emerg Med* 23:1229, 1994.

Holmes JF, Goodwin HC, Land C et al: Coagulation testing in pediatric blunt trauma patients, *Pediatr Emerg Care* 17:324, 2001.

Hooker EA, Miller FB, Holanderi R et al: Do all trauma patients need early crossmatching for blood? *J Emerg Med* 12:447, 1994.

Ivatury RR, Kazigo J, Rohman M et al: Directed emergency room thoracotomy: a prognostic prerequisite for survival, *J Trauma* 31:1076, 1991.

Jaffe D, Wesson D: Emergency management of blunt trauma in children, *N Engl J Med* 324:1477, 1991.

Kevill K, Wong M, Goldman HS et al: Is a complete trauma series indicated for all pediatric trauma victims? *Pediatr Emerg Care* 18:75, 2002.

King BR, Baker MD, Braitman LE et al: Endotracheal tube selection in children: a comparison of four methods, *Ann Emerg Med* 22:530, 1993.

Nakayama DK, Waggoner T, Venkataraman ST et al: The use of drugs in emergency airway management in pediatric trauma, *Ann Surg* 216:205, 1992.

Newgard CD, Lewis RJ, Jolly BJ: Use of out-of-hospital variables to predict severity of injury in pediatric patients involved in motor vehicle crashes, *Ann Emerg Med* 39:481, 2002.

Orsborn R, Haley K, Hammond S et al: Pediatric pedestrian versus motor vehicle patterns of injury: debunking the myth, *Air Med J* 18:107, 1999.

Osberg JS, Kahn P, Rowe K et al: Pediatric trauma: impact on work and family finances, *Pediatrics* 98:890, 1996.

Pearlman MD, Tintinalli JE, Lorenz RP: Blunt trauma during pregnancy, *N Engl J Med* 323:1609, 1990.

Phillips S, Rond PC, Kelly SM et al: The need for pediatric-specific triage criteria: results from the Florida Trauma Triage Study, *Pediatr Emerg Care* 12:394, 1996.

Scales TM, Todriquez A: Focused assessment with sonography for trauma (FAST): results from an international consensus conference, *J Trauma* 47:632, 1999.

Stewart G, Meert K, Rosenberg N: Trauma in infants less than three months of age, *Pediatr Emerg Care* 9:199, 1993.

Teech SJ, Antosia RE, Luno DF et al: Prehospital fluid therapy in pediatric trauma patients, *Pediatr Emerg Care* 17:5, 1995.

Thomas B, Falcone RE, Vasquez D et al: Ultrasound evaluation of blunt abdominal trauma: program implementation, initial experience, and learning curve, *J Trauma* 42:384, 1997.

Trunkey D: Initial treatment of patients with extensive trauma, *N Engl J Med* 324:1259, 1991.

Walls RM: Rapid-sequence intubation in head trauma, *Ann Emerg Med* 22:1008, 1993.

Weesner CL, Hargarfen SW, Aprakamian C et al: Fatal childhood injury patterns in an urban setting, *Ann Emerg Med* 23:231, 1994.

Woolard DJ, Terndrup TE: Sedative-analgesic agent administration in children: analysis of use and complications in the emergency department, *J Emerg Med* 12:453, 1994.

Yamamoto LG, Yim GK, Britten AG: Rapid sequence anesthesia induction for emergency intubation, *Pediatr Emerg Care* 6:200, 1990.

Yen K, Gorelick MH: Ultrasound applications for the pediatric emergency department: a review of the current literature, *Pediatr Emerg Care* 18:226, 2002.

Yurt RW: Triage, initial assessment and early treatment of the pediatric trauma patient, *Pediatr Clin North Am* 39:1083, 1992.

57 Head Trauma

PETER T. PONS

ALERT Any patient with head trauma must be considered to have spinal trauma and other associated injuries until they are excluded. Initial evaluation must focus on airway, ventilation, circulation, and immobilization of the cervical spine. Head injury as an isolated finding very rarely causes shock.

Auto accidents account for most traumatic brain injuries (TBIs). The *primary insult* is the injury to the brain that occurs at the time of impact. This results from translational or rotational forces. Translational forces produce compressive and tensile strains on the skull and brain, leading to focal brain injuries such as linear skull fractures, cerebral contusions, epidural hematomas, acute subdural hematomas, and contrecoup cerebral contusions. Rotational forces can be more devastating, resulting in a shearing stress that causes diffuse brain injuries, including mild contusion, cerebral concussion, and diffuse cerebral injury. Significant distortion of the skull can occur in infants younger than 2 years because of the open sutures and the relative elasticity of the skull. This distortion can be transmitted to the underlying meninges, cortical vessels, and brain, leading to a high incidence of hematomas, tentorial and dural lesions, and shearing.

The *secondary insult* is the progressive deficit caused by cerebral ischemia, hypoxia, hypercapnia, hypotension, and increased intracranial pressure (ICP). Brain swelling is the most common cause of death in patients with severe head injuries. Brain swelling compromises delivery of oxygen and glucose to neurons.

Child abuse should be considered in cases of intracranial injuries or skull fractures in children younger than 1 year if there is no history of significant accidental trauma, such as a motor vehicle accident.

Aggressive early resuscitation, encompassing the establishment of the integrity of the airway, ventilation, and circulation, and the immobilization of the spine, largely determines the outcome. Careful examination, evaluation, and treatment of associated injuries is crucial. This is followed by systematic, definitive care of neurologic and other injuries.

Minor head trauma is associated with normal mental status without abnormal or local neurologic findings and no evidence of skull fracture. The Glasgow Coma Scale (GCS) score for such patients is 13 to 15 or 14 to 15, depending upon the study. *Moderate* head trauma is associated with a GCS score of 9 to 12 or 9 to 13, and patients with *severe* head trauma have a GCS score lower than 8.

DIAGNOSTIC FINDINGS

History

The mechanism of trauma and associated signs and symptoms must be determined after initial resuscitation:

1. Mechanism of injury: direct blow (define implement) or acceleration-deceleration
2. Circumstances of accident: motor vehicle accident, sports injury, diving accident,

fall, or blow (any inconsistencies that might suggest abuse)

3. Chronology:
   a. Loss of consciousness immediately or shortly after accident
   b. Period of lucidity
   c. Progression of deficits
4. Associated findings:
   a. Amnesia
   b. Disorientation
   c. Sensorimotor abnormalities
   d. Visual disturbances
   e. Dizziness
   f. Vomiting or nausea
   g. Seizures
5. Medications in effect at the time of the incident, including alcohol, drugs, and prescribed treatments
6. Medical history and allergies
7. Coagulopathy

Associated injuries, especially facial and neck, are often present.

General Physical Examination

In addition to specific evaluation of the head and back, examination of the cervical spine and other areas of trauma should be performed. In infants and children younger than 2 years, a specific examination for scalp hematomas should be performed.

Frequent repetition of the examination is essential to detect any signs of deterioration as well as to monitor improvement. Specific consideration must be given to determining the extent of neurologic injury, the presence of a mass lesion effect, and the course of the injury.

Vital Signs

1. Airway: Often occluded by blood, mucus, fractures, or foreign bodies, leading to respiratory distress.
2. Hypotension: Acute head trauma does not produce hypotension except in infants with open sutures and massive intracranial bleeding or in individuals with large scalp lacerations. If shock is present, look for other associated injuries.
3. Dysrhythmias: ventricular and atrial. Prolonged QT interval and large T and prominent U waves have been noted without cardiac abnormality.
4. Cushing's reflex: Produces elevated blood pressure, slowed pulse, and irregular respirations. Usually a late finding of increased ICP.
5. Cheyne-Stokes respiration: Characterized by crescendo-decrescendo patterns of hyperventilation followed by periods of apnea. Often accompanies decorticate posturing caused by cerebral hemispheric lesions and incipient temporal lobe herniation. May be seen during normal infant sleep.
6. Central neurogenic hyperventilation with deep, rapid ventilation. May accompany decerebrate posturing and indicates brainstem dysfunction, either as a primary injury or secondary to supratentorial herniation.

Neurologic Examination (see Table 15-3)

Level of consciousness

1. Maximal depression in the level of consciousness usually occurs at the time of impact and should subsequently improve. Failure to improve indicates that additional or massive injury has occurred.
2. The level of consciousness may be recorded in a descriptive narrative indicating the patient's response to stimuli; the mnemonic is "AVPU":
   - A: awake verbal child
   - V: in a nonverbal child, denotes a child who is responsive to verbal stimuli; clues include behavioral signs such as eye opening, quieting, and calming
   - P: response to painful stimuli, such as moaning or crying
   - U: unresponsive to any stimuli

   Another descriptive approach consists of *alert* (awake and responds verbally to questions), *lethargic* (sleeps when undisturbed but is incoherent when awakened), *semicomatose* (responds to painful stimuli in a purposeful, decorticate, or decerebrate posture), and *comatose* (no response to stimuli).

3. The GCS for responsiveness (Table 57-1) standardizes assessment, predicts outcome, and is useful in monitoring patients. A pediatric modification has been developed.

 A GCS score of 3 to 8 upon presentation to the emergency department (ED) indicates severe head trauma and is predictive of past traumatic seizures. Children with a GCS score of 15 and normal neurologic findings are generally not reported to have significant intracranial hemorrhage.

Posturing. Decerebrate posturing (extension) and flaccidity are associated with the worst prognosis. Decorticate posturing manifests as flexion.

Pupils: Size, Equality, and Reactivity

1. Unilateral pupillary dilation strongly suggests a mass lesion with actual or incipient herniation requiring immediate intervention. A dilated and fixed pupil is the most reliable sign of the side of the lesion. It usually results from pressure on the ipsilateral third cranial nerve (oculomotor).
2. Venous pulsations on examination of the fundus indicate an ICP lower than 15 mm Hg. However, they may be absent in patients with normal ICP.

TABLE 57-1 Pediatric Modification of Glasgow Coma Scale (GCS) by Age of Patient*

GCS Score	Pediatric Modification	
EYE OPENING		
≥1 year	**0-1 year**	
4 Spontaneously	4 Spontaneously	
3 To verbal command	3 To shout	
2 To pain	2 To pain	
1 No response	1 No response	
BEST MOTOR RESPONSE		
≥1 year	**0-1 year**	
6 Obeys		
5 Localizes pain	5 Localizes pain	
4 Flexion withdrawal	4 Flexion withdrawal	
3 Flexion abnormal (decorticate)	3 Flexion abnormal (decorticate)	
2 Extension (decerebrate)	2 Extension (decerebrate)	
1 No response	1 No response	
BEST VERBAL RESPONSE		
>5 years	**0-2 years**	**2-5 years**
5 Oriented and converses	5 Cries appropriately, smiles, coos	5 Appropriate words and phrases
4 Disoriented and converses	4 Cries	4 Inappropriate words
3 Inappropriate words	3 Inappropriate crying/screaming	3 Cries/screams
2 Incomprehensible sounds	2 Grunts	2 Grunts
1 No response	1 No response	1 No response

* Score is the sum of the individual scores from eye opening, best verbal response, and best motor response, using age-specific criteria. GCS score of 13-15 indicates mild head injury, GCS score of 9-12 indicates moderate head injury, and GCS score of ≤8 indicates severe head injury.

3. Examination must exclude previous eye trauma, topical medications, and congenital anisocoria.

   NOTE: Retinal hemorrhage in children younger than 1 year is usually associated with shaking injuries.
4. Hemorrhaging into the retina with a decrease in visual acuity may be noted after trauma.

Eye movements

1. Destructive lesions in the occipital or frontal lobes cause deviation of the eyes toward the lesion. Injury to the brainstem causes deviation away from the lesion.
2. Oculocephalic reflex (doll's eye) demonstrates intactness of the brainstem, as does the oculovestibular reflex. These should be tested only after the cervical spine has been cleared.
   a. Oculocephalic reflex (doll's eye reflex) is performed with the patient's eyes held open and the head turned quickly from side to side. A comatose patient with an intact brainstem responds by moving the eyes in the direction opposite to the direction in which the head is turned, as if still gazing ahead in the initial position. Comatose patients with midbrain or pons lesions have random eye movements.
   b. Oculovestibular reflex with caloric stimulation is performed with the patient's head elevated 30 degrees in a patient with an intact eardrum. Iced water is then injected through a small catheter lying in the ear canal (up to 200 ml is used in an adult). Comatose patients with an intact brainstem respond with conjugate deviation of the eyes toward the irrigated ear, whereas those with a brainstem lesion show no response.
   c. Corneal reflex is elicited by gently stroking the cornea with sterile cotton. A blink response demonstrates intactness of the brainstem and nuclei of cranial nerves V, VI, and VII.

Sensory and motor responses

1. Motor responses may be determined from the response to verbal commands, painful stimuli, and spontaneous movements. Tone, any posturing, and symmetry should be evaluated.
2. Sensory examination should include light touch and pain.

Reflexes

1. Presence, absence, and equality of reflexes should be ascertained.
2. The presence of Babinski's reflex (dorsiflexive plantar response) indicates an upper motor neuron lesion.

Rectal examination. A rectal examination must be performed to check for spinal cord integrity, which is indicated by the presence of sphincter tone.

Other Findings.

For a careful assessment, the following signs are important:

1. Bulging fontanelle
2. Palpable depression or crepitus of skull; unusual hematoma, particularly a longitudinal one
3. Evidence of basilar skull fracture:
   a. Battle's sign (ecchymosis posterior to ear) or raccoon eyes sign (bilateral black eyes)
   b. Cerebrospinal fluid (CSF) rhinorrhea or otorrhea
   c. Hemotympanum or bleeding from the middle ear
4. Diabetes insipidus; polyuria, nocturia, and polydipsia
5. Cortical blindness may occur after minor head injury from vascular hyperactivity (similar to migraine equivalent). Typically, children sustain trauma without loss of consciousness. Blindness develops after a latent period of 15 to 45 minutes and may last for a few hours up to 10 days, usually with total recovery. Pupillary light reflexes are normal.

Increased intracranial pressure. Increased ICP should be suspected in patients with trauma who have a GCS score less than 8, seizures that are difficult to control, abnormal vital signs (hypertension, bradycardia, abnormal respirations), dilated and unreactive pupils, and decerebrate or decorticate posturing.

As the ICP rises, a relatively well-defined series of events occurs, leading ultimately to the patient's death unless appropriate actions are taken to slow or reverse the process. As the pressure rises in the supratentorial compartment, the brain (usually the uncus or medial temporal lobe) is pushed against and through the opening of the tentorium. This produces compression of the ipsilateral third cranial nerve, leading to a fixed, dilated pupil. Occasionally, the contralateral third nerve is compromised.

Progression of the herniation leads to compression of the pyramidal tract, usually resulting in contralateral weakness or paralysis. Simultaneously, pressure on the reticular activating system leads to impaired consciousness, which may be the first sign of deterioration.

In the infant with an open fontanelle, initial findings include a bulging fontanelle, irritability, and listlessness, eventually progressing to focal findings. Patients with closed fontanelles and increased ICP present a more classic picture.

In patients with cerebellar tonsillar herniation, the midline force causes the low brainstem and cerebellar tonsils to herniate through the foramen magnum, leading to Cushing's reflex (bradycardia, hypertension, and apnea).

Prognostic Factors

Prognostic factors in severe head trauma may be useful in the management of children's injuries. Severe head trauma is defined as unconsciousness for more than 6 hours and inability to obey commands, utter recognizable words, or open the eyes.

Children younger than 10 years generally have the best prognosis, according to the literature. Those with a GCS score of 5 to 8 usually do not die, and only 20% have permanent focal deficits. Those with GCS scores of 3 to 5 can achieve independent function. Higher scores are associated with even fewer sequelae. The recovery to consciousness and function is usually complete within 3 weeks, and 77% of the children in one study returned to a regular school setting.

The worst prognosis is for those children with flaccidity or decerebrate posturing. Children with prolonged coma tend to have a poor outcome, but in one study, 9 of 14 children in coma for more than 2 weeks had little or no handicapping neurologic sequelae.

Complications

Several other findings secondary to complications of the initial mechanical injury, as well as hypoxia, increased ICP, hypotension, and hypercapnia, may be noted:

1. Altered neurologic findings, as noted.
2. Seizures within 1 week of injury occur in approximately 5% of children hospitalized after head trauma; another 5% have a seizure after the first week. Half of the children eventually stop having seizures; 25% have occasional seizures; and the remainder have more than 10 per year. Patients in coma longer than 6 hours have almost a 50% incidence of seizures. Other findings associated with seizures are a GCS score of 3 to 8 and abnormality on computed tomography (CT) scans. Children with these findings have a 35% to 40% incidence of seizure, whereas in those without such abnormalities, the incidence is approximately 5%.
3. Psychosocial and behavioral findings after mild head trauma include disinhibition, depression, emotional lability, and irritability.
4. Noncardiogenic pulmonary edema.
5. Apnea. Posttraumatic apnea is due to transient impairment of the reticular activating system along the brainstem. Usually, it is self-limited or requires minimal stimulation. Prolonged apnea implies a more serious injury.

6. Shock is generally not associated with isolated head trauma. However, in children younger than 1 year, an expanding epidural hematoma may lead to significant blood loss. A subgaleal hematoma or scalp avulsion may also cause major blood loss.
7. Death resulting from the primary process or secondary complications.

Ancillary Data

X-Ray Film of the Cervical Spine. (See Chapter 61.) An x-ray film of the cervical spine should be obtained routinely in all patients older than 3 years with a posttraumatic altered mental status, neurologic deficit, neck or back pain, and a mechanism of injury consistent with causing a spine injury and in patients who give incomplete histories, such as younger children and drug abusers. Younger infants should undergo radiographic study selectively.

A cross-table lateral cervical spine view should be the first radiograph obtained.

Skull X-Ray Film. An x-ray study of the skull is usually not needed in the initial management because a bone fracture is not the critical injury; intracranial injury must be defined. Thus, CT scanning is the preferred diagnostic study. Plain film x-rays may be useful in tracking a bullet or other object if there is penetrating trauma as well as to document child abuse.

Patients for whom there is a high risk of fracture include those with the following factors:

1. Documented loss of consciousness for longer than 5 minutes or lack of consciousness at the time of the evaluation.
2. The possibility of a depressed skull fracture (palpable defect, crepitus) or a suggestive history (blunt injury from the head of a hammer or the heel of a high-heeled shoe). Tangential views may be required.
3. Focal neurologic signs.
4. Penetrating trauma.
5. Evidence of basilar skull fracture (Battle's or raccoon eyes sign, CSF leaking from nose or ear, hemotympanum).
6. Head trauma in which child abuse is suspected, particularly in children younger than 1 year.

Important findings on a skull x-ray film are as follows:

1. Fracture that crosses the middle meningeal artery groove, which is associated with higher incidence of epidural hematoma
2. Depressed skull fracture
3. Open fracture

The absence of a fracture does not exclude significant intracranial pathologic conditions. The presence of a skull fracture may be a valuable marker in the early identification of pediatric patients with moderate head injury who are at greatly increased risk of an intracranial injury.

Computed Tomography Scan or Magnetic Resonance Imaging. CT scanning is the definitive diagnostic procedure of choice. A noncontrast CT scan of the *acutely* traumatized patient, including bone and subdural windows, is usually sufficient, but a contrast CT scan (using a dose of contrast agent at 3 ml/kg) may be useful for chronic subdural hematoma (7 days of age or older). Generalized cerebral swelling is common. If a CT scan is immediately available, a skull x-ray film may be selectively omitted.

Indications for obtaining a CT scan include but are not limited to the following:

1. Unconsciousness at the time of evaluation
2. Focal neurologic deficits
3. Depressed skull fracture or fracture crossing the middle meningeal artery groove; suspicion of a depressed skull fracture
4. Deterioration of mental status or neurologic function
5. Delayed posttraumatic seizure
6. Children younger than 1 year who have bradycardia, diastasis of sutures on skull x-ray study, or a full fontanelle
7. Progressive or ongoing symptoms, such as headache and vomiting

8. Scalp hematoma (infants and children younger than 2 years)

However, no clinical findings accurately identify all patients with abnormal CT findings. Clinical findings that have been associated with abnormal CT findings include a GCS score of 12 or less, altered mental status on admission, and focal abnormalities detected on neurologic examination.

Another study has shown that four variables (nausea, vomiting, severe headache, and skull depression) identified patients with minor head trauma and a GCS score of 15 who ultimately required neurosurgical intervention. These clinical parameters may be useful in identifying patients who require CT scans. Prospective studies are still required.

Assessing the patient with head trauma requires a systematic approach to radiologic evaluation. Magnetic resonance imaging (MRI) may offer detection of more subtle changes indicating contusions and nonhemorrhagic injuries. Diffuse axonal injury or isodense subdurals are useful in detecting sequelae of child abuse but the MRI is ideal for acute bleeding or fractures. More planes of visualization are available in MRI without patient manipulation, and evaluation of extracerebral fluid collections is improved. Time availability and patient instability usually preclude the use of MRI in the emergency setting.

Other Data

1. Arterial blood gas (ABG) analysis and oximetry are important to ensure that the patient is being adequately ventilated and oxygenated and that hyperventilation is maintaining $PaCO_2$.
2. Lumbar puncture (LP) is not indicated. If infection is being considered, LP should be performed only after CT findings are normal in a patient with preceding trauma. Empiric administration of antibiotics after collection of appropriate culture specimens should be considered.
3. An electroencephalogram (EEG) rarely provides any information that is useful either therapeutically or prognostically.
4. Check electrolyte levels if there is evidence of diabetes insipidus.
5. The serum cleaved tau protein may be a marker for traumatic brain injury. When detected within 10 hours of the head injury, it is associated with a risk of increased ICP. Other serum markers have been studied as well.
6. Perform a chest x-ray study to exclude pulmonary edema.

INITIAL MANAGEMENT

The initial management of severe head trauma is directed not at therapy of the head trauma itself but rather at immediate or potential life threats. The goal is to maintain adequate cerebral perfusion and oxygenation. Minimal head trauma requires a careful examination, appropriate laboratory studies, a short period of observation, and good follow-up observation and instructions.

Airway

1. Oxygenate the patient and keep PaO_2 above 60 mm Hg.
2. Suction blood and secretions, and remove foreign material from the airway.
3. If the patient is unable to maintain a patent airway, active management is essential but attempts must be made to maintain cervical spine precautions, if necessary. Some authorities recommend endotracheal intubation when the GCS score is less than 8 or when there is persistent hypoxia. Orotracheal intubation with maintenance of in-line cervical spine immobilization may be attempted.
4. Patients who are acutely unconscious secondary to trauma, particularly those requiring prolonged diagnostic evaluation or transport, should generally be considered for intubation on a prophylactic basis as well as for initiation of hyperventilation.

5. If time permits, administer lidocaine (1.5 mg/kg IV) 1 minute before intubation to prevent an acute rise in ICP. Administration of atropine (0.01 mg/kg/dose; minimum: 0.1 mg; maximum: 1 mg) may reduce potential bradycardia. Rapid-sequence induction is outlined in Chapter 56.

Respirations.

Supplemental oxygen and assisted ventilation should be administered as necessary.

Circulatory Status. (See Chapter 5)

Volume resuscitation with restoration of normal intravascular volume is essential to maintain cerebral perfusion pressure (CPP). Intake and output must be closely monitored. CPP depends on an adequate blood pressure.

Shock must be managed aggressively with crystalloid infused through large-bore IV lines. If shock is present, associated injuries should be delineated while hemodynamic stability is being achieved.

Immobilization of Cervical Spine

See Chapter 61.

Reduction of Intracranial Pressure

1. Hyperventilation is the most rapid method of decreasing ICP and is usually indicated if the GCS score is less than or equal to 8 (see Table 57-1).
   a. Avoid prophylactic hyperventilation ($Paco_2$ ≤35 mm Hg) during the first 24 hours after severe TBI because cerebral perfusion may be compromised at a time when cerebral blood flow is reduced.
   b. Reducing the ICP below 25 mm Hg may cause vasoconstriction and cerebral ischemia. Decreasing the $Paco_2$ from 40 to 20 mm Hg reduces cerebral blood flow to nearly 60% of normal. Hyperventilation to $Paco_2$ below 35 mm Hg may be useful for brief periods in the patient with an acute neurologic deterioration or for longer periods if the increased ICP is refractory to other measures.
   c. Maintain Pao_2 of at least 90 mm Hg. Supplemental oxygen and positive end-expiratory pressure (PEEP) may be required.
2. Elevate head to approximately 30 degrees if the patient is not in shock.
3. Administer one or more of the following:
   a. Furosemide (Lasix), 1 mg/kg/dose q4-6hr IV (adult: 20 to 40 mg/dose q4-6hr IV)
   b. Mannitol:
      (1) Dosage: 0.25 g/kg/dose over 10 to 15 minutes q3-4hr IV prn.
      (2) Not used in routine management but useful if there are signs of increased ICP.
      (3) Risks: fluid and electrolyte imbalance, hyperosmolality, volume overload, and rebound cerebral edema. Not to be used for patients with renal failure. Role in patients with evidence of shock is controversial.
4. Monitor ICP in consultation with a neurosurgeon in cases of severe head trauma (GCS score 3 to 8), particularly in patients with abnormal CT findings (hematoma, contusion, edema, compressed basal cistern). Optimally, maintain ICP at 20 mm Hg or less and CPP at 50 mm Hg or more. An ICP above 40 mm Hg is associated with a poor outcome.
5. Barbiturates are useful for significant cerebral edema associated with elevated and poorly responsive ICP. These agents decrease ICP and cerebral metabolism and stabilize cell membranes. Because the ability to evaluate neurologic status is lost with their use, barbiturates should be given only in consultation with a neurosurgeon.

- Pentobarbital (Nembutal) dosage is 3 to 20 mg/kg IV slow push while blood pressure is monitored. Infusion is kept at 1 to 2 mg/kg/hr to maintain a serum drug level of 25 to 40 μg/ml. Levels above 30 μg/ml may be associated with hypotension in as many as 60% of cases.

6. The prophylactic use of anticonvulsants such as phenytoin and phenobarbital is controversial and should be discussed with the consultant neurosurgeon. Anticonvulsant therapy should be initiated if there is seizure activity and should be considered in patients with severe TBI, significant neurologic deficit, penetrating brain injuries, or depressed fractures with true penetration, at least in the acute period.
7. Maintain hypothermia if already present. Induce hypothermia (see Chapter 51) only as a last resort in patients whose ICP remains elevated despite other measures and after consultation.
   a. It reduces cerebral metabolism and vulnerability to hypoxemia.
   b. In consultation with a neurosurgeon, temperature may be gradually reduced to 32° to 33° C.
8. The potential role of calcium channel blockers is under investigation; these agents may help reduce cerebral damage after head trauma. Studies are also exploring the effects of a vasoactive analogue of adrenocorticotropic hormone (GMM_2).

SPECIFIC CLINICAL ENTITIES (Fig. 57-1)

Minor Head Trauma (GCS score higher than 13 or 14)

The diagnosis of minor head trauma requires an unremarkable history and normal findings. Neurologically normal children with normal CT findings are at very low risk for deterioration. Minor head trauma should be treated as follows:

1. Children 2 to 20 years old:
   a. With no loss of consciousness: Observation. CT or MRI is often not performed because the marginal benefits are outweighed by the cost, inconvenience, and logistics as well as the potential risks of sedation.
   b. With brief (<1 minute) loss of consciousness: Observation often combined with CT. If CT is not readily available, skull radiographs may assist in defining a high-risk population.
2. Children younger than 2 years:
   a. In younger children, a lower threshold for performing imaging studies is needed.
   b. High-risk group includes children who have depressed mental status, focal neurologic findings, signs of depressed or basilar skull fracture, irritability, or vomiting that occurs five or more times or persists longer than 6 hours, and children younger than 3 months.
   c. Intermediate-risk group consists of children with three or four episodes of vomiting, transient (<1 minute) loss of consciousness, history of lethargy or irritability, abnormal behavior, and no acute (>24 hour) skull fracture. Also in this group are children with a higher-force mechanism of injury (high-speed motor vehicle accident or fall of more than 3 or 4 feet), fall onto a hard surface, large and boggy scalp hematoma particularly if in the temporoparietal area, or unwitnessed trauma that is potentially a major mechanism, and those for whom there are concerns about abuse.
   d. Low-risk group consists of those with no signs or symptoms at least 2 hours after the incident and a low-force mechanism of injury.

Disposition of the child with minor head trauma should reflect the nature of the findings, concerns about child abuse, and follow-up and compliance with the necessity for observation.

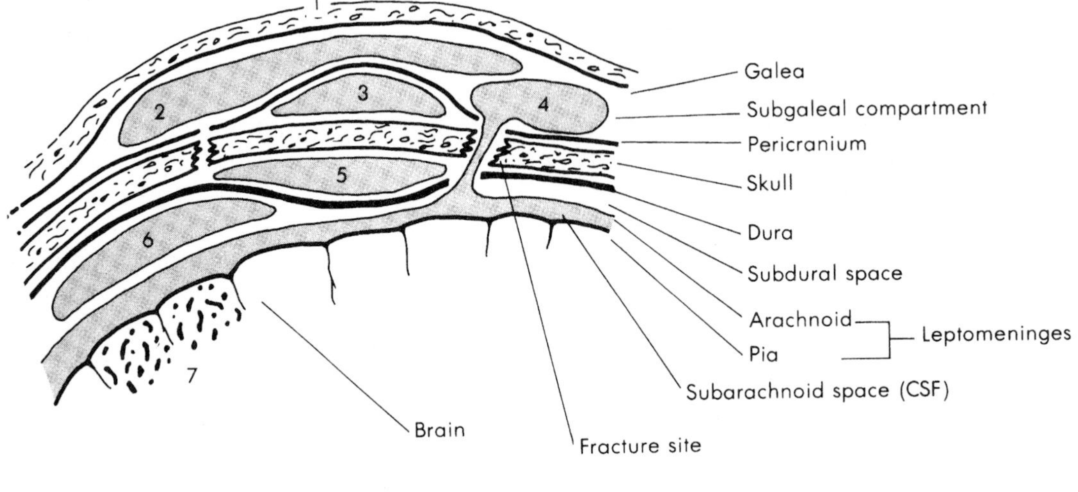

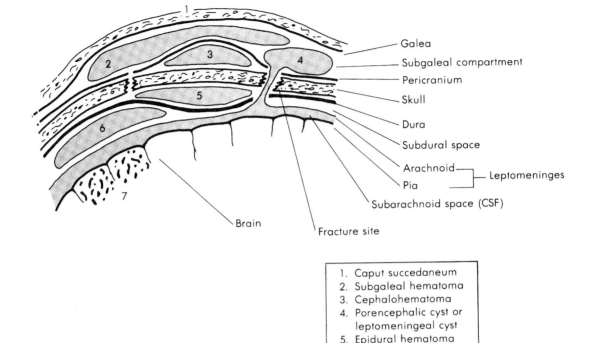

Fig. 57-1 Traumatic head injuries.

Discharge instructions as outlined later should be given.

Contusion of Scalp, Forehead, or Face

Diagnostic Findings

1. Localized swelling and tenderness; variable hematoma or ecchymosis.
2. No neurologic deficit.
3. Subgaleal hematoma may follow minor head trauma, extending across suture lines and the attachment of the galea aponeurosis laterally at the zygomatic arch, auricular muscle, and tissues of the posterior cervical angle and encroaching anteriorly on the orbital ridges of the frontal bones and under the frontal and occipital bellies of the occipitofrontal muscles. Significant blood loss may occur.

Management

1. Discharge the patient.
2. Prescribe ice packs for swelling and analgesia (aspirin or acetaminophen) for pain.
3. Discuss head injury precautions.
4. Do not aspirate the contusion (commonly liquefies in children).

Concussion

Diagnostic Findings

1. Transient neurologic dysfunction, which disappears within minutes to days, leaving a neurologically normal patient.
2. May include transient loss of consciousness as well as findings such as dizziness, nausea, vomiting, amnesia, or confusion.
3. CT is indicated in a patient with dysfunction for longer than 5 minutes.

Management

1. Observation. When symptoms have been persistent or home environment seems inadequate for close monitoring, hospitalization is recommended.
2. Aspirin or acetaminophen analgesia. Narcotics should be avoided.
3. Specific criteria for return to sports activities are listed later (Disposition).

Skull Fracture

Diagnostic Findings

1. Pain, tenderness, and swelling over the fracture site. Isolated skull fractures rarely manifest without local signs, such as palpable fracture, soft tissue swelling, and indications of basilar skull fracture. May be associated with other severe injuries.
2. Significance related not to bony defect but to intensity of injury and possible damage to underlying structures.
3. Basilar skull fracture is suggested by findings of hemotympanum, Battle's sign (bilateral postauricular ecchymoses), raccoon eyes sign (bilateral periorbital ecchymoses), or CSF rhinorrhea or otorrhea. Anosmia may indicate involvement of cranial nerve I via damage to the cribriform plate. The risk of intracranial bleeding is three times greater in the presence of a skull fracture.
4. Clinical characteristics suggesting an intracranial injury associated with a parietal skull fracture include neurologic dysfunction and a bilateral, depressed, or diastatic skull fracture.
5. X-ray study (p. 422). CT is preferred because it can demonstrate intracranial injury as well as the skull fracture.
   a. Linear fractures involving the flat bones of the skull (frontal, temporal, parietal, or occipital) may be noted:
      (1) Fractures crossing the middle meningeal artery have the potential of causing epidural hematoma.
      (2) Fractures of the occiput, particularly if stellate or comminuted, are associated with a child's being repeatedly swung so as to strike the head against an object (child abuse).
   b. Depressed fractures are recognized on skull x-rays as areas of lucency adjacent to an area of increased density. This represents a double density of bone caused by overlapping of a depressed segment on a nondepressed segment. Tangential views or CT scan may be helpful to distinguish this entity.
   c. Basilar skull fracture is commonly not detectable on plain x-ray films. Rarely, a blood-air level may be noted in the sphenoid sinus (with patient supine as film is taken), often visualized on a cross-table lateral cervical spine x-ray. CT scan is the most sensitive diagnostic tool.
6. A local swelling with increased transillumination overlying a fracture suggests a porencephalic or leptomeningeal cyst associated with a "growing" fracture.

Management

1. Generally, hospitalize all patients with skull fractures for observation, with neurosurgical consultation.
2. Perform CT early in patients with fractures detected on plain x-ray films or if there is any neurologic dysfunction, especially if progressive.
3. Prescribe aspirin or acetaminophen analgesia (no narcotics).
4. Use of antibiotics for patients with basilar skull fractures is controversial, and the ultimate decision should rest with the neurosurgeon. Empiric antibiotic therapy may select out resistant organisms, and there is no clear evidence that their use decreases the risk of meningitis. Intracranial contamination by foreign bodies is often treated with ampicillin and chloramphenicol or

other agents that provide coverage for gram-positive and anaerobic organisms.

5. Depressed fractures often require surgical elevation of a fragment.

Cerebral Contusion

Diagnostic Findings

1. Decreased level of consciousness is usually present.
2. Associated neurologic deficits, if any, reflect the contused area of brain. Pathologically, this represents an injury to the brain and is marked by hemorrhage and swelling.
3. CT scan demonstrates an area of cortex with both increased density and decreased density.

Management

1. Hospitalization and close observation are required.
2. Principles of head trauma management, including stabilization of airway, ventilation, circulation, and cervical spine, should be used, depending on the extent of injury and neurologic impairment. Other measures outlined previously should be implemented when appropriate.

Intracranial Hemorrhage

Diagnostic Findings (see Fig. 57-1)

1. *Subdural hematomas* are more common than epidural hematomas and usually result from laceration of bridging veins.
2. *Epidural hematoma* is usually associated with a skull fracture and meningeal artery bleeding. The classic history of loss of consciousness followed by a lucid period and then deepening coma is rare (10%). In children younger than 5 years, epidural hemorrhage usually follows a fall.
3. *Intracerebral hemorrhage* is usually associated with a brain laceration. The anterior frontotemporal region is most common. Progression of findings may be gradual.

Because the clinical presentations of these entities are similar, it is impossible to differentiate them clinically without radiologic confirmation. They show signs of a space-occupying lesion, with progressive increase in ICP. Hemiparesis, unequal pupils, hyperactive deep tendon reflexes, and presence of Babinski's reflex may be noted. Drowsiness may progress to stupor, coma, and convulsions. In rare cases, the signs and symptoms progress insidiously, with irritability, anorexia, and failure to thrive.

Ancillary data. An x-ray film may demonstrate a fracture, particularly with epidural hematomas, whereas a CT scan differentiates the location of hemorrhage.

1. Subdural hematomas appear as an increased density spread over the entire cerebral cortex. There is often cerebral edema on the side of the injury, with a midline shift.
2. Epidural hematoma appears as a lens-shaped (biconvex) area of increased density. The size of the hematoma is limited by the dural attachments at the sutures.
3. Intracerebral hemorrhage has increased density within the cortex and is surrounded by small areas of decreased density that represent edema.

An individual with a history of head trauma and coma or abnormal neurologic findings should be presumed to have an intracranial injury even if the initial CT scan does not confirm its presence. Follow-up scanning may be required.

Management

1. Resuscitation and head trauma management are urgently required. Emergency intervention is mandatory. Suspicion and recognition of skull fracture determine the ultimate outcome.
2. Neurosurgical consultation is required, with an immediate CT scan to define the lesion; generally evacuate the hematoma.
3. On occasion, emergency trephination without CT scanning is required. It may be performed by trained physicians in the

patient with a "coning syndrome" and a dilated pupil who show no response to intubation and hyperventilation or who have other injuries that need operative intervention.

DISPOSITION

Obviously, the decision about discharge or admission of a patient with head trauma must be individualized, reflecting the mechanism of injury, clinical condition, progression of findings, home situation and compliance with therapy, and follow-up observation. Children with a GCS score of 14 or 15, minor head trauma, and normal CT findings can usually be observed at home. Those with a lower GCS score are usually observed in the hospital.

The criteria for hospitalization must be individualized, but indications may include the following:

1. Documented, prolonged loss of consciousness
2. Coma, altered mental status, or seizure
3. Focal neurologic deficit
4. Persistent vomiting or severe and persistent headache
5. Abnormal CT findings
6. Presence of recent linear skull fracture
7. Alcohol or drug intoxication that interferes with a reliable examination
8. Suspicion of child abuse or unreliable caregiver
9. High-risk individuals, including children younger than 2 years and patients with underlying hydrocephalus or coagulopathy

Studies of children with less significant head trauma indicate that some may be observed at home by a responsible adult after a period of monitoring. Criteria for such a disposition include the following:

1. Loss of consciousness for less than 5 minutes
2. Normal examination
3. Absence of severe or progressive symptoms of headaches or vomiting
4. Absence of clinical evidence of basilar skull fracture

Follow-up observation should be arranged because even a minor head trauma may cause mild, long-term problems, such as inability to learn new material or behavioral problems (increased irritability and wide emotional swings).

Recommendations for return of a patient to sports activities after a concussion, according to grade of injury, are as follows:

- *Grade 1:* transient confusion, no loss of consciousness and duration of mental status abnormalities less than 15 minutes. Patient may return to sports activity on the same day only if all symptoms resolve within 15 minutes. If a second grade 1 concussion occurs, no sports activity is allowed until the patient is asymptomatic for a week.
- *Grade 2:* transient confusion, no loss of consciousness, and duration of mental status abnormalities 15 minutes or longer. No sports activity is allowed until patient is asymptomatic for a week. If a grade 2 concussion occurs on the same day as a grade 1 concussion, no sports activities are allowed for 2 weeks.
- *Grade 3:* concussion involving loss of consciousness. No sports activity until the patient is asymptomatic for 1 week if the loss of consciousness was brief (seconds), or for 2 weeks if the loss of consciousness was prolonged (minutes or longer). For a second grade 3 concussion, no sports activity until the patient is asymptomatic for 1 month.

If intracranial disease is detected on CT or MRI, the patient may participate in no sports activity for the remainder of season and should even be discouraged from future return to contact sports.

Parental Education

All children who are discharged from the hospital after head trauma must be released to the care of a responsible adult who has been carefully and explicitly instructed in head precautions:

1. Limit activities and restrict the patient to a light diet. If trauma is recent, apply an ice pack to reduce swelling.
2. Awaken the child every 2 hours and observe.
3. Call your physician immediately if any of the following occurs:
   a. Increasing sleepiness, drowsiness, or inability to be awakened from sleep
   b. Change in equality of pupils (black center of eye) or development of blurred vision, peculiar movements of the eyes, or difficulty focusing
   c. Stumbling, unusual weakness, difficulty using arms or legs, or a change in normal gait or crawl
   d. Seizures
   e. Change in personality or behavior, such as increasing irritability, confusion, unusual restlessness, or inability to concentrate
   f. Persistent vomiting (more than three times)
   g. Drainage of blood or fluid from nose or ears
   h. Severe headache
4. Aspirin or acetaminophen may be given for pain. Do not use narcotics.

BIBLIOGRAPHY

American Academy of Pediatrics, Committee on Quality Improvement: The management of minor closed head injury in children, *Pediatrics* 104:1407, 1999.

Ampel L, Hott KA, Sielaff GW et al: An approach to airway management in the acutely head-injured patient, *J Emerg Med* 6:1, 1988.

Bernard B, Zimmerman RA, Bilaniuk LT: Neuroradiologic evaluation of pediatric craniocerebral trauma, *Top Magn Reson Imaging* 5:161, 1993.

Brock BF, Krause GS, White BC et al: Neurotrauma: concepts, current practice, and emergency therapies, *Ann Emerg Med* 22:957, 1993.

Davis RL, Hughes M, Gubler D et al: The use of cranial CT scans in the triage of pediatric patients with mild head injury, *Pediatrics* 95:345, 1995.

Davis RL, Mullen N, Makela M et al: Cranial computed tomography scans in children after minimal head injury with loss of consciousness, *Ann Emerg Med* 24:640, 1994.

Dietrich AM, Bowman MJ, Ginn-Pease ME et al: Pediatric head injures: can clinical factors reliably predict an abnormality on computed tomography? *Ann Emerg Med* 22:1535, 1993.

Dolan M: Head trauma. In Barkin RM, editor: *Pediatric emergency medicine: concepts and clinical practice,* ed 2, St Louis, 1997, Mosby.

Duhaime AC, Alario AJ, Lewander WJ et al: Head injury in very young children: mechanisms, injury types and ophthalmologic findings in 100 hospitalized patients younger than 2 years of age, *Pediatrics* 90:179, 1992.

Feldman JA, Fish S: Resuscitation fluid for a patient with head injury and hypovolemic shock, *J Emerg Med* 9:465, 1991.

Goldman H, Morehead M, Murphy S: Use of adrenocorticotrophic hormone analog to minimize brain injury, *Ann Emerg Med* 22:1035, 1993.

Greenes DS, Schutzman SA: Clinical indicators of intracranial injury in health-injured infants, *Pediatrics* 104:861, 1999.

Greenes DS, Schutzman SA: Clinical significance of scalp abnormalities in asymptomatic head-injured infants, *Pediatr Emerg Care* 17:88, 2001.

Greenes DS, Schutzman SA: Infants with isolated skull fracture: what are their clinical characteristics and do they require hospitalization? *Ann Emerg Med* 30:253, 1997.

Grushkin KD, Schutzman SA: Head trauma in children younger than 2 years: are there predictors for complications? *Arch Pediatr Adolesc Med* 153:15, 1999.

Hamill JF, Bedford RF, Weaver DC et al: Lidocaine before endotracheal intubation: intravenous or laryngotracheal? *Anesthesiology* 55:578, 1981.

Harrison DW, Walls RM: Blindness following minor head trauma in children: a report of two cases with a review of the literature, *J Emerg Med* 8:21, 1990.

Kadish HA, Schunk JE: Pediatric basilar skull fracture: do children with normal neurologic findings and no intracranial injury require hospitalization? *Ann Emerg Med* 26:37, 1995.

Kraus JF, Fife D, Conroy C: Pediatric brain injuries: the nature, clinical course, and early outcomes in a defined U.S. population, *Pediatrics* 79:501, 1987.

Kraus JF, Rock A, Hemyari P: Brain injuries among infants, children, adolescents, and young adults, *Am J Dis Child* 144:684, 1990.

Kuban K, Winston K, Bresnan M: Childhood subgaleal hematoma following minor head trauma, *Am J Dis Child* 137:637, 1983.

Lewis RJ, Yee L, Inkelis SH et al: Clinical predictors of posttraumatic seizures in children with head trauma, *Ann Emerg Med* 22:1114, 1993.

Lieh-Lai MW, Theodorou AA, Sarnaik AP et al: Limitations of the Glasgow Coma Scale in predicting outcome in children with traumatic brain injury, *J Pediatr* 120:195, 1992.

Lloyd DA, Carty H, Patterson M et al: Predictive value of skull radiography for intracranial injury in children with blunt head injury, *Lancet* 349:821, 1997.

Mahoney WJ, D'Souza BJ, Haller JA et al: Long-term outcome of children with severe head trauma and prolonged coma, *Pediatrics* 71:756, 1983.

Marik P, Chen K, Voron J et al: Management of increased intracranial pressure: a review for clinicians, *J Emerg Med* 17:712, 1999.

Miller EC, Holmes JF, Derlet RN: Utilizing clinical factors to reduce head CT ordering for minor head trauma patients, *J Emerg Med* 15:453, 1997.

Ramundo ML, McKnight T, Kempf J et al: Clinical predictors of computed tomographic abnormalities following pediatric traumatic brain injury, *Pediatr Emerg Care* 11:1, 1995.

Rhee KJ, Muntz CB, Donald PJ et al: Does nasotracheal intubation increase complication in patients with skull bone fracture? *Ann Emerg Med* 22:1145, 1993.

Roddy SP, Cohn SM, Moller BA et al: Minimal head trauma in children revisited: is routine hospitalization required? *Pediatrics* 101:575, 1998.

Ros SP, Ros MA: Should patients with normal cranial CT scans following minor head injury be hospitalized for observation? *Pediatr Emerg Care* 5:216, 1989.

Rosenthal BW, Bergman I: Intracranial injury after moderate head trauma in children, *J Pediatr* 115:346, 1989.

Schunk JE, Rodgerson JD, Woodward GA: The utility of head computed tomographic scanning in pediatric patients with normal neurologic examination in the emergency department, *Pediatr Emerg Care* 12:160, 1996.

Schutzman SA, Barnes PD, Mantello M et al: Epidural hematomas in children, *Ann Emerg Med* 22:535, 1993.

Schutzman SA, Barnes P, Duhaime AC et al: Evaluation and management of children younger than two years old with apparently minor head trauma: proposed guidelines, *Pediatr* 107:983, 2001.

Schutzman SA, Greenes DS: Pediatric minor head trauma, *Ann Emerg Med* 37:65, 2001.

Shahar E, Sagy M, Koren G et al: Calcium block agents in pediatric emergency care, *Pediatr Emerg Care* 6:52, 1990.

Shane SA, Fuchs SM: Skull fracture in infants and predictors of associated intracranial injury, *Pediatr Emerg Care* 13:198, 1997.

Shaw GJ, Jauch EP, Zelman FP: Serum cleaved tau protein levels and clinical outcome in adult patients with closed heat injury, *Ann Emerg Med* 39:254, 2002.

Stein SC, O'Malley KF, Ross SE: Is routine computed tomography scanning too expensive for mild head injury? *Ann Emerg Med* 20:1286, 1991.

Stein SC, Ross SE: Mild head injury: a plea for routine early CT scanning, *J Trauma* 33:11, 1992.

Stein SC, Ross SE: The value of computer tomography scans in patients with low-risk head injuries, *Neurosurgery* 26:638, 1990.

Tannebaum RD, Sloan EP: Non-hemorrhagic pontine infarct in a child following mild head trauma, *Acad Emerg Med* 2:523, 1995.

Tecklenburg FW, Wright MS: Minor head trauma in the pediatric patient, *Pediatr Emerg Care* 7:40, 1991.

Tempkin NR, Dikmen SS, Wilensky AJ et al: A randomized, double-blind study of phenytoin for the prevention of posttraumatic seizures, *N Engl J Med* 323:497, 1990.

Woodward GA: Posttraumatic cortical blindness: are we missing the diagnosis in children? *Pediatr Emerg Care* 6:289, 1990.

58 Facial Trauma

ALERT Protection of the airway is essential after facial trauma and often requires active intervention. Cervical spine and other associated injuries must be excluded.

Facial trauma in children is most commonly associated with vehicular accidents, usually because of failure to use restraints, as well as falls and child abuse. Home accidents, athletic injuries, bites (animal and human), playground accidents, and altercations are also sources of facial trauma.

As a result of the disproportionate size of the cranium with respect to the face, skull fractures are more common than facial fractures in children younger than 12 years. The period of maximal enlargement of the face occurs during the sixth and seventh years. Facial proportions at that time are influenced primarily by the development of the midface and the eruption of teeth. Therefore the development and treatment of the preadolescent must reflect the stage of facial development.

DIAGNOSTIC FINDINGS

Patients with facial trauma often have involvement of other organ systems, especially the head, chest, and abdomen. Facial trauma rarely represents a life threat, and therefore its evaluation and treatment should be deferred until the other, more serious injuries are evaluated and treated.

1. A complete appraisal of facial trauma consists of careful evaluation of soft tissue, bony structures, innervation, eyes, ears, and mouth. Specific attention to the eye is required as outlined in Chapter 59.
2. Inspection of the face must include assessment for deformity, asymmetry, dental malocclusion or displacement, cerebrospinal fluid (CSF) rhinorrhea, nasal septal hematoma, and examination of any obvious wounds.
3. Palpation of the face should include the infraorbital and supraorbital ridges, zygomas and zygomatic arches, nasal bones, maxilla (grasp the upper central incisors and attempt to move them), and mandible. Examine for tenderness, bony defects, crepitus, and false motion.
4. Neuromuscular evaluation assesses the facial nerves, trigeminal nerves, extraocular movements, visual acuity, and hearing. The facial nerves may be tested by having the patient wrinkle the forehead, smile, bare the teeth, and tightly close the eyes. All three branches of the trigeminal nerve (sensory) should be tested on each side of the face. Anesthesia in any area implies a disruption of that branch until proven otherwise. Extraocular movements are tested to uncover diplopia or entrapment, both signs of a blowout fracture.
5. Twenty percent to 50% of children with significant facial fractures have concurrent intracranial findings, and 1% to 4% have cervical spine injuries.

Complications

1. Disfigurement
2. Loss of function
3. Infection

4. Airway obstruction
5. Hemorrhage
6. Ocular injuries, which occur in as many as 67% of facial fractures, especially those that are midfacial.

Ancillary Data

X-Ray Study. The selection of radiographic studies should be based on physical findings, the clinician's suspicions, and the patient's overall status. If there is any possibility of cervical spine trauma, cervical spine x-ray films must be ordered and evaluated to exclude abnormalities before any other radiographic investigations.

Computed tomography (CT) is the preferred modality and is useful in defining fractures and facial injuries and intracranial injuries.

A *Waters' view* is the single most helpful x-ray film for the evaluation of facial fractures; the physician should specifically look at the infraorbital floor, orbital rim, maxilla, and maxillary sinus. The *Towne view* is useful to view the zygoma and mandibular ramus, and *Caldwell films* allow evaluation of the frontal bones and sinuses, orbit, and mandibular symphysis. Specific views for common facial injuries are listed in Table 58-1. Findings include fractures, air-fluid levels in the sphenoid sinus (implies basilar skull fracture), opacification or air-fluid levels in the maxillary sinus (implies blowout fracture), and subcutaneous air (implies occult fracture until proved otherwise).

TABLE 58-1 Optimal Views for Specific Facial Injuries

Injury	Radiologic View(s)
Nasal	Waters', lateral nose
Orbital	Caldwell, Waters', lateral and oblique facial CT scan
Zygomatic/maxillary	
Tripod	Waters', CT scan
Zygomatic arch	Towne, Waters', PA facial, CT scan
LeFort	CT scan
Mandible	Towne, Caldwell, panoramic, CT scan
Alveolar arch	Panoramic
Temporomandibular joint	Oblique and lateral (open and closed mouth), Towne
Teeth	Panoramic, bite wings

From Rahman WM, O'Connor TJ: Facial trauma. In Barkin RM, editor: *Pediatric emergency medicine: concepts and clinical practice*, ed 2, St Louis, 1997, Mosby.
CT, Computed tomography.

MANAGEMENT

Management procedures for specific soft tissue and bony injuries follow. However, several general principles must be carefully considered, as partially outlined in Chapter 65:

1. Provide adequate airway and ventilation. Administer oxygen at 3 to 6 L/min while determining the necessity for active intervention. Intubation may be required on either an emergency or a prophylactic basis. Cricothyrotomy is necessary with massive facial injury and airway obstruction because of the risk of intracranial intubation, which is especially associated with cribriform plate fracture. Nasotracheal intubation is usually avoided.
2. Evaluate cervical spine (see Chapter 61).
3. Begin stabilization of the cardiovascular system. Control hemorrhage.
4. Administer tetanus prophylaxis as indicated.
5. Arrange for specific management of the fracture in consultation with otolaryngologists, oral surgeons, or plastic surgeons.
6. Initiate antibiotic therapy in patients with open facial fractures. Penicillin and cephalosporins are often used unless there is central nervous system (CNS) involvement (orbital floor or maxillary or frontal sinuses), in which case nafcillin (or equivalent) and chloramphenicol or alternative agents are used.
7. Stimulate prevention programs that encourage the use of seat belts and motorcycle full-face helmets.

SPECIAL CONCERNS IN THE MANAGEMENT OF FACIAL SOFT TISSUE INJURIES

The general principles of management of soft tissue injuries are summarized in Chapter 65. Bony injuries usually require attention first, followed by management of soft tissue damage. All involved structures must be identified, and bleeding controlled. The injury should be repaired within 24 hours. Anesthesia (local or regional), cleansing with copious irrigation, debridement, and removal of all imbedded particles are imperative.

Lip Lacerations

Lacerations of the lips require extra attention because a displacement of 1 to 2 mm in the vermilion border (the mucocutaneous junction) is quite noticeable. Little, if any, wound revision should be performed in this area. If there is significant loss of tissue, the patient should be referred to a plastic surgeon.

1. The vermilion border, if violated, should be marked on both sides of the laceration before injection of anesthetic, because injection causes distortion of landmarks. This marking may be made with a needle scratch or a needle dipped in methylene blue. Unless the laceration is very superficial, the closure should be layered to prevent tissue defects.
2. The first skin stitch placed to repair a facial laceration extending beyond the vermilion border should be at the vermilion border. The cutaneous component is then closed with nonabsorbable synthetic suture. The vermilion section is closed with 5-0 or 6-0 silk for patient comfort.
3. Lower lip anesthesia may be achieved by injecting 1 to 2 ml of 2% lidocaine with epinephrine in close proximity to the neurovascular bundle of the mental nerve intraorally at the point just posterior to the first premolar.

Lip Burn, Electrical

Burns to the lips from biting power cords deserve special consideration. They may initially appear localized but may become more extensive over the subsequent 3 to 5 days.

Lip burns should not be debrided. Hemorrhage may occur in the subsequent 5 to 10 days, and close observation is essential, often in the hospital. Bleeding is controlled by pressure, with the area kept clean. Special feeding devices and arm splints may be necessary. Delayed revision may be required after 6 to 12 months.

Mouth and Tongue

1. Through-and-through lacerations of the mouth require a careful, layered closure. The inner mucosa is closed first with 4-0 or 5-0 absorbable suture to give a watertight seal. The wound is then irrigated from the exterior and closed in layers. Some authorities recommend that these lacerations be covered with antibiotics because of the level of contamination. Penicillin VK, 40,000 units (25 mg)/kg/24 hr q6hr PO for 10 days, is adequate for these wounds.
2. With lacerations in the area of the submandibular or parotid salivary ducts, the physician must demonstrate patency of these structures before closure. If there is any doubt, an ENT consultant should be contacted.
3. Superficial lacerations of the tongue need not be closed. However, larger lacerations should be repaired in a layered fashion, the mucosal layer being closed with a synthetic absorbable suture so it need not be removed later. Exposure of a tongue laceration may be improved by having an assistant grasp the tongue with a piece of gauze and apply gentle traction. Anesthesia is difficult for these lacerations, and sedation may be required (p. 515).
4. Local care for mouth wounds should include rinsing of the mouth three

or four times a day with a mild antiseptic such as half-strength hydrogen peroxide.

Nose

Any nasal injury requires an examination for a septal hematoma, a large, purple, grapelike swelling over the septum, which should be drained through a vertical incision to avoid eventual septal necrosis. An anterior nasal pack should then be placed to prevent reaccumulation of blood. The patient should be treated with penicillin and referred to a consultant for follow-up observation.

Through-and-through lacerations of the nose require a careful layered closure and antibiotic treatment.

Ear

1. Adequate anesthesia of the ear may be achieved by raising a wheal with lidocaine (Xylocaine) 1% without epinephrine around the entire base of the ear. Injuries to the ear require approximation of the cartilaginous structures with fine absorbable suture. The lateral skin should be closed with fine nonabsorbable suture; the medial skin may be closed with absorbable suture to prevent bending of the ear back for suture removal. Ear canal injuries require alternative anesthesia.
2. All significant injuries to the cartilage of the ear should be splinted with moist cotton balls placed medially and laterally and then dressed with a circumferential bandage around the head. These injuries, if at all contaminated, should be treated with antibiotics to prevent the complication of a smoldering chondritis.
3. Subperichondrial hematomas of the ear, which are usually caused by direct blunt trauma, often need aspiration and application of a compression dressing to avoid the development of a "cauliflower ear." Careful follow-up and, possibly, reaspiration are indicated.

Eyelid (see Chapter 59)

1. Lacerations involving the lid margin should be referred to an ophthalmologist. If the injury prevents the cornea from being bathed by tears, artificial tears should be instilled on a regular basis until repair is achieved.
2. Lacerations not involving the lid margin should be carefully closed in layers, the skin being sutured with fine silk for comfort.
3. Wounds near the medial canthus may violate the lacrimal apparatus and require probing of the tear duct by an ophthalmologist to demonstrate its integrity.

Eyebrow

1. Debridement of lacerations to the eyebrow should be kept to an absolute minimum and should be performed parallel to the hair follicles, not perpendicular to the skin, to minimize the scar.
2. The eyebrow should not be shaved, because the margins are important landmarks to observe in the closure.

Scalp

It is imperative to explore all scalp lacerations with the finger to exclude fractures and debris. There may be a great deal of blood loss. Lacerations may involve the skin, subcutaneous tissue, galea, subgalea, and periosteum or pericranium. Anesthetic agents should be administered above the galea, where most of the nerves and vessels rest. When involved, the galea is closed separately.

Neck

Penetrating injuries of the neck involving the platysma or deeper structures or extensive blunt soft tissue damage require surgical consultation and in-hospital observation for a minimum of 24 to 48 hours.

Missile injuries to the neck produce major injury. High-velocity bullets cause significant disorder in 90% of victims, whereas buckshots or birdshots inflicted at a distance less than 5 meters, as well as high-velocity shrapnel, routinely cause major damage.

Three zones of the anterior neck are commonly identified:

- Zone I: below the level of the top of the sternal notch
- Zone II: between the angle of the mandible and the sternal notch
- Zone III: the region cephalad to the angle of the mandible

Airway stabilization and ventilation must be considered along with fluid resuscitation and direct pressure (not clamping) for control of hemorrhage. Anterior neck injuries from striking the steering wheel or a wire or board cause laryngotracheal damage, making airway management difficult. Chest x-ray films, arteriography, endoscopy, and water-soluble contrast studies may help define the extent of the injury. In the stable patient, cervical spine films and soft tissue films of the neck may be useful. Angiography often is indicated in asymptomatic zone I injuries to identify damage to thoracic outlet vessels, whereas it may be performed in zone III wounds to exclude a high internal carotid injury at the base of the skull.

The necessity for mandatory versus selective surgical exploration is controversial. Findings requiring surgery include shock; active bleeding; moderate, large, or expanding hematomas; pulse deficits; bruits; neurologic deficits; dyspnea; hoarseness; stridor; dysphonia; hemoptysis; difficulty or pain with swallowing; subcutaneous crepitations or air; and hematemesis. If none of these findings is present, the edges of the wound can be spread apart gently to prevent dislodging a clot. If the platysma has been penetrated, the patient should be admitted for observation. The need for surgical exploration and repair must reflect individual experience and preference and the ability of the facility to provide close monitoring and timely intervention if the patient's condition deteriorates.

FACIAL FRACTURES AND DISLOCATIONS

Facial fractures are rare in the pediatric age group because of the elasticity of the child's facial bones and the protection offered by the child's relatively large skull. Any facial fractures in children should increase the physician's suspicion of child abuse (see Chapter 25).

Facial fractures are often associated with other, more severe injuries that require emergent attention of a higher priority (e.g., closed-head and cervical spine injuries) (see Chapter 56). As many as 55% of facial fractures have associated closed-head injuries.

The emphasis here is on diagnosis. Manual palpation of the facial skeleton is particularly helpful, especially of the orbital rim, zygomatic arch, nasal bridge, and inferior border of the mandible. Ocular injuries are often associated with facial fractures, and it is imperative to exclude injuries to the eye as well as associated injuries to the head, cervical spine, and so on.

Facial fractures cannot be definitively treated in the emergency department (ED) but instead require referral to a consultant. If a facial fracture is not initially diagnosed, however, the child may suffer permanent impaired function, disability, and disfigurement. Delay in treatment may be required because of the patient's general condition and associated injuries. The outcome can still be excellent without extensive complications. Appropriate antibiotic therapy should be considered. Uncomplicated mandibular and maxillary fractures can be managed by routine methods with good outcome even after a delay of weeks. Cosmetic complications, however, are more likely to occur with prolonged delay in treatment of zygoma fractures.

Nasal Fractures

Nasal fractures may be difficult to diagnose in children because of the relative immaturity of the nasal pyramid, which makes an adequate physical examination difficult. X-ray films may be of help in the diagnosis, especially if there is a displaced fracture. Intranasal inspection should be performed, with a search for a septal hematoma or a fracture-dislocation of the septal cartilage. A septal hematoma should be treated as outlined on p. 435 to avoid a "saddle nose" deformity.

1. Any continuing epistaxis should be controlled by an anterior nasal pack.
2. Because of the growth potential of a child's nose, any fracture should be reduced accurately to avoid future disfigurement. Therefore any child with significant posttraumatic epistaxis, tenderness, and swelling is assumed to have a nasal fracture until proven otherwise.
3. Any child with a documented or suspected nasal fracture should be referred to a consultant for reevaluation in 4 to 6 days (after the swelling has subsided).
4. Trauma to the bridge of the nose may result in an ethmoidal fracture with possible violation of the cribriform plate followed by CSF rhinorrhea. This may be disguised by epistaxis. Patients with ethmoidal fractures and suspected CSF rhinorrhea should be admitted for observation and kept in a head-up position. If a CSF leak is proved, prophylactic antibiotics may be used according to the recommendation of the neurosurgical consultant.

Mandibular Fractures

Because of inherent weakness from multiple tooth buds, the child's mandible is more susceptible to fracture than the adult's mandible. The subcondylar area is the most common site of fracture, especially in children younger than 10 years.

1. Patients with mandibular fractures have mandibular pain and tenderness, which are often exacerbated by movement of the mandible. Presence of a malocclusion, a step-off in dentition, or a sublingual hematoma is highly suggestive of a mandibular fracture. Patients with malocclusion after trauma should be assumed to have a mandibular fracture. Ecchymosis on the floor of the mouth is pathognomonic. Laceration of the chin associated with hyperextension may also be noted. Crepitus, felt by the examiner's fingers placed in the auditory meatus during mandibular movement, may indicate a condylar fracture.
2. Because the mandible is a ring structure, multiple mandibular fractures are very common, with the fracture sites possibly distant from the point of trauma. Mandibular fractures involving the teeth are considered open fractures.
3. Mandibular x-ray films, especially a panoramic view, assist in the diagnosis.
4. Most patients with mandibular fracture must be admitted to undergo fixation by a consultant. Usually, closed immobilization for 3 to 4 weeks is adequate.

Zygomatic Fractures

In children, the frontozygomatic suture is weak and may be a common site of fracture. Severe trauma may result in a tripod or trimalar fracture with fracture lines at the frontozygomatic suture, at the temporozygomatic suture, and through the infraorbital foramen. Patients with this complex fracture often have flatness of the cheek, anesthesia over the infraorbital nerve (cheek and ala of nose and upper lip), a palpable step defect, or change in consensual gaze.

A zygomatic arch fracture may be caused by lateral force over the area of the arch. The patient with such a fracture may have a palpable defect over the arch or difficulty with mandibular movement, caused by impingement of the defect on movement of the coronoid process of the mandible. X-ray studies, specifically Waters' (occipitomental) and submental-vertex views, are helpful in diagnosis of these fractures.

The patient with a zygomatic arch fracture usually does not need to be hospitalized immediately, but the case should be discussed with a consultant because open reduction and fixation are frequently required.

Orbital Floor Fractures (Blow-Out Fractures) (see Chapter 59)

Isolated fractures of the orbital floor are most often caused by the direct application of pressure to the globe of the eye with subsequent fracture at the weakest area of the orbit, the floor. This pressure often results in herniation of orbital contents and flow of blood into the maxillary sinus.

Patients with orbital floor fracture have impaired ocular motility with diplopia, secondary to entrapment of the inferior rectus muscle, infraorbital hypesthesia (ipsilateral cheek and lip), and enophthalmos. The motility impairment may be difficult to see in a child and may require a forced-traction examination by a consultant with the patient under anesthesia. Periorbital crepitus is highly suggestive of a fracture.

Medial wall fractures may manifest as epistaxis, emphysema of the lips or conjunctiva, and, rarely, limitation of lateral gaze because of entrapment of the medial rectus muscle.

- The Waters' view and CT scans are most helpful in radiographic diagnosis of this injury. Presence of orbital contents or opacification of the maxillary sinus is presumptive evidence of an orbital floor fracture until proven otherwise. An exaggerated Waters' view may be helpful. The patient's head is angled so that the orbitomeatal line forms a 37-degree angle with the plane of the cassette. The beam is angled at 10 degrees, 20 degrees, and 30 degrees caudad.

Patients with orbital floor fractures do not usually need to be admitted but should be referred to a consultant for follow-up observation in 3 to 5 days. Ocular injuries should be excluded. Decongestants and prophylactic antibiotics may be used, and patients are advised to avoid Valsalva's maneuvers (i.e., blowing the nose). Definitive therapy of these fractures remains controversial. Many authorities delay the decision about selective repair for 10 to 14 days.

Maxillary Fractures

Maxillary fractures are most often the result of massive facial trauma, such as that caused by a deceleration injury. The patient has midface mobility, as demonstrated by movement of the hard palate and upper incisors during examination, as well as massive facial soft tissue injury and malocclusion. In addition, CSF rhinorrhea may be present.

An idealized classification scheme for maxillary fractures follows (however, fractures rarely appear in pure form).

- LeFort I: horizontal fracture at the level of the nasal fossa. Fracture of maxilla at level of nasal fossa. This separates the hard palate from its bony frame.
- LeFort II: pyramidal dysjunction involving fractures of the maxilla, nasal bones, and medial aspects of the orbits.
- LeFort III: craniofacial disjunction involving fractures of the maxilla, zygomas, nasal bones, ethmoids, and vomer.

Because of the configuration of the child's head, LeFort II and III fractures are rare in children, and when present, they are usually accompanied by other head trauma inconsistent with survival. LeFort I fractures may often be seen in conjunction with dentoalveolar injuries. Radiographically, these fractures are diagnosed from the lateral facial bone and Waters' views.

Immediate care of maxillary fracture requires aggressive airway maintenance and intensive care monitoring. Cervical spine injuries must also be suspected in patients with these injuries, especially those with an altered sensorium. In such cases, a CT scan is indicated, and a consultant should be contacted immediately (e.g., a neurosurgeon if the patient is comatose).

Temporomandibular Joint Dislocations

Dislocation of the temporomandibular joint (TMJ) may be the result of trauma or may be caused merely when the patient opens the mouth widely. In these cases, the mandible dislocates forward and superiorly. The dislocation may be unilateral or bilateral.

Patients with TMJ dislocation have moderate discomfort and are unable to close the mouth. If the dislocation is posttraumatic, x-ray films are indicated before reduction, to rule out fracture.

1. The physician performs reduction of a TMJ dislocation by placing the thumbs (wrapped in gauze for protection) on the third molars of the mandible with the fingers curled under the mandibular symphysis. He or she then levers the condyles downward and posteriorly by applying downward pressure on the molars and slight upward pressure on the symphysis. In cases of severe spasm, IV diazepam may facilitate reduction.
2. Postreduction x-ray studies are indicated for the first occurrence of this dislocation if it is not related to trauma.

The patient should be admitted for occlusal fixation if severe pain, tenderness, or spasm is present after reduction. Otherwise the patient may be discharged after being told to eat a soft diet and to avoid yawning or otherwise stressing the temporomandibular joints for several days.

BIBLIOGRAPHY

Ellis E, Scott K: Assessment of patients with facial fractures, *Emerg Med Clin North Am* 18:411, 2000.

Hung RH, Foss J: Maxillofacial injuries in the pediatric patient, *Oral Surg Oral Med Oral Pathol* 99:126, 2000.

Keene J, Doris PE: A simple radiographic diagnosis of occult blow-out fracture, *Ann Emerg Med* 14:335, 1985.

Kendall JL, Anglin D, Demetriades D: Penetrating neck trauma, *Emerg Med Clin North Am* 16:85, 1998.

Rahman WH, O'Connor TJ: Facial trauma. In Barkin RM, editor: *Pediatric emergency medicine: concepts and clinical practice,* ed 2, St Louis, 1997, Mosby.

Schwab RN, Genners K, Robinson WA: Clinical predictors of mandibular fractures, *Am J Emerg Med* 16:304, 1998.

Sinclair D, Schwartz M, Gruss J et al: A retrospective review of the relationship between facial fractures, head injuries and cervical spine injuries, *J Emerg Med* 6:109, 1988.

59 Eye Trauma

ALERT Visual acuity must be screened. If it is found to be abnormal, referral to an ophthalmologist is essential. Associated injuries, especially facial fractures, must be excluded.

Eye injuries in children commonly result from sports injuries or projectiles. Baseball is the leading cause of sports-related injuries, followed by basketball. There are often associated facial fractures. Injuries to the eye may be classified as follows:

Eyeball	Sclera and cornea
Closed-globe injury:	Partial-thickness wound
Contusion	No corneal or scleral wound
Split-thickness (lamellar) laceration	Partial-thickness laceration of the eyewall
Open-globe injury:	Eyewall has full-thickness wound:
Rupture	Full-thickness wound of the eye caused by blunt impact; results from globe deformation, increased intraocular pressure, and finally rupture; inside-out mechanism
Laceration:	Full-thickness wound caused by a sharp object; outside-in mechanism
Penetrating	Laceration of a single eyewall
Perforating	Laceration of two eyewalls (entrance and exit)
Intraocular foreign body	Retained foreign body with penetrating laceration

The traumatized eye needs prompt attention because of potential damage and the high level of anxiety for the patient. Both can be reduced by a systematic approach emphasizing visual acuity and external examination. Visual acuity determination is often neglected or is performed in a cursory fashion. It is helpful to remember that an injured eye with good acuity, regardless of its appearance, is unlikely to have sustained an injury requiring immediate referral or surgery.

The following equipment facilitates examination and treatment of the eye:

1. Visual acuity chart
2. Bright penlight
3. Ophthalmoscope
4. Irrigation setup, including irrigating ocular lens, saline solution, and intravenous (IV) tubing
5. Fluorescein strips (and Wood's or cobalt blue light)
6. Topical anesthetics
7. Topical antibiotics
8. Lid retractor
9. Foreign body spud
10. Patch (gauze and fox metal)
11. Paper or plastic tape
12. Contact lens removal suction cup
13. Slit lamp

GENERAL EXAMINATION

Visual Acuity

Visual acuity should be assessed first. The only exception is an acute chemical injury to the eye, which requires immediate irrigation.

1. By 6 weeks, an infant's eyes can fixate, and by 10 to 12 weeks, fixation is associated with smooth pursuit (fix and follow).
2. For children younger than 3 years, use HOTV letter charts, a picture-card test that is easy to administer. Older preschool children can usually do the "E"

test. By 7 years, most children can use the Snellen chart.

3. Each eye should be checked individually, with the patient wearing eyeglasses if previously prescribed.

Many preschool children do not have 20/20 visual acuity, despite normal physical findings. Some may have delayed myelination of the optic nerve. Useful age-specific acuity levels for screening are as follows:

Age	Visual Acuity
3 yr	20/40
4 yr	20/30
5 yr	20/20

The numerator in a visual acuity value is the distance in feet at which the patient reads the chart, and the denominator is the distance at which a normal adult reads the same line.

A difference of more than two lines between the eyes is probably more significant than the absolute acuity and suggests unequal refractive error, amblyopia, or trauma. A pinhole testing device may compensate for visual acuity impairment caused by a refractive error.

In patients who are unable to cooperate in reading an eye chart, the following assessments may be helpful: testing of light perception by watching response to light source (blinking, aversion, discomfort, identifying of two lights) or of the ability to recognize movement of an object, count fingers, distinguish faces, or recognize objects or pictures. These subjective responses should be recorded.

External Examination

1. Lid and orbit:
   a. Orbital bones: Palpate the orbital rim for a step-off or marked local tenderness. Press on the zygomatic arch; if it is not tender, it is usually intact.
   b. Infraorbital nerve: Compare sensation on the two cheeks. Hypesthesia points to a fracture of the orbital floor, which the nerve traverses.
   c. Lids: Retract lids with a lid retractor. If a retractor is unavailable, use two paper clips shaped like a U. Instill topical anesthetic drops to anesthetize the cornea.
   d. Position of the globe: exophthalmos or enophthalmos.
2. Anterior segment:
   a. Sclera, conjunctiva.
   b. Cornea: clarity and absence of fluorescein staining.
   c. Anterior chamber: clarity and depth.
   d. Iris, lens.
3. Pupil: size, reactivity, symmetry, regularity.
4. Ocular motility: Test in all nine positions (primary, up, down, down to both sides, and up to both sides) for limitation and diplopia.
5. Posterior segment: vitreous, retina, optic nerve.
6. Intraocular pressure.

Funduscopic Examination

The funduscopic examination is performed to evaluate for optic nerve pallor, papilledema, retinal or vitreous hemorrhage, and macular abnormalities.

Fluorescein Stains

Fluorescein stain shows corneal epithelial defects and should be used if there is a question of abrasion. A fluorescein strip is moistened (with sterile saline or water) and applied to the conjunctiva. A staining area appears green under white light. A cobalt blue flashlight or Wood's light causes the dye to fluoresce, facilitating the examination.

X-Ray Studies

1. Waters' view to evaluate the orbital rim and maxillary sinus.
2. Computed tomography (CT) scan for localization of a foreign body and for facial fractures. Can also allow evaluation for choroidal detachment, fracture, lens dislocation, and globe rupture.

Magnetic resonance imaging (MRI) may be an adjunct to exclude a metabolic foreign body.

3. Tomography of the orbital floor to define an orbital floor blowout fracture, if surgery is contemplated.
4. Ultrasonography is of growing utility in evaluation of eye injuries.

TOPICAL MEDICATIONS

1. Mydriatics and cycloplegics (red-topped bottle):
   a. Tropicamide (Mydriacyl): onset, 15 to 20 minutes; duration, 2 to 6 hours (useful for ocular examination).
   b. Homatropine 2% to 5%: onset, 30 minutes; duration, 24 to 48 hours (useful for more prolonged action, as with corneal abrasion).
2. Anesthetic (clear or white top): proparacaine 0.5% (Alcaine, Ophthaine, Ophthetic); 1 to 2 drops provides immediate corneal anesthesia. Not for home use.
3. Topical steroids: indicated for some allergic conditions, iritis, and phlyctenular disease. Should be prescribed in consultation with an ophthalmologist if available. Complications include exacerbation of herpes, glaucoma, and impaired healing.
4. Nonsteroidal antiinflammatory topical agents: diclofenac or ketorolac.
5. Topical antibiotics for bacterial conjunctivitis are normally given four times per day for 3 days (a patient in whom there is no response should be seen again):
   a. Sulfa (sulfisoxazole 4% [Gantrisin], sulfacetamide 10% [Sodium Sulamyd]): may cause burning.
   b. Polymyxin B–bacitracin (Polysporin): if patient is allergic to sulfa.
   c. Polymyxin B-bacitracin-neomycin (Neosporin): may cause local sensitization with prolonged use.
   d. Erythromycin: minimal corneal activity.

   NOTE: Pilocarpine (for pupil constriction, miosis) is bottled with a green top, and timolol has a yellow top. Irrigating and lubricating solutions have blue-topped bottles.

EYE PATCHES

An eye patch keeps the lid closed over a corneal surface defect and promotes healing. Use two patches or pads to fill the depth of the orbital recess. Secure with a single piece of paper tape. Place strips of tape from the hairline to the angle of the jaw. Patching is indicated for treatment of corneal epithelial defects of any cause. Do not patch eye infections.

Although the pressure eye patch has traditionally been used in management of traumatic corneal defects, a number of studies have not substantiated a difference between patching and not patching in treatment of such defects.

Because corneal abrasions can become infected, a patched eye should be examined every 24 hours; patching should be continued until fluorescein staining is gone. Usually the patch should be left in place for that time without supplemental medication; removal of the patch to instill topical medication usually results in inadequate patching. In addition, children can lose central nervous system (CNS) fusional mechanisms rapidly. After only 1 to 2 days, esotropia may develop. Therefore long-term, unsupervised patching of children is ill advised.

Cycloplegic agents may be useful in reducing photophobia and surface pain caused by secondary iritis and ciliary spasm. Medium-acting cycloplegics prevent pupillary movement and put the ciliary body to rest. Cyclogen 2%, homatropine 2% to 5%, and scopolamine 0.25%, usually last 24 hours or longer. Atropine 1% lasts 7 to 10 days and should be avoided.

Antibiotic ointment such as erythromycin is usually recommended.

TYPES OF INJURIES

Corneal Abrasion, Foreign Body, Radiation or Solar Keratitis, Chemical Burn (Table 59-1)

Most ocular injuries damage the corneal epithelium with resulting pain and photophobia. Frequently, the pain is so intense that examination is difficult or impossible without topical anesthetics.

Chemical Injuries

Chemical injuries are a true ophthalmologic emergency and must undergo triage for immediate care. Alkali burns are usually much worse than acid injuries; it is important to find out the pH of the chemical agent. The eye should be lavaged as soon as possible, preferably at the site of injury. If the pH of the tears is abnormal, lavage should be continued in the emergency department (ED) with normal saline solution. Extensive lavage is easier with an irrigating contact lens (Mediflow lens). Lavage should be continued until tear pH is normal. The cul-de-sacs must be swept to ensure that foreign material is not left in contact with the globe. Referral to an ophthalmologist is usually indicated unless the history suggests only minimal exposure, the vision is completely normal, and there is no corneal staining or corneal clouding.

Foreign Bodies

Corneal foreign bodies typically are painful but may be asymptomatic for a prolonged time. Long-standing ferrous foreign bodies usually rust, leaving a "rust ring" when removed. The rust is usually easier to remove in 24 to 48 hours. Many children are difficult enough to examine at the slit lamp, let alone to approach with a needle or foreign body spud. Such children are best managed with immobilization (often with a papoose board), a topical anesthetic, and a lid speculum. When restrained, many children watch the physician, and a foreign body can be quickly removed. While the child is still restrained, topical antibiotic can be instilled, and the eye patched. It is important to remember that the topical anesthetic will wear off in 15 to 30 minutes and that systemic analgesics and ice packs will help relieve discomfort.

Perforation or Rupture

Ocular perforation usually causes decreased vision and intraocular hemorrhage. If the anterior chamber has been entered, it is often flat or shallow compared with the chamber in the uninjured eye. The pupil is often irregular. To minimize further injury, the patient should be moved with the eye shielded to prevent pressure on the globe and with instructions to avoid any Valsalva's maneuvers, which increase intraocular pressure. If x-ray films are obtained to enable a search for a retained foreign body, the patient should be helped to sit up on the stretcher or on the x-ray study table, to avoid increasing the intraocular pressure with such movements.

Rupture must be recognized because pressure on the eyeball can cause extrusion of intraocular contents. With such injuries, intraocular blood appears as a brown/blue spot or line on the white of the eye, which may plug the wound and preserve the appearance of the eye. A teardrop pupil may be noted. Patients with these injuries need immediate ophthalmologic evaluation, but their eye should be shielded and they should be kept in bed with the head elevated 40 degrees until treatment is initiated.

Hyphema

Hyphema is blood in the anterior chamber rather than the subconjunctival space and represents a severe ocular injury. Although it may complicate a penetrating injury, it usually follows blunt trauma with an object small enough to fit within the ocular rim, such as a knuckle, bottle, small ball, or pool cue.

Diagnostic Findings. Vision is impaired immediately but may have returned to normal by the time the patient enters the ED. After

TABLE 59-1 Corneal Abrasion, Burn, and Foreign Body

	Corneal Abrasion	Foreign Body	Radiation Burn	Chemical Burn
CAUSE	Direct trauma, contact lens, foreign body		Sun lamp, snow reflection	Alkali much worse than acid
DIAGNOSTIC FINDINGS	Pain, photophobia, lacrimation, fluorescein positive; small, vertical linear abrasion suggests foreign body beneath upper lid	Pain, photophobia, lacrimation, fluorescein finding positive; may see foreign body*	Pain, photophobia, lacrimation, fluorescein positive Punctate keratitis or diffuse abrasion; stain may be difficult to see without magnification	Pain, photophobia, lacrimation Cornea: hazy to opacified Conjunctiva/sclera: no ischemic change to blanched
VISUAL ACUITY	WNL	Usually WNL	Decreased	Markedly decreased
COMPLICATIONS	Infection	Penetration, infection	Infection	Corneal opacification, necrosis
TREATMENT	Remove contact lens, if present Visual acuity check Topical anesthetic† Topical antibiotic with topical NSAID drops Cycloplegic (homatropine 5%) if >40% involved Eye patch‡ Systemic analgesia Recheck in 24 hr§ Avoid contact lens for 4-5 days	Visual acuity check Topical anesthetic† Remove with spud or 25-gauge needle if superficial; otherwise refer Topical antibiotics Topical cycloplegic Eye patch Recheck in 24 hr	Visual acuity check Topical anesthetic,† eye patch, analgesia Recheck in 24-48 hr	Irrigate with 1-2 L saline solution per eye *immediately* Evert eyelids Clear fornices Refer to ophthalmologist

NSAID, nonsteroidal antiinflammatory drug; *WNL*, within normal limits.

* If there is any question of intraocular foreign body, particularly after hammering metal on metal, orbital x-ray studies and direct ophthalmoscopy should be performed. Penetrating injuries require immediate repair by an ophthalmologist.

† Topical anesthetics facilitate examination. They should not be dispensed for prn use.

‡ Although traditionally recommended, efficacy is controversial.

§ On reevaluation in 24 hr, check to make certain that staining and edema have decreased. If not, refer.

recording the visual acuity, the examiner should look at the iris for blood or a meniscus. Unclotted blood in suspension in the aqueous humor may be suspected if the iris color or the detail of the iris stroma is not the same as that in the uninjured eye. If a patient has been supine, the blood may not layer out until x-ray studies in the seated position are performed, leading to a distinct meniscus. However, the most common cause of overlooking the diagnosis of hyphema is failure to look carefully, particularly in patients with a brown iris.

Complications. Complications include the following:

1. Associated injuries, such as corneal abrasion, orbital rim or floor fracture, vitreous hemorrhage, and retinal edema, may be present.
2. Increased intraocular pressure may be present initially and requires careful monitoring. This examination should not be done with the Schiotz tonometer; the applanation unit should be used. Patients with sickle cell disease may have dramatic glaucomatous changes with a mild pressure increase.
3. Secondary hemorrhage occurs in as many as 30% of patients with a hyphema and is associated with glaucoma, corneal blood staining, and optic atrophy. It typically occurs 3 to 5 days after injury.

Management. Care of the patient with hyphema is directed to reducing the incidence of secondary hemorrhage. There are many treatment regimens, choice of which depends on the patient's general health, age, family availability, and physician preference.

1. Bed rest with no Valsalva's maneuvers: This treatment can be given at home if social circumstances allow it. No reading is allowed, although television is permitted. The head of the bed is elevated. Sedation is given as needed.
2. Metal shield for the involved eye: Patch under the shield for comfort or treatment of an associated corneal abrasion. Bilateral patching is not required.
3. Pupillary dilation may be necessary to see the fundus. If so, the pupil can be kept dilated with 0.25% scopolamine, 5% homatropine, or 1% atropine. Allowing the pupil to constrict and then dilating it may cause secondary hemorrhage.
4. Oral prednisone, 1 mg/kg/24 hr, may decrease the incidence of secondary hemorrhage.
5. Prophylactic therapy with aminocaproic acid may reduce secondary hemorrhage. The initial dosage of 200 mg/kg/dose (maximum: 6 g) PO is followed by 50 to 100 mg/kg/dose q6hr PO for 3 to 7 days.
6. Intraocular pressure must be carefully monitored in patients with sickle cell disease.
7. The anterior chamber angle should be examined by gonioscopy 4 to 6 weeks after injury. If there is an angle recession, annual examinations for late-onset glaucoma are indicated. Dilated fundal examination with scleral depression ideally should be performed when possible to rule out a traumatic retinal tear or detachment; these two conditions are rare in children.

Blow-Out Fracture

Blunt trauma may fracture the orbital floor as a result of being hit with something small enough to enter between the orbital rims. The eyeball absorbs the force of the blow and is compressed backward into the orbit. The marked increase in intraorbital pressure results in a blow-out fracture of the orbital floor, which is thin.

Diagnostic Findings

1. Pain is related to the injury, periorbital swelling and ecchymosis, subcutaneous emphysema, and ipsilateral epistaxis.
2. Associated injuries include corneal abrasions, traumatic cataracts, hyphema,

vitreous hemorrhage, and retinal damage in 15% to 40% of patients.

Complications. Several problems may be noted:

1. Hypesthesia in the distribution of the intraorbital nerve, which is best tested by evaluating sensation of the upper lip and cheek. Regeneration usually occurs.
2. Limitation of upward gaze with vertical diplopia, caused by entrapment of the inferior rectus muscle and orbital fat in the orbital floor break.
3. Enophthalmos of the injured eye, which becomes obvious as the swelling resolves.

Ancillary Data. Helpful imaging studies include the following:

1. X-ray film: Waters' view shows antral clouding.
2. Tomograms may be needed.

Differential Diagnosis

1. Restriction of vertical motion may result from mechanical entrapment of the inferior rectus muscle or damage to the nerve of that muscle. This distinction can be made by a forced traction test.
2. Posttraumatic diplopia occurring with entrapment must be considered in the differential diagnosis of a number of entities:
   a. Orbital fracture
   b. Extraocular muscle avulsion, contusion, transection, or hematoma
   c. Palsy of the third, fourth, or sixth cranial nerves

Management

1. A careful examination to exclude intraocular damage and other entities in the differential diagnosis must be conducted.
2. An ophthalmologist should be involved in the acute and long-term care of the patient.
3. If the vision is normal and there are no associated facial or other major injuries, the patient can usually be followed as an outpatient. Analgesics, ice packs, elevation, and bed rest are indicated.
4. If the motility defect persists or there is frank enophthalmos initially, surgical exploration is usually necessary. The timing of surgery is controversial. Some of the restrictions in eye movement may result from hemorrhage and edema in the orbital fat, which typically resolve and may not require surgery. However, some authorities consider it important to explore the orbital floor early and remove any orbital material in the defect.

Subconjunctival Hemorrhage

The subconjunctival space is defined by the conjunctiva anteriorly, the sclera posteriorly, the cul-de-sacs above and below, and the limbus centrally. The conjunctiva lines the inside of the eyelid and then is reflected in the cul-de-sac before it spreads over the globe and inserts at the corneal-scleral limbus. This space is therefore extraocular. Subconjunctival hemorrhage is associated with trauma, coughing, Valsalva's maneuver, or a coagulation disorder.

Diagnostic Findings

1. The symptoms are usually those associated with the initial trauma.
2. Vision is normal if there is no damage to the intraocular contents. The hemorrhage spreads out as a thin sheet and appears bright red and homogeneous. It comes up to the limbus. Usually conjunctival vessels are not involved in areas where hemorrhage is not present.
3. The condition resolves in 1 to 2 weeks without sequelae.
4. Cases of trauma to the eye followed by a 360-degree subconjunctival hemorrhage should be referred to an ophthalmologist, especially if there is associated anterior chamber or vitreous hemorrhage, because of the potential of posterior rupture of the globe.

Management. If there is conjunctival prolapse, sterile ointment prevents keratinization.

Lid and Lacrimal Laceration

Lid lacerations may be associated with ocular injuries and may lead to other complications if improperly treated. The eyelids provide protection and lubrication of the eye.

1. Full-thickness lacerations of the lid may be associated with perforating injuries of the globe.
2. Improper repair of the eyelid may result in poor lacrimal function, with secondary irritation and lacrimation.
3. Laceration of the medial aspect of the lid may involve the lacrimal system, which, if not treated, may result in poor lacrimal drainage and epiphora.

Management

1. Examine the eye. Be certain there is no penetration of the globe. If there is any suspicion of globe penetration, avoid direct pressure and excessive manipulation. Immediate ophthalmologic consultation is indicated. If there is any doubt, treat as a globe penetration injury. In general, start systemic antibiotics, keep the patient in a fasting state (NPO), and apply a loose patch and metal shield until the patient can be seen by the ophthalmologist. With question of a foreign body penetration, obtain a CT scan or soft tissue x-ray film of the globe.
2. Irrigate all wounds carefully. Minimize debridement.
3. Careful apposition of the lid margins is essential in vertical lacerations, usually requiring general anesthesia in children and involvement of an ophthalmologist.
   a. Lid avulsion requires reattachment of the eyelid to the canthal tendons.
   b. Interruption of the lacrimal system necessitates intubation of the lacrimal system and suturing of the canaliculus. The medial portion of the lid includes the lacrimal drainage canaliculi, whereas the lacrimal duct runs along the outer third of the upper lid.
4. Horizontal lacerations may disrupt the levator palpebra, causing ptosis. Careful apposition is essential. A through-and-through laceration requires a three-layered closure (conjunctiva, levator aponeurosis, and skin). Consult an ophthalmologist.

Ecchymosis of the Eyelid ("Black Eye")

An eye with ecchymosis must be examined to exclude more significant abnormalities, such as an orbital fracture or hyphema. It is treated with cold compresses, analgesics, and head elevation.

Other Blunt Ocular Injuries

Several other findings may be noted. Traumatic iritis may manifest as photophobia, blurred vision, or headache. Traumatic cataracts, subluxation and dislocation of the lens, and retinal tears, detachment, and hemorrhage are reported after trauma and require referral.

BIBLIOGRAPHY

Alfaro DV, Roth DB, Laughlin RM et al: Paediatric post-traumatic endophthalmitis, *Br J Ophthalmol* 79:888, 1995.

Campanile TM, St. Clair DA, Benaim M: The evaluation of eye patching in the treatment of traumatic corneal epithelial defects, *J Emerg Med* 15:769, 1997.

DeRespinis PA, Caputo AR, Fiore PM et al: A survey of severe eye injuries in children, *Am J Dis Child* 143:711, 1989.

Farber MD, Fiscella R, Goldberg MF: Aminocaproic acid versus prednisone for the treatment of traumatic hyphema, *Ophthalmology* 98:279, 1991.

Juang PSC, Rosen P: Ocular examination techniques for the emergency department, *J Emerg Med* 15:793, 1997.

Klein BR, Sears MZ: Pediatric ocular injuries, *Pediatr Rev* 13:422, 1992.

Kraft SP, Christianson MD, Crawford JS et al: Traumatic hyphema in children, *Ophthalmology* 94:1233, 1987.

Linden JA, Renner GS: Trauma to the globe, *Emerg Med Clin North Am* 13:581, 1991

Michael JG, Hug D, Dowd MD: Management of corneal abrasion in children: a randomized clinical trial, *Ann Emerg Med* 40:67, 2002.

Nelson LB, Wilson TW, Jeffers JB: Eye injuries in childhood: demography, etiology and prevention, *Pediatrics* 84:438, 1989.

Rittichier KK, Roback MG, Bassett KE: Are signs and symptoms associated with persistent corneal abrasions in children? *Arch Pediatr Adolesc Med* 15:370, 2000.

Rychwalski PJ, O'Halloran HS, Cooper HM et al: Evaluation and classification of pediatric ocular trauma, *Pediatr Emerg Care* 15:277, 1999.

Shingleton BJ: Eye injuries, *N Engl J Med* 325:408, 1991.

Szucs PA, Nashed AH, Allergra JR et al: Safety and efficacy of diclofenac ophthalmic solution in the treatment of corneal abrasions, *Ann Emerg Med* 35:131, 2000.

60 Dental Injuries

GARY K. BELANGER

ALERT After management of associated injuries, traumatic dental problems usually require referral.

The examination of the oral cavity requires a systematic approach to the soft tissues and teeth. The mechanism and time of traumatic injuries must be determined, as must the onset and nature of other complaints and complicating medical problems (e.g., cardiac disease, which may require antibiotic prophylaxis, or bleeding diatheses). The status of tetanus immunizations should be assessed.

BASIC CONSIDERATIONS

Soft Tissues

1. Lips:
   a. Normal: pink, moist, continuous vermilion border, possible glandular inclusions (Fordyce's granules)
   b. Abnormal: tenderness, ulcers, swelling, lacerations, hemorrhage, hematoma, burn
2. Mucosa:
   a. Normal: pink, moist, possible glandular inclusions, major salivary duct openings, possible areas of hyperkeratosis associated with chewing
   b. Abnormal: same as for lips; possible torn frenulum
3. Tongue:
   a. Normal: pink, papillated dorsum (possibly coated), smooth ventral surface, normal range of motion and strength
   b. Abnormal: same as for lips; weakness, loss of function
4. Palate:
   a. Normal: *hard palate*—pink, firm, rugae normal in anterior half; *soft palate*—pink, mobile, functional
   b. Abnormal: same as for lips; *soft palate*—abnormal function or loss of function
5. Floor of the mouth:
   a. Normal: pink with areas of high vascularization (varices) appearing blue-gray; moist, major salivary duct openings, tissue tags
   b. Abnormal: same as for lips; excessive firmness or elevation may indicate cellulitis or mucus-retention phenomenon

Teeth (See Fig. 60-1)

1. Color:
   a. Normal: white (permanent [secondary] teeth can appear slightly more yellow than primary teeth)
   b. Abnormal: caries, pulp degeneration; environmental and genetic defects can cause a range of color changes
2. Integrity:
   a. Normal: complete crown without interruptions of surface structure
   b. Abnormal: caries, fractures, hypoplasias, anomalous crown forms

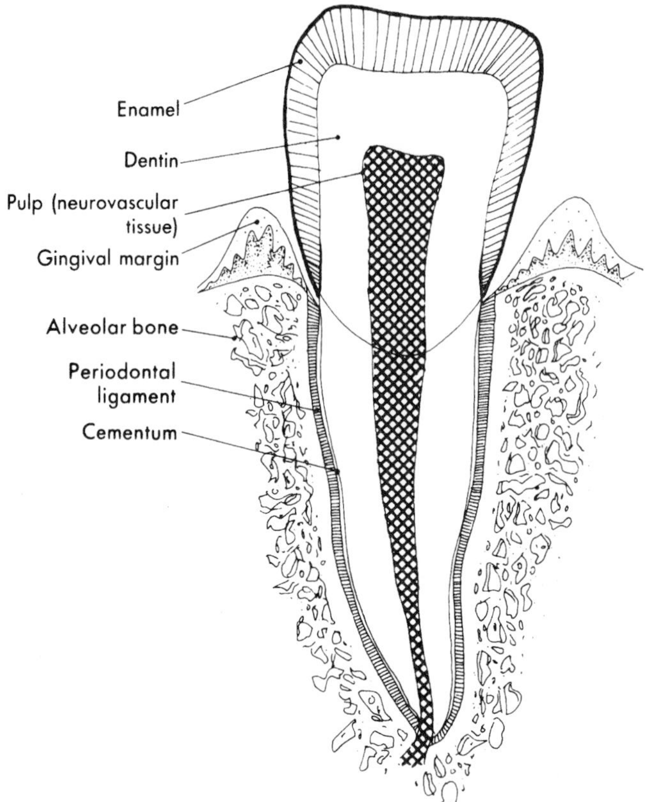

Fig. 60-1 Basic dental anatomy.

3. Mobility:
   a. Normal: lateral and anteroposterior (AP) movement slight to imperceptible; vertical movement nonexistent; exfoliating primary teeth may normally be very mobile
   b. Abnormal: displacement by light finger pressure
4. Position:
   a. Normal: upper teeth overlap lower teeth; mirror imaging of teeth left to right; teeth in each arch arranged in arch form
   b. Abnormal: asymmetry and obvious displacements
5. Pain and sensitivity can be ascertained by questioning patient about abnormal pain on percussion or sensitivity to air, cold, heat, or chewing in both involved and uninvolved areas
6. Development status (Fig. 60-2). Abnormality of development is defined as more than a 1-year deviation from the figure.

Mandible (See Chapter 58)

1. Observe opening and closing of mouth.
2. Check bite for malocclusion.
3. Palpate for tenderness, crepitus, deformity, asymmetry, and mental nerve anesthesia.

TRAUMATIC INJURIES TO THE TEETH

Tooth fractures are usually caused by a blow to the tooth from a fall, sports activity, a fight, or abuse. It is important to define whether the

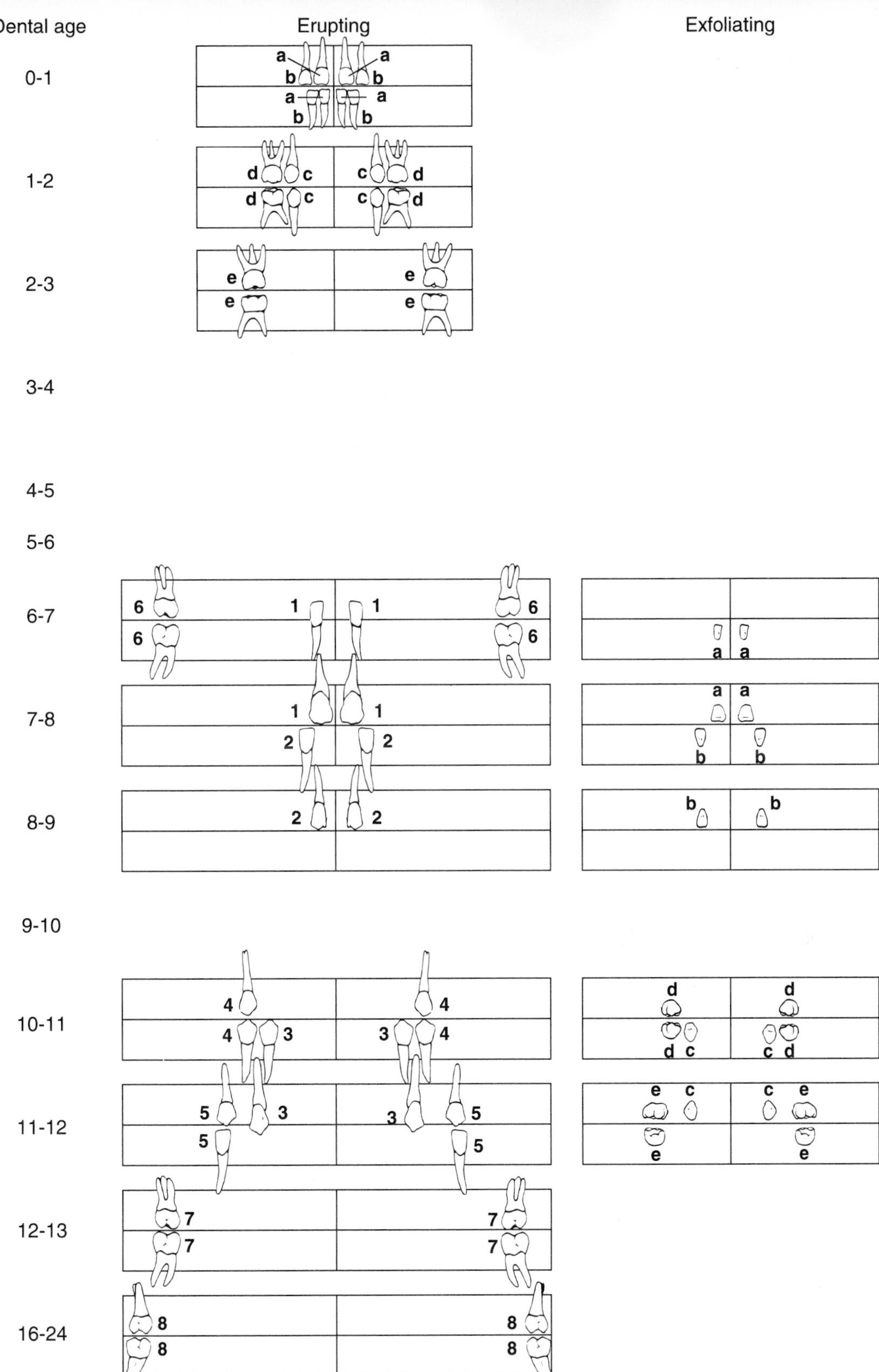

Fig. 60-2 Most common pattern of dental development. *a* to *e*, A quadrant's primary teeth. *1* to *8*, A quadrant's secondary (permanent) teeth. Within each age box, the vertical line represents the dental midline, and the horizontal line represents upper and lower dentitions.

injury is to a primary or secondary (permanent) tooth (possible after about age 6 years).

Diagnostic Findings

The signs and symptoms vary with the site of fracture. Cracks, loss of tooth structures, hemorrhage at the gingival margin or from an exposed pulp, pain, and sensitivity to stimuli can all result.

1. Crown cracks (crazing), which are incomplete fractures of the enamel without loss of tooth structure, may be associated with other injuries to the tooth.
2. Uncomplicated crown fractures involve the enamel or dentin. If the dentin is involved, a yellow area appears at the center of the fracture site and may demonstrate sensitivity to thermal or direct stimuli (air, heat, cold) because of proximity of the pulp.
3. Complicated crown fractures extending through the pulp almost uniformly produce sensitivity to thermal or direct stimuli (e.g., touch, air, ice). There is usually hemorrhage from the exposed dental pulp. Pulp injuries may lead to subsequent inflammation, necrosis, and abscess formation.
4. A crown-root fracture appears as a "split tooth" and involves the enamel, dentin, cementum, and almost always the pulp. There is usually hemorrhage at the gingival margin, and if the fracture extends through the pulp, there is bleeding along the fracture line as well.
5. Root fractures are rare in the anterior primary teeth before 18 months of age. They involve the cementum, dentin, and pulp and, on physical examination, may be associated with movement of the tooth.
6. Periodontal injuries are often found with dental fractures.

Complications

1. Embedding of tooth fragments into the soft tissue (tongue, lips)
2. Aspiration of tooth fragment
3. Damage to the pulp, resulting in subsequent inflammation, necrosis, or abscess formation; may be secondary to initial injury to the neurovascular bundle at time of trauma or to secondary bacterial contamination and inflammatory response
4. Dentoalveolar abscess
5. Damage to underlying permanent tooth bud
6. Death of tooth nerve or eventual loss

Ancillary Data. Dental x-ray films, if available, are particularly important in the evaluation of all injuries involving fractures of the dentin, pulp, or roots. Radiographic evaluation is required modality for diagnosis of root fractures.

Differential Diagnosis

1. Dental attrition (normal wear)
2. Loss or fracture of a previously placed restoration

Management

Life-threatening conditions must be stabilized and take precedence over dental injuries. Management of specific dental injuries reflects the nature of the findings and whether a primary or secondary tooth is involved.

1. Uncomplicated crown fractures or cracks not involving the pulp:
   a. Primary tooth: nonurgent referral to a dentist for follow-up for definitive treatment
   b. Secondary tooth: dental referral within 24 hours for the following reasons:
      (1) Smoothing of sharp, jagged edges of the remaining surface to prevent damage to soft tissues
      (2) Restoring tooth appearance with the use of composite resin material
      (3) Initial data gathering for long-term follow-up to monitor for pulp death
2. Complicated crown fracture involving the pulp:
   a. Primary tooth: urgent dental referral within 24 hours

b. Secondary tooth: immediate referral to minimize bacterial contamination of the pulp, minimize pain, and provide subsequent endodontic therapy and crown restoration

3. Crown-root fracture:
   a. Primary tooth: urgent referral within 24 hours, usually for extraction
   b. Secondary tooth; immediate referral
4. Root fractures: immediate referral to a dentist for stabilization or extraction of the fracture segment; primary teeth may be removed
5. Long-term goals of the dentist include the following:
   a. Maintenance of vitality of the tooth, if possible
   b. Treatment of the pulp and its complications, often requiring root canal therapy and a crown
   c. Restoration of a clinical crown
   d. Extraction and prosthesis, if other goals are not achieved

Disposition

Close dental follow-up is essential for all patients with dental trauma and for any findings on physical examination—for both acute management and long-term monitoring of dental health. Some dental injuries cause signs or symptoms years after the original trauma.

TRAUMATIC PERIODONTAL INJURIES

Periodontal injuries involving the alveolar bone or socket and the periodontal ligament are almost always caused by a blow. Teeth are abnormally mobile or displaced.

Diagnostic Findings

The extent of mobility or displacement reflects the severity of the injury. Pain and increased sensitivity are commonly present.

1. Concussion results in minimal damage to the periodontal ligament. The tooth is sensitive to percussion or pressure such as from chewing, biting, or mobility testing but is not displaced or excessively mobile.
2. Subluxation produces abnormal looseness and mobility (<2 mm of displacement) of the tooth because of moderate damage to the periodontal ligament with slight displacement. The tooth is displaced out of the socket. Hemorrhage at the gingival margin may be noted.
3. Intrusive or traumatic impaction displacement is common in a primary tooth, which has been driven into the socket. The tooth may appear avulsed. Compression fractures of the alveolar socket are common.
4. Extrusive displacement occurs with relocation of the tooth from out of the alveolar socket into an abnormal position and is often associated with a fracture of the alveolar socket and tear of the periodontal ligament.
5. Avulsion of a tooth is common, particularly in 7- to 10-year-old children. The tooth is completely detached from the alveolar socket and the periodontal ligament is severed.
6. Periodontal injuries may be associated with dental fractures.

Complications

1. Complications involving traumatic injuries to the teeth
2. Pathologic root resorption
3. Ankylosis (fusion of tooth to bone)
4. Eruption problem for a permanent successor tooth (i.e., delays, displacement, space loss)

Ancillary Data. Dental radiographs, if available, are particularly important to identify associated root fractures.

Differential Diagnosis

1. Root fracture
2. Normally exfoliating primary tooth (variably mobile, possibility of slight bleeding)

3. Newly erupting primary and secondary teeth (slightly mobile, possibility of being malpositioned)
4. Dentoalveolar infection
5. Systemic disease with bone loss (e.g., hypothyroidism, diabetes, leukemia)

Management

First priority must be given to stabilization of life-threatening conditions.

1. Concussion: No immediate therapy indicated but long-term follow-up observation is required to ensure that complications of root resorption, pulp injury, and ankylosis do not occur.
2. Subluxation: Usually requires immobilization with an acrylic splint and long-term follow-up observation.
3. Intrusive displacement:
   a. Primary tooth: urgent referral to dentist within 24 hours. Unaffected permanent tooth will be allowed to erupt with careful observation and close follow-up observation.
   b. Secondary tooth: Initial caregiver should attempt to reposition, particularly in adolescents. Younger patients' secondary teeth may be allowed to erupt. Immediate dental referral for stabilization.
4. Extrusive displacement.
   a. Primary tooth: urgent referral to dentist within 24 hours (usually extracted).
   b. Secondary tooth: immediate dental referral for stabilization and positioning:
      (1) Initial caregiver should attempt to reposition using gentle pressure.
      (2) Delays in repositioning the tooth increase the chance that the tooth will stabilize in an ectopic position.
5. Avulsion:
   a. Primary tooth: nonurgent dental referral (do not replace the tooth).
   b. Secondary tooth: immediate dental referral and careful handling of the tooth and rapid reimplantation to maximize the success of replacement. Periodontal ligament fibers are best preserved if reimplanted within 15 minutes. Dentist immobilizes the tooth with nonrigid acrylic splint and arranges close follow-up observation.
      (1) Hold the tooth carefully by the crown. Do not touch the roots!
      (2) Wash the tooth with saline solution or milk (plug the sink's drain to prevent loss of the tooth). Rinse off foreign material.
      (3) Irrigate the socket and suction lightly to remove clots. Insert the tooth slowly but firmly into the socket as soon as possible (lacerations should be cared for after reimplantation if bleeding is controlled). Maintain compression for several minutes.
      (4) Arrange for the patient to see a dentist immediately. In the interim, have the child hold the tooth in place with a finger or bite on a gauze to stabilize the tooth.
      (5) If immediate reimplantation is impossible, place the tooth under the child's or parent's tongue to bathe it in saliva until the patient is seen by a dentist. Other options are soaking the tooth in milk or normal saline solution until reimplanted by a dentist.
6. Long-term goals of dentist include the following:
   a. Maintaining the tooth in the dentition; stabilizing the tooth via interdental acrylic splinting immediately after the injury
   b. Monitoring and treating later pulp and root resorption problems
   c. Considering possible later orthodontic repositioning

d. Extracting tooth and inserting prosthesis if other goals are not achieved

Disposition

Dental follow-up observation is essential.

BIBLIOGRAPHY

Andreasen JO, Andreasen FM, editors: *Textbook and color atlas of traumatic injuries to the teeth,* ed 3, St Louis, 1994, Mosby.

Crona-Larsson G, Noren JG: Luxation injuries to permanent teeth: a retrospective study of etiological factors, *Endodont Dent Traumatol* 5:176, 1989.

Harding AM, Camp JH: Traumatic injuries in the preschool child, *Dental Clin North Am* 39:817, 1995.

Harrington MS, Eberhart AF, Knapp JF: Dentofacial trauma in children, *J Dent Child* 55:334, 1988.

Josell SD, Abrams RG: Managing common dental problems and emergencies, *Pediatr Clin North Am* 38:1325, 1991.

Krasner P, Rankow HJ: New philosophy for the treatment of avulsed teeth, *Oral Surg* 95:616, 1995.

Wilson CFG: Management of trauma to primary and developing teeth, *Dent Clin North Am* 39:133, 1995.

61 Spine and Spinal Cord Trauma

ALERT Extreme caution must be exercised when the type and mechanism of injury are sufficient to cause spinal or spinal cord trauma.

Most trauma spinal cord injuries are partial or incomplete. With care from the onset of trauma, substantial recovery may ensue, thereby preventing the catastrophic physical and psychologic disorders associated with major neurologic involvement. Motor vehicle accidents remain the single most common cause of spinal and spinal cord trauma, followed by falls, diving accidents, electrical injuries, and, in newborns, birth trauma.

Initial stabilization of the spine in all major trauma events, particularly of the head and face, with collar, sandbags, and tape is imperative in the interval before the cervical spine can be evaluated. This stabilization is maintained until x-ray studies have excluded injury or appropriate intervention for an abnormality has been initiated.

The case-fatality rate for cervical spine injuries is 59%, in contrast to a 6% rate for head injuries. Children younger than 8 years tend to sustain injury to the upper (C1-C3) cervical spine.

ETIOLOGY

Mechanisms of Injury

1. Flexion:
   a. Stretching of the posterior ligamentous complex produces tears or spinous process avulsions.
   b. Wedge fractures of vertebral bodies result from mechanical pressure of one vertebral body on the next with most of the force exerted on the anterior part of the vertebral body. They are usually stable.
   c. Ligamentous disruptions result in variable extent of subluxation and dislocation of bony spinal elements. These injuries are potentially unstable.
   d. Clay shoveler's fracture is an avulsion fracture of C7, C6, or T1 spinous process because of sudden flexion. It is mechanically stable.
   e. Flexion teardrop and bilateral facet dislocations are extremely unstable.
2. Flexion-rotation:
   a. Simultaneous flexion and rotation around one of the facet joints may cause unilateral facet-joint dislocation.
   b. Rotational forces produce unstable articular process fractures in the lumbar region.
3. Extension:
   a. With extension, compression of the posterior neural arch of C1 or the pedicles of C2 secondary to the heavy occiput above can result in fractures of these elements. The latter is known as a hangman's fracture and is unstable.
   b. Stretching of the anterior longitudinal ligament can produce ligamentous tears or avulsion (teardrop) fractures of the vertebral body.
   c. Buckling of the ligamentum flavum into the posterior spinal canal can

produce central or posterior cord syndromes.

4. Vertical compression/axial loading:
   a. Jefferson fracture of C1 results in its shattering into several parts with widening of the predental space and prevertebral hematoma. This fracture is extremely unstable.
5. The cervical and lumbar spines straighten at the time of impact from above or below, potentially compressing the nucleus pulposus (disc matter) into the vertebral body, with compromise of the anterior spinal canal, causing the anterior cord syndrome.
6. Generally, children younger than 6 years who fall less than 5 feet have clinical evidence of injury upon history or physical examination, if significant injury exists.

DIAGNOSTIC FINDINGS

At high risk for spinal injuries are patients with the following findings:

1. Injury compatible with causing spinal injury as outlined previously
2. Posttraumatic neck or back pain
3. Posttraumatic neurologic complaints or deficits, whether stable or progressive
4. Posttraumatic impaired level of consciousness or an inability to give an accurate history (e.g., infants, alcohol or drug abusers, patients who have had a concussion or are postictal)
5. Breathing difficulty
6. Presence of severe associated injuries or shock

The ability to ambulate after an accident does not exclude spine or spinal cord trauma, because 15% to 20% of patients may be able to walk initially. Severe head and facial injuries carry a 15% to 20% risk of concomitant spine or spinal cord trauma. Other associated injuries must be defined. The neck and back should be palpated for tenderness, step deformity, crepitus, and paraspinous spasm.

Vital Signs

1. Breathing pattern may indicate loss of diaphragmatic breathing and hypoventilation or apnea with injuries to C3, C4, and C5, which supply the phrenic nerve. Although lower cervical lesions preserve diaphragmatic function, there may be a loss of abdominal and intercostal breathing.
2. Hypotension may exist with spinal shock. Hypovolemic shock must be excluded.
3. Temperature regulation is impaired with associated hypothermia or hyperthermia.

Neurologic Findings
(see Chapters 15 and 57)

1. Determine mental status and level of consciousness.
2. Cranial nerves: Assess for associated intracranial injury.
3. Motor:
   a. Tone:
      (1) Flaccid: lower motor neuron (LMN) lesion or spinal shock (with areflexia)
      (2) Spastic: upper motor neuron (UMN) lesion (with hyperreflexia)
   b. Power (Table 61-1):
      (1) Compare strength of upper with lower extremities and right side with left side. Muscles that are essential for maintaining normal posture usually have bilateral innervation and are not useful in lateralizing weakness. The best muscle groups to use for rapid examination are the following:
         (a) Upper extremity: dorsiflexion of wrist and extension of forearm
         (b) Lower extremity: dorsiflexion of great toe and flexion of lower leg at knee
      (2) Mass flexion withdrawal movements in response to stimulation

TABLE 61-1 Spinal Cord Injuries: Motor, Sensory, and Reflex Deficits

Level of Lesion	Motor Function Lost	Sensation Lost At and Below	Reflex
C2	Breathing	Occiput	
C3	Spontaneous breathing and trapezius function	Thyroid cartilage	
C4		Suprasternal notch	
C5	Shoulder flexion and abduction	Infraclavicular ± lateral arm sparing	Biceps brachialis*
C6		Infraclavicular ± lateral arm, forearm sparing	Brachioradialis*
C7	Elbow and wrist extension	Infraclavicular with sparing as above to middle finger	Triceps*
C8	Small muscles of hand (lumbricales and interossei)	Infraclavicular with sparing as above to little finger	
T1		Infraclavicular with upper extremity sparing to axilla	
T4		Nipple line	
T7	Intercostal and abdominal musculature	Inferior costal margin	Upper abdominal†
T10		Umbilicus	Lower abdominal†
T12			
L1	Hip flexion	Groin	
L2		Anteromedial thigh	
L3	Hip adduction and knee extension	Medial knee	Knee/patellar*
L4	Hip abduction and knee extension	Anterior knee and medial calf	
L5	Foot and great toe dorsiflexion	Lateral dorsum foot and lateral sole foot	
S1	Foot and great toe plantar flexion	Lateral dorsum foot and lateral sole foot	Ankle/Achilles*
S2			
S3	Perianal and rectal sphincter tone	Perianal and rectal sensation	
S4			

* Deep tendon.
† Superficial.

may occur in infants with paralyzed limbs and may be indistinguishable from normal movements.

4. Sensation. Upper level of sensory impairment is best guide to accurate localization (see Table 61-1 and Fig. 61-1):
   a. Light-touch sense tests ipsilateral posterior spinal column and contralateral anterior column.
   b. Pain sense (pinprick) tests contralateral anterolateral spinal column.
   c. Position sense tests ipsilateral posterior spinal column.
5. Reflexes:
   a. Deep tendon, superficial (see Table 61-1).
   b. Primitive: Babinski's reflex, Hoffmann's reflex, and others, if present beyond 4 weeks of life, may indicate a UMN lesion.
   c. Rectal: Very important prognostically to assess rectal tone in children with quadriplegia or paraplegia. If rectal tone is present, sacral sparing is implied, with subsequent partial or complete neurologic recovery in up to 30% to 50% of cases. Absence of rectal tone implies only a 2% to 3% chance of partial or complete recovery.
   d. Bulbocavernous reflex testing is performed by pressing the glans penis or pulling on the urinary catheter. An intact reflex results in distinct contraction of the rectal sphincter. The absence of an intact reflex indicates the presence of spinal shock. No accurate estimate of prognosis can be made until this reflex has returned.
   e. Autonomic reflex paralysis produces vasomotor paralysis with flushed, warm, dry skin, loss of temperature regulation (if lesion above T8), hypotension, and bradycardia.
6. Mental status changes, craniofacial injuries, range of motion abnormalities, and focal neurologic findings are not always present in acute cervical spine injuries.

Stability of Cervical Spine Injury

1. Intact anterior structures with disrupted posterior elements are often unstable.
2. Intact posterior elements with disrupted anterior elements are occasionally unstable.
3. Disruption of both anterior and posterior structures usually causes instability.
4. Mechanically stable fractures may still coexist with neurologic defects.

Spinal stability can be assessed by using a **three-column technique**: The *anterior* column consists of the anterior longitudinal ligament, the anterior two thirds of the vertebral body, the anulus fibrosus, and the disc. The *middle* column contains the posterior one third of the vertebral body, the anulus fibrosus, the disc, and the posterior longitudinal ligament. The *posterior* column comprises the remaining posterior components: the pedicles, lateral masses, intertransverse ligaments, facet capsular ligaments, lamina, ligamentum flavum, spinous processes, interspinous and supraspinous ligaments, and ligamentum nuchae. To be unstable, the injury generally involves two of these columns.

Spinal Cord Injury without Radiographic Abnormality

Spinal cord injury without radiographic abnormality (SCIWORA) may occur in as many as 50% to 60% of children with traumatic spinal cord injuries, not commonly in children younger than 8 years. Ir results from a nondisruptive and self-reducing intersegmental deformation as a result of the relative elasticity of the spinal cord in this age group. Hyperextension with inward bulging of interlaminal ligaments, reversible disc prolapse, flexion compression of the cord, longitudinal distraction of the cord, and vertebral artery spasm or thrombosis may all contribute.

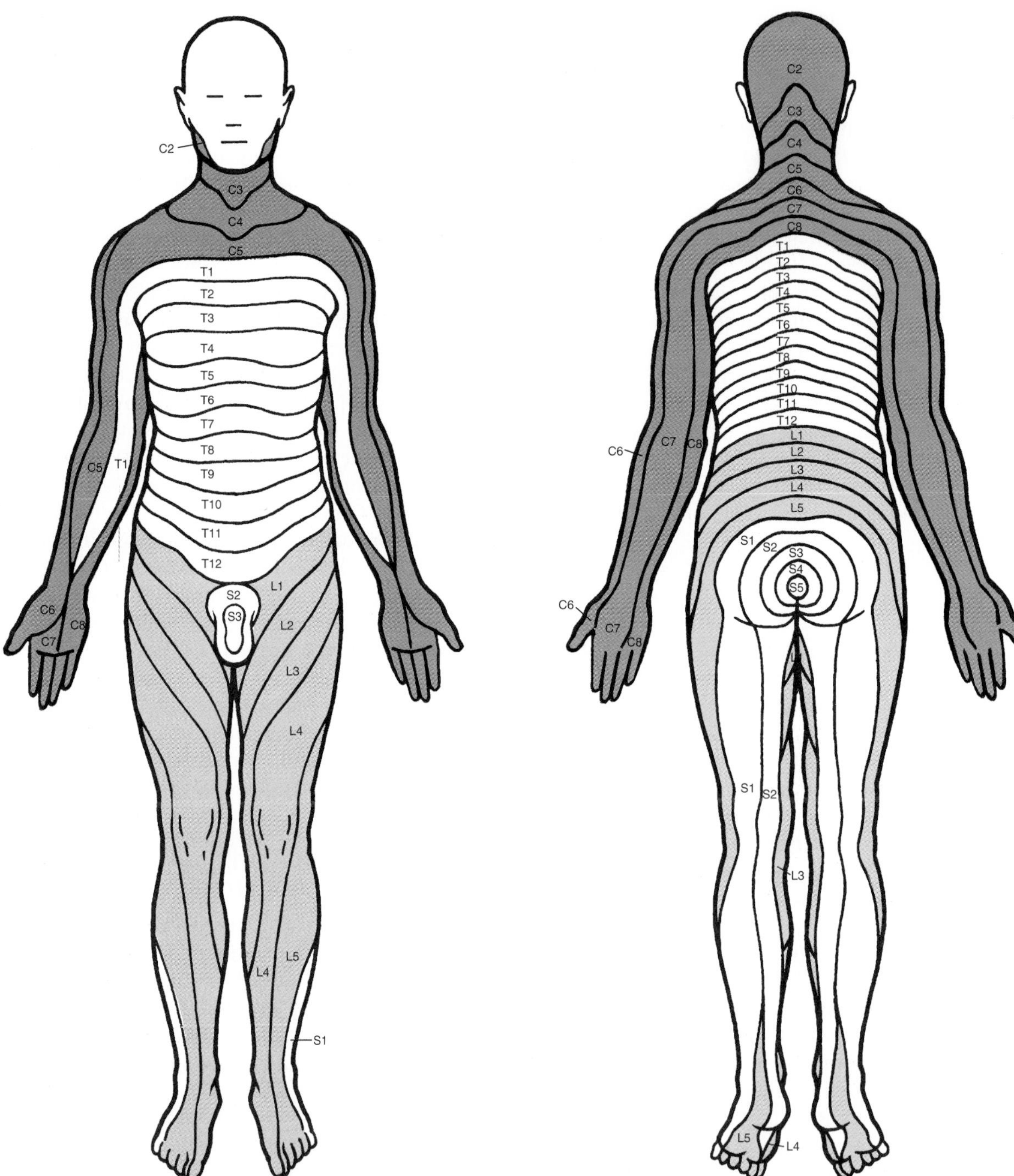

Fig. 61-1 Segmental area of innervation of the skin. Overlapping of one segment occurs between adjacent dermatomes.

(From Marx JA, Hockberger RS, Walls RM et al: *Rosen's emergency medicine: concepts and clinical practice,* ed 5, St Louis, 2002, Mosby.)

Paresthesia may be the only clinical finding, and it is essential to address the presence of transient paresthesias at the time of the accident. The diagnosis can then be made only after occult fractures and ligament or disc damage have been excluded by computed tomographic (CT) scanning, flexion-extension x-ray studies, and myelography.

Patients with a complete injury of the spinal cord have a poor prognosis whereas those with a mild deficit generally do well. Magnetic resonance imaging (MRI) findings are usually abnormal. If they are normal, the prognosis is excellent, but if there is a major cord hemorrhage or transsection, the outcome is poor.

Spinal cord injuries may have a delayed onset of deficit, manifesting as central cord, partial cord, and complete cord syndromes days after the event. The prognosis reflects the abnormality.

Complications

1. Quadriplegia or paraplegia; paralysis.
2. Spinal shock: Flaccid paralysis, areflexia, and sensory loss distal to lesion. Impaired temperature control. Hypotension with bradycardia. Skin is warm, flushed, and dry as a result of loss of sympathetic tone and decreased peripheral vascular resistance. Priapism. Occurs with all types of cord injuries, irrespective of permanency of deficits.
3. Acute urinary retention or incontinence.
4. Paralytic ileus with potential for aspiration.
5. Gastric stress ulcer.
6. Incomplete spinal cord syndromes:
   - **a.** Any amount of neurologic function below the level of the lesion, no matter how minor, implies an incomplete lesion and bodes a reasonably good prognosis.
   - **b.** Anterior cord (contusion of the anterior cord or laceration/thrombosis of the anterior spinal artery): Complete paralysis and hypalgesia with preservation of touch and proprioception. Flexion or vertical compression injury with anterior spinal cord compressed by bony fragments, disc material, or hematoma.
   - **c.** Central cord (damage to central gray matter and most central regions of the pyramidal and spinothalamic tracts): Motor weakness in arms greater than in legs, with variable bladder and sensory involvement. Extension injury, with buckling of the ligamentum flavum into posterior spinal canal causing transient cord compression and microhemorrhage of the central cord.
   - **d.** Posterior cord: Loss of proprioception with variable paresis. Extension injury as in (b). Rare.
   - **e.** Brown-Séquard syndrome: Cord hemisection with ipsilateral motor, proprioception, and light-touch deficit, with contralateral pain and temperature impairment. Usually, penetrating injury.
   - **f.** Horner's syndrome: Unilateral ptosis, miosis, anhidrosis, facial flushing with apparent enophthalmos. Disruption of the cervical sympathetic chain arising at C7-T2.
7. Vertical trauma in addition to spinal injury may have associated pelvic fractures as well as urinary and thoracic injuries.
8. Death secondary to respiratory failure, cardiovascular collapse, hypothermia or hyperthermia, or associated injuries.
9. Long-term sequelae, including psychologic trauma, repeated pulmonary and genitourinary infections, muscle contractures, progressive spinal deformity, and decubitus ulcers.

Ancillary Data

Cervical X-Ray Studies. (See Fig. 61-2.) The criteria for obtaining a cervical spine series in the traumatized child are undefined.

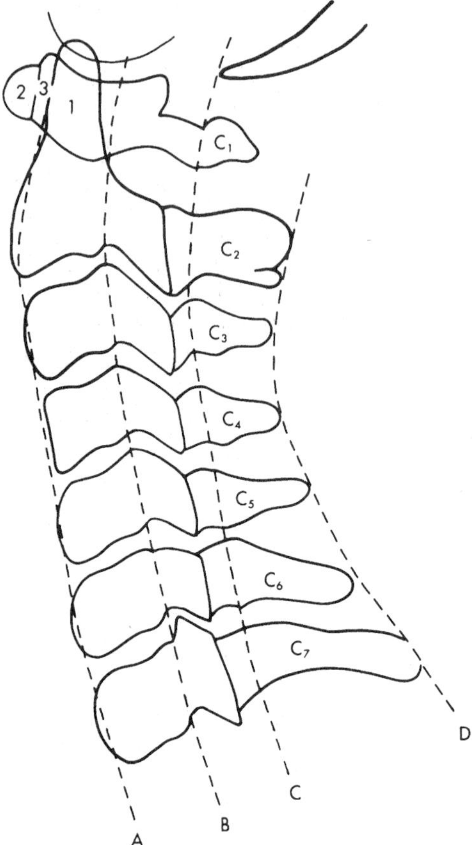

Fig. 61-2 Cervical vertebrae. Lateral cervical spine: *A*, Anterior vertebral bodies; *B*, posterior vertebral bodies and anterior spinal canal; *C*, spinolaminal line and posterior spinal canal; *D*, spinous process tips C2-C7. *1*, Odontoid process of dens of C2; *2*, anterior arch of C1; *3*, predental space between posterior surface of anterior arch of C1 and anterior surface of odontoid process.

Indications for radiography after spinal trauma generally include the following:

1. Acute neurologic deficit or altered mental status
2. Intoxication from alcohol or drugs
3. Head or back and neck pain or tenderness
4. High-risk mechanism of injury: high-speed motor vehicle accident, fall of more than 10 feet, or injury associated with near-drowning
5. Severe associated injuries of head, face, or musculoskeletal system
6. Competitive pain from a nonspinal injury

All cervical vertebrae except C1 have a body. C1 moves in union with the occiput. C1 (axis) has the odontoid process (dens) protruding from its body to rest posterior to the anterior arch of C1 and anterior to the transverse atlantal ligament, allowing for rotation of the neck. The atlas is formed from three ossification centers (body and two neural arches), whereas the axis forms from four centers (odontoid, body, and two neural arches).

The most important initial x-ray film is the *cross-table lateral cervical spine view.* This film identifies more than 75% to 95% of cervical spine fractures, dislocations, and subluxations. It should be obtained early in the resuscitation, and the cervical spine should be immobilized during this phase.

All seven cervical vertebrae must be included. To visualize C7-T1, it may be necessary to have one person hold the patient's head, applying in-line traction, while another pulls gently down on the arms from the foot of the bed. This maneuver is particularly useful in heavy patients. Lead aprons should be worn by care providers.

Swimmer's (transaxillary) view should be obtained if C7-T1 is not visualized by the preceding technique.

A complete cervical spine trauma series must consist, at a minimum, of the cross-table lateral view, anteroposterior (AP) view, and open-mouth odontoid study. Some authorities recommend oblique views as well.

Assessment of the Lateral Cervical Spine (ABCDS)

1. *A*lignment: four continuous curvilinear lines without step-offs. Loss of the normal lordotic curve is seen in 20% of normal patients with spasm, or it may be the only evidence of severe spinal injury (see Fig. 61-2).
2. *B*ony integrity: Compare uniformity, shape, mineralization, density. Look for

fracture lines, displacements, subluxations, or dislocations in systematic manner by first assessing each vertebral body and then each pedicle, facet joint, lamina, and spinous process.

3. Cartilaginous spaces:
   a. Assessment of disc-space uniformity. Isolated disc-space narrowing in a child with the appropriate type and mechanism of injury is suggestive of acute disc herniation. Lengthening of the disc space implies disruption of the anulus fibrosus and possibly the longitudinal ligaments.
   b. The inferior articular facets above and the superior facet below articulate and must line up in parallel. Widening, facet overriding, or vertebral body rotation more than 11 degrees above the facet joint is pathologic.
   c. Interspinous widening is suggestive of ligamentous disruption of the interspinous and supraspinous ligaments.
4. Dens: Assess integrity.
5. Soft tissue spaces:
   a. Predental space (space between the posterior aspect of the anterior arch of C1 and the anterior aspect of the odontoid process of C2 on a lateral view) should be 5 mm or less in children younger than 8 years and 3 mm or less in adults. Greater distance may represent odontoid fractures with posterior displacement or transverse atlantal ligament tear.
   b. Normal prevertebral spaces:
      (1) Anterior to C2: 7 mm or less in children and adults
      (2) Anterior to C3, C4: 5 mm or less in children and adults or less than 40% of the AP diameter of the C3 and C4 vertebral bodies
      (3) Between C6 and trachea: 14 mm or less in children (younger than 15 years) and 22 mm or less in adults

      NOTE: In children younger than 2 years, the retropharyngeal space may normally appear widened during expiration, suggesting the importance of obtaining an inspiratory film. Nasogastric (NG) or endotracheal (ET) tubes may invalidate these measurements. Soft tissue swelling may be secondary to hemorrhage, abscess, infection, foreign body, tumor, air, or bony injury. Using these measurements as sole criteria for determination of injury is not reliable.
   c. Because the retropharyngeal space may be widened during expiration, an inspiratory film should be attempted.
   d. The body of the hyoid bone should normally lie entirely below a line that is parallel to the top of C3. The hyoid bone crosses the epiglottis and is helpful in identifying an inflamed epiglottis.

Other Considerations

1. The odontoid film (open-mouth view preferable) ensures that the dens is centered between the lateral masses of the atlas, and the AP view is useful in assessing C3-C7. Both should be obtained after initial stabilization of the patient and after confirmation that the lateral view is normal.
2. Oblique, flexion, and extension views and tomograms are occasionally required although practice varies. They should be obtained with supervision in the cooperative patient. Flexion films are useful in excluding ligamentous injury in patients with normal mental status and minor malalignment with cervical spine series or if there is severe persistent neck pain or spinal tenderness.
3. Epiphyseal growth plates may resemble fractures. Other developmental changes must be considered in interpreting films:
   a. Pseudosubluxation of C2 occurs anterior to C3, particularly in children

younger than 8 years, and in rare cases at C3-C4. Maximum normal is 2.7 mm, although it is more than 3 mm and up to 5 mm in 20% in children younger than 8 years. If the posterior cervical line (the line [cervical line, spinolaminar line, line of Swischuk] drawn from the anterior aspect of the spinous process of C1 to the anterior aspect of the spinous process of C3) misses the anterior aspect of the C2 spinous process by 2 mm or more, a hangman's fracture with subluxation may be present. This finding is useful only if C2 is displaced anterior to C3. Normally, the posterior cervical line misses the anterior aspect of the C2 spinal process by 2 mm or more.

   b. The posterior arch of C1 (three ossification centers) fuses around 3 years, and the anterior arch at 7 to 10 years.

   c. The epiphyseal plate at the base of the odontoid fuses with the body of C2 at 3 to 6 years.

4. Widening of the anteroposterior dimension of C2 in relation to C3 may indicate a fracture.
5. The minimal wedge shape of the body of C3 may be normal. The anterior wedging of immature vertebral bodies may look like compression fractures. Similar-appearing adjacent vertebral bodies suggest a normal variant.
6. A CT scan often is preferred in selected circumstances when routine film findings are normal and a fracture is still suspected, the plain films are inadequate, or there is a suspicious finding on plain film. The anatomy can be well documented by CT without unnecessary movement of the patient, and obtaining a CT scan can be particularly important in patients with abnormal neurologic findings who have normal cervical x-ray studies.
7. MRI is superior to CT in demonstrating spinal cord injury (edema, hemorrhage, compression, and transection) and intervertebral disc herniation. CT is better in defining bony injury. Limitations of availability and the image degradation caused by resuscitation and monitoring equipment restrict MRI's usefulness in evaluating acutely injured patients. Experience with the modality in pediatric trauma is limited.

Thoracic and Lumbar Spine X-Ray Studies

1. A cross-table lateral view of the thoracic or lumbar spine should be obtained first, with the patient immobilized on a firm backboard.
2. An AP view is taken next (oblique views sometimes needed).
3. Interpedicular space must be assessed, as well as the *ABCs* previously described for cervical x-rays.
4. The distance between the medial aspects of the two pedicles overlying each vertebral body (on the AP view) gradually increases in a caudal (cervical-to-lumbar) direction. A marked increase in this distance is indicative of posterior disruption and probable instability.
5. Most fractures of the lower spine occur in the region of T10-L4 although in the multiply injured patient, injuries are common at T2-T7. In multiple-level, noncontiguous fractures, the secondary lesions commonly occur at L4-L5 and C1-C2.
6. Fractures of T1-T5 may produce mediastinal hematomas with widening of the mediastinum.
7. Thoracolumbar compression fractures in children may appear as beaklike projections on the anterior margin of the vertebral body, usually superior.

DIFFERENTIAL DIAGNOSIS

1. Hysterical paralysis
2. Trauma:
   - **a.** Bilateral brachial plexus injury
   - **b.** Nerve root injury
   - **c.** Cauda equina syndrome

3. Vascular: ischemia resulting from atherosclerosis, thromboembolic disease, thoracic aorta dissection, or epidural hematoma
4. Spinal tumor

MANAGEMENT

Initial attention must be paid to resuscitation and support while the spine is immobilized at the levels of suspected injury. Immediate consultation with a neurosurgeon is necessary.

1. Airway stabilization, with ventilatory support as necessary and administration of oxygen:
   a. Bag-valve-mask ventilation, nasotracheal intubation, or cricothyroidotomy in patients with severe respiratory compromise.
   b. Oral ET intubation may be contraindicated because it may cause excessive cervical spine motion.
   c. Forced vital capacity determination may be useful in the evaluation.
2. Circulation (see Chapter 5):
   a. If shock is present, treat initially as hypovolemic shock. Look for a source of internal hemorrhage. Excessive transfusion of crystalloid in the presence of spinal shock may precipitate pulmonary edema. Urinary output rather than blood pressure is the best monitor.
   b. Once hypovolemic shock has been excluded, neurogenic shock should be considered. Patients with neurogenic shock are hypotensive with bradycardia and have warm, flushed, dry skin—in contrast to those with hypovolemic shock.
      (1) To treat decreased sympathetic tone: low-dose norepinephrine (Levophed), drip infusion at 0.1 to 1.0 μg. To treat increased parasympathetic tone: atropine, 0.01 to 0.02 mg/kg/dose IV repeated q5-10min as necessary, used alternatively or concurrently with norepinephrine.
      (2) Insert NG tube once neck is stabilized and a Foley catheter is in place. Consider cimetidine, 20 to 40 mg/kg/24 hr (maximum: 300 mg) q6hr IV.
3. Immobilization and stabilization of neck from the outset:
   a. Place the neck in neutral position with sandbags and 1- to 2-inch tape across the forehead and chin with the patient on a rigid backboard or scoop.
   b. Apply gentle in-line traction with neurologic abnormalities. Cervical spine stabilization can be achieved with a semi-hard Stif Neck, Philadelphia collar, or four-poster collar. Tape and sandbags or a supplemental device in combination with an immobilizer is most effective. Soft collars offer no demonstrable stability.
   c. Much attention is given to the cervical spine; thoracic and lumbar fractures are equally possible, even in the young child. These must be diligently sought.
4. When there is cervical neurologic impairment, skeletal traction is indicated on an emergent basis. Traction can be applied by using halo, Gardner-Wells, Crutchfield, or Vinke tongs. A neurosurgeon is best involved in these procedures.
   a. The patient is then transferred to a suitable frame, and 1 to 5 lb of weight per interspace (adult) is applied. Further lateral spine x-ray films are obtained to assess alignment. If alignment is not achieved, muscle relaxants are often required.
   b. Thoracic and lumbar injuries are treated by immobilizing the patient to allow for postural reduction. Concurrent stabilization of other life-threatening injuries with appropriate consultations is essential.

5. Steroids have generally been demonstrated to reduce neurologic function at all levels of injury when begun within 8 hours. Very-high-dose methylprednisolone, 30 mg/kg IV, followed by an infusion of 5.4 mg/kg/hr for the subsequent 23 hours, appears to be beneficial. However, children younger than 13 years were excluded from the initial studies of the use of steroids for this purpose, as were patients with gunshot wounds, nerve root impairment, and cauda equina syndrome. Significant improvement in motor function and in pin and touch sensations were seen in treated patients at 6 weeks and 6 months after injury.
6. Gangliosides are a complex acidic glycolipid present in the central nervous system (CNS) as a component of the cell membrane. Administration of ganglioside GM_1 may enhance recovery after injury.
7. Surgical decompression, when required, should be performed in a timely fashion. When performed more than 8 hours after injury, it is significantly less successful. The indications include progressive neurologic deterioration, penetrating injuries of the spinal cord, and a foreign body within the spinal canal. Surgical stabilization and realignment may be necessary for potentially unstable injuries or for relief of pain.

DISPOSITION

All patients with spine or spinal cord injury require hospitalization and immediate neurosurgical consultation. A team approach to the management of such patients is mandatory. After they are stabilized, patients often must be transferred to neurosurgical spinal trauma centers.

Parental Education

Prevention

1. Automobile restraints should always be used.
2. Swimming and diving in uncontrolled areas should be avoided.
3. Trampolines should be forbidden.

BIBLIOGRAPHY

Anderson DK, Hall ED: Pathophysiology of spinal cord trauma, *Ann Emerg Med* 22:987, 1993.

Bohn D, Armstrong D, Becker L et al: Cervical spine injuries in children, *J Trauma* 30:463, 1990.

Bracken MB, Shepard MJ, Collins WF et al: A randomized controlled trial of methylprednisolone or naloxone in the treatment of acute spinal cord injury: results of the Second National Acute Spinal Cord Injury Study, *N Engl J Med* 322:1405, 1990.

DeBehn DJ, Havel CG: Utility of pre-cervical soft tissue measurements in identifying patients with cervical spine fracture, *Ann Emerg Med* 24:1119, 1994.

El-Khoury GY, Kathol MH, Daniel WW: Imaging of acute injuries of the cervical spine: value of plain radiography, CT and MR imaging. *Am J Roentgenol* 164:43, 1995.

Felsberg GJ, Tien RD, Osumi AK et al: Utility of MR imaging in pediatric spinal cord injury, *Pediatr Radiol* 25:131, 1995.

Fesmire FM, Luten RC: The pediatric cervical spine: developmental anatomy and clinical aspects, *J Emerg Med* 7:133, 1989.

Geisler FH, Dorsey FC, Coleman WP: Past and current clinical studies with GM-1 ganglioside in acute spinal cord injury, *Ann Emerg Med* 22:1041, 1993.

Geisler FH, Dorsey FC, Coleman WP: Recovery of motor function after spinal cord injury: a randomized placebo controlled trial with GM-1 ganglioside, *N Engl J Med* 324:1829, 1991.

Hockberger RS, Kirshenbaum K, Doris PE: Spinal injury. In Rosen P, editor: *Emergency medicine: concepts and clinical practice*, ed 5, St. Louis, 2002, Mosby.

Kriss VM, Kriss TC: Imaging of the cervical spine in infants, *Pediatr Emerg Care* 13:44, 1996.

Kriss VM, Kriss TC: SCIWORA: spinal cord injury without radiographic abnormality in infants and children, *Clin Pediatr* 35:199, 1996.

Pang D, Pollack IF: Spinal cord injury without radiographic abnormality in children: the SCIWORA syndrome, *J Trauma* 29:654, 1989.

Prendergast MA, Saxe JM, Ledgerwood AM et al: Massive steroids do not reduce the zone of injury after penetrating spinal cord injury, *J Trauma* 37:576, 1994.

Schwartz GR, Wright SW, Fein JA et al: Pediatric cervical spine injury sustained in falls from low heights, *Ann Emerg Care* 30:249, 1997.

Stieu IG, Wells GA, Wandembeen KL et al: The Canadian C-spine rule for radiography in alert and stable trauma patients, *JAMA* 286:1840, 2001.

Turetsky DB, Vines FS, Clayman DA et al: Technique and use of supine oblique views in acute cervical spine trauma, *Ann Emerg Med* 22:685, 1993.

62 Thoracic Trauma

VINCENT J. MARKOVCHICK and BENJAMIN HONIGMAN

ALERT Blunt or penetrating thoracic trauma requires a rapid assessment of pulmonary, cardiac, and mediastinal injuries. These may necessitate lifesaving procedures without a complete database.

Traumatic injuries of the chest are common and require urgent attention to therapy and diagnosis. More than with injuries in any other anatomic area, the physician must rapidly assess the patient's status and may have to intervene without a full diagnosis. Delays in management are often life threatening, whereas lifesaving procedures such as pericardiocentesis and the insertion of a chest tube are associated with relatively minimal complications.

The initial evaluation of the patient must take into consideration all aspects of the injuries (see Chapter 56). The airway, ventilation, and circulation are of primary concern. Specific attention must be focused on the mechanism and severity of the injury and the progression of signs and symptoms since the trauma.

1. *Blunt trauma* is associated with chest wall injuries (rib fractures or flail chest), hemothorax, pneumothorax, pulmonary contusion, myocardial contusion, aortic tears, diaphragmatic rupture, and esophageal rupture (Box 62-1).
2. *Penetrating injuries* cause hemothorax, pneumothorax, penetrating cardiac injuries and tamponade, direct vessel damage, esophageal, and diaphragmatic injuries. The amount of time elapsed since injury and the patient's current status provide some indication of the urgency of intervention.

Diagnostic findings detected with a quick physical examination must include blood pressure (BP) (including an evaluation for pulsus paradoxus), respiratory rate and pattern, and heart sounds. Evidence of upper airway obstruction must be sought, including stridor and facial and neck injuries, and active intervention initiated when indicated. If the upper airway appears intact, lower airway compromise must be excluded through evaluation of chest wall stability, symmetry and adequacy of air movement, and presence or absence of subcutaneous emphysema.

Predictors of thoracic injury in children suffering blunt torso trauma have been reported to include low systolic BP, elevated respiratory rate, abnormal thoracic findings including auscultation findings, femur fracture, and a Glasgow Coma Scale (GCS) score lower than 15.

If the patient is in obvious respiratory distress, immediate therapy is required. Oxygen should be administered by a nonrebreathing bag reservoir mask, and simultaneously, an airway ensured. Unilateral or bilateral chest tubes may be required, often solely on the basis of the physical examination.

Shock must be treated. With isolated thoracic injuries, shock is most commonly caused by massive pulmonary hemorrhage, pericardial tamponade, or tension pneumothorax.

Box 62-1

BLUNT THORACIC INJURIES

IMMEDIATELY LIFE-THREATENING

Upper airway obstruction
Tension pneumothorax (p. 472)
Open pneumothorax (p. 472)
Massive hemothorax (p. 475)
Pericardial tamponade (p. 480)
Flail chest (p. 470)

POTENTIALLY LIFE-THREATENING

Pulmonary contusion (p. 474)
Myocardial contusion (p. 479)
Bronchial disruption
Diaphragmatic rupture (p. 478)
Aortic injury (p. 482)
Esophageal rupture

SERIOUS

Simple pneumothorax (p. 472)
Simple hemothorax (p. 475)
Rib fractures (p. 469)
Traumatic asphyxia

With multiple trauma, other causes must be excluded.

Ancillary data that are mandatory in any thoracic injury are chest x-ray film (supine view obtained with portable machine if the patient is unstable), electrocardiogram (ECG), arterial blood gas (ABG) analysis, oximetry, and complete blood count (CBC) (hematocrit [Hct] measured in the emergency department [ED]). In patients with major injuries, blood typing and cross-match should also be performed immediately. However, these studies should not delay interventions in the patient with respiratory distress after a traumatic injury.

RIB FRACTURE

ALERT Rib fractures are rare in children because of the highly elastic chest wall; therefore, when a rib fracture is noted, significant underlying organ injury (e.g., liver, lung, spleen) must be suspected. Upper rib fractures are associated with pulmonary and major vessel injuries; lower rib injuries are associated with potential liver, spleen, lung, and kidney injury. Conversely, the absence of a rib fracture does not preclude serious injury to the underlying soft tissue structures. Child abuse may have to be considered.

Fractured ribs are caused by blunt trauma resulting from motor vehicle accidents, falls, blows with blunt objects, child abuse, and athletic injuries and are the most common significant findings after blunt trauma. Rib fracture is unlikely in minor trauma; however, a rib fracture from major trauma may lacerate underlying structures. Child abuse may have to be considered, particularly in children younger than 12 months.

Diagnostic Findings

The mechanism of injury and an estimate of the force of impact may predict the type of injury:

1. Dyspnea and chest pain are common symptoms with isolated rib fractures.
2. Point tenderness over the rib is uniformly present. Anterior-posterior and lateral-lateral compression is painful. Referred pain is present on proximal or distal compression of the fractured rib.
3. Tachypnea, tachycardia, and shock are associated with underlying organ damage and respiratory failure.

Complications

1. Pneumothorax occurs in more than one third of patients.
2. Hemothorax is noted in 13% of patients.
3. Pulmonary laceration or contusion.
4. Myocardial contusion.
5. Solid visceral damage (liver, spleen, kidney), particularly with fractures of ribs 9 to 12.
6. Neurovascular tears (e.g., subclavian, brachial plexus, aorta) with fractures of ribs 1 and 2.

Ancillary Data

1. Chest x-ray studies. Most useful in evaluating status of pulmonary parenchyma and mediastinum. More than 50% of single-rib fractures are overlooked on the initial chest x-ray film.
2. Hct measurement (to be done in ED) and urinalysis.
3. Continuous oxygen saturation monitoring and ABG analysis, if pulmonary contusions are evident.
4. ECG for major blunt chest injury.
5. Dynamic computed tomography (CT) scan as an initial screen before angiogram for widened mediastinum (aortic tear) or fractures of the first or second rib, particularly if displaced (vascular injury).

Differential Diagnosis

1. Infectious/inflammatory: pleurisy, pneumonia, perichondritis, pericarditis
2. Trauma: rib contusion, costochondral separation (snapping sound with breathing)

Management

1. Treatment of any complications.
2. Simple rib fractures without complications:
   a. Analgesia.
   b. Intercostal nerve block using long-acting local anesthetic agent such as bupivacaine (Marcaine) with epinephrine. Inject 1 to 2 ml in the subcostal space at the posterior axillary line. The intercostal nerves above and below the fracture should be blocked.
3. Instructions to patients:
   a. Patients should be taught deep-breathing exercises.
   b. Patients should not use binders or rib belts, which would inhibit adequate ventilation.

Disposition

1. Hospitalization should be strongly considered for young children and infants with any rib fracture because of the extreme force necessary to break a rib in this age group and, therefore, the high probability of complications and the high possibility of child abuse if the mechanism is inconsistent with the injury.
2. Hospitalization for observation should be strongly considered for older children and adolescents who sustain multiple (more than two) fractures.
3. All children with any complications should be hospitalized.

Parental Education

1. Continue deep-breathing exercises.
2. Call your physician if cough, fever, dyspnea, or increased pain develops.

FLAIL CHEST

ALERT Flail chest is invariably associated with pulmonary contusion and abnormal respiratory physiology.

Flail chest results from blunt trauma when three or more adjacent ribs are fractured at two points, leading to a freely movable chest wall segment. This results in paradoxic movement on respiration (inward with inspiration and outward with expiration), which may compress lung tissue, decrease ventilation on the ipsilateral side, and cause the mediastinum to shift to the other side. Venous return is decreased secondary to lung compression. More important, the underlying pulmonary contusion contributes to hypoxia and increasing respiratory distress.

Diagnostic Findings

1. Usually associated with multiple trauma.
2. Tenderness over ribs with crepitus and ecchymoses.
3. Commonly associated with increased heart and respiratory rates. Shock may occur secondary to complications or related injuries.
4. Visible or palpable paradoxic movement, which may require a tangential

light to see. Up to 30% of cases are missed on the initial examination in the first 6 hours.

5. Decreased oxygen saturation, as indicated by oximetry, secondary to underlying pulmonary contusion.

Complications. Complications are commonly associated with flail chest. Respiratory insufficiency is caused by pulmonary contusion, atelectasis, and decreases in tidal volume and vital capacity, with resultant hypoxia, atrioventricular (AV) shunting, and, ultimately, shock. Mortality is higher when associated head injuries are present.

The respiratory embarrassment results primarily not from the paradoxic movement of the chest but from the underlying injury to lung parenchyma.

Ancillary Data. Chest x-ray studies, oximetry, and ABG analysis are required.

Management

1. For management of multiple trauma, treat and diagnose complications and associated life-threatening injuries: give oxygen, establish intravenous (IV) access, obtain chest x-ray film, and obtain ABG analysis and Hct determination.
2. Connect patient to bag reservoir mask, oxygen, and oxygen saturation monitor.
3. Stabilize flail chest with sandbags and pressure over the unstable segment, or position the patient on the side of injury, if possible.
4. Correct associated respiratory complications (e.g., thoracostomy for pneumothorax or hemothorax). If respiratory distress continues, intubate the patient and stabilize internally with positive-pressure ventilation.
5. Intubate the patient if flail chest is associated with the following conditions:
   a. Shock
   b. Three or more related injuries
   c. Five or more rib fractures
   d. Underlying pulmonary disease
   e. Respiratory failure, with $Pa{O_2}$ less than 50 mm Hg and $Pa{CO_2}$ greater than 50 mm Hg:
      (1) Relative indications include increasing respiratory rate, restlessness, anxiety, abnormal alveolar-to-arterial oxygen gradient (A–$a{O_2}$) or decreasing $Pa{O_2}$ or oxygen saturation.
      (2) Some clinicians recommend intubation only when flail chest is associated with respiratory failure.
6. Strongly consider thoracostomy if the patient either is to have general anesthesia or if the patient needs ventilator support (especially if positive end-expiratory pressure [PEEP] is to be used). In addition, thoracostomy is required for hemothorax or pneumothorax (see Appendix A-9).
7. Do not give antibiotics prophylactically. Steroids are not indicated.

Disposition

All patients with flail chest must be admitted to an intensive care unit (ICU).

STERNAL FRACTURE

ALERT Sternal fractures and dislocations in children are unusual but when present suggest underlying myocardial contusion, cardiac rupture, pericardial tamponade, pulmonary contusion, or aortic rupture. The mortality rate is 25% to 45%.

Diagnostic Findings

Simple sternal fractures, which are unusual, are accompanied by anterior chest pain with point tenderness and ecchymoses over the sternum. More commonly, there are associated problems.

Complications

1. Flail chest and other contiguous injuries
2. Myocardial contusion or rupture, pericardial tamponade, or vascular injury

3. Pulmonary contusion
4. Traumatic aortic dissection

Ancillary Data

1. Chest x-ray study reveals fractures on lateral view, although special sternal views may be necessary. Differentiate sternal fracture from nonossified cartilage of sternum. Fractures are not seen on posteroanterior (PA) or rib views.
2. ECG shows nonspecific ST-T wave changes and a persistent tachycardia. Dysrhythmias may be seen.

Management

1. Treat life-threatening injuries and complications with oxygen, IV lines, cardiac monitoring, and specific intervention.
2. Give analgesia.
3. Surgery may be required if the fracture is displaced.

Disposition

All patients with sternal fracture must be admitted to an ICU for continuous monitoring.

TRAUMATIC PNEUMOTHORAX

ALERT A simple pneumothorax may cause respiratory distress. Bilateral or tension pneumothorax is life threatening and requires immediate intervention.

A *simple* pneumothorax occurs when air accumulates in the pleural space without mediastinal shift. It is invariably present with penetrating chest injuries and in 15% to 50% of patients with blunt trauma chest injury.

A *tension* pneumothorax is produced when there is progressive accumulation of air in the pleural space with shift of mediastinal structures to the opposite hemithorax and compression of the mediastinum and contralateral lung. Tension pneumothorax can progressively decrease cardiac output. Massive shunting of blood occurs from perfused but nonventilated areas because of lung compression, atelectasis, and collapse.

Open pneumothorax accompanies sucking chest wounds when there is a free bidirectional flow of air between the atmosphere and the pleural space. It requires a large enough penetrating wound to result in a loss of a portion of the chest wall that approaches the size of the bronchial lumen.

Etiology

1. Blunt trauma: complication of fractured ribs, cardiopulmonary resuscitation, violent chest impact with closed glottis, or bronchial disruption
2. Penetrating trauma: complication of stab, gunshot, or other penetrating wound, or complication of insertion of a central venous catheter

Diagnostic Findings

1. Patients have dyspnea, chest pain, and a history of trauma.
2. The patient with a small, uncomplicated pneumothorax has normal vital signs, although respiratory and heart rates may be increased. Large defects are associated with respiratory distress and sometimes cyanosis.
3. Tension pneumothorax is accompanied by respiratory distress, hypotension, tachycardia, and absence of breath sounds. Other signs that may be present are pulsus paradoxus, increased jugular venous pressure (JVP), tracheal shift, altered mental status, and, at times, cyanosis. Air hunger is usually marked.
   a. If the patient is being ventilated with bag-valve-mask apparatus, an early indication of tension pneumothorax is a growing resistance to bag ventilation. If the patient is being mechanically ventilated, increasing airway pressure may be needed to deliver the same volume of air.
   b. Other clues are increased central venous pressure (CVP), decreased BP, electromechanical dissociation, and

marked intercostal and supraclavicular retractions.

4. Absence or marked decrease of breath sounds and hyperresonance to percussion may be present. Subcutaneous emphysema with crepitus is common and increases rapidly if positive-pressure ventilation is being used.

   NOTE: Soon after penetrating injuries, and in children with small chests, transmission of breath sounds from the unaffected lung may simulate normal breath sounds, making clinical diagnosis more difficult.

5. Pneumomediastinum may accompany pneumothorax.

Complications. Complications include respiratory distress, hypotension, and cardiac arrest.

Ancillary Data

1. Chest x-ray film for simple pneumothorax:
   a. Is the definitive diagnostic procedure.
   b. On occasion, pneumothorax may be found only on an expiratory view, because expiration increases intrapleural pressure, pushing the lung and visceral pleura away from the chest wall.
   c. Classification: small, less than 10% of lung volume; moderate, 10% to 50%; large, more than 50%.

      NOTE: Tension pneumothorax should be a clinical diagnosis and should not await x-ray confirmation. X-ray film shows marked lung compression with mediastinal shift away from the affected side.
2. ABG analysis and oximetry after patient is stabilized.

Differential Diagnosis

Many other entities besides trauma cause pneumothorax:

1. Asthma and other reactive airway diseases with hyperexpansion
2. Spontaneous pneumothorax secondary to apical blebs in adolescents
3. Meconium aspiration and hyaline membrane disease in the newborn (see Chapter 11)

Management

Life-threatening injuries must be treated immediately.

1. Tube thoracostomy is the treatment of choice for pneumothorax, sometimes before a definitive diagnosis is made (see Appendix A-9).
   a. Indications for insertion of a chest tube include the following:
      (1) Tension pneumothorax
      (2) Traumatic cause, especially penetrating injuries
      (3) Any pneumothorax with respiratory symptoms
      (4) Increasing pneumothorax after initial conservative therapy
      (5) Pneumothorax with need for mechanical ventilation or general anesthesia
      (6) Associated hemothorax
      (7) Bilateral pneumothorax

      NOTE: A symptom-free patient with a small (<10%), simple pneumothorax—one that shows no increase on second x-ray study—who does not need general anesthesia or mechanical ventilation may be observed in the hospital without a chest tube.
   b. Position for chest tube:
      (1) Insert in fourth or fifth intercostal space in midaxillary line directed posteriorly and apically.
      (2) Insert superior to rib because neurovascular bundle runs inferior to rib in the lateral interspaces.
   c. Size: As large a tube as possible should be inserted, particularly with a hemothorax:

Age	Tube Size
Newborn	10 to 12 Fr
Infant	14 to 20 Fr

Child	20 to 28 Fr
Adolescent	28 to 42 Fr

d. Use a tube with a radiopaque line (for placement verification by x-ray film), and make certain that the last hole in the tube is within the pleural cavity.
e. Drainage: All chest tubes should be connected to an underwater seal drainage. Patients with continuous air leaks or associated hemothorax may require suction (15 to 25 cm H_2O).

2. Chest venting may be required as an initial, transient therapeutic maneuver when tension pneumothorax is suspected and there is some delay in placement of a chest tube.
   a. Venting can be done with a needle, angiocatheter, or one-way flutter valve.
   b. Venting necessitates the eventual use of a chest tube.
   c. Venting should be done in the second or third intercostal space at the midclavicular line of the anterior chest wall or in the fourth or fifth intercostal space at the midaxillary line. Care must be taken to keep the vent from being dislodged before the chest tube is placed.
3. Emergency management focuses on conversion to a simple pneumothorax, followed by immediate evacuation of entrapped air and reexpansion of the lung by means of a tube thoracostomy. This approach is usually effective.

Disposition

All patients with traumatic pneumothorax must be hospitalized. The level of monitoring depends on the severity of respiratory distress and associated injuries.

PULMONARY CONTUSION

ALERT Pulmonary contusion is a significant cause of respiratory failure after major blunt trauma injury in children, particularly rapid deceleration injuries.

Pulmonary contusion occurs when there is lung parenchymal damage with intraalveolar hemorrhage and edema. It occurs secondary to increased capillary membrane permeability, which impairs gas exchange.

Pulmonary contusion is usually associated with high-impact trauma; most cases occur at age 5 years or older. Most patients have multiple trauma and involvement of at least one other major organ system. There is often a relative absence of external chest wall injury.

Diagnostic Findings

Patients who have experienced a rapid-deceleration injury may arrive with dyspnea and cyanosis, particularly those older than 5 years. Hemoptysis is rare in children. Tachycardia, tachypnea, anxiety, restlessness, labored respiration, and hypotension may be present. Localized rales or wheezing, with decreased breath sounds, may also be present. Significant hypoxia may be delayed 4 to 6 hours from the time of injury.

Obvious evidence of external trauma may not be present. Approximately 80% to 90% of patients have associated injuries.

Complications. Pneumonia is a complication. Intrathoracic effusion and hemothorax may develop over 48 hours.

Ancillary Data

1. Chest x-ray film: For all patients with increased respiratory or heart rate after trauma even if there is no external evidence of injury. Serial x-ray studies may be required.
   a. Findings vary from patchy areas of alveolar infiltrates to frank consolidation. They may be delayed 4 to 6 hours or they may be rapid in onset. CT scan may demonstrate contusion earlier.
   b. X-ray findings usually clear in 48 to 60 hours.

2. ABG analysis:
   a. Hypoxemia is invariable but may be delayed in onset for 4 to 6 hours (deteriorates over the ensuing 24 hours). Continuous oximetry is appropriate.
   b. The $A\text{–}aO_2$ difference (gradient) at room air ($A\text{–}aO_2 = 150 - PaO_2 - 1.2\ PaCO_2$), which is normally 15 or less, is the first to increase.
   c. Respiratory rate also increases and is a noninvasive clue to onset of insufficiency when monitored.
   d. Chest CT: Pulmonary contusions are evident on this study earlier than on a standard chest x-ray film.

Differential Diagnosis

1. Trauma: Multiple causes of acute respiratory distress syndrome (ARDS) in children include smoke inhalation and fat emboli (fracture, penetrating chest wound). ARDS is usually delayed in onset, beginning 24 to 48 hours after the injury, and it has diffuse involvement (p. 41).
2. Medical causes of infiltrates and hypoxia: congestive heart failure (CHF), embolism, pneumonia.

Management

1. Treat associated life-threatening injuries.
2. Maintain oxygenation and ventilation:
   a. Intubation and ventilation are indicated if PaO_2 is less than 50 mm Hg at 100% O_2 (sea level).
   b. PEEP or continuous positive airway pressure (CPAP) may shorten the length of ventilatory assistance. Begin at 5 cm H_2O and increase slowly, monitoring oxygenation and cardiac output.
3. Give IV fluids:
   a. Patients with pulmonary contusion benefit from low levels of fluid administration. However, associated injuries may require high volumes of crystalloid solution. This infusion may increase pulmonary interstitial fluid, worsening the respiratory status.
   b. Ideally, the goal is to combine blood products and crystalloid solution to maintain adequate perfusion, CVP, and urinary output.
4. Steroids should not be used.
5. Analgesics may be required but must be used sparingly in view of their potential for respiratory compromise. Intercostal nerve blocks may produce comfort and allow easier respirations in patients with rib fractures.
6. Antibiotics are reserved for demonstrated infections.

Disposition

All patients with pulmonary contusion must be admitted to an ICU.

HEMOTHORAX

ALERT Hemothorax can cause hypovolemic shock and respiratory failure from compression of the lung.

As a result of blunt or penetrating trauma, large amounts of blood can accumulate in the pleural space, secondary to injury to intercostal and internal mammary arteries, the heart, the great vessels, or the hilar vessels. Lung lacerations usually have self-limited bleeding. Hemostasis eventually occurs in hemothorax as a result of low pulmonary arterial pressures, large concentrations of thromboplastin in lung tissue, and the compressive effects of the pleural blood volume.

Diagnostic Findings

1. With small amounts of blood loss ($<10\%$ of blood volume), diagnosis may be difficult in an isolated injury; however, more than 75% of cases of blood loss are associated with extrathoracic injuries. The physical examination usually demonstrates evidence of trauma.

2. Larger accumulations of blood (>25% of blood volume) produce pallor, restlessness, anxiety, tachycardia, vasoconstriction, and, eventually, orthostatic and resting hypotension.
3. Chest examination demonstrates evidence of external trauma and decreased breath sounds. Pneumothorax is often an associated finding.

Complications

1. Respiratory failure, hypotension, and shock
2. Infection with empyema

Ancillary Data

1. Chest x-ray study:
   a. An upright film shows blunting of the costophrenic angle when more than 175 ml of blood accumulates in the adolescent.
   b. A supine chest film demonstrates haziness of the affected side.
   c. Pneumothorax may be present.
   d. A lateral decubitus film may be helpful if an upright film cannot be obtained or interpreted.
2. ABG analysis and oximetry reflect the degree of respiratory compromise.
3. Bedside ultrasonography in the ED has been reported to be extremely sensitive and specific in detecting the presence of fluid in the pleural cavity.

Differential Diagnosis

1. Pleural effusion of any origin, for example, CHF, pneumonia, empyema, chylothorax, or hydrothorax (from improperly placed CVP catheter)
2. Trauma: pulmonary contusion (upright or decubitus chest x-ray film should differentiate the two)

Management

1. Priorities should be established with respect to concurrent life-threatening injuries—that is, maintenance of oxygenation and ventilation. Fluid resuscitation is commonly needed.
2. Tube thoracostomy is the treatment required immediately, sometimes solely on the basis of respiratory distress and physical examination (see Appendix A-9).
   a. Indications:
      (1) Penetrating injury with obvious or suspected hemothorax, respiratory distress, or shock. Treatment is required immediately, before chest x-ray film is obtained.
      (2) Blunt injuries with suspected hemothorax (e.g., decreased breath sounds, multiple rib fractures), respiratory failure, or shock. Treatment is required immediately.
      (3) Unsuspected thoracic injuries in a child with multiple trauma. A chest x-ray film is usually indicated before intervention but may not always be possible.
      (4) The child in hemorrhagic shock with no evidence of either internal blood loss from the abdomen, retroperitoneal space, or pelvis, or external blood loss. In such a patient bilateral chest tubes may be required as a diagnostic and therapeutic modality if hemothorax is present on the chest x-ray film or if instability prevents performance of a chest x-ray film.
   b. Size: Large-bore polymeric silicone (Silastic) tubes should be used for blood drainage: newborn, 8 to 12 Fr; infant, 16 to 20 Fr; children, 20 to 28 Fr; adolescents, 28 to 42 Fr.
   c. Position: in the fourth or fifth intercostal space in midaxillary line and directed superiorly and posteriorly. If large amounts of blood return or if the tube becomes clotted, a second chest

tube inserted one or two interspaces below the first may be required.

NOTE: The chest tube should be connected to an underwater seal drain and 15 to 25 cm H_2O suction.

3. Autotransfusions are useful if appropriate equipment is available.
4. Thoracotomy is only rarely needed but may be lifesaving in rare circumstances:
   a. When the blood drainage from the initial thoracostomy tube is more than one third of the patient's blood volume (blood volume in child, 80 ml/kg; in adult, 70 ml/kg)
   b. With persistent bleeding of more than 10% blood volume per hour
   c. With increasing hemothorax on chest x-ray film, despite therapy
   d. With persistent hypotension despite adequate crystalloid solution and blood replacement and when other areas of blood loss have been excluded
   e. If vital signs deteriorate after initial successful resuscitation
5. Salvage is greatest in patients with penetrating chest injuries whose condition does not deteriorate until arrival in the ED or is stable throughout.

Disposition

All patients require admission to an ICU.

SUBCUTANEOUS EMPHYSEMA AND PNEUMOMEDIASTINUM

ALERT The presence of subcutaneous emphysema or pneumomediastinum in a patient with trauma requires a careful search for laryngeal fracture, esophageal tear, and tracheobronchial injury as well as pneumothorax.

Air in the subcutaneous tissue or mediastinum after trauma may be caused by an underlying intrapleural leak from a pneumothorax or bronchial tear or may be secondary to a penetrating injury with spread through the fascial planes.

Traumatic bronchial disruption is rare but may result from chest compression during expiration against a closed glottis or direct shearing associated with a crushing injury. Although also rare, esophageal rupture can result from a blow to the upper abdomen forceful enough to eject gastric contents into the lower esophagus under high pressure.

Etiology

1. Trauma: blunt or penetrating (usually secondary to laryngeal tear). May involve pulmonary or mediastinal structures. May be secondary to foreign body.
2. Infection: respiratory.
3. Allergy: asthma.
4. Intoxication: marijuana inhalation, smoking or inhalation of cocaine, or heroin injection may cause increased intrathoracic pressure from Valsalva's maneuver and bronchial tear.
5. Valsalva's maneuver from any mechanism, including yelling, coughing, emesis.
6. Iatrogenic: after intubation of trachea or esophagus.

Diagnostic Findings

1. History of trauma or excessive Valsalva's maneuver
2. Pain and crepitus overlying the upper thorax and neck
3. Hamman's crunch on auscultation in 50% to 80% of patients

Complications. Complications are directly related to the cause (e.g., mediastinitis from perforation of esophagus secondary to contamination with gastrointestinal contents)—in contrast to the benign course of only a pneumomediastinum caused by a simple Valsalva maneuver.

Ancillary Data

1. Chest x-ray film reveals air in the tissue planes of the thorax, neck, or mediastinum.

2. Laryngoscopy, bronchoscopy, or an esophagram may be indicated to determine the cause.

Differential Diagnosis

There may be infection by gas gangrene.

Management

1. Treat the underlying cause. Surgical intervention may be needed with certain entities. Bronchial disruption may require thoracostomy or intrathoracic control of the airway, reflecting the stability of the patient. Esophageal rupture necessitates a transthoracic exposure and mediastinal drainage.
2. Administer 100% oxygen to facilitate resorption secondary to nitrogen washout.
3. Administer antibiotics (penicillin or cephalosporin) if an esophageal tear is present.

Disposition

1. Hospitalize the patient with subcutaneous emphysema and pneumomediastinum to evaluate causes and facilitate nitrogen washout.
2. Monitor patients with benign causes as outpatients (e.g., marijuana, simple Valsalva's maneuver) if there are no complications.

DIAPHRAGMATIC RUPTURE

ALERT Often overlooked, diaphragmatic rupture may be an asymptomatic lesion or a large herniation accompanied by severe respiratory distress. Presentation may be acute or delayed in onset. The possibility of a diaphragmatic injury should be considered in any penetrating injury to the lower chest or upper abdomen.

Diaphragmatic tears may result from blunt or penetrating forces and most often (in more than 90% of cases) are on the left side. Blunt abdominal compression generates increased intraabdominal pressure, which can tear the diaphragm, with herniation of the stomach, colon, small bowel, spleen, or liver. The negative intrathoracic pressures create a gradient that keeps the diaphragmatic rupture open and facilitates herniation of abdominal contents into the thorax.

Diagnostic Findings

1. Presentation varies considerably, depending on whether the signs and symptoms are acute or delayed in onset, on the side of the defect, and on the severity of herniation of abdominal organs.
2. In acute cases, patients complain of pain in the abdomen and chest with dyspnea, nausea, and vomiting. Delayed presentation may be accompanied by nausea, vomiting, abdominal pain, and intermittent episodes of abdominal cramping and colic, with radiation to the associated shoulder.
3. Vital signs may be normal, or there may be tachycardia, hypotension, and tachypnea.
4. A large herniation produces cardiac dullness, with displacement of the point of maximal impulse (PMI) to the right, decreased breath sounds and tympany in the left chest, and bowel sounds or borborygmi in the chest. The abdomen may be distended with obstruction or scaphoid if large amounts of abdominal contents are in the thoracic cavity.

Complication. The complication is bowel obstruction with strangulation of herniated bowel and compromise of ventilation. This may be delayed in the patients with a small diaphragmatic defect secondary to a penetrating injury.

Ancillary Data

1. Chest x-ray film demonstrates an elevated diaphragm (usually on the left), pleural effusion, silhouetting of the diaphragm, and bowel or viscus in the chest. There

may be a mediastinal shift to the right, atelectasis, and an air-fluid bubble, or the nasogastric (NG) tube may be above the diaphragm.

NOTE: From 20% to 40% of films are read as normal because of misinterpretation of the findings. A common error is to misread the herniated bowel and other abdominal organs as a hemopneumothorax.

2. Laparotomy for associated injuries may reveal an unsuspected diaphragmatic tear.
3. Contrast studies (diluted upper gastrointestinal [GI] or barium enema study) may show intrathoracic abdominal contents. They are usually performed in stable cases with delayed presentation.
4. Peritoneal lavage: A low red blood cell (RBC) count (>5000 RBCs/ml) in the peritoneal fluid indicates diaphragmatic injury associated with a penetrating wound of the lower thorax and is considered a positive finding (see Chapter 63).

Differential Diagnosis

See Chapters 14, 20, and 63.

Management

1. Stabilize the patient, giving particular attention to airway management, oxygen, IV lines, and cardiac monitoring. Treat life-threatening conditions and hypovolemic shock.
2. Place an NG tube for decompression of the stomach. The tube may also be a useful aid in diagnosis if it is visualized within the chest on x-ray films.
3. Surgery is the definitive treatment. Acute herniated bowel must be reduced, and vascular compromise prevented. With delayed presentation, resection for strangulated bowel is commonly needed. The diaphragmatic surface should be explored at surgery for blunt trauma to the chest.

Disposition

Patients must be hospitalized for fluid resuscitation and surgery.

MYOCARDIAL CONTUSION

ALERT Children with major blunt trauma to the chest and persistent tachycardia or other ECG changes must be monitored and admitted for cardiac evaluation.

Myocardial contusion results from blunt trauma to the anterior midchest from auto accidents, falls, or blunt objects. Most myocardial contusions involve the right ventricle. The injury may cause a cardiac concussion with sudden disruption of cardiac activity, ventricular fibrillation, or dysrhythmias and cellular injury from edema, leading to necrosis, ischemia, valvular or ventricular rupture, or pericardial tamponade.

In the multiply traumatized patient, the diagnosis can be difficult or impossible because of the more obvious presentation of associated problems such as hypovolemic shock, pneumothorax, and head trauma. The condition must be suspected in any young patient without previous heart disease who has sustained chest trauma and has a persistent, unexplained tachycardia or dysrhythmia.

Diagnostic Findings

1. Chest pain is often present with associated chest wall trauma. Unfortunately, the pain may be delayed until several days after the injury, when cellular swelling and ischemia ensue. Chest pain is unrelieved by nitrates.
2. Patients have a persistent tachycardia and may have tachypnea caused by associated pulmonary injuries or hypotension from ventricular dysfunction.
3. Contusions or tenderness over the precordium may be present, but associated rib and sternal fractures are unusual in children because of the compliance of a child's chest wall.

4. A new murmur, secondary to disruption of the septum, cardiac valve, or papillary muscle, may be present. Rales may be a later finding associated with left ventricular failure or pulmonary contusion.

Complications

1. Low cardiac output state secondary to ventricular dysfunction
2. Increased sensitivity to fluid overload
3. Cardiac tamponade (muffled sounds, hypotension, and pulsus paradoxus)
4. Dysrhythmias

Ancillary Data

1. ECG:
   a. Any new findings, including persistent unexplained sinus tachycardia and nonspecific ST-T wave changes.
   b. Acute ST segment elevation or T wave inversion.
   c. Any dysrhythmia (e.g., premature atrial or ventricular contractions, atrial fibrillation, atrial flutter).
   d. New bundle branch block.
2. Chest x-ray studies: May demonstrate rib or sternal fracture and associated pulmonary injury. A lateral chest view must be obtained.
3. Isoenzyme measurements: The creatine phosphokinase (CPK-MB) band peaks within 24 hours but may not rise until days after injury, at the point at which edema and ischemia occur; therefore, this finding is not very useful and not diagnostic.
4. Radionuclide studies (ventricular angiography) have been inconsistently demonstrated to be useful in detecting myocardial dysfunction after blunt trauma to the chest.
5. Echocardiography (two-dimensional) is useful to assess wall motion and exclude pericardial effusion.

Management

1. Stabilize life-threatening conditions. Administer oxygen and fluids, and initiate cardiac monitoring. Prevent overzealous fluid administration, which may precipitate left ventricular failure.
2. Give analgesics as required.
3. Treat dysrhythmias (see Chapter 6).
4. Treat cardiogenic shock if present (see Chapter 5).

Disposition

1. Patients with myocardial contusion should be hospitalized for at least 24 to 72 hours for monitoring in the following situations:
   a. Anterior chest wall injury secondary to violent blunt trauma
   b. Persistent tachycardia when other causes have been ruled out
   c. Any changes on ECG or signs of dysrhythmia
   d. As required by associated injuries
2. If tachycardia has subsided and if the home environment is adequate, the patient with no signs of cardiac dysfunction need not be hospitalized.
3. Long-term resolution usually occurs within a year of injury.

PERICARDIAL TAMPONADE

ALERT With an overlying penetrating wound, the presence of hypotension, distended neck veins (increased CVP), tachycardia, and muffled or faint heart sounds requires immediate pericardiocentesis after tension pneumothorax has been ruled out. If vital signs are unstable, thoracotomy should be considered.

Penetrating wounds of the chest may injure the pericardium or myocardium, resulting in pericardial pressure and volume with resultant impaired diastolic filling, increased CVP, hypotension, and tachycardia.

Diagnostic Findings

Patients are agitated and hypoxic and have poor peripheral circulation, elevated CVP, tachycardia, and hypotension. A penetrating wound to any area of the thorax, epigastrium, or supraclavicular area may result in tamponade.

1. A paradoxic pulse greater than 10 mm Hg is usually present. Pulsus paradoxus may also be caused by constrictive pericarditis, asthma, pulmonary embolism, and so on.
2. If hypovolemic shock is present, the neck veins may not be distended until the patient has been resuscitated with fluid.
3. Beck's triad (hypotension, increased venous pressure with distended neck veins, and muffled, distant heart sounds) is not usually present in the acutely traumatized patient.
4. If bradycardia occurs, cardiac arrest is imminent. Tamponade must be relieved immediately.

Complications. Complications of pericardial tamponade are hypovolemic shock, cardiogenic shock, and death.

Ancillary Data

1. Chest x-ray film is usually nondiagnostic.
2. Bedside cardiac ultrasonography or echocardiography demonstrates pericardial fluid. It is often useful to diagnose the tamponade on an emergency basis and to provide bedside guidance for the pericardiocentesis needle.
3. ECG may show nonspecific ST-T wave changes and low voltage. ECG has no pathognomonic changes. In rare cases, pulsus alternans may be seen with chronic effusion.

Differential Diagnosis

1. Constrictive pericarditis
2. Tension pneumothorax

Management

1. Initiate resuscitation, including oxygen, fluids, and cardiac monitoring. Consider active airway and ventilatory support.
2. Obtain immediate bedside cardiac ultrasonography in the ED if available.
3. Insert a CVP catheter.
4. An initial fluid push of 0.9% normal saline (NS) solution, 10 to 20 ml/kg over 20 minutes, may provide support of BP during preparations for a pericardiocentesis.
5. Pericardiocentesis may be a lifesaving procedure that permits temporary improvement in cardiac output; it is performed as follows:
   a. Under bedside ultrasonographic guidance, an 18-gauge needle attached to a syringe by a three-way stopcock is introduced into the left subxiphoid area and is aimed cephalad and back toward the tip of the right scapula.
   b. When the tip of the needle enters the fluid within the pericardial space, fluid is aspirated.
   c. Aspiration of a few millimeters of blood may promote temporary dramatic improvement.
   d. Rarely is a patient stable enough to permit a diagnostic evaluation such as an echocardiogram before pericardiocentesis; this technology is becoming increasingly available on an emergency basis (see Appendix A-5).
   e. On contact of the needle with the epicardium, the ECG will demonstrate an injury current, and the needle should be withdrawn slightly. It should then be in the pericardial space.
   f. A negative pericardiocentesis (no aspiration of blood) does not exclude the possibility of a pericardial tamponade.
6. Thoracotomy is indicated in the patient with cardiac arrest, particularly in the presence of electromechanical dissociation, or in the patient who has become bradycardic or has lost vital signs. The pericardial sac may be very tense if it is filled with blood and may require pericardiotomy with a scalpel rather than a scissors.

NOTE: A tense tamponade should not be mistaken for adhesive pericarditis.

7. Definitive surgical care is the ultimate treatment. The patient should be moved expeditiously to the operating room once the diagnosis is made and the patient is temporarily stabilized.
8. If pericardiocentesis is positive (blood is aspirated), it may help to leave a catheter in the pericardial space. Even if the catheter does not drain, it may relieve the pressure in the pericardial space. If the patient's condition deteriorates again, pericardiocentesis should be repeated immediately, and subxiphoid pericardiotomy considered.

Disposition

1. Transport the patient to the operating room immediately.
2. If a thoracic surgeon or trauma surgeon is not available, repeated pericardiocentesis may be needed to allow transfer of the patient to an appropriate facility.

AORTIC INJURY

ALERT Violent acceleration-deceleration injuries with associated chest trauma, upper rib fractures, or widened mediastinum require emergent evaluation.

Injury to the aorta may occur from acceleration-deceleration injuries occurring in an automobile accident (usually in front seat occupants), fall from a height, or sudden massive compression injury, any of which results in a shearing force on the mobile aorta at points of fixation, most commonly at the isthmus distal to the left subclavian artery. Injury may also result from pressure waves generated in the aorta by the compression and decompression.

High-risk injuries include those that occur at high speeds (auto accident occurring at more than 45 mph) and those in which there is chest trauma, fracture of the first or second ribs, or damage caused by the steering wheel.

Diagnostic Findings

1. Patients complain initially of retrosternal or interscapular pain, although the location may change with progression of the dissection. Dyspnea, stridor, and dysphagia occur secondary to pressure of a hematoma on the left recurrent laryngeal nerve, trachea, and esophagus. Ischemic extremity pain may be present.
2. A harsh systolic murmur of the precordium and interscapular area develops.
   a. A pseudocoarctation syndrome with upper extremity hypertension and decreased femoral pulses may be noted. Carotid bruits may be present with decreased carotid pulse and a pulsatile mass at the base of the neck.
   b. Generalized hypertension may occur.

Complications. Hypovolemic shock and death secondary to rupture are common (80% to 90% of cases).

Ancillary Data

1. Standard upright chest x-ray film if the patient is stable enough:
   a. Supine chest film findings may be falsely positive and normalize when films are repeated with the patient upright.
   b. Widened or indistinct mediastinum (in adult, >8 cm at superior margin of anterior fourth rib and proportionately less in children) is present in 50% to 85% of patients; if so, upper thoracic spinal fracture must be excluded.
   c. Blurring of the aortic knob with loss of sharp aortic outline.
   d. Depression of the left main-stem bronchus.
   e. Left pleural effusion.
   f. Deviation of an NG tube to the right at the T4 level.
   g. A left apical pleural cap.
2. CT scan: A dynamic CT scan of the chest may be performed when a traumatic aortic dissection is suspected. This study is

very sensitive but is nonspecific unless an intimal flap can be visualized. It may also be useful to detect a periaortic hematoma.

3. Aortography is the definitive study for establishing the diagnosis. It is indicated if the patient is stable enough to tolerate it. If the patient is hemodynamically unstable from intraperitoneal hemorrhage, aortography is usually not done until after laparotomy.
4. Transesophageal ultrasonography may be helpful in the diagnosis of aortic dissection.

Management

1. Supportive resuscitation measures, including oxygen, fluids, blood.
2. Immediate thoracic surgical consultation:
   a. Obtain thoracic aortogram or dynamic chest CT scan.
   b. If the patient is unstable, immediate surgery is indicated, sometimes without aortography.
3. Exclusion of concomitant intraabdominal injuries. If findings of ultrasonography, peritoneal lavage, or abdominal CT scanning are positive, the abdomen should be explored before aortography.
4. Problem of concomitant head injury. Aortic evaluation must be performed after resuscitation of the abdomen and head.

BIBLIOGRAPHY

Bonodio WA, Hellmich T: Post-traumatic pulmonary contusion in children, *Ann Emerg Med* 18:1050, 1989.

Bulloch B, Schubert CJ, Brophy PD et al: Cause and clinical characteristics of rib fractures in infants, *Pediatrics* 105:851, 2000.

Cooper A, Foltin GL: Thoracic trauma. In Barkin RM, editor: *Pediatric emergency medicine: concepts and clinical practice, ed 2*, St Louis, 1997, Mosby.

Dyer DS, Moore EE et al: Thoracic aortic injury: how predictive is mechanism and is chest computed tomography a reliable screening tool? *J Trauma* 48:673, 2000.

Eckstein M, Henderson S, Markovchick VJ: Thorax. In Marx J, Hockberger R, Walls R, editors: *Emergency medicine: concepts and clinical practice, ed 5*, St Louis, 2002, Mosby.

Eddy AC, Rusch VW, Fligner CL et al: The epidemiology of traumatic rupture of the thoracic aorta in children: a 13-year review, *J Trauma* 30:989, 1990.

Garcia VF, Gotschall LS, Eichelberger MR et al: Rib fractures in children: a marker of severe trauma, *J Trauma* 30:695, 1990.

Helling TS, Duke P, Beggs CW et al: A prospective evaluation of 68 patients suffering blunt chest trauma for evidence of cardiac injury, *J Trauma* 29:961, 1989.

Holmes JF, Sokolove PE, Brant WE et al: A clinical decision rule for identifying children with thoracic injuries after blunt torso trauma, *Ann Emerg Med* 39:492, 2002.

Kearney PA, Rouhana SW, Burney RE: Blunt rupture of the diaphragm: mechanism, diagnosis and treatment, *Ann Emerg Med* 18:1326, 1989.

Ma JO, Mateer JR: Trauma ultrasound examination versus chest radiography in the detection of hemothorax, *Ann Emerg Med* 29:312, 1997.

Marnocha KE, Maglinte DDT, Woods J et al: Blunt chest trauma and suspected aortic rupture: reliability of chest radiograph findings, *Ann Emerg Med* 14:644, 1985.

Mellner JL, Little AG, Shermata DW: Thoracic trauma in children, *Pediatrics* 74:813, 1984.

Nakayama DK, Ramenofsky ML: Chest injuries in children, *Ann Surg* 210:770, 1989.

Shapiro MJ, Yanofsky SD, Trupp J et al: Cardiovascular evaluation in blunt thoracic trauma using transesophageal echocardiography (TEE), *J Trauma* 31:835, 1991.

Tenzer ML: The spectrum of myocardial contusion: a review, *J Trauma* 25:620, 1985.

63 Abdominal Trauma

ALERT Intraabdominal trauma poses an immediate threat to life. Aggressive volume resuscitation and timely evaluation, surgical consultation, and possible laparotomy are the foundations of therapy. Multisystem involvement is common.

In 80% to 90% of trauma cases, intraabdominal injuries are the result of blunt trauma. Hypovolemia in the presence of significant blunt trauma requires that intraperitoneal hemorrhage be excluded.

MECHANISM OF INJURY

Blunt Trauma

Blunt trauma injuries are caused primarily by motor vehicles, falls, contact sports, and child abuse. With infants and small children, pedestrian accidents predominate because of a child's limited ability to avoid or respond to potentially dangerous traffic situations. Passenger injuries are more common among adolescents. Auto accidents in which patients were wearing shoulder-lap seat belts have been reported to cause rib and lumbar spine fractures and duodenal and jejunal perforations; injuries in a person wearing a lap belt only produce contusion or perforation of the intestine or mesentery, but these findings may be inconsistent. The use of motor bikes poses a growing hazard. Inflicted injury may present a diagnostic dilemma.

The spleen and then the liver are the most likely organs to be injured, whereas small bowel contusions and perforations are the most common type of damage to the hollow viscus. The rib cage in the child, although resilient and less prone to fracture than that in the adult, affords only partial protection for the liver and spleen. Intraabdominal injuries are often part of a multisystem involvement resulting from vehicular accidents. Injury to two or more intraabdominal organs occurs in up to 30% of patients with blunt trauma.

Findings associated with serious injuries include gross hematuria, abdominal tenderness, hematocrit (Hct) level less than 25%, lap belt injury, assault or abuse as a mechanism, rib fractures, shock, and hypovolemia.

Type of Injury in Blunt Trauma

1. Crush injuries occur with compression of organs between external forces and the posterior thoracic cage or spine, resulting in contusions, lacerations, or disruption.
2. Shear injuries occur when acceleration and deceleration forces cause tearing of viscera and vascular pedicles, particularly at relatively fixed points of attachment.
3. Burst injury of hollow viscera follows the generation of sudden and pronounced increases in intraabdominal pressure (e.g., by seat belts).

Penetrating Trauma

In children younger than 13 years, penetrating injuries are likely to be caused by accidental impalement on objects such as scissors and picket fences or by accidental discharge of a weapon. In patients older than 13 years, 75% of penetrating trauma injuries are knife or handgun wounds inflicted by an assailant.

1. *Stab wounds* to the abdomen cause intraperitoneal organ damage in 30% of

cases. Penetration of the peritoneum occurs 50% to 60% of the time.

2. *Gunshot wounds* enter the peritoneal cavity in 85% of cases, causing visceral injury in 95% to 99% of patients with intraperitoneal penetration.
3. Penetrating trauma to the lower chest (below the fourth intercostal space anteriorly or the sixth to the seventh space laterally and posteriorly) places the abdomen and diaphragm at risk. Coincident injury to the diaphragm or peritoneal cavity occurs in 25% to 40% of patients with lower chest penetration. The peritoneal cavity may also be entered via back or flank wounds.

DIAGNOSTIC FINDINGS

The ability to obtain an accurate history may be compromised by the urgency of the situation, communication skills of the child, concomitant intracranial injuries, reluctance of parents, and interfering toxic agents (e.g., drugs or alcohol). Information about underlying cardiorespiratory disease, coagulopathies, and medication usage will help guide volume resuscitation.

In a child with vehicular trauma, it is helpful to know the amount of damage to the automobile and what, if any, restraint systems were used for the child. For penetrating injuries the type of weapon, number of shots or stabs inflicted, and amount of blood loss at the scene should be ascertained.

Child abuse should be suspected when the child has difficulty with or shows fear about relating the circumstances of the injury or if the history is inconsistent with the injuries.

1. Volume loss secondary to acute hemorrhage (solid viscera or vascular) or later development of bacterial or chemical peritonitis (hollow viscus or pancreas) leads to inadequate perfusion, causing dizziness and confusion. With orthostatic hypotension these findings may be seen only with the assumption of upright posture.
2. Pain is usually caused by hematic, infectious, or enzymatic irritation of the peritoneum. It may be localized or diffuse. Diminished ability to sense pain (e.g., because of alcohol, concussion, or spinal injury), ineffectual communication, or significant injury elsewhere may impair the recognition of abdominal pain.
   - Splenic and liver injury can cause diaphragmatic irritation and radiation of pain to the ipsilateral shoulder, especially when the patient is in the Trendelenburg position.
3. Nausea and vomiting are nonspecific (e.g., peritoneal irritation or obstruction caused by a duodenal hematoma).

Physical Findings. Physical findings are unreliable in 30% to 40% of cases, particularly in those in which central nervous system (CNS) trauma coexists. Serial examinations by a single observer are invaluable, especially with the patient whose sensorium is clearing.

1. All clothing must be removed to allow careful inspection of axilla, skin folds, and scalp for entrance and exit wounds.
2. Inspection may reveal superficial abrasions or contusions, which are deceptively unremarkable in most cases of intraabdominal injury.
3. Acute hypotension is caused by hemorrhage from a solid organ or by major vessel injury. Hypotension may be delayed when there is third spacing or significant vomiting with pancreatitis or damage to a hollow viscus. Findings may be delayed for hours to days after trauma. Splenic injuries are usually obvious immediately but in rare cases may also have delayed presentation.
4. Tenderness is found in up to 90% of patients with intraabdominal abnormality and alert mental status. It may be localized to the quadrant of injury (e.g., spleen, liver), or it may be diffuse. Abdominal rebound, tenderness, and rigidity are more specific but less common.

5. Bowel sounds may be decreased or absent, and either finding can be helpful in predicting intraperitoneal injury. However, bowel sounds may be present with significant injury or absent as a result of vertebral fractures, electrolyte disturbances, or other pathologic conditions.
6. Gastrointestinal (GI) hemorrhage may follow blunt or penetrating trauma and is identified with nasogastric (NG) tube placement and rectal examination. A study in adults suggested that the digital rectal examination need be done only selectively in the following situations: penetrating trauma in proximity to the rectum, pelvic fractures, in anticipation of rapid-sequence intubation, and when neurogenic shock from a spinal cord injury cannot be entirely excluded or verified by the remainder of the examination.
7. Acute distension secondary to hemorrhage requires extreme loss of intravascular volume and is accompanied by profound shock. It may occur gradually when secondary to third spacing from peritonitis.
8. Pregnant patients with major trauma or obstetric problems, such as vaginal bleeding, uterine tenderness, uterine contractions, or ruptured membrane, should be observed for at least 24 hours with cardiotocographic monitoring. The pregnant patient in whom gestational age of the fetus is more than 24 weeks and who has experienced deceleration injuries, falls, or abdominal trauma should undergo cardiotocographic monitoring for at least 4 hours.

Ancillary Data. Laboratory evaluation should reflect routine management of multisystem trauma as outlined in Chapter 56.

1. The Hct level must be measured early and followed throughout the period of observation. If hemorrhage has been acute, a normal initial Hct value may be misleading. Changes reflect the baseline Hct, volume, and rate of blood loss, endogenous plasma refill, and parenteral fluid administration.
2. White blood cell (WBC) elevation occurs within several hours and may last for several days; it is a nonspecific response to injury. A prolonged leukocytosis may be seen with visceral injury and bacterial or chemical peritonitis.
3. Elevated serum amylase concentration is an insensitive and nonspecific marker of pancreatic or proximal small bowel injury. Persistently high or rising values may be suggestive.
4. Other routine laboratory studies should reflect clinical condition and mechanism of injury but may include blood type and cross-match, platelet count, measurement of electrolytes, blood urea nitrogen (BUN), and liver enzymes, arterial blood gas (ABG) analysis, and toxicologic screen. Hematuria should be excluded (see Chapter 64).

Diagnostic Peritoneal Lavage. Diagnostic peritoneal lavage (DPL) is a safe and extremely sensitive (98%) method of detecting intraperitoneal hemorrhage. However, it is neither organ nor injury specific and is not useful in assessing retroperitoneal injury. It is particularly valuable in judging whether the patient with blunt trauma and hemodynamic instability should undergo urgent laparotomy. DPL is reliable in clinical settings in which imaging or monitoring capacity is limited or personnel are without experience in the nonoperative management of trauma. A positive DPL finding, as defined by red blood cell (RBC) criterion or gross appearance of the aspirate, should be supplemented by abdominal computed tomography (CT) if the patient is stable and the institution is capable of expectant (i.e., nonoperative) management.

DPL is also useful in patients who are unconscious, are intoxicated, or require immediate general anesthesia for repair of life-threatening intracranial or axial skeletal injury. Patients in whom the integrity of the bowel is at risk, usually as a result of a penetrating mechanism, may be accurately and expeditiously evaluated by DPL. The procedure is relatively insensitive for small bowel and pancreatic injuries. A positive DPL result is often supplemented by abdominal CT in stable patients.

1. Indications for DPL:
   a. Blunt trauma in acutely injured and unstable patients with multiple trauma who have sustained a major mechanism of injury:
      (1) Unreliable physical findings because of CNS or spinal cord injury, alcohol or drug intoxication, or communication barriers.
      (2) Unexplained hypotension in the field or emergency department (ED).
      (3) General anesthesia is required for immediate repair of life-threatening intracranial or axial skeletal injury.
   b. Penetrating injury:
      (1) Local stab wound exploration that is:
         (a) Positive or equivocal.
         (b) Contraindicated or technically difficult because of low chest penetration or multiple stab wounds.
      (2) Gunshot wound with questionable peritoneal cavity penetration.
2. Contraindications to DPL:
   a. Absolute: Indications for laparotomy already exist.
   b. Relative: DPL would be technically difficult because of previous abdominal surgery or intraperitoneal infection and adhesions, pregnancy, or massive obesity.
3. Procedure:
   a. A decompressive NG tube and urinary catheter are placed.
   b. Percutaneous entry via the Seldinger (guide wire) technique is more rapidly performed, may have comparable accuracy and incidence of complications, and is becoming more popular in the evaluation of children.

      The semiopen method involves establishing a sterile field and injecting local anesthesia. Entry is made infraumbilically through the anterior rectus sheath. The catheter tip is directed through the peritoneum toward the pelvis. The fully open technique requires direct visualization of the peritoneum and is used to ensure safety and accuracy when technical obstacles are considerable.

      Aspiration of 10 ml or more of free blood in adults (lesser amounts in pediatric patients) is positive. If this does not occur, 15 ml/kg (adult: 1 L) of normal saline solution (NS) should be instilled and recovered by gravity drainage. This procedure is usually performed after surgical consultation.
4. Results of studies on the recovered peritoneal fluid that constitute a "positive tap" and presence of an intraperitoneal hemorrhage in adults are as follows:
   a. RBC criterion is the most accurate parameter of peritoneal lavage fluid:

Type of Trauma	RBCs/mm^3 in Peritoneal Fluid
Blunt	>100,000 (20,000-100,000 equivocal)
Penetrating stab wound:	
Anterior abdomen*	>100,000 (20,000-100,000 equivocal)
Lower chest†	>5,000 (1,000-5,000 equivocal)
Flank/back	>100,000 (20,000-100,000 equivocal)
Penetrating gunshot wound	>5000 (1,000-5,000 equivocal)

* Inferior to costal margin to groin creases between anterior axillary lines.

† Between the fourth intercostal space anteriorly; seventh intercostal space posteriorly; and the costal margins. This incorporates the area of possible diaphragmatic excursion. DPL in patients with possible diaphragmatic injury is considered to yield a positive finding at more than 5000 RBCs/mm^3.

b. Elevations of lavage amylase (>20 IU/L) and alkaline phosphatase (>3 IU/L) may occur immediately after injury of the small bowel. A positive lavage WBC count (>500/mm^3) is insensitive for 4 to 6 hours after injury, is nonspecific, and should not be the sole indicator for laparotomy. Bile and Gram stains are of relatively little use in acute trauma.

c. If the initial results are equivocal, a CT scan may be useful. A second lavage procedure in 4 to 6 hours may be diagnostic.

NOTE: Few data exist for the use of DPL in children. These guidelines minimize missed significant injury, accepting a low rate of negative laparotomy findings.

Radiologic Studies. X-ray studies should be performed only after initial stabilization and when additional diagnostic data are necessary for management. Patients in whom serious injuries are suspected must be monitored by experienced personnel while in the radiology suite.

1. Plain films are useful for detection of small quantities of free intraperitoneal air, but normal findings do not exclude a perforation. Patients should be maintained in the upright or left-lateral decubitus position, if possible, for 10 to 15 minutes before the x-ray film is taken to mobilize air. Peritoneal lavage causes iatrogenic pneumoperitoneum. Retroperitoneal rupture of a hollow viscus reveals a stippling pattern, outlining the duodenum, kidney, or psoas margins. Foreign bodies and missiles, hemoperitoneum, and skeletal fractures may be visualized or localized.

   NOTE: The incidence of free air caused by acute injury is so rare that one need not delay peritoneal lavage merely to obtain a "negative" preliminary x-ray film.

2. Ultrasonography is of value in quickly discerning free intraperitoneal hemorrhage. It is particularly useful because it can be performed rapidly and in the resuscitation area of the ED. A focused examination of Morison's pouch, the splenorenal recess, and the pouch of Douglas is useful in this evaluation because blood is likely to accumulate in these dependent portions of the intraperitoneal cavity. More complete examinations may identify other lesions, including pancreatic pseudocyst, viable fetus, and enlargement of the pancreas, liver, or spleen. Ultrasonography is more limited in defining solid visceral injury, retroperitoneal injury, and bowel injury. It may be of value in evaluating cardiac function. It does not show anatomic detail.

3. CT scanning offers simultaneous visualization of all organs in the peritoneal cavity and retroperitoneum. It defines intraabdominal hemorrhage and the extent of damage to solid viscera. It may also facilitate concurrent intracranial evaluation.

   A double-contrast (intravenous [IV] and enteral) CT scan provides a valuable adjunct in determining the presence and extent of hepatosplenic and retroperitoneal compartment injury and is commonly performed when CT is selected. Use of an oral contrast agent may improve sensitivity for pancreatic injury but does not help identify injuries requiring surgical treatment; however, it is insensitive for GI perforation and intraluminal lesions. The benefit of an oral contrast agent in this situation is controversial, given the potential time delay and risk of aspiration. Diaphragmatic injury and significant pancreatic disease can also be missed with this procedure.

   CT alone is probably sufficient in patients with hemodynamic stability and no alteration in responsiveness. It may also be useful in stable patients undergoing DPL in whom the lavage RBC count is positive and who have an associated pelvic fracture or suspected isolated solid visceral injury, equivocal DPL results, or in whom there are technical difficulties in performing the DPL.

On CT scan, solid organ injuries appear as a loss of homogeneity or disruption of the cortex. Hematoma appears as a nonenhanced collection of fluids that displaces normal anatomic relationships. Hollow-organ perforation may be identified from intraabdominal free air or extravasated contrast. An organ's failure to be enhanced with IV contrast material may suggest that a vascular injury has occurred.

4. Contrast studies may be useful in stable patients without life-threatening conditions. Intramural duodenal hematomas are best diagnosed with barium. A water-soluble contrast medium (e.g., Gastrografin) should be used for suspected gastric, duodenal, and rectal perforations. An intravenous pyelogram (IVP) is indicated in the blunt trauma patient with significant posttraumatic hematuria if CT has not been performed or is unavailable. With a penetrating mechanism, an IVP may help define entry proximate to the genitourinary (GU) tract irrespective of the presence of hematuria (see Chapter 64). Only limited studies may be indicated before laparotomy in the compensated but unstable patient.
5. Radionuclide studies: Liver-spleen studies are accurate in detecting subcapsular hematomas, parenchymal damage, lacerations, and intraparenchymal hematomas and may be particularly useful in the stable patient with these suspected injuries. However, CT, because of the additional information it provides, has largely supplanted radionuclide studies for acute evaluation. Ongoing management of conservatively managed splenic injuries may be monitored with radionuclide studies.
6. Angiography is the most accurate method for visualizing vascular injury and active bleeding but has limited application in acute trauma.
7. Laparoscopy is a promising tool in experienced hands for the investigation of penetrating trauma, particularly to the low chest, flank, and back.

MANAGEMENT

General Principles

Resuscitation of the injured child must be tailored to the specific requirements of the patient and the nature of the trauma. Aggressive and systematic treatment, as outlined in Chapter 56, becomes crucial in view of the frequency of associated injuries in abdominal trauma. Delivery of adequate replacement fluid is critical. In the stable patient, extensive evaluation and diagnostic studies may be appropriately performed to establish the nature of the injuries and the status of the patient. Immediate thoracotomy or laparotomy may be indicated under the following circumstances:

1. Blunt trauma:
   - a. Hemodynamic instability despite adequate volume resuscitation with strongly suspected or documented intraperitoneal hemorrhage
   - b. Transfusion requirement greater than 50% of estimated blood volume with suspected intraperitoneal injury
   - c. Physical signs of peritonitis
   - d. Positive peritoneal lavage result (see earlier discussion)
   - e. Radiologic evidence of pneumoperitoneum, diaphragmatic injury, intraperitoneal bladder rupture, or renovascular pedicle injury
2. Penetrating trauma:
   - a. Gunshot wounds with hemodynamic instability or suspected intraperitoneal penetration
   - b. All stab wounds with hemodynamic instability; positive DPL result; GI blood; radiologic evidence of

retroperitoneal air; implement in situ; positive laparoscopy. Evisceration is a relative indication for operation.

Findings that have been significantly associated with intraabdominal injury include low systolic blood pressure, abdominal tenderness, femur fracture, serum glutamate oxaloacetate transaminase (SGOT) level higher than 200 U/L or serum glutamate pyruvate transaminase (SGPT) level higher than 125 U/L, urinalysis (UA) showing more than 5 RBCs per high-power field (HPF), and an initial Hct value lower than 30%.

Certain general principles apply. The emergency physician must make the initial assessment and stabilization while organizing resources within the ED. Assignment of specific tasks to members of the team should be rapid, preferably before the patient's arrival. Surgical staff should be contacted as early as possible to assist in the management of the patient.

Primary Assessment

The primary assessment must ensure an adequate airway and ventilation and treatment of shock, when appropriate. The spine must be immobilized in the multiply traumatized patient with suspected spinal injury and in the patient with altered mental status from blunt trauma injuries (pending spine films) (see Chapter 61).

1. All patients need oxygen administration and cardiac monitoring upon arrival. Initiate airway intervention, as appropriate.
2. Remove clothing while vital signs are being obtained.
3. Hemorrhage is the immediate threat to life. Place large-bore catheters as dictated by the clinical situation. A central line may be required for monitoring if there is intercurrent cardiothoracic disease or if it is necessary to gain rapid venous access.

   Initially, give a rapid bolus of 0.9% NS or lactated Ringer's (LR) solution, 20 ml/kg IV. Additional administration of crystalloid solution must reflect the response to the initial infusion and the presence of ongoing hemorrhage. In general, once 40 to 50 ml/kg of crystalloid solution has been infused during the initial resuscitation, blood should be administered if evidence of hypovolemia persists.
4. Initial laboratory studies are required. Hematocrit should be measured in the ED, and a clot of blood sent for type and cross-match. An ABG determination may be helpful.
5. Other considerations:
   a. Placement of an NG tube will decompress the stomach, permitting improved ventilation and a more reliable examination. It will assist in determining whether there is upper GI hemorrhage.
   b. A urinary catheter is required to monitor urinary output and to help monitor fluid management. The urethral meatus should be examined for blood, the presence of which precludes insertion of the catheter.
   c. Reassessment is constantly required, with ongoing measures of vital signs and serial examinations by the same examiner. Once the primary assessment has been completed, a more extensive physical examination should be made, and history obtained.
6. Perform a rectal examination early to assess the integrity of spinal cord function, exclude GI bleeding, and evaluate the prostate.
7. It is easy to overlook trauma to the thoracic or lumbar spine and the bony pelvis. These structures should be evaluated with chest, abdomen, and pelvic x-ray studies as required.

Blunt Trauma (Fig. 63-1)

Certain victims of blunt trauma are candidates for immediate laparotomy after the initial resuscitation. In hemodynamically stable patients, further diagnostic evaluations and expectant management may be suitable.

1. Perform urgent laparotomy (as mentioned previously) after stabilizing measures have been taken.
2. Conservative management is appropriate when physicians experienced in pediatric abdominal trauma are present and the facilities and personnel necessary for intensive observation of the child are available. Onset of instability, progression of abdominal findings, or the need for extensive blood transfusions (>40 ml/kg) to supplement crystalloid solution mandate operative intervention. Criteria for observation in a nontrauma center should be more stringent, favoring earlier surgical intervention or transfer with trained personnel to a better-equipped facility.
3. Pregnancy presents unique problems. By 12 weeks of pregnancy, the uterus has grown out of the protective pelvis. Unique complications include uterine rupture and abruptio placentae. Management should consist of resuscitation of the patient and prolonged fetal monitoring, usually in consultation with an obstetrician.

Splenic Injury. Injury to the spleen is associated with variable intraabdominal bleeding. Some patients have massive bleeding. Left upper quadrant pain, guarding, and rigidity as well as left shoulder pain may be present.

1. Splenectomy increases a patient's risk of overwhelming infection 65-fold. Therefore, maximal splenic preservation is attempted whenever possible through the use of splenoplasty, partial splenectomy, hemostatic agents, and, more recently, autotransplantation. Stable patients with defined injuries after blunt trauma may be managed in a nonoperative fashion with close monitoring. Serial clinical evaluations are indicated; serial CT scans are recommended by some but have not proved to change management. Patients with penetrating abdominal trauma are not candidates for nonoperative management because of the high incidence of associated injuries. Total splenectomy is rarely required and is reserved for the pulverized, nonsalvageable organ.
2. Laparotomy is indicated for the unstable patient with suspected splenic trauma.
3. A CT scan should be obtained in the stable patient with suspected splenic trauma. The need for laparotomy (major laceration or hematoma), for close intensive observation with serial Hct determinations (minor laceration), or for minimal observation (normal CT findings), is dictated by the clinical status of the patient and findings of the scan.

   NOTE: Children with positive scan findings who do not require surgery should be maintained at bed rest with daily Hct determinations for 1 week. During this period, the rate of bleeding and the results of physical examination and monitoring parameters are the main determinants of the need for laparotomy.

   It is essential not to be lulled into a false sense of security; splenic lacerations that have ceased active bleeding and previously contained subcapsular hematomas may subsequently leak or rupture, classically on day 3 to 5 after injury.

   The need for more than 4 units of blood in adults (or relative equivalent in children) over 48 hours or progressive peritoneal irritation necessitates consideration for laparotomy. Patients may return to full activity after 2 to 6 months of convalescence and a normal CT exam or liver-spleen scan.
4. If splenectomy must be performed, it should optimally be accompanied by

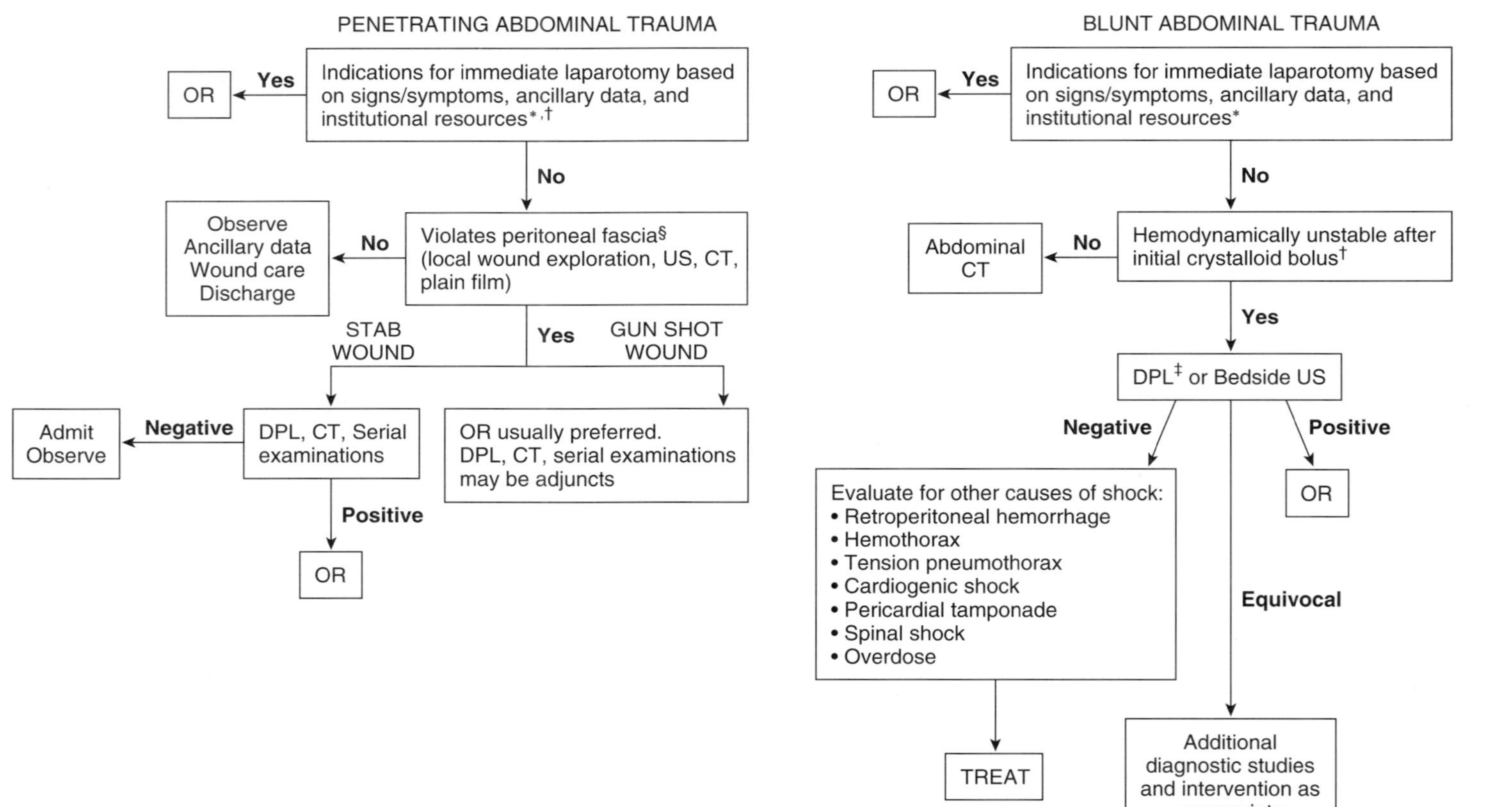

Fig. 63-1 Management protocol for acute abdominal trauma. Assumes optimal resuscitation (see Chapters 4 and 56). Associated injuries may modify protocol. *Laparoscopy may be useful. †Flank and back do not include areas overlying the thoracic cage. ‡Ancillary studies include plain abdominal film (upright), computed tomography, serial Hct, etc. §Level of significance reflects the actual abnormality as well as the ability of the facility to monitor patient and intervene in an emergency, if necessary. Peritoneal lavage before surgery may be indicated. On discharge, all patients require close follow-up observation. **In patients with significant closed-head injury, DPL may be required to exclude hollow viscus perforation. ***NOTE:*** Patients with major blunt trauma and positive peritoneal lavage findings should undergo laparotomy if in unstable condition but may be considered for observation and ancillary studies if in stable condition and adequate support services are available.

omental implantation of splenic remnants. Patients should receive vaccine to provide prophylaxis against *Streptococcus pneumoniae* and *Haemophilus influenzae* as soon as possible before (or after, if necessary) operation.

Liver Injury. The liver is the second major source of hemorrhage from blunt trauma but tends to result in more massive hemorrhage; one third of patients die before transport. It is the major cause of immediate mortality related to abdominal trauma. With significant liver injury, the patient may be in shock or have a protuberant abdomen and right upper quadrant or diffuse abdominal pain.

The same basic principles of splenic management apply to injuries to the liver, although there is rarely time for diagnostic studies beyond peritoneal lavage.

Pancreatic and Duodenal Injuries. Because the pancreas and duodenum are located retroperitoneally, signs and symptoms of their injury may be obscure and delayed.

Pancreatic contusions, the most common type of injury to the pancreas, cause variable levels of midepigastric, diffuse abdominal, or back pain. Lacerations cause focal hemorrhage and release of enzymatic contents toxic to the surrounding tissues. If this contamination is contained within the lesser sac, severe localized abdominal and back pain may be present. With leakage, there is diffuse chemical peritonitis. Elevated or rising serum or peritoneal lavage amylase levels may be seen. Conservative therapy with NG suction and parenteral nutrition is helpful. Worsening clinical signs may prompt surgical exploration.

Trauma is the leading cause of pancreatic pseudocysts in children, which may occur days to months after injury. Capsulized collections of pancreatic secretions and debris form in the lesser sac, causing chronic, intermittent attacks of abdominal pain, nausea, vomiting, and weight loss. Ultrasonography and CT are valuable in securing the diagnosis. Pseudocysts may resolve spontaneously. Otherwise, surgery is required.

Duodenal intramural hematoma causes signs and symptoms of proximal intestinal obstruction. The diagnosis is confirmed by barium contrast studies. Transection of the duodenum should be specifically considered if the barium does not at least partially pass, if extravasation has occurred, or if there is unexplained diffuse abdominal tenderness. The hematoma often resolves after 8 to 10 days of conservative management, which consists of placement of an NG tube and parenteral nutrition. Surgery is necessary if this approach fails. Duodenal perforations cause a range of abdominal pain and tenderness, often developing hours after injury. Intraabdominal or retroperitoneal free air may be demonstrated radiographically. Surgery is necessary.

Bowel Injuries. Injury to the remainder of the small bowel or colon may also lead to subtle or delayed findings. Perforation usually results in signs of peritonitis 4 to 12 hours after injury and radiologic evidence of free air. Elevations in peritoneal lavage enzymatic markers may be diagnostic immediately after injury.

Penetrating Wounds (see Fig. 63-1)

Stab Wounds

1. Immediate exploration is required for hemodynamically unstable patients or for those with clear physical or radiographic evidence of intraperitoneal injury (peritoneal irritation, significant GI bleeding, evisceration, evidence of diaphragmatic injury, or positive peritoneal lavage finding).
2. In the stable, cooperative child, local wound exploration with meticulous hemostasis and possible extension of the wound to facilitate inspection are used to assess the extent of the penetration. An equivocal examination finding must be considered positive:
   a. If the end of the wound tract is clearly demonstrated to be superficial to the posterior rectus fascia, wound care is

provided and the patient may be safely discharged if the stab wound was an isolated injury.

b. If the end of the wound tract cannot be seen clearly or the peritoneum is violated, peritoneal lavage or laparoscopy should be performed. If findings are negative or equivocal, observation for 12 to 24 hours with additional studies and possibly a second DPL procedure are indicated. Positive lavage results are an indication for laparotomy.

3. The care of flank and back wounds (excluding areas overlying the thoracic cage) should be individualized. Because retroperitoneal structures are at greater risk, peritoneal lavage may not be diagnostic, and other ancillary diagnostic techniques, such as CT with a contrast agent or laparoscopy, may be helpful. Local wound exploration is useful for superficial entry wounds.
4. Penetrating injury of the lower chest (below the fourth intercostal space anteriorly or sixth to seventh posteriorly) places the abdomen at risk. However, deep local wound exploration over the ribcage is hazardous and is contraindicated because of the risk of causing a pneumothorax. Peritoneal lavage is the most accurate determinant of diaphragmatic injury and should be performed unless other clinical evidence dictates the need for laparotomy.

Gunshot Wounds. The incidence of intraabdominal injury exceeds 95% if the missile has entered the peritoneal cavity. Therefore the criteria for selective management are greatly restricted compared with those for stab wounds.

1. Unstable patients undergo immediate surgical exploration. When peritoneal violation is suspected on the basis of entrance and exit wounds or radiographic findings, or if other evidence of intraabdominal injury exists (peritoneal irritation, evisceration, evidence of diaphragmatic injury, free intraperitoneal air, or positive peritoneal lavage finding), laparotomy should be performed.
2. Local wound exploration is technically more difficult and less reliable. It is not generally used. Observe patients with obviously superficial injuries. For those in whom an intraabdominal penetration is unclear, perform peritoneal lavage or additional studies.
3. If the situation permits, perform DPL and potentially other studies in the patient with gunshot wound of the lower chest to look for concomitant diaphragmatic or intraabdominal injury. Such patients often need immediate thoracic surgery, which precludes peritoneal lavage.
4. There is limited experience with laparoscopy in gunshot wounds. It may be useful in the determination of intraperitoneal penetration and injury as well as entry of the diaphragm.

BIBLIOGRAPHY

Foltin GL, Cooper AP: Abdominal trauma. In Barkin RM, editor: *Pediatric emergency medicine: concepts and clinical practice*, ed 2, St Louis, 1997, Mosby.

Graham JS, Wong AT: A review of computed tomography in the diagnosis of intestinal and mesenteric injury in pediatric blunt abdominal trauma, *J Pediatr Surg* 31:754, 1996.

Harris BH, Barlow BA, Ballantine TV et al: American Pediatric Surgical Association: principles of trauma care, *J Pediatr Surg* 27:423, 1992.

Healy M, Simon R, Winchell R et al: A prospective evaluation of abdominal ultrasound in blunt trauma: is it useful? *J Trauma* 42:220, 1996.

Holmes JF, Sokolov PE, Brant WE et al: Indentification of children with intra-abdominal injuries after blunt trauma, *Ann Emerg Med* 39:500, 2002.

Katz S, Lazar L, Rathaus V et al: Can ultrasonography replace computed tomography in the initial assessment of children with abdominal trauma? *Pediatr Surg* 31:649, 1996.

Konradsen HB, Hemrichsen J: Pneumococcal infections in splenectomized children are preventable, *Acta Paediatr Scand* 80:423, 1991.

Konstantakos AK, Barnoski AL, Plaisier BR et al: Optimizing the management of blunt splenic injury in adults and children, *Surgery* 126:805, 1999.

Marx JA: Abdominal injuries. In Mark JA, Hockberger RS, Walls RM et al, editors: *Rosen's Emergency medicine: concepts and clinical practice,* ed 5, St Louis, 2002, Mosby.

McAnena OJ, Marx JA, Moore EE: Contribution of peritoneal lavage enzyme determinations to the management of isolated hollow visceral abdominal injuries, *Ann Emerg Med* 20:834, 1991.

Nordenholz KE, Rubin MA, Gularte GG et al: Ultrasound with evaluation and management of blunt abdominal trauma, *Ann Emerg Med* 29:357, 1997.

Pearl WS, Todd KH: Ultrasonography for the initial evaluation of blunt abdominal trauma: a review of prospective trials, *Ann Emerg Med* 27:353, 1996.

Porter JM, Ursic CM: Digital rectal examination for trauma: does every patient need one? *Am Surg* 67:438, 2001.

Porter RS, Nester BA, Dalsey WC et al: Use of ultrasound to determine need for laparotomy in trauma patients, *Ann Emerg Med* 29:323, 1997.

Reid MM: Splenectomy, sepsis, immunization, and guidelines, *Lancet* 344:970, 1992.

Saladino R, Lund D, Fleisher G: The spectrum of liver and spleen injuries in children: failure of the pediatric trauma score and clinical signs to predict isolated injuries, *Ann Emerg Med* 6:636, 1991.

Shafi S, Gilbert JC, Irish MS et al: Follow-up imaging studies in children with splenic injuries, *Clin Pediatr* 38:273, 1999.

Sievers EM, Murray JA, Chen D et al: Abdominal computed tomography scan in pediatric blunt abdominal trauma, *Am Surg* 65:968, 1999.

Sivit CJ, Taylor GA, Newman KD: Safety belt injuries in children with lap-belt ecchymoses, *Am J Radiol* 157:111, 1991.

Taylor GA, Eichelberger MR, O'Donnel R et al: Indications for computed tomography in children with blunt abdominal trauma, *Ann Surg* 213:212, 1991.

Tsang BD, Panacek EA, Brant WE et al: Effect of oral contrast administration for abdominal computed tomography in the evaluation of acute blunt trauma, *Ann Emerg Med* 30:7, 1997.

Turnock RR, Sprigg A, Lloyd DA: Computed tomography in the management of blunt abdominal trauma in children, *Br J Surg* 80:982, 1993.

64 Genitourinary Trauma

ALERT Anyone with trauma to the perineum, back, abdomen, flank, or genitalia should be suspected of having genitourinary (GU) trauma. Hematuria, oliguria, tenderness, pain, masses, or lower rib fractures must be carefully evaluated for associated abnormality.

Automobile accidents, sports injuries, and falls cause 75% of genitourinary (GU) trauma. After the brain, the kidney is the most commonly injured internal organ in children. The kidney, primarily an intraabdominal organ in younger children, is more mobile and is not protected by perinephric fat and fascial layers. Other factors predisposing to renal injury after blunt trauma in a child are the flexible thoracic cage, the poorly developed abdominal and thoracic musculature, and the relatively large size of the kidney. Up to 10% of patients with blunt abdominal trauma have renal injuries. Although most urogenital injuries are caused by blunt trauma, the incidence of penetrating trauma in the pediatric population has increased dramatically in the past several years.

The diagnosis of GU trauma must be entertained anytime a patient has hematuria (more than 5 red blood cells/high-powered field [RBCs/HPF]), decreased urinary output, an unexplained abdominal mass or pain and tenderness, penetrating trauma, a fractured pelvis, fractures of the lower ribs or thoracic or lumbar vertebrae, blood at the urethral meatus, or scrotal swelling and hematoma.

Preexisting congenital anomalies such as hydronephrosis and polycystic disease make renal injury more likely and are present in 10% of children evaluated for renal trauma. Other causes of hematuria (see Chapter 37) and infection (p. 833) must also be considered in the initial evaluation. Epididymitis, testicular torsion, and penile disorders are discussed in Chapter 77.

EVALUATION

Evaluation of a child in whom GU trauma is possible must include a careful physical examination as well as urinalysis and radiographic studies when appropriate. The physical examination should focus on a search for flank pain or tenderness, flank hematoma (Grey Turner's sign), periumbilical ecchymoses (Cullen's sign), low posterior rib fracture, abdominal tenderness, and pelvic instability. Indications for imaging and choice of radiographic study are still somewhat controversial. The most commonly used modalities are computed tomography (CT) and intravenous pyelography (IVP).

1. Urinalysis:
   a. Urine dipstick tests show positive results if the urine contains hemoglobin or myoglobin. False-positive results occur when urine is contaminated with povidone-iodine (Betadine) or hexachlorophene. Drugs and chemicals may turn the urine dark or red (p. 365).
   b. Microscopic examination of the urine for red cells is mandatory if the test strip result is positive.

c. The absence of hematuria does not exclude significant renal injury. Renal vascular thrombosis, renal pedicle injury, and complete transection of the ureter are common causes of false-negative test strip results.

2. Abdominal flat plate and chest x-ray film. A variety of findings that require further evaluation may be associated with GU injuries:
   a. Fracture of lower rib.
   b. Fracture of vertebrae or transverse processes in lower thoracic or lumbar vertebrae.
   c. Pelvic fracture.
   d. Other findings, including ileus, scoliosis of vertebral column toward the injured side, unilateral enlarged kidney shadow, loss of psoas muscle margin, displaced bowel secondary to hemorrhage or urine extravasation, and elevated ipsilateral hemidiaphragm.

3. CT scan enhanced by intravenous (IV) contrast medium can be useful in the identification of renal injuries as well as pelvic, peritoneal, and retroperitoneal structures. Some studies suggest that the sensitivity of this modality may approach that of IVP. Contrast-enhanced CT clearly has the benefit of identifying associated abdominal injuries in the multiply injured patient (see Chapter 63). It provides good anatomic detail and does not depend on renal vasculature. It is useful for staging of renal injuries in blunt trauma. The modality has limited sensitivity in identifying minor parenchymal fractures and minimal degrees of extravasation seldom critical to accurate therapeutic decisions.
   a. Indications for use of this modality include a stable patient with blunt trauma with any one of a number the following findings:
      (1) Gross or microscopic hematuria (>20-50 RBC/HPF)
      (2) Multiple trauma
      (3) Flank pain or fullness, hematoma or ecchymoses
      (4) Mechanism suggesting intraabdominal or renal injury
   b. The exact indications for CT study are controversial. Studies have suggested hematuria cutoff values of 20 RBCs/HPF and 50 RBCs/HPF, although some clinicians have expressed concern about the existence of significant injuries without any hematuria. A growing body of data suggests that routine CT evaluation of children with only microscopic hematuria and no other suggestive findings is probably not justified solely to evaluate traumatic injuries, because of the low incidence with which problems requiring surgical intervention are detected (i.e., an imaging study demonstrates either contusion or normal kidneys and only rarely more significant injuries). Another group of physicians have suggested that clinical judgment based on the presence of pelvic fractures and abdominal or chest injuries helps identify patients with potential significant renal injuries.
   c. Reactions to IV contrast material may be reduced in patients with a questionable history of reaction by pretreatment with corticosteroids. Optimally, give methylprednisolone (Solu-Medrol), 0.5-1 mg/kg/dose (adult: 32 mg/dose), 12 and 2 hours before contrast material is injected or one dose 2 hours after challenge. Obviously, in the emergent setting pretreatment is unrealistic.

4. Excretory urography (IVP) is a common method for initial appraisal of suspected renal injury or traumatic hematuria,

although it provides less information than a CT scan with respect to associated problems. Its sensitivity has been reported to be as high as 90%. It can provide a determination of urologic function. The study cannot provide imaging of other intraabdominal organs, which may have associated injuries.

a. The presence of urologic function, regardless of delay or diminution, usually indicates that the injury is amenable to self-repair. Parenchymal laceration or urinary extravasation usually resolves in patients uncompromised by hemorrhagic complications, with the exception of apparent polar or hemirenal nonfunction; this finding suggests a parenchymal avulsion, which requires surgery or selective embolization.
b. Persistent urographic nonfunction reflects either parenchymal shattering or pedicle interruption (avulsion, thrombosis).
c. Indications for excretory urography after trauma are similar to those discussed previously for CT.

5. Retrograde urethrogram should be performed before urethral instrumentation or catheterization, if appropriate.
   a. Indications include the following:
      (1) Blood at meatus
      (2) Significant scrotal or perineal hematoma
      (3) Obvious urethral trauma (penetrating or foreign body)
   b. Procedure: 10 to 30 ml of standard water-soluble Renografin is drawn into a catheter-tipped syringe, the tip of which is inserted into the urethral meatus. Anterior, posterior, and oblique x-ray films are obtained as the dye is injected. Patient sedation may be required.
6. Cystogram is indicated when the injury and findings are consistent with bladder injury, pelvic fracture, inadequate urine production, or gross hematuria.
   a. If indicated, a cystogram is performed after a urethrogram.
   b. Procedure: 150 to 300 ml (depending on size of child) of 10% solution water-soluble contrast agent (Renografin) is placed in the bladder through urethral catheter by gravity. Smaller volumes may be required to fill the bladder in an infant. Anteroposterior (AP) and oblique views are required with filled and postevacuation films.
7. Isotopic renal scanning has limitations similar to those of CT. It may be used to monitor patients with known renal injury and to detect recovery or loss of function of renal parenchyma.
8. The renal arteriogram has been largely supplanted by CT. Indications for an arteriogram include assessment of the nature of persistent, fresh hemorrhage or of delayed or intermittent hematuria and evaluation of renal shattering. Digital subtraction angiography is preferable for evaluation of renovascular injury.
9. Ultrasonography has been studied as a modality for evaluation of GU trauma and has been found to have sensitivity of only 40% to 70% compared with CT. It may also not detect associated injuries and is therefore rarely used in the acute trauma setting. Ultrasonography may be useful for follow-up studies of patients with previously diagnosed and staged renal injury.
10. Magnetic resonance imaging (MRI) has been shown to be very similar to CT in evaluation of renal trauma. Because it is not readily available, the use of MRI in the acute trauma setting is limited, although it may be useful for follow-up. It may also have a role in staging the renal injuries of the patient with iodine

allergy who is unable to undergo contrast-enhanced CT.

RENAL TRAUMA

More than 90% of direct renal trauma is caused by blunt injuries from auto accidents or significant falls. Males, particularly those younger than 30 years, are at greatest risk. The kidney can move on the pedicle and can therefore be contused or lacerated by ribs or a spinal transverse process. Gerota's fascia surrounding the kidney may restrict bleeding.

Diagnostic Findings

Signs or symptoms, such as abrasion, ecchymosis, and pain or tenderness of the chest, back, abdomen, or flank should raise suspicion of renal injury.

Classification of Degree of Renal Trauma

Class I: renal contusions or hematomas that are small, subcapsular, and nonexpanding. Hematuria with no evidence of decreased renal function, extravasation, or pelvicaliceal injury on IVP.

Class II: shallow, nonexpanding renal cortical lacerations less than 1 cm in depth and hematomas confined to the retroperitoneum without urinary extravasation.

Class III: deep lacerations into the perirenal fat, more than 1 cm in depth but not penetrating into the collecting system. No urinary extravasation.

Class IV: deep lacerations into the cortex, medulla, and collecting system, or renal vascular injury with contained hemorrhage.

Class V: shattered or fractured kidney and renal pedicle injuries that devascularize the kidney.

Complications

1. Extravasation of urine is variably associated with infection or obstruction.
2. Vascular compromise of the kidney.
3. Acute tubular necrosis (ATN) with renal failure.
4. Hemorrhage with hypovolemic shock.
5. Delayed complications, including hypertension, chronic infection, hydronephrosis, calculus formation, chronic renal failure, arteriovenous fistula, pseudocyst formation, and nonfunction.

Ancillary Data. Procedures include complete blood count (CBC), urinalysis, abdominal flat plate, and IVP or contrast-enhanced CT scan. If the renal unit is not seen, selective arteriogram is performed and then, for follow-up evaluation, renal scan and sonography.

The urinalysis result may be normal, especially in pedicle injury or renal vascular thrombosis.

Management (Fig. 64-1)

1. Class I, II, and III injuries account for about 85% of renal injuries. Conservative treatment is appropriate, and the patients do well with good follow-up care. Patients are started on bed rest with frequent monitoring of vital signs and urinalysis.
2. Moderate injuries noted in class IV injuries may require surgical intervention. Surgery is generally indicated if there is an expanding or pulsatile retroperitoneal hematoma, renovascular injury, extensive extravasation of contrast in a patient with a high-grade renal injury, or hemodynamic instability in a patient with renal injury.

   Many other patients with Class IV injuries are managed nonsurgically with close monitoring of vital signs and serial hematocrit measurements while they are treated with IV antibiotics. It is crucial that such a patient is attended to by a surgeon who is capable of intervening surgically if the patient's condition deteriorates. These patients must be followed closely after discharge for the development of hypertension or the need for delayed nephrectomy.
3. Severe class V injuries are rare (3%). Exploration and either nephrectomy of

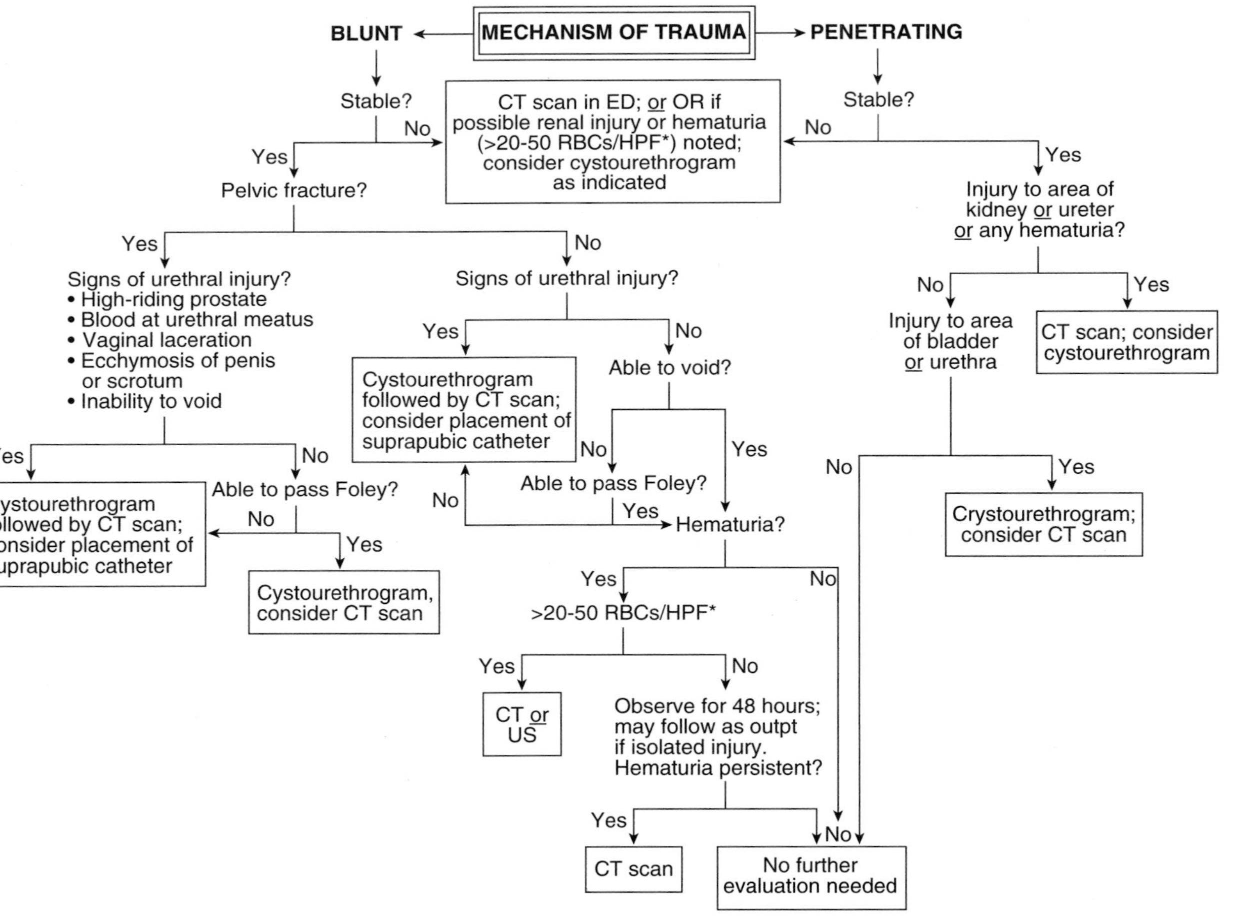

Fig. 64-1 Algorithm for evaluating the trauma patient for genitourinary injury. *US*, Ultrasonography.
* See text for disscussion of degree of hematuria (p. 496).

(Modified from Barkin RM: Pediatric emergency medicine: concepts and clinical practice, ed 2, St Louis, 1997, Mosby.)

the fractured kidney or repair of the renal pedicle injury are recommended. Results of revascularization are usually poor. Penetrating renal trauma is generally treated surgically.

URETERAL TRAUMA

Blunt injuries result from a hyperextension, with bowstringing of the ureter, that causes complete or partial laceration. Although rare, ureteral injury is more common in children than adults. Ureteral injuries are common in children after auto-pedestrian accidents because of the flexibility of their torsos and their limited retroperitoneal fat for protection. The tear almost always occurs at the ureteropelvic junction (UPJ). Penetrating ureteral injuries and surgical damage are more common in adults.

Diagnostic Findings

Patients may have lumboiliac pain from a blow, a flank mass from extravasated urine or blood, frequency of urination, hematuria, or pyuria. The diagnosis is often missed because of the severity of other associated multiple injuries and the subtlety of the findings. The prognosis is better with early repair.

Delayed retroperitoneal mass, back pain, unexplained fever, or urine drainage from a wound or surgical incision site may be noted. More than 50% of patients with delayed repair lose ureter and kidney function.

Complications

1. Extravasated urine may cause peritonitis if the peritoneum is damaged, or empyema if the diaphragm is involved.
2. Ureteral strictures secondary to obstruction or infection may occur.

Ancillary Data

1. Hematuria is present in 66% of cases but may not be noted with complete transection of the ureter.
2. IVP demonstrates extravasation of dye. If the injury is near the UPJ, the dye may travel up and around the kidney, simulating a lacerated renal cortex or pelvis. A retrograde pyelogram may later be performed to more accurately diagnose the level of injury to the ureter.
3. A CT scan may be used in multiple trauma cases but is no better than IVP in demonstrating ureteral injuries.

Management

1. A urologist should be consulted for primary repair and cutaneous ureterostomy as indicated. A nephroureterectomy may be necessary if the diagnosis is delayed.
2. Long-term follow-up observation must include monitoring of blood pressure and ensuring that a ureteral stricture or obstruction does not develop.

BLADDER TRAUMA

Most bladder ruptures result from blunt trauma to patients with full bladders, often during automobile or auto-pedestrian accidents. Bladder rupture is rarely an isolated finding, 90% of cases being associated with significant visceral or bony injury. Seventy-five percent of patients with ruptured bladder have a pelvic fracture. Inappropriate use of lap seat belts may increase the risk of bladder injury. Penetrating injuries may be caused by guns, knives, or fractured pelvic bones.

Diagnostic Findings

1. The bladder may demonstrate irritability (frequency, hesitancy) or the patient may have suprapubic or generalized abdominal pain or tenderness or an acute surgical abdomen.
2. Bladder contusion is a bruise to the bladder wall.
3. Intraperitoneal bladder rupture is more common in younger children than in adults because the pediatric bladder is an abdominal organ. The break is usually at the bladder dome:
   a. Suprapubic tenderness, abdominal pain, ileus, extreme desire but inability

to void, hematuria, pallor, tachycardia, hypotension

b. Delayed symptoms, which appear 24 to 72 hours after rupture, including fever, abdominal tenderness, and vomiting

4. Extraperitoneal bladder rupture is less common, occurring more often in the older child and adolescent with pelvic injury:
   a. Symptoms are similar to those associated with intraperitoneal injury, except that the patient may pass a small amount of urine, and a hematoma may be palpated in the suprapubic region. Urine can dissect up to the kidney or down into the legs, scrotum, and buttock.
   b. A red, indurated suprapubic area may develop if diagnosis is delayed.
5. Intraperitoneal and extraperitoneal rupture may occur.
6. Urethral injuries and associated abdominal or pelvic abnormalities are common.

Complications. Complications of bladder rupture include peritonitis, abscess, sepsis, ileus, osteomyelitis, bladder neck contractures, and poor bladder muscle function.

Ancillary Data. Hematuria is present in more than 95% of patients. The degree of hematuria does not correlate with the severity of injury.

1. Retrograde cystogram:
   a. A cystogram is indicated when penetrating trauma and suspicion of lower GU injury, pelvic fracture, lower abdominal or perineal trauma with hematuria, or inability to void are present. The upper urinary system must first be evaluated. Care must be exercised in the patient with gross hematuria because of concern for a urethral injury.
   b. Contused bladder will show normal vesicle outline and a teardrop shape with bilateral hematomas or a half-moon shape with unilateral hematoma.
2. With intraperitoneal rupture, intraperitoneal organs may be outlined by dye.
3. Extraperitoneal rupture demonstrates dye in contact areas after the dye is drained from bladder on postevacuation film.
4. A CT scan may be useful in multiple trauma but may not detect bladder injury because distension of the bladder is usually inadequate.

Management

1. Bladder contusion is treated by hospitalizing the patient and placing an indwelling catheter for 7 to 10 days. Patients with minor contusions can be observed at home without catheter placement. Close follow-up observation is essential. Contact sports should be avoided for 2 to 6 weeks. Prognosis is good.
2. Bladder rupture may be evaluated with cystoscopy and, if small, treated with an indwelling catheter for 7 to 14 days. Larger deficits require operative repair and suprapubic cystoscopy.
3. A urologist should be consulted when the diagnosis is first suspected.

URETHRAL INJURIES

Urethral injuries commonly occur after blunt trauma and are associated with pelvic fractures. The most common mechanism is a direct blow to the perineum because of a "straddle" injury. Pelvic fractures, however, are rare in children and generally not as severe as in adults. They may be a complication of urethral catheterization. Injury of the urethra is uncommon in females and if present is often associated with pelvic ring disruption.

Diagnostic Findings

1. Injury to the urethra in children most commonly occurs at the bladder neck. Although injury at the prostate membranous location is common in men, there is

laxity in this region in young boys, so injury to this site is much less common. Signs are as follows:

a. Blood at urethral meatus and inability to void.
b. In patients close to adulthood, the prostate may be boggy and high riding.

2. Injury to the bulbous and pendulous or penile urethra may result from a straddle fall or from foreign bodies; findings are:
   a. Perineal pain
   b. Blood at the meatus, but a good urinary stream when voiding.
   c. If patient is seen late after injury, penile and perineal edema, necrosis, and ecchymosis may be present.

Complications. Complications of urethral injuries include stricture, impotence, and urinary incontinence.

Ancillary Data. Urinalysis should be performed, as should retrograde urethrogram before a urinary catheter is placed.

Management

1. A urologist must be consulted immediately when blood is identified at the meatus or the abnormality is defined.
2. Anterior injuries, if small, may be treated with a urethral catheter; otherwise operative repair is needed.
3. Posterior injuries are controversial. There is question about whether immediate or delayed intervention provides the best repair.
4. Because urethral injuries may be iatrogenic, careful technique in urinary catheterization is advisable. The catheter should never be forced.

EXTERNAL GENITALIA TRAUMA (p. 672)

Penile, scrotal, and testicular injuries may result from missiles (bullet or knife); from strangulation secondary to a condom, string, hair, or constricting metal band; from blunt injury to an erect penis during intercourse or a fall; from being caught in a zipper; or from amputation. Vulvar lesions usually occur after blunt trauma. The presence of vaginal injuries in a girl must raise suspicion of child abuse.

Diagnostic Findings

Penile swelling, ecchymosis, and other direct injury can be present. With a constricting band, close inspection is necessary because edema can hide a small constricting band such as hair.

Ancillary Data. Ancillary procedures to be performed include urinalysis to evaluate for blood, which indicates urethral injury requiring a retrograde urethrogram. Ultrasonography may be useful in the assessment of significant blunt scrotal and testicular trauma.

Management

Urology consultation is necessary.

Lacerations of the Penile Skin. Lacerations of the penile skin can be sutured with absorbable suture.

1. If the wound is not deep, or beyond the Colles' fascia, it can be closed in the emergency department (ED) with two layers of polyglactin 910 (Vicryl) or Dexon sutures. If deeper, the wound should be explored in the operating room.
2. If the corpus cavernosum penis is violated, the wound should be explored in the operating room.
3. Constricting devices should be removed as soon as possible. The distal penis that appears necrotic should be treated conservatively. Often, an apparently nonviable penis survives.

Zipper Injuries. Zipper injuries to the external genitalia are best treated by breaking or cutting the small bridge (U-shaped bar) between the anterior and posterior faceplates of the zipper fastener with a bone cutter. Others recommend local anesthetic of the involved skin and then unzipping the zipper by moving one tooth at a time, alternating sides.

Amputation of the Penis. Amputation of the penis requires immediate consultation.

Lacerations of the Scrotum

1. Laceration of scrotal skin alone: debridement and closure with absorbable suture.
2. Scrotal skin and dartos layer only: debridement and two-layered closure with absorbable suture to reduce the chance of hematoma formation.
3. Penetrating wound or major blunt trauma needs surgical exploration. Conservative treatment leads to a high incidence of atrophied testes and loss of viability.

Blunt Injuries to the Scrotum. Usually, blunt scrotal injuries can be managed with ice, elevation, and analgesia.

Scrotal ultrasonography should be performed if a testicular rupture is suspected. This modality is highly accurate. It can differentiate testicular rupture, scrotal hematoma, extratesticular fluid collection, and epididymal hematomas. A ruptured testicle requires surgical repair. The other injuries are often treated conservatively.

If there is a large or expanding hematoma, it may have to undergo surgical exploration. A urology consultation must be obtained.

Injury to the Vulva. Vulvar injury must be examined (often with the patient under anesthesia) to exclude extension of injury to the vagina, rectum, bladder, and urethra. Lacerations in the perineal area in prepubertal girls are more likely to involve the vagina. Because the extent of the injury is easily underestimated, examination with the use of anesthesia must be considered if there is any concern about vaginal trauma.

Vulvar hematomas are usually treated conservatively and commonly result from handlebar or crossbar injuries. Treatment consists of strict bed rest, ice packs, analgesia, stool softener, and close monitoring of urinary output. Rarely is a urinary catheter needed. Abuse should be excluded in a patient with vulvar hematomas.

BIBLIOGRAPHY

Abou-Jaoude WA, Sugarman JM, Fallat ME et al: Indicators of genitourinary tract injury or anomaly in cases of pediatric blunt trauma, *J Pediatr Surg* 31:86, 1996.

Fleisher G: Prospective evaluation of selective criteria for imaging among children with suspected blunt renal trauma, *Pediatr Emerg Care* 5:8, 1989.

Gausche M: Genitourinary trauma. In Barkin RM, editor: *Pediatric emergency medicine: concepts and clinical practice*, ed 2, St Louis, 1997, Mosby.

Guerriero WG: Etiology, classification and management of renal trauma, *Surg Clin North Am* 68:1071, 1988.

Kane NM, Cronan JJ, Dorfman GS et al: Pediatric abdominal trauma: evaluation by computed tomography, *Pediatrics* 82:11, 1988.

Lappaniemi A, Lamminen A, Tervanartiala P et al: Comparison of high field magnetic resonance imaging with computed tomography in the evaluation of blunt renal trauma, *J Trauma* 38:420, 1995.

Lasser EC, Berry CC, Talner LB et al: Pretreatment with corticosteroids to alleviate reaction to intravenous contrast material, *N Engl J Med* 317:845, 1987.

Margenthaler JA, Weber TR, Keller MS: Blunt renal trauma in children: experience with conservative management at a pediatric trauma center, *J Trauma* 52:928, 2002.

Mayor B, Gudinchet F, Wicky S et al: Imaging evaluation of blunt renal trauma in children: diagnostic accuracy of intravenous pyelography and ultrasonography, *Pediatr Radiol* 25:214, 1995.

McAleer IM, Kaplan GW: Pediatric genitourinary trauma, *Urol Clin North Am* 22:177, 1995.

McAleer IM, Kaplan GW, Scherz HC et al: Genitourinary trauma in the pediatric patient, *Urology* 42:563, 1993.

Miller Ks, McAninch JW: Radiographic assessment of renal trauma: our 15-year experience, *J Urology* 154:352, 1995.

Morey AF, Bruce JE, McAninch JW: Efficacy of radiographic imaging in pediatric blunt renal trauma, *J Urol* 156:2014, 1996.

Munter DW, Faleske EJ: Blunt scrotal trauma: emergency department evaluation and management, *Am J Emerg Med* 7:227, 1989.

Nolan JF, Stillwell TJ, Sands JP: Acute management of the zipper-trapped penis, *J Emerg Med* 8:305, 1990.

Palmer JK, Benson GS, Corriere JN: Diagnosis and initial management of urologic injuries associated with 200 consecutive pelvic fractures, *J Urol* 130:712, 1983.

Stein JP, Kaji DM, Eastham J et al: Blunt renal trauma in the pediatric population: indications for radiographic evaluation, *Urology* 44:406, 1994.

65 Soft Tissue Injuries

VINCENT J. MARKOVCHICK

Soft tissue injuries are common in children. They often are caused by falls, contact with sharp objects, or motor vehicle accidents. Because many involved areas are visible, such as the face (see Chapter 58), it is imperative that the principles of meticulous wound care and repair be practiced to maximize cosmetic and functional results.

DIAGNOSTIC FINDINGS

The following facts should be ascertained: the mechanism (cut, fall, crush, bite, or electrical injury) and the time of injury, whether the wound was clean or dirty, the amount of blood lost, the history of a foreign body sensation, and the level of paresthesia or motor function impairment distal to the wound. Child abuse must be considered when the history and injury are inconsistent.

The status of the patient's tetanus immunization as well as allergies to antibiotics, local anesthetic agents, and other medications, in addition to underlying medical problems, should be noted. True allergies to local anesthetics are extremely rare.

Local pain and swelling are common with all soft tissue trauma. Furthermore, children tend to be fearful and anxious.

All wounds must be carefully inspected to determine the depth of injury and involvement of underlying tissues, including vessels, nerves, muscles, tendons, ligaments, bone, joints, and ducts.

1. Attention must be given to the physical examination and to documentation of an accurate description of the wound for the record. The wound may be described with respect to location, length, depth, nature of the edges, cleanliness, and involvement of any underlying structures.
2. The integrity of arterial circulation is determined from palpation of peripheral pulses, skin color, temperature, and capillary filling. Contusions over the forearm or leg may lead to delayed onset of compartment syndrome.
3. Sensory deficits are tested by determination of distal sensation, often requiring measurement of two-point discrimination distal to the lesion. This can easily be performed with a paper clip whose ends have been separated by 8 mm. Nerve injuries are classified as follows:
   a. Neuropraxia: nerve continuity maintained and no axonal degeneration secondary to compression or contusion
   b. Axonotmesis: preservation of anatomic continuity of nerve with axonal degeneration
   c. Neurotmesis: complete division of nerve
4. After a careful sensory examination, application of or infiltration with local anesthesia may be provided for a painless yet accurate examination, cleansing, debridement, and definitive treatment.
5. Tendons, ligaments, and muscles should be tested distal to the injury individually and by muscle group.

6. Foreign bodies should be identified and removed.
7. Injuries of the hand or foot require very careful assessment. The examination of the hand, which is commonly injured in children, is outlined in Chapter 68. Open wounds require direct visualization with hemostasis. The tendons, if exposed, must be visualized throughout their full range of motion because motor function may remain normal with partial laceration of tendons or ligaments.

Complications. Infections can be minimized by meticulous wound preparation, irrigation and debridement, careful closure of the wound, and application of appropriate dressings and splints.

Other complications include the following:

1. Failure to recognize deep structure injury to nerve, tendon, bone, or joint capsule with sensory or motor deficits (fractures underlying lacerations must be considered open fractures)
2. Delayed recognition of a foreign body
3. Cosmetic deformity

Ancillary Data. X-ray studies should be obtained when appropriate before motor function or range of motion is tested:

1. For injuries secondary to blunt trauma or crush injury.
2. To exclude a radiopaque foreign body. The relative qualities of wound contaminants are as follows:
   a. Highly radiopaque: bone, metal (lead, steel, copper), gravel, or stone chips
   b. Slightly radiopaque: bone (birds), metal (aluminum), glass, some plastics
   c. Water density: plants, wood in situ more than 24 hours, some plastics
   d. Radiolucent: air, gas, wood in situ less than 24 hours, some plastics

   NOTE: Glass fragments can usually be seen on a standard x-ray film. Small (0.5- to 1-mm) or thin glass fragments are more difficult to see but can be detected if no underlying bone is present.

MANAGEMENT (See Appendix to this chapter and Chapter 58)

Although unusual, massive hypovolemia from a vascular injury or extensive laceration of the scalp or face may cause hypotension, which is usually responsive to administration of crystalloid solution (0.9% normal saline [NS] or lactated Ringer's [LR] solution at 20 ml/kg over 20 to 30 minutes). Stabilization of life-threatening conditions has the greatest priority.

1. If hypotension is present, other injuries, in addition to the soft tissue damage, should be considered.
2. Hemorrhage can usually be controlled by direct pressure or local injection of lidocaine with epinephrine if there are no contraindications to their use. If placement of hemostats is required for control of hemorrhage, this must always be performed under direct vision (never blindly) to prevent iatrogenic injury to nerves, vessels, or tendons. Uncontrolled ongoing hemorrhage from an extremity should be controlled by application of a tourniquet and not by hemostats.
3. Tetanus immunizations must be updated (p. 734).

Immediate consultation should be requested if the injury is beyond the expertise of the evaluator or if extensive follow-up evaluation will be required.

Analgesia and Sedation

Appropriate attention must be directed to reducing discomfort and anxiety as discussed in the Appendix to this chapter.

Restraint, Position, and Draping

Wounds in small children are most easily repaired if the child is appropriately sedated (see Appendix to this chapter) or restrained. Sedation must be individualized and necessitates careful attention to the child's respiratory status and the potential for aspiration of vomitus. A sterile field should be created by the use of drapes. However, the face generally should not be totally draped.

If extensive bleeding is associated with a finger laceration, an excellent field and tourniquet can be achieved by cleansing the patient's finger and then slipping the hand into a sterile glove, snipping the end of the glove on the involved finger, and rolling the finger of the glove back to provide exposure and tourniquet. Careful scrubbing is then performed.

Wound Exploration

Wound exploration should be performed on all injuries so that the extent of the damage may be fully appreciated, violation of underlying structures realized, undetected fractures and tendon lacerations discovered, and removal of all foreign bodies ensured. Optimally, the wound is explored after injection of local anesthesia, hemostasis is obtained, and sensory examination is completed.

Embedded, inert foreign bodies such as glass or metal should be removed if possible. X-ray films are often helpful in their localization. The precise location of an embedded object can be identified by taping paper clips or a flexible radiopaque marker such as wire to the skin overlying the suspected location and obtaining anteroposterior (AP) and lateral views at 90 degrees to each other. However, if foreign bodies are small and embedded deeply into muscle and so cannot be easily removed, they may be left in place. The patient should be informed of the presence of the foreign body, and follow-up observation should be arranged.

NOTE: Organic foreign bodies such as wood should be removed whenever possible to prevent local inflammatory reactions. Xeroradiography may be necessary to localize some foreign bodies not seen on standard soft tissue radiographs. Surgical consultation should usually be obtained unless the material is superficial; deeper objects may require controlled removal in the operating room.

Wound Cleansing and Irrigation

Cleansing and irrigation are best performed after local anesthesia has been injected; 1% povidone-iodine solution (Betadine) is an excellent cleansing agent. The "scrub" should not be used because it causes extensive tissue necrosis. If hair must be removed, it is ideally done by clipping rather than shaving, because the latter increases the incidence of wound infections. Moistening the hair with lubricating jelly (K-Y or Surgilube) may keep it out of the way. Eyebrows should not be shaved or clipped; they are important landmarks for aligning the wound.

Irrigation assists in the removal of particulate material from a *contaminated* wound. The efficacy is related to the force of the irrigating stream: A higher pressure is more efficient. Larger particles are more easily removed than smaller ones. High-pressure irrigation is accomplished by attaching an 18-gauge angiocatheter or 18- or 19-gauge needle to a 35-ml syringe and pressing down firmly on the plunger while keeping the tip 3 to 4 mm above the wound during flushing. A 500- to 1000-ml bag of normal saline solution fitted with blood administration tubing in a pressure sleeve may facilitate this process. Saline solution in pressurized canisters delivering 8 to 10 pounds per square inch (psi) is also effective. Irrigation before primary closure of a *clean, noncontaminated* facial or scalp laceration is of less importance.

Foreign material in an abrasion must be removed within 24 hours to prevent the creation of a permanent traumatic tattoo, particularly in such cosmetically important areas as the face. Anesthesia of the abrasion may be achieved by direct application of a cotton ball or swab to the wound that has been saturated in 4% lidocaine, 2% viscous lidocaine, or LET (lidocaine, epinephrine, tetracaine). The abrasion should then be scrubbed with a scrub brush or toothbrush. A No. 11 scalpel blade or 18-gauge needle may be used for material not removed by the scrubbing process.

Hemostasis

Direct pressure and tourniquets are occasionally needed for hemostasis. Vessels should not be sutured or clamped blindly because of the risk of injury to other underlying tissues.

Wound Revision and Debridement

Very conservative debridement, after anesthesia, of devitalized or severely contaminated tissue may be required. Ragged and uneven edges may have to be incised with a scalpel or iris scissors to improve the wound configuration. Most wounds do well with little or no revision. It should be explained to the parents that the wound may leave a noticeable scar, which may be further revised by a consultant after 18 to 24 months of healing.

Residual pigment in abrasions can lead to permanent tattooing if foreign particulate material is not removed. Scrubbing and selective debridement are important.

Wound Closure

Wounds should be closed as soon as possible. In general, wounds more than 8 to 12 hours old should not be closed. Clean wounds on the face and scalp may be closed, if necessary, up to 24 hours after the injury because of the excellent vasculature.

1. Contaminated or dirty wounds (i.e., those with a high level of bacterial inoculum) are optimally treated with vigorous cleansing, appropriate dressing, and a delayed primary closure at 72 to 96 hours. Other wounds that should be considered for delayed closure are those associated with extensive tissue damage, retained foreign body, borderline ischemic tissue, prolonged interval (generally >6 hours) between injury and attempted closure except in well-vascularized areas, those with acute infection, and those in which closure can be done only with excessive tension.
2. Puncture wounds should not be closed. Debridement and irrigation with close follow-up evaluation are essential.
3. Most bites on the face should be closed primarily after careful cleansing, irrigation, and debridement. Serious consideration should be given to delayed primary closure for bites in other areas of the body. However, if in the judgment of the clinician delayed closure would result in a serious cosmetic or functional deficit, such wounds may be closed primarily (p. 308).

Wound Closure Techniques
(Table 65-1)

The location of the injury and the objective of closure influence techniques. If the primary goal is a good cosmetic closure, deep or large wounds often require multilayered closure. The top sutures should be removed within 3 to 7 days to minimize the possibility that suture marks will be part of the scar.

If a good functional result is the primary goal, as on the head, arm, or leg, then a single-layer closure is usually adequate.

A sterile scalpel blade or stitch cutter facilitates removal, which must be performed at the appropriate time to reduce suture marks.

Specific suturing techniques are beyond the scope of this book, but several principles are important to emphasize:

1. Subcutaneous sutures should be placed equal in depth and distance from the wound edges.
2. Extrinsic tension should be reduced with the use of buried sutures or undermining of the subcutaneous layers. This step is often required in cases of extensive loss of tissue because of trauma or revision. Undermine areas of loose tissue at the level of subcutaneous fat or fascia to a width equal to the gap of the wound at its widest point.
3. To aid edge eversion, the base of the suture loop should be as wide as or wider than the top of the suture loop. Enter the skin perpendicular to the skin plane rather than tangentially (less important with shallow sutures).

TABLE 65-1 Suture Repair of Soft Tissue Injuries

Location	Anesthetic†	Suture Material*	Technique of Closure and Dressing	Suture Removal	Pitfalls
Scalp	Lidocaine 1% with epinephrine	3-0 or 4-0 nonabsorbable monofilament	Interrupted in galea; single tight layer in scalp—horizontal mattress if bleeding not well controlled by simple sutures; hair apposition	7-12 days	Failure to explore wound for fracture; hematoma formation secondary to "loose" closure
Face	Lidocaine 1% with epinephrine or use field block†	4-0 or 5-0 synthetic absorbable or 6-0 nonabsorbable monofilament	If full-thickness laceration, layered closure is desirable	3-5 days	Failure to recognize and examine for damage to underlying structures, i.e., facial nerve or parotid duct
Pinna (ear)	Lidocaine 1% (field block)	6-0 nonabsorbable monofilament or 5-0 synthetic absorbable	Close perichondrium with 5-0 synthetic absorbable; close skin with nonabsorbable interrupted sutures—stint dressing	4-6 days	Hematoma formation secondary to improper or no dressing
Eyebrow	Lidocaine 1% with epinephrine†	4-0 or 5-0 synthetic absorbable and 6-0 nonabsorbable monofilament	Layered closure	4-5 days	Perpendicular excision rather than one parallel to direction of hair follicles; shaving of eyebrows not indicated
Eyelid	Lidocaine 1%†	6-0 nonabsorbable monofilament	Single-layer horizontal mattress, interrupted or running	3-5 days	Failure to examine for globe injury or to appreciate injury to tarsal plate
Lip	Lidocaine 1% with epinephrine or use field block	4-0 or 5-0 synthetic absorbable in mucosa, muscle and intradermal layer; 6-0 nonabsorbable monofilament	Three layers (mucosa, muscle, and skin) if through-and-through, otherwise two layers	3-5 days	1-mm or greater malalignment of the vermilion border, causing cosmetic deformity

Continued

TABLE 65-1 Suture Repair of Soft Tissue Injuries—cont'd

Location	Anesthetic	Suture Material*	Technique of Closure and Dressing	Suture Removal	Pitfalls
Oral cavity	Lidocaine 1% with epinephrine; may use field block; IV sedation may be necessary in children	4-0 synthetic absorbable	Simple interrupted or horizontal mattress: layered closure if muscularis of tongue involved	7-8 days or allow to dissolve	Inadequate sedation and exposure (particularly in children) for necessary procedure
Neck	Lidocaine 1% with epinephrine	4-0 synthetic absorbable intradermal 5-0 nonabsorbable monofilament	Two-layered closure for best cosmetic results	4-6 days	Failure to appreciate implication of zone I or zone III injuries; delay in airway management
Abdomen	Lidocaine 1% with epinephrine	4-0 synthetic absorbable 4-0 or 5-0 nonabsorbable monofilament	Single or layered closure	6-12 days	Failure to use local wound exploration as an initial screen and aggressively follow up with further diagnostic procedures
Back	Lidocaine 1% with epinephrine	4-0 synthetic absorbable 4-0 or 5-0 nonabsorbable monofilament	Single or layered closure	6-12 days	Failure to appreciate possibility of renal or diaphragmatic injury
Chest	Lidocaine 1% with epinephrine	4-0 synthetic absorbable 4-0 or 5-0 nonabsorbable monofilament	Single or layered closure	6-12 days	Exploration of wound may cause hemorrhage or pneumothorax; failure to consider possibility of diaphragmatic penetration in low chest wounds and pericardial tamponade in wounds near midline
Extremity	Lidocaine 1% with epinephrine†	3-0 or 4-0 synthetic absorbable (muscle) 4-0 or 5-0 nonabsorbable monofilament	Single-layered closure is adequate although layered or running SC closure may give better cosmetic result; apply splint if wound over a joint	6-14 days	Failure to make sensory examination before anesthesia; failure to explore wound visually after hemostasis; unrecognized foreign body left in wound

Hands and feet	Lidocaine 1% (if field block, use 2% lidocaine or 0.25% bipivacaine)	4-0 or 5-0 nonabsorbable monofilament	Single-layered closure only with simple or horizontal mattress interrupted suture, at least 5 mm from cut wound edges; horizontal mattress sutures should be used if tension on wound edges; apply splint if wound over a joint	7-12 days	Use of subcuticular sutures; failure to explore wound visually with digit in original position at time of injury
Nailbeds	Lidocaine 2% or bipivacaine 0.25% digital nerve block	5-0 synthetic absorbable	Gentle, meticulous placement to obtain even edges; stint dressing with original nail or aluminum foil between cuticle and nail matrix to prevent adhesions	Allow to be absorbed	Loss of suture by tying too tightly and having it cut through friable nailbed suture; adhesions caused by failure to place stint between cuticle and matrix

* Tape may be used for surface or epidermal closure if buried intradermal closure results in perfectly even wound edges and no propensity for differential swelling of wound edges exists. Tape or tissue adhesive may also be used for tiny laceration with minimal or no tension on wound edges.
† Topical anesthetic agents (LET [lidocaine, epinephrine, tetracaine], EMLA) may be alternative or adjunct for superficial injuries.
Synthetic absorbable sutures: polyglycolic acid, polyglactin 910, polydiaxone, glycolide trimethylene carbonate.
Synthetic nonabsorbable monofilament: nylon, polypropylene, polybutester.

4. The closer the suture is to the wound edge, the better the control of the edge. Space the sutures equal distances apart at the same depth on both sides of the wound. Tighten sutures to bring edges of the skin together; do not strangulate the skin edges.
5. Achieve longitudinal alignment of relatively straight lacerations by selecting the midpoint of the laceration for the first suture and continuing to bisect each section. Place the sutures at the same depth on both sides, and close the wound with the least amount of tension.
6. For management of a flap, if it is proximal to the blood supply, especially on an extremity, the tip usually survives unless the base is narrow. A proximal flap usually survives if its base is three times as long as its height. Distally based flaps have a higher risk of necrosis.
7. Horizontal mattress sutures should be considered for all wounds with significant tension that are to be closed in a single layer (i.e., wounds overlying joints).
8. Butyl-2-cyanoacrylate adhesive (Dermabond, Indermil) is suitable for closure of small lacerations with minimal tension and may replace tape and sutures for closure of these small wounds. It has been found to be useful in facial lacerations less than 4 cm long and less than 0.5 cm wide. Care must be taken to avoid interposing the adhesive between cut edges of the wound and to make the wound edges perfectly even. This adhesive should not be used for wounds that are deep, require multiple closure layers, result from animal bites, or involve mucocutaneous or hair-containing surfaces.
   a. The adhesive is applied with the applicator. A high-viscosity Dermabond may be easier to apply.
   b. The wound's edges are held together for approximately 30 seconds. Commonly, the physician uses the fingers or forceps to tightly approximate the wound edges.
   c. The wound should be kept dry with a protective dressing for 48 hours.
9. Cutaneous tape closure may occasionally be used for superficial wounds in areas without motion, for which meticulous closure is not required. The area should be dried, tincture of benzoin applied, and the edges approximated without tension or underlying dead space.
10. Staples may be used for lacerations of the scalp, trunk, or extremity.
11. Considerations regarding lacerations of the lip, eyelid, eyebrow, nose, ear, scalp, and neck are discussed in Chapter 58.
12. The hair apposition technique has proved to be useful in linear scalp lacerations less than 10 cm:
    a. Four to five strands of hair (>3 cm) are bundled on each side of the laceration and twisted to appose the wound.
    b. This twist is then secured with tissue glue.

Primary Repair of Nerve Injuries

Repair of nerve injuries is more effective in children than in adults. Neuropraxia or axonotmesis should be observed for 3 to 6 months along with electrodiagnostic studies before surgical repair is performed. Neurotmesis requires an early epineural repair by a surgeon.

Dressing and Splints of the Hands and Feet

1. A large bulky dressing of the hand or foot is optimal for most children, particularly when immobilization will be necessary for only a few days.
2. Injuries of the hand requiring immobilization usually involve wounds over the joints and are best dressed in the "hooded cobra" position. The wrist is in neutral position, the metacarpophalangeal (MCP) joints are flexed at about 60 to 70 degrees, the interphalangeal (IP) joints are flexed at

10 to 20 degrees, and the thumb is abducted. A volar plaster splint may be incorporated over the dressing for additional immobilization.

3. The foot may need to be immobilized temporarily if extensive injuries are present, particularly those involving tendons. Immobilization may be achieved by maintaining the ankle at 90 degrees with a posterior plaster splint.
4. Strong consideration should be given to splinting all full-thickness lacerations over joints for 1 to 2 weeks.

Antibiotics

Antibiotics are not required for clean, noncontaminated lacerations. Grossly contaminated wounds are best left open and treated with delayed closure after copious irrigation.

The use of prophylactic antibiotics in animal bites and other contaminated wounds remains controversial. Their use should be left to the judgment and discretion of the treating physician. If an antibiotic is used, it should be inexpensive and broad spectrum (see Chapter 45).

Oral penicillin may reduce the incidence of infection of intraoral and through-and-through lip lacerations. Topical antibacterial ointment may be used.

Puncture Wounds

Puncture wounds, usually of the foot, are common in children. Such an injury has a higher infection rate because foreign material is easily trapped within it and the small size of the wound impedes irrigation. Simple puncture wounds can usually be treated with simple local irrigation with normal saline solution, blind probing of the wound with fine forceps, and close observation.

Wounds that possibly have a retained foreign material, are grossly contaminated, or show local tenderness 2 to 3 days after the injury often need more aggressive medical and surgical therapy. After local anesthesia (without epinephrine), enlargement of the wound up to 4 to 5 mm using a No. 11 scalpel blade may be helpful in removing foreign material and irrigating the wound.

Osteomyelitis, a very rare complication of puncture wounds of the foot (usually through a sneaker), is most commonly due to *Pseudomonas aeruginosa* (see p. 769).

Fishhooks

Fishhooks commonly become embedded in fingers and other areas. Techniques for their removal after anesthesia is achieved include:

1. Advance the tip of the hook through the skin past the barb and cut the distal hook and barb off. The remaining hook can be removed along its track of entry.
2. An 18-gauge needle is introduced along the barbed side of the hook at the entrance side of the wound, with the bevel toward the inside of the hook curve. Apply slight pressure upward on the hook shank to disengage it from the soft tissues. Push the needle upward and rotate until the lumen locks firmly over the barb. Keep the needle locked on the barb with gentle pressure. Then, with a slight rotation of the hook shank upward, the hook and needle can be removed through the original wound with a slight downward movement.
3. Devices specifically designed to remove fishhooks are available.

Splinters, Subungual Hematomas, and Paronychia

See discussion on these problems in Chapter 68, p. 551.

PARENTAL EDUCATION

Parental education and follow-up should be specifically delineated on a printed instruction sheet.

1. Mild bleeding and some discomfort may occur after suturing as anesthesia wears off.
2. Keep the wound clean and dry for 2 days. Then begin gentle cleaning of the wound

with soap and water. If scab formation is significant, peroxide may be useful to facilitate removal of sutures.
3. Call your physician if the wound becomes red, painful, or swollen, if it drains pus, or if red streaks appear in the skin around it.
4. Change the dressing as directed.
5. Return for suture removal as instructed.
6. Apply sunscreen (sun-protective factor [SPF] 15 or greater) over the scar for 6 months after injury.

BIBLIOGRAPHY

Applebaum JS, Zalut T, Applebaum D: The use of tissue adhesion for traumatic laceration repair in the emergency department, *Ann Emerg Med* 22:1190, 1993.

Berk WA, Welch RD, Bock BF: Controversial issues in clinical management of the simple wound, *Ann Emerg Med* 21:72, 1992.

Brinkman KR, Lambert RW: Evaluation of skin stapling for wound closure in the emergency department, *Ann Emerg Med* 18:1122, 1989.

Chisholm CD, Cordell WH, Rogers K et al: Comparison of a new pressurized saline canister versus syringe irrigation for laceration cleansing in the emergency department, *Ann Emerg Med* 21:1364, 1992.

Doser C, Cooper WL, Ediger WM et al: Fishhook injuries: a prospective evaluation, *Am J Emerg Med* 9:413, 1991.

Grisham JE, Zukin DD: Suture selection for the pediatrician, *Pediatr Emerg Care* 6:301, 1990.

Hollander JE, Richman PB, Werblud M et al: Irrigation in facial and scalp lacerations: does it alter outcome? *Ann Emerg Med* 31:73, 1998.

Hunt TK: The physiology of wound healing, *Ann Emerg Med* 17:1265, 1988.

Inaba AS, Zukin DD, Perro M: An update on the evaluation and management of plantar puncture wounds and *Pseudomonas* osteomyelitis, *Pediatr Emerg Care* 8:38, 1992.

Jacobs RF, McCarthy RE, Elser JM: *Pseudomonas* osteochondritis complicating puncture wounds of the foot in children: a 10-year evaluation, *J Infect Dis* 160:657, 1989.

Markovchick V: Soft tissue injury and wound repair. In Reisdorff EJ, Roberts MR, editors: *Pediatric Emergency Medicine*, Philadelphia, 1993, WB Saunders.

Ong Eng Hock, M, Oui SBS, Saw SM et al: A randomized controlled trial comparing the hair apposition technique with tissue glue to standard suturing in scalp lacerations, *Ann Emerg Med* 40:19, 2002.

Osmond MH: Pediatric wound management: the role of tissue adhesives, *Pediatr Emerg Care* 15:137, 1995.

Quinn JV, Drzewieck A, Limm et al: A randomized controlled trial comparing a tissue adhesive with suturing in the repair of pediatric facial lacerations, *Ann Emerg Med* 22:1130, 1993.

Simon HK, McLaird DJ, Bruns TB et al: Long-term appearance of lacerations repaired using tissue adhesive, *Pediatrics* 99:193, 1997.

Singer AJ, Hollanger JE, Quinn JV: Evaluation and management of traumatic lacerations, *N Engl J Med* 337:1142, 1997.

Zukin DD, Inaba AS, Wuerker C: Minor wounds. In Barkin RM, editor: *Pediatric emergency medicine: concepts and clinical practice*, ed 2, St Louis, 1997, Mosby.

65 Appendix to Chapter: Procedural Analgesia and Sedation

The child who needs analgesia or sedation for a procedure must be approached systematically, with a number of factors taken into consideration:

1. What response is required—analgesia, sedation, or both?
2. What level of titration of analgesia or sedation is required? Intravenous (IV) administration provides the most rapid onset of activity and controlled titration of effect. The efficacy of other routes reflects mucosal absorption and gastrointestinal absorption and motility.
3. What routes are available or potentially available?
4. Is immediate reversal of potential side effects necessary? Agents are available for narcotics (naloxone) and benzodiazepines (flumazenil).
5. Is the child at particular risk for a specific side effect? Infants younger than 1 month are particularly sensitive to morphine-induced respiratory depression. Do underlying medical problems or medications enhance the risk in the specific patient?
6. What monitoring equipment, personnel, and capabilities are available? Many agents have a dose-dependent relationship with ventilation. The P_{CO_2} may rise before the P_{O_2} drops.
7. What level of resuscitation capabilities is available?
8. What is the clinician's personal experience with the agent?

The answers to these questions will largely determine the therapeutic alternative that is chosen. It is essential to be sensitive to the needs of the child in providing optimal analgesia and sedation within the bounds of an appropriate balance between the risks and benefits. Children receiving systemic agents require monitoring if risk of a negative effect on the airway, breathing, or circulation is anticipated.

In addition to pharmacologic approaches, psychologic measures such as hypnosis and distraction may be useful with appropriate preparation. Parental participation can be helpful in reducing anxiety, communicating truthfully with the patient, and supporting the child through the procedure. A positive attitude will also lessen anxiety. Letting children make choices (e.g., site of IV access, selection of stickers) is important.

A number of measurement tools are available to assess pain in adults and children older than 7 years. They include the use of cognitive (i.e., self-reporting, faces) and behavioral scales (Children's Hospital of Eastern Ontario Pain Scale [CHEOPS]).

Administration of sucrose with such vehicles as Sweet-Ease has been shown to be useful in pain relief for venipunctures and circumcision in neonates.

ANALGESIA (Table 65-2)

Pain control may be achieved with systemic narcotic and other agents for longer or more complicated procedures while the patient is monitored. Localized analgesia may be useful for procedures involving only limited areas through various routes: topical (LET [lidocaine, epinephrine, tetracaine], EMLA, cryoanesthesia),

TABLE 65-2 Recommended Sedative and Analgesic Agents for Pediatric Emergency Department Patients*

Indication	Agent	Route	Initial Dosage (mg/kg)	Maximum Initial Dose†	Onset	Duration
ANALGESIA						
Mild-moderate	Acetaminophen	PO, PR	10-15	1000 mg		
Moderate	Ibuprofen	PO	10	800 mg		
Severe	Morphine sulfate	IV, SC	0.1	10 mg	5-6 min	3-4 hr
	Ketorolac	IM, IV	0.5-1	60 mg		
	Meperidine	IM	2	100 mg	30-60 min	2-3 hr
	plus promethazine	IM	1	50 mg		
SEDATION						
Moderate	Midazolam	PO, PR, IN	0.5	10 mg	10-20 min	1 hr
	Chloral hydrate	PR, PO	50-80	2000 mg	30-90 min	2-4 hr
Deep	Midazolam	IV	0.1	5 mg	2-5 min	30 min
	Diazepam	IV	0.2	10 mg	5-10 min	1-2 hr
	Lorazepam	IV	0.02-0.05	2 mg	5-6 min	2-3 hr
	Pentobarbital	IV	2-5	200 mg	1 min	15 min
ANALGESIA AND SEDATION						
No IV	Codeine	PO	1-2	60 mg	1 hr	3-4 hr
	Hydrocodone	PO	0.2	7.5 mg	1 hr	3-4 hr
	Morphine	IM	0.1	10 mg	5-10 min	4-5 hr
	plus midazolam	IM	0.1	5 mg		
	Ketamine‡	IM	4	50 mg	2-10 min	1 hr
	Meperidine	IM	2	50 mg	30-60 min	1-3 hr
	plus promethazine	IM	1	25 mg		
	plus chlorpromazine (MPC/DPT)§	IM	1	25 mg		
With IV	Morphine	IV	0.1	10 mg	5-6 min	3-4 hr
	Morphine	IV	0.1	10 mg		
	plus midazolam	IV	0.1	5 mg		
	Fentanyl‖	IV (slow)	0.001-0.002	0.005 mg/kg (0.05-0.1 mg)	2-3 min	1 hr
	Fentanyl‖	IV	0.001-0.002	0.005 mg/kg (0.05-0.1 mg)	2-3 min	1 hr
	plus midazolam	IV	0.1	5 mg	2-5 min	30 min
	Ketamine‡	IV	1	100 mg	1 min	10 min

IN, intranasal; *PO*, oral; *PR*, rectal.

* Use of these agents requires monitoring, in accordance with prescribed guidelines, of blood pressure, pulse, respirations, and oximetry.

† Therapeutic doses may vary with individual patients. If higher dosages are required, they should be titrated while patient is monitored.

‡ Atropine is often given in the same syringe to reduce excess secretions associated with ketamine. Administer slowly (<0.5 mg/kg/min).

§ Rarely used combination.

‖ One-third dose in children <6 mo.

local infiltration (subcutaneous [SC], intradermal, field), regional block, or nerve block.

Topical

Topical mixtures may be useful for superficial injuries, particularly in young children. Do not use on mucosal lesions or where epinephrine is contraindicated.

1. LET (topical lidocaine 2% to 4%, epinephrine 1:1000, and tetracaine 0.5% to 2%): Has been shown to be an effective topical anesthetic preparation. For anesthesia, 2 to 3 ml of LET is instilled within the inner margins of the laceration until the cavity is filled. An equal amount of LET is applied by using a cotton ball or swab (not gauze) over the wound for 10 to 15 minutes. The individual holding the cotton ball or swab should wear gloves. Mixing 3 ml of LET with 150 mg of methylcellulose creates a "slurry" that may easily be applied. After 10 to 15 minutes, excellent local anesthesia and vasoconstriction are achieved. LET appears to be as effective as TAC (see number 2) and to lack some of the latter's reported complications.
2. TAC (topical tetracaine 1%, topical adrenaline [epinephrine] 1:4000, cocaine HCl solution 4%): Is less commonly used than LET because of the potential complications of cocaine; many studies have proven TAC's efficacy and safety when it is utilized in appropriate clinical situations. It should *never* be used on mucosal injuries because of the potential absorption of cocaine. TAC is most effective on the face and inconsistently useful on extremities. Cardiac arrest has been reported. TAC is applied in a manner similar to LET.
3. EMLA (*e*utectic *m*ixture of *l*ocal *a*nesthetics) cream: A commercially available mixture of lidocaine 2.5% and prilocaine 2.5% suspended in an oil-in-water emulsion that is effective on uncomplicated extremity wounds; 2.5 to 5 g is applied on the skin and sealed at least 1 hour before any procedure. It is particularly effective on extremity wounds.
4. Transient anesthesia can be obtained with topical application for 5 to 15 minutes of gauze saturated with 2% to 4% lidocaine.
5. Other transdermal drug delivery systems are being developed, including some that enhance penetration with a liposomal delivery system (ELA-Max, 4% lidocaine cream [Ferndale Laboratories]).

Infiltrative

Lidocaine (Xylocaine) 1% or 2% is adequate for most cases requiring infiltrative and regional anesthesia. It is infiltrated with a small needle (25- or 27-gauge) directly through the wound margins. Onset of anesthesia is 5 to 15 minutes with a duration of 1 to 2 hours.

1. Discomfort may be reduced by *buffering* the lidocaine. Sodium bicarbonate is added to the lidocaine in a ratio by volume of 1:10 to neutralize the pH. The shelf life of buffered lidocaine is 1 week. *Slow injection* (30 seconds) through a 27-gauge needle minimizes pain. *Warming* the lidocaine (storing in a fluid warmer at 98.6° F) may also be helpful. A slow rate of administration probably has the greatest effect in reducing pain.
2. Before injection, a small amount of 4% lidocaine or other topical anesthetic may be applied to the wound to decrease the pain of injection.
3. Toxic levels may result from local administration of more than 4 mg/kg plain lidocaine or more than 7 mg/kg of lidocaine with epinephrine. Toxicity includes sinus arrest, bradycardia, hypotension, atrioventricular (AV) block, irritability, respiratory depression, seizures, and coma.
4. Lidocaine containing epinephrine at a ratio of 1:100,000 may assist with hemostasis but should be used only in

areas of good perfusion and should *never* be used on the digits, hands, feet, ear, tarsal plate of the eye, bridge of the nose, nipple, or penis.

5. Regional anesthesia may be achieved by using proper anatomic landmarks but may require additional local infiltration as well. It minimizes distortion.
6. The ear may be adequately anesthetized by raising a wheal with lidocaine 1% without epinephrine around the entire base of the ear. This procedure will anesthetize all but the external canal.
7. Bupivacaine (Marcaine) is an alternative agent with onset of 10 to 30 minutes and a duration of anesthesia of 4 to 6 hours. The maximum dose (bupivacaine without epinephrine) is 2 to 3 mg/kg/dose.

Systemic Nonnarcotic

1. Aspirin and acetaminophen.
2. Nonsteroidal antiinflammatory drugs (NSAIDs) are potent analgesic and antiinflammatory agents:
   a. Ibuprofen is widely used. It may be a more effective antipyretic than acetaminophen.
   b. Ketorolac is the only available parenteral NSAID available in the United States. Available PO, IM, and IV; dosage is 0.5 mg/kg q6hr IV for 48 to 72 hours (maximum: 30 mg q6hr IV).

Systemic Narcotic

Selection of systemic narcotic agents should be made on the basis of the required duration of action, dose, route of administration, patient's weight and clinical stability, and use of narcotic potentiators. Appropriate monitoring is required.

1. Fentanyl (Sublimaze), 1 to 2 μg/kg up to a total dose of 5 μg/kg IV slowly over 3 to 5 minutes, has been used with great success. It has a half-life of 20 minutes and can be easily reversed with naloxone (Narcan). Older children often need less than the calculated dose. Oral transmucosal fentanyl incorporated into a candy matrix may be a useful premedication, although findings for this agent have not been consistent.
2. Meperidine (Demerol) is used in a number of mixtures, but other agents may be preferred.
   a. Dosage:
      - Meperidine, 1 mg/kg/dose (maximum: 50 mg/dose) IM; *or*
      - Meperidine, 1 mg/kg/dose (maximum: 50 mg/dose), and hydroxyzine (Atarax, Vistaril), 0.5 to 1 mg/kg/dose IM; *or*
      - Meperidine, 1 to 2 mg/kg/dose (maximum: 50 mg/dose), and promethazine (Phenergan), 0.25 to 0.5 mg/kg/dose (maximum: 12.5 mg/dose), and chlorpromazine (Thorazine), 0.25-0.5 mg/kg/dose (maximum: 12.5 mg/dose) IM. Usually mixed in ratio of 1:0.25:0.25 (DPT cocktail).
   b. Repeated use of meperidine is associated with an increased risk of seizures.
3. Morphine, 1 mg/kg/dose IV, is a potent narcotic that should be titrated slowly. It should not be used in hemodynamically or neurologically unstable patients.
4. Codeine is an oral opioid with a potency one-sixth that of parenteral morphine.
5. Patient-controlled analgesia (PCA), although not typically begun in the emergency department (ED) setting, may be considered on admission for children who will be in substantial ongoing pain.

SEDATION (see Table 65-2)

Sedation is not required for most injuries and procedures. There are, however, specific circumstances in which it is appropriate and will expedite the procedure. If a child is sedated, the face and chest should be uncovered (if not directly involved in procedure) when possible during the procedure to permit monitoring of color and respiratory effort. Oximetry and other vital signs must be monitored concurrently.

1. Midazolam (Versed), 0.05 to 0.10 mg/kg/dose IV over 1 to 2 minutes up to a maximum dose of 4 to 5 mg, may be given to an endpoint of drowsiness with slurred speech in the patient. Efficacy of more than 98% causing antegrade amnesia. Flumazenil is a specific antagonist of benzodiazepines. Midazolam is often used in combination with fentanyl.
   a. Intranasal (IN) administration of the parenteral solution in a dose of 0.3 to 0.5 mg/kg/dose IN is effective.
   b. Oral midazolam, 0.3 to 0.7 mg/kg/dose PO, may reduce anxiety when given 30 to 45 minutes before a procedure.
   c. Rectal (PR) midazolam, 0.45 mg/kg/dose PR, may be useful when given 15 minutes before a procedure.
2. Chloral hydrate is an effective oral agent, particularly for nonpainful procedures such as radiologic imaging or electroencephalography (EEG). The duration is variable but is generally 2 to 3 hours when this agent is given in a dose of 50 to 80 mg/kg/dose (maximum: 2000 mg) PO. Lower dosages are usually inadequate; higher dosages are more than 90% successful in children younger than 4 years and more than 80% in older children.
3. Pentobarbital (Nembutal) has been particularly effective in imaging and other nonpainful procedures. The starting dose is generally 2.5 mg/kg IV with supplemental doses of 1.25 mg/kg IV as needed up to a total maximum dose of 10 to 12 mg/kg IV.
4. Etomidate, 0.2 mg/kg, is a short-acting sedative that is often used with an analgesic such as fentanyl. It is primarily a sedative agent. May be associated with myoclonus and has little associated respiratory depression. This agent was traditionally used for rapid sequence induction.

Often sedation can be avoided by creating a positive environment for the child. Avoid verbal and nonverbal communication that adds to the child's anxiety. Distracting the child may be useful.

OTHER AGENTS

1. Ketamine sedation may be used for facial lacerations requiring the patient's cooperation when close monitoring and observation are possible. A dosage of 1 to 5 mg/kg/dose IM is given 10 minutes after atropine, 0.01 mg/kg, the latter to reduce secretions. The ketamine IV dose is 0.5 to 1 mg/kg/dose IV. The oral dose of 10 mg/kg/dose PO may reduce anxiety. Patients must be observed carefully until fully awake, with equipment to manage the airway and ventilation if necessary. Combined ketamine (1-2 mg/kg/dose IV) and midazolam (0.05-0.10 mg/kg/dose IV) have been effectively used in procedures such as lumbar punctures and imaging studies.

   Ketamine should not be used in patients 3 months or younger, children who are to have procedures requiring stimulation of the posterior pharynx, or patients with acute pulmonary infection or disease, cardiovascular disease, head injury, glaucoma, or psychosis. Those older than 1 to 5 years are more likely to have psychosis; the ideal age for use of ketamine is 3 months to 10 years.
2. Propofol is a parenteral ultra-short-acting sedative-hypnotic with antiemetic, antipruritic, anticonvulsant, anxiolytic, hypnotic, and analgesic properties. There is very limited experience in children, and the drug is not FDA approved for youngsters. The suggested dosage in children is 0.5 to 2 mg/kg/dose IV followed by an infusion of 0.025 to 0.1 mg/kg/min IV because of the rapid clearance. Patients generally regain consciousness within 8 minutes of cessation of the drug.

Because this agent is a potent general anesthetic agent, the risk of respiratory depression or apnea is significant and this agent should generally be used by clinicians with experience and expertise in its use. Hypotension may occur.

3. Nitrous oxide (30% to 50% mixture) is a useful supplement to local anesthetics.

SEQUENTIAL COMBINATION THERAPY: MIDAZOLAM AND FENTANYL

The sequential combination therapy using midazolam, 1 mg/ml, and fentanyl, 50 μg/ml, given systematically provides analgesia and sedation. Additional medication is then given if the previous step was not effective. Continuous monitoring of individual responses is required. Oxygen should generally be administered. Pharmacologic antagonists should be readily available.

Step 1: Give fentanyl, 1 μg/kg IV, over 60 to 90 seconds.

Step 2: Give midazolam, 0.035 mg/kg IV.

Step 3: Repeat fentanyl, 1 μg/kg IV over 2 minutes, if patient is not drowsy and tranquil.

Step 4: Repeat one half of the first dose of midazolam if adequate sedation is not achieved.

Step 5: Consider additional slow bolus of midazolam, 0.017 mg/kg IV.

The maximum doses are fentanyl, 5 μg/kg/hr IV, and midazolam, 0.15 mg/kg given stepwise with careful monitoring.

REVERSAL AGENTS

Naloxone (Narcan) is an opioid antagonist. The dosage is 0.1 mg/kg/dose IV or IM up to 2 mg/dose; it may be repeated every 2 to 3 minutes to a maximum total dose of 10 mg. Onset of action for naloxone when administered IV is 1 to 2 minutes with a duration of 20 to 40 minutes.

Flumazenil (Romazicon) is a pure benzodiazepine antagonist. The dosage is 0.02 mg/kg/dose IV or IM up to 0.2 mg/dose over 15 seconds. Dose may be repeated at 60-second intervals to a maximum total dose of 1 mg. Onset of action for flumazenil when administered IV is 1 to 2 minutes with a duration of 20 to 40 minutes.

DISCHARGE GUIDELINES

After sedation and completion of the procedure, the child should be monitored until all vital signs are normal, mental status and muscular control and function have returned to baseline, and no support is required.

Specific instructions are required to be followed by a responsible person:

- Monitor change in mental status and motor function. Watch for any difficulty with breathing.
- Provide dietary instructions, if any. Limit eating for the first 1 to 2 hours after discharge.
- Ensure that responsible person knows how to reach the contact person at the ED.
- Arrange for observation. Have the patient return if any concerns, including recurrent vomiting, change in behavior, or other new problems, arise.
- Set activity limitations. Generally, no playing that requires coordination (biking, skating, swimming) for next 24 hours.

BIBLIOGRAPHY

Algren JT, Algren CC: Sedation and analgesia for minor pediatric procedures, *Pediatr Emerg Care* 12:435, 1996.

American Academy of Pediatrics, Committee on Drugs: Guidelines for monitoring and management of pediatric patients during and after sedation for diagnostic and therapeutic procedures, *Pediatrics* 89:1110, 1992.

American Academy of Pediatrics, Committee on Drugs: Reappraisal of lytic cocktail (Demerol, Phenergan and Thorazine [DPT]) for sedation of children, *Pediatrics* 95:598, 1995.

American College of Emergency Physicians: Clinical policy for procedural sedation and analgesia in the emergency department, *Ann Emerg Med* 31:663, 1998.

Bonadio WA: Safe and effective method for application of tetracaine, adrenaline and cocaine to oral lacerations, *Ann Emerg Med* 28:396, 1996.

Brogan GX, Giarrusso E, Hollander JE et al: Comparison of plain, warmed and buffered lidocaine for anesthesia of traumatic wounds, *Ann Emerg Med* 26:2, 1995.

Connors K, Terndrup T: Nasal versus oral midazolam for sedation of anxious children undergoing laceration repair, *Ann Emerg Med* 24:1074, 1994.

Emslander HC: Local and topical anesthesia for pediatric wound repair: a review of selected aspects, *Pediatr Emerg Care* 14:123, 1998.

Fatovich DM, Jacobs IG: A randomized controlled trial of oral midazolam and buffered lidocaine for suturing lacerations in children, *Ann Emerg Med* 215:209, 1995.

Gamis AS, Knapp IF, Glenski JA: Nitrous oxide analgesia in a pediatric emergency department, *Ann Emerg Med* 18:177, 1989.

Green SM, Krauss BN: Procedural sedation terminology moving beyond "conscious sedation," *Ann Emerg Med* 3:433, 2002.

Green SM, Rothrock SG, Lynch EL: Intramuscular ketamine for pediatric sedation in the emergency department: safety profile in 1,022 cases, *Ann Emerg Care* 31:688, 1998.

Houck CS, Wilder RT, McDermott IS et al: Safety of intravenous ketorolac therapy in children and cost savings from a unit dosing system, *J Pediatr* 129:292, 1996.

Luhmann JD, Kennedy RM, Porter FL et al: A randomized clinical trial of continuous nitrous oxide and midazolam for sedation of young children during laceration repair, *Ann Emerg Med* 37:20, 2001.

Offman GM, Nowakowski R, Troshynski TJ et al: Risk reduction in pediatric procedural sedation by application of an American Academy of Pediatrics/American Society of Anesthesiologists process model, *Pediatrics* 109:236, 2002.

Parker R, Mahan RA, Giugliano D et al: Efficacy and safety of intravenous midazolam and ketamine for therapeutic and diagnostic procedures in children, *Pediatrics* 99:427, 1997.

Parshad J, Palmisano P, Nichols M: Chloral hydrate: the good and the bad, *Pediatr Emerg Care* 15:432, 1999.

Scarfone RJ, Jasani M, Gracely EJ: Pain of local anesthetics: rate of administration and buffering, *Ann Emerg Med* 31:36, 1998.

Schechter NL, Weisman SI, Rosenblum M et al: The use of oral transmucosal fentanyl citrate in children, *Pediatrics* 95:335, 1995.

Schilling CG, Bank DE, Borchart BA et al: Tetracaine, epinephrine (adrenaline) and cocaine (TAC) versus lidocaine, epinephrine and tetracaine (LET) for anesthesia of lacerations in children, *Ann Emerg Med* 25:203, 1995.

Shane JA, Fuchs SM, Khine H: Rectal midazolam for the sedation of preschool children undergoing laceration repair, *Ann Emerg Med* 24:1065, 1994.

Singer AJ, Stark MJ: LET versus EMLA for pretreating lacerations: a randomized trial, *Acad Emerg Med* 8:223, 2001.

Smith GA, Strausbaugh SD, Harbeck-Weber C et al: New non-cocaine containing topical anesthetics compared with tetracaine-adrenaline-cocaine during repair of lacerations, *Pediatrics* 100:825, 1997.

Smith GA, Strausbaugh SD, Harbeck-Weber C: Comparison of topical anesthetics without cocaine to tetracaine-cocaine and lidocaine infiltration during repair of lacerations: bupivacaine-norepinephrine is an effective new topical anesthetic agent, *Pediatrics* 97:301, 1996.

Steinberg AD: Should chloral hydrate be banned? *Pediatrics* 92:442, 1993.

Steward DI: Management of childhood pain: new approaches to procedure related pain, *J Pediatr* 122:51, 1993.

Terndrup TE, D'Agostino I: Pain control, analgesia and sedation. In Barkin RM, editor: *Pediatric emergency medicine: concepts and clinical practice*, ed 2, St Louis, 1997, Mosby.

Terndrup TE, Dire DJ, Madden CM et al: Comparison of intramuscular meperidine and promethazine with and without chlorpromazine: a randomized, prospective double-blind trial, *Ann Emerg Med* 22:206, 1993.

Theroux MC, West DW, Corddry DH et al: Efficacy of intranasal midazolam in facilitating suturing of lacerations in preschool children in the emergency department, *Pediatrics* 91:624, 1993.

Waldbilig DK, Quinn JV, Stiell IG et al: Randomized double-blind controlled trial comparing room temperature and heated lidocaine for digital nerve block, *Ann Emerg Med* 26:677, 1995.

Yaster M, Tobin JR, Fisher QA et al: Local anesthetics in the management of acute pain in children, *Pediatrics* 124:165, 1994.

Zempsky WT, Karasic RB: EMLA versus TAC for topical anesthesia of extremity wounds in children, *Ann Emerg Med* 30:163, 1997.

X

Orthopedic Injuries

66 Management Principles

ALERT Management of orthopedic injuries must follow stabilization of the patient. The unique growth characteristics of the child affect the nature of potential injuries.

Most orthopedic injuries seen in the emergency department (ED) are not life threatening. However, those involving multiple trauma must be appropriately prioritized, and when the pelvis or femur is broken, vascular support may be required (spinal injuries are discussed in Chapter 61). For all patients, the diagnosis and management must be precise to maximize permanent function.

Children's bones differ from those of adults, having a physis or growth plate. The physis between the metaphysis and epiphysis consists of proliferating cartilaginous cells. This growth plate is weak, often separating more easily than the adjacent tendon or ligament tears. The bones are pliable and less dense, allowing bending, buckling, and greenstick fractures; fractures heal rapidly, and nonunions are rare. A child's periosteum is thicker and more resistant to disruption, potentially reducing the extent of displacement and serving as a hinge to assist in reduction. Ligaments are more resistant to injury than are growth plates. Injury of the growth plate and buckle fractures are by far more common than sprains, which are uncommon in children.

The elasticity of children's bones allows the bones to deform before breaking and may result in a greenstick or torus fracture. Children's bones are able to absorb more energy and force before breaking compared with a mature adult skeleton.

Greenstick fracture involves the diaphysis of one side of a long bone, thus resulting in a fracture of one side of the cortex with an intact opposite side.

Torus (buckle) fracture is a buckling of one side of the cortex without an actual fracture line. It is usually seen in the metaphysis. The cortex in the developing skeleton and the microstructure and macrostructure dictate that the pattern of failure will be a torus deformation rather than a complete transverse fracture. A torus fracture is one of the most common patterns affecting the developing skeleton.

DIAGNOSTIC FINDINGS

An accurate history of the time of the event, mechanism of injury, and direction of forces and any history of previous injury and aggravating disease processes or bleeding diatheses should be obtained. The mechanism of injury is particularly important in defining the potential and type of injury and may assist in development of treatment plans—reduction of the fracture or dislocation using a force opposite to the force that led to the injury. Often, the injury was not witnessed and the child may be either unable (because of age) or too frightened to give a reliable history. Pseudoparalysis secondary to pain is common in the younger child. Children rarely complain persistently unless there is an abnormality. It is particularly important to recognize that pain may be referred, the classic example being a hip injury manifesting as knee pain. Histories that are vague or inconsistent with injuries and a delay in seeking medical care suggest child abuse. Approximately 15% to 25% of fractures in children younger than 3 years are caused by nonaccidental trauma (see Chapter 25).

Observation and examination for obvious deformities, swelling, ecchymoses, and point tenderness should be performed. In addition, evaluation of skin integrity, neurovascular status, muscle and tendon function, and pretreatment x-ray films are required.

Because of difficulty with physical evaluation and the lack of history in many cases, x-ray studies should be obtained if there is any suspicion of an underlying fracture (Box 66-1). Routine anteroposterior (AP) and lateral views, with inclusion of the joints above and below the suspected fracture site, help ensure that all potentially involved areas are studied. If any doubt exists because of the growth plates, *comparison views* may be obtained on a selective basis. Gonadal shields should be used. The fractures most commonly missed by x-ray study are fractures of the ribs, the elbow, and the periarticular regions of the phalanges. Other problem areas are fractures of the navicular and calcaneus.

Box 66-1

DIAGNOSTIC FINDINGS SUGGESTIVE OF A PATIENT HAVING A POSITIVE EXTREMITY RADIOGRAPH

UPPER EXTREMITY	LOWER EXTREMITY
Gross deformity	Gross deformity
Activity restricted	Activity restricted
Bone point tenderness	Bone point tenderness
Pain on motion	Pain on motion
Swelling moderate or severe	Knee injury
Time since injury >6 hr	Foot injury

The age of fractures may be estimated by the following radiologic guidelines:

Age (days)	X-ray Findings
4-10	Resolution of soft tissues
10-14	Periosteal elevation
14-21	Soft callus
21-4	Hard callus
1 year	Remodeling

Compartment syndrome may result from crush, burns, bleeding, seizures, swelling, muscle hypertrophy, dressings, cases, or snakebites. It results from an increase in an intracompartmental pressure within a fascial sheath, which causes compromise of the circulation within the compartment. Compartments commonly affected by compartment syndrome are the volar and dorsal compartments of the forearm, anterior compartment of the leg, peroneal and deep posterior compartments of the leg, interossei of the hand, gluteus medius, and the biceps and deltoid of the upper arm. Pain (with passive stretching of the involved muscle), pallor, paralysis, paresthesias, and pulselessness (5 Ps) may occur. Irreversible injury can occur after 5 to 6 hours of ischemia, often in association with rhabdomyolysis and infection. Elevation, removal of a constrictive dressing, and fasciotomy may be appropriate.

MANAGEMENT

Fracture remodeling and growth are rapid with particular stimulation of longitudinal growth and therefore may lead to overgrowth of an extremity when they occur when a child is between 2 and 10 years old. Greater degrees of angulation are accepted in the pediatric population when it involves metaphyseal fractures. However, angulation should be reduced as much as possible. Angulation is tolerated better in children younger than 2 years with fractures near the ends of bones, where there is bayonet opposition, or if the deformity is in the plane of motion of the joint. Accurate reduction is required for displaced intraarticular fractures; fractures that are grossly shortened, angulated, or rotated; fractures at marked angles to the plane of motion of a joint; and fractures that cross the growth plate. It is unusual for children to need open reductions, but early orthopedic consultation is usually desirable.

Dislocations are rare, and when they do occur, they most commonly involve the radial head or patella. *Fractures often accompany dislocations because the ligamentous structures are more resistant to trauma than the epiphyseal plates.* In general, the dislocation should be reduced before the fracture is treated. An orthopedist should be involved. Neurologic function should be evaluated and, in most instances, x-ray studies obtained before and after reduction. Dislocations that are open or involve neurovascular compromise are true emergencies. A deformity is best corrected with the assistance of an orthopedic consultant, with application of gentle, steady, inline traction, if such traction does not further impede circulation, increase pain significantly, or result in increased resistance with correction.

Patients with any fracture or dislocation involving a potential for vascular compromise (e.g., supracondylar, humerus, posterior knee dislocation) should generally be admitted to the hospital after immediate ED orthopedic consultation and management. If there is any suggestion of vascular compromise, it is also wise to have an immediate vascular consultation to assist in making a decision about angiography or surgery. The absence of a pulse does not always indicate that the vascular status is compromised, nor does the presence of a pulse ensure adequate circulation. Severe pain in the forearm or calf, pain with passive stretching of the fingers or toes, and a sensory deficit in the distal extremity are more sensitive indicators of ischemia, which may be caused by arterial injury or a compartment syndrome.

Analgesia

Analgesia is usually required before reduction in treatment of dislocations or poorly aligned fractures. Appropriate training, monitoring, and equipment are essential. As discussed in the Appendix to Chapter 65, there are many alternatives, partially reflecting the clinician's preference. Analgesia should be provided only after careful evaluation of the entire patient and the injured site. There is no reason to withhold analgesia after evaluation for isolated orthopedic injuries. The primary concern with good reduction of pain should be to immobilize and stabilize a fracture site. The use of any analgesic requires careful monitoring of the patient.

- Fentanyl (Sublimaze), 1 to 5 μg/kg over 1 to 2 minutes up to a total dose of about 100 μg, may be given, with the upper limit requiring titration. Older children may need a smaller dose than calculated. The half-life is 20 minutes.
- Midazolam (Versed), 0.05 to 0.10 mg/kg/dose (max: 2.5 mg/dose) IV, may be used as the sole agent or as an adjunct to fentanyl because of its rapid onset of action and short half-life. Midazolam, 0.3 to 0.7 mg/kg, may also be used orally and 0.4 mg/kg intranasally.

Some clinicians routinely use a combination therapy as described on page 516.

- Midazolam ≤0.1 mg/kg (max: 2.5 mg) IV repeated every 3 min until the speech is slurred or eyes glassy up to a dose of 0.3 mg/kg (max: 5 mg) combined with fentanyl ≤0.001 mg/kg IV every 3 min until there is a decreased response up to 0.005 mg/kg (max: 100 μg).
- Midazolam as above may also be combined with ketamine ≤0.5 mg/kg IV q3min until response. Flumazenil (Romazicon) should be available.

Conscious sedation protocols and guidelines need to be followed judiciously. Nitrous oxide may be used. Patient-controlled anesthesia (PCA) may be useful in the postoperative setting under institutional specific protocols.

The Bier block has been used for upper extremity reductions, usually in cooperation with an orthopedist:

1. A double-cuff pneumatic pressure cuff is placed above the elbow on the affected arm.

2. The limb is exsanguinated by means of a pneumatic splint or an Esmarch bandage on the affected limb, and the upper cuff is inflated to 200 to 250 mm Hg.
3. A 0.5% solution of lidocaine, 1.5 to 3 mg/kg, is administered intravenously in the involved limb over 30 to 60 seconds.
4. The lower cuff is inflated to 100 mm Hg above systolic pressure, and the upper cuff is deflated. Anesthesia is generally achieved in 5 minutes. The tourniquet may be left in place for 60 to 90 minutes or 15 minutes after infusion of lidocaine.
5. The block is terminated by slow deflation of the upper cuff.

A second IV line should be placed in the patient's unaffected arm in case dysrhythmias are noted as a result of systemic absorption of lidocaine; monitoring is essential.

Local analgesia may be achieved for closed reduction by "hematoma" block with 1% to 2% lidocaine solution injected directly into the hematoma.

Long-Term Follow-Up

Although stiffness is unusual, long-term care for children is essential to monitor growth and development. Communication with parents regarding treatment, home care, and possible complications is central to initiating the management plan. In general, sprains and strains should be elevated, with use of ice packs for 12 to 24 hours. Elevation can reduce swelling and pain. Ice packs are best prepared by crushing ice and placing it with some water in a plastic bag; they should be applied for 15 to 20 minutes every 3 to 4 hours with continuing use of an elastic bandage in between. An elastic (Ace) bandage, if used, should be rewrapped as necessary if it is too loose or too tight. If a cast is applied, it should be kept dry. Parents should call immediately if there is severe pressure or pain within the cast, increasing blueness, coldness, tingling, swelling, or decreased motion of the toes or fingers. Oral analgesics and antiinflammatory agents may be useful for ongoing care.

Long-term sequelae of fractures that should be monitored include nonunion, avascular necrosis, angulation deformities, shortening, overgrowth, infection, joint stiffness, and post-traumatic arthritis.

SPLINTS

All suspected fractures should be splinted when the patient arrives at the ED. Splinting can be performed in the position of function with firm materials, slings, and tape and is used primarily as an initial treatment to rest an injured area. Casts are often not applied for at least 48 hours after acute injuries because of swelling. Acute injuries should be splinted over adequate padding (e.g., Webril, stockinette) with plaster or fiberglass (10 layers for upper extremities and 20 layers for lower extremities). The splint is affixed with cotton or elastic bandages. An alternative is to place a circular cast and immediately bivalve it. Commercial splints and fiberglass casting material are also available.

Swelling during this period can cause neurovascular compromise if confined to a compartment. One joint above and one joint below the fracture should be incorporated into the splint. Delayed casting is particularly important in children, who are often unable to follow after-care instructions for elevation, rest, and cool packs. They can then be immobilized and monitored by an orthopedist.

Patients with obvious deformities should be stabilized on arrival at the ED, before complete evaluation, unless there is compromise of sensation or circulation distal to the injury, which is indicated by pain, pallor, pulselessness, paralysis, paresthesias, and pain with passive movement. If neurovascular deficits exist, gentle longitudinal traction in line with the extremity should be performed.

Fractures of the femur are usually immobilized with a Thomas splint or Hare or Buck traction.

Arm Splints

Splints commonly used for arm fractures include the following:

Sling and Swathe. A sling and swathe are used for injuries between the sternoclavicular joint and elbow. The arm is placed at 90 degrees of flexion with a sling and immobilized against the chest with a swathe wrapped around the body.

Long-Arm Splint. The long-arm splint is used for injuries between the elbow and wrist, most commonly involving fractures of the forearm and distal radius.

Posterior Long-Arm Splint. The posterior long-arm splint is used for elbow and forearm injuries as well as wrist injuries, in which forearm rotation and elbow flexion must be eliminated. The plaster is applied from the dorsal aspect of the mid-upper arm, across the olecranon, and down the ulnar aspect of the forearm to the distal palmar flexion crease. In addition, seven to eight layers of plaster are positioned from the upper part of the humerus across the radial side of the elbow as a cross support. The elbow should be at 90 degrees of flexion with the forearm in neutral position.

Sugar-Tong Splint. The *brachial humerus* splint is applied from above the acromioclavicular (AC) joint, over the humerus, around the elbow, and up to the axillary crease. A collar and cuff provide support. The *forearm* splint goes from the distal palmar flexion crease to the elbow. The plaster is brought around the elbow to the dorsum of the hand just proximal to the metacarpophalangeal (MCP) joints.

Hand and Wrist Splints

Hand and wrist splints are used for injuries between the wrist and the tips of the fingers. In general, the position of function is the "hooded cobra": The wrist is in neutral position (the long axis of the forearm roughly lines up with the long axis of the thumb), the MCP joints are flexed to about 60 to 70 degrees, the interphalangeal (IP) joints are flexed 10 to 20 degrees, and the thumb is widely abducted (p. 543). The tips of the fingers must be visible for neurovascular examination. Other types of hand-wrist splints include the following:

Ulnar Gutter Splint. Ulnar gutter splints are useful for nondisplaced fractures of the fourth and fifth digits. The fourth and fifth fingers should be kept at about 35 to 40 degrees of flexion at the MCP joint and 20 to 30 degrees at the IP joints.

Dorsal Extension Splints. The dorsal extension splint is used for nonrotated finger injuries involving the phalanges, metacarpals, MCP joints and proximal interphalangeal (PIP) joints. A foam-padded aluminum splint is taped to the dorsum of the hand and wrist and bent to keep the MCP joint at 90 degrees of flexion. The PIP joint is bent to 45 degrees.

Thumb Spica. Thumb spicas are used for scaphoid injuries to the wrist, for ligamentous damage, and for injuries to the thumb. Plaster is cut in half longitudinally into two tails. The splint is applied to the radial aspect of the forearm, and one tail is wrapped around the thenar eminence and onto the palm and hand across the distal palmar crease. The second tail is wrapped around the thumb and up to the base of the nail.

Leg Splints

Long-Leg Posterior Splint. For injuries between the knee and ankle, the long-leg posterior splint is applied from the groin to the toes, with the ankle in neutral position of function.

Short-Leg Posterior Splint. The short-leg posterior splint is used for injuries between the ankle and tips of the toes. It is applied from just below the knee over the back of the leg to the toes, with the ankle at a 90-degree angle. The toes must remain visible. A stirrup or air splint, available commercially, provides support along the lateral and medial aspects of the ankle and distal leg.

SPRAINS AND STRAINS

The diagnosis of sprain or ligamentous tears, as an isolated injury, is unusual in children.

A *sprain,* a tear of a ligament joining bone to bone around the joint, is most commonly caused by outside forces, especially contact sports. *Strains* are tears of the muscle or of fascia joining muscle to bone (musculotendinous unit), often resulting from a dynamic injury and usually not a contact sport.

Buckle fractures or epiphyseal injuries, rather than sprains and ligamentous injuries, often occur in young children because of the ease of injury to the epiphysis. However, adolescents do suffer ligamentous injuries.

First-Degree Sprain

First-degree sprain consists of minimal tearing of a ligament. There is point tenderness with neither abnormal motion nor joint instability and little or no swelling. The patient can bear weight on a leg with a first-degree sprain.

Second-Degree Sprain

Second-degree sprain consists of appreciable tearing of a ligament (5% to 99% of fibers disrupted). There is point tenderness with moderate loss of function and variable presence of abnormal motion and joint instability. Weight bearing is painful, there is localized soft tissue hemorrhage, and hemarthrosis is present. Pain is evoked by testing of joint stability, and instability may be persistent.

Third-Degree Sprain

In third-degree sprain, there is complete disruption of the ligament surrounding a joint. Extreme pain, loss of function, abnormal motion with absolute joint instability, deformity with tenderness and swelling, and diffuse hemorrhage are present. The patient is unable to bear weight, and there is persistent instability without surgical repair.

The patient may complain of little discomfort after the initial insult, and testing of the stability of the joint may cause little pain. Dislocations may have reduced spontaneously (common in fracture-dislocation of the knee). The only clue may be the patient's unwillingness or inability to bear weight across the joint.

Strains

Strains are classified in a manner similar to sprains. First-degree strains involve minimal tearing of a musculotendinous unit, whereas second-degree strains involve more significant tears. Third-degree strains are marked by complete tears and may initially be painless. Injuries are marked by tenderness and pain, usually accompanied by no evidence of joint instability.

Management

Elevation, ice, and analgesia may reduce symptoms of strains and sprains. Splint immobilization may be used after x-ray studies have excluded a fracture and before consultation for second- and third-degree injuries. Support and crutches may be helpful.

EPIPHYSEAL FRACTURES (Fig. 66-1)

A long bone can be divided into four parts. The first part is the shaft of the bone, known as the *diaphysis.* The second part, the *metaphysis,* is adjacent to the growth plate. The third part is the *growth or epiphyseal plate,* a radiolucent horizontal line near the end of the bone where longitudinal growth occurs. The fourth part, the *epiphysis,* is the end of the bone near a joint; it is separated from the metaphysis by the epiphyseal plate.

Five types of epiphyseal fractures are identified by Salter and Harris, with the risk of growth disturbance lowest with a type I fracture and highest with a type V fracture.

Type I

Type I epiphyseal fracture consists of separation of the epiphysis from the metaphysis without displacement or injury to the growth plate. There is tenderness and pain at the point of the growth plate without other findings. The x-ray film result is initially normal but films obtained 7 to 10 days later may show calcification and new bone formation at

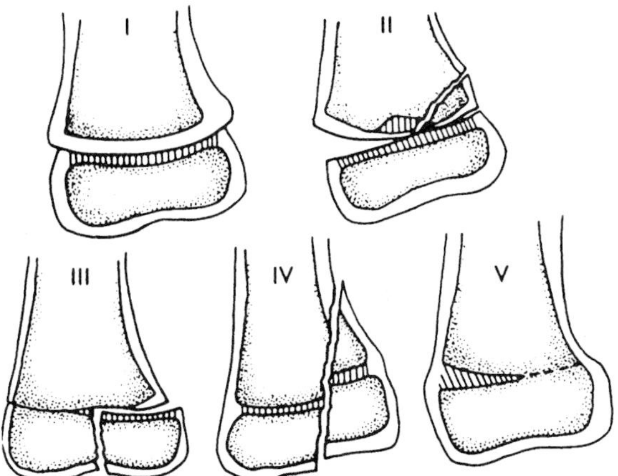

Fig. 66-1 Epiphyseal fractures: Salter classification.

the site of injury. The fracture should be immobilized for 3 weeks. Growth disturbance is rare.

Type II

Type II fracture consists of an epiphyseal plate slip with fracture through the metaphysis, producing a triangular metaphyseal fragment. It is the most common type of fracture. Treatment is achieved with a closed reduction and immobilization for 3 weeks (upper extremity) to 6 weeks (lower extremity). Growth disturbances are rare.

Type III

Type III epiphyseal fracture consists of an epiphyseal plate slip with an intraarticular fracture involving the epiphysis. The most common site is the distal tibial epiphysis. Accurate reduction (often surgical) with maintenance of blood supply is essential to reducing the risk of growth disturbance.

Type IV

In type IV epiphyseal fracture, an intraarticular fracture extends through the epiphysis, epiphyseal plate, and metaphysis. The lateral condyle of the humerus is the most common site. It requires surgical open reduction and internal fixation, and the prognosis for growth is guarded.

Type V

Type V epiphyseal fracture consists of a crush injury to the epiphyseal plate, producing growth arrest. It usually occurs in joints that move in one plane (flexion-extension), such as a knee, when a force in another plane is applied (abduction or adduction), such as smashing into an automobile dashboard or a direct-crush injury. The x-ray film may initially be normal. Despite treatment (no weight bearing for 3 weeks), the prognosis for normal growth is poor. Therefore, this type of injury must be treated with immobilization and early follow-up. Parents must be advised of growth problems the fracture will cause. Early orthopedic consultation is vital.

OPEN FRACTURES

Open fractures need immediate treatment unless life-threatening injuries supersede. It is important to note how much bone is exposed and whether it is comminuted, the severity of soft tissue damage, and the extent of contamination and bleeding. The only clue to an open fracture may be the collection of blood with fat globules from what is thought to be a small puncture wound. Regardless of the exposure of bone, the injury should be considered an open fracture and cleaned, debrided, sampled for culture, covered, and immobilized. A sterile dressing soaked in antiseptic solution is applied to the wound. Tetanus toxoid or antitoxin should be given, when appropriate (p. 734). Therapy with cefazolin (Ancef), 75 to 125 mg/kg/24 hr q6-8hr IV, should be initiated, with an initial dose of 25 to 50 mg/kg IV. Anaerobic coverage may have to be considered.

The goal is to convert an open wound to a clean, closed wound as much as possible before definitive surgery.

BIBLIOGRAPHY

Berde CB, Lehn BM, Yee YD et al: Patient controlled analgesia in children and adolescents: a randomized, prospective comparison with intramuscular administration of morphine for post-operative analgesia, *J Pediatr* 118:460, 1991.

Cramer KE: Orthopedic aspects of child abuse, *Pediatr Clin North Am* 43:1035, 1996.

England SP and Sundberg S: Management of common pediatric fractures, *Pediatr Clin North Am* 43:991, 1996.

Hodge D III: Management principles: musculoskeletal and soft tissue injuries. In Barkin RM, editor: *Pediatric emergency medicine: concepts and clinical practice,* ed 2, St Louis, 1997, Mosby.

Kennedy RM, Porter FL, Miller JP et al: Comparison of fentanyl/midazolam with ketamine/midazolam for pediatric orthopedic emergencies, *Pediatrics* 102:956, 1998.

67 Upper Extremity Injuries

CLAVICULAR FRACTURE

Clavicular fracture is the most common fracture in children, including newborns. It may be associated with chest or shoulder trauma. In preschool children it is usually a greenstick fracture, with middle-third fracture most common.

Mechanism of Injury

A fall or blow to the shoulder or extended arm is the common cause.

Diagnostic Findings

1. Pain on movement of the affected arm or shoulder.
2. Fracture most common in middle third of clavicle.
3. Tenderness and, possibly, deformity at the point of fracture. Comparison examination of the normal contralateral side may be useful.
4. Possible injury of the subclavian vessels. It is important to examine for this possibility. Clues include the presence of an unusual amount of swelling or ecchymosis, pulse changes, and occasionally a bruit over the involved vessel, which may radiate down the arm or to the heart.

X-Ray Film. A clavicular anteroposterior (AP) view is indicated. If x-ray findings are negative but there is a strong clinical suspicion of fracture, a 30-degree cephalic view may be useful.

Management

1. Fractures should generally be immobilized for 3 to 6 weeks in a figure-of-eight splint to maintain abduction of the shoulder. A commercial clavicular strap or a strap made of tubular stockinette filled with felt or cotton padding may be used. A sling may provide additional comfort. Some clinicians believe that there is little significant difference in the outcome between treatments with a figure-of-eight splint and a simple sling, the latter avoiding the potential complication of brachial plexus palsy. Remember:
   - **a.** Prevent skin maceration by placing a powdered pad in the axilla.
   - **b.** Tighten to maintain abduction of the shoulder (occasional adjustment may be necessary).
   - **c.** Observe frequently for axillary artery or brachial plexus compression.
   - **d.** Caution parents that a residual bump will develop as the clavicle heals, which will subside in 6 to 12 months.
2. Fractures of the distal (outer) tip of the clavicle should be treated as acromioclavicular separations.
3. A simple sling may avoid distraction of the pieces of fractures of the proximal (inner) third.
4. Follow-up visits every 2 to 3 weeks, with further radiographs to assess callus formation when clinical healing is achieved.
5. Orthopedic referral if there is neurovascular or soft tissue compromise.

ACROMIOCLAVICULAR SEPARATION

Acromioclavicular separation is partial to complete disruption of the acromioclavicular (AC) ligaments.

Mechanism of Injury

Falling or a blow to the point of the acromion of the shoulder produces the injury.

Diagnostic Findings

1. Tenderness over the AC articulation
2. Limited abduction of the arm
3. In third-degree separation, stepoff with upward displacement of the clavicle, representing complete rupture of the sternoclavicular and costoclavicular ligaments

X-Ray Film. An AC joint view is indicated. Traditionally, this view is obtained initially without weights; some authorities obtain weight-bearing films if findings of the first film are normal. Comparison views of the other shoulder are necessary in all but third-degree separations. AC separation is classified as follows:

1. *First-degree:* no evidence of displacement or joint subluxation
2. *Second-degree:* with weight bearing, there is less than 1 cm of upward displacement of the distal clavicle, indicating partial subluxation
3. *Third-degree:* with weight bearing, there is more than 1 cm of upward displacement

With the increasingly conservative approach to even the most significant AC injuries, some clinicians have suggested that weight-bearing films are no longer essential, preferring the following new classification:

1. *First-degree:* less than 3-mm (or less than 50%) increase in AC joint width compared with the uninjured side, and normal coracoclavicular (CC) distance (less than 5 mm or less than 50% difference between injured and uninjured sides)
2. *Second-degree:* 3-mm or greater (or greater than 50%) increase of AC joint width compared with the uninjured side, and normal CC distance
3. *Third-degree:* 5-mm or greater (or 50% or more) increase of CC distance compared with uninjured side, with or without AC widening and with or without clavicular elevation

Management

1. First- and second-degree separations need immobilization with sling and swathe or shoulder immobilizer and follow-up with an orthopedist.
2. For third-degree separation, orthopedic consultation in the emergency department (ED) is needed.

SHOULDER DISLOCATION: ANTERIOR

Anterior dislocation accounts for 95% of cases of shoulder dislocations.

Mechanism of Injury

A blow to or fall on the arm while it is in external rotation, abduction, and extension produces this dislocation.

Diagnostic Findings

1. Prominent acromion process with flattening of the deltoid muscle
2. Head of the humerus palpable anterior, inferior, and medial to the glenoid fossa
3. Limitation of abduction and absence of external rotation

Complications

1. Fracture of greater tuberosity or other bones secondary to manipulation
2. Associated abnormality of the glenoid (labrum detachment, tear of anterior capsule and subscapularis muscle, or Hill-Sachs lesion, the latter representing a compression fracture of the posterior humeral head)
3. Compromise of axillary nerve (lack of sensation over the lateral portion of the shoulder and upper arm with deltoid muscle palsy) and distal blood vessels

X-Ray Films. AP and axillary views are indicated. The humeral head lies inferior to the coracoid process. Fractures should be excluded. Postreduction x-ray films may reveal a fracture that either was not seen initially (prereduction) or is secondary to reduction.

Management

1. Provide intravenous narcotic analgesia and muscle relaxation for patient comfort; also optimize the patient's condition for reduction. Morphine, 0.1 mg/kg/dose, or meperidine, 1 mg/kg/dose, may be used with diazepam (Valium), 0.1 mg/kg/dose, as discussed in the Appendix to Chapter 65.
2. Reduction of dislocation:
   - **a.** With the patient prone and the involved arm and shoulder hanging in a dependent position over the table, have the patient hold a weight (about 1 lb of weight per 7 kg of body weight). Reduction is usually achieved in 20 to 30 minutes. With younger children, the weight may have to be taped.
   - **b.** In older children, especially when it is desirable to avoid large doses of opiates (e.g., long trip from the point of injury to definitive medical care), or in recalcitrant dislocations, an alternative reduction technique is to help the child reach behind the head (as if to scratch the head). Then, with an assistant supporting the trunk, apply outward traction in the line of the long axis of the humerus while pushing the head of the humerus up into the fossa using pressure applied in the axilla.
   - **c.** Another method is to have the child sit and have an assistant apply countertraction with a sheet by pulling with the sheet from the axilla toward the child's opposite shoulder. Then reduce the shoulder with a gentle, constant traction in a longitudinal manner with the shoulder abducted approximately 45 degrees. If this is unsuccessful, the abduction may be increased to 90 degrees while traction is maintained.
   - **d.** Scapular manipulation has been used as well, with either of two approaches:
     - **(1)** With the patient prone and the arm hanging down, exert traction on the affected extremity scapula manipulated by pushing the inferior tip medially, using thumb pressure while stabilizing or laterally rotating the superior aspect.
     - **(2)** Two-person approach: With the patient seated, the unaffected shoulder is placed against an immobile support such as a wall or the raised head of a stretcher. Facing the patient, one person grasps the wrist of the patient's affected side and slowly raises the arm to the horizontal plane. Firm but gentle forward traction is applied, with counterbalance provided by placing the palm of the extended free arm over the patient's midclavicular region. The force required in applying the traction is not great. Once traction is applied, the other person manipulates the scapula as described in (1).
3. Other considerations:
   - **a.** The arm should be examined by physical assessment, and x-ray films should be taken before and after reduction.
   - **b.** After reduction, treat any fractures. These often require surgery.
   - **c.** Have patient use a sling and swathe or shoulder immobilizer (splinted in internal rotation) for 4 weeks to allow the capsule to heal.
   - **d.** There is a 70% recurrence rate for anterior shoulder dislocation in patients younger than 20 years. Surgery may be required.

SHOULDER DISLOCATION: POSTERIOR

Posterior dislocations are uncommon.

Mechanism of Injury

Violent internal rotation motion of the shoulder, such as a seizure or electrical shock, or direct trauma to the shoulder joint when the arm is outstretched can produce a posterior dislocation.

Diagnostic Findings

1. The patient is unable to abduct or externally rotate the arm.
2. The affected shoulder is flat anteriorly or full posteriorly. There is a defect in the position of the humeral head, which is felt as a vague prominence behind and below the acromion. The injury may be bilateral.
3. There may be associated fracture.

X-Ray Films. The AP view may be normal, but the dislocation is apparent on an axillary or transthoracic view. The humeral head may overlie the glenoid rim. Prereduction and postreduction x-ray studies should be obtained.

Management

1. Muscle relaxation and analgesia are usually required, sometimes necessitating general anesthesia.
2. Reduction of dislocation:
   a. Orthopedic consultation is advisable.
   b. Exert pressure on the posterior aspect of the shoulder joint with the arm in external rotation.
   c. Two-person approach: One person applies traction along the long axis of the humerus while it is in 45 degrees of abduction or backward extension with the elbow flexed to 90 degrees; the second person then pushes on the humeral head from behind.
   d. Reduction techniques used for anterior shoulder dislocation may also be used.
3. Other considerations:
   a. Treat any associated fractures after reduction.
   b. Reexamine by physical assessment and x-ray film after reduction.
   c. Immobilize with sling and swathe for 4 to 6 weeks.

ROTATOR CUFF INJURY

Mechanism of Injury

Strenuous shoulder motion, such as in throwing, heavy lifting, or falling on the shoulder, causes injury to the rotator cuff.

NOTE: The rotator cuff ("SIT": *s*upraspinatus, *i*nfraspinatus, and *t*eres minor) stabilizes the shoulder in the glenoid fossa in abduction and allows the shoulder to abduct and externally rotate.

Diagnostic Findings

1. Severe pain worsening with attempts at abduction or external rotation. Abduction of the shoulder may not be possible. Passive range of motion of the shoulder joint may be normal.
2. Tenderness over the insertion of the rotator cuff into the tuberosities.
3. Tear may be only partial, with painful, weak abduction and a lack of endurance.

X-Ray Films. AP and lateral views of the shoulder may be normal or show a fracture of tuberosity. If significant with persistent weakness, magnetic resonance imaging (MRI) scan demonstrates soft tissue shoulder joint injury.

Management

1. Treat minimal tears with initial immobilization while maintaining good passive range of motion. Give analgesia.
2. Large tears need surgical intervention after confirmation of diagnosis. Early repair also is required in cases of an avulsion fracture of the tuberosity.

BRACHIAL PLEXUS INJURY

Mechanism of Injury

The brachial plexus can be injured by traction during delivery, particularly in a large baby born to a nulliparous mother. This injury may also result from major trauma, such as a fall from a height or a motor vehicle accident, whereby traction forces the head and neck laterally and the shoulder is forced downward.

Diagnostic Findings

1. The patient holds the arm loosely at the side of the thorax in internal rotation with extension of the elbow, pronation of the forearm, and flexion at the wrist.
2. There is swelling in the region of the shoulder.

X-Ray Films. Upper extremity and clavicle views are indicated to exclude a fracture of the clavicle or humerus, or shoulder dislocation. Cervical spine injury is also a consideration.

Management

1. Prescribe physical therapy to prevent contractures.
2. Consider neurosurgical consultation.

Most children injured during birth have at least partial recovery by 18 months of age; injury in older children may respond less fully.

SCAPULAR FRACTURE

Mechanism of Injury

Severe blunt trauma produces scapular injuries.

Diagnostic Findings

1. Swelling and localized tenderness are seen.
2. Severe associated injuries to the head, neck, and intrathoracic structures are possible because of the force required to produce this injury.

X-Ray Films. Scapular views are indicated. A chest x-ray film and other indicated studies are important in cases of severe trauma (see Chapter 56).

Management

A sling and swathe are indicated after caring for other injuries. Orthopedic follow-up is recommended.

PROXIMAL HUMERAL EPIPHYSEAL FRACTURE

Mechanism of Injury

Blunt trauma to the arm or shoulder may cause the fracture.

Diagnostic Findings

1. Shoulder deformed by pain and tenderness
2. Possible associated neurovascular injury

X-Ray Films. A Salter type II epiphyseal slip is most commonly seen. With infants, a Salter type I slip may be found. Such fractures may be classified from the amount of displacement.

Management

1. Treat separation (<1 cm) with angulation of less than 40 degrees and absence of malrotation with a shoulder immobilizer or sling and swathe. Greater angulation requires closed reduction.
2. Surgical correction is needed for three-piece fractures; four-piece fractures often require replacement with a prosthesis.
3. Arrange orthopedic consultation.

HUMERAL SHAFT FRACTURE

A middle-third fracture is the most common humeral fracture.

Mechanism of Injury

1. Spiral fractures result from a twisting motion. Consider nonaccidental trauma when a young child presents with this injury.
2. Transverse fractures result from a direct blow.

Diagnostic Findings

Tenderness with or without deformity is noted.

Complications. Complications are associated with arterial and radial nerve injury, particularly middle- or distal-third humeral shaft injuries. Sensation (first dorsal web space) and motor function (extension of wrist and metacarpophalangeal [MCP] joint) should be assessed.

X-Ray Films. AP and lateral views of the humerus, including the shoulder and elbow, are indicated.

Management

1. In the younger child with minimal displacement and angulation, sling and swathe immobilization may be sufficient. In the older child, immobilization in a long-arm (sugar-tong) splint from the axilla to the wrist with flexion of the elbow at 90 degrees may be required; place arm in a sling and swathe.
2. Radial nerve involvement mandates early and frequent reassessment. Splint patients in position of function. May need traction or surgical repair to release entrapped radial nerve.

CONDYLAR AND SUPRACONDYLAR FRACTURES OF DISTAL HUMERUS

Condylar and supracondylar fractures of the distal humerus are the most common fractures of the elbow in children younger than 8 years.

Mechanism of Injury

1. A fall on the outstretched hand with the elbow extended or a fall on the flexed elbow
2. May also occur from snapping force, as in throwing a baseball too hard

Diagnostic Findings

1. Tenderness and deformity of the distal humerus. Distal fragment displaced upward, posteriorly, and medially.
2. Pain with flexion of the elbow.
3. May have associated dislocation of the elbow (see next section).
4. Lateral condyle fracture is more common than medial type, which is commonly associated with ulnar nerve injury.

Complications

1. Nerve injury is associated with 20% of supracondylar fractures.
2. Pain with extension of fingers is an early sign of Volkmann's ischemia, which results from a volar compartment syndrome of the forearm, leading to permanent hand disability.
3. In addition to neuromuscular complications, condylar fractures pose a risk for malunion and nonunion.

X-Ray Films. AP, lateral, and possibly oblique views are indicated. Posterior displacement is recognized by extending a line down the anterior of the cortex of the distal humerus on the lateral x-ray film. Normally, this line intersects the middle third of the capitellum. With posterior displacement accompanying a supracondylar fracture, the line intersects anterior to the capitellum or the anterior third.

A subtle sign of a nondisplaced fracture is the "fat pad sign." The sign is nonspecific and reflects hemorrhage into the elbow joint. This sign may be related to injury of the radial head, capitellum, trochlear, olecranon, or coronoid process. The fat pad sign is an area of radiolucency seen on the lateral x-ray view of the elbow just above the olecranon process posteriorly or above the radial head anteriorly. The *posterior fat pad sign* is of greatest importance because it predicts an occult fracture of the elbow; anterior sign may be seen normally (see next section on posterior elbow dislocation).

Management

1. Orthopedic consultation in the ED. Urgency of treatment reflects the extent of displacement and neurovascular status.
   a. Early reduction if necessary, and immobilization with the elbow held at 90 degrees of flexion. Test radial pulse before and after flexion.
   b. If there is any question of neurovascular compromise, immediate reduction is mandatory (traction, supination of the forearm, and flexion with direct pressure to align the displaced segment).
   c. Open reduction may be required with condylar fracture.
2. Hospitalization. Neurovascular compromise must be closely monitored for at least 24 hours. Patients with undisplaced

supracondylar fractures may be monitored as outpatients if flexion is adequate and good follow-up and observation are feasible.

ELBOW DISLOCATION: POSTERIOR

Posterior dislocation of the elbow is the second most common dislocation in children.

Mechanism of Injury

A fall on a hyperextended arm causes the dislocation.

Diagnostic Findings

There is obvious deformity, swelling, and effusion. The two epicondyles and the tip of the olecranon normally form an isosceles triangle. In a dislocation, the sides of the triangle are unequal, whereas in a nondisplaced supracondylar fracture, they remain equal.

There may be associated fracture, often supracondylar (see preceding topic).

Complications

Neurovascular compromise is common. There is nerve injury (median) in as many as 5% to 10% of patients.

X-Ray Films. AP, lateral, and oblique views of the elbow are indicated. There may be an associated fracture. A posterior fat pad sign is pathognomonic of elbow injury (dislocation, fracture, or possibly a sign of spontaneous reduction of elbow). An anterior fat pad sign may be normal or pathologic (see condylar and supracondylar fractures of distal humerus).

Management

1. Administer analgesia and sedation (p. 527 and Appendix to Chapter 65) and possibly muscle relaxation (diazepam [Valium]) (p. 515).
2. With the patient prone and the arm in a dependent position over the edge of the bed, apply gentle traction, with guidance of the olecranon process into normal position.

   NOTE: A trapped medial epicondyle fracture, which requires open surgery, must be ruled out.
3. Order postreduction x-ray films, and perform a physical examination to check neurovascular and motor function and to exclude fractures.
4. Immobilize the arm in a splint with the elbow flexed 90 degrees for 14 to 16 days. Test the radial pulse before and after flexion.
5. Arrange for close follow-up to monitor range of motion and to exclude compartment syndrome and myositis ossificans.
6. Arrange for orthopedic consultation in the ED.

RADIAL HEAD DISLOCATION OR SUBLUXATION (NURSEMAID'S ELBOW)

Dislocation or subluxation of the radial head occurs more often in younger (<5 years) than in older children. Recurrent radial head subluxation occurs frequently, with patients 24 months or younger at great risk.

Mechanism of Injury

1. Sudden longitudinal pull on the forearm while the arm is pronated
2. Reported after rolling over in children younger than 6 months

Diagnostic Findings

1. The arm is in passive pronation. The child usually will not move the arm.
2. Resistance to the pain with full supination.
3. Pain over the head of the radius.
4. In rare cases, the anterior dislocation of the radial head is associated with a fracture of the proximal ulna *(Monteggia's fracture)*.

X-Ray Films. Radiographic findings are usually normal. X-ray diagnosis is usually not required unless the mechanism of injury is unusual, the physical findings are atypical, or the arm does not become rapidly asymptomatic after attempts at reduction. In fact, if prereduction films are obtained, reduction is usually achieved by the radiology technician in the process of supinating the forearm for the films.

1. A line drawn on the x-ray film along the proximal shaft of the radius should pass through the capitellum. If it does not, there is a dislocation.
2. If x-ray films are obtained, the forearm should be evaluated to rule out Monteggia's fracture.

Management

Orthopedic consultation is usually unnecessary.

1. Reduce the dislocation or subluxation by supinating the forearm while feeling the head of the radius (anulus) and, in a continuous motion, flexing the elbow. There is usually a palpable click over the radial head.
   a. The patient should be asymptomatic after 5 to 10 minutes, although if the subluxation has been present for several hours, return of function may take 6 to 12 hours.
   b. Patients in whom symptoms do not rapidly subside should undergo x-ray study.
2. An alternative reduction technique is to pronate the forearm with flexion at the elbow.
3. A sling is usually not required except for comfort.
4. After reduction in a patient with Monteggia's fracture, the forearm is casted in neutral position with flexion of more than 90 degrees at the elbow; the cast remains for at least 6 weeks. Orthopedic consultation should be obtained for this fracture.

RADIAL HEAD FRACTURE

Mechanism of Injury

A fall on an outstretched hand produces a fracture of the radial head. This injury is relatively uncommon in children.

Diagnostic Findings

1. There may be tenderness over the radial head.
2. Injury may be associated with supracondylar, olecranon, or epicondyle fracture.
3. Compartment syndrome of the forearm has been described with minimally displaced or angulated radial head fractures.

X-Ray Films. AP and lateral views are indicated.

Management

1. For nondisplaced fracture: long-arm splint, including immobilization of wrist, and a sling.
2. If more than one third of the articular surface is displaced, excision is needed. Angulation does not require reduction with displacement of less than 20 degrees. With greater angulation, reduction is required to prevent limitation of movement.

DISTAL-THIRD FRACTURES OF RADIUS AND ULNAR

Fracture of the distal third of the radius and ulna is common in school-age children and adolescents.

Mechanism of Injury

A fall on the palm of the hand or a blow to the forearm causes forearm fractures.

Diagnostic Findings

There is swelling and tenderness over the fracture site.

1. If a single bone is fractured and there is overriding, radial head dislocation with fracture of the proximal ulna *(Monteggia's fracture)* or a distal radioulnar dislocation with radial fracture *(Galeazzi's fracture)* is present.
2. *Torus fracture:* common in children—a buckling or angulation of the cortex with no actual fracture line. A torus fracture is usually seen in the metaphyseal area.

3. *Greenstick fracture* involves the diaphysis of a long bone—a fracture of one side of the cortex.
4. *Colles' fracture:* transverse fracture of the distal radius with dorsal angulation and loss or reversal of volar tilt of distal radial articular surface; patient may have an accompanying fracture of the ulnar styloid. Usually, a Salter type II epiphyseal injury.
5. *Smith's fracture:* fracture of distal radius with increase in the volar tilt of the distal radial articular surface; the reverse of Colles' fracture. Caused by a blow on the dorsum of the wrist or distal radius with the forearm in pronation.
6. *Barton's fracture:* marginal fracture of the dorsal or volar surface of the radius with dorsal or volar (corresponding to involved surface) dislocation of the carpal bones and hand.
7. *Hutchinson's or chauffeur's fracture:* fracture of the radial styloid process secondary to direct trauma or from impact of the styloid process against the navicular bone. Typically nondisplaced.

Occasionally, median or ulnar nerve injury occurs, with self-limited neuropraxia.

Management

Rotational deformities must be eliminated. Fractures that are angulated more than 15 degrees (especially proximal) in children lead to decreased function. The potential for longitudinal bone growth depends on the distance of the fracture from the growth plates, especially the distal plate, where 80% of forearm growth occurs. Most pediatric distal forearm fractures can be treated nonoperatively. The fracture should be immobilized for 4 to 6 weeks. If both the radius and ulna are broken or dislocated, alignment is more difficult to attain and hold; therefore surgical stabilization may be necessary. Indirect or limited open reduction with fixation tools, such as Kirschner's wires, is very successful, as is open reduction with internal fixation.

Torus Fracture. It is immobilized for 4 to 6 weeks in a long-arm splint.

Colles' Fracture

1. Reduce by traction in the line of the deformity to disimpact the fragments; follow with pressure on the dorsal aspect of the distal fragment and volar aspect of the proximal fragment. Also apply pressure on the radial aspect of the distal fragment to correct radial deviation.
2. Test for reduction by palpation, lack of recurrence of deformity, and x-ray film.
3. Immobilize the hand in maximum ulnar deviation, the wrist neutral, and the forearm in full pronation. (If the fracture was markedly displaced, immobilization in supination may be helpful.) Use anterior and posterior splints wrapped in place or an immediately bivalved cast. The cast should extend from the knuckles to the midhumerus. Some orthopedists prefer a short-arm cast. Once swelling resolves, a circular cast may be applied.
4. Ensure that there is no neurovascular compromise.
5. Consult with an orthopedist in the ED.

Smith's Fracture

1. Reduce by applying longitudinal traction until the fragments are distracted. Supinate and apply dorsal pressure on the distal fragment.
2. Immobilize the arm with an anterior and posterior (sugar-tong) splint, with the forearm in supination and the wrist in extension.
3. Consult with an orthopedist in the ED.

Barton's Fracture. Open reduction is usually required.

BIBLIOGRAPHY

Chacon D, Kissoon N, Brown T et al: Use of comparison radiographs in the diagnosis of traumatic injuries with the elbow, *Ann Emerg Med* 21:895, 1992.

Cheng JC, Shen WY: Limb fracture pattern in different pediatric age groups: a study of 3350 children, *J Orthop Trauma* 7:15, 1993.

Hendley GE: Necessity of radiographs in the emergency department management of shoulder dislocations, *Ann Emerg Med* 36:108, 2000.

Hendley GW, Kinlaw K: Clinically significant abnormalities in post reduction radiographs after anterior shoulder dislocation, *Ann Emerg Med* 28:399, 1996.

McDonald J, Whitelaw C, Goldsmith LJ: Radial head subluxation: comparing two methods of reduction, *Acad Emerg Med* 6:715, 1999.

McNamara EM: Reduction of anterior shoulder dislocation by scapular manipulation, *Emerg Med* 21:1140, 1993.

Schunk JE: Radial head subluxation: epidemiology and treatment of 87 episodes, *Ann Emerg Med* 19:1029, 1990.

Skaggs D, Mirzayan R: The posterior fat pad sign in association with occult fracture of the elbow in children, *J Bone Joint Surg* 81-A:1429, 1999.

Skaggs D, Pershad J: Pediatric elbow trauma, *Pediatr Emerg Care* 13:425, 1997.

Snyder HS: Radiographic changes of radial head subluxation in children, *J Emerg Med* 8:265, 1990.

68 Hand and Wrist Injuries

Hand and wrist injuries are common in children, and it is imperative to recognize their extent. A seemingly benign injury, if inappropriately managed, can lead to significant functional deficit. Historical data must include the time and mechanism of injury, defining whether it was a crush or puncture wound, whether it is dirty or clean, whether there is tissue loss, the location of the injury, whether it is the patient's dominant hand, immunization status, allergies, history of previous hand injuries, and if possible, a subjective description of motor and sensory deficits.

The physical examination is often more difficult because of decreased cooperation by the frightened child as well as the size of the structures. Skin, nerves, vessels, tendons, bone, joints, and ligaments must be evaluated. The nomenclature of the fingers is thumb, index, long, ring, and little fingers. The bones of the hand are depicted in Fig. 68-1.

BASIC HAND EXAMINATION

Hand examination must be systematically and rapidly performed.

Observation

Observe the hand at rest, looking for tendon injuries and obvious deformities. Fingers on flexion should normally point toward the scaphoid tubercle. If they deviate, there is a rotational injury. Digital cyanosis and capillary filling should be assessed.

Sensation

The hand should be observed for sweating, which should be present if the digital nerve (sympathetic) is intact. Finger skin should wrinkle in warm water. This does not require the active participation of the young or intoxicated patient. Systematically assess sensation:

1. Radial nerve: dorsal thumb–web space
2. Median nerve: tip of the index finger
3. Ulnar nerve: tip of the little finger

Sensation distal to the injury should be examined. Two-point discrimination is particularly useful. It can be performed by determining discrimination at 8-mm separation, using a paper clip.

Motor Function

Each tendon should be checked individually for function in the fingers and as part of the group in the hand and wrist:

1. Flexor digitorum profundus: Stabilize the proximal interphalangeal (PIP) and metacarpophalangeal (MCP) joints while asking the patient to flex the distal interphalangeal (DIP) joint.
2. Flexor digitorum sublimis: Hold the fingers extended and ask the patient to flex only the PIP joint. Some clinicians recommend that for testing of the small finger, the index and longer fingers can be held extended, and the MCP joints of the ring and small finger can be flexed at least 45 degrees. The PIP joints of the ring and small fingers are flexed to test the flexor function.
3. Extensor tendons: Extend each joint individually.
4. Flexor tendons: Flex each joint individually.

The following nerves should be checked:

1. Radial nerve: Have the patient extend the wrist and the digits at the MCP joints.

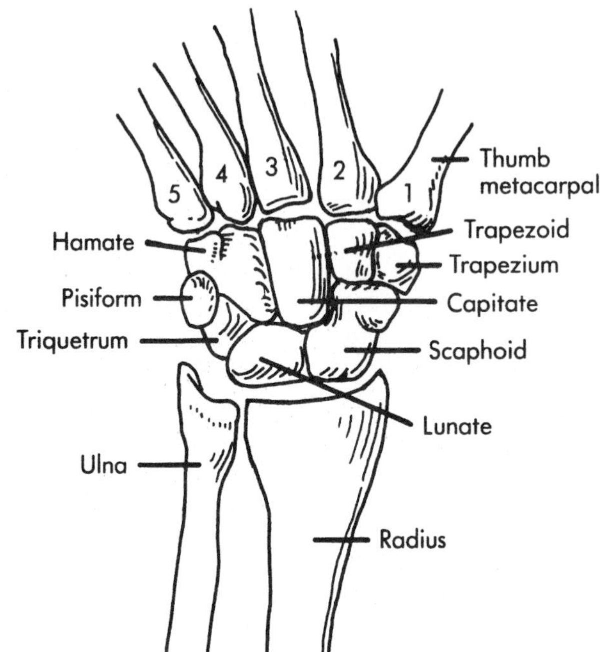

Fig. 68-1 Normal carpal bones.

(From Rosen P et al: *Diagnostic radiology in emergency medicine*, St Louis, 1992, Mosby.)

2. Median nerve: Have the patient point the thumb upward or pinch the tips of the thumb and little finger together.
3. Ulnar nerve: Interossei muscles are tested by having patient abduct and adduct the long finger from the midline.

Other Considerations

1. If there is injury around a joint, check it for stability.
2. X-ray films are useful in showing fractures, foreign bodies, and air in the joint. A true anteroposterior view (AP) and a lateral view of involved digits must be obtained, with the fingernail used as a landmark.
3. Fractures of the hand or wrist are less common in children than in adults. In children, fractures usually heal rapidly because of the thick periosteum. Surgical repair is rarely needed, and early functional use is essential.
4. Distal radius point tenderness and a decrease of 20% or more in grip strength is associated with a fracture.

PERILUNATE DISLOCATION

Mechanism of Injury

A fall on an outstretched hand produces the dislocation.

Diagnostic Findings

There is pain and tenderness in the wrist, possibly accompanied by minimal swelling or deformity.

X-Ray Films. On a lateral radiograph, the long finger metacarpal, capitate, lunate, and radius normally line up in a straight line, and the lunate and navicular form an angle no greater than 50 degrees. This normal alignment is disrupted with a dislocation. A true lateral x-ray film is necessary because dislocation is easily missed on an AP view (Fig. 68-2).

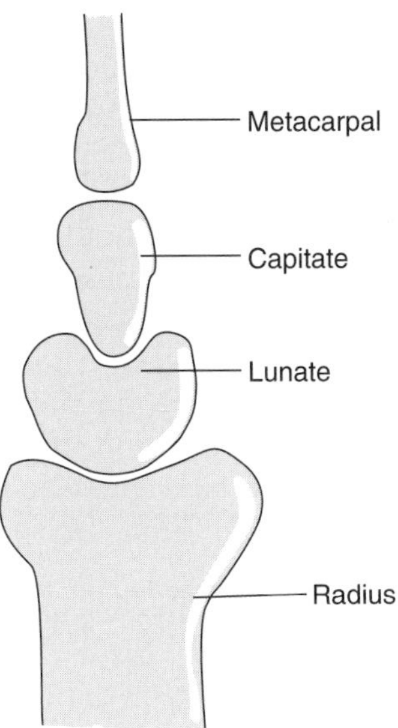

Fig. 68-2 Normal wrist lateral view. The long finger metacarpal, capitate, lunate, and radius normally line up. If the lunate is dislocated, this alignment is disrupted.

If the dislocation is missed, the patient will have long-term disability. Thus, the injury must not be passed off as a sprain.

Management

1. Immediate orthopedic consultation should be arranged.
2. Open reduction is often required.

NAVICULAR (SCAPHOID) BONE FRACTURE

Fracture of the navicular bone is the most common carpal fracture as well as the orthopedic injury most commonly misdiagnosed in the emergency department (ED). Other fractures of the carpal bones are rare in children.

Mechanism of Injury

Falling on an outstretched (dorsiflexed) hand results in navicular fractures.

Diagnostic Findings

1. Tenderness over the anatomic snuffbox and clinical suspicion. The scaphoid compression test may be more sensitive than presence or absence of snuffbox tenderness. For the test, inward longitudinal pressure is applied along the axis of the thumb metacarpal. Pain in the wrist suggests scaphoid tenderness.
2. Decrease in grip strength.

X-Ray Films. A study of the wrist, including the navicular view, is indicated. The x-ray findings may be normal, but if the patient has clinical snuffbox tenderness, the injury should be treated as a fracture.

Management

Nondisplaced fracture should be treated with a long-arm cast, which includes the thumb, MCP joint, and elbow. Immobilization lasts for 7 to 8 weeks unless no fracture was seen on the initial x-ray film, in which case the wrist should be reevaluated by x-ray examination in 7 to 10 days.

Even though nonunion and avascular necrosis of the navicular bone are rare in children, it is wise to have an orthopedist monitor the child. If the fracture is displaced, an orthopedic consultation should be obtained in the ED.

METACARPAL BONE FRACTURE

Mechanism of Injury

A direct blow to the hand produces fracture of a metacarpal bone.

Diagnostic Findings

1. Swelling and point tenderness
2. Deformity with displacement (extent of rotation and angulation must be assessed)
3. Types of fracture:
   a. *Boxer's fracture*: fracture of the little finger's metacarpal head. Patient usually has good functional result with up to 35 to 40 degrees of volar angulation.

   b. *Bennett's fracture*: fracture of the thumb metacarpal base into the joint. Unusual in children.

X-Ray Films. AP and lateral views of the hand are indicated.

Management

1. Immobilize the hand and arm for 3 to 4 weeks with splinting (often casting) from the midforearm to the distal phalanges. Splint the MCP joint at 45 to 90 degrees of flexion (to prevent MCP contracture) with the wrist in extension.
2. Once the fracture is reduced and immobilized, recheck the fracture with x-ray examination to ensure that rotation and alignment have been corrected.
3. Bennett's fractures, even if reduced, usually need internal fixation to hold reduction because of the opposing forces of the abductor pollicis longus and adductor pollicis muscles.

In general, more deformity is tolerated in the metacarpals of the ring and little fingers than in those of the thumb and index and long fingers.

PHALANGEAL FRACTURE

The phalanx is the bone most commonly fractured in children.

Mechanism of Injury

There is a direct blow to the tip of the finger, such as being caught in a car door.

Diagnostic Findings

1. Swelling and point tenderness of the phalanx.
2. Deformity with displacement. On flexion, the fingernails normally point toward the scaphoid tubercle. If they do not, there may be a rotational injury.

X-Ray Films. AP and lateral views are indicated. A true lateral view of the individual digits must be obtained, with the fingernail used as a landmark.

Management

1. With fracture of the middle or distal phalanx, immobilize the phalanx of the involved digit and the neighboring digit in a finger splint. If involved, the long and ring fingers should always be splinted together because their lumbricales are mutually dependent.
2. If the proximal phalanx is fractured, use a dorsal splint that incorporates the wrist at 30 degrees of extension, the MCP joint flexed at 30 to 50 degrees, and the interphalangeal (IP) joint flexed at 10 to 15 degrees.
3. For open and intraarticular fractures, with or without displacement, that involve a large portion of the joint space, refer the patient to a hand or orthopedic surgeon.
4. Rotational or angulation deformities are difficult to correct and require orthopedic consultation. A fracture of the phalangeal neck is a transverse fracture through the neck of either the proximal or middle phalanx. Maintaining reduction is difficult, and loss of reduction may be functionally significant.
5. Epiphyseal fractures usually occur in the proximal phalangeal base of the little fingers—usually Salter type II fractures. They require reduction and splinting to a neighboring phalanx, with flexion at the joint. Open reduction is required for complete separation of the epiphyseal plate.

FINGER DISLOCATION

In children, ligaments and capsular structures are stronger than epiphyseal plates. Trauma that might dislocate a finger in an adult may instead produce a fracture in a child. Dislocations are rare in children.

Mechanism of Injury

There is a blow to the tip of the finger that produces a dislocation.

Diagnostic Findings

1. Obvious deformity and tenderness at the joint
2. Swelling and inability to flex the finger
3. Complex dislocation if the MCP joint involved:
   a. Phalanx displaced on metacarpal—not at 90 degrees, as in a simple dislocation, but more parallel, with slight displacement and less angulation
   b. Dimpling of palmar skin

X-Ray Films. X-ray films should be obtained before reduction is attempted because there may be an underlying fracture. Dislocated bones are usually at 90 degrees to each other.

A complex fracture has widened joint space and parallel position. The sesamoid bone may be in the joint space, a finding that often signifies the need for surgery.

Management

1. Refer the patient to an orthopedist.
2. Reduce the dislocation by hyperextending the joint while pushing the distal bone over into position from above. Do not pull. Immobilize the finger for 1 to 2 weeks.
3. After reduction, check for ligamentous instability, and immobilize the finger with splinting for 1 to 2 weeks.

BOUTONNIÈRE DEFORMITY

Boutonnière deformity is a rupture of the central slip of the extensor tendon at the PIP joint, with volar subluxation of the lateral bands.

Mechanism of Injury

A direct blow or laceration produces a boutonnière deformity.

Diagnostic Findings

1. Tenderness and swelling over the dorsal PIP joint may make diagnosis clinically difficult.
2. The distal IP joint is held in extension, whereas the proximal IP joint is held in flexion.

X-Ray Film. Fracture should be excluded by x-ray study.

Management

If fracture is not present, splint the finger in extension, and arrange for follow-up with a hand surgeon. Patients seen days after injury without treatment probably need surgical repair.

MALLET FINGER

Mallet finger is a fracture of the base of the distal phalanx with disruption of the extensor tendons at the DIP joint. It is common in adolescents and may be a Salter type III epiphyseal injury. Younger children typically have a Salter type I or II injury.

Mechanism of Injury

There is blunt trauma, such as a blow to the tip of the finger from a softball or football that strikes the finger ("jammed finger").

Diagnostic Findings

1. The patient is unable to extend the distal phalanx because of terminal slip rupture, laceration of the terminal slip, or an avulsion fracture.
2. There is tenderness and swelling of the DIP joint.
3. The finger is held with the distal phalanx flexed.

X-Ray Films. AP and lateral views of the digit are indicated. These views may show a chip fracture of the distal phalanx at the DIP joint.

Management

1. Fracture involving less than 25% of the joint surface (without subluxation) is splinted in hyperextension, and the patient is referred for follow-up. The finger may be splinted on either the dorsal or the volar surface, but the tape must be

changed daily while the fingers are held in extension. Use foam and aluminum splints.

2. With fracture of more than 25% of the joint surface or a subluxed joint, operative reduction and fixation are required.
3. In older adolescents, injury may occur without fracture and the finger may be splinted with the DIP joints in hyperextension. Strict immobilization for 6 weeks is necessary.

GAMEKEEPER'S THUMB (SKIER'S THUMB)

Gamekeeper's or skier's thumb consists of injury to the ulnar collateral ligament of the thumb.

Mechanism of Injury

There is hyperextension of the MCP joint of the thumb (a common ski-pole injury, with a fall on an outstretched hand that is clasping the pole).

Diagnostic Findings

1. Swelling and tenderness over the ulnar aspect of the MCP joint of the thumb with increased pain on radial deviation of this joint
2. Laxity of the joint with stressing

X-Ray Films. AP and lateral views are indicated to exclude an avulsion fracture of the proximal phalanx.

Management

1. Apply a thumb spica splint with the thumb in extension; splint remains in place for 6 weeks. Arrange for follow-up with a hand surgeon.
2. With stress instability greater than 30% to 45%, initial surgical repair is needed.

LACERATION

See also Chapter 65.

Diagnostic Findings

1. Evaluate the wound to determine the depth of injury and involvement of underlying tissues, including vessels, nerves, muscles, tendons, ligaments, bones, and joints.
2. Sensation and motor function must be specifically tested, with focus on the three major nerves (radial, median, and ulnar) as well as sensation distal to the injury. Two-point discrimination is particularly useful. Each tendon must be evaluated. Consider the stance of the fingers when the tendon was lacerated (p. 543).

Management

1. Use direct pressure and elevation to obtain hemostasis. Never use a clamp, hemostat, or deep suture. If extensive bleeding is associated with a finger laceration, an excellent field tourniquet can be achieved by cleansing the patient's finger and then slipping the hand into a sterile glove, snipping the end of the glove on the involved finger, and then rolling back the finger of the glove to provide exposure and tourniquet. Devices are also available commercially. Careful scrubbing is then done.
2. After sensory examination, infiltrate the wound with lidocaine (Xylocaine) without epinephrine to facilitate cleansing and laceration repair. Epinephrine-containing medications should *not* be used. Slow infiltration and buffered lidocaine reduce pain (see Appendix to Chapter 65).
3. Partial tendon tears may or may not cause functional deficits; tears with deficits as well as complete lacerations require referral. Partial tendon lacerations may be associated with pain on use of the tendon, decreased tone (often with altered stance), weakness, or evidence of laceration of the tendon sheath.

Extensor tendon repairs have an excellent prognosis, whereas flexor tendon injuries, even with meticulous surgical technique, have a poorer prognosis.

4. Repair lacerations using either 4-0 or 5-0 nylon (e.g., Prolene, Ethilon, Surgilon) suture material on a P3 needle. Never use deep sutures.

   Do not suture a wound that is more than 8 hours old. Arrange for delayed closure at 48 to 72 hours if indicated.
5. Children require extensive dressing and splints to maintain position and thereby minimize further injury and facilitate repair. Even minor lacerations over joints should be splinted to facilitate healing.

   In children with extensive injuries, particularly when there is associated tendon damage, the best position for splinting is the "hooded cobra": The wrist is in neutral position (long axis of forearm roughly lines up with long axis of thumb), the MCP joints are flexed to about 60 to 70 degrees, the IP joints are flexed 10 to 20 degrees, and the thumb is widely abducted. The first layer of dressing, when required, is a nonadherent material. The second layer maintains the position of the hand and is a noncircumferential, noncompressible material (e.g., fluffs or sponges), mostly occupying the palm and the dorsum of the hand, wrist, and forearm. In the final layer, tension and compression should decrease as one moves from the distal end proximally. A plaster splint of 10 to 15 layers (or fiberglass) may be incorporated into the volar (palmar) side of the dressing.

FINGERTIP INJURIES

Crush injuries are common in children and may be associated with tuft fracture.

Mechanism of Injury

There is a blow to the distal phalanx between two firm objects.

Diagnostic Findings

1. Discoloration, swelling, local tenderness
2. Often, associated subungual hematoma
3. Possibility of associated nail bed injury

X-Ray Films. X-ray films should be obtained to exclude underlying fracture.

Management

1. *Subungual hematoma:* Drain with electric cautery or a red-hot paper clip. Exclude fractures.
2. If there is a laceration, cleanse it thoroughly and use sutures sparingly, with only loose approximation of the skin.
3. If the nail bed is injured, with partial avulsion, or if it is lacerated, the nail should be left on to act as a splint and to protect the nail bed. If the nail is avulsed at the base and there is a transverse fracture of the distal phalanx, there is usually a laceration of the nail bed. Under these circumstances, the nail should be removed and the nail bed repaired to prevent distortion. Use 5-0 fine absorbable sutures (Vicryl, Dexon). Use stint dressing with original nail or aluminum foil between cuticle and nail matrix to prevent adhesions.
4. Distal tuft injuries usually heal without treatment other than good wound cleansing, dressing, and splinting.

AMPUTATION OF FINGERTIPS

Fingertip amputation is common in children.

Management

1. If the subcutaneous tissue is intact, initial cleaning and debridement with a bulky dressing are adequate. It will heal well by secondary intention.
2. If there is partial laceration of the fingertip, it should be loosely approximated. Children heal remarkably well, and little is lost if the tissue becomes necrotic and demarcates and subsequently must be removed.
3. X-ray examination is necessary to ensure that there is no bony involvement. Consult a hand surgeon.

4. Amputation at or distal to the distal half of the fingernail may be treated nonoperatively, with careful cleansing and debridement, covering with ointment and gauze, and immobilization. Antibiotics are indicated if significant contamination is present. Such conservative treatment also may be useful in very distal (distal to insertion of extensor and flexor tendons of distal phalanx) amputations. Obtain consultation.
5. For the completely amputated digit, treatment depends on the availability of microsurgery. Wrap the amputated part in sterile gauze that has been soaked in lactated Ringer's solution, put the part in a plastic bag, seal the bag, and place the bag in iced water. This approach prevents immersion and water-logging. Rapid transport is essential.

WRINGER OR DEGLOVING INJURY

Mechanism of Injury

With a wringer or degloving injury, the involved limb is caught in a roller, producing a crushing friction burn. A shearing force component is added if the individual attempts to pull the hand away. This injury may also be seen when an extremity is run over by a car.

Diagnostic Findings

1. There is swelling of the involved soft tissue area.
2. Fractures are uncommon and depend on the type of force applied. Dislocations may occur.
3. Degloving and crushing injuries may coexist, resulting in deep soft tissue damage.

Complications

1. Extensive hematoma and compartmental swelling are present with neurovascular compromise.
2. Skin slough is common if there is loss of vascular supply or a compartment syndrome.

Management

1. Control swelling by applying a sterile occlusive dressing after cleansing the extremity.
2. Elevate the extremity, and hospitalize the patient for 24 hours of observation.
   - In rare circumstances, with mild injury and assurance of good follow-up and compliance, the patient may be discharged, after reexaminations every 12 hours have been arranged. In such cases, splint the arm.
3. Fasciotomy of the forearm or carpal tunnel decompression may be needed because of neurovascular compromise.
4. Skin graft may be needed.

AMPUTATION OF THE HAND OR ITS PARTS

Management

1. Examine the hand completely. Preserve any viable tissue.
2. Clean the hand, wrap in sterile gauze, soak in lactated Ringer's solution, place it in a plastic bag, seal the bag, and then put it on ice.
3. X-ray the hand to determine integrity.
4. Immediately refer the patient to a center capable of reimplantation.

RING ON A SWOLLEN FINGER

Management

There are several alternative methods of removing the ring:

1. Place a piece of string under the ring. Then, from the distal end of the finger, wrap the string around the finger in close loops. Exert a slow pull on the proximal end, gently pulling the ring distally as the string unwinds.
2. Alternate at 5-minute intervals between soaking the finger in cold water and elevating the fingers. Perform these maneuvers for 30 minutes, and apply oil (mineral or cooking) while the hand is

elevated. Then, with a steady motion, push the ring off the finger.
3. Cut the ring with a ring cutter.

SUBUNGUAL SPLINTER

Management

A splinter under the nail can be removed by gently shaving the nail over the distal end of the splinter until the splinter is exposed. A single-edge razor or scalpel can be used.

INFECTIONS

Felon

Mechanism of Injury. Improper trimming of nails or puncture wound to the volar aspect of the distal phalanx causes felons.

Diagnostic Findings. Swelling, erythema, and tenderness of the volar aspect of the distal phalanx are present.

Management

1. Drainage: Incision can be made at the site of maximum tenderness or laterally, with care taken to avoid the neurovascular bundle. A Penrose drain promotes drainage. Incision and drainage should be carried out before the wound becomes fluctuant, because intercompartmental pressure will produce ischemic necrosis.
2. Elevation and soaks.

Paronychia

Mechanism of Injury. Hangnail or any bacterial inoculum causes irritation, leading to infection.

Diagnostic Findings. There is swelling, erythema, and tenderness alongside the nail, all of which may extend under it.

Management

1. Digital block is essential. Do *not* use epinephrine-containing anesthetics.
2. If infection is relatively acute, lift the cuticle up around the entire nail to relieve pus, and insert a cotton wick to promote drainage. Continue treatment with soaks.
3. If the condition is chronic, excise the medial or lateral edge of the nail to permit drainage. Make a longitudinal cut in the outer portion of the nail, and then grasp the free edge with a hemostat to remove the nail. Cover with petroleum jelly-impregnated gauze.
4. Antibiotics may be used.

Acute Suppurative Tenosynovitis

Mechanism of Injury. Extension of local infection can involve the synovium.

Diagnostic Findings

1. Erythema and tenderness along the tendon sheath, often with maximal pain over metacarpal head.
2. Finger held in flexed position. Passive extension of DIP joint causes severe pain.

Management

1. Hospitalize the patient.
2. Immobilize the entire length of the tendon.
3. Consider incision and drainage by an orthopedist.
4. Give high-dose antibiotics: nafcillin (or equivalent), 100 mg/kg/24 hr q4hr IV, in absence of penicillin allergy.

Palmar (Thenar and Midpalmar) Space Infection

Mechanism of Injury. Extension of a localized puncture wound, laceration, or an animal bite leads to infection.

Diagnostic Findings. Swelling, tenderness, and erythema are present.

Management

1. Hospitalize the patient.
2. Arrange for incision and drainage by a hand surgeon.
3. Administer antibiotics: nafcillin (or equivalent), 100 mg/kg/24 hr q4hr IV, in the absence of a penicillin allergy, unless Gram stain or culture results indicate other choices.

4. Injection injuries from a paint gun usually need decompression by a hand surgeon.

Herpetic Whitlow

Etiology. Herpes simplex I virus is usually acquired from oral lesions.

Diagnostic Findings

1. In contrast to bacterial paronychia, the lesions in herpetic whitlow are more blistered, the exudate is serous, and the pain is described as burning. The lesions may be subungual and difficult to see.
2. Gram staining of the exudate may show giant cells but no bacteria. If the lesion is recurrent, viral cultures are useful.

Complications. Complications of herpetic whitlow are superimposed bacterial infection, recurrence, and a long, indolent course.

Management

1. Splint the involved digit.
2. Oral analgesics may be useful.
3. In general, surgery is avoided because it spreads the infection. However, if the lesions are subungual, incision and drainage with decompression may increase the patient's comfort.
4. Topical acyclovir (Zovirax) 5% ointment may shorten the course and diminish recurrences.

BIBLIOGRAPHY

Bhende MS, Dandrea LA, Davis HW: Hand injuries in children presenting to a pediatric emergency department, *Ann Emerg Med* 22:1519, 1993.

Brook I: Aerobic and anaerobic microbiology of paronychia, *Ann Emerg Med* 19:994, 1990.

Lewis HG, Clarke P, Kneafsey B et al: A 10-year review of high pressure injection injuries to the hand, *J Hand Surg* 23B:479, 1998.

Pershad J, Monroe K, King W et al: Can clinical parameters predict fractures in acute pediatric wrist fractures? *Acad Emerg Med* 7:1152, 2000.

Seaberg DC, Angelos WJ, Paris PM: Treatment of subungual hematomas with nail trephination: a prospective study, *Am J Emerg Med* 9:209, 1991.

Stein A, Lemos M, Stein S: Clinical evaluation of flexor tendon function in the small finger, *Ann Emerg Med* 19:991, 1990.

69 Lower Extremity Injury

PELVIC FRACTURE

Fracture of the pelvis is usually incurred in a patient who is a pedestrian or a passenger in an automobile collision. There are often major associated injuries, and the mortality rate is high.

Mechanism of Injury

Pelvic fracture results from blunt trauma to the pelvic area.

Diagnostic Findings

1. Local tenderness. Excessive movement or crepitus on pelvic rocking or pressure on the symphysis.
2. Because the pelvis is a bony ring, fractures of one part are usually associated with fractures elsewhere in the ring, particularly if the fracture is displaced. The ischiopubic ring follows this ring concept independently.
3. Blood loss. May be significant, with up to 2500 ml of hemorrhage common in adults. Massive retroperitoneal hematoma can occur with shock and vascular collapse.
4. Injuries to the bladder or urethra (see Chapter 64).
   a. If there is blood at the meatus or inability to void with a distended bladder, obtain a retrograde urethrogram before passing a catheter.
   b. If the urethra is intact, perform a cystogram followed by an intravenous pyelogram (IVP).
   c. Hematuria is present in 50% to 60% of patients, but only 10% have significant injuries.
5. Rectal and vaginal examination. Direct vaginal and perineal injuries may occur, or the examination may demonstrate communication with an open fracture.
6. There is a high association between pelvic fracture and head trauma.
7. Infrequently, there are also injuries to the obturator, femoral, or sciatic nerves.

X-Ray Films. Anteroposterior (AP) and frog-leg projections should be obtained. Multiple ossification sites are present in the pelvic ring and must not be confused with a fracture.

Management

1. Manage life-threatening injuries first (see Chapter 56).
2. Initiate intravenous (IV) fluids with normal saline or lactated Ringer's (LR) solution and, shortly thereafter, blood, if indicated. Massive hemorrhage is less common in pediatric pelvic fractures but ultimately determines the mortality rate.
3. Involve general surgery, orthopedic, and urology consultants as needed.
4. Pneumatic military antishock trousers (MASTs) may be helpful in both the initial immobilization of the patient and subsequent therapy. Pediatric MAST suits are available.
5. If profuse bleeding is present, angiography may be required to localize the site.
6. Pelvic fracture in a woman with a gravid uterus presents a major risk of fetal injury and death. Obstetrics consultation is necessary. Fetal distress must be assessed by monitoring scalp pH and heart tones. If evidence of distress is present, an emergency cesarean section may have to be

considered. The mother and child must be cared for at an appropriate institution.

APOPHYSEAL INJURIES OF THE PELVIS

Normal pelvic apophyses, along the inferior aspect of the ischium and the superior aspect of the iliac wing, can mimic nondisplaced avulsion fractures. These apophyses stay open until approximately 21 years of age. Sudden movement involving abduction or adduction of the thigh, as in sprinting, can cause injury to one or more of these apophyses.

HIP FRACTURE

Hip fracture is rare in children.

Mechanism of Injury

A fall onto the hip region with transmission of a large energy force causes a hip fracture.

Diagnostic Findings

1. Leg is externally rotated and shortened.
2. Localized swelling and tenderness are present, with pain on movement of leg.
3. There is a large potential for loss of blood.
4. In children who have severe falls, the hips should be checked for range of motion and pain.

Management

1. Immobilization
2. Orthopedic consultation in the emergency department (ED)

HIP DISLOCATION: POSTERIOR

Posterior hip dislocation is rare in children, and there is usually an associated fracture. Anterior and obturator dislocations are less common.

Mechanism of Injury

Longitudinal forces applied to the knee with the hip and knee in 90-degree flexion and slight abduction (knee hits dashboard in car) produce a posterior hip dislocation.

Diagnostic Findings

1. The leg is shortened, internally rotated, and slightly adducted.
2. There may be associated fractures, especially of the posterior wall of acetabulum, and sciatic nerve injury (10%).

Complication. Avascular necrosis of the femoral head may follow posterior hip dislocation, particularly if reduction is delayed.

X-Ray Films. AP and lateral views of the hip are indicated. A computed tomography (CT) scan of articular surfaces is excellent for spatial resolution.

Management

1. Reduction without delay, preferably by an orthopedist, with the use of spinal or general anesthesia. If transfer of the patient is necessary, with a long transit time, reduce the dislocation to prevent aseptic necrosis. Traction in the line of deformity should be followed by gentle flexion of the hip to 90 degrees and then internal-to-external rotation.
2. Bed rest and long-term follow-up observation are essential.

HIP DISLOCATION: CONGENITAL

Also known as developmental dysplasia of the hip, congenital dislocation of the hip should be diagnosed in infancy, when prognosis for recovery is excellent. The presentation may be variable, reflecting the severity of the dysplasia and the child's age at diagnosis.

Diagnostic Findings

1. Children younger than 6 months may have asymmetries of leg length, skinfolds, and range of motion of the hip. Ortolani's and Barlow's maneuvers are abnormal.
2. An older child in whom the diagnosis has been delayed may limp or may be unable to walk and should be referred to an orthopedist for care. Abduction may be limited.

Complications

1. Limited range of motion may develop with inadequate or delayed treatment.
2. Avascular necrosis of the femoral head may occur.

X-Ray Films. AP pelvis radiographs are indicated in older children. Prior to ossification of the femoral head at 3 to 6 months of age, ultrasonography may be diagnostic.

Management

Orthopedic referral is indicated for intervention and follow-up.

TOXIC SYNOVITIS OF THE HIP

Because of its self-limited nature and its peak in children 3 to 6 years old, toxic synovitis of the hip is also called "transient synovitis." It often follows an upper respiratory tract infection.

Diagnostic Findings

1. Toxic synovitis of the hip is a diagnosis of exclusion.
2. Patient is unable to bear full weight. The child may limp and complain of knee pain (see Chapter 40).
3. Minimal (or no) pain occurs on abduction and external rotation, with variably limited range of motion. It is usually unilateral.
4. Complete blood count (CBC) is usually normal; erythrocyte sedimentation rate (ESR) is normal or slightly elevated.

X-Ray Films. X-ray findings are usually normal or show small effusion.

Management

1. This disorder is self-limited. Symptomatic treatment with ibuprofen, 10 mg/kg/dose q6hr PO, or naproxen, 7.5 mg/kg/dose q12hr PO, and follow-up observation are all that is required.
2. Septic arthritis must be excluded clinically or by arthrocentesis or incision and drainage, if necessary. If there is any question about the diagnosis, the patient should be admitted for evaluation.

LEGG-CALVÉ-PERTHES DISEASE (AVASCULAR NECROSIS OF THE FEMORAL HEAD)

Legg-Calvé-Perthes disease is a common cause of limp in 4- to 10-year-old children.

Diagnostic Findings

1. Hip movement is limited, particularly, internal rotation and abduction. Limp is common (see Chapter 40).
2. Tenderness is found over the anterior capsule.

X-Ray Films. There is widened joint space between the ossified head and acetabulum, progressing to collapse of the head, increased neck width, and head demineralization. Radionuclide bone scintigraphy can evaluate for avascular necrosis of the bone.

Management

1. Bracing and protection of the hip
2. Orthopedic monitoring

EPIPHYSEAL SEPARATION OF THE HEAD OF THE FEMUR (SLIPPED CAPITAL FEMORAL EPIPHYSIS)

Slipped capital femoral epiphysis is usually seen in obese or rapidly growing adolescent boys (12 to 15 years old) and may be bilateral.

Mechanism of Injury

1. Upward blow transmitted through the shaft of the femur.
2. The patient may have no history of trauma.

Diagnostic Findings

1. The leg may be shortened, externally rotated, and adducted. The patient may stand on the toes with the heel off the ground on one side to compensate for the discrepancy in leg length. Pain is felt

with movement. Internal rotation and abduction are limited.

2. Weight bearing is impaired and limp is present (see Chapter 40).
3. There is pain on palpation. Pain may be referred to the knee, groin, or hip.

X-Ray Films. AP and frogleg views are indicated. Widening and irregularity of the epiphyseal plate are noted. If the plate is displaced, it usually is downward and posterior.

Management

1. Surgical reduction and immobilization for 12 weeks are often required.
2. Follow-up observation is important to watch for avascular necrosis of the femoral head.

FEMORAL SHAFT FRACTURE

Mechanism of Injury

A direct blow to the thigh (bumper injury) produces fracture of the femoral shaft.

Diagnostic Findings

1. Swelling, deformity, tenderness, and pain on movement.
2. Impaired weight bearing.
3. Possible significant blood loss, although a transfusion is rarely required.
4. Possible neurovascular compromise.
5. Rare fat embolus, especially with associated injuries of the hip, knee, or pelvis.
6. Epiphyseal-metaphyseal fractures may be the result of child abuse. Spiral fractures, especially in the prewalking child, should raise a concern about child abuse.

X-Ray Films. AP and lateral views to cover entire femur, including hip, are indicated.

Management

1. Immediate reduction of the fracture with Hare or Thomas traction splinting
2. Orthopedic consultation for long-term therapy with traction, external fixation, or internal rod, depending on the age of the child

THIGH MUSCLE INJURY OR MYOSITIS OSSIFICANS

Mechanism of Injury

1. Most commonly, a direct blow to or tear of the muscle is responsible.
2. More common with repetitive trauma.
3. Common in the quadriceps muscle.

Diagnostic Findings

1. Firm mass present in muscle after the acute hematoma phase.
2. Progressive contracture of muscle.
3. With quadriceps muscle involvement, passive knee flexion may be decreased.

X-Ray Films. Early fluctuant calcification is seen in soft tissues, which later becomes mature, woven bone superficial to the periosteum.

Management

1. Avoid reinjury and limit activity until the muscle is pain free and nontender with normal motion. Ambulation using crutches to reduce weight bearing.
2. Obtain orthopedic consultation for long-term therapy.

INJURY TO COLLATERAL LIGAMENT OF KNEE

The medial collateral ligament is most commonly affected.

Mechanism of Injury

A twisting injury or blow to the outer aspect of the knee causes ligamentous injury. A varus stress commonly involves the lateral collateral ligament, whereas valgus stress often injures the medial collateral ligament.

Diagnostic Findings

1. Pain on flexion and palpation.
2. Knee effusion.
3. Pain and instability with varus and valgus stress testing: With the knee extended, stress is applied to one side of the knee joint while counterpressure is applied against the other side:

a. Valgus stress testing, in which a lateral-to-medial force is applied on the lateral aspect of the knee, is used to detect medial collateral ligament stability.
b. Varus stress testing, in which a medial-to-lateral force is applied on the medial aspect of the knee, checks for lateral collateral ligament integrity.

The degree of ligamentous laxity varies, especially in children. Use the other knee for comparison.

X-Ray Films. AP and lateral views of the knee are indicated. Arthroscopy and magnetic resonance imaging (MRI) may be needed.

MANAGEMENT

1. Immobilize with knee immobilizer.
2. Avoid weight bearing.
3. Refer the patient to an orthopedist.

INJURY TO MENISCUS OF KNEE

The medial meniscus is most commonly affected. Meniscus injury is uncommon in children but does occur in adolescents.

Mechanism of Injury

Meniscus injury occurs with a squatting or twisting injury. While the knee is bearing weight and is slightly flexed, a twisting motion is applied. Internal rotation injures the medial meniscus, whereas external rotation damages the lateral meniscus.

Diagnostic Findings

1. Pain on flexion of the joint. The knee may lock in flexion or the leg may not extend fully.
2. Knee effusion, with tenderness over the involved meniscus.
3. McMurray's maneuver: In a supine patient, hold the foot under the arch with one hand, and cup the knee with the other. Flex the knee. Then extend the knee with the leg in internal or external rotation. A clicking or rattling on extension in internal rotation indicates a tear of the lateral meniscus and, on external rotation, involvement of the medial meniscus.

X-Ray Films. AP and lateral views of the knee are indicated. Arthroscopy and MRI may be needed.

Management

1. Orthopedic consultation for immobilization, arthroscopy, and possible removal of the meniscus.
2. Definitive care is needed within 1 to 2 days.

INJURY TO CRUCIATE LIGAMENT OF KNEE

The anterior cruciate ligament is most commonly affected, with injury usually occurring in children older than 8 years.

Mechanism of Injury

Forcible hyperextension or abduction and external rotation of the leg damages the ligament, often in association with acceleration or deceleration.

Diagnostic Findings

1. Patient may feel or hear a pop of the knee if the anterior cruciate ligament is ruptured.
2. Effusion.
3. AP drawer sign: The patient is supine with the hip flexed 45 degrees, the knee flexed 90 degrees, and the foot resting on the table in external rotation. Pushing or pulling produces a sliding motion, indicative of ligamentous injury. If there is increased anterior mobility, anterior cruciate ligament instability is present; if there is increased posterior mobility, posterior cruciate ligament damage has occurred.
4. Lachman's test is the most sensitive test; it consists of testing for the anterior drawer sign with the knee in 15 to 20 degrees of flexion and then anterior stability test.

X-Ray Films. AP and lateral views of the knee are indicated. Small avulsion fragment of tibial spine should be excluded. Arthroscopy and MRI may be needed.

Management

1. Immobilization and orthopedic referral for evaluation for surgical repair
2. With associated tibial spine fracture, hospitalization and orthopedic consultation

PATELLAR DISLOCATION

Dislocation of the patella is most common in adolescent girls.

Mechanism of Injury

1. Internal rotation of the leg or a direct blow to the outer aspect of the knee
2. Rare occurrence with forcible contraction of the quadriceps muscle

Diagnostic Findings

1. Displaced patella palpated lateral to its normal position.
2. Effusion and tenderness over medial collateral ligament and along articular surface of patella.
3. Subluxation of patella usually reduces spontaneously. Sense of knee "giving out" or buckling.
4. The pain can be reproduced when the examiner pushes the patella laterally with the knee flexed at 30 degrees and the foot supported (patellar apprehension).
5. Possibility of associated fracture of medial border of patella or osteochondral fracture of the lateral condyle.

X-Ray Films. AP and lateral views of the knee and tangential (sunrise) view of the patella are indicated.

Management

1. Reduction is achieved by extending the knee and flexing the hip (relaxing quadriceps). Apply slight medial pressure to the patella. Reduction often happens spontaneously.
2. Immobilize the knee in extension for 6 weeks, and have the patient avoid weight bearing.
3. If patellar dislocation is recurrent, the patellar tendon should be surgically reimplanted.

PATELLAR FRACTURE

Mechanism of Injury

Blunt force over the anterior aspect of the knee can fracture the patella.

Diagnostic Findings

1. Effusion and tenderness. Fracture may be palpable.
2. Extension of the knee is limited if the fracture is transverse with complete transection of the extensor tendon. The patient may also lose extensor function as a result of rupture of the patellar or quadriceps tendon or fracture of the tibial tubercle.
3. If the fracture was caused by pressure applied through the femur, such as the knee's hitting a dashboard, posterior dislocation of the hip must also be excluded.

X-Ray Films. AP and lateral views of the knee and tangential (sunrise) view of the patella are indicated.

Management

1. Immobilization of the knee in extension and orthopedic referral
2. Possibility of hospitalization and surgery with complete fracture

DISTAL FEMUR OR TIBIAL PLATEAU FRACTURE

Mechanism of Injury

A direct blow or indirect valgus or varus stress is the cause of a distal femur or tibial plateau fracture.

Diagnostic Findings

A knee effusion is commonly present.

X-Ray Films. AP and lateral views are indicated. Stress films may be needed after consultation with an orthopedist.

Management

Temporary immobilization and referral to an orthopedist are required.

KNEE DISLOCATION

Dislocation of the knee is usually associated with a fracture and is rare in childhood.

Mechanism of Injury

Severe trauma disrupting all ligaments permits the dislocation.

Diagnostic Findings

An obvious deformity of the knee is present.

Complication. Neurovascular compromise is common. With absence of peripheral pulse, immediate reduction (without x-ray studies) is required.

X-Ray Films. AP and lateral views are required before and after reduction if neurovascular status is intact before reduction.

Management

1. Immediate orthopedic referral and reduction, usually with internal fixation
2. Possible immediate vascular consultation

OSGOOD-SCHLATTER DISEASE

Osgood-Schlatter disease is usually seen in active children 11 to 15 years old during a rapid growth period. Boys are more often affected.

Mechanism of Injury

Constant pulling of the patellar tendon on its insertion causes this partial separation of the tibial tubercle. Predisposing factors include patellar malposition and extensor mechanism malalignment.

Diagnostic Findings

1. Localized swelling, pain, and tenderness over the tibial tuberosity
2. Possibility of a partial avulsion of the tubercle

X-Ray Films. AP and lateral knee views are required. The tibial tuberosity is normally irregular in adolescents.

Management

1. Restrict activity in mild cases; immobilize the knee in extension for 2 to 4 weeks for all others.
2. With avulsed fracture, there is a possibility of nonunion or avascular necrosis, requiring surgery at later date.
3. Patients with this disease are best monitored by an orthopedist.

CHONDROMALACIA PATELLAE

Chondromalacia patellae is softening of the patella.

Mechanism of Injury

A fall on a flexed knee or chronic, strenuous exercise such as jogging causes the damage.

Diagnostic Findings

1. Pain after exercise, with a sensation that the knee is grating or giving out
2. Pain when child sits for long periods with the knee flexed or when the patient walks up or down stairs
3. Pain and crepitus with palpation of the patella as it moves over its articular surface

X-Ray Film of Patella. The x-ray findings are normal.

Management

Restriction of activity with strengthening of the quadriceps muscles is indicated. Antiinflammatory agents such as ibuprofen may be useful.

BURSITIS

Inflammation of any of the various bursae around the knee, evidenced by swelling or pain.

Mechanisms of Injury

1. Usual mechanism is overuse.
2. Bursitis may be secondary to direct blow with bleeding into the bursa.

Diagnostic Findings

Localized swelling and tenderness in prepatellar region (for prepatellar bursitis), in distal patellar tendon region (for deep infrapatellar bursitis), in proximal medial tibia (for pes anserinus bursitis), or over the medial joint line (for tibial collateral ligament bursitis).

X-Ray Films. The film is normal.

Management

1. Varies according to location
2. Includes ice, nonsteroidal antiinflammatory drugs (NSAIDs), compression, and restriction of activity
3. Referral to orthopedist for possible aspiration or steroid injection

TIBIAL OR FIBULAR FRACTURE (BOOT-TOP FRACTURE)

Mechanism of Injury

A direct blow or indirect stress to the bone produces a tibial or fibular fracture.

Diagnostic Findings

1. Tenderness, swelling, deformity, and impaired weight bearing.
2. Spiral and oblique fractures are usually located at the junction of the middle and distal thirds, the weakest region of the tibia. Tibial shaft fractures associated with a reciprocal fibular fracture are considered eccentric if the fibular site is subcapital or malleolar in location. Children rarely have an eccentric fibular fracture, perhaps reflecting the greater flexibility of the ligamentous structures anchoring the proximal and distal fibula in children.

Complications

1. Open fractures.
2. Distal neurovascular injuries are common (e.g., compartment syndrome). If the proximal third of the tibia is fractured, there may be injury at the bifurcation of the anterior and posterior tibial arteries.

X-Ray Films. AP and lateral views are indicated. Even if a fracture is not seen on radiographs, epiphyseal separation may have occurred. Toward the end of adolescence, the medial aspect of the distal tibial epiphysis closes first.

Management

1. Isolated fibular fractures are managed with a short-leg walking cast. Undisplaced tibial fractures can be immobilized in a long-leg posterior splint; the patient is told not to bear weight on the leg and is monitored as an outpatient for 4 to 6 weeks. Early orthopedic consultation.
2. Displaced closed tibial fractures require hospitalization for observation of circulatory status. Orthopedic consultation in the ED should be obtained.
3. Open fractures require immediate consultation for surgical cleansing and stabilization.

BIBLIOGRAPHY

Barkin RM, Barkin SZ, Barkin AZ: The limping child, *J Emerg Med* 18:331, 2000.

Ciarallo L, Fleischer G: Femoral fractures: are children at risk for significant blood loss? *Pediatr Emerg Care* 12:343, 1996.

Del Beccaro MA, Champoux AN, Bockers T et al: Septic arthritis versus transient synovitis of the hip: the value of screening laboratory tests, *Ann Emerg Med* 21:1418, 1992.

Eckerwall G, Wingstrand H, Hagglund G et al: Growth in 110 children with Legg-Calvé-Perthes disease: a longitudinal infancy-childhood-puberty growth model study, *J Pediatr Orthop* 5:181, 1996.

Koop S, Quanbeck D: Three common causes of childhood hip pain, *Pediatr Clin North Am* 43:1053, 1996.

70 Ankle and Foot Injuries

ANKLE SPRAIN

Ankle sprain is a ligamentous injury. The talus articulates primarily with the tibia. The medial and lateral malleoli provide horizontal stability. On the medial side of the ankle, the deltoid ligament binds the medial malleolus to the talus and calcaneus. On the lateral side, stability is achieved by three ligaments (anterior talofibular, posterior talofibular, and calcaneofibular ligaments).

Mechanism of Injury

Twisting of the foot produces ankle sprains. Inversion (supination) and eversion (pronation) injuries are more common than plantarflexion and dorsiflexion injuries. Inversion is the most common.

Diagnostic Findings

Local swelling, discoloration, and tenderness with impaired weight bearing are present.

1. Tenderness anterior and inferior to the lateral malleolus (attachment of talofibular and calcaneofibular ligaments) is common with inversion injuries.
2. Eversion injuries damage the deltoid ligament, which is important for ankle stability. Separation greater than 5 mm between the medial malleolus and talus is evidence of deltoid ligament injury. Deltoid ligaments, which almost never tear without associated fracture, have accompanying local tenderness.

X-Ray Films. Anteroposterior (AP), lateral, and mortise views are indicated. With severe sprain, after routine films rule out fractures, the ankle should be stressed to demonstrate stability of the ankle mortise.

Management

1. First-degree (mild sprain): ice and elevation; no weight bearing for 3 to 4 days; once swelling is resolved, passive exercises are started; once patient starts walking, support with ankle wrap or stirrup splint. Early mobilization and weight bearing are acceptable in first-degree sprain.
2. Second-degree (partial tear): immobilization in plaster splint, cast, or stirrup splint for 3 to 4 weeks. Adolescents: no weight bearing; preadolescents: limited activity and use of a short walking cast.
3. Third-degree (complete tear): often requires surgical repair. Refer patient to orthopedic consultant.

ANKLE FRACTURE

Lateral malleolus is the most common type of ankle fracture.

Mechanism of Injury

Usually an inversion or eversion injury is the cause of an ankle fracture.

Diagnostic Findings

1. Swelling, ecchymosis, and tenderness over the malleolus with impaired weight bearing.
2. Pain when the foot is directed toward the tibial surface.
3. Inversion injury produces oblique fracture of the medial malleolus and either horizontal fracture of the lateral malleolus or a tear of the lateral ligament. Eversion injury causes opposite damage.

X-Ray Films

1. AP and lateral ankle views.
2. Mortise view if there is a question of instability.
3. Diagnostic yield from x-ray films is greatest in the presence of localized bone pain.
4. In adults, the predictability of an abnormality is greatest when there is pain near the malleolus and either an inability to bear weight or bone tenderness at the posterior tip or edge of a malleoli. This observation may be applicable in children.

Management

1. Lateral malleolus: immobilization for 4 weeks and no weight bearing.
2. Medial malleolus: immobilization and orthopedic referral. Size of fragment determines therapy.

ANKLE FRACTURE-DISLOCATION

Mechanism of Injury

Severe force applied to the area of the tibiotalar interface causes the fracture-dislocation.

Diagnostic Findings

Obvious deformity and swelling are present.

X-Ray Films

1. AP, lateral, and mortise ankle views
2. Displaced talus (posterior and lateral to the tibia)
3. Prereduction and postreduction films

Management

1. Rapid reduction to reduce swelling and neurovascular compromise
2. Open reduction and internal fixation are usually required for associated fractures

CALCANEAL FRACTURE

Fracture of the calcaneus is associated with a spinal compression injury and with fractures of the hip and knee in as many as 50% of cases.

Mechanism of Injury

A fall from a height on extended legs can produce a fracture of the calcaneus.

Diagnostic Findings

1. Local swelling, tenderness, impaired weight bearing, ecchymosis on the posterior sole of the foot.
2. Frequent associated injuries, especially vertebral.
3. Puncture wounds are discussed in Chapter 65.

X-Ray Films. AP, lateral, and calcaneal views are indicated. Bohler's angle (the angle described by anterior and posterior halves of the superior cortex of the bone) is flattened. Spinal films may be indicated.

Management

Compression dressing, immobilization, and orthopedic consultation are necessary.

SEVER'S DISEASE (CALCANEAL APOPHYSITIS)

Sever's disease is a common entity occurring in children 9 to 11 years old during rapid growth.

Mechanism of Injury

Mechanical stress and excessive tension on the growing calcaneal apophysis cause Sever's disease.

Diagnostic Findings

1. Calcaneal apophysis is very tender to palpation, especially to transverse compression.
2. Achilles–plantar fascia complex may be tight.

X-Ray Films. X-ray films are typically not helpful because the calcaneal apophysis is often fragmented and dense in normal children.

Management

1. Rest the heel.
2. In very symptomatic patients, prescribe a short-leg walking cast for 10 to 14 days.
3. Refer the patient to an orthopedist.

METATARSAL FRACTURE

Mechanism of Injury

The base of the fifth metatarsal is fractured as a result of inversion, with avulsion of the insertion of the peroneus brevis tendon. Fractures of the metatarsal midshaft are usually crush injuries.

Diagnostic Findings

1. Local swelling with impaired weight bearing.
2. March fractures: hairline stress fractures at the base of the metatarsal, often after hiking, jogging, or jumping. Pain is usually over the second, third, or fourth metatarsals. X-ray film findings may initially be normal.

X-Ray Films. AP, lateral, and oblique views are indicated.

Management

1. Immobilization in a posterior short-leg splint or short-leg walker cast for 5 to 6 weeks.
2. March fractures of the fifth metatarsal: wearing of hard-soled shoes or, with significant pain, immobilization in a short-leg walking cast.
3. For displaced fracture, possible surgery. Refer the patient to an orthopedic consultant.

PHALANGEAL FRACTURES

Mechanism of Injury

"Stubbing" of toe on an immovable object produces the fracture.

Diagnostic Findings

Local swelling and tenderness are present over the involved phalanx. Subungual injuries are discussed in Chapter 68.

X-Ray Films. AP and lateral views of the toe are indicated.

Management

The injury is managed by splinting the injured toe to the adjacent toe for 2 to 3 weeks with tape.

DISLOCATIONS OF BONES OF FOOT

Dislocations of bones of the foot are uncommon but may occur at the phalangeal, metatarsophalangeal, talonavicular, subtalar, or tarsometatarsal joints.

Mechanism of Injury

A twisting movement with associated force applied to the foot causes a foot bone dislocation.

Diagnostic Findings

Obvious deformity, tenderness, and decreased motion are characteristic.

X-Ray Films. AP, lateral, and oblique views are indicated.

Management

1. Phalangeal and metatarsophalangeal dislocations can usually be reduced by manual manipulation. After infiltration with local anesthetic, a compression splint is useful for several days before mobilization.
2. Other dislocations require either closed reduction with the patient under general anesthesia or open reduction; the patient should be referred to an orthopedist.

BIBLIOGRAPHY

Annis AH, Stiell IG, Stewart DG et al: Cost effectiveness analysis of the Ottawa ankle rules, *Ann Emerg Med* 26:422, 1995.

Chande VT: Decision rules for roentgenography of children with acute ankle injuries, *Arch Pediatr Adolesc Med* 149:255, 1995.

Griffin LY: Common sports injuries of the foot and ankle seen in children and adolescents, *Orthop Clin North Am* 25:83, 1994.

Plint AC, Bulloch B, Osmond AH et al: Validation of the Ottawa Ankle Rules in children with ankle injuries, *Acad Emerg Med* 6:1005, 1999.

Schnaue-Constantouris EM, Birrer RB, Grisafi PJ et al: Digital foot trauma: emergency diagnosis and treatment, *J Emerg Med* 22:163, 2002.

Wedmore IS, Charette J: Emergency department evaluation and treatment of ankle and foot injuries, *Emerg Med Clin North Am* 18:85, 2000.

XI

Diagnostic Categories

71 Cardiovascular Disorders

Also See Chapters 11 (Chest Pain), 16 (Congestive Heart Failure), 17 (Cyanosis), 18 (Hypertension), 19 (Pulmonary Edema), 23 (Syncope), and 62 (Thoracic Trauma)

Bacterial Endocarditis

Reginald L. Washington

ALERT In high-risk children, blood cultures are diagnostic in patients with a new murmur; treatment for children with predisposing factors should be initiated. Prevention is essential during procedures in patients with increased risks.

Bacterial endocarditis is a microbial infection of the endocardial surface of the heart, most commonly involving a heart valve. The frequency of endocarditis among children seems to have increased in recent years. This change is due in part to improved survival among children who are at risk for endocarditis, such as those with congenital heart disease and hospitalized newborn infants.

Congenital heart defects such as ventricular septal defects, patent ductus arteriosus, aortic valve abnormalities, and tetralogy of Fallot are common underlying conditions in 90% of cases of bacterial endocarditis. A growing proportion of children with endocarditis have undergone previous corrective or palliative surgery for congenital heart disease with or without implantation of vascular grafts, patches, or prosthetic cardiac valves. Infective endocarditis in the absence of congenital heart disease is often associated with central indwelling venous catheters.

In general, congenital cardiac lesions involving high-velocity jets of blood flow, foreign material, or both are associated with the highest risk for the development of endocarditis. Any lesion associated with turbulence of flow, with or without shunting, can be a substrate for endocarditis.

Neonatal endocarditis commonly occurs on the right side of the heart and is associated with a disruption of endothelium or valvular endothelial tissue produced by catheter-induced trauma.

Bacteremia and infective carditis are associated with many predisposing events:

1. Dental cleaning, irrigation, or extractions, particularly with gingival bleeding.
2. Tonsillectomy.
3. Bronchoscopy.
4. Cystoscopy or urethral catheterization.
5. Sigmoidoscopy.
6. Intravenous drug abuse.
7. Manipulation of a suppurative focus.

ETIOLOGY

Bacterial Infection

Endocarditis resulting from bacterial infection is caused by the following organisms:

1. *Streptococcus viridans* in 32% to 43% of cases.
2. *Staphylococcus aureus* is causative in 27% to 33%.
3. The HACEK organisms *(Haemophilus, Actinobacillus, Cardiobacterium, Eikenella,* and *Kingella)* in 5%.

4. *Streptococcus faecalis, Streptococcus pneumoniae, Haemophilus influenzae,* enterococci, and gram-negative organisms in less than 5%.

Culture-negative endocarditis occurs in 5% to 20% of cases. It is commonly due to current or recent antibiotic therapy or a fastidious organism. Diagnosis may require direct culture of the vegetation.

DIAGNOSTIC FINDINGS

Clinically apparent features are related to hemodynamic compromise caused by local involvement of a valve, peripheral embolization (hema- turia or neurologic changes), or immunologic reaction (fever or myalgia). The common clinical and laboratory findings in endocarditis include:

Very common: Fever (87% of patients), positive blood culture results, and elevations in acute inflammatory markers (erythrocyte sedimentation rate [ESR], C-reactive protein). A heart murmur is present in 90% of cases.

Common: Nonspecific symptoms (headache, anorexia, myalgias, malaise), anemia, hematuria, leukocytosis, and rheumatoid factor.

Infrequent: New or changing murmur, congestive heart failure, petechiae, peripheral emboli, splenomegaly (65% of patients), neurologic changes, and echocardiographic vegetations.

Rare: Osler's nodes (small, tender, intradermal nodules in the pads of the fingers and toes), Janeway lesions (painless erythematous hemorrhagic maculae on the palms or soles), Roth spots, and splinter hemorrhages under the nails (uncommon in children).

Persistent fever is almost universal but varies with the responsible organism. Streptococcal endocarditis tends to cause low-grade fevers, whereas *Staphylococcus* produces high spiking fevers. A new or changing murmur can be difficult to elicit, particularly in children with preexisting murmurs. In adults, murmur is now considered a minor criteria in the diagnosis.

Complications

1. Congestive heart failure (CHF) most commonly occurs with the involvement of the aortic or mitral valves. Pericardial effusion is noted in 21% of patients.
2. Neurologic complications occur in 34% of patients, including mycotic, embolic, and cerebral abscesses. *S. aureus* endocarditis presents the greatest risk.
3. Diffuse glomerulonephritis and renal failure resulting from an embolic or immune complex–mediated process.
4. Abdominal viscera from emboli.
5. Progressive cardiac destruction, including mycotic aneurysm, pericarditis, rupture of sinus of Valsalva, obstructive heart disease, acquired ventricular septal defect, and conduction defects.

Ancillary Data

1. A complete blood count (CBC) demonstrates a leukocytosis and mild hemolytic anemia. The ESR is elevated in 71% to 90% of cases. Urinalysis shows microscopic hematuria. An electrocardiogram (ECG) may show prolonged PR interval or bundle block. Chest x-ray findings may be abnormal.
2. Blood cultures are indicated for all patients with fever of unexplained origin and a pathologic heart murmur, a history of heart disease, or previous endocarditis. Because bacteremia in patients with infective endocarditis is usually continuous, it is not necessary to obtain culture specimens at any particular phase of the fever cycle. It is important, however, to obtain adequate volumes of blood for cultures. Usually, three culture specimens are obtained by separate venipunctures on the first day. There is usually no value in

obtaining more than five blood culture specimens over 2 days unless the patient received antibiotic therapy. Because therapy should not be delayed in patients with acute endocarditis, three separate venipunctures for blood culture specimens may be performed over a short time.

3. Echocardiography has become increasingly important in the diagnosis of endocarditis. The improved resolution combined with increased vigilance has resulted in a detection rate as high as 70% to 80%. Transesophageal echocardiography is more sensitive than transthoracic imaging in adults and in patients with prosthetic valves. In younger children, transthoracic imaging and transesophageal echocardiography have equal resolution, but in infants with prosthetic aortic-pulmonary shunts, echocardiographic findings may be normal because the shunt is often difficult to image. Small thrombi on indwelling catheters are common and difficult to distinguish from true vegetations.

MANAGEMENT

Initial stabilization of the cardiac and respiratory status must be achieved immediately with oxygen and therapy for congestive heart failure.

Antibiotics

1. Antibiotics must be compatible with suspected or proven organisms, and the agent may have to be changed once sensitivity data are available. Bactericidal antibiotics are preferred.
2. Antibiotic levels must achieve at least a 1:8 serum-to-bactericidal level at all times. Antibiotic serum levels (peak and trough) and potential toxicity must be constantly assessed.
3. Penicillin-type antibiotics have a synergistic effect with aminoglycosides.
4. *Streptococcal endocarditis on native cardiac valves:*
   a. A 4-week regimen of intravenous aqueous crystalline penicillin G achieves a high cure rate.
   b. A 2-week course of therapy with penicillin, ampicillin, or ceftriaxone combined with gentamicin has become increasingly popular and results in bacteriologic cure rates in up to 98% of adults.
5. *Streptococcal endocarditis on prosthetic cardiac valves or other prosthetic material:*
   a. Penicillin-susceptible strains should be treated for 6 weeks with penicillin, ampicillin, and ceftriaxone combined with gentamicin for the first 2 weeks of therapy.
   b. For patients unable to tolerate beta-lactam antibiotic therapy, a combination of vancomycin for 6 weeks with gentamicin for the first 2 weeks is recommended.
6. *Enterococcal endocarditis on native cardiac valves or prosthetic material:* Enterococcal endocarditis is rare in children. Treatment is difficult because of the relative resistance of enterococci to penicillin and ampicillin and their variable resistance to aminoglycosides and vancomycin. The treatment regimen for native valve endocarditis caused by susceptible strains requires a combination of penicillin G or ampicillin together with gentamicin for 4 to 6 weeks.
7. *Staphylococcal endocarditis on native valves:* Therapy for methicillin-susceptible *S. aureus* endocarditis consists of semisynthetic beta-lactamase–resistant penicillin given intravenously for a minimum of 6 weeks. The addition of gentamicin for the first 3 to 5 days is optimal and may accelerate the killing of the staphylococci.
8. *Staphylococcal endocarditis on prosthetic material:* Staphylococcal endocarditis

on prosthetic cardiac valves or prosthetic materials is usually caused by coagulase-negative staphylococci that are methicillin resistant, especially if the endocarditis develops within one year of cardiac surgery. Treatment should consist of vancomycin plus rifampin with the possible addition of gentamicin.

9. *Gram-negative endocarditis:* The gram-negative bacteria that most often cause endocarditis include the HACEK group of fastidious coccobacilli. The recommended therapy is a 4-week course of ceftriaxone or another third-generation cephalosporin alone or ampicillin plus gentamicin.
10. Fungal endocarditis usually requires a combination of antifungal agent and surgery.
11. Infectious disease consultation is recommended with respect to ideal agents, monitoring, and duration of therapy.

Surgical Intervention

Surgical intervention is indicated for the following conditions:

1. CHF is increasing
2. The infection is uncontrolled by antibiotics
3. The vegetation enlarges during prolonged (4 weeks) therapy
4. New heart block develops
5. Recurrent septic emboli or extensive cardiac destruction appear

If a conduit or prosthesis is present and medical management is not effective, surgical removal and replacement of the conduit or prosthesis may be required for adequate sterilization and control.

Prevention

Endocarditis prophylaxis is mandatory in high-risk patients and recommended in high or moderate-risk patients; risk is determined by the presence of the following conditions (negligible risk is defined as same risk as the general population):

High risk	Prosthetic cardiac valve (including biosynthetic and homograft valves), cyanotic congenital heart disease (i.e. single ventricle, transposition of great arteries, tetralogy of Fallot)
	Prior history of bacterial endocarditis
	Surgically created systemic-pulmonary shunt or conduit
Moderate risk	Other congenital cardiac malformation, not in other categories
	Acquired valvular dysfunction (i.e., acute rheumatic disease)
	Hypertrophic cardiomyopathy
	Mitral valve prolapse with valvular regurgitation and/or thickened leaflet
Negligible risk	Functional or innocent murmurs
	Cardiac pacemakers (intravascular or epicardial)
	Implanted defibrillators or stents
	History of Kawasaki's disease or rheumatic fever without valvular dysfunction

Procedures placing children at greatest risk are noted in Table 71-1. Specific regimens for prophylaxis are outlined in Table 71-2.

DISPOSITION

All patients with bacterial endocarditis must be hospitalized in an intensive care unit (ICU) for monitoring and immediate laboratory evaluation and initiation of antibiotic therapy. Mortality rate, especially with conduits or prosthetic valves, is as high as 50%.

BIBLIOGRAPHY

Brook MM: Pediatric bacterial endocarditis treatment and prophylaxis, *Pediatr Clin North Am* 46:275, 1999.

Committee on rheumatic fever, endocarditis, and Kawasaki's disease of the American Heart Association Council on Cardiovascular Disease in the Young, *Circulation* 105:2115, 2002.

Dajani AS, Taubert KA, Wilson W et al: Prevention of bacterial endocarditis: Recommendations by the American Heart Association, *JAMA* 277:1794, 1997.

Ferrieri P, Gewitz MH, Gerber MA et al: Unique features of infective endocarditis in childhood, *Pediatrics* 109:931, 2002.

TABLE 71-1 Common Invasive Procedures and Antibiotic (Endocarditis) Prophylaxis

Procedure	Endocarditis Prophylaxis Recommended	Endocarditis Prophylaxis Not Recommended
DENTAL PROCEDURES	Dental extractions	Restorative dentistry
	Periodontal procedures	Local anesthetic injections (nonintraligamentary)
	Dental implant placement and reimplantation of avulsed teeth	Intracanal endodontic treatment; postplacement and buildup
	Root canal instrumentation	Placement of rubber dams
	Prophylactic cleaning of teeth or implants where bleeding is anticipated	Postoperative suture removal
		Placement of removable prosthodontic or orthodontic appliances
		Taking of oral impressions
		Fluoride treatments
		Taking of oral radiographs
		Orthodontic appliance adjustment
		Shedding of primary teeth
ORAL, RESPIRATORY, ESOPHAGEAL, OTHER PROCEDURES	Tonsillectomy or adenoidectomy	Endotracheal intubation
	Surgical operations involving respiratory mucosa	Flexible bronchoscopy (without biopsy)
	Rigid bronchoscopy	Tympanostomy tube insertion/removal
	Flexible bronchoscopy with biopsy	Transesophageal echocardiography
		Cardiac catheterization including device placement
		Skin biopsy
GASTROINTESTINAL, GENITOURINARY PROCEDURES	Biliary tract surgery	Gastrointestinal endoscopy without biopsy
	Surgical operations involving intestinal mucosa	Vaginal delivery
	Cystoscopy	Cesarean section
	Urethral dilation	Urinary catheterization without infection
		Circumcision

Data modified from Dajani AS, Taubert KA, Wilson W et al: Prevention of bacterial endocarditis: recommendations by the American Heart Association, JAMA, 277:1794, 1797, 1997.

TABLE 71-2 Prophylactic Regimens for Procedures Associated with Endocarditis

Patient Situation	Agent	Regimen (Maximum Dose)
DENTAL, ORAL, RESPIRATORY TRACT, OR ESOPHAGEAL PROCEDURES		
Standard general prophylaxis	Amoxicillin	50 mg/kg PO 1 hr before procedure (2.0 g)
Unable to take oral medications	Ampicillin	50 mg/kg IM/IV 30 min before procedure (2.0 g)*
Allergic to penicillin	Clindamycin *or*	20 mg/kg PO 1hr before procedure (600 mg)
	Cephalexin *or* cefadroxil *or*	50 mg/kg PO 1 hr before procedure (2.0 g)
	Azithromycin *or* clarithromycin	15 mg/kg PO 1 hr before procedure (500 mg)
Allergic to penicillin *and* unable to take oral medications	Clindamycin *or*	20 mg/kg IV 30 min before procedure (600 mg)*
	Cefazolin	25 mg/kg IM/IV 30 min before procedure (1.0 g)*
GASTROINTESTINAL (EXCEPT ESOPHAGEAL) AND GENITOURINARY PROCEDURES		
High risk	Ampicillin plus gentamicin	30 min before procedure: Ampicillin: 50 mg/kg IM/IV (2.0 g)* plus Gentamicin: 1.5 mg/kg IM/IV (120 mg)* 6 hr after procedure: Ampicillin: 25 mg/kg IM/IV (1.0 g)* *or* Amoxicillin: 25 mg/kg PO (1.0 g)
High risk *and* allergic to penicillin	Vancomycin plus gentamicin	30 min before procedure: Vancomycin: 20 mg/kg IV (1.0 g)* plus Gentamicin: 1.5 mg/kg IV (120 mg)*
Moderate risk	Ampicillin *or*	50 mg/kg IM/IV (2.0 g) 30 min before*
	Amoxicillin	50 mg/kg po (2.0 g) 1 hr before
Moderate risk *and* allergic to penicillin	Vancomycin	20 mg/kg IV (1.0 g) 30 min before*

Modified from Dajani AS, Taubert KA, Wilson W et al: Prevention of bacterial endocarditis: recommendations by the American Heart Association, *JAMA* 277:1794, 1997.
* All IV infusions should be completed 30 minutes before procedure.
IM, Intramuscularly; *IV*, intravenously; *PO*, by mouth.

Myocarditis

Reginald L. Washington

ALERT Cardiac dysfunction after an infectious illness requires rapid evaluation.

Myocarditis is an inflammatory lesion characterized by cellular infiltrate of the myocardium, usually predominantly mononuclear. Because of decreased myocardial contractility, CHF often results. Viral agents are the most common cause.

ETIOLOGY

1. Rheumatic fever (p. 575)
2. Infection:
   a. Viral:
      (1) Enterovirus; coxsackievirus A and B, echovirus, and poliomyelitis

(2) Influenza A and B
(3) Other: mumps, variola, vaccinia, varicella-zoster, rubella, hepatitis

b. Bacterial: diphtheria, β-hemolytic streptococci, meningococci, staphylococci, salmonellae, tuberculosis
c. *Mycoplasma pneumoniae*
d. Fungal
e. Congenital syphilis
f. Parasitic: toxoplasmosis, trichinosis, Chagas' disease

3. Drugs: antibiotics, indomethacin
4. Other: collagen vascular disease, substance abuse

DIAGNOSTIC FINDINGS

The onset is usually gradual and is preceded by an upper respiratory infection (URI) or a "flu-like" syndrome. The early symptoms may mimic those of a severe URI, and only after cardiac decompensation does the diagnosis become obvious. In rare cases, the myocarditis is isolated without preceding illness. The onset may be acute.

Cardiac examination may demonstrate tachycardia with a gallop rhythm, atypical systolic murmur, weak or distant heart sounds, and hepatomegaly. Evidence of CHF with pulmonary edema may be present with tachypnea, wheezing, rale, and respiratory distress. Infants may have nonspecific findings such as poor feeding and irritability.

There are also signs and symptoms associated with the specific etiologic agent or condition.

Complications

1. Congestive cardiomyopathy and CHF
2. Constrictive pericarditis
3. Hemopericardium
4. Cardiac arrest and death

Ancillary Data

1. Chest x-ray film shows cardiomegaly. Pericardial effusion may be present.
2. ECG.
   a. Tachycardia
   b. Decreased QRS complex voltages
   c. Nonspecific elevation of ST segment and flattening or inversion of T waves
3. Arterial blood gas (ABG) analysis, with cardiac decompensation.
4. Echocardiogram reveals dilated cardiac chambers with decreased function. Pericardial effusion may be present.
5. Other studies as indicated by etiologic considerations.

DIFFERENTIAL DIAGNOSIS

1. Infection: pericarditis (p. 574)
2. Autoimmune disease: acute rheumatic fever (ARF) (p. 575)
3. Vascular disorder: congenital heart disease
4. Other: endocardial fibroelastosis, glycogen storage disease

MANAGEMENT

1. Stabilize the cardiac and respiratory status in symptomatic patients.
2. Give oxygen at 3 to 6 L/min to all symptomatic patients. Assess airway patency and initiate intervention if necessary. Monitor ABGs if indicated.
3. Improve cardiac contractility while reducing workloads in patients with CHF (see Chapter 16).
   a. Digoxin may be helpful but must be used with extreme caution because the inflamed myocardium is sensitive, and signs of toxicity appear with low dosages (see Table 16-2). In acute situations, pressor agents (see Table 5-2) may be required.
   b. Vasodilators such as nitroprusside may be used if cardiac function is not improved by digoxin and the preload is adequate.
   c. β-Blocking agents should not be used.
   d. Diuretic therapy: furosemide (Lasix), 1 mg/kg/dose q6-12hr prn IV (see Table 16-3).

4. Dysrhythmia and conduction disturbances are common and need treatment (see Chapter 6).
5. Give antibiotics for defined bacterial causes.

DISPOSITION

The patient should be admitted to the hospital and monitored closely until the cardiovascular status has stabilized. The clinical course may be erratic. A cardiologist should be involved in initial care and follow-up observation.

BIBLIOGRAPHY

Martin AB, Webber S, Fricker FJ et al: Acute myocarditis: rapid diagnosis by PCR in children, *Circulation* 90:330, 1994.

Press S, Lipkind R: Acute myocarditis in infants, *Clin Pediatr* 29:73, 1990.

Pericarditis

Reginald L. Washington

ALERT The possibility of cardiac tamponade must be ruled out.

A broad spectrum of inflammatory diseases involve the pericardium and the pericardial space. Fluid accumulation may rapidly cause cardiac decompensation. Viral and autoimmune causes are most common, although pericarditis is often considered idiopathic.

ETIOLOGY

1. Infection
   a. Viral: coxsackievirus, influenza
   b. Bacterial: *S. aureus, S. pneumoniae,* β-hemolytic streptococci, *H. influenzae, Escherichia coli, Pseudomonas,* and meningococci
   c. Other: fungal, tuberculosis, parasitic
2. Autoimmune: ARF, polyarteritis nodosa, systemic lupus erythematosus
3. Metabolic: uremia
4. Postpericardiotomy syndrome

DIAGNOSTIC FINDINGS

A pericardial friction rub is often associated with sharp, stabbing pain located in the midchest with radiation to the shoulder and neck. The rub is best heard at any point between the apex and left sternal border. It is intensified with deep inspiration and decreased when the patient sits up and leans forward. It is differentiated from pleural friction rubs when the patient holds the breath.

If a pericardial effusion is present, the heart may seem big on percussion, and auscultation reveals distant, muffled heart sounds. Friction rub may be present. The presence of pulsus paradoxus (decrease in amplitude of blood pressure on inspiration—significant if more than 15 mm Hg) indicates at least a moderate accumulation of pericardial fluid. This may indicate a cardiac tamponade, particularly if there is distension of the jugular veins, tachycardia, enlargement of the liver, peripheral edema, and, in rare cases, hypotension. Urgent intervention is required.

1. Dyspnea and fever may be present.
2. Associated signs and symptoms of the causative entity may be present.

Complication

Cardiac decompensation, often from cardiac tamponade, is a common complication of pericarditis.

Ancillary Data

1. Chest x-ray film: Findings vary with the amount of pericardial fluid. As accumulation increases, the cardiopericardial silhouette enlarges, and the contours become obscured, often in the shape of a water bottle. Fluoroscopy demonstrates the absence of pulsations of the cardiac borders.
2. ECG:
   a. ST-T wave elevation with inverted T waves.
   b. Decreased QRS complex and T wave voltages.

3. Echocardiogram: pericardial effusion is diagnostic.
4. CBC, ESR, and cultures as indicated by potential etiologic agents.

MANAGEMENT

Cardiac function must be rapidly assessed, and decompression of the pericardium achieved if necessary. If there is a large volume of pericardial fluid, a pericardiocentesis should be performed for diagnostic and therapeutic objectives (see Appendix A-5).

1. Fluid should be sent for cell count, measurements of glucose, protein, and lactate dehydrogenase (LDH), Gram staining, and culture.
2. Rapid infusion of fluids may be necessary if the removal of pericardial fluid results in hypotension.
3. Resection of the pericardium through a surgical incision is often required after needle aspiration.

Treatment of the underlying disorder should be initiated:

1. Give antibiotics as appropriate for bacterial, fungal, tuberculosis, or parasitic disease. If a bacterial cause is likely and initial Gram stain result is nondiagnostic, initiate nafcillin (or equivalent), 150 mg/kg/24 hr q4hr IV, and cefuroxime, 100 to 150 mg/kg/24 hr q8hr IV (or equivalent), pending culture results. A surgical pericardial window may be required.
2. Dialysis, if uremia is the cause.

Antiinflammatory agents are useful for autoimmune or idiopathic causes. They improve long-term resolution but are not helpful in the immediate situation if there is evidence of cardiac decompensation. Alternative regimens include the following:

1. Aspirin:
   a. Load with 100 mg/kg/24 hr q4hr PO for 1 to 2 days and then reduce the dosage to 60 mg/kg/24 hr q6hr PO for 4 to 6 weeks.
   b. Ideal serum drug level: 15 to 25 mg/dl.
2. Indomethacin, 1.5 to 2.5 mg/kg/24 hr q6-8hr PO (maximum: 100 mg/24 hr), may be used instead of aspirin in older patients.
3. If there is no resolution with aspirin or indomethacin, initiate prednisone, 1 to 2 mg/kg/24 hr q6hr PO, for 5 to 7 days, and slowly taper the dosage. This treatment should be given only in consultation with a cardiologist.

DISPOSITION

The patient should be hospitalized for observation. If there is any evidence of cardiac decompensation, intensive care and evaluation for potential pericardiocentesis are necessary. In rare early cases without evidence of cardiac decompensation, treatment on an outpatient basis with close follow-up may be attempted after a cardiology consultation.

Acute Rheumatic Fever

Acute rheumatic fever is a delayed, nonsuppurative, autoimmune disease occurring as a sequela of group A streptococcal infections. Skin infections do not generally place a child at risk. The incidence of rheumatic fever peaks in 6- to 15-year-old children and is more common in inner cities and black populations. The average annual incidence is declining. However, there has been a resurgence in many areas of the United States.

DIAGNOSTIC FINDINGS

The Jones criteria are the basis for making the diagnosis during the initial attack, which is based on two major manifestations *or* one major and two minor manifestations. Their presence indicates a high probability of ARF, if supported by evidence of a preceding group A streptococcal infection if documented by rising streptococcal antibody levels or a positive throat culture result. A useful mnemonic is "CASES": *c*arditis, *a*rthritis, *S*Q nodules, *e*rythema marginatum, and Sydenham's chorea.

Major Manifestations

1. Carditis: Usually associated with a murmur of valvulitis. New murmur, tachycardia disproportionate to fever, and in rare cases, pericarditis and CHF. Mitral and aortic valves are most commonly involved. Some clinicians believe the diagnosis can be made in the presence of active carditis, even if it is the only manifestation of the initial attack.
2. Polyarthritis: Most common but benign major manifestation. Two or more joints are involved, most commonly the ankles, knees, wrists, or elbows. Usual findings are swelling, heat, redness, severe pain, tenderness to touch, and limitation of motion. Lasts about 4 weeks in untreated patients. Dramatic response to salicylates.
3. Subcutaneous nodules: Variably sized, hard, painless nodes that are rare and are seen most frequently in patients with carditis. Commonly found overlying joints, scalp, and spine. Also seen in rheumatoid arthritis and erythema nodosum.
4. Erythema marginatum: Rapidly spreading, ringed eruption, forming serpiginous or wavy lines primarily over the trunk and extremities. Transient and migratory. The rash is not pruritic or indurated, and it blanches with pressure.
5. Sydenham's chorea: Marked emotional lability with involuntary motor movements. Usually self-limited but may last several months.

Minor Manifestations

1. Clinical findings:
   a. Arthralgia with pain in one or more joints without objective evidence of inflammation. Should not be used as additional criterion if arthritis is present.
   b. Fever (temperature >39° C) present early.
2. Laboratory findings:
   a. Elevations of acute-phase reactants (ESR or C-reactive protein) are usually noted in patients who have polyarthritis or acute carditis. These values are often normal in patients who have chorea alone.
   b. Prolonged PR interval occurs frequently but does not constitute adequate criteria for carditis.
   c. Supportive evidence of group A streptococcal infection. The antistreptolysin O (ASO) titer is the most widely used streptococcal antibody test. Elevated or rising ASO titers provide reliable evidence of a recent group A streptococcal infection. A single titer is considered to be modestly elevated if it is at least 240 Todd units in adults and 320 Todd units in children. A positive culture result is suggestive.

The diagnosis of rheumatic fever can be made without strict adherence to the criteria in three circumstances: chorea, indolent carditis, and recurrent attacks of rheumatic fever.

Complications

1. Cardiac:
   a. Dysrhythmias (see Chapter 6)
   b. Mitral or aortic valvular disease. ARF is the most common cause of chronic aortic regurgitation and aortic stenosis, as well as mitral stenosis
   c. Pericarditis (p. 574)
   d. CHF (see Chapter 16)
2. Rheumatic lung disease: pleurisy or pneumonia
3. Renal disease: glomerulonephritis or interstitial nephritis
4. Recurrence

Ancillary Data

1. CBC, ESR, and C-reactive protein measurement

2. Streptozyme measuring antistreptolysin (ASO), antihyaluronidase (AH), antistreptokinase (ASK), antideoxyribonuclease (ADNase), and antinicotinamide-adenine dinucleotidase (ANA-Dase)
3. Throat culture
4. ECG and chest x-ray film

DIFFERENTIAL DIAGNOSIS

See Chapters 16 and 27.

MANAGEMENT

1. Initial management must focus on cardiac stabilization, if necessary (see Chapter 16).
   a. Digoxin is the drug of choice (see Table 16-2).
   b. Furosemide (Lasix), 1 mg/kg/dose IV, may be useful (see Table 16-3).
2. Acute-phase reactions should be monitored throughout the course of disease for an indication of resolution.
3. Antibiotics should be given to all patients:
   - Penicillin V, 25,000 to 50,000 units/kg/24 hr q6hr PO for 10 days, *or*
   - Benzathine penicillin G alone (or with procaine) in the dosages specified in the following table:

Weight (lb)	Benzathine Penicillin G (units) (Bicillin)
<30	300,000
31-60	600,000
60-90	900,000
>90	1,200,000

4. Antiinflammatory agents:
   a. Aspirin for fever and joint pain:
      (1) Initially give 100 mg/kg/24 hr q4-6hr PO for a maximum of 5000 mg/24 hr.
      (2) Maintain levels at 20 to 25 mg/dl.
      (3) After 1 week, decrease dosage to 50 mg/kg/24 hr q6hr PO for 4 to 6 more weeks of therapy.
   b. Steroids with evidence of carditis or CHF:
      (1) Begin prednisone, 2 mg/kg/24 hr q12-24hr PO.
      (2) After 1 week, decrease to 1 mg/kg/24 hr for 1 week, and begin aspirin at 50 mg/kg/24 hr.
      (3) Taper prednisone dosage over the next 2 weeks.
5. For chorea: Haloperidol, 0.01 to 0.03 mg/kg/24 hr q6hr PO (adult dose: 2 to 5 mg/24 hr q8hr PO), may be useful.
6. Bed rest.
7. Prevention: prophylactic antibiotics:
   - Oral penicillin VK, 250,000 to 400,000 units q12hr PO, *or*
   - Benzathine penicillin (1.2 million units IM) injections every 3 weeks

Prophylactic antibiotics are given indefinitely to patients with cardiac involvement and to those with chorea initially. Patients without cardiac involvement should receive antibiotics for at least 5 years. For penicillin-allergic patients, erythromycin (250 mg PO BID) or sulfadiazine (weight ≤27 kg: 0.5 gm/day PO; weight >27 kg: 1 g/day PO) may be used.

The duration of prophylaxis for persons who have had ARF is as follows:

- Rheumatic fever without carditis: 5 years or until 21 years old, whichever is longer
- Rheumatic fever with carditis but no residual heart disease: 10 years or well into adulthood, whichever is longer
- Rheumatic fever with carditis and residual heart disease: at least 10 years since last episode and at least until 40 years of age, sometimes lifelong

DISPOSITION

1. Admit patients to the hospital for stabilization and initiation of treatment.
2. On discharge, emphasize the importance of prophylactic antibiotics as well as the increased risk of endocarditis for the patient with abnormal heart valves.

BIBLIOGRAPHY

American Heart Association: Guidelines for the diagnosis of rheumatic fever, *JAMA* 268:2069, 1992.

Dajani A, Taubert K, Ferrieri P et al: Treatment of adult streptococcal pharyngitis and prevention of rheumatic fever: a statement for health professionals. Committee on Rheumatic Fever, Endocarditis, and Kawasaki Disease of the Council on Cardiovascular Disease in the Young, the American Heart Association, *Pediatrics* 96:758, 1995.

Kaplan EL, Berrios K, Speth J et al: Pharmacokinetics of benzathine penicillin G: serum levels during the 28 days after intramuscular injection of 1,200,000 units, *J Pediatr* 115:146, 1989.

Lue HC, Wu MH, Wong JK et al: Three versus four week administration of benzathine penicillin G: effects on incidence of streptococcal infections and recurrences of rheumatic fever, *Pediatrics* 975:984, 1996.

Deep Vein Thrombosis

Although uncommon in children and adolescents, deep vein thrombosis does occur in the presence of one of a number of predisposing factors.

ETIOLOGY

Predisposing Factors

1. Trauma: injury to the endothelium:
   a. Leg injury
   b. Pelvic injury
2. Vascular: stasis or reduction in venous return:
   a. Extended bed rest or immobilization
   b. Cyanotic heart disease or CHF
3. Endocrine: hypercoagulability:
   a. Pregnancy
   b. Birth control pills
4. Osteomyelitis
5. Hypercoagulability associated with conditions such as nephrotic syndrome

DIAGNOSTIC FINDINGS

The clinical diagnosis of deep vein thrombosis is unreliable, but several findings should be sought:

1. Leg warmth, tenderness, or swelling.
2. Homans' sign (unreliable): With the patient's knee extended, dorsiflex the foot. Pain or soreness in the calf or increased muscular resistance to dorsiflexion is considered positive for presence of the sign.
3. Pulmonary embolism in the absence of other sources.

Complications

Pulmonary Embolism. Clinically, pulmonary embolism (PE) is accompanied by dyspnea (58% to 81% of patients), pleuritic pain (72% to 84%), hemoptysis (30%), cough (50%), and anxiety. Only 20% of patients have hemoptysis, dyspnea, and chest pain. Physical examination shows tachypnea, tachycardia, rales and increased secondary heart sound (pulmonary component); of these patients, 32% to 58% have evidence of deep vein thrombosis.

There may be few symptoms. The classic triad (hemoptysis, pleuritic chest pain, and dyspnea) is seen in only 28% of patients.

Helpful laboratory tests include the following:

1. ABG analysis may show hypoxia, although 10% to 20% of patients with severe PE have normal ABG findings.
2. ECG may demonstrate nonspecific ST-T changes (SIQ3T3, RV1, S1, S2, S3).
3. Chest x-ray film findings may be normal, or elevated hemidiaphragm, infiltrate, effusion, and segmental or subsegmental atelectasis may be seen.
4. Ventilation-perfusion scan is diagnostic.
5. Definitive diagnosis may require pulmonary arteriography.

Ancillary Data

1. CBC, platelet count, prothrombin time (PT), partial thromboplastin time (PTT) and INR.
2. Venogram (usually indicated only in patients with uncertain diagnosis) to define the location, extent, and age of the thrombus. Doppler ultrasonography and plethysmography are useful techniques that may provide definitive or confirmatory diagnostic information.

DIFFERENTIAL DIAGNOSIS

1. Infection: cellulitis (p. 582)
2. Trauma:
   a. A sudden onset of leg tenderness, redness, swelling, and a palpable venous cord with superficial thrombophlebitis. Pulmonary embolism can occur if the thrombus is in the proximal saphenous vein.
   b. Muscle contusion.
   c. Compartment syndrome.
   d. Torn medial head of the gastrocnemius muscle. History of acute onset of pain during exercise, usually while the patient is up on the toes (basketball, tennis, or skiing).

MANAGEMENT

1. Elevation of the leg.
2. Application of heat packs to the leg.
3. Bed rest.
4. Anticoagulation (an important part of therapy):
   a. Heparin is given as a continuous intravenous infusion:
      (1) Initial dose is 50 units/kg IV.
      (2) Continuous drip is 10 to 15 units/kg/hr IV.
      (3) Goal is to maintain PTT at two times control value.
      (4) Heparin therapy should be given for 7 to 10 days, for the last 4 days, concurrent with the administration of warfarin (Coumadin).
      (5) Antidote: protamine sulfate (1 mg IV for each 100 units of heparin given concurrently; 0.5 mg IV for each 100 units of heparin given in preceding 30 minutes, and so on); maximum: 50 mg/dose.

      NOTE: No heparin effect is present in normal patients 4 hours after cessation of therapy.
   b. Oral warfarin (Coumadin) should be initiated 4 to 5 days after anticoagulation is begun with heparin:
      (1) Dosage is 0.1 mg/kg/24 hr PO (adult: 2 to 10 mg/24 hr PO).
      (2) Dosage should be titrated to maintain PT at two times control value. The international normalized ratio value (INR) is usually monitored.
      (3) Duration of effect is 4 to 5 days.
      (4) Therapy should be continued for 4 to 6 weeks.
      (5) Antidote: vitamin K (infants: 1 to 2 mg/dose IV; children and adults: 5 to 10 mg/dose). Fresh-frozen plasma may be given for a more immediate effect.
   c. Contraindications to anticoagulation therapy are as follows:
      (1) Active bleeding or blood dyscrasia
      (2) Cerebrovascular hemorrhage
      (3) Pregnancy
      (4) Poor compliance
   d. Drugs that interact with warfarin include antibiotics, barbiturates, thyroid medications, prostaglandin inhibitors (aspirin), and alcohol.
5. Fibrinolytics: Their use should be initiated only after consultation with the admitting physician and consulting hematologist.

DISPOSITION

All patients in whom the diagnosis is proven or suspected should be hospitalized, the latter group until diagnostic studies have excluded the diagnosis.

BIBLIOGRAPHY

Bernstein B, Coupey S, Schonberg SK: Pulmonary embolism in adolescents, *Am J Dis Child* 140:667, 1986.

David M, Andrew M: Venous thromboembolic complications in children, *J Pediatr* 123:337, 1993.

Hirsh J: Heparin, *N Engl J Med* 324:1565, 1991.

72 Dermatologic Disorders

Also See Chapter 42 (Rash)

Acne

Acne vulgaris occurs in as many as 85% of children, with the onset between 8 and 10 years of age in 40%. Neonates may demonstrate a self-limited form of acne in the first 4 to 6 weeks of life in response to maternal androgens; this form requires no treatment.

Acne results from outlet obstruction of the follicular canal with accumulation of sebum and keratinous debris. Sebaceous follicles are primarily located on the face, upper chest, and back. Acne is a multifactorial process involving anaerobic pathogens such as *Propionibacterium acnes*.

DIAGNOSTIC FINDINGS

Obstruction of the follicle leads to a wide, patulous opening filled with stratum corneum cells known as open comedones or "blackheads," which are commonly seen early in adolescent acne. Obstruction beneath the opening of the neck of the sebaceous follicle produces cystic lesions known as closed comedones or "whiteheads," which can progress to inflammatory acne with papules, pustules, cysts, and also draining sinus tracts that result in permanent scarring.

MANAGEMENT

Mild to Moderate Acne

Topical keratolytic agents are usually adequate in 80% to 85% of adolescents. These agents inhibit bacterial growth and have a comedolytic and sebostatic effect. The two most commonly used are benzoyl peroxide gel in 5% concentration and retinoic acid 0.05% cream. Either agent may be used once a day, or if there is significant inflammation, retinoic acid cream may be applied to acne-bearing skin in the evening and the benzoyl peroxide gel may be applied in the morning. If necessary, the frequency may be increased to twice a day.

Moderate to Severe Acne

In the presence of marked disease with tremendous inflammation, oral antibiotics should be initiated. Tetracycline, 0.5 to 1 g/24 hr PO, is given for 2 to 3 months until lesions are suppressed. This therapy should not be given to children younger than 9 years or to an adolescent girl who might be pregnant.

Severe Cystic Acne

Severe cystic disease may additionally need treatment with oral retinoids; 13-cis-retinoic acid (isotretinoin [Accutane]) may be started at an initial dose of 40 mg once or twice daily PO. It should not be used in women of childbearing age and requires careful monitoring.

DISPOSITION

All patients may be monitored on a regular basis to ensure compliance with the treatment regimen and to monitor progress. The management is directed at control and not eradication, with a response expected in 4 to 8 weeks.

Atopic Dermatitis (Eczema)

Atopic dermatitis is both an acute and a chronic dermatologic problem, often associated with asthma or allergic rhinitis. There is often a family history of allergic disorders.

DIAGNOSTIC FINDINGS

The severity of the disease varies tremendously. Exacerbations are associated with erythema and edema as well as crusting and weeping. Lesions are often intensely red at the center, gradually tapering out at the periphery and fading into normal skin. Patients have thickened, lichenified skin areas. Some have symmetrically distributed coin-shaped patches of dermatitis, primarily in the extremities. This is called *nummular eczema.*

Intense itching is often present, causing excoriation and secondary bacterial infection. In the absence of acute dermatitis, children with eczema often have dry skin with a fine, gritty feel.

Most children have the initial episode in the first few months of life, with the condition resolving by 2 years of age. Recurrences occur between 5 and 8 years and again at puberty.

The pattern varies with the age of the child:

1. Infants typically have fine, scaly erythematous patches on the extensor surface and face, which are generally symmetric in location but not in severity.
2. Children primarily have symmetric involvement of the flexor surfaces. The lesions may be papules with plaques.
3. Adolescents have dry, scaly lesions over the hands, feet, and genitalia.

Complications

1. Secondary bacterial infection from *Staphylococcus aureus.*
2. Secondary infection from herpes simplex virus (eczema herpeticum).

Ancillary Data

Cultures of the infected sites are useful.

DIFFERENTIAL DIAGNOSIS

Eczema must be differentiated from superficial infections and inflammatory processes caused by the following:

1. Seborrheic dermatitis (p. 595)
2. Contact dermatitis (p. 586)
3. Tinea corporis (p. 586)

Other unusual conditions that may be considered in children are psoriasis (thick, reddened, well-defined plaques with silvery scales on the exterior surface of the arms, legs, and pressure areas), Wiskott-Aldrich syndrome (eczema, thrombocytopenia, purpura, and immunodeficiency), and acrodermatitis enteropathica (zinc deficiency).

MANAGEMENT

Acute Exacerbation

Mild Disease

1. If there is no significant weeping or crusting, hydration is required. This is best achieved by bathing the child in water with an emollient (e.g., Alpha Keri oil) and then applying an emollient such as Eucerin to the involved areas without drying off the youngster. Do not use soap because it is drying; a soap substitute such as Cetaphil cleanser may be used.
2. If there are well-circumscribed areas with marked erythema, hydrocortisone cream 1%, applied four times a day, is useful for short periods and should be applied before the Eucerin.

Moderate to Severe Disease

1. For significant weeping and crusting, hydration is essential. The parent should use the following schedule for 2 to 3 days:
   a. During the day, apply wet compresses (gauze or soft dishtowels) that are damp but not soaking with warm water. Keep them wet and remove them every 5 minutes, reapplying damp ones for a total of 15 minutes of treatment. Repeat three to five times a day.

b. At night, bathe the child. Have the child wear cotton pajamas that are wet (not soaked) with warm water. Then put a pair of dry pajamas over the wet ones. If disease is severe, apply wet dressings over topical steroids at night for 5 to 7 nights.

c. Do not use soap.

2. Topical steroids are usually necessary. They should be applied after the wet-compress treatment, before putting on the child's pajamas.
   a. Fluorinated steroids are particularly effective but should not be used on the face or intertriginous areas:
      (1) Fluocinolone acetonide cream, 0.01% (Synalar)
      (2) Triamcinolone cream, 0.01% (Kenalog)
   b. Hydrocortisone cream (1%) may be used on facial areas.
3. Antipruritic (antihistamine) agents are useful to reduce scratching and may produce some sedation:
   a. Diphenhydramine (Benadryl), 5 mg/kg/24 hr q6hr prn PO (over the counter), or
   b. Hydroxyzine (Atarax, Vistaril), 2 mg/kg/24 hr q6hr prn PO
4. Antibiotics are often indicated if evidence of secondary bacterial infection is present:
   a. Dicloxacillin, 50 mg/kg/24 hr q6hr PO for 10 days, or
   b. Cephalexin (Keflex) or cephradine (Velosef), 25 to 50 mg/kg/24 hr q6hr PO for 10 days
   c. Mupirocin 2% (Bactroban) may be a topical alternative for treatment of small areas of group A streptococcal infection

Ongoing Management

Ongoing management is crucial to minimizing acute problems:

1. Hydration of skin should be maximized with daily baths and with application of Eucerin to the wet skin without drying off the child. If the problem is mild, lubricating creams such as Nivea may be easier to use. Hydration is particularly important in dry areas or areas that are recurrent problems. Some clinicians recommend placing bath oils, such as Alpha Keri, in the water.
2. Use of soap should be discouraged because it is a drying agent. Cetaphil lotion cleanser may be used as a soap substitute.
3. Occlusive ointments such as petroleum jelly should not be used.
4. Fingernails should be kept short to minimize scratching.

DISPOSITION

Most children can be sent home with appropriate management as described previously. Hospitalization is indicated for severe disease, particularly if there is evidence of bacterial infection, eczema herpeticum, or poor compliance, or if the child shows no response to home management.

Parental Education

1. Maintain skin hydration and reduce scratching. Patience and persistence are required.
2. Avoid skin-sensitizing agents that cause contact dermatitis: wool, soaps, chlorine, detergents, etc.
3. Call your physician if any of the following occurs:
   a. There is increasing redness, crusting, pustules, large blisters, or evidence of fever or toxicity.
   b. No response is seen in 2 to 3 days.
4. Follow-up observation is essential. Keep health care appointments.

Cellulitis and Periorbital Cellulitis

Cellulitis is an acute suppurative infection of the skin and the subcutaneous tissue.

TABLE 72-1 Cellulitis: Etiologic Characteristics and Treatment

Etiology	Special Clinical Characteristics	Antibiotics
Streptococcus pneumoniae	Facial	Penicillin G, 25,000-50,000 units/kg/24 hr q4hr IV*; **if PO**: penicillin V, 25,000 units (40 mg)/kg/24 hr q6hr PO
Staphylococcus aureus	Often preexisting break in skin	Nafcillin, 100-150 mg/kg/24 hr q4hr IV; **if PO**: dicloxacillin, 50 mg/kg/24 hr q6hr PO (*or* cephalosporin: cephradine/cephalexin, 25-50 mg/kg/24 hr q6hr PO)
Group A streptococci	Often preexisting break in skin; rapidly spreading erythema, induration, pain, lymphadenitis	Penicillin G, as above
Haemophilus influenzae	Facial; periorbital; purplish swelling; <9 yr	Cefotaxime, 50-150 mg/kg/24 hr q6-8hr, *or* ceftriaxone, 50-75 mg/kg/24 hr q12hr IV, *or* cefuroxime, 50-100 mg/kg/24 hr q6-8hr IV
Anaerobes *(Clostridium perfringens)*	Possibly preexisting injury with necrotic tissue; dirty, foul-smelling, seropurulent discharge	Penicillin G, as above

* If toxic, consider addition of vancomycin, 40 mg/kg/24 hr q6-8hr IV to cover resistant organisms.

ETIOLOGY

Cellulitis is caused by bacterial infection (Table 72-1). Streptococcal organisms are common because the incidence of *Haemophilus influenzae* has decreased as a result of widespread immunizations.

DIAGNOSTIC FINDINGS

The lesions are generally erythematous, with swelling, tenderness, and edema. The edges are indefinite:

1. Common sites of involvement are the face and periorbital region, neck, and extremities.
2. Often, a preexisting break exists in the skin, caused by an animal or insect bite, laceration, abrasion, or chickenpox.
3. The violaceous (purplish) swelling associated with facial cellulitis can be caused by most pathogens, not only H. *influenzae.*
4. *Lymphangitis* appears as red lines spreading rapidly from the focus of infection in the direction of regional lymph nodes. It is most common with group A streptococci.
5. *Erysipelas* manifests as a small deeply erythematous area of the skin; borders are irregular and raised. An elevated advancing edge is painful to touch. The area is indurated, and lymphangitis may be present. Group A streptococci is usually causative.

Often, concomitant fever, malaise, and regional lymphadenopathy are present. Periorbital cellulitis is often accompanied by otitis media and systemic bacterial infection at other sites. Sinusitis, especially ethmoiditis, may be a predisposing condition.

Complications

1. Bacteremia with secondary focus.
2. Infection of underlying joint or bone. Subcutaneous air implies myonecrosis secondary to clostridial infection.
3. Deeper involvement of the orbit (Table 72-2).

Ancillary Data

Although empiric treatment is usually appropriate, additional data are useful when

TABLE 72-2 Periorbital Cellulitis: Differentiating Clinical Features

	CLINICAL FEATURE			
Condition	**Lid Erythema with Swelling**	**Ophthalmoplegia**	**Proptosis**	**Acuity**
Periorbital cellulitis	Common	Absent	Absent	Absent
Orbital cellulitis	Common	Common	Common	Variable
Subperiosteal abscess	Absent	Absent	Lateral	Absent
Orbital abscess	Common	Common	Common	Common
Cavernous sinus thrombosis*	Common	Common	Common	Common

Modified from Barkin RM, Todd JK, Amer J: *Pediatrics* 62:390, 1978.
* Plus papilledema, meningismus, prostration, and cranial nerve involvement.

widespread cellulitis involves the face or periorbital region or in cases of systemic toxicity:

1. Blood culture in the toxic child. Results are commonly positive with facial cellulitis, whereas they are usually negative in patients with extremity cellulitis.
2. White blood cell (WBC) count is elevated with a shift to the left.
3. Needle aspiration of the edge of the lesion with a 23- to 25-gauge (face) or 18-gauge (extremity) needle, after thorough povidone-iodine preparation of the insertion site, may be considered in very toxic children or children without rapid response to appropriate antibiotic management. The needle is inserted at an angle while negative pressure is maintained with a 10 ml syringe. If no material is obtained, 0.5 ml of nonbacteriostatic saline solution is injected, and the material withdrawn. The aspirate is sent for Gram stain and culture. Aspiration of periorbital cellulitis should be performed only if the edge extends beyond the orbit.
4. Urine counterimmune electrophoresis (CIE) may be a useful diagnostic adjunct, if results of Gram stain and culture are negative.
5. Computed tomography (CT) scan of the orbit may be necessary to determine the extent of the infection, thereby differentiating periorbital or preseptal cellulitis from deep orbital cellulitis. Evaluation of the sinuses may be useful in excluding an accompanying sinus infection.

DIFFERENTIAL DIAGNOSIS

Infection

1. Erysipelas is an infection with acute lymphangitis of the skin that must be differentiated from less invasive group A streptococcal infections. There is erythema with marked induration. The margins are raised and clearly demarcated. Fever, vomiting, and irritability may be present.
2. Osteomyelitis or septic arthritis is difficult to differentiate from simple cellulitis. Bone scans and aspiration are useful.
3. Lymphadenitis or abscess (particularly cervical) may have an overlying cellulitis. With appropriate treatment, the cellulitis resolves rapidly, leaving a clearly defined lymph node. Abscesses should demonstrate fluctuance.
4. Periorbital or preseptal cellulitis must be distinguished from other infections of the orbit (see Table 72-2). Spread to deeper structures is rare. Although the CT scan gives a definite answer about the extent of involvement, the physical examination should delineate the structures involved.

Allergy

Insect bites may cause a tense, warm, erythematous area. The history of insect exposure, presence of an entry point, and partial response to antihistamines is helpful in differentiation of allergy from cellulitis.

Trauma

After known or unknown trauma, contusions or hematomas may develop. In addition, environmental stresses such as hypothermia (frostbite), sunburn, and chemical burns may produce tissue injury.

MANAGEMENT

Antibiotics are the major form of treatment for cellulitis. The choice of antibiotics must reflect the likely etiologic agents, the immunization status of the child, the toxicity of the patient, and the involved site as well as results of Gram stain and culture of the needle aspirate. A total treatment course of 10 days is required, often with a combination of parenteral and oral medications.

1. Patients with only a localized cellulitis (not involving the face and with no evidence of systemic toxicity) can usually be treated as outpatients with antibiotics chosen on an empiric basis:
   a. Dicloxacillin, 50 mg/kg/24 hr q6hr PO, or cefazolin (Ancef) or cephradine (Velosef), 25 to 50 mg/kg/24 hr q6hr PO for 10 days
   b. For lymphangitis consistent with a group A streptococcal infection, penicillin alone: penicillin V, 25,000 units (40 mg)/kg/24 hr q6hr PO for 10 days
2. Patients with systemic toxicity or facial involvement need parenteral therapy. If the organism is unknown, the following guidelines are used:
   a. For patients younger than 9 years with toxicity or with large areas of involvement or facial location:
      (1) Cefotaxime, 50 to 150 mg/kg/24 hr q6-8hr IV, or ceftriaxone, 50 to 75 mg/kg/24 hr q12hr IV, *or* cefuroxime, 50 to 100 mg/kg/ 24 hr q6hr IV.
      (2) If there is a break in the skin, thereby increasing the likelihood of *S. aureus,* nafcillin (as previously described) may be used in addition to one of the cephalosporins suggested, the latter to cover *H. influenzae* in unimmunized children.
   b. For patients older than 9 years: nafcillin as previously described.
   c. For erysipelas, penicillin G, 50,000 to 100,000 units/kg/24 hr q4hr IV may be required initially in addition to the previous therapy. Resolution of fever occurs in 24 hours.
   d. After resolution of the cellulitis and defervescence: Therapy is changed to oral medications for a total course of 10 days. Agents that may be used include amoxicillin, amoxicillin-clavulanate (Augmentin), cephalosporin, dicloxacillin, or trimethoprim-sulfamethoxazole, depending on presentation, identity of culture isolates, and sensitivity.

DISPOSITION

Patients with only localized cellulitis and no involvement of the face or systemic toxicity may be monitored closely as outpatients. Nontoxic patients with periorbital cellulitis may be discharged with appropriate antibiotic therapy, with arrangements for reevaluation for improvement in 6 to 12 hours; others must be hospitalized.

Parental Education

1. See that the child takes all medications and keeps appointments for follow-up observation.
2. Call your physician if any of the following occurs:
   a. Fever rises.
   b. The area of cellulitis increases or becomes fluctuant.

c. The underlying joint or bone remains tender or painful once cellulitis has resolved.

BIBLIOGRAPHY

Powell KR: Orbital and periorbital cellulitis, *Pediatr Rev* 16:163, 1995.

Schwartz GR, Wright SW: Changing bacteriology with periorbital cellulitis, *Ann Emerg Med* 28:617, 1996.

Contact Dermatitis

Contact irritant dermatitis results from contact with an exogenous substance. It may be caused primarily by an irritant, such as an alkali or a detergent, or by prolonged contact of the skin with urine and feces as in diaper dermatitis (p. 588). It is usually mild in nature.

Allergic contact dermatitis is lymphocyte-mediated and caused by a variety of substances, including plants (poison ivy or poison oak), topical medications, shoes, nickel, and cosmetics.

DIAGNOSTIC FINDINGS

1. The distribution and pattern of the lesions as well as the history of contact are diagnostic. The lesions are often limited to exposed contact surfaces, and they may be sharply delineated or have bizarre symmetric distribution.
2. The dermatitis is initially erythematous with edema but may progress to vesicle formation, weeping, and crusting.

MANAGEMENT

The offending allergen or irritant, if identifiable, should be removed.

Severe, Generalized, Allergic Contact Dermatitis

A short course of systemic steroids is indicated if there is extensive involvement over the body, face, or genitalia, especially if edema is significant. Exacerbation may occur if duration of therapy is not sufficient.

1. Prednisone, 1 to 2 mg/kg/24 hr q6-24hr PO, is given for 1 week and then the dosage is tapered over the next 2 weeks for a total therapeutic period of 3 weeks.
2. Therapy may be initiated parenterally: dexamethasone (Decadron), 0.25 mg/kg/dose IV or IM.

Moderate Allergic Contact Dermatitis

Topical steroids and compresses are adequate as described for atopic dermatitis (p. 581).

Mild Allergic or Irritant Contact Dermatitis

1. Topical steroids are usually adequate.
2. Hydration of the involved area may be useful and, after baths, application of Eucerin or Nivea. Other clinicians prefer application of compresses of tepid water, saline, or Burow's solution to weeping areas to dry up the involved region.

DISPOSITION

1. Patients may be discharged but should be monitored until the dermatitis resolves.
2. Patch testing may be useful in defining potential allergens that should be avoided.

Dermatophytosis

See Table 72-3.

ANCILLARY DATA

1. Wood's light examination: In dark room, shine a Wood's light. Dermatophysis lesions should fluoresce.
2. Potassium hydroxide (KOH) preparation: Place a specimen taken from just inside the advancing border of the infection on a slide. Add 1 to 2 drops of 10% to 20% KOH; place a cover glass on the slide and heat gently (do not boil); examine slide under a microscope. Ideally, the hyphae can be seen branching.

TABLE 72-3 Dermatophytoses: Clinical Characteristics

	Location	Diagnostic Findings	Differential Diagnosis	Management
Tinea capitis	Scalp, hair	Initially, noninflammatory—bald, scaly patch; 2-8 wk; inflammatory phase—edematous nodule with pustule (kerion); rare if adenopathy or alopecia is present	Alopecia areata (scalp within normal limits); trichotillomania; pyoderma	Griseofulvin
Tinea corporis	Nonhairy parts of body	Dry, scaly, annular lesion with clear center	Pityriasis rosea, atopic dermatitis	Topical
Tinea pedis	Feet	Vesicle, erosion of fourth and fifth toes, extending to other toe and arch of foot; adolescent	Atopic or contact dermatitis	Topical
Tinea fachei	Face	Erythematous, scaly lesion; butterfly distribution	Systemic lupus erythematosus	Topical
Tinea cruris	Groin	Sharply demarcated erythematous, scaly lesion; scrotum not involved; adolescent		Topical
Tinea unguium	Nails	Nail is thickened, friable; subungual debris; nail discoloration; adolescents	Psoriasis	Griseofulvin and topical; possibly surgery (if poor response)

3. Culture: The specimen should be plated on Sabouraud's agar or dermatophyte test medium (DTM). The latter turns red if a dermatophyte is present. Incubate the culture for up to 4 weeks. The cotton swab method of specimen collection is performed by moistening a sterile cotton-tipped applicator with tap water and vigorously rubbing and rotating it over the affected area of the scalp for 15 seconds. Inoculate the applicator into Mycosel medium, which may be transported in a routine bacterial culturette transport medium.

MANAGEMENT (see Table 72-3)

1. Topical: Apply cream or solution two to three times per day for at least 1 week after the eruption has cleared. Clearing may take 2 to 4 weeks:
   a. Tolnaftate (Tinactin)
   b. Clotrimazole (Lotrimin) (over-the-counter)
   c. Miconazole (MicaTin)
   d. Haloprogin (Halotex)
2. Tinea capitis and tinea unguium:
   a. Terbinafine has proved to be effective in the treatment of *tinea capitis.* The oral daily dose is 62.5 mg/24 hr for children weighing less than 20 kg, 125 mg/24 hr for those weighing 20 to 40 kg, and 250 mg/24 hr for those weighing more than 40 kg; therapy is given for a total of two weeks.
   b. Oral griseofulvin (microsize: 10 mg/kg/24 hr; or ultramicrosize: 5-10 mg/kg/24 hr) given PO for 6 weeks (hair) or 3 months (nails). Ultramicrosize is better absorbed. Culture should be obtained before griseofulvin therapy is started. Supplement griseofulvin with twice-weekly

shampooing with selenium sulfide suspension.

c. Selenium sulfide, 1% to 2.5%, may be adjunctive therapy for tinea capitis.

3. Kerion: Requires prednisone, 1 to 2 mg/kg/24 hr for 1 month, usually in consultation with a dermatologist.

BIBLIOGRAPHY

Friedlander SF, Aly R, Krafchik B et al: Terbinafine in the treatment of *Trichophyton* tinea capitis: a randomized double-blind, parallel-group, duration finding study, *Pediatrics* 109:602, 2002.

Friedlander SF, Bickering B, Cummingham BB et al: Use of the cotton swab method in diagnosing tinea capitis, *Pediatrics* 104:276, 1999.

Hubbard TW: The predictive value of symptoms in diagnosing childhood tinea capitis, *Arch Pediatr Adolesc Med* 153:1150, 1999.

Diaper Dermatitis and Candidiasis

Diaper dermatitis is a result of prolonged contact with urine or feces, leading to chemical irritation and associated dampness and maceration. Candidiasis, secondary to *Candida albicans* infection, is usually associated with prolonged dermatitis in the diaper region; 80% of diaper dermatitides that last more than 4 days are colonized with *Candida,* even before the classic rash appears.

DIAGNOSTIC FINDINGS

Clinical presentation of diaper dermatitis consists of diffuse erythema with vesiculation and isolated erosions in the diaper area. Satellite papules on an erythematous base caused by *C. albicans* usually develop when the dermatitis has been present for more than 3 days (also called *Monilia*). This may be associated with white plaques on an erythematous base on the buccal mucosa, which is known as *thrush.*

DIFFERENTIAL DIAGNOSIS

Other entities that must be distinguished are contact dermatitis (p. 586), atopic dermatitis (p. 581), and bullous impetigo (p. 591).

MANAGEMENT

1. Instruct the parents to remove the irritant, as follows:
   a. Change diapers frequently.
   b. Leave the baby without a diaper as much as possible. Naps are a particularly good time. Overnight, put three diapers on the baby and use a rubber pad on the bed.
   c. Fasten diapers loosely:
      (1) If cloth diapers are used, double-rinse them. Alkalinity may be reduced by adding dilute vinegar (1 cup in washer tub of water or 1 oz in 1 gallon). Do not use plastic pants.
      (2) If disposable diapers are used, punch a few holes in the plastic liner. Newer superabsorbent diapers may reduce dermatitis.
   d. Keep the skin clean, washing gently with warm water. Superfatted or nonirritating soaps (Neutrogena, Basis, Lowila) may be used sparingly. Cetaphil lotion cleanser may also be used.
2. If there is any evidence of satellite lesions associated with candidiasis, initiate application of nystatin cream to the involved area during diaper changes. Continue for 2 to 3 days after resolution of the diaper dermatitis:
   a. With marked erythema, mix hydrocortisone cream (1%) with the nystatin and instruct that it be applied to the diaper area until the erythema has decreased. Other alternatives to nystatin are miconazole and clotrimazole. Do not use fluorinated steroid preparations.
   b. Treat oral white plaques (thrush) with nystatin oral suspension: 1 ml in each

side of the mouth qid for 2 to 3 days after clearing.
3. An alternative is fluconazole (load of 6 mg/kg/dose followed by 3 mg/kg/dose once a day orally).

Complication

A complication of diaper dermatitis is secondary bacterial infection.

DISPOSITION

Patients may be sent home.

Parental Education

1. Initiate more frequent diaper changes and avoid skin-sensitizing agents.
2. Expose the diaper area to air when possible, and avoid airtight occlusion caused by such things as rubber pants.
3. Do not use cornstarch or ointments in the diaper area.
4. Call your physician if any of the following occurs:
   a. Satellite lesions develop in the diaper area.
   b. White plaques develop in the mouth.
   c. You see evidence of bacterial infection, such as crusting, pustules, or large blisters.
   d. The rash has not resolved in 1 week.

BIBLIOGRAPHY

Janniger CK, Thomas I: Diaper dermatitis: an approach to prevention employing effective diaper care, *Cutis* 52:153, 1993.

Ward DB, Fleischer AB JR, Feldman SR et al: Characterization of diaper dermatitis in the United States, *Arch Pediatr Adolesc Med* 154:943, 2000.

Wolf R, Wolf D, Tuzun B et al: Diaper dermatitis, *Clin Dermatol* 18:657, 2000.

Eczema

See p. 581.

Erythema Multiforme

Erythema multiforme is a self-limited, hypersensitivity reaction with a broad spectrum of presentations, including toxic epidermal necrolysis and Stevens-Johnson syndrome.

ETIOLOGY: PRECIPITANTS

1. Infections:
   a. Viral: herpes simplex, Epstein-Barr (EB) virus—infectious mononucleosis, enterovirus
   b. Other: group A streptococci, *Mycoplasma pneumoniae*
2. Intoxications: sulfonamides, penicillin, barbiturates, phenytoin

DIAGNOSTIC FINDINGS

Classically, erythema multiforme is a monomorphous eruption.

1. Initially it manifests as symmetric, concentric, and erythematous lesions, primarily on the dorsal surfaces of the hand and extensor surfaces of the extremities. The palms and soles are often involved while the trunk is spared. The lesions become papular with an intense erythematous periphery and cyanotic center, appearing as *target* or iris lesions. They may become bullous.
2. There may be a prodrome of fever, headache, sore throat, cough, rhinorrhea, and lymphadenopathy.
3. The skin lesions evolve over 3 to 5 days with resolution over 2 to 4 weeks. They may recur.

Toxic Epidermal Necrolysis (Lyell's Disease)

1. Drug-induced, toxic epidermal necrolysis represents a severe form of erythema multiforme with cleavage of the skin below the epidermis and dermal layer resulting in full-thickness necrosis of the epidermis. Occurs primarily in adults.

2. Rarely, the lesions progress to produce severe confluent erythema and bullae with subsequent shedding of the epidermis, predominantly over the extremities, face, and neck.
3. Nikolsky's sign is present at the site of the lesions, whereby minor rubbing results in desquamation of underlying skin.
4. Extensive loss of superficial epidermis may occur, with subsequent fluid losses and complications paralleling those of a second-degree burn.
5. Patients are usually toxic, with high fever, malaise, and anorexia.
6. Long-term sequelae may involve the eyes, skin, and nails.

Stevens-Johnson Syndrome

1. A variant of erythema multiforme. The cutaneous lesions extensively involve the mucosal membranes and affect at least two sites (conjunctivae or mucosa of mouth, genitalia, or nose).
2. Blisters form and subsequently unroof with formation of extensive hemorrhagic crusts on the mucosal surface.
3. Patients are usually toxic and have difficulty with fluid intake.
4. A prodrome 1 to 14 days before the onset of mucocutaneous lesions is noted, consisting of malaise, nausea, vomiting, sore throat, cough, myalgia, and arthralgia.

Complications

1. Dehydration from surface losses or poor fluid intake
2. Secondary bacterial infections
3. Chronic dry eye or mild chronic symblepharon

Ancillary Data

1. Throat culture to rule out group A streptococci
2. Data related to fluid status if dehydration is present (see Chapter 7)
3. Other tests related to defining precipitants

DIFFERENTIAL DIAGNOSIS

1. Differential consideration of toxic epidermal necrosis: staphylococcal scalded-skin syndrome and Ritter's syndrome in a newborn (pp. 589 and 595). Patients are sick with fever.
2. Differential consideration of Stevens-Johnson syndrome: Kawasaki's disease (mucocutaneous lymph node syndrome) (p. 726).

MANAGEMENT

1. Supportive care is essential: fluid management, antipruritics, and analgesics.
2. Toxic epidermal necrolysis: See Chapter 46 on burns for discussion of management of fluids, etc. (steroids have no value in therapy).
3. Stevens-Johnson syndrome: Careful attention should be given to fluid management, oral hygiene, and eye care.
   a. If fluid intake is a problem, discomfort may be decreased by having patient gargle with a solution containing equal parts of Kaopectate, diphenhydramine (Benadryl), and 2% viscous lidocaine (Xylocaine). The dose of the 2% viscous lidocaine (Xylocaine) should not exceed 15 ml q3hr or 120 ml in 24 hours in the adult (proportionately less in child). The patient should not eat or drink for 1 hour after application because of the danger of aspiration. Antacids such as Maalox and Mylanta are equally effective.
   b. Mouth washes with half-strength peroxide, if tolerated, are useful.
   c. If there is extensive involvement of the eye, consult an ophthalmologist.
   d. If possible the precipitant should be identified. There is *no* clear role for steroids.

DISPOSITION

Patients with uncomplicated illness may be monitored as outpatients, with instructions to watch for more extensive involvement.

Patients with toxic epidermal necrolysis should be hospitalized for fluid and skin management unless there is very minimal involvement and follow-up observation is excellent. Dermatologic consultation should be obtained.

The ability to maintain hydration and the extent of involvement dictate the disposition of patients with Stevens-Johnson syndrome.

BIBLIOGRAPHY

Assier H: Erythema multiforme with mucous membrane involvement and Stevens-Johnson syndrome are clinically different disorders with distinct causes, *Arch Dermatol* 131:539, 1995.

Prendiville JS, Hebert AA, Greenwald MJ et al: Management of Stevens-Johnson syndrome and toxic epidermal necrolysis in children, *J Pediatr* 115:881, 1989.

Sheridan RL, Schultz JT, Ryan CM et al: Long-term consequences of toxic epidermal necrolysis in children, *Pediatrics* 109:74, 2002.

Impetigo

ETIOLOGY: INFECTION

Impetigo is a bacterial infection caused by group A streptococci or *S. aureus* (bullous impetigo).

DIAGNOSTIC FINDINGS

An erythematous area evolves into numerous thin-walled vesicles, often overlying areas of abrasion or trauma. The vesicles are quickly unroofed, leaving a superficial ulcer that becomes covered with a thick, honey-colored crust. These spread centrifugally and may coalesce into larger lesions.

Less commonly, the vesicles become bullae that coalesce. When ruptured, they leave a discrete round lesion. This is *bullous impetigo,* usually caused by *S. aureus.*

Lesions most commonly occur on the face and extremities or in areas of trauma.

Complications

1. Acute glomerulonephritis secondary to nephrogenic strains of streptococci
2. Ecthyma: streptococcal infection with extension through all layers of the epidermis, resulting in a firm, dark crust with surrounding erythema and edema

Ancillary Data

Very rarely, a culture of the lesion is indicated if there is doubt about the diagnosis.

MANAGEMENT

Local skin care may be helpful. Soaking with water combined with some abrasion is useful in removing the crusts.

Antibiotics are indicated for all patients:

1. For lesions that consist primarily of erythema and crusts (the most likely causative organism is group A streptococci):
   a. Penicillin V, 25,000 to 50,000 units/kg/24 hr q6hr PO for 10 days, *or*
   b. Benzathine penicillin G (Bicillin C-R), usually given 900,000:300,000 IM as a single injection according to Table 72-4, although this is infrequently utilized.
2. For bullous impetigo (resulting from *S. aureus* infection): dicloxacillin, 50 mg/kg/24 hr q6hr PO for 10 days.
3. Alternative antibiotics:
   a. Erythromycin, 30 to 50 mg/kg/24 hr q6hr PO for 10 days, *or*

TABLE 72-4 Schedule of Benzathine for Impetigo

Weight (lb)	Benzathine Penicillin G (units)	Bicillin C-R (units) (900,000 benzathine: 300,000 procaine)
<30	300,000	300,000:100,000
31-60	600,000	600,000:200,000
61-90	900,000	900,000:300,000
>90	1,200,000	NA

b. Cephalexin (Keflex) or cephradine (Velosef), 25 to 50 mg/kg/24 hr q6hr PO for 10 days, which may be particularly useful because of the potential significance of *S. aureus* in poorly responsive infections, *or*
c. Mupirocin 2% (Bactroban) ointment, a topical treatment equal to oral medication.

DISPOSITION

All patients with uncomplicated disease may be sent home.

Parental Education

1. Have your child take all medication.
2. Remove the crust with soaking and minimal abrasion.
3. Minimize sharing of towels, sheets, etc.
4. Bring any other children with similar lesions in for treatment.

Patients are not infectious 24 hours after treatment is initiated.

BIBLIOGRAPHY

Demidovich CW, Wittler RR, Ruff ME et al: Impetigo: current etiology and comparison of penicillin, erythromycin and cephalexin therapy, *Am J Dis Child* 144:1313, 1990.

Mertz PM, Marshall DA, Eaglstein WH et al: Topical mupirocin treatment of impetigo is equal to oral erythromycin, *Arch Dermatol* 125:1069, 1989.

Rice RD, Duggan AK, DeAngelis C: Cost-effectiveness of erythromycin versus mupirocin for the treatment of impetigo in children, *Pediatrics* 89:210, 1992.

Lice (Pediculosis)

Lice or crabs primarily affect the head or pubic areas and are transmitted by person-to-person spread. They cannot live beyond 3 days without human contact.

DIAGNOSTIC FINDINGS

Excoriated papules or pustules are noted in the scalp or perineum. A louse is often seen in the hair or on hats or underwear. Gelatinous nits are often noted as tightly adherent white specks on the shaft of the hair.

Intense nocturnal pruritus may be present.

Complications

Complications consist of secondary bacterial infections such as impetigo (discussed previously).

MANAGEMENT

1. Several pediculicides are commonly available; children may return to school after one treatment:
   a. RID (purified pyrethrins): Apply about 1 oz undiluted to infested area until entirely wet, and allow to remain for 10 minutes. Wash thoroughly. A second treatment is usually needed in 7 to 10 days. Available over the counter.
   b. NIX (permethrin 1%) creme rinse: After washing hair, saturate with creme rinse, allow to remain for 10 minutes, then rinse. Single application is usually adequate, although most clinicians recommend a second treatment 7 days later. Available over the counter. The hair should be combed with a nit comb.
   c. Kwell (Lindane): Apply about 1 oz (adult) of Kwell shampoo to either the scalp or the pubic region and work into a lather, frequently adding small amounts of water. Scrub the hair well for 4 minutes and rinse thoroughly. Removal of the shampoo must be thorough because of the potential for contact dermatitis or central nervous system (CNS) toxicity. One treatment is usually adequate, but some clinicians prefer to repeat treatment in 10 days. For an adult, 1 to 2 oz is enough; prescribe smaller amounts for children. Do not give extra medication or use in pregnant women.
   d. Other preparations are available as well.

2. Mechanical removal of nits using wet combing is 38% effective when done every 3 to 4 days for several weeks.
   a. Some clinicians suggest applying olive oil or petrolatum to the hair to kill the nits in conjunction with the preceding medications. If the nits are present in the eyelashes or eyebrows, apply petrolatum (Vaseline) carefully to the area overnight once. Do not have the parents mechanically remove the nits, because this tends to produce eye trauma.
   b. Although the nits are dead in the hair, they may stay tightly adherent. Remove by washing the hair with warm vinegar for about 30 minutes to loosen the nits and then mechanically remove them with a fine-toothed comb.
3. Treat symptomatic contacts; for example, treat all nonpregnant sexual contacts.
4. All the child's bed linens and clothes that have recently been worn should be machine washed and dried using the hot cycle of dryer for at least 20 minutes. Hats and other headgear that are difficult to wash should be put in a sealed plastic bag for 10 to 14 days.
5. Antihistamines may be necessary for pruritus, which may continue for several weeks: diphenhydramine (Benadryl), 5 mg/kg/24 hr q6hr PO, or hydroxyzine (Atarax, Vistaril), 2 mg/kg/24 hr q6hr PO.

Pinworms

Enterobius vermicularis are ½-inch, white, threadlike worms that infect the perianal region.

DIAGNOSTIC FINDINGS

1. Children complain of perianal itching. In rare cases, with persistent irritation, an associated vulvovaginitis may be present.
2. Worms may be seen by parents.

Ancillary Data

A piece of transparent adhesive tape or tape from a special kit is gently touched to the perianal region. The sticky side is applied to a glass slide for examination for ova by light microscopy. The highest yield is from specimens collected at night.

DIFFERENTIAL DIAGNOSIS

Pinworms should be distinguished from irritation, fissures, and contact dermatitis in the perianal region.

MANAGEMENT

1. One of two drugs should be used:
   a. Mebendazole (Vermox) for children older than 2 years, 100-mg chewable tablet PO once (repeat in 1 week), *or*
   b. Pyrantel (Antiminth), 11 mg (0.2 ml)/kg/dose (maximum: 1 g) PO once (repeat in 1 week)
2. Family members or contacts with perianal irritation or itching should be similarly examined and treated. Asymptomatic contact need not be treated.

Parental Education

Children are usually infected by other children, many of whom carry pinworms but are asymptomatic. Good personal hygiene, with particular attention to handwashing, may reduce the chance of infection.

Pityriasis Rosea

Pityriasis rosea affects children and adolescents and is of unknown cause.

DIAGNOSTIC FINDINGS

1. Initially, a round, scaly, erythematous patch (2 to 4 cm) with central clearing develops, usually on the trunk. This herald patch precedes the generalized eruption by an average of 10 days and may be confused with tinea corporis.

2. Multiple erythematous macules develop and progress to small, rose-colored papules, primarily over the trunk. The individual lesions are oval, are 1 to 2 cm in size, and follow the wrinkle or cleavage lines of the skin. This creates a "Christmas tree" distribution on the back.
3. In black children, distribution varies, being primarily on the proximal extremities, inguinal and axillary areas, and the neck.
4. Patients may initially have pruritus but later become asymptomatic.
5. The rash may last for several months, marked by resolution and recurrences.

MANAGEMENT

1. Reassurance is of primary importance. Contact irritants should be avoided.
2. Antihistamines may be useful if itching is severe:
   a. Diphenhydramine (Benadryl), 5 mg/kg/24 hr q6hr PO, *or*
   b. Hydroxyzine (Atarax, Vistaril), 2 mg/kg/24 hr q6hr PO
3. Exposure to ultraviolet (UV) light (either natural or sunlamp) may hasten the resolution.

Scabies

Scabies is caused by the mite *Sarcoptes scabiei* and requires close person-to-person contact for transmission. The female mite cannot live beyond 2 to 3 days without human contact.

DIAGNOSTIC FINDINGS

1. Lesions appear as erythematous papules associated with S-shaped linear burrows.
   a. They are located primarily on the dorsum of the hand, interdigital web spaces, elbows (extensor surface), wrists, anterior axillary folds, abdomen, and genitalia. The head and neck are rarely involved.
   b. There is intense nocturnal pruritus, which may continue for up to 1 week after successful treatment.
2. Infants often have an associated acute dermatitis with excoriations and crusting. In addition to the normal distribution, they have involvement of the head, neck, palms, and soles.

Complication

Impetigo (p. 591) is a secondary bacterial infection.

Ancillary Data

Microscopic examination for mites, eggs, or feces may be made by placing a drop of mineral oil at the advancing end of a burrow and unroofing the burrow with a scalpel. The specimen is then placed on a microscope slide, a cover glass is applied, and the material is examined by light microscopy.

MANAGEMENT

1. Two scabicides are primarily used, although lindane is preferred. After one treatment, children can return to school:
   a. Lindane (Kwell lotion) is applied to dry skin in a thin layer from the neck down. The lotion is left on for 8 hours, and the patient is then bathed thoroughly to remove residual lotion. Removal must be complete because of the potential of contact dermatitis and CNS toxicity. Lindane should not be used in pregnant women or children younger than 1 year. One treatment is usually adequate, although a retreatment is sometimes necessary 1 week later, particularly in infants and children with many lesions. In adults, 1 to 2 oz is usually adequate, with proportionately smaller volumes in children.
   b. Crotamiton 10% (Eurax cream) is applied from the neck down, with particular attention to folds and creases; application is repeated in 24 hours.

After 48 hours, the child should be thoroughly bathed.

c. Permethrin topical cream (Elimite) has low toxicity and is effective; 1 to 2 oz is applied to the entire body and left on for 12 hours before being rinsed off. A second treatment in 7 to 10 days is suggested but is not always needed.

2. All members of the household and sexual contacts should be treated. (Lindane should not be used in pregnant women.) All the child's bed linens and clothes that have recently been worn should be machine washed. Blankets and other items that are difficult to clean should be put away for 4 days.
3. Antihistamines may be necessary for prolonged pruritus: diphenhydramine (Benadryl), 5 mg/kg/24 hr q6hr PO, or hydroxyzine (Atarax, Vistaril), 2 mg/kg/24 hr q6hr PO. Itching may continue for 1 week after treatment.

BIBLIOGRAPHY

Rasmussen JE: Scabies, *Pediatr Rev* 15:110, 1994.

Seborrheic Dermatitis

Seborrheic dermatitis is caused by the overproduction of sebum in areas rich with sebaceous glands, including the scalp, face, midchest, and perineum. It is commonly seen during the first few months of life and in adolescents at puberty.

DIAGNOSTIC FINDINGS

1. The involved areas are minimally erythematous, dry, and scaly with a greasy sensation. Lesions have more intense color at the periphery, with clearing at the center. Edges are sharply demarcated. Weeping and edema are not present.
2. Newborns particularly have problems with the scalp and may develop "cradle cap."

MANAGEMENT

1. In infants the scalp may be treated by washing with minimal abrasion (washcloth or soft brush) in an effort to remove the scales. Do not use oils.
2. In children and adolescents, shampoos such as Sebulex and those containing selenium sulfide, combined with abrasion, may be helpful.
3. Hydrocortisone cream (1%) is used in markedly involved areas, except for the scalp.
4. Resolution usually occurs within 1 week. Recurrences may be noted.

Staphylococcal Scalded Skin Syndrome

ETIOLOGY

Infection

S. aureus, phage group II, produces an exotoxin (exfolitin) in the patient. The bacteria typically colonize in the patient without overt infection.

DIAGNOSTIC FINDINGS

1. Staphylococcal scalded skin syndrome may be generalized in the newborn (Ritter's disease) and the child. Patients may be febrile and irritable.
2. An erythematous eruption develops primarily on the face (perioral and periorbital), the flexor area of the neck, and the axilla and groin, with accompanying tenderness of the skin, progressing to a tender scarlatiniform rash over 1 to 2 days:
   a. Edema of the face develops, with crusting around the eyes and mouth and sparing of mucous membranes.
   b. Patients have Nikolsky's sign, whereby the epidermis separates with only minor trauma.
3. If the erythema does not progress but desquamates, the patient merely has a scarlatiniform rash.

4. Some patients experience only a localized involvement with the evolution of large bullae with clear or purulent fluid. This is bullous impetigo (p. 591).

Complications

1. Dehydration from fluid losses
2. Systemic infection with *S. aureus*
3. Toxic shock syndrome (p. 736)

Ancillary Data

Bacterial culture of involved areas may be performed.

DIFFERENTIAL DIAGNOSIS

1. Erythema multiforme, toxic epidermal necrolysis (p. 589)
2. Group A streptococcal infection: impetigo or scarlatiniform rash (p. 591)

MANAGEMENT

1. Patients need support with fluids and analgesia.
2. Local treatment with warm compresses may be helpful. However, if the loss of epidermis is extensive, the protocol for management of burns should be implemented (see Chapter 46).
3. Antibiotics should be initiated for all patients:
   a. Dicloxacillin, 50 mg/kg/24 hr q6hr PO for 10 days
   b. Parenteral antibiotics (nafcillin or equivalent) for toxic patients

DISPOSITION

Most patients should be hospitalized for local skin care, monitoring of fluids, and antibiotic therapy.

BIBLIOGRAPHY

Ladhani L: Recent developments in staphylococcal scalded skin syndrome, *Clin Microbiol Infect* 7:301, 2001.

Sunburn

Sunburn results from overexposure to UV light. Phototoxic agents that sensitize skin to sun include sulfonamides, tetracycline, hydantoin, barbiturates, chlorpromazine, chlorothiazide, coal tar derivatives, perfumes, celery, and parsnips.

DIAGNOSTIC FINDINGS

1. The exposed skin is erythematous and tender in the first few hours. With significant burns, it will become erythematous and edematous over the next 6 to 12 hours and ultimately blister by 24 hours.
2. Patients may have concomitant chills, headache, and malaise (see Chapter 50).
3. Photosensitizing agents should be considered, including sulfonamides, diphenhydramine, phenothiazines, and tetracyclines.

MANAGEMENT

1. Cool baths or wet compresses are helpful in relieving the pain and burning; they may be used three to four times per day for 10 minutes each. Bland emollients (Eucerin, Nutraderm, Lubriderm) may be helpful.
2. Aspirin or indomethacin (1 to 3 mg/kg/24 hr q6-8hr PO in children older than 14 years) is useful in the management of severe sunburn if begun within 12 hours.
3. Steroids have no proven role.

DISPOSITION

Patients may be sent home.

Parental Education

1. Avoid overexposure in the future, particularly if the child is taking a photosensitizing agent.
2. Use sunscreens with a sun protective factor (SPF) of at least 15 before exposure in

the future. SPF 30 is generally advised for direct, prolonged exposure. Sunscreen should be reapplied after swimming or active sweating.

3. Push fluids to maintain hydration.

BIBLIOGRAPHY

Hebert AA: Photoprotection in children, *Adv Dermatol* 8:309, 1993.

Urticaria

ETIOLOGY

1. Allergy:
   a. Drugs: penicillin, salicylates, narcotics
   b. Foods: nuts, shellfish, eggs
   c. Inhalants
   d. Insect bites (p. 310)
2. Infections:
   a. Viral: hepatitis, EB virus (infectious mononucleosis)
   b. Parasites
3. Trauma: mechanical, thermal (cold and heat), sun or solar
4. Autoimmune: systemic lupus erythematosus, inflammatory bowel disease
5. Neoplasms

DIAGNOSTIC FINDINGS

1. Eruption is a rapidly evolving, erythematous, raised wheal with marked edema. The edema is well circumscribed and tense. The lesions are markedly pruritic.
2. Subcutaneous extension of the edema, known as *angioedema,* occurs in as many as 50% of children with acute urticaria.
3. If urticaria is associated with anaphylaxis, there may be respiratory or circulatory compromise (see Chapter 12).

Ancillary Data

No tests are indicated initially except to define the cause.

MANAGEMENT

1. Avoid etiologic conditions.
2. Ensure that there is no associated respiratory compromise. If it is present, begin therapy immediately as outlined in Chapter 12.
3. Antihistamines and epinephrine are the hallmarks of therapy:
   a. Diphenhydramine (Benadryl), 5 mg/kg/24 hr q6hr PO, IM, or IV, *or*
   b. Hydroxyzine (Atarax, Vistaril), 2 mg/kg/24 hr q6hr PO (causes less associated fatigue).
   c. With poor response, pseudoephedrine (Sudafed), 4 to 5 mg/kg/24 hr q6hr PO, may be added.
   d. An alternative for recurrent or persistent allergic urticaria is histamine (H_2) blockers such as cimetidine (Tagamet), 20 to 30 mg/kg/24 hr q4-6hr PO (adult: 300 mg q6hr PO).
   e. Epinephrine (1:1000), 0.01 ml/kg/dose (maximum: 0.35 ml/dose) SC q20min prn, up to three doses, may be given if rapid clearing of rash is desired.
4. Refer patients with recurrent or persistent (beyond 4 to 6 weeks) urticaria for a more complete evaluation.

BIBLIOGRAPHY

Mahwood T, Janniger CK: Childhood urticaria, *Cutis* 52:78, 1993.

Moscati RN, Moore GP: Comparison of cimetidine and diphenhydramine in the treatment of acute urticaria, *Ann Emerg Med* 19:12, 1990.

Warts and Molluscum Contagiosum

Warts are viral-induced, intraepidermal tumors caused by human papovavirus. They are often asymptomatic, although those on pressure-bearing surfaces may be painful. Spontaneous resolution occurs in 9 to 24 months. Warts may be categorized on the basis of their appearance and location (Table 72-5).

TABLE 72-5 Categories of Warts and Appropriate Management

Common	Filiform	Flat	Plantar	Venereal
DIAGNOSTIC FINDINGS				
Solitary papule, irregular scaly surface; found anywhere	Projection from skin on narrow stalk; lip, nose, or eyelids	Flat-topped, skin-colored papule; face or extremity	Smooth papule level with skin surface on weight-bearing surfaces	Multiple confluent papules, irregular surface; genital mucosa or adjacent skin (condylomata acuminata)
MANAGEMENT				
Cryotherapy, salicylic acid paint (periungual: cantharidin, salicylic acid paint)	Surgery	Retinoic acid, salicylic acid paint	Salicylic acid plaster, salicylic acid paint	Podophyllin, cryotherapy

MANAGEMENT TECHNIQUES (listed in Table 72-5)

1. Cryotherapy: Cotton swab is dipped in liquid nitrogen, applied to the center of the wart until it is white, and maintained for 20 to 30 seconds.
2. Salicylic acid paint: Salicylic acid in concentration above 10% is applied to the wart twice a day for 2 to 4 weeks. On thick surfaces salicylic acid, 16.7%, and lactic acid, 16.7%, in flexible collodion are used. A weaker concentration (10%) is used on flat warts.
3. Salicylic acid plaster: Cotton plaster with salicylic acid (40%) is cut to size of wart and taped to skin; it remains for 3 to 5 days and is then replaced. Wart is treated for 2 to 3 weeks.
4. Retinoic acid (0.1% cream) is applied once or twice a day, with resolution in 2 to 4 weeks.
5. Cantharidin is applied directly to periungual warts, and the warts are then covered with tape for 24 hours.
6. Podophyllin (25%) is applied to venereal warts and washed off thoroughly in 4 hours. Treatment may have to be repeated in 1 week. Because this agent is neurotoxic, it must not be used on an extensive area or at home.

Molluscum contagiosum is a white or whitish-yellow papule with central umbilication caused by a poxvirus. Grouped genital lesions are common, often surrounded by an area of dermatitis. Wright's stain of the contents of the papule reveals epidermal cytoplasmic viral inclusions.

Sharp dermal curettage is the treatment of choice if removal is desired. This may leave a small scar. Spontaneous resolution occurs in 2 to 3 years.

BIBLIOGRAPHY

Rosekrans JA: Dermatologic disorders. In Barkin RM, editor: *Pediatric emergency medicine: concepts and clinical practice,* ed 2, St Louis, 1997, Mosby.

Weston WL, Lane AT, Morelli JC: *Color textbook of pediatric dermatology,* ed 2, St Louis, 1996, Mosby.

73 Ear, Nose, and Throat Disorders

Dentoalveolar Infections

Toothaches and associated dentoalveolar infections are usually caused by untreated dental caries, although they may be related to failing dental restorations. Visits to the emergency department (ED) are related primarily to dental caries, abscess, or pain.

DIAGNOSTIC FINDINGS

1. Patients usually complain of local or generalized dental or facial pain, often exacerbated by heat, cold, sweets, air, and chewing pressure.
2. The affected tooth usually has an obvious defect, such as dental caries or broken or lost restoration.
3. Facial swelling is commonly noted. Dentoalveolar swelling or fistula also may be present.

Complications

1. Facial cellulitis (p. 582)
2. Bacteremia
3. Loss of tooth

Ancillary Data

Dental x-ray films, if available, are helpful.

DIFFERENTIAL DIAGNOSIS

1. Dentoalveolar or periodontal abscess.
2. Newly erupting tooth.
3. Traumatic dental injury.
4. Broken dental restoration.
5. Foreign object embedded in tissue.
6. *Dental stains* may be mistaken for caries in a tooth. Normal teeth have some color variation. Stains also may be caused by external agents that can be removed with cleaning; such stains (green, orange, or black) result from poor hygiene or from excessive use of certain foods or beverages, smoking, or liquid medications (iron). Intrinsic conditions that lead to dental staining include problems in the neonatal period (biliary atresia, hepatitis, erythroblastosis, and maternal tetracycline ingestion), trauma, excessive fluoride, and tetracycline ingestion between 3 months and 8 years of age.

MANAGEMENT

Toothache without Infection

1. Evaluation of legitimate need for analgesics (ibuprofen often effective), which children rarely require
2. Dental referral within 24 hours

Toothache with Localized Infection

1. Initiation of antibiotics: penicillin V, 25,000 to 50,000 units (15-30 mg)/kg/24 hr q6hr PO for 7 to 10 days
2. Consideration of analgesics (ibuprofen often effective)
3. Dental referral within 24 hours

Dental Infection with Cellulitis

1. Hospitalize the patient.
2. Initiate antibiotic therapy:
   a. Give nafcillin (or equivalent), 150 mg/kg/24 hr q4hr IV.
   b. Switch to dicloxacillin once parenteral therapy is no longer indicated, at a dosage of 50 mg/kg/24 hr q6hr PO for a total course of 10 days.

3. Consult with a dentist to evaluate the need for incision and drainage, extraction of tooth, or open drainage. Dentist will attempt to relieve pain, treat infection, and provide appropriate follow-up as necessary for extraction or root canal treatment, restoration, or dental prosthesis.

BIBLIOGRAPHY

Dorfman DH, Kastner B, Vinci RJ: Dental concerns unrelated to trauma in the pediatric emergency department, *Arch Pediatr Adolesc Med* 155:699, 2001.

Josell SD, Abrams RE: Common oral and dental emergencies and problems, *Pediatr Clin North Am* 29:705, 1982.

Kureishi A, Chow AW: The tender tooth: dentoalveolar, pericoronal and periodontal infections, *Infect Dis Clin North Am* 2:163, 1988.

Epistaxis (Nosebleed)

Nasal bleeding normally originates in the anterior portion of the nasal septum (Kiesselbach's plexus), which accounts for 90% of cases.

ETIOLOGY

1. Trauma: nose picking, foreign body, repeated hard blowing with associated upper respiratory infection, nasal fracture
2. Allergic rhinitis or polyp
3. Bleeding dyscrasia, aspirin ingestion, anticoagulants, leukemia
4. Vascular: telangiectasia, hemangioma; hypertension is an unusual association

DIAGNOSTIC FINDINGS

Active bleeding from one or both nostrils is present. Examination of the nose reveals an inflamed area at Kiesselbach's plexus for anterior epistaxis. Posterior epistaxis involves the posterior branch of the sphenopalatine artery. Predisposing causes should be defined.

Complication

Although epistaxis is usually self-limited, extensive bleeding may cause anemia or shock.

Ancillary Data

Rarely are any laboratory data indicated unless there are suggestions of systemic disease. A bleeding screen (complete blood count [CBC], platelet count, prothrombin time [PT], partial thromboplastin time [PTT], and bleeding time) for recurrent epistaxis is indicated if there is a history of significant bleeding with lacerations, circumcision, and so on, spontaneous bleeding at other sites, or a family history of bleeding (see Chapter 29).

MANAGEMENT

1. Apply constant pressure over the anterior nares for a minimum of 10 minutes. Preceding this step, the patient should blow the nose to remove clots. Optimally, have the patient remain sitting with the head forward to avoid draining blood posteriorly into the airway or esophagus.
2. If pressure is unsuccessful, place a piece of cotton soaked in 0.25% phenylephrine (Neo-Synephrine), or epinephrine (1:1000) and 1% cocaine in the nose, and then apply pressure for 10 minutes.
3. If anterior bleeding continues or the problem is recurrent, cauterize the bleeding site with application of a silver nitrate stick for 3 seconds. Do not use cautery in children with bleeding problems.
4. Apply petrolatum (Vaseline) daily for 4 to 5 days to decrease friability of the anterior nasal mucosa.

If posterior bleeding is present, a posterior pack (and Foley catheter) may be inserted by an otolaryngologist.

DISPOSITION

Patients with epistaxis can usually be discharged. If a posterior pack is inserted, the patient must be admitted to the hospital. Hospitalization should be seriously considered if bilateral anterior packs are used. Appropriate allergy management, if indicated, should be instituted. Hematologic or otolaryngologic consultation is rarely necessary.

Parental Education

1. Increase home humidity. Minimize nose trauma and picking.
2. Apply petrolatum daily to the anterior nares for 4 to 5 days.
3. If bleeding recurs, apply pressure for a full 10 minutes, compressing the soft and bony parts of the nose and pressing downward toward the cheeks with thumb and forefinger.
4. Call your physician if there are unexplained bruises, if large amounts of blood are lost, or if bleeding cannot be controlled by pressure.

BIBLIOGRAPHY

Padgam N: Epistaxis: anatomical and clinical correlates, *J Laryngol Otol* 104:308, 1990.

Foreign Bodies in the Nose and Ear

Foreign bodies found in the nose or ear commonly include inanimate objects (e.g., toys, earrings), vegetable materials, and insects. The nose is a common site in children younger than 3 years; the ear is a common site in those younger than 8 years.

DIAGNOSTIC FINDINGS

1. A patient with a *nasal* foreign body has nasal obstruction or unilateral foul-smelling discharge. The object may be visualized.
2. A patient with a foreign body in the *ear* often has pain or discharge from the external ear canal. There may be a history either of inserting an object into the ear or of a buzzing sound associated with an insect. The object may be visualized.

MANAGEMENT

The patient's cooperation is essential and may be achieved through immobilization, sedation, or anesthesia. Good visualization, an excellent light source, and proper equipment are necessary. Button batteries should be promptly removed.

Nasal Foreign Bodies

Have the child blow the nose vigorously; then try suction. If this is unsuccessful, proceed with other techniques:

1. Vasoconstriction. Use topical epinephrine (1%) applied with a cotton-tipped swab, sprayed phenylephrine (0.25%), or cocaine (1%) before instrumentation, either individually or in combination.
2. Use forceps if the object can be grasped. Suction and hook or loop may be useful for larger objects.
3. If these maneuvers are unsuccessful and there is room, a lubricated No. 8 Foley catheter may be passed beyond the object, inflated with 2 to 3 ml water (with the patient in reverse Trendelenburg position), and withdrawn.

Ear Foreign Bodies

Several techniques are useful in attempting to remove objects.

1. If the object is an insect, kill it before removal by inserting alcohol.
2. Irrigation: Direct the stream of water beyond the object to flush it out. Do not use irrigation with vegetable matter (the material may swell) or if the tympanic membrane (TM) is perforated.

   NOTE: A useful irrigation technique is to cut off the needle of a large butterfly (18-gauge) catheter, leaving the pliable section of tubing. The ear is then easily irrigated with water and the fluid aspirated from the canal. A pulsating water device may also be used.
3. Mechanical removal: Use forceps for small objects, hooks, or loops.

DISPOSITION

If the foreign body cannot be removed, the patient should be referred to an otolaryngologist for ambulatory management.

BIBLIOGRAPHY

Baker MD: Foreign bodies of the ears and nose in childhood, *Pediatr Emerg Care* 3:67, 1987.

Brownstein DR, Hodge D III: Foreign bodies of the eye, ear and nose, *Pediatr Emerg Care* 4:215, 1988.

Kavanagh KT, Litovitz T: Miniature battery foreign bodies in auditory and nasal bodies, *JAMA* 255:1470, 1986.

Acute Necrotizing Gingivitis

Acute necrotizing gingivitis is an acute, contagious oral infection involving the gingival tissues of adolescents and young adults.

ETIOLOGY: INFECTION

This disease is caused by the spirochete *Borrelia vincentii.*

DIAGNOSTIC FINDINGS

1. History of recent emotional or physical stress (rarely epidemic). Fatigue may be a factor.
2. The classic symptom triad is intense, unremitting pain; punched-out interdental papillae covered with a white pseudomembrane; and foul odor from the mouth.
3. Acute necrotizing gingivitis is rarely associated with regional lymphadenopathy, malaise, and fever.

Complications

Without treatment, bone loss and loosening of teeth occur.

DIFFERENTIAL DIAGNOSIS

1. Infection: acute viral and bacterial infections
2. Leukemic gingivitis

MANAGEMENT

1. Give penicillin V, 25,000 to 50,000 units (15 to 30 mg)/kg/24 hr q6hr PO for 10 days.
2. Refer the patient to a dentist, and follow up with observation for tissue debridement. Surgery may be necessary.

Cervical Lymphadenopathy

The cervical lymph nodes course along the carotid sheath and drain the head and neck. The superior node group has afferents from the tongue, tonsils, nose, teeth, and the back of the head and neck. It becomes inflamed with potential suppuration from infections in these areas.

ETIOLOGY: INFECTION

1. Bacterial: group A streptococci, *Staphylococcus aureus,* typical and atypical mycobacteria
2. Viral: infectious mononucleosis, enterovirus, rubella
3. Other: cat-scratch fever (see p. 307), toxoplasmosis, histoplasmosis, tuberculosis, mucocutaneous lymph node syndrome (Kawasaki's disease)

   NOTE: Lymphadenopathy may be an early finding in patients with human immunodeficiency virus (HIV).

DIAGNOSTIC FINDINGS

1. History should be obtained about the rapidity of disease progression, recent travel, exposure to tuberculosis, contact with cats, and concurrent systemic signs and symptoms.
2. Pyogenic lesions have a unilateral, visible, firm, tender, discrete swelling early in the disease, which may progress to generalized swelling, erythema, and tenderness that becomes fluctuant. Patients usually are febrile and become increasingly toxic with extension of the process. There may be pain on neck movement.
3. Nonpyogenic organisms have a more insidious course. Tuberculosis, histoplasmosis, or toxoplasmosis should be considered for a mass in a child older than 10 years; for persistent, unexplained fever or weight loss; or for fixation of the mass with overlying skin, skin ulceration, supraclavicular location, no local tenderness,

or increase in size to 3 cm or more in diameter.

4. Cat-scratch fever (see p. 307) is caused by a small, pleomorphic gram-negative bacterium. Regional lymphadenopathy of an extremity occurs about 14 days (range: 3 to 50 days) after the scratch.
5. Palpable head and neck nodes are detected in 45% of normal children and 34% of neonates. Nodes are most commonly palpable in the occipital and postauricular areas in younger children, and in the cervical and submandibular regions in older children.

Complications

Suppuration and spontaneous drainage of the lymph node occurs.

1. Exterior drainage is a problem for cosmetic reasons.
2. Nodes caused by atypical mycobacteria may have chronic drainage.
3. Interior drainage may involve multiple neck structures, with significant morbidity.

Ancillary Data

1. White blood cells (WBC) with differential (shift to left).
2. Throat culture for group A streptococci.
3. Tests for mononucleosis (Monospot) and streptococci (Streptozyme).
4. Intermediate-strength purified protein derivative (PPD) test (reaction usually <10 mm with atypical disease but may be normal).
5. Aspiration of the node with an 18-gauge needle if there is no resolution of signs and symptoms after 48 hours of appropriate antibiotic therapy. Biopsy may also be considered, particularly if nonpyogenic organism is suggested:
   a. Care should be exercised if atypical mycobacteria are considered because of the potential for chronic drainage.
   b. Culture for bacteria and mycobacteria, as well as Gram and acid-fast stains, should be obtained for the aspirate.
   c. If a formal surgical incision and drainage (I & D) is performed, the same cultures should be performed as for an aspirate.
6. Computed tomography (CT) scan of the neck may be indicated in toxic patients and patients with large nodes that are not rapidly responsive to therapy. Ultrasonography is useful in defining the nature of a neck mass.

DIFFERENTIAL DIAGNOSIS

Considerations must include those entities that cause *stiff neck* (p. 741). Differential considerations of neck masses include:

1. Infection: parotitis (most commonly mumps). This infection obliterates the angle of the jaw, is associated with parotid tenderness, and is often bilateral.
2. Neoplasm: lymphoma, leukemia, metastatic carcinoma.
3. Congenital anomalies in the development of muscles, vessels, lymphatics, and bronchials:
   a. Thyroglossal duct cyst: midline mass without external sinus. Requires surgery.
   b. Bronchial cleft cyst: sinus (vestigial cleft or pouch with opening into skin or pharynx), fistula, cyst (trapped portion of cleft or pouch that enlarges gradually and requires surgery).
   c. Teratoma: tissue from all three general layers.
   d. Laryngocele.
4. Hemangioma or cystic hygroma.

MANAGEMENT

Management of cervical lymphadenopathy must proceed in an orderly fashion, and other causes should be considered if the patient's initial response is slow. Total resolution may occur over many weeks.

1. Prescribe antibiotics for at least 10 days after appropriate culture specimens are obtained:
   a. Cephalexin (Keflex) or cephradine (Velosef) or equivalent, 25 to 50 mg/kg/24 hr q6hr PO, *or*
   b. Erythromycin, 30 to 50 mg/kg/24 hr q6hr PO, *or*
   c. Dicloxacillin, 50 mg/kg/24 hr q6hr PO
   d. Some clinicians prefer a more limited coverage initially: penicillin V, 80,000 units (50 mg)/kg/24 hr q6hr PO, given for 48 hours if the node is not fluctuant initially. This is a relatively high dosage.
   e. If clinical improvement is noted, the therapy is continued.
   f. If the patient is toxic or the lymph node is fluctuant, large, or markedly tender, initiate parenteral antibiotics (nafcillin [or equivalent], 150 mg/kg/24 hr q4hr IV). I & D may be required, depending on the child's toxicity and comfort, and the node's size, warmth, fluctuance, and localization. This is often done in the operating room.
2. If the lymphadenopathy is slow to resolve with routine antibiotics, clindamycin, 10 to 25 mg/kg/24 hr q6hr PO (or 15 to 40 mg/kg/24 hr q6-8hr IV), may be initiated to ensure coverage of gram-positive and anaerobic organisms.
3. Consider other antibiotics if the Gram stain or culture of the node aspirate shows a less common organism, such as *H. influenzae*.
4. Treatment of atypical mycobacterial infections is controversial. Excision provides the best cure rate. Some clinicians treat with rifampin after surgery. Infectious disease consultation is indicated.

DISPOSITION

1. The patient may be monitored at home unless he or she has significant toxicity, the node has marked fluctuance, tenderness, or erythema, or I & D is required. Close follow-up observation is essential.
2. Surgical consultation is necessary for patients with fluctuant or unresponsive nodes.

Parental Education

Complete resolution of lymphadenopathy may take several months. The parent of a child monitored at home should understand the following:

1. Treatment requires very-high-dose antibiotics. The child should take all doses.
2. Call your physician if any of the following occurs:
   a. Swelling increases or becomes more red, tender, or fluctuant.
   b. Systemic toxicity develops.

BIBLIOGRAPHY

English CK, Wear DT, Margileth AM et al: Cat-scratch disease, *JAMA* 259:1347, 1988.

Wright JE: Cervical lymphadenitis in childhood: which antibiotic agent? *Med J Aust* 150:150, 1989.

Acute Mastoiditis

The middle ear communicates with the mastoid air cells, leading to concurrent infections if acute otitis media (AOM) is improperly treated.

ETIOLOGY

Acute mastoiditis is caused by bacterial infection identical to the organisms that cause AOM, most commonly *Streptococcus pneumoniae, H. influenzae,* group A streptococci, *Staphylococcus epidermidis,* and a number of anaerobes. *H. influenzae* is less common in children older than 8 years.

DIAGNOSTIC FINDINGS

AOM is followed by pain, edema, and tenderness over the mastoid area. Postauricular swelling, resulting from a subperiosteal abscess, may cause severe pain and displace the pinna forward, making the ear prominent.

Complications

1. Infection: meningitis and intracranial abscess
2. Paralysis of facial nerve
3. Sensorineural hearing loss

Ancillary Data

1. Mastoid x-ray film shows clouding of the septa of the mastoid bone (48%). Bony destruction and resorption of air cells eventually occur (12%). CT may provide definitive anatomic data.
2. Tympanocentesis, culture, and Gram stain of aspirated material may be useful.

DIFFERENTIAL DIAGNOSIS

Acute mastoiditis should be differentiated from other infections. Postauricular lymphadenitis may be difficult to differentiate.

1. Postauricular tenderness and erythema overlie a distinct node and do not diffusely involve the mastoid.
2. External otitis media is often associated.
3. Differentiation may require a CT scan in confusing or poorly responsive cases.

MANAGEMENT

1. Initiate antibiotic therapy pending results of culture and sensitivity testing:
   a. Cefotaxime, 50 to 150 mg/kg/24 hr q6-8hr IV, *or* cefuroxime, 100 mg/kg/24 hr q6-8hr IV, *or* ceftriaxone, 50 to 75 mg/kg/24 hr q12hr IV.
   b. Vancomycin may need to be considered if *S. pneumoniae* is a concern. *S. pneumoniae* is most common in children younger than 2 years.

      NOTE: Once the illness begins to resolve, oral antibiotics may be used for a total course of 4 weeks of treatment.
   c. Many clinicians use clindamycin, 15 to 40 mg/kg/24 hr q6-8hr IV, and ultimately, 10 to 25 mg/kg/24 hr q6hr PO to ensure coverage for gram-positive and anaerobic organisms, the route reflecting response and toxicity. This approach is particularly important in patients with poorly responsive or chronic disease.
2. Analgesia may be given, with codeine, 0.5 mg/kg/dose q4-6hr PO, or meperidine (Demerol), 1 mg/kg/dose q3-4hr IM, as indicated.
3. If the patient's condition worsens or a subperiosteal abscess develops, a postauricular I & D with a mastoidectomy should be performed by an otolaryngologist.

DISPOSITION

Hospitalization and consultation with an otolaryngologist are usually required.

BIBLIOGRAPHY

Ogle JW, Lauer BA: Acute mastoiditis: diagnosis and complications, *Am J Dis Child* 140:1178, 1986.

Scott TA, Jackler RK: Acute mastoiditis in infancy: a sequela of unrecognized acute otitis media, *Otolaryngol Head Neck Surg* 101:683, 1989.

Ward SL, Mason EO, Ward ER et al: Pneumococcal mastoiditis in children, *Pediatrics* 106:695, 2000.

Acute Otitis Media

ALERT Extreme irritability or lethargy may imply concurrent meningitis or other systemic infection.

AOM is a suppurative effusion of the middle ear that accounts for one third of office visits by children who are ill.

ETIOLOGY: INFECTION

Infection often follows evidence of eustachian tube dysfunction caused by either obstruction or abnormal patency. Pathogens include the following:

1. Bacteria (Table 73-1): No bacteria are isolated in up to 30% of patients studied;

TABLE 73-1 Acute Otitis Media: Common Pathogens and Treatment

Age Group/ Condition	Common Pathogens	Antibiotics[a]	Daily Dosage[b] (mg/kg/24 hr)	Frequency/Route	Minimum Duration	Comments
<2 mo	*S. pneumoniae, H. influenzae,* group A streptococci, *S. aureus,* gram-negative enteric	Ampicillin; *and*	100-200	q4hr IV	3-7 days, then appropriate PO	Appropriate if signs of systemic illness; tympanocentesis may be indicated; hospitalize; if no signs, symptoms, or toxicity, use regimen for older child
		gentamicin **or**	5.0-7.5	q8hr IV		
		cefotaxime	50-100	q8hr IV		
Infants, toddlers, and adolescents[f]	*S. pneumoniae, H. influenzae, M. catarrhalis,* group A streptococci	Amoxicillin; **or**	30-50[g]	q8hr PO	10-14 days	
		erythromycin *and*	30-50	q6hr PO	10-14 days	
		sulfisoxazole[c]; **or**	100-150	q6hr PO	10-14 days	
		erythromycin *and*	30-50	q6hr PO	10-14 days	
		trimethoprim-sulfamethoxazole;	8.0 40	q12hr PO	10-14 days	
		or Augmentin[d];	20-40 (amox)	q8hr PO	10-14 days	
		or cefaclor; **or**	20-40	q8hr PO	10-14 days	
		cefixime[e]; **or**	8	q24hr PO	10-14 days	
		azithromycin; **or**	10 mg (day 1) 5 mg (days 2-5)	q24hr PO	5 days[h]	
		clarithromycin	15	q12hr PO	10 days	
Refractory		Sulfisoxazole; **or**	100-150	q12hr PO	14 days	Use after initial course; if no resolution, consider tympanocentesis
		trimethoprim-sulfamethoxazole;	8.0 40	q12hr PO	14 days	
		or amoxicillin	20	q8hr PO	14 days	
Recurrent		Sulfisoxazole, **or**	50-75	q12hr PO	2-4 mo	Otolaryngologist and audiologist may be helpful
		trimethoprim-sulfamethoxazole	4.0 20	q24hr PO	2-4 mo	

[a] Additional acceptable antibiotics are available but are either broader in spectrum or more costly.
[b] See Formulary (p. 878) for adult (maximum) doses.
[c] Available as a single combination (Pediazole).
[d] Amoxicillin-clavulanate.
[e] Other cephalosporins are cefpodoxime, cefprozil, and cefuroxime. Cefuroxime (30 mg/kg/24 hr) may be efficacious with 5 days of therapy.
[f] There is growing evidence that *H. influenzae* is an important pathogen in this age group; therefore broader-spectrum antibiotics are also appropriate therapies.
[g] Double the standard dose, administering 80-90 mg/kg/24 hr bid PO, has been recommended to reduce problem of bacterial resistance.
[h] A three-day regimen has also been approved. Some suggest that a single dose may be effective.

when bacteria are isolated, *S. pneumoniae, H. influenzae,* and *Moraxella catarrhalis* are the most common pathogens identified.

2. Viral: parainfluenza, respiratory syncytial virus, rhinovirus, influenza, adenovirus, and enterovirus.
3. *Mycoplasma pneumoniae*: associated with bullous myringitis, as are other pathogens.
4. Other: tuberculosis.

Predisposing factors include associated upper respiratory infection, nasotracheal intubation, and Down syndrome. American Indians, Eskimos, and infants with straight eustachian tubes also are at higher risk. A genetic component has been suggested.

DIAGNOSTIC FINDINGS

1. Lethargy, irritability and other behavioral changes, ear pain, fever, and accompanying respiratory symptoms. Drainage may be present if the TM has ruptured. In the older child, hearing loss may occur.
2. TM findings:
   a. Full visualization of the TM is essential, often necessitating the removal of cerumen and debris by means of irrigation (provided no perforation is present) or a cerumen spoon. The presence of cerumen does not preclude the diagnosis of AOM:
      (1) A useful irrigation technique is to cut the needle off a large butterfly catheter (18 gauge), leaving only the pliable tubing. The ear then can be easily irrigated through the catheter with subsequent aspiration of the fluid from the canal.
      (2) A pulsating water device may also be effective.
      (3) Ceruminolytic agents such as sodium docusate may also be useful.
   b. TM has increased vascularity and erythema with obscured landmarks.
   c. Pneumatic otoscopy is a reliable means of determining whether an effusion is present. Decreased mobility accompanies AOM, often with bulging or retraction unless the TM is perforated.
   d. The optimal position of the child for the examination varies with the examiner and the child. Many prefer to have the child supine on the examining table, restrained by an adult or by specific pediatric restraints. The partially cooperative child may be seated in the parent's lap, face-to-face, and hugged tightly, with the child's legs wrapped around the parent's waist. One of the parent's arms embraces the child while the other holds the child's head.

Complications

1. Persistent AOM after an initial course of antibiotics is seen in 25% of patients. A second course of antibiotics is appropriate. If AOM persists after completion of a second or third course, referral to an otolaryngologist and tympanocentesis may be indicated for diagnostic and therapeutic purposes. On the basis of culture results, an additional course of antibiotics is initiated and follow-up observation is arranged. Many clinicians prefer inserting tympanometry tubes after a third course of antibiotic therapy if there has been little response.
2. Recurrent AOM occurs when a child has had three episodes of AOM in 6 months or four episodes in 12 months.
   a. Recurrent AOM is particularly common in children who had their first episode of AOM before 1 year of age. In children who have six or more episodes of AOM before 6 years of age, 49% have had the initial episode during the first year of life.
   b. Prophylactic antibiotics (especially after episodes of otitis media) or pressure-equalizing tubes are indicated.

3. Perforations occur when sufficient pressure in the middle ear develops, which may produce external otitis media (p. 610) or a transient conductive hearing loss. Local and systemic therapy is indicated.
4. Serous otitis media (SOM) occurs in 42% of children after an episode of AOM and usually resolves without intervention. Temporary hearing losses may occur; if the hearing loss persists beyond 3 months, the patient should be referred for audiologic evaluation.
5. Conductive hearing loss may be present with AOM and SOM. If hearing loss is persistent, intervention with pressure-equalizing tubes may be appropriate.
6. Mastoiditis, common before the antibiotic era, is now rare (p. 604).
7. Cholesteatoma, a saclike structure lined by keratinized, stratified, squamous epithelium with accumulation of desquamating epithelium or keratin in the middle ear, may be caused by recurrent AOM. It may result in erosion of the bone and progressive enlargement of the otic antrum.

Ancillary Data

1. Generally, no studies beyond a good physical examination are required for AOM.
2. Tympanocentesis is indicated in symptomatic patients younger than 8 weeks (particularly if toxic), in immunocompromised children, and in patients with AOM that persists after multiple courses of treatment. It is useful in defining pathogens, and the material recovered should undergo Gram stain and culture. In rare cases, tympanocentesis may be used to relieve severe pain. Puncture of the bullae associated with tense bullous myringitis results in immediate relief.
   - a. The procedure is performed as follows
     - (1) A slightly bent 3-inch, 18-gauge spinal needle attached to a 1-ml syringe is used.
     - (2) The TM is visualized with an otoscope, and the lens of the otoscope is moved sideways to allow access.
     - (3) The needle is inserted with aspiration into the inferior, posterior portion of the membrane.
   - b. Tympanocentesis may also be performed through a binocular scope, often with the assistance of an otolaryngologist.
3. Tympanometry with an electrical acoustic impedance bridge measures compliance of the TM and middle ear. It is useful in confirming the physical findings in children older than 7 months.
4. Audiologic evaluation is indicated in children with persistent or recurrent otitis media, especially if there has been an effusion for more than 3 months.
5. Nasopharyngeal and throat cultures are not helpful.

DIFFERENTIAL DIAGNOSIS

AOM should be differentiated from ear pain caused by the following:

1. Infection
   - a. External otitis media (p. 610)
   - b. Mastoiditis (p. 604)
   - c. Dental abscess (p. 599)
   - d. Peritonsillar abscess
   - e. Sinusitis
   - f. Lymphadenitis
   - g. Parotitis
2. Trauma: foreign body perforating the TM or, if still present, external otitis media; barotrauma; instrumentation
3. Serous otitis media or eustachian tube dysfunction
4. Impacted third molar
5. Temporomandibular joint dysfunction

Heavy (≥20 cigarettes/day) smoking by a mother increases the risk of recurrent AOM in the first year of her child's life.

MANAGEMENT

The patient must be evaluated to ascertain that a more significant infection, such as meningitis, is not present.

1. Antibiotics are generally used for children with AOM. However, meta-analysis has suggested that symptoms may resolve spontaneously. The choice of antibiotics varies with the child's age and allergies, the seriousness of the infection, the likelihood of compliance, and the etiologic agent (see Table 73-1).
   a. Children younger than 2 months require broad-spectrum coverage, usually administered parenterally to a hospitalized patient if there is any evidence of systemic illness.
   b. A single dose of ceftriaxone, 50 mg/kg/dose IV or IM, is efficacious and may be useful in selected children, especially those with acute gastroenteritis.
   c. Children with bullous myringitis, which is frequently associated with *M. pneumoniae*, also need treatment for other organisms considered to be pathogens in the age group. If pain is severe, myringotomy may be indicated.
   d. From 60% to 90% of patients improve within 72 hours of the start of therapy.
2. Decongestants and decongestant-antihistamine combinations given either systemically (antihistamines or vasoconstrictors) or nasally are not effective in altering the course.
3. Eardrops may be useful in the treatment of external otitis media resulting from perforation (polymyxin B [Lidosporin] or neomycin-polymyxin B [Cortisporin] suspension) or to relieve pain (glycerin [Auralgan] or mineral oil).
4. Antipyretics and analgesics such as acetaminophen or aspirin should be given.
5. Recurrent AOM is initially treated prophylactically with low-dose antibiotics, such as amoxicillin, 20 mg/kg/24 hr q12-24hr PO, *or* sulfisoxazole, 50 to 75 mg/kg/24 hr q12hr PO, *or* trimethoprim-sulfamethoxazole, 4/20 mg/kg/24 hr q24hr PO.
6. Tympanostomy ventilation tubes may be considered in children with bilateral effusions if prolonged prophylactic antibiotics are unsuccessful or there is a bilateral conductive hearing loss. Duration of ventilation tubes is 6 to 18 months with a mean of 13 months. Adenoidectomy may have an additional benefit if tubes do not reduce the incidence of recurrent AOM, although this issue is controversial. Antihistamines and decongestants do not have proven efficacy.
7. The role of steroids in AOM is under investigation.

DISPOSITION

1. Children may be monitored at home if no other serious systemic infection is present, with a follow-up appointment in 2 to 3 weeks.
2. Children younger than 2 months and those with significant toxicity or immunodeficiencies should be hospitalized.
3. Patients with persistent (after two courses) or recurrent AOM may benefit from otolaryngologic consultation.

Parental Education

1. The entire course of antibiotics should be taken even if the child is better.
2. Antipyretics (acetaminophen or aspirin) may make the child feel better.
3. A return appointment in 2 to 3 weeks should be made for evaluation of response to treatment.
4. Call your physician if any of the following occurs:
   a. There is no improvement in 36 hours or the fever continues beyond 72 hours. If the signs and symptoms continue, the antibiotic may have to be changed

to ensure treatment of resistant organisms.

b. The child becomes increasingly irritable or lethargic.

c. The child has vomiting or diarrhea.

BIBLIOGRAPHY

American Academy of Pediatrics Otitis Media Guideline Panel: managing otitis media with effusion in young children, *Pediatrics* 94:766, 1994.

American Academy of Pediatrics Section on Otolaryngology: follow-up management of children with tympanostomy tubes, *Pediatrics* 109:328, 2002.

Bernard PAM, Stenstrom RJ, Feldman W et al: Randomized controlled trial comparing long-term sulfonamide therapy to ventilation tubes for otitis media with effusion, *Pediatrics* 88:215, 1991.

Casselbram ML, Mandel EM, Fall PA et al: The heritability of otitis media, *JAMA* 282:2125, 1999.

Celin SE, Bluestone CD, Stephenson J et al: Bacteriology of acute otitis media in adults, *JAMA* 266:2249, 1991.

Cohen R, Navel M, Grumberg J et al: One dose ceftriaxone vs ten days of amoxicillin/clavulanate therapy for acute otitis media: clinical efficacy and change in nasopharyngeal flora, *Pediatr Infect Dis* 18:403, 1999.

Committee on Drugs, American Academy of Pediatrics: Guidelines for monitoring and management of pediatric patients during and after sedation for diagnostic and therapeutic procedures, *Pediatrics* 89:1110, 1992.

Culpepper L, Froom J: Routine antimicrobial treatment of acute otitis media: is it necessary? *JAMA* 278:1643, 1997.

Del Mar C, Glasziou P, Hayem M: Are antibiotics indicated as initial treatment for children with acute otitis media? a meta-analysis, *BMJ* 314:1526, 1997.

Dowell SF, Butler JC, Giebink GS et al: Acute otitis media management and surveillance in an era of pneumococcal resistance: a report of the drug-resistant *Streptococcus pneumoniae* therapeutic working group, *Pediatr Infect Dis J* 18:1, 1999.

Gates GA, Avery CA, Prihoda TJ: Effectiveness of adenoidectomy and tympanostomy tubes in the treatment of chronic otitis media with effusion, *N Engl J Med* 317:1444, 1987.

Giebink GS, Canafax DM, Kempthorne J: Antimicrobial treatment of acute otitis media, *J Pediatr* 119:495, 1991.

Green SM, Rothrock SE: Single dose of intramuscular ceftriaxone for acute otitis media in children, *Pediatrics* 91:23, 1993.

Isaacson E, Rosenfield RM: Care of the child with tympanotomy tubes: a guide for the pediatrician, *Pediatrics* 93:924, 1996.

Mandel EM, Casselbrant ML, Rockette HE et al: Efficacy of 20 versus 10-day antimicrobial treatment for acute otitis media, *Pediatrics* 96:5, 1995.

McCracken GH: Diagnosis and management of acute otitis media in the urgent care setting, *Ann Emerg Med* 39:413, 2002.

Paradise JL, Bluestone CD, Rogers KD et al: Efficacy of adenoidectomy for recurrent otitis media in children previously treated with tympanostomy tube placement: results of parallel randomized and non-randomized trials, *JAMA* 263:2066, 1990.

Singer A, Sauris E, Viccellioi AW et al: Ceruminolytic effects of docusate sodium: a randomized controlled trial, *Ann Emerg Med* 36:3, 2000.

External Otitis Media

External otitis media is an inflammatory reaction of the external ear canal.

ETIOLOGY

1. Infection
   a. Perforated TM with drainage of pus
   b. Impetigo
   c. Herpes simplex
   d. Furunculosis associated with *S. aureus*
2. Dermatitis, referred to as "swimmer's ear," causing irritation and damage
3. Foreign body

DIAGNOSTIC FINDINGS

1. Severe pain (particularly on movement of the tragus) and drainage are common.
2. Systemic signs are uncommon.
3. The external ear canal is swollen with drainage, erythema, and edema. The TM is intact and mobile with normal color (unless caused by perforation).

Complications

Malignant external otitis media (caused by *Pseudomonas* organisms) is uncommon.

Ancillary Data

Culture of the discharge is not helpful because it often grows *Pseudomonas* or *S. aureus* organisms, not necessarily reflecting the true pathogens.

DIFFERENTIAL DIAGNOSIS

Ear pain from external otitis media should be differentiated from pain caused by infections such as the following:

1. AOM (p. 605)
2. Dental infection (p. 599)
3. Mastoiditis (p. 604)
4. Posterior auricular lymphadenopathy

MANAGEMENT

1. If no perforation is present, the ear may be irrigated with saline.
2. Eardrops (suspension if perforated) such as polymyxin B (Lidosporin or Cortisporin) should be initiated: 2 to 3 drops, four to six times a day inserted into the ear. If significant swelling is present, a cotton wick should be inserted after being soaked in an otic-drop suspension until direct application of the drops is possible. Many ear solutions and suspensions contain neomycin, which may cause contact dermatitis in 1 of every 1000 patients. If burning is noted and problematic, ophthalmologic drops such as gentamicin or tobramycin may be used as eardrops.
3. Systemic antibiotics are not indicated unless the underlying condition requires such treatment.
4. Foreign bodies, if present, should be removed.

DISPOSITION

Children may be monitored at home and reevaluated if there is no resolution in 4 to 5 days.

Acute Parotitis

ETIOLOGY: INFECTION

1. Viral (nonsuppurative):
   a. Mumps (the most common etiologic agent)
   b. Other: coxsackievirus and parainfluenza virus
2. Bacterial (suppurative):
   a. *S. aureus* or *S. pneumoniae*
   b. Obstruction from stricture, calculi, or foreign material (food) often present
3. Fungal: *Candida* organisms

DIAGNOSTIC FINDINGS

1. Nonsuppurative parotitis (e.g., mumps) is an insidious disease with slow onset of fever and earache accompanied by tenderness and enlargement of the parotid gland.
   a. The ear lobe is pushed upward and outward, and the angle of the mandible is obscured.
   b. The orifice of Stensen's duct is edematous and erythematous and exudes a clear fluid.
2. Suppurative parotitis is caused by an anatomic stricture.
3. Systemic toxicity is present.
4. The area of the parotid gland is painful and tender with overlying erythema.
5. A purulent discharge is noted at Stensen's duct.

Complications

1. Mumps may be associated with encephalitis or orchitis.
2. Suppurative parotitis may follow an episode of nonsuppurative infection.

Ancillary Data

1. Serum amylase value is elevated in acute infectious parotitis and normal in recurrent parotitis.
2. Culture of the drainage from Stensen's duct may be helpful if the suppurative parotitis is unresponsive to antibiotics.
3. Sialogram is rarely helpful.

DIFFERENTIAL DIAGNOSIS

1. Infection: cervical lymphadenopathy (p. 602)
2. Recurrent parotitis: usually unilateral and may occur as many as 10 times before spontaneously resolving

3. Neoplasm
4. Hemangioma

MANAGEMENT

1. Nonsuppurative parotitis, most commonly mumps, resolves without therapy. Discomfort may be reduced by avoiding citrus fruits such as oranges and lemons.
2. Suppurative parotitis requires antibiotic therapy:
   a. For nontoxic children: dicloxacillin, 50 mg/kg/24 hr q6hr PO
   b. For systemically ill children: nafcillin (or equivalent), 100 mg/kg/24 hr q4hr IV
3. If suppurative parotitis is present, surgical consultation should be sought early. Often, probing of Stensen's duct or early I & D is desirable to avoid damage to the facial nerve and to facilitate resolution.

DISPOSITION

All patients may be monitored at home unless they are toxic or have fluctuant parotitis, which requires parenteral therapy.

Parental Education

Mumps is contagious until the swelling has disappeared, usually 6 days into the illness.

1. Avoid citrus fruits because they stimulate the parotid gland with resultant pain.
2. Call your physician if any of the following occurs:
   a. The swelling has not resolved in 7 days.
   b. Erythema, increasing tenderness, or pain develops over the parotid gland.

BIBLIOGRAPHY

Meyer C, Cotton RT: Salivary gland disease in children: a review, *Clin Pediatr* 26:314, 1986.

Peritonsillar Abscess

Tonsillar infections occasionally suppurate beyond the tonsillar capsule into surrounding tissues.

ETIOLOGY

Bacterial infection often involving multiple organisms:

1. Group A streptococci common
2. Uncommonly *H. influenzae, S. pneumoniae, S. aureus*
3. Normal mouth flora, including anaerobes

DIAGNOSTIC FINDINGS

These infections have a rapid onset.

1. Toxicity accompanied by fever, severe sore throat, progressive trismus, drooling, alteration in speech ("hot potato voice"), and dysphagia are common.
2. Tonsil is unilaterally displaced medially with erythema and edema of the soft palate. Palpation may be useful. Uvula deviates to the opposite side. The abscess may be fluctuant.
3. Differentiating between abscess and cellulitis may be difficult. In 24 hours, a cellulitis is usually better or has progressed to a true abscess.
4. May occur concurrent with infectious mononucleosis.

Complications

1. Extension beyond the tonsillar regions into the retropharyngeal or mediastinal spaces
2. Upper respiratory obstruction as a result of edema and swelling
3. Aspiration pneumonia secondary to spontaneous rupture

Ancillary Data

1. Needle aspiration with culture and Gram stain

2. WBC count usually elevated with a shift to the left
3. Throat culture for group A streptococci
4. CT scan
5. EB virus

DIFFERENTIAL DIAGNOSIS

Peritonsillar abscess should be differentiated from infection caused by the following:

1. Severe pharyngotonsillitis from group A streptococci or infectious mononucleosis.
2. Parapharyngeal abscess with erythema and swelling of the lateral pharyngeal wall and brawny induration of the neck. Neck spasms and torticollis occur in children, usually those younger than 5 years.
3. Peritonsillar cellulitis without definite abscess or displacement of the uvula. This disorder can often be treated with high doses of penicillin and close follow-up observation.
4. Tetanus.
5. Dental infection.

MANAGEMENT

If there is any compromise of the airway, intervention to protect it should be an immediate priority.

1. Antibiotics should be initiated early in treatment: ampicillin, 100 to 200 mg/kg/24 hr q4hr IV.
   a. If resolution is slow: nafcillin (or equivalent), 100 to 150 mg/kg/24 hr q4hr IV, should be started. An alternative or adjunct is clindamycin, 15 to 40 mg q6-8hr IV, especially in toxic children.
   b. The antibiotic agent may be changed when results of culture and sensitivity testing are available.
2. Analgesia may be given: meperidine (Demerol), 1 to 2 mg/kg/dose q4-6hr IM.
3. I & D is required if the abscess is fluctuant, the child is toxic, or there is no resolution after 48 hours of therapy:
   a. Needle aspiration may initially be both diagnostic and therapeutic.
   b. Definitive I & D should be carried out in the operating room.
4. Tonsillectomy is indicated on an elective basis 3 to 4 weeks after resolution of the inflammation unless improvement is slow, in which case it may be performed on an emergent basis.

DISPOSITION

Patients with peritonsillar abscess should be admitted to the hospital for antibiotic therapy and drainage. An otolaryngologist should be involved in the management.

BIBLIOGRAPHY

Hardingham M: Peritonsillar infections, *Otolaryngol Clin North Am* 20:273, 1987.

Pharyngotonsillitis (Sore Throat)

Acute pharyngitis is commonly associated with tonsillitis resulting from inflammation of the throat, with associated soreness, fever, and minimal nasal involvement.

ETIOLOGY: INFECTION

1. Bacterial:
   a. Group A streptococci
   b. Less common pathogens, including *Neisseria gonorrhoeae, H. influenzae, Neisseria meningitidis*, other streptococci, and *Corynebacterium diphtheriae*
2. Viral:
   a. Adenovirus: patient may have accompanying conjunctivitis.
   b. Enterovirus: herpangina with associated fever, sore throat, dysphagia,

vomiting, and small vesicles on the soft palate, tonsil, or pharynx.

c. Influenza, parainfluenza, Epstein-Barr (EB) virus (infectious mononucleosis), and herpes simplex (less frequent); 15% of patients with infectious mononucleosis also have group A streptococcal infection.

3. *M. pneumoniae*: common in school-age children.

DIAGNOSTIC FINDINGS (Table 73-2)

Clinically, patients have a range of symptoms, making it difficult to differentiate group A streptococcal infections from viral infections on the basis of the signs and symptoms alone.

1. Infants with streptococcal infections commonly have excoriated nares and are listless.
2. A viral cause is generally more likely in children up to 6 years of age.
3. Children younger than 3 years with group A streptococcal infection typically have chronic, mucopurulent rhinitis, low-grade fever, and cervical adenitis.
4. Streptococcal infections in school-age children produce complaints of sore throat, accompanied by headache, vomiting, and abdominal pain. The peak age is 5 to 12 years.
5. Adults with streptococcal infection have tonsillar findings similar to those in school-age children but rarely have

TABLE 73-2 Pharyngotonsillitis: Diagnostic Signs and Symptoms

	GROUP A STREPTOCOCCI			
	Infant	**School-Age**	**Adult**	**Viral**
ONSET	Gradual	Sudden	Sudden	Gradual
CHIEF COMPLAINT	Anorexia, rhinitis, listlessness	Sore throat	Sore throat	Sore throat, cough, hoarseness, rhinitis, conjunctivitis
DIAGNOSTIC FINDINGS				
Sore throat	+	+++	+++	+++
Tonsillar erythema	+	+++	+++	++
Tonsillar exudate	+	++	+++	+
Palatal petechiae	+	+++	+++	+
Adenitis	+++	+++	+++	++
Excoriated nares	+++	+	+	+
Conjunctivitis	+	+	+	+++
Cough	+	+	+	+++
Congestion	+	+	+	+++
Hoarseness	+	+	+	+++
Fever	Low grade	High	High	Rare or low grade
Abdominal pain	+	++	+	+
Headache	+	++	++	+
Vomiting	+	++	++	+
Scarlatiniform rash	+	+++	+++	+
Streptococcal contact	+++	+++	+++	+
ANCILLARY DATA				
Positive streptococcal culture	+++	++	+++	+
Elevated white blood cell count	++	++	+++	+

+ to +++, Relative of finding.

abdominal pain or a history of contact. This infection is uncommon in adults except during epidemics.
6. A scarlatiniform rash is diagnostic of streptococcal infection (infants rarely have the eruption).
7. Weighing against the possibility of group A streptococcal infection in a child is the presence of rhinorrhea, cough, or hoarseness as well as the absence of fever, tonsillopharyngeal erythema or exudate, and cervical adenitis.
8. Exudative pharyngitis accompanies infection with group A streptococci, EB virus (infectious mononucleosis, p. 730), *Corynebacterium diphtheriae,* or adenoviruses. Exudative pharyngitis is commonly caused by a virus in children younger than 3 years and frequently caused by group A streptococci in children older than 6 years. In children younger than 6 years, group A streptococci account for 10% to 20% of cases. Soft palate petechiae are found with group A streptococcal and EB virus infections; vesicles or ulcers on the posterior tonsillar pillars with enterovirus infection; and ulcers on the anterior palate with adenopathy in herpes infections.

Complications

1. Group A streptococci: acute rheumatic fever (ARF) (p. 575) and acute glomerulonephritis (p. 817). Half of children with these sequelae have no history of an antecedent pharyngitis. ARF may be prevented if therapy is started within 7 to 9 days of onset of symptoms.
2. Otitis media (p. 605).
3. Cervical lymphadenopathy (p. 602).
4. Recurrent streptococcal pharyngitis (histories rarely reliable). Culture documentation is important.
5. Chronic adenotonsillar hypertrophy may lead to upper airway obstruction.

Ancillary Data

Throat cultures are indicated for the patient who has a sore throat with or without fever to help exclude group A streptococci as the cause.

1. Culture specimens should normally be evaluated only for group A streptococci, optimally with the use of selective media, anaerobic methodology, bacitracin "A" discs, or antigen testing techniques. Swab specimens are best obtained by rotating the swab over both tonsillar areas. Repeat swabbing twice. Culture of a single specimen may miss a small number of patients in whom culture of duplicate specimens identifies group A streptococcal infection.
2. In an infant, nasal rather than throat specimens should be cultured.
3. Positive culture results with low colony counts may indicate the carrier state. To investigate this possibility, a serum streptococcal antigen (Streptozyme) test must be ordered. Low titers are consistent with the chronic carrier state.
4. Symptomatic family members should undergo culture.
5. If symptoms are suggestive, culture for *C. diphtheriae.*
6. Rapid simple diagnostic tools to identify group A streptococci make immediate diagnosis possible, simplifying management. A number of these assays appear to be more sensitive and specific than culture of a single throat specimen, thereby omitting the need for concurrent cultures in patients with negative rapid streptococcal test results. If other tests with significant false-negative rates are used, it is essential to confirm negative test results with a routine throat culture.

MANAGEMENT

Symptomatic relief may be obtained by gargling with warm water, sucking hard candy, and taking aspirin or acetaminophen (40 to 50 mg/kg/24 hr q6hr PO).

1. If the infection is streptococcal, antibiotic therapy should be administered for a total of 10 days of continuous therapy (unless given IM):
   a. Penicillin VK, 25 to 50 mg (40,000 to 80,000 units)/kg/24 hr q6hr PO, *or*
   b. Benzathine penicillin G administered IM once (usually given as 900,000: 300,000 Bicillin C-R, which is 75% benzathine, because it hurts less). Dosage should be calculated by the amount of benzathine required:

Weight (lb)	Benzathine Penicillin G (units)	Bicillin C-R (units) (900,000 Benzathine: 300,000 Procaine)
>30	300,000	300,000:100,000
31-60	600,000	600,000:200,000
61-90	900,000	900,000:300,000
>90	1,200,000	NA

2. Alternative antibiotics.
   a. Erythromycin, 30 to 50 mg/kg/24 hr q8hr PO. Erythromycin estolate (30-50 mg/kg/24 hr q6-8hr PO) has fewer gastrointestinal symptoms and the additional benefit of treating other potential pharyngeal pathogens, such as *Chlamydia* organisms.
   b. Clarithromycin (Biaxin), 15 mg/kg/24 hr q12hr PO for 10 days.
   c. Azithromycin (Zithromax), 10 mg/kg/24 hr q24hr PO first day, then 5 mg/kg/24 hr q24hr PO on days 2 through 5.
3. Evidence suggests that 5 days of amoxicillin-clavulanate, cefuroxime, or clarithromycin are equivalent to 10 days of penicillin.

Symptomatic improvement is noted after early therapy with antibiotics. Treatment also allows children to return to school or daycare sooner, thereby decreasing the associated family disruption. Patients may return to school (work or daycare) 24 hours after beginning medication. The risk of acute rheumatic fever and acute glomerulonephritis is not increased if antibiotics are started within 7 days of the onset of symptoms.

Preliminary studies have shown that equivalent cure rates may be achieved by a dosage in children of penicillin VK, 250 mg q12hr PO, or erythromycin, 20 mg/kg/24 hr q12hr PO for 10 days. Another alternative is cefadroxil (Duricef), 30 mg/kg/24 hr q24hr PO for 10 days (expensive).

Indications for tonsillectomy for recurrent sore throats are controversial, and the procedure should be considered only in selected cases. Symptomatic chronic adenotonsillar hypertrophy may require removal of the tonsils and adenoids. A 30-day course of amoxicillin-clavulanate, in a dose of 40 mg amoxicillin/kg/24 hr q8hr PO, may reduce the need for surgery.

Evidence suggests that the child with *problematic* group A streptococcal carriage may be treated with benzathine penicillin G as outlined *plus* rifampin, 10 mg/kg/dose q12hr for eight doses PO. Clindamycin, 20 mg/kg/24 hr (maximum: 450 mg/24 hr) q8hr PO for 10 days, may be substituted for rifampin. Another regimen is to use penicillin V, 250 to 500 mg q8-12hr for 10 days, and to add rifampin, 20 mg/kg/24 hr q24hr, for the last 4 days of the penicillin course.

DISPOSITION

Patients may be monitored at home.

Parental Education

1. Medication should be taken for the full 10 days (unless given IM).
2. Symptomatic treatment may be helpful:
   a. Gargle with warm salt water (1 tsp salt in 8-oz glass of water).
   b. Suck hard candy.
   c. Take aspirin or acetaminophen (10 to 15 mg/kg/dose q6hr prn PO).

3. Family members who are symptomatic with fever, sore throat, anorexia, or headache should undergo throat or nasal culture.
4. Children may return to school in 24 hours.
5. Call your physician if any of the following occurs:
   a. Severe pain, drooling, difficulty swallowing or breathing, or big, swollen lymph nodes develop.
   b. There is evidence of infection elsewhere.
   c. The fever lasts longer than 48 hours.

BIBLIOGRAPHY

Bass JW: A review of the rationale and advantages of various mixtures of benzathine penicillin G, *Pediatrics* 97:960, 1996.

Bisno AT: Acute pharyngitis: etiology and diagnosis, *Pediatrics* 97:949, 1996.

Doctor A, Harper MB, Fleisher CR: Group A beta-hemolytic streptococcal bacteremia: historical overview, changing incidence and recent association with varicella, *Pediatrics* 96:428,1995.

Gerber MA, Randolph MF, DeMeo KK et al: Lack of impact of early antibiotic therapy for streptococcal pharyngitis on recurrence rates, *J Pediatr* 117:853, 1990.

Green SM: Acute pharyngitis: the case for empiric antimicrobial therapy, *Ann Emerg Med* 25:404, 1995.

Hofer C, Binns HJ, Tanz RR: Strategies for managing streptococcal pharyngitis, *Arch Pediatr Adolesc Med* 151:824, 1997.

Nawaz H, Smith DS, Mazhari R et al: Concordance of clinical findings and clinical judgment in the diagnosis of streptococcal pharyngitis, *Acad Emerg Med* 7:1104, 2000.

Pichichero ME: Group A streptococcal tonsillopharyngitis: cost-effective diagnosis and treatment, *Ann Emerg Med* 25:390, 1995.

Portier H, Chavenet PK, Waldner A et al: Five versus 10 day treatment of streptococcal pharyngotonsillitis: a randomized controlled trial comparing cefpodoxime proxetil and phenoxymethylpenicillin, *Scand J Infect Dis* 26:591, 1994.

Selafani AP, Ginsburg J, Shah MK et al: Treatment of symptomatic chronic adenotonsillar hypertrophy with amoxicillin/clavulanate potassium: short- and long-term results, *Pediatrics* 101:675, 1998.

Tanz RR, Poncher JR, Corydon KE et al: Clindamycin treatment of chronic pharyngeal carriage of group A streptococcus, *J Pediatr* 119:123, 1991.

Retropharyngeal Abscess

ALERT Retropharyngeal abscess needs immediate intervention to prevent respiratory obstruction.

Otitis media and nasopharyngeal infections may lead to suppurative adenitis of the small lymph nodes between the buccopharyngeal and prevertebral fascia. If untreated, this condition can lead to abscess formation, particularly in children younger than 5 years.

ETIOLOGY

Retropharyngeal abscess results from bacterial infection commonly caused by group A streptococci, *S. aureus, Haemophilus* species (71% beta-lactamase producer), and anaerobes (*Bacteroides, Peptostreptococcus,* and *Fusobacterium* species). It occurs by direct spread from nasopharyngitis, otitis media, vertebral osteomyelitis, or wound infection after a penetrating injury of the posterior pharynx or palate.

DIAGNOSTIC FINDINGS

1. Nasopharyngitis or otitis media usually precedes the development of fever, difficulty swallowing, drooling, and severe throat pain. Patients may have a muffled voice, dysphagia or trismus, or stridor or swelling of the posterior wall of the pharynx and cervical nodes.
2. Meningismus may result from irritation of the paravertebral ligaments. Some patients complain of pain in the back of the neck or shoulder that is precipitated or aggravated by swallowing.
3. Labored respirations with gurgling and hyperextension of the head are evidence of potential respiratory obstruction.
4. A definite unilateral posterior pharyngeal wall mass is present, often becoming fluctuant.

Complications

1. Obstruction of the trachea, esophagus, or nasal passages.

2. Aspiration pneumonia if abscess ruptures. Possible dissection of purulent material into mediastinum.
3. Sudden death if abscess erodes into major blood vessel.

Ancillary Data

1. Lateral neck x-ray film. Demonstrates increased soft tissue mass between the anterior wall of the cervical spine and the pharyngeal wall. In a child the retropharyngeal soft tissue should not be greater than 5 mm at the level of C3 or 40% of the anteroposterior (AP) diameter of the body at C4 at that level. CT, ultrasonography, or magnetic resonance imaging (MRI) are more sensitive in characterizing soft tissue swelling and defining the anatomy.
2. WBC: Increased with shift to left.
3. Cultures and Gram stain of purulent material. Obtained from I & D.

DIFFERENTIAL DIAGNOSIS

1. Infection: croup or epiglottitis
2. Trauma: foreign body

MANAGEMENT

1. Stabilize the airway, if necessary. Monitor.
2. Initiate antibiotics immediately: nafcillin (or equivalent), 100 to 150 mg/kg/24 hr q4hr IV. Clindamycin, 15 to 40 mg q6-8hr IV, may also be considered.
3. Give analgesia: meperidine (Demerol), 1 to 2 mg/kg/dose q4-6hr IM.
4. I & D is indicated immediately if obstruction is present or an evolving abscess becomes fluctuant:
   a. Normally performed in the operating room.
   b. The head is positioned down and hyperextended to minimize aspiration.

DISPOSITION

All patients with retropharyngeal abscess need hospitalization, antibiotics, and immediate otolaryngologic consultation.

BIBLIOGRAPHY

Asmar BI: Bacteriology of retropharyngeal abscess in children, *Pediatr Infect Dis* 9:595, 1990.

Brook I: Microbiology of retropharyngeal abscesses in children, *Am J Dis Child* 141:202, 1987.

Morrison JE, Pashley NRT: Retropharyngeal abscesses in children: a 10-year review, *Pediatr Emerg Care* 4:9, 1988.

Rhinitis (Common Cold)

Nasopharyngitis, or rhinitis, is common among children and represents what is usually a self-limited process. Nasal rhinitis may be allergic in origin as well as infectious.

ETIOLOGY: INFECTION

1. Viral: rhinovirus, respiratory syncytial virus (RSV), adenovirus, influenza, parainfluenza
2. Bacterial: *C. diphtheriae, H. influenzae, S. pneumoniae, N. meningitidis*

DIAGNOSTIC FINDINGS

Patients have nasal congestion, sneezing, and, commonly, a clear watery discharge. Throat irritation and pharyngitis may be associated. There are minimal constitutional symptoms.

Associated clinical findings include lymphadenopathy, otitis media, sinusitis, pneumonia, croup, and bronchiolitis. Allergic rhinitis is usually accompanied by pale, swollen, and boggy nasal mucosa.

Ancillary Data

Nasal cultures should not be done because there is no way to interpret the results unless nares are excoriated (group A streptococci).

MANAGEMENT

Symptomatic therapy is indicated by removing the discharge and attempting to decrease congestion:

1. In younger children, use a bulb syringe. Neo-Synephrine nosedrops (0.25% phenylephrine) may also be used q4hr.

2. In older children, use a bulb syringe or prescribe nose blowing and decongestants. Oxymetazoline (Afrin) nosedrops (0.025% to 0.05%) q8-12hr may be helpful. Routine antibiotic treatment of purulent nasopharyngitis is not useful. Antihistamine-decongestant combinations have little impact on the common cold.
3. Allergic rhinitis may be treated with antihistamines. The first choice is the inexpensive alkylamines such as chlorpheniramine (0.35 mg/kg/24 hr q6hr PO). Another alternative is clemastine (Tavist). Some clinicians use a nasal spray such as oxymetazoline or Nasalcrom.
4. Antiviral agents may be useful in selected circumstances:
   a. Amantidine (Symmetrel) is active against influenza A. Suggested pediatric dosage for prophylaxis and active treatment is 5 mg/kg/24 hr bid PO to a maximum of 150 mg in children 1 to 9 years old for 3 to 5 days in treatment for active disease.
   b. Rimantidine (Flumadine) is also active against influenza A. The dosage is identical to that for amantidine.

Parental Education

1. Place 2 to 3 drops of water or fresh salt water (tsp of salt in a cup of water) in each nostril with the child lying on the back.
2. If old enough, have the child blow the nose.
3. With a baby, use a rubber bulb syringe to remove the mucus.
4. Use a vaporizer in the child's room during napping and sleeping.
5. For children older than 18 months, use decongestants such as pseudoephedrine and chlorpheniramine (can be obtained over the counter without prescription).
6. Call your physician if any of the following occurs:
   a. Child has a fever and is younger than 3 months.
   b. The fever lasts longer than 24 to 48 hours.
   c. Child has difficulty breathing, is wheezing, or has croup or any other evidence of infection, such as red eye or ear pain.
   d. The skin under the nose becomes crusty.

BIBLIOGRAPHY

Arora A, Magee L, Peck J et al: Antiviral therapeutics for the pediatric population, *Pediatr Emerg Care* 27:369, 2001.

Hutton N, Wilson MH, Mellits ED et al: Effectiveness of antihistamine-decongestant combination for young children with the common cold: a randomized, controlled clinical trial, *J Pediatr* 118:125, 1991.

Todd JK, Todd N, Damato J et al: Bacteriology and treatment of purulent nasopharyngitis: a double blind, placebo controlled evaluation, *Pediatr Infect Dis* 3:226, 1984.

Acute Sinusitis

ALERT Sinusitis may be associated with intracranial and extracranial infections.

Swelling of the nasal mucosa and obstruction of the meatus result in an acute inflammatory reaction within the sinuses.

ETIOLOGY

1. Infections:
   a. Common bacteria infections: *H. influenzae* accounts for 19% to 32% of positive aerobic cultures; *S. pneumoniae*, 9% to 28%; group A streptococci, 17% to 27%; *S. aureus*, 6% to 21%; and *Moraxella catarrhalis*.
   b. Fungal infections in diabetic and immunocompromised patients.
   c. Up to 93% of patients with chronic sinusitis have infection with anaerobic organisms (*Bacteroides* species and *Fusobacterium* species).

      NOTE: Culture results are nondiagnostic in as many as a third of patients.

2. Impairment of normal nasal physiologic processes with poor ventilation and increased secretions secondary to adenoidal hypertrophy, polyps, cleft palate, or allergies.
3. Trauma.
4. Dental infections with contiguous spread.

DIAGNOSTIC FINDINGS

1. Rhinorrhea is present in 78% of patients, 64% having a purulent discharge. Cough, often worse at night (50%), sinus pain or headache (12%), and temperatures over 38.5° C (101° F) (19%) are reported. Concurrent upper respiratory tract infections are common; signs and symptoms are insidious. Malodorous breath *(fetor oris)* may be noted.
2. Only 8% of patients have tenderness overlying the frontal, ethmoid, or maxillary sinuses, whereas transillumination of the sinuses is unequal or poor in 76%. Transillumination is of limited value in children because of the variable development of sinuses before age 8 to 10 years. Sphenoid sinusitis is associated with occipital or retroorbital pain and is rare in children. Swelling may be present over an involved sinus.
3. Chronic sinusitis may have variable findings. Malaise, fatigability, and anorexia may be noted.

Complications

Complications occur in 4.5% of patients with sinusitis:

1. Periorbital infections, particularly ethmoid (p. 583)
2. Osteomyelitis of the sinus wall, most commonly the frontal (this appears as Pott's puffy tumor, a midfrontal swelling)
3. Brain, subdural, or epidural abscesses
4. Meningitis

Ancillary Data

1. X-ray film studies have variable reliability in young children and are not routinely recommended in children <6 years or younger. Normal sinus film findings are helpful. Abnormal sinus film findings are difficult to interpret, although in children older than 6 years, the interpretation can be more definitive. The ethmoid sinuses develop completely by 7 years, and the maxillary sinuses shortly thereafter, whereas the frontal and sphenoid sinuses develop after puberty.

   Sinusitis appears as clouding, mucosal thickening, or air-fluid levels within the sinuses, the last being most helpful in defining an acute infection. CT (coronal, without a contrast agent) is the standard of diagnosis and may obviate plain films.

   X-ray films are indicated if the child is seriously ill, has had recurrent episodes, or has chronic disease or suspected suppurative complications.
2. Antral puncture with aspiration by an otolaryngologist is indicated for severe pain unresponsive to medical management; sinusitis in a seriously ill, toxic child; an unsatisfactory response; suppurative complications; or sinusitis in an immunocompromised host. Gram stain and aerobic and anaerobic cultures should be performed on the aspirated material.

DIFFERENTIAL DIAGNOSIS

1. Allergy
2. Foreign body in the nose (p. 601)
3. Neoplasm or polyp
4. Functional organic causes of headache (see Chapter 36)

MANAGEMENT

The symptoms in bacterial sinusitis usually resolve in 48 to 72 hours. Up to 20% of patients have a persistent nasal discharge after a 2-week course of antibiotics:

1. Antibiotic treatment for 2 to 3 weeks:
   a. Augmentin (amoxicillin with clavulanic acid), 20 to 40 mg amoxicillin/kg/24 hr q8hr PO, *or*
   b. Amoxicillin, 50 mg/kg/24 hr q8hr PO, *or*
   c. Cefuroxime (Ceftin), 8 mg q24hr PO

   NOTE: Empiric recommendations for length of therapy range from 10 to 28 days. An alternative is to treat for 7 days after the patient becomes symptom free. Failure of response justifies the addition of specific coverage for *S. aureus* (dicloxacillin, 50 mg/kg/24 hr q6hr PO) and anaerobic organisms.
2. Decongestants and antihistamines are commonly used. Afrin or Neo-Synephrine nosedrops may be used for 2 days. Topical nasal steroids can help if an allergic component is suspected.
3. Desensitization rarely may be helpful if allergies are a contributory factor.
4. Sphenoid sinusitis requires aggressive antibiotic therapy (often parenteral), sometimes in conjunction with surgical drainage.
5. For management of chronic sinusitis, another antibiotic should be used after the previously described standard regimen:
   a. Clindamycin, 25 to 40 mg q6-8hr IV or 20 mg/kg/24 hr q8hr PO, *or*
   b. Cefoxitin (Mefoxin), 80 to 160 mg/kg/24 hr IV

DISPOSITION

1. Patients can usually be discharged and instructed to take oral antibiotics at home for 2 to 3 weeks. If symptoms do not resolve, patients should be referred to an otolaryngologist for assessment and possible irrigation of the antrum.
2. Patients with sphenoid sinusitis are usually hospitalized for parenteral therapy.

Parental Education

Call the physician if any of the following occurs:

1. Symptoms worsen or the patient has a fever or toxicity.
2. Symptoms have not improved markedly in 1 week and disappeared in 2 to 3 weeks.

BIBLIOGRAPHY

American Academy of Pediatrics Subcommittee on Management of Sinusitis: Clinical practice guidelines: management of sinusitis, *Pediatrics* 108:798, 2001.

Goldenhersh MJ, Rachelefsky GS: Sinusitis: early recognition, aggressive treatment, *Contemp Pediatr* 6:22, 1989.

Hnatuk LAF, Macdonald RE, Papsin BL: Isolated sphenoid sinusitis, *J Otolaryngol* 23:36, 1994.

Johnson DL, Markle BM, Wiedermann BL: Treatment of intracranial abscesses associated with sinusitis in children and adolescents, *J Pediatr* 113:15, 1988.

Kovatch AL, Wald ER, Ledesma-Medina J et al: Maxillary sinus radiographs in children with nonrespiratory complaints, *Pediatrics* 73:306, 1984.

Lew D, Southwick FS, Montgomery WW et al: Sphenoid sinusitis: a review of 30 cases, *N Engl J Med* 309:1149, 1983.

O'Brien KL, Dowell SF, Schwartz B et al: Acute sinusitis: principles of judicious use of antimicrobial agents, *Pediatrics* 101:174, 1998.

Tinkelman DG, Silk HJ: Clinical and bacteriologic features of chronic sinusitis in children, *Am J Dis Child* 143:938, 1989.

Wald ER: Chronic sinusitis in children, *J Pediatr* 127:339, 1995.

Wald ER: Sinusitis in children, *Pediatr Infect Dis J* 7:S150, 1988.

Williams JW, Simel DC: Does this patient have sinusitis? *JAMA* 270:1242, 1993.

Acute Stomatitis

Acute stomatitis is generalized inflammation of the oral mucosa.

ETIOLOGY AND DIAGNOSTIC FINDINGS

Infection

1. Herpes simplex causes distinct multiple small ulcers of the oral mucosa and generalized inflammation. In rare cases, other viruses (e.g., coxsackievirus) may cause diffuse ulceration,

primarily on the palate, that lasts 7 to 10 days.
2. Thrush is caused by *Candida albicans*. The white plaques are predominantly on the buccal mucosa and tongue with generalized erythema.

Aphthous Stomatitis or "Canker Sores"

"Canker sores" are erythematous, indurated papules that quickly erode to become painful circumscribed necrotic lesions of the mucosa that do not involve the lips. Their onset is often related to physical or emotional stress, and they resolve spontaneously in 1 to 2 weeks.

Complication

Dehydration may result if oral intake is impaired by painful ulcers.

DIFFERENTIAL DIAGNOSIS

1. Infection: necrotizing ulcerative gingivitis (Vincent angina) (p. 602)
2. Trauma:
   a. Acid, alkali, or other caustic agents (p. 372)
   b. Mechanical or thermal injuries

MANAGEMENT

1. These entities are self-limited but occasionally cause discomfort and interfere with intake so that some intervention is appropriate. Approaches to local analgesia include the following:
   a. Antacid (Maalox or Mylanta) gargled or swallowed to coat the mucosa, *or*
   b. 1% to 2% viscous lidocaine (Xylocaine) gargled or applied directly prn, *or*
   c. Mixture (1 part each) of lidocaine (2% viscous Xylocaine), diphenhydramine (Benadryl), and kaolin-pectin (Kaopectate), gargled prn

   NOTE: The dosage of the 2% viscous lidocaine (Xylocaine) should not exceed 15 ml q3hr or 120 ml in 24 hours in the adult (proportionately less in children). The patient should not eat or drink for 1 hour after application because of the danger of aspiration.
2. Frequent mouthwashes and alteration of diet to bland foods may help.
3. Thrush may be treated with nystatin (100,000 units/ml), using 1 ml (dropper) in each side of mouth four times a day, and continued for 3 to 4 days after resolution.

DISPOSITION

Patients should be followed at home unless the hydration status requires inpatient therapy.

74 Endocrine Disorders

Also See Chapter 38 (Hypoglycemia)

Adrenal Insufficiency

ETIOLOGY

1. Congenital: enzymatic defects, hemorrhage (birth injury), and hypoplasia
2. Infection:
   a. Waterhouse-Friderichsen syndrome (adrenal hemorrhage), *Neisseria meningitidis, Streptococcus pneumoniae*
   b. Tuberculosis, histoplasmosis
3. Autoimmune disease
4. Withdrawal of steroid therapy or unusual stress in patient taking pharmacologic dosage of glucocorticosteroids (e.g., surgery, infection)

DIAGNOSTIC FINDINGS

See Table 74-1.

DIFFERENTIAL DIAGNOSIS

1. Acute insufficiency: infection, poisoning, diabetic ketoacidosis, hemorrhage
2. Addison's disease: central nervous system (CNS) disease such as tumor or anorexia nervosa

MANAGEMENT

1. Initial management: Restore intravascular volume with normal saline (0.9% NS), initially 20 ml/kg and then at a rate reflecting vital signs. When appropriate, correct levels of electrolytes and glucose and achieve acid-base balance. Hypotension may require pressor agents.
2. Adrenal corticosteroid replacement therapy (Table 74-2):
   a. Acute crises:
      (1) Hydrocortisone (Solu-Cortef), 2 mg/kg/dose q4-6hr intravenously (IV), *and*
      (2) Cortisone, 1 to 5 mg/kg/24 hr q12-24hr PO, to allow tapering of intravenous medications. Intramuscular cortisone therapy often is recommended initially to facilitate the transition to oral therapy once stabilization has occurred.
   b. Addison's disease:
      (1) Glucocorticoids:
         - Hydrocortisone, 0.5 mg/kg/24 hr (15-20 mg/m^2/24 hr) q6-8hr PO; *or*
         - Cortisone, 0.5 to 0.75 mg/kg/24 hr (20 mg/m^2/24 hr) q6-8hr PO; *or*
         - Prednisone, 0.1 to 0.15 mg/kg/24 hr (4-5 mg/m^2/24 hr) PO
      (2) Mineralocorticoids:
         - Fludrocortisone (Florinef), 0.05 to 0.1 mg/24 hr PO; *or*
         - Desoxycorticosterone, 1 to 5 mg per 24-48 hr intramuscularly (IM)
3. Give antibiotics when indicated.

TABLE 74-1 Distinguishing Acute from Chronic Adrenal Insufficiency

Clinical Manifestation	Acute	Chronic (Addison's Disease)
Nausea/vomiting	+++	+++
Abdominal pain	++	++
Hypothermia	+	±
Hypotension	+++	+++
Dehydration	++	±
Failure to thrive	–	+
Fatigue/weakness	+++	+++
Confusion, coma	+	–
Hyperpigmentation	–	++
Hypoglycemia	++	++
↓ Na^+/↑ K^+	+++	+++

4. Give corticosteroids for patients with adrenal insufficiency who are undergoing surgery:
   a. Administer hydrocortisone (Solu-Cortef), 1 to 2 mg/kg IV (or equivalent), before surgery. In an emergency, administer as preanesthetic drug. If surgery is elective, administer in four doses over 48 hours.
   b. During anesthesia, administer hydrocortisone, 25 to 100 mg IV.
   c. After surgery, give hydrocortisone, 0.5 to 1.0 mg/kg/dose q6hr IV, for 3 days and then taper to presurgical levels (if any).

DISPOSITION

Patients with acute adrenal crisis should be admitted to an intensive care unit (ICU). In cases of chronic illness, disposition must be determined by clinical status and ease of follow-up, which is essential.

BIBLIOGRAPHY

Urban MD, Kogut MD: Adrenocortical insufficiency in the child, *Curr Ther Endocrinol Metab* 5:131, 1994.

Diabetic Ketoacidosis

ALERT Start treatment early with hydration. Insulin may be given once a glucose determination has been made. Always look for a precipitating cause. Monitor vital signs, intake and output, and mental status.

Diabetes mellitus has certain unique features in the pediatric age group. Children are more subject to infection, emotional and environmental stresses, increased caloric requirements, and extremes of activity and dietary patterns. These features put the child with diabetes at risk of development of ketoacidosis.

Diabetic ketoacidosis (DKA) requires urgent attention when a patient is hyperglycemic (serum glucose >300 mg/dl), ketonemic (serum ketones large level at >1:2 dilution), or acidotic (pH <7.1 or serum bicarbonate [HCO_3] value <12 mEq/L) and is experiencing glycosuria and ketonuria.

ETIOLOGY: PRECIPITATING FACTORS

A number of conditions cause DKA in a patient with well-controlled diabetes:

1. Infection: virus, bacteria (group A streptococci or abscess is common).
2. Intrapsychic: emotional or environmental stresses at home or school. Adolescents often manipulate their surroundings by becoming ill.
3. Drugs and diet: alteration of normal insulin dosage (poor compliance); ingestion of steroids, birth control pills; major change in diet.
4. Trauma: major trauma or surgery.
5. Endocrine: pregnancy, puberty, Cushing's syndrome, hyperthyroidism.

DIAGNOSTIC FINDINGS (Box 74-1)

DKA is marked by tachypnea with Kussmaul's respiration (deep, rapid pattern), tachycardia, orthostatic blood pressure changes, acetone on the breath, vomiting, dehydration, and mental

TABLE 74-2 Adrenal Corticosteroids

Drug	Availability	Dose*	Frequency	Gluco-corticoid Effect†	Mineralo-corticoid Effect†
GLUCOCORTICOIDS					
Cortisone	IM: 25, 50 mg/ml	0.25 mg/kg/24 hr	q12-24hr	100 mg	100 mg
	PO: 5, 25 mg	0.5-0.75 mg/kg/24 hr	q6-8hr		
Hydrocortisone (Solu-Cortef)	PO: 5, 10, 20 mg	0.5 mg/kg/24 hr	q8hr	80 mg	80 mg
	IV/IM: 100, 250, 500 mg	Asthma§: 4-5 mg/kg/dose	q6hr		
Prednisone	PO: 1, 5, 10, 20 mg, 5 mg/5 ml‡	0.1-0.15 mg/kg/24 hr	q12hr	20 mg	Little effect
		Asthma§: 1-2 mg/kg/24 hr	q6hr		
Methylprednisolone (Solu-Medrol)	IV: 40, 125, 500,1000 mg	Asthma§: 1-2 mg/kg/dose	q6hr	16 mg	No effect
Dexamethasone (Decadron)	IV/IM: 4, 24 mg/ml	Croup: 0.60 mg/kg/dose	q6hr	2 mg	No effect
	PO: 1, 2, 4, 6 mg; 0.5 mg/ml	Meningitis: 0.15 mg/kg/dose	q6hr (16 doses)		
MINERALOCORTICOIDS					
Fludrocortisone (Florinef)	PO: 0.1 mg	0.05-1 mg/24 hr	q24hr	5 mg	0.2 mg
Desoxycorticosterone (DOCA)	IM: 5 mg/ml (in oil)	1-5 mg/24-48 hr	q24-48hr	No effect	2 mg

With long-term therapy, dose requires adjustment. Attempt QOD dosing when using pharmacologic doses. Long-acting preparation for physiologic replacement are available with monthly (or longer) activity.

* Physiologic replacement unless otherwise indicated.

† Equivalent doses of different drugs required for same clinical effect.

‡ Also available as prednisolone (Orapred) 15 mg/ml.

§ Asthma, status asthmaticus.

status changes, which may lead to obtundation and coma. Abdominal pain is a common finding, often mimicking an acute surgical condition that resolves with treatment of the acidosis.

It is imperative to document the history of diabetes mellitus, standard insulin regimen, past management, duration of symptoms, estimated weight loss, and presence of precipitating factors.

Patients not previously diagnosed may give a history of excessive or poor food intake, weight loss, or dehydration in the presence of a large urinary output. A dehydrated child with a normal or large urine flow must be considered diabetic until proven otherwise.

Box 74-1

DIAGNOSTIC FINDINGS IN DIABETIC KETOACIDOSIS

EARLY

Due to hyperglycemia:
 Polyuria, polydipsia, polyphagia, visual disturbance
Due to muscle breakdown and dehydration:
 Weight loss, weakness

LATE

Due to ketonemia:
 Anorexia, nausea, vomiting, fruity acetone breath
Due to hyperosmolality:
 Altered mental status
Due to acidosis:
 Abdominal pain, Kussmaul's respiration
Due to hypokalemia:
 Ileus, muscle cramps, dysrhythmia

Those whose diabetes is in poor control have polyuria, polydipsia, polyphagia, and weight loss. Recurrent episodes of DKA are often associated with psychosocial dysfunction.

Complications

1. Dehydration with metabolic acidosis (differential of metabolic acidosis, p. 365).
2. Cerebral edema is unpredictable in onset, usually occurring within 8 to 12 hours after initiation of treatment. Seizures may be noted. Abrupt changes in mental status, pupillary changes, and posturing progressing to coma are associated with a mortality rate of 21%; 27% of survivors are left with neurologic sequelae.

   Retrospective studies have suggested that the development of cerebral edema was associated with lower initial partial pressure of CO_2, higher blood urea nitrogen (BUN) concentration, and treatment with bicarbonate. The risk of cerebral edema may indeed be more closely related to the duration and severity of DKA.
3. Adult respiratory distress syndrome (p. 41).
4. Death caused by CNS or metabolic complications.

   Hyperglycemic hyperosmolar nonketotic coma (HHNC), with a glucose level of 800 to 1200 mg/dl, rarely occurs in children; it occurs more often in adults. Patients may not be acidotic, but they do have hyperglycemia, hyperosmolality, and dehydration. They also may be comatose, presumably because of a relative water deficiency. Ketosis and acetones are minimal or absent. HHNC has been reported in children younger than 2 years and in children with preexisting neurologic damage.

Ancillary Data

1. Electrolytes may be abnormal with an anion gap (p. 76) and must be monitored every 2 to 4 hours during stabilization:
   a. Hyponatremia resulting from urinary losses: Sodium level may be artificially depressed by hyperglycemia and hyperlipidemia. An estimate of the true serum sodium level may be derived as follows:

$$\text{Corrected serum Na}^+ \text{ (mEq/L)} = \text{Measured serum Na}^+ \text{ (mEq/L)} + [(\text{Plasma glucose [mg/dl]} - 100) \times 0.016]$$

   b. A total body potassium deficit (the serum level may be normal): Serum potassium rises by 0.5 mEq/L for each 0.1 decrease in pH.
   c. Acidosis with a low bicarbonate level and pH, the size of the decrease reflecting the severity of disease.
   d. BUN level is usually elevated.
2. Glucose level is elevated above 300 mg/dl with glucosuria and must be monitored every 1 to 2 hours until stable. Screening

with reagent strips (Dextrostix or Chemstrip) may provide a bedside estimate. Serum osmolarity should be determined if the glucose level is above 1000 mg/dl. Home blood glucose monitoring facilitates glucose control over the long term and during illness.

3. Serum ketones are large at a dilution of 1:2 or above with ketonuria. Ketone measurements reflect acetoacetate but not beta-hydroxybutyrate. Because the latter dissociates to acetoacetate with clinical improvement, ketonemia may persist despite clinical resolution and should be checked every 2 to 4 hours until clear.
4. Urinalysis reveals glucosuria and ketonuria. The normal renal glucose threshold is about 180 mg/dl, but variability does exist.
5. Arterial blood gas (ABG) analysis demonstrates a respiratory alkalosis superimposed on a metabolic acidosis.
6. Amylase level may be elevated; white blood cell (WBC) count is variable.
7. Electrocardiogram (ECG) may be used for rapid assessment of serum potassium levels.
8. Cultures of throat, blood, urine, and cervix are performed as indicated.
9. Glycosylated hemoglobin level gives an excellent measure of the degree of long-term control.

MANAGEMENT

Initial Management

Initial stabilization must include intravenous administration of fluids, cardiac monitoring, and determination of serum electrolyte, glucose, acetone, and BUN levels and venous (or arterial) pH. A bedside reagent strip test may facilitate management. Laboratory data should be determined every 1 to 2 hours during the initial treatment periods. Vital signs, fluids, insulin level, and urinary output must be monitored and followed on a flow sheet.

Initial therapy should begin with aggressive hydration: infusion of 0.9% NS solution at a rate of 20 ml/kg over 30 minutes, which should be repeated until partial reconstitution of vascular space and stabilization of blood pressure, pulse, and respiration have been achieved.

After the initial bolus, fluid and electrolyte therapy must reflect maintenance and deficit requirements. Patients typically have an isotonic 10% dehydration (see Chapter 7). Deficits are calculated and carefully replaced on the basis of serum concentration with 0.45% NS with potassium salts:

- If the corrected sodium is 140 mEq/L or less, replace half of the deficit over first 16 hours and restore total deficit over 36 hours.
- If the corrected sodium is 140 mEq/L or more, restore total deficit evenly over 48 hours.

The rates often must be increased because of the obligate excessive urinary losses and hemodynamic considerations.

Normally, the pH does not need to be actively corrected because correction of intravascular volume facilitates the return to normal values; excessive administration of sodium bicarbonate may lead to alkalosis, a shift of the oxyhemoglobin dissociation curve, and paradoxic cerebrospinal fluid (CSF) acidosis. Evidence would indicate that correction of severe acidosis with administration of bicarbonate does not affect outcome. With severe acidosis, the bicarbonate deficit may be partially (50%) corrected with administration of bicarbonate, 1 to 2 mEq/kg over 30 minutes, while the response is monitored.

If neurologic changes are noted, infusion should be slowed, and other monitoring and measurements initiated. Potassium must be added to the infusion early (after initial flush) because of the total body deficit. Potassium acetate may be substituted for potassium chloride if the patient is highly acidotic. Some clinicians prefer KPO_4 because of a relatively common phosphorus depletion:

Serum K^+ (mEq/L)	Potassium Infusate (mEq/L)
<3	40-60*
3-4	30
4-5	20
5-6	10

* Many patients may not tolerate infusion peripherally. Significant risk for dysrhythmia.

Glucose should be added to the IV fluid infusion when the glucose level is less than 250 mg/dl (without stopping the infusion of insulin). One unit of insulin causes intracellular movement of 2 to 4 g of glucose.

Patients with mild to moderate disease who show rapid response to the initial fluid management can be given oral hydration if vomiting has ceased and vital signs are stable with normovolemia.

Patients with only mild diabetes and without significant acidosis may be managed with oral hydration if vomiting is not a problem. Patients with nonketotic hyperosmolar diabetic coma show response to hydration, replacement of electrolyte deficits, and reduction of serum glucose level and hyperosmolarity. Fluid therapy is primary.

Although the mechanism of evolution of cerebral edema is unknown, several observations about its management should be considered. The expansion of the treatment plan to 48 hours and early use of fluid containing Na^+ at 125 mEq/L may be protective. The failure of the serum sodium concentration to rise as glucose concentration declines is a marker of excessive administration of free water. A total fluid dose higher than 4 L/m^2/day may correlate with greater risk. Further data are required.

Insulin

Insulin is the second major component of therapy. Infusion must be related to the state of hydration, fluid management, and laboratory data. Several routes of administration are available.

Many insulin preparations are available, including semisynthetic human insulins. Regular crystalline insulin has an onset of 30 minutes, peaks at 2 to 4 hours, and has a duration of 6 to 8 hours. U100 preparations are commonly used.

1. Continuous IV infusion of regular insulin causes a smooth fall in glucose level, with lower incidence of hypoglycemia and hypokalemia and better ongoing control of therapy. Optimally, glucose level falls 50 to 100 mg/dl/hr.

   Method: 50 units of regular insulin are mixed in 250 ml of 0.9% NS (0.2 units/ml) and infused at a rate of 0.1 to 0.2 units/kg/hr. Run insulin solution through IV tubing before initiating therapy.
2. Intramuscular injection of regular insulin is an acceptable alternative, 0.1 to 0.2 units/kg/hr injected intramuscularly.

Insulin administration should not be stopped when the glucose level is less than 250 mg/dl. The hourly insulin dose is lowered and glucose (5% to 10%) is added to the fluid to maintain a serum glucose level around 200 to 250 mg/dl. Insulin should be stopped, and subcutaneous (SC) insulin begun, when the patient has negative serum acetone at a dilution of 1:2.

If an infusion is used, administer SC insulin 30 minutes before stopping the IV infusion. SC insulin is initiated at the rate of 0.25 to 0.5 units/kg q4-6hr. It is based on the serum glucose acetone value. Rapid glucose monitoring devices facilitate this process.

As mentioned, regular insulin administered subcutaneously has an onset of 30 to 60 minutes, peaks at 2 hours, and has a duration of 6 to 12 hours, requiring administration on a routine basis before meals. A synthesized insulin analogue called lispro (Humalog) has an earlier onset (5 to 15 minutes) and shorter duration (≤4 hr).

Long-acting insulin should be initiated as soon as possible. This therapy should be coordinated with the primary care provider. The sum of the short-acting insulin administered in the previous 24-hour period gives an approximation of the following day's requirement. Typically, patients require 0.6 to 0.8 unit/kg/24 hr divided so that two thirds of the dose is administered in the morning and one third in the evening. A common insulin mixture is two-thirds isophane insulin suspension (NPH) and one-third regular insulin to provide a smooth pattern. NPH has an onset of 2 hours, peaks at 8 to 10 hours, and has a duration of 16 to 20 hours.

NOTE: Patients with newly diagnosed diabetes have a low initial insulin requirement. At the time of initial diagnosis, insulin requirement is high (≥1 unit/kg/24 hr). This requirement falls rapidly ("honeymoon period") to as little as 0.1 to 0.3 units/kg/24 hr for the next few weeks to months.

Insulin pumps provide markedly improved control in selected patients.

DISPOSITION

Patients with significant DKA need to be hospitalized unless prolonged observation with monitoring equipment, personnel, and expertise is available in the ambulatory setting. Patients with pH less than 7, serum HCO_3 values lower than 10 mEq/L, or altered mental status should be hospitalized early in treatment. In addition, those with intercurrent infections often need to be admitted. Patients having a first episode usually should be hospitalized for control and education, although ambulatory education may be used after stabilization.

Insulin therapy on discharge should be coordinated with the primary care provider. All diabetic patients need close follow-up observation with frequent blood glucose level monitoring at home. These must be ensured before discharge.

BIBLIOGRAPHY

Bonadio WA: Pediatric diabetic ketoacidosis: pathophysiology and potential for outpatient management of selected children, *Pediatr Emerg Care* 8:287, 1992.

Felner EI, White PC: Improving management of diabetic ketoacidosis in children, *Pediatrics* 108:735, 2001.

Finberg L: Why do patients with diabetic ketoacidosis have cerebral swelling and why does treatment sometimes make it worse? *Arch Pediatr Adolesc Med* 150:785, 1996.

Glaser N, Barnett P, McCaslin I et al: Risk factors for cerebral edema in children with diabetic ketoacidosis, *N Engl J Med* 344:264, 2001.

Green SM, Rothrock SG, Ho JD et al: Failure of adjunctive bicarbonate to improve outcome in severe pediatric diabetic ketoacidosis, *Ann Emerg Med* 31:41, 1998.

Harris GD, Fiordalisi I, Harris WL et al: Minimizing the risk of brain herniation during treatment of diabetic ketoacidemia: a retrospective and prospective study, *J Pediatr* 117:22, 1990.

Klekamp J, Churchwell KB: Diabetic ketoacidosis in children: initial clinical assessment, *Pediatr Ann* 25:387, 1996.

Rosenbloom A: Intracerebral crisis during treatment of diabetic ketoacidosis, *Diabetes Care* 13:22, 1990.

Rosenbloom AL, Schatz DA: Diabetic ketoacidosis in childhood, *Pediatr Ann* 23:284, 1994.

Failure to Thrive

ALERT Although feeding problems are often causative, organic conditions must be excluded. Prolonged delay in diagnosis and active intervention may result in long-term neurologic delays.

Growth failure in children occurs when the rate of weight gain is below that anticipated for a peer age group. Although a single measurement below the third or fifth percentile is suggestive, a decrease in the velocity of growth is diagnostic.

The most common pattern occurs when the weight is reduced out of proportion to the height; head circumference is normal. This situation is usually due to inadequate intake or malabsorption. Proportional reduction in weight and height with a normal or increased head circumference is associated with constitutional dwarfism and endocrinopathies. When the head is small and the weight and height are similarly reduced, the cause is usually related to CNS disease or intrauterine growth retardation.

ETIOLOGY

1. Inadequate caloric intake is usually primary, accounting for more than one half of cases.
2. Psychosocial problems are present in nearly one half of children:
   - **a.** Parent-child dysfunction:
     - **(1)** Perinatal and neonatal factors related to bonding and emotional support
     - **(2)** Developmental delays
   - **b.** Family dysfunction:
     - **(1)** Socioeconomic limitations
     - **(2)** Child abuse or neglect
     - **(3)** Family discord
3. Organic conditions:
   - **a.** Congenital: anatomic problems or inborn errors of metabolism
   - **b.** Gastrointestinal:
     - **(1)** Malabsorption
     - **(2)** Liver disease
     - **(3)** Obstructive disease
     - **(4)** Gastroesophageal reflux (GER)
     - **(5)** Food allergies
   - **c.** Cardiopulmonary:
     - **(1)** Congenital or acquired heart disease
     - **(2)** Cystic fibrosis
     - **(3)** Chronic lung disease
   - **d.** Renal:
     - **(1)** Renal failure or infection
     - **(2)** Renal tubular acidosis
   - **e.** CNS: congenital, perinatal, or acquired disease
   - **f.** Endocrine or metabolic:
     - **(1)** Thyroid, pituitary, diabetes mellitus, adrenal, parathyroid
     - **(2)** Inborn errors of metabolism
   - **g.** Immunologic/infectious:
     - **(1)** Acquired immunodeficiency syndrome (AIDS); severe combined immunodeficiency
     - **(2)** Chronic infections: tuberculosis (TB), human immunodeficiency virus (HIV), parasites
   - **h.** Toxic: heavy metal (lead), etc.

DIAGNOSTIC FINDINGS

1. Feeding technique, efficacy, pattern, and problems must be clearly defined. Calorie count may be useful.
2. Growth charts, including weight, height, and head circumference (see p. 857), to determine patterns of growth and relationships among these three parameters. Physical, environmental, and social changes should be temporally noted on the chart.
3. Perinatal history, developmental milestones, family history including growth patterns and inherited diseases, and psychosocial issues and family function may be suggestive.
4. Beyond specific evaluation of growth parameters, the physical examination should focus on excluding potential causes. Neglect or abuse should be excluded.

Complications

1. Neurologic delays accompanying inadequate intake
2. Malnutrition, dehydration, anemia

Ancillary Data

1. Screening studies, including urinalysis and urine culture, electrolyte and glucose measurements, WBC, and erythrocyte sedimentation rate (ESR). Stool specimen to test for pH, reducing substances, blood, fat, and infectious agents.
2. Radiologic evaluation for bone age.
3. Chest x-ray study if there is any indication of cardiac or pulmonary disease.
4. Selective studies to exclude organic causes.

DIFFERENTIAL DIAGNOSIS

The important consideration is whether the changing velocity pattern reflects potential organic or nonorganic problems or the normal growth pattern for the child.

Potential causes beyond feeding and family problems should be excluded as suggested by the presenting findings and the pattern of relationship between growth patterns.

MANAGEMENT

1. Assuming that acute fluid problems are corrected, the initial screening studies are obtained. If their results are normal, a trial of feeding is usually initiated, focusing on techniques when caloric intake is thought to be inadequate. Measurement of intake and output and adjustments to formula, solids, and so on, to maximize calories should be initiated.

   Close follow-up and monitoring is essential. Family support must be initiated.

   If this is unsuccessful, admission and inpatient feeding and observation may be required.
2. If no improvement is noted or initial examination suggests an organic cause, other diagnostic considerations must be excluded and treated.

DISPOSITION

1. Outpatient management is usually appropriate while feeding techniques are adjusted. Close follow-up and support are essential.
2. Admission may be required if the child is unstable, markedly malnourished, compliance uncertain, suspected to have been abused, or likely to have a significant organic etiology.
3. Referral is appropriate for all patients to ensure continuity.

BIBLIOGRAPHY

Maggioni A, Lifshitz F: Nutritional management of failure to thrive, *Pediatr Clin North Am* 42:791, 1995.

Thyroid Disease

THYROIDITIS

Chronic lymphocytic thyroiditis (Hashimoto's disease) is an autoimmune disease. It accounts for most nontoxic goiters, with a peak incidence between 8 and 15 years and a female predominance of 4:1.

Diagnostic Findings

Thyroid enlargement is noted in more than 85% of patients—the thyroid is usually firm and nontender and has a cobblestone sensation. Patients are rarely symptomatic.

Ancillary Data (Table 74-3)

Serum thyroglobulin and microsomal antibodies may be elevated. Results of function studies are usually normal.

Differential Diagnosis

1. Simple colloid goiter.
2. Infection: Suppurative thyroiditis has an acute onset of fever, dysphagia, sore throat, and painful, tender swelling in the area of the thyroid. Commonly it results from mixed aerobic and anaerobic organisms; *S. aureus* is rarely grown in culture. Antibiotics (penicillin or dicloxacillin) or surgical drainage is required.

Management

Patients with documented hypothyroidism should be treated with replacement doses of sodium l-thyroxine (100 $\mu g/m^2/24$ hr). Patients with euthyroidism are usually treated because in some, hypothyroidism develops. Such treatment ordinarily reduces the goiter size.

Disposition

All patients should be monitored at home for at least 6 months. If treatment was not initiated, they should be reevaluated at 6-month intervals to assess thyroid function.

TABLE 74-3 Thyroid Function Tests: Common Disorders of Thyroid Function

Disorder	Serum Thyroxine (T_4)	Triiodothyronine (T_3) Resin Uptake	Serum Thyrotropin (TSH)	Comments
Chronic lymphocytic thyroiditis				Thyroid antibody increased
Euthyroid	WNL	WNL to ↑	WNL to ↑	
Hypothyroid	↓	WNL to ↓	↑	
Hyperthyroid	↑	↑	↓	
Hyperthyroid	↑*	↑	↓	
Hypothyroid				
Primary	↓	↓	↑	
Secondary	↓	↓	↓	Decreased response to TRH
TBG				
↓ TBG	↓	↑	WNL	Free thyroxine index normal
↑ TBG (pregnancy, birth control pills)	↑	↓	WNL	Free thyroxine index normal

Modified from Fisher DA: *J Pediatr* 82:187, 1973.
* May be normal or low in triiodothyronine toxicosis.
TRH, Thyroid-releasing hormone; *TBG*, thyroid-binding globulin.

HYPERTHYROIDISM

Etiology

1. Autoimmune (Graves' disease). Often associated with other autoimmune diseases. In about 10% of patients with chronic lymphocytic thyroiditis, hyperthyroidism develops.
2. Hypothalamic or pituitary dysfunction. Rare.
3. Congenital. Present in children of mothers who have or have had Graves' disease. May persist to 6 to 12 months and may have postneonatal onset.

Diagnostic Findings

Patients usually have a gradual onset of symptoms, with an enlarged thyroid gland and associated decreasing school performance, weight loss, tachycardia, eye prominence and exophthalmos, motor hyperactivity with tremor, and increased sweating. Atrial fibrillation can be present.

Thyroid storm is very rare in children. It manifests as acute onset of hyperthermia, tachycardia, sweating, and nervousness. It occurs almost exclusively in patients with preexisting hyperthyroidism, secondary to a diffuse toxic goiter (Graves' disease).

Complications. Hyperthyroidism can cause an elevated metabolic rate, with delirium, coma, and potentially, death.

Ancillary Data. See Table 74-3.

Differential Diagnosis

Hyperthyroidism should be differentiated from a neoplasm such as pheochromocytoma.

Management

There are several management options:

1. Most clinicians inhibit synthesis of thyroid hormone and initiate oral antithyroid medication (propylthiouracil [PTU], 5 mg/kg/24 hr up to 300 mg/24 hr) for 3 to 4 years unless remission occurs earlier. Lugol's solution (5 drops q8hr PO) is usually begun 1 hour after PTU.
2. Surgery is indicated for patients whose compliance is poor, for those whose glands are three to four times normal size, and for

those with adenomas or carcinomas. Patients must be euthyroid before surgery. The use of radioactive iodides in children is controversial.

3. Propranolol, 10 to 20 mg/dose q6-8hr PO, is useful initially for patients in a hypermetabolic state. In patients with thyroid storm, immediate therapy with propranolol, 1 to 2 mg/dose IV initially, followed by oral therapy, is indicated. Propranolol is contraindicated in patients with congestive heart failure. Fluid deficits, hyponatremia, and hyperthermia should be corrected.
4. Congenital hyperthyroidism may initially be treated with Lugol's solution, 1 drop q8hr PO.

Disposition

Patients generally can be monitored clinically and chemically at home, with frequent office visits for at least 3 to 4 years. Patients with thyroid storm must be hospitalized.

HYPOTHYROIDISM

Etiology

1. Congenital: aplasia, hypoplasia, errors of metabolism, autoimmune disease, maternal ingestion of drugs or goitrogens during pregnancy
2. Autoimmune: chronic lymphocytic thyroiditis (Hashimoto's thyroiditis)
3. Intoxication: iodides, radiation
4. Hypothalamic or pituitary dysfunction
5. Trauma: neck injury or surgery
6. Infection: viral (rarely aerobic or anaerobic bacteria)
7. Neoplasm: primary (carcinoma) or secondary infiltration

Diagnostic Findings

Clinical presentation varies according to the patient's age and duration of illness. Although most patients with congenital hypothyroidism are asymptomatic, they may be lethargic and may eat poorly. Less commonly, hypotonia, prolonged jaundice, umbilical hernia, wide fontanel, or delayed growth is noted. Most states require neonatal screening for hypothyroidism, and the diagnosis should be made early.

In later childhood, patients exhibit growth retardation, delays in dentition, edema, poor performance (in school and play), hoarseness, delayed tendon reflexes with flabby muscles, and a dull, placid expression.

Complications. Myxedema coma (usually caused by autoimmune [Hashimoto's] thyroiditis, therapy with radioactive iodine [^{131}I], or surgery), is extremely rare but may accompany coma, hypothermia, hypoglycemia, and respiratory failure. Therapy is initiated parenterally.

Ancillary Data. See Table 74-3.

Management

Hormone replacement is initiated after laboratory specimens are obtained to evaluate function. Levothyroxine (Synthroid) is a stable, synthetic hormone that can be given once a day. Dosage should be adjusted to maintain the serum thyroxine (T_4) level between 10 and 12 µg/dl:

Age	Dosage (µg/kg/24 hr)	Average Levothyroxine Dose (µg/24 hr)
<6 mo	8-10	25-50
6-12 mo	6-8	50-75
1-5 yr	5-6	75-100
6-12 yr	4-5	100-150
>12 yr	2-3	100-200

In the older child, there is usually less urgency, and the child should be started on a low dosage (25 µg/24 hr), which is increased every 2 to 4 weeks until full replacement is achieved. Patients should be monitored closely.

Therapy for myxedema coma should be initiated parenterally. The adult dose is 200 to 500 µg levothyroxine IV, followed by 50 µg/24 hr IV.

Disposition

In patients without complications, therapy should be initiated, and the patients should be monitored as outpatients, with laboratory tests repeated in 2 weeks. Serum thyroxine and serum thyrotropin measurements are the tests of choice. Because excessive therapy in the infant may cause craniosynostosis and brain dysfunction, infants should be monitored at 3-month intervals in the first year of life.

BIBLIOGRAPHY

Lafranchi S: Thyroiditis and acquired hypothyroidism, *Pediatr Ann* 21:29, 1992.

Zimmerman D, Gan-Gaisand M: Hyperthyroidism in children and adolescents, *Pediatr Clin North Am* 37:1273, 1990.

75 Eye Disorders

Also See Chapter 59 (Eye Trauma)

Chalazion and Hordeolum

A *chalazion* is an inflammatory granulomatous nodule of the meibomian gland on an otherwise normal eyelid. It results from retained secretions of a gland. Physical discomfort, as well as some disfigurement from the mass effect of the nodule, may be present.

Hot compresses are used initially to encourage drainage. The chalazion may be treated with incision and curettage by an ophthalmologist. It also may respond to steroid injection.

A *hordeolum (stye)* is a painful, tender, erythematous infection of the hair follicle of the eyelashes, usually resulting from *Staphylococcus aureus*. A hordeolum usually points and drains and may occur in multiple sites. Very rarely is it complicated by periorbital cellulitis (p. 582).

Hot compresses are useful; if a stye does not drain spontaneously, incision and drainage may be performed. Topical medications are probably not helpful, and recurrent multiple lesions may respond to systemic antistaphylococcal agents.

Conjunctivitis

Infectious conjunctivitis is the most common cause of "red eye" in children and is usually benign and self-limited in older children. Bacterial conjunctivitis typically produces purulent discharge with polyps in the smear. The cornea is not involved, and vision is unaffected; there is little pain. Viral disease causes keratoconjunctivitis with corneal involvement. Affected patients have pain, photophobia, and mildly decreased vision. The discharge is classically mucoid with mononuclear cells on the smear. Chlamydial disease may cause symptoms similar to those of viral keratoconjunctivitis. Diagnostic findings are summarized in Table 75-1.

ETIOLOGY AND DIAGNOSTIC FINDINGS

1. Infection:
- **a.** Bacterial:
  - **(1)** *Haemophilus influenzae*: bilateral and purulent
  - **(2)** *Streptococcus pneumoniae*: purulent
  - **(3)** *Neisseria gonorrhoeae*: usually occurs in the first days of life; large amount of hyperacute mucopurulent discharge; also occurs in sexually active individuals
  - **(4)** *S. aureus*: rare
  - **(5)** *Pseudomonas* organisms secondary to contact lens
- **b.** Viral:
  - **(1)** Adenovirus: mucopurulent discharge; associated pharyngitis in some
  - **(2)** Herpes simplex: Dendritic pattern with corneal ulcer and keratitis; unilateral; vesicle on eyelid may be present; herpes type 1 is more common, although type 2 can occur through spread from genital lesions
  - **(3)** Varicella: vesicle on lid; conjunctivitis

TABLE 75-1 Infective Conjunctivitis: Diagnostic Findings and Management

Cause	Epidemiology	DIAGNOSTIC FINDINGS						
		Vision	**Pain**	**Photophobia**	**Discharge/ Microscopic**	**Cornea**	**Conjunctiva**	**Management**[*,‖]
BACTERIA[†,‖] *S. pneumonia* *H. influenzae*	Bilateral, history of exposure	WNL	None	None	Purulent; PMN on smear	WNL	Injected papillary	Topical antibiotics
VIRAL								
Adenovirus[‡] types 8, 19, 3, and 7	Incubation: 5-14 days; history of exposure; systemic symptoms; preauricular node	Often decreased	FBS	±	Mucoid; mononuclear on smear	Punctate keratopathy	Injected follicles	Topical antibiotics for secondary bacterial infection
Herpes[§]	Unilateral; often secondary	±	FBS	+	Mucoid; mononuclear on smear	Dendrite	Injected follicles	Refer to ophthalmologist
Varicella (chickenpox)	"Pox" may involve lid, rarely cornea	WNL	±	±	Mucoid; mononuclear on smear	±	Injected follicles	Follow
CHLAMYDIA	May be recurrent if inadequately treated	WNL	±	±	Inclusion bodies (Giemsa); fluorescent antibody	WNL	Injected follicles	Erythromycin for 2-3 wk

FBS, Foreign body sensation; *PMN*, polymorphonuclear neutrophil; *WNL*, within normal limits.

* Do not prescribe topical analgesics for *prn* use.

† "Bacterial" conjunctivitis unresponsive to topical antibiotics more often results from viral agents or iritis than from insensitivity to antibiotics.

‡ Adenoviral conjunctivitis also is known as epidemic keratoconjunctivitis. Children should be kept out of school or daycare until resolution.

§ Herpes simplex can be difficult to diagnose. Because steroids dramatically worsen herpes keratitis, they should not be prescribed without clear indications.

‖ Prolonged treatment with neomycin-containing antibiotics can cause local sensitivity.

c. *Chlamydia trachomatis*: purulent discharge beginning at 5 to 15 days of life; possible associated pneumonia

2. Allergy:
   a. Watery discharge with chemosis and edema of the conjunctiva, pruritic
   b. Bulbar conjunctivitis
   c. Rhinorrhea
   d. Seasonal allergy
3. Chemical: may occur bilaterally in newborns after delivery if silver nitrate drops are not well irrigated; in older children, secondary to cosmetics, drugs, eyedrops, or aerosols
4. Ophthalmia neonatorum (Table 75-2): In babies with conjunctivitis, cultures and a "stat" Gram stain should be obtained to exclude *N. gonorrhoeae*. If the baby has gonorrhea or *Chlamydia*, systemic treatment must be given, and the mother and her sexual partner evaluated.

DIFFERENTIAL DIAGNOSIS

In addition to the various distinguishing etiologic agents that cause infectious or allergic conjunctivitis, a number of other entities must be considered (see Tables 75-1 and 75-2):

1. Trauma:
   a. Foreign body, usually associated with pain, photophobia; vision may be normal; fluorescein finding positive (p. 444)
   b. Corneal abrasion (p. 444)
   c. Traumatic iritis, which is accompanied by blurred vision with severe acute unilateral pain; photophobia; flush around limbus
   d. Traumatic hyphema (p. 443)
2. Congenital:
   a. Nasolacrimal duct obstruction
   b. Congenital glaucoma, which causes visual impairment with conjunctival

TABLE 75-2 Neonatal Ophthalmia: Diagnostic Findings

Etiology	Incubation Period	Diagnostic Findings	Management
CHEMICAL			
Silver nitrate	24 hr	Diffuse injection; culture: negative	Wait and watch
GONOCOCCAL			
Neisseria gonorrhoeae	24-72 hr	Hyperpurulent; history of infected birth canal or infected contact; smear: typical gonococcus	Systemic and topical antibiotics; hospitalize
CHLAMYDIA			
(inclusion conjunctivitis) *Chlamydia trachomatis*	7-10 days	Indolent, although often purulent; history of infected birth canal; may have had partial response to topical antibiotics; no follicles in infant; smear: cytoplasmic inclusion; culture: negative	Systemic erythromycin or sulfonamides; exclude systemic disease
OTHER BACTERIA	2-5 days	Purulent or hyperpurulent	Topical antibiotics

injection, photophobia, and a small or midsize, fixed pupil; rare

3. Systemic disease: ataxia-telangiectasia, Kawasaki's disease, juvenile rheumatoid arthritis

MANAGEMENT

1. Remove any foreign bodies (p. 443).
2. Treat allergic conjunctivitis, if significantly symptomatic, with systemic antihistamines: diphenhydramine (Benadryl), 5 mg/kg/24 hr q6hr PO for 3 to 5 days, or hydroxyzine (Vistaril, Atarax), 2 mg/kg/24 hr q6hr PO.
3. Infectious conjunctivitis:
   a. Treat *Chlamydia* disorders with oral erythromycin, 30 to 50 mg/kg/24 hr q6-8hr PO, or sulfisoxazole (Gantrisin), 150 mg/kg/24 hr q6hr PO.
   b. Refer patients with herpes conjunctivitis to an ophthalmologist. Topical antiviral agents such as 1% trifluridine drops and 5% vidarabine ointments may be used.
   c. Treat bacterial and viral conjunctivitis with ophthalmic ointment or solution for 2 days beyond clearing:
      (1) Sulfacetamide (10% to 15%) or sulfisoxazole (4%) solution (drops) q2-4hr in eye; *or*
      (2) Sulfacetamide (10%) or sulfisoxazole (4%) ointment q4-6hr in eye; *or*
      (3) Polymyxin B-bacitracin (Polysporin) ointment q4-6hr in eye
      (4) Tobramycin and gentamicin preparations are preferred by some clinicians
   d. Gonococcal ophthalmia requires hospitalization, consultation, and systemic antibiotics. Term infants may be treated with aqueous penicillin G, 50,000 units/kg/24 hr q8hr IV for 7 days. An alternative antibiotic is ceftriaxone, 125 mg intramuscularly (IM).
   e. Management tips:
      (1) Always exclude herpes simplex (fluorescein stain may be helpful).
      (2) Exclude corneal foreign body.
      (3) Warn parents to handle towels and pillowcases of the infected child with care.
      (4) Consider adenovirus in children who show no response in 3 to 4 days.
      (5) Consider *Chlamydia* in patients with a history of recurrence.
      (6) Consider intraocular disease (iritis, glaucoma) for "deep" pain unrelieved by topical anesthetics and for decreased vision and photophobia.
      (7) Think of allergy if the main symptom is itching. Look for modest discharge and thickened conjunctiva at the limbus.
      (8) Chlamydial conjunctivitis can be diagnosed with direct monoclonal fluorescent antibody testing, enzyme-linked immunosorbent assay (ELISA), or nucleic acid probe.
      (9) Topical steroids are best prescribed by an ophthalmologist.
      (10) Topical anesthetics should never be prescribed for prn use.
      (11) Bacterial cultures are rarely useful in older children.

DISPOSITION

Parental Education

1. Before using topical medication, remove the yellow discharge and dried matter from the eye with a wet cotton ball and warm water.
2. Place 2 drops of eyedrops in each eye every 2 to 4 hours (or as often as possible) while your child is awake until the eye is improving; then decrease the frequency.

a. For younger children, only an eye ointment will be provided; it may be used four times per day, but blurs vision. It also may be used for bad infections at bedtime in conjunction with the drops.
b. Continue the medication until your child has awakened for two mornings without an eye discharge.

3. Your child may infect other people. Use of separate towels and washcloths, as well as careful hand washing, prevents infection.
4. Call your physician if any of the following occurs:
   a. The infection has not responded in 72 hours.
   b. The eyelids become red or swollen.
   c. The eyeball becomes cloudy or sores develop on it.
   d. Vision becomes blurred.
   e. The eye becomes painful or develops photophobia.

BIBLIOGRAPHY

Beinfang DC, Kelly LD, Nicholson DH et al: Ophthalmology, *N Engl J Med* 323:956, 1990.

Levin AV: Eye emergencies: acute management in the pediatric ambulatory care setting, *Pediatr Emerg Care* 7:367, 1991.

Maller JS: Eye disorders. In Barkin RM, editor: *Pediatric emergency medicine: concepts and clinical practice*, ed 2, St Louis, 1997, Mosby.

Powell KR: Orbital and periorbital cellulitis, *Pediatr Rev* 16:163, 1995.

76 Gastrointestinal Disorders

Also See Chapters 24 (Acute Abdominal Pain), 30 (Constipation), 32 (Diarrhea), 33 (Dysphagia), 35 (Gastrointestinal Hemorrhage), 44 (Vomiting), and 63 (Abdominal Trauma)

Acute Infectious Diarrhea

ALERT Rapid assessment of the patient's state of hydration, complications, and likely etiologic agents is imperative. Fluid resuscitation may be required.

Acute infectious diarrhea is accompanied by an increase in stool number or water content. Commonly, a host of viral and bacterial agents and parasites is associated with unique epidemiologic and clinical characteristics (see Chapter 32).

ETIOLOGY AND DIAGNOSTIC FINDINGS

Rotavirus

Rotavirus accounts for 39% of cases of diarrheal disease requiring hospitalization. Antibody to the virus indicating past infection is noted in up to 90% of 2-year-old children. Rotavirus infection commonly occurs in the cooler months, usually affecting children 6 to 18 months old. Vomiting is a prominent early symptom, often preceding the onset of diarrhea, which is loose, relatively frequent (>5 stools/day), and rarely associated with mucus or blood. Respiratory symptoms may accompany the gastrointestinal (GI) symptoms that last for 2 to 3 days.

A rotavirus vaccine has been studied extensively, but further studies are still under way.

Other Viral Agents

Astrovirus causes findings similar to those of rotavirus but has about one half the incidence. Children from infancy to 7 years are predominantly affected. A winter peak in incidence is noted. Transmission is from person to person, and contaminated water and shellfish have been reported vehicles. Asymptomatic shedding has been noted.

Adenovirus-induced diarrhea lasts longer than that caused by rotavirus, having an incubation period of 3 to 10 days and lasting 5 to 12 days. Patients have watery diarrhea with vomiting, fever, and dehydration.

Calicivirus (Norwalk-like or snow mountain–like virus) is also similar to rotavirus, commonly occurring in children 3 months to 6 years old. In developing countries, children often acquire the infection after the first decade of life. The illness lasts about 4 days after a 1- or 2-hour to 4-day incubation period. Person-to-person and fecal-oral transmissions occur; drinking water, cold food, and shellfish have also been implicated.

Salmonella Organisms

Multiple animal reservoirs (cattle, poultry, shellfish, rodents, and turtles) facilitate transmission of *Salmonella*. Infection with this organism is more common in warm months.

1. Gastroenteritis is the most common clinical presentation:
   a. Children younger than 5 years of age are primarily affected.
   b. Symptoms of fever, vomiting, and diarrhea begin 24 to 48 hours after exposure, diminishing over 3 to 5 days.

Older children may have abdominal pain, which is often mistaken as indicating acute appendicitis.

c. The stool is commonly loose and slimy with a foul odor. The green diarrhea variably contains mucus, rarely is bloody, and usually contains polymorphonuclear (PMN) leukocytes.

d. The reservoirs are animals, contaminated food or water, and humans. Animals that have frequently been incriminated include poultry, pet turtles, and livestock. Foods such as chicken, eggs, unpasteurized milk, and cantaloupes have been linked to outbreaks.

2. The white blood cell (WBC) count is usually elevated with a variable shift to the left.
3. Septicemia may occur because of the potential of penetrating the lamina propria. Meningitis, osteomyelitis, septic arthritis, endocarditis, pneumonia, and urinary tract infections (UTIs) have been reported. Children who are younger than 1 year and those who have sickle cell disease or other hemoglobinopathies or who are immunocompromised are at increased risk of bacterial infection; for such patients, a blood culture should generally be part of the evaluation.
4. *Salmonella typhi* causes severe, prolonged disease with gastroenteritis associated with fever, malaise, headache, and myalgias. Hepatosplenomegaly and rose spots (2-mm maculopapular lesions) may appear.

Prolonged shedding of *Salmonella* organisms in the stool is a common finding; stool results are positive for several months.

Shigella Organisms

1. *Shigella* organisms are commonly spread by person-to-person transmission, occurring most often in children younger than 5 years. Commonly (in >50% of cases), other members of the patient's household also have diarrhea.
2. Patients have rapid onset of fever, crampy abdominal pain, and diarrhea. Stools are watery and usually contain mucus, blood, and PMN leukocytes.
3. Febrile convulsions are common, with a peak between 6 months and 3 years, particularly in children with a family history of seizures or a high peak temperature (p. 754). Meningismus and respiratory symptoms may be present.
4. WBC count usually is less than 10,000 cells/mm^3 with a marked shift to the left. Blood culture results are usually negative.

Campylobacter Organisms

1. *Campylobacter* organisms are transmitted by contaminated food and person-to-person contact. Incubation period is 2 to 7 days, with a peak in children younger than 6 years during warm months. Transmission occurs from person to person and from pet to person.
2. Although the patient may be asymptomatic, the onset of illness can be marked by high fever, myalgia, headache, abdominal cramps, and vomiting. Diarrhea is profuse, watery, mucousy, and bloody. Leukocytes are common. Resolution occurs in 2 to 5 days.

Yersinia enterocolitica

1. *Yersinia enterocolitica* occurs sporadically in toddlers and teenagers during the cooler months, after exposure to contaminated food or water or by person-to-person transmission. Incubation is 3 to 4 days.
2. In younger children, acute diarrhea with fever and abdominal pain is common. Stools contain rare leukocytes and blood. Older children with mesenteric adenitis have fever and right lower quadrant (RLQ) pain.

Enterotoxigenic or Invasive *Escherichia coli*

1. *Escherichia coli* may cause disease by production of an enterotoxin or by tissue invasion. Classification of the mechanism according to serogroup of the organism is unreliable. *E. coli* serotype 0157.H7 is associated with hemolytic-uremic syndrome.
2. Diarrhea is particularly severe in infants and young children with *E. coli* infection. It may produce symptoms similar to those caused by cholera (profuse, watery diarrhea) or *Shigella* organisms (fever and systemic symptoms). Mucus, blood, and PMN leukocytes are found in the stool.

Food Poisoning

1. Staphylococcal food poisoning results from a common-source food that usually was poorly refrigerated. Vomiting, marked prostration, and diarrhea occur within 12 to 16 hours of ingestion.
2. *Clostridium perfringens* may produce abdominal pain and diarrhea within 8 to 24 hours of ingestion of contaminated food. Fever, nausea, and vomiting are rare. The disease resolves in 24 to 48 hours.
3. *Clostridium botulinum*, although it does not cause diarrhea, may produce clinical symptoms within 12 to 36 hours (range: 6 hours to 8 days) of ingestion of foods—usually home-preserved vegetables, fruit, or fish. Honey may cause infantile botulism in children younger than 1 year. Patients have nausea, vomiting, diplopia, dysphagia, dysarthria, and dry mouth. Ptosis, mydriasis, nystagmus, and paresis of extraocular muscles may also be noted (p. 723).
4. Symptoms may occur after ingestion of selected fish.
   a. Scombroid poisoning is associated with eating dark-fleshed fish that was improperly preserved, resulting in the degradation of histidine to histamine. Patients have facial flushing, a peppery taste in the mouth, epigastric pain, and headache beginning right after the ingestion. Treatment is with antihistamines.
   b. Ciguatera, which occurs 1 to 6 hours after ingestion and results from the release of a neurotoxin. Patients have unusual neurologic findings, including reversal of hot-cold discrimination, transient blindness, and a metallic taste in the mouth. Support is needed for this condition, which is usually self-limited.

Parasites

1. *Giardia lamblia* is the most commonly identified intestinal parasite. Its presence is usually asymptomatic but may cause nausea, flatulence, bloating, epigastric pain or cramps, and watery diarrhea. The patient rarely has right upper quadrant (RUQ) pain and tenderness. There is no consistent eosinophilia.
2. *Cryptosporidium* is associated with malabsorption or secretory diarrhea that is usually self-limited. Spread is via contaminated water supply or person-to-person transmission, or from infected animals. Although no treatment is usually required, paromomycin may be effective. This infection is a serious illness in immunocompromised patients.
3. *Isospora belli* is usually due to contaminated food and water and may be treated with trimethoprim-sulfamethoxazole. Like *Cyclospora*, *I. belli* usually causes a self-limited disease in immunocompromised hosts.
4. Diarrheal diseases associated with parasites are usually chronic in nature and are associated with multisystem disease and weight loss.

Clostridium difficile

Clostridium difficile is associated with pseudomembranous colitis and with many cases of antibiotic-related diarrhea in adults and children. The most common agents are amoxicillin, ampicillin, the cephalosporins, and clindamycin. Tetracycline, erythromycin, sulfonamides, and trimethoprim are less often associated. Children may be asymptomatic or may have chronic diarrhea, often with abdominal cramping. Stools are bloody with very rare leukocytes.

This organism is commonly cultured from the intestines of newborns without consistent clinical significance. *C. difficile* is an uncommon cause of enterocolitis in children in the first year of life.

Traveler's Diarrhea

Traveler's diarrhea is a nonspecific term used to define diarrhea that often occurs during travel in foreign countries and that is not associated with a known pathogen. *E. coli* that produces a heat-labile enterotoxin is probably the cause. Symptoms consist of abdominal cramps, tenesmus, vomiting, nausea, chills, anorexia, and watery diarrhea.

Complications

1. Dehydration (see Chapter 7)
2. Postinfectious malabsorption

   NOTE: Children often experience a temporary lactose intolerance and develop watery diarrhea when challenged with lactose (dairy) products. Lactose-free soy formulas should be used for 2 to 4 weeks.
3. Hemolytic-uremic syndrome (p. 819)
4. Acute tubular necrosis (p. 828)
5. Systemic extension of infection (e.g., meningitis, septic arthritis)

Ancillary Data

Cultures of the Stool. Cultures are useful in determining the bacterial cause of the acute diarrhea but should be reserved for patients in whom the results will have a therapeutic or epidemiologic impact. Rectal swabs handled expeditiously provide a good culture source if stool is unavailable. Cultures should be routinely performed in children younger than 1 year who are febrile or toxic on arrival with diarrhea and whose stool contains PMN leukocytes. Cultures are also important for cases in which multiple members of the same family are ill, when any member of the patient's family is a food handler, if the patient has recently traveled extensively, or if a symptomatic child is immunosuppressed or has a hemoglobinopathy.

Fecal Leukocytes (Methylene Blue Smear of Stool). Ninety percent of patients with diarrhea resulting from *Salmonella* or *Shigella* organisms have PMN leukocytes in the stool. Fecal leukocytes also are often found in patients with *Campylobacter* organisms, *Y. enterocolitica*, invasive *E. coli*, *C. difficile*, or *Vibrio parahaemolyticus*. This test is an excellent screen to identify the group of patients at greatest risk of having a bacterial pathogen. It is performed as follows:

1. A small amount of mucus is placed on a clear glass slide and mixed with 2 drops of methylene blue.
2. A coverglass is placed on the slide. Nuclear staining occurs over 2 minutes.
3. Microscopic examination for PMN leukocytes is performed; the finding is positive when there are 5 or more WBCs per high-powered field (WBCs/HPF).

Rotavirus Test. Rotavirus may be identified by electron microscopy, radioimmunoassay, or the easier enzyme-linked immunosorbent assay (ELISA) test, which is commercially available. Similar technology exists for adenovirus infection and cryptosporidiosis.

Blood Tests. Blood tests are important if a significant abnormality of intake or output is present. Testing should include measurements of electrolytes and blood urea nitrogen (BUN) as well as a complete blood count (CBC) with differential. These studies should be performed in all patients with any degree of dehydration or a prolonged course.

When the ratio of band forms over total neutrophils (segmented plus bands) is more than

0.10, *Shigella, Salmonella,* or *Campylobacter* organisms should be suspected. The WBC count is usually less than 10,000 cells/mm^3 with a marked shift to the left in patients with *Shigella* infection. In *Salmonella* infection, the WBC count is increased, with a mild shift to the left. A high WBC count is also found in patients with *Campylobacter* and *Yersinia* infections.

Testing for Ova and Parasites. Cultures are important if *Giardia* or other parasites are suspected. With *Giardia* organisms, cysts are present in formed stools and trophozoites in watery stool or duodenal aspirates.

Blood Cultures. In infants and young children with high fever and significant toxicity, as well as in immunocompromised patients, blood cultures should be performed.

DIFFERENTIAL DIAGNOSIS

See Chapter 32.

MANAGEMENT

The initial assessment of the patient must focus on the magnitude and type of dehydration. Rapid correction of deficits as outlined in Chapter 7 is imperative.

Antibiotics (Table 76-1)

Antibiotics must be restricted to specific etiologic agents, especially *Shigella* infection. In general they are not useful in most diarrheal illnesses. The ultimate choice should reflect results of culture and sensitivity testing, the patient's clinical status, and epidemiologic considerations.

TABLE 76-1 Antibiotic Indications in Infectious Diarrhea

Etiologic Agent	Drug of Choice	Dose: mg/kg/ 24 hr (Adult: g/dose)	Route/ Frequency	Comments
Salmonella	Ampicillin **and** gentamicin*	200-400 (1 g) 5-7.5 (80 mg)	IV q4-6hr IV q8hr	Only in toxic patient when bacteremia is a concern; prolongs carrier status
Shigella	Trimethoprim-sulfamethoxazole; **or**	8-10/40-50 (double strength)	PO q12hr	Preferred, depending on sensitivity; treat 5 days
	Ceftriaxone; **or**	50-100	IV/IM q12-24hr	Treat for 5 days
	Ampicillin	50-100 (0.5 g)	PO q6-8hr	Do not use amoxicillin; may be given parenterally to very toxic patients
Campylobacter	Erythromycin	30-50 (0.5 g)	PO q6-8hr	Effectiveness unproven; reduces duration of excretion
Yersinia enterocolitica	Trimethoprim-sulfamethoxazole	8-10/40-50	PO q12hr	With severe toxicity, tetracycline (>8 yr old) and aminoglycoside may be used; controversial
Giardia	Furazolidone; **or**	6-8 (0.1 g)	PO q6hr	7-10 days; suspension available
	Metronidazole	15 (0.25 g)	PO q8hr	5 days

* Controversial. Generally, antibiotics are indicated only for invasive disease or in patients at risk of invasive disease. Other approaches are third-generation cephalosporin (ceftriaxone, cefotaxime); ampicillin and chloramphenicol; trimethoprim-sulfamethoxazole (IV). Drug must reflect local sensitivity patterns and treatment approaches.

Antibiotic therapy in patients with proven or suspected *Salmonella* infection is controversial because it prolongs the carrier state; however, it should be initiated in toxic patients younger than 6 months, in those with suspected bacteremia, and in children who are immunosuppressed or have a hemoglobinopathy.

The symptoms of *Campylobacter* disorders may resolve more rapidly after treatment with erythromycin.

Ciprofloxacin, 500 mg BID PO for 3 to 5 days, may be an alternative treatment in children older than 17 years with *Campylobacter, Shigella*, or *Salmonella* infection.

C. difficile pseudomembranous colitis rarely requires antibiotic therapy but often actually responds to cessation of previous antibiotics. If indicated by either significant or ongoing symptoms, vancomycin, 40 mg/kg/24 hr q6hr PO (adult maximum: 2 g/24 hr), or metronidazole, 15 to 40 mg/kg/24 hr q8hr PO, for 10 days may be useful.

Antidiarrheal Agents

Agents like kaolin and pectin suspensions have no defined value. Diphenoxylate and atropine (Lomotil) cause segmental contraction of the intestines, retarding movement of intestinal contents; its use may have a detrimental effect on recovery from infections by *Shigella* organisms. Special care is required because of the frequency of overdose in children.

Loperamide (Imodium) may have a similar role by decreasing peristalsis. The initial oral dose of loperamide, given on the first day, for a 13- to 20-kg child is 1 mg TID; for a 20- to 30-kg child, 2 mg BID; for a child weighing more than 30 kg, 2 mg TID. After the first day, the child is given a 0.1 mg/kg/dose after each unformed stool, up to the maximum daily dose noted above. Another dosage regimen is 0.4 to 0.8 mg/kg/24 hr q6-12hr PO in children older than 2 years up to a maximum of 2 mg/dose.

Antispasmodics

The role of antispasmodic agents in diarrhea is controversial, and they are rarely indicated.

Bile Acid Treatment

In children with prolonged diarrhea, primarily of a secretory nature that does not respond to a clear liquid or NPO (nothing by mouth) regimen, bile acids may contribute to GI irritation; stools are usually green. A short course of aluminum hydroxide (Amphojel), 2.5 to 5 ml (to 1 tsp) q6hr or with meals PO for 2 to 4 days, may be useful in recalcitrant diarrhea. Cholestyramine (Questran), available in 4-g packages, also absorbs and combines with bile acids when 1 g/24 hours is administered to infants younger than 1 year (up to 4 g/24 hours in older children). Both agents also bind bacterial enterotoxins and fatty acids.

Prostaglandin Inhibitors

Hormone- or prostaglandin-mediated secretory diarrhea may be treated pharmacologically if traditional dietary manipulations are ineffective. Aspirin, indomethacin, and nonsteroidal antiinflammatory agents may be indicated empirically.

Prophylaxis for Traveler's Diarrhea

Prevention of traveler's diarrhea through attention to strict sanitary guidelines is mandatory. If necessary, treatment should focus primarily on support, including fluid management and restricted diet. Recent guidelines recommend against routine prophylaxis because adverse reactions occur in 2% to 5% of patients. The decision to use prophylaxis must be individualized, reflecting the underlying health of the patient and the circumstances of the prospective travel. For mild diarrhea in adolescents and adults, antimotility agents such as diphenoxylate with atropine (Lomotil) may have a very limited role, despite the drug's potential problems, supplementing fluid therapy. More severe diarrhea (>3 stools in 8 hours with nausea, vomiting, or fever) is treated with doxycycline (children >8 years) or trimethoprim-sulfamethoxazole. Reduction in diarrhea may also be achieved with use of bismuth subsalicylate, 2 tablets QID or 30 ml q30min for 3 hours. Loperamide, 4 mg (adult) initially, then a 2-mg (adult) capsule after each unformed stool for 2 days (maximum: 8 capsules/day), may also be effective.

Drugs are normally prescribed for the patient, who carries them along in the event of illness. They are not given prophylactically. Oral hydration must be instituted simultaneously.

DISPOSITION

All patients with serious toxicity, dehydration, abnormal electrolyte levels, or a history of significant noncompliance should be hospitalized for intravenous (IV) therapy. In addition, admission should be sought for patients with sickle cell disease, hemoglobinopathies, or compromised immune systems. Oral rehydration may be attempted under close observation in nontoxic children.

Once the deficit has been restored and abnormal losses reduced, clear liquids (Pedialyte, Ricelyte, or Lytren) should be initiated slowly. If an adequate response is noted, a soy formula can be tried with slow progression.

Patients with minimal or no dehydration may be monitored at home with careful fluid management and close follow-up observation.

Parental Education

1. Give only clear liquids; give as much as the child wants. The following liquids may be used during the first 24 hours:
   a. Rehydralyte, Ricelyte, or Lytren
   b. Defizzed, room-temperature soda for older children (>2 years) if diarrhea is only mild
   c. Gatorade
2. If your child is vomiting, give clear liquids slowly. In younger children, start with a teaspoonful and slowly increase the amount. If vomiting occurs, let the child rest for awhile and then try again. About 8 hours after vomiting has stopped, your child can gradually return to a normal diet.
3. After 24 hours, your child's diet may be advanced if the diarrhea has improved. If only formula is being taken, mix the formula with twice as much water to make up half-strength formula, which should be given over the next 24 hours. Applesauce, bananas, rice, and toast may be given if your child is eating solids. If this is tolerated, your child may be advanced to a regular diet over the next 2 to 3 days.
4. If your child has had a prolonged course of diarrhea, it may be helpful in the younger child to advance from clear liquids to a soy formula (Isomil, ProSobee, or Soyalac) for 1 to 2 weeks.
5. Do not use boiled milk. Kool-Aid and soda are not ideal liquids, particularly for younger infants, because they contain few electrolytes.
6. Call the physician if any of the following occurs:
   a. The diarrhea or vomiting is increasing in frequency or amount.
   b. The diarrhea does not improve after 24 hours of clear liquids or resolve entirely after 3 to 4 days.
   c. Vomiting continues for more than 24 hours.
   d. The stool has blood or the vomited material contains blood or turns green.
   e. Signs of dehydration develop, such as decreased urination, less moisture in diapers, dry mouth, no tears, weight loss, lethargy, and irritability.

BIBLIOGRAPHY

Cohen MB: Etiology and mechanisms of acute infectious diarrhea in infants in the United States, *J Pediatr* 118:534, 1991.

DuPont HL, Ericsson CD, Johnson DC et al: Prevention of travelers' diarrhea by the tablet formulation of bismuth subsalicylate, *JAMA* 257:1347, 1987.

Herrmann JE, Taylor DN, Echeverria P et al: Astroviruses as a cause of gastroenteritis in children, *N Engl J Med* 324:1757, 1991.
Kelly CP, Pothoulakis C, LaMont JT: *C. difficile* colitis, *N Engl J Med* 330:257, 1994.
Krajden M, Brown M, Petrasek A et al: Clinical features of adenovirus enteritis: a review of 127 cases, *Pediatr Infect Dis J* 9:636, 1990.
Pickering LK: Therapy of acute infectious diarrhea in children, *J Pediatr* 118:S119, 1991.
Varsana I, Eidlitz-Marcus T, Nussinovitch M et al: Comparative efficacy of ceftriaxone and ampicillin for treatment of severe shigellosis in children, *J Pediatr* 118:627, 1991.

Gastrointestinal Foreign Bodies

Although most foreign bodies inadvertently swallowed by the inquisitive child pass without incident, they may lodge at points of physiologic narrowing, including the cricopharyngeal muscle, the carina or aortic arch, Schatzki's ring, or the cardioesophageal junction. They may also become stuck at the ligament of Treitz. Children rarely insert foreign bodies into the rectum.

DIAGNOSTIC FINDINGS

Most patients are asymptomatic, and the foreign body passes without difficulty. When the foreign body does lodge in the esophagus, the patient may be anxious and may have difficulty swallowing.

Physical findings are usually unremarkable. It is important to be certain that there is no evidence of a foreign body in the airway.

X-ray films are indicated if there is any question of an airway foreign body or if the patient is symptomatic. Some clinicians recommend that an x-ray film be taken in asymptomatic patients at 24 hours to ensure that the object has passed and thereby minimize the number of x-ray films obtained.

1. Coins that are in the esophagus lie in the frontal plane (full circle can be seen), whereas those in the trachea lie sagittally and appear end-on in a posteroanterior (PA) chest film.
2. Objects commonly become lodged at the proximal thoracic inlet; the cricopharyngeus muscle, the aortic arch, or the carina.
3. A lateral chest view supplementing the AP view may be helpful if there is any question of localization.
4. If the foreign body is not found on the chest films, an abdominal film should be obtained. If it still cannot be located, a contrast study may be indicated.
5. For reference: a dime measures 17 mm in diameter, a penny 18 mm, a nickel 20 mm, and a quarter 23 mm.

More recently, investigators have been studying the reliability of metal detectors in defining the location of a metallic foreign body.

DIFFERENTIAL DIAGNOSIS

Foreign bodies in the trachea are differentiated by history, physical examination, and x-ray film (p. 808).

MANAGEMENT

Historically, asymptomatic patients have been managed without intervention or diagnostic studies and with reassurance. Most foreign bodies, whether round, irregular, or sharp (e.g., pins) pass without difficulty. Evidence has suggested, however, that 17% of patients with coin ingestions may have no symptoms. Therefore it is appropriate to consider chest radiographs that include the cervical esophagus in patients who have ingested coins if there is any question of symptoms, if compliance is likely to be poor, or if follow-up observation will be difficult.

All patients should be instructed to watch for fecal passage of the object and to report any symptoms, such as pain, tenderness, obstruction, or signs of perforation, immediately to permit further diagnostic and therapeutic steps.

1. Esophageal foreign bodies:
   a. If the object is sharp or has sharp projections and it is lodged, remove it via

endoscopy. Endoscopy may be used for other types of objects as well. Obtain an x-ray film before attempting retrieval.

b. Other foreign bodies (e.g., coins) that have been lodged in the distal esophagus in the asymptomatic patient for less than 24 hours may be observed during the first 24 hours, assuming the child remains asymptomatic. If such objects do not subsequently move over the first 24 hours, they may be removed via endoscopy. Some institutions with radiologic assistance pass a Foley catheter beyond the foreign body, blow the balloon up with a radiopaque substance, and gently pull the material out. The procedure should be performed under fluoroscopic control, and a nasogastric (NG) tube should be passed beforehand to empty the stomach. Preparations should be made in the event that the patient aspirates the foreign body, a risk that is minimized by placing the patient in Trendelenburg's position.

   If a single coin was ingested in the preceding 24 hours by a patient without prior esophageal disease or surgery and no respiratory distress, a single pass of a Hurst bougie dilator may be effectively passed through the mouth with the patient in an upright position.

   Dilator size is chosen according to age, as follows:

Age (yr)	Dilator Size (French)
1-2	28
2-3	36
4-5	36
>5	40

2. Foreign bodies lodged in the stomach (usually distal antrum) can usually be watched for 2 to 3 weeks unless they have corrosive potential, such as button batteries (p. 374).
3. Foreign bodies lodged at the ligament of Treitz:
   a. Round objects may be watched for up to 1 week, awaiting passage, unless the patient shows evidence of obstruction or perforation.
   b. Elongated objects such as pencils should be observed for 6 to 8 hours and, if no movement is noted, removed either endoscopically or surgically.
4. Rectal foreign bodies:
   a. If large, they usually require general anesthesia to facilitate removal.
   b. Small objects can be removed through an anoscope. Preparation of the patient with oral (PO) or rectal (PR) mineral oil may be useful.
5. Button batteries lodged in the esophagus should be removed endoscopically. If they have passed beyond the pylorus, the patient may be observed if asymptomatic. Batteries less than 15 mm in diameter in the stomach may also be observed; batteries more than 15 mm in diameter should be viewed on x-ray film again in 48 hours and, if still in the stomach, retrieved at that time (see Chapter 55).
6. Although efficacy has not been proven, some clinicians continue to believe that glucagon (0.03 to 0.1 mg/kg/dose IV; adult: 1 mg/dose) may have some value in the management of esophageal foreign bodies.

DISPOSITION

An asymptomatic patient may be discharged with close follow-up observation if the foreign body is lodged in an anatomic site not requiring urgent removal. Symptomatic patients and patients with foreign bodies requiring removal should be hospitalized.

BIBLIOGRAPHY

Ros SP, Cetta F: Successful use of a metal detector in locating coins ingested by children, *J Pediatr* 120:753, 1992.

Sacchetti A, Carraccio C, Lichtenstine R: Hand-held metal detection identification of ingested foreign bodies, *Pediatr Emerg Care* 10:204, 1994.

Schunk JE, Harrison AM, Correl HM et al: Fluoroscopic Foley catheter removal of esophageal foreign bodies in children: experience with episodes, *Pediatrics* 94:709, 1994.

Sheizh A: Button battery ingestions in children, *Pediatr Emerg Care* 9:224, 1993.

Soprano JV, Fleisher GR, Mandl KD: The spontaneous passage of esophageal coins in children, *Acta Pediatr Adolesc Med* 153:1073, 1999.

Viral Hepatitis

Acute viral hepatitis is commonly classified as hepatitis A (predominantly fecal-oral transmission), hepatitis B (largely parenteral), and hepatitis C, D, and E (non-A/non-B [transfusion related]), on the basis of serologic and clinical data (Table 76-2).

What used to be called "non-A, non-B hepatitis" is caused by three specific viruses, hepatitis C, D, and E.

1. Hepatitis C is the most common form of non-A, non-B posttransfusion hepatitis. Perinatal and sexual transmission is uncommon. Vertical transmission occurs in high-risk mothers (IV drug abuse, sexually transmitted disease [STD], human immunodeficiency virus [HIV]). It is characterized by an acute infection after an incubation period of 6 to 12 weeks. Disease is mild or subclinical. Chronic disease may occur, producing chronic active hepatitis in 35% to 50% of patients and cirrhosis in 20%.
2. Hepatitis D may cause epidemics in high-risk patients. Coinfection with hepatitis B may occur; 5% of cases progress to chronic disease. Superinfection with hepatitis B may also occur.
3. Hepatitis E is enterically transmitted and has an incubation period of 6 weeks. It occurs more commonly in males, most notably in those 15 to 39 years old. The incubation is 6 weeks.

Patients may have variable types of hepatitis, including acute icteric, anicteric, acute fulminant, and subacute. Most infections are self-limited.

DIAGNOSTIC FINDINGS

(see Table 76-2)

Epidemiologic and diagnostic findings vary.

1. Patients generally have a prodromal, preicteric phase with malaise and anorexia.
2. Jaundice develops, accompanied by scleral icterus (serum bilirubin >2.5 mg/dl) and pruritus.
3. The abdomen may be distended. Palpation of the RUQ over the liver demonstrates the greatest tenderness. Splenomegaly is variably present.
4. Evidence of serum sickness is present with hepatitis B. Arthralgia, myalgia, erythematous or maculopapular rash, and fever are noted. Patients may have myocarditis or pericarditis, with symptoms of pleuritic chest pain and friction rubs.

Complications

1. Fulminant hepatitis: A poor prognosis is seen with hepatitis B when it is associated with a prolonged prothrombin time (PT) (>4 higher than control) that is unresponsive to large doses of vitamin K, serum bilirubin elevation (>20 mg/dl), leukocytosis (>12,500 WBCs/mm^3), and hypoglycemia.
2. Chronic active hepatitis.
3. Hepatorenal syndrome with edema and ascites.
4. Hepatic encephalopathy marked by altered mental status, seizures, and coma. Tremor, asterixis, and hyperreflexia may be present.
5. Bleeding diathesis.

Ancillary Data

1. WBC count usually is normal.
2. Prothrombin time is prolonged. Other bleeding studies are normal.
3. Liver functions are elevated. Transaminase and bilirubin levels are elevated

TABLE 76-2 Hepatitis: Characteristics of Virus Types

	A	B	C	D	E
Virus type	RNA	DNA	RNA	RNA	RNA
Antigen	HAVAg	HBsAg, HBcAg, HBeAg	HCVAg	HDVAg	HEVAg
Serologic diagnosis	Anti-HAV IgM (may persist 4 mo)	HBsAg Anti-HBc IgM Anti-HBe/HBeAg	Anti-HCV	Anti-HDV (IgM, IgG)	Anti-HEV
Epidemiology					
Transmission	Fecal-oral, contaminated water/food, oral-anal sex	Parenteral blood products, sexual, IV drug use, perinatal, child to child in household	Parenteral, perinatal, sexual, IV drug use	Parenteral, coinfection or super infection with HBV	Fecal-oral (see A); travel to endemic area
Onset	Acute	Insidious	Insidious with relapse	Coinfection	Acute
Incubation period	2-6 wk	2-6 mo	6-12 wk	2-8 wk	6 wk
Chronicity	No	Infants: 90% Adults: 6%-10%	50%-80%	2%-70%	No
Symptoms	90%-95% children <5 yr asymptomatic; flulike symptoms early; jaundice may last 1-3 wk; may be fulminant	Asymptomatic to fulminant; insidious onset with prolonged jaundice	Acute or chronic; more mild than B; often anicteric	Acute or chronic	Icteric or anticteric hepatitis; usually self-limited
Management	Supportive Prevent spread (hygiene, IG)	Supportive	Supportive May be role for α-interferon with chronic hepatitis C	Supportive α-interferon may be beneficial	Supportive
Vaccine	Yes	Yes	No	No	No

for weeks in hepatitis A and months in hepatitis B. Bilirubin level greater than 20 mg/dl is consistent with severe disease. Glutamyl transferase level greater than 300 units/L is consistent with biliary atresia or alpha$_1$-antitrypsin deficiency.

4. Urine is dark with urobilinogen and bilirubin.

5. Serologic studies are important in differentiating the type of hepatitis. Patients with hepatitis and no other risk factors most likely have HAV and the first screening test would probably be Anti-HAV IgM. First-line, cost-effective screening tests if history is compatible are HbsAG for HBV or Anti-HCV for HCV.

a. Hepatitis A antibody (IgM) is diagnostic of an acute infection.
b. Serologic tests for hepatitis B are listed below.

Hepatitis B Antigen/Antibody	Interpretation
Surface antigen (HBsAg)	Earliest indicator of the presence of acute HBV infection. Does not differentiate between acute and chronic infection.
Antibody to surface antigen (Anti-HBs)	Prior infection with HBV and clinical recovery; immunity after vaccine.
Early (e) antigen (HBeAg)	Early indicator of acute infection from active viral replication; most infectious period; persistence indicates higher risk of progression of disease with chronic infection.
Antibody to e antigen (Anti-HBe)	Seroconversion from HBeAg to Anti-HBe during acute phase suggests resolving HBV infection.
Antibody to core antigen (Anti-HBc)	Antibody found in high titer in acute, resolved or chronic HBV infection. Not present after immunization.
IgM antibody to HBcAg (IgM Anti-HBc)	Acute or recent HBV infection, including infection in HBsAg-negative persons during this transient "window" phase of infection.

6. Detection of HCV-RNA is the best means of confirming hepatitis C. Anti-HCV is suggestive of infection with hepatitis C (current or past). Qualitative RNA polymerase chain reaction (PCR) testing is diagnostic.
7. Hepatitis D is detected from the presence of hepatitis D antigen. Chronic illness may be indicated by the finding of high titer levels at 2 to 4 weeks.
8. Serologic evaluation may be diagnostic for hepatitis E virus antigen. IgM Anti-HEV is present during acute HEV infection. Electron microscopy of infected stools may be useful.
9. If indicated, other studies should be performed to exclude other causes of hepatitis.

DIFFERENTIAL DIAGNOSIS

1. Infection or inflammation:
   a. Viral: infectious mononucleosis (Epstein-Barr [EB] virus), cytomegalovirus, herpes simplex
   b. Toxoplasmosis
   c. Cholangitis
2. Metabolic disorders:
   a. Cholelithiasis
   b. Wilson's disease
   c. Gilbert's disease and Dubin-Johnson syndrome
3. Drugs:
   a. Alcohol
   b. Analgesic: aspirin, acetaminophen
   c. Anesthetic: halothane
   d. Antibiotic: erythromycin estolate, sulfonamides, tetracycline, rifampin, carbenicillin
   e. Antituberculosis: isoniazid, rifampin
   f. Others: phenytoin, phenothiazine, morphine
4. Congenital disorder: biliary atresia (infants)

MANAGEMENT

Most patients need careful follow-up observation and monitoring to ensure that their liver functions are normalizing and that hydration is maintained.

Patients with impending liver failure need a host of supportive measures:

1. Respiratory and cardiovascular support:
   a. Oxygen and active airway management if necessary
   b. Maintenance of intravascular volume

2. Central nervous system (CNS) support, if encephalopathy is present:
   a. Decrease of protein intake
   b. NG tube with administration of neomycin, 50 to 100 mg/kg/24 hr q6hr, via the tube
   c. Treatment of cerebral edema:
      (1) Fluid restriction: 75% of maintenance level
      (2) Steroids: dexamethasone, 0.25 mg/kg/dose q6hr IV; their use is controversial
      (3) Mannitol, 0.25 to 1.0 g/kg/dose q6hr IV
      (4) Hyperventilation (if ventilatory support is necessary)
3. Other:
   a. Give diuretics for fluid overload:
      (1) Furosemide (Lasix), 1 to 2 mg/kg/dose q2-6hr IV or PO
      (2) Spironolactone (Aldactone), 1 to 3 mg/kg/24 hr q6-8hr PO
   b. Maintain serum glucose level at 100 to 150 mg/dl.
   c. Support nutrition.
   d. For bleeding, administer fresh-frozen plasma (10 ml/kg/dose q12-24hr IV) and vitamin K (infants: 1-2 mg/dose IV slowly; children and adults: 5-10 mg/dose IV).
   e. Treat infections and GI bleeding appropriately.
   f. Isolate the patient.

      NOTE: Other modalities that have been attempted without proven benefit include exchange transfusions and dialysis.
4. Trials of α-interferon have demonstrated normalized liver function in patients with chronic hepatitis C; 50% of patients showing response to the therapy experienced relapse when it ceased. α-Interferon may produce transient beneficial effects for hepatitis D.
5. Immunization against hepatitis B may be useful.

Preventive Measures

Hepatitis A. Hepatitis A vaccine is currently available for children 2 years or older. It is recommended for the following people:

1. Travelers to areas with intermediate to high rates of endemic hepatitis A
2. Children living in defined or circumscribed communities with high endemic or periodic outbreaks of HIV infection
3. Patients with chronic hepatitis

Patients with *household contacts* should receive 0.02 ml/kg intramuscularly (IM) of immune serum globulin (IG) as soon after exposure as possible. IG is not indicated beyond 2 weeks after exposure. Administration of IG should also be considered in the following circumstances:

1. In daycare centers with children older than 2 years who are toilet trained: Give IG to all children in the daycare room when there is a case of hepatitis in an employee or child of an employee in contact with index case.
2. In daycare centers with children who are not toilet trained: Give IG to all employees and children if there is a case of hepatitis in an employee or child or in the household contacts of two enrolled children.
3. If recognition of the outbreak is delayed by 3 weeks or there are cases in three or more families, consider administering IG to all staff and children and household contacts of children 3 years or younger.
4. Give IG to those who have personal contact with individuals with hepatitis in an institutional setting.
5. Exposure in classrooms or other places in schools has not generally posed a significant risk of infection. Hospital personnel caring for patients with hepatitis A are not routinely treated. Emphasis should be given to good handwashing technique.
6. Preexposure prophylaxis for travelers to areas where hygiene is poor may be achieved by giving a dose of IG immediately before departure as follows: 0.02 ml/kg for children who are staying in the

area less than 3 months, and 0.06 ml/kg for children who are staying 3 months or longer; 2 ml IM to adults staying in such areas less than 3 months, and 5 ml to those staying longer.

Hepatitis B. *Preexposure* prophylaxis is available from a vaccine prepared from formalin-inactivated subunits derived from hepatitis B surface antigen (HBsAg) from plasma of carriers or genetically engineered recombinant HB vaccine. A three-dose series is recommended, with administration of the vaccine at days 1, 30, and 180 to high-risk individuals.

For children younger than 10 years, give 10 μg of plasma-derived HB vaccine (0.5 ml) or 5 μg (0.5 ml) of recombinant vaccine; older children and adults should be given 20 μg (1 ml) of plasma-derived HB vaccine or 10 μg (1 ml) of recombinant vaccine. Immunosuppressed patients may receive twice the recommended dose of plasma-derived HB vaccine. Children in this group include those from families with hepatitis B virus infection or chronic carriers, those in institutions for the mentally retarded, and those receiving large amounts of blood and blood products.

Postexposure prophylaxis must reflect the type of exposure (blood or percutaneous needlestick or mucosal membrane) and HBsAg of the donor:

1. For those who have been exposed to blood known to be HBsAg positive; exposure may be percutaneous, ocular, or through mucosal membrane: A single dose of hepatitis B immunoglobulin (HBIG) (0.06 ml/kg or 5 ml for adult) should be given as soon as possible after exposure and within 24 hours if possible. Hepatitis B vaccine 1 ml (20 μg children younger than 10 years: 0.5 ml) should be given as an IM injection at a separate site as soon as possible but within 7 days of exposure, with second and third doses given at 1 month and 6 months after the first dose. If HB vaccine is refused, repeat HBIG in 1 month.
2. For those who have been exposed to blood of unknown HBsAg status:
   a. High-risk patients (e.g., patients with Down syndrome who are institutionalized, patients undergoing dialysis, drug abusers). Initiate hepatitis B vaccine three-dose regimen. Consider HBIG, 0.06 ml/kg (adult: 5 ml), as well.
   b. Treatment of exposed low-risk patients should be individualized. Vaccine should be considered. Therapy may be delayed if status can be determined within 7 days of exposure.

Sexual contacts of persons with acute hepatitis B infections are at higher risk of acquiring the disease. A single dose of HBIG, 0.06 ml/kg (5 ml in adult), should be given to susceptible individuals who have had sexual contact with an HBsAg-positive person if it can be given within 14 days of the last sexual contact. A second HBIG dose should be given in cases of heterosexual exposures if the index patient remains HBsAg positive 3 months after detection. Subsequent doses of hepatitis B vaccine should be given at 1 and 6 months.

Newborns of mothers who are HBsAg positive are at risk for transmission of hepatitis B virus. HBIG (0.5 ml) IM should be administered within 12 hours of birth. In addition, HB vaccine (0.5 ml) should be given at the time of administration of HBIG and 1 month and 6 months later. HBsAg testing should be performed at 6 months in consultation with appropriate experts. Infants born to mothers who have not been screened for HBsAg should receive vaccine and HBIG at birth, and the vaccine schedule should be completed as provided in routine immunization.

Routine immunization of infants is recommended against hepatitis B. Immunization is done during the first few days of life, and subsequently at 1 to 2 and 18 months of age. Routine immunization of older children is also feasible.

Hepatitis Non-A/Non-B. Management is the same as for hepatitis A, although some recommend IG, 0.06 ml/kg IM, after exposure to blood.

BIBLIOGRAPHY

American Academy of Pediatrics, Committee on Infectious Diseases: Prevention of hepatitis A infections: guidelines for use of hepatitis A vaccine and immune globulin, *Pediatrics* 98:1207, 1996.

Clemens RM, Safary A, Hepburn A et al: Clinical experience with an inactivated hepatitis A vaccine, *J Infect Dis* 171:514, 1995.

Morton TA, Kelen GD: Hepatitis C, *Ann Emerg Med* 31:381, 1998.

Report of the committee on infectious diseases, 25 ed, Elk Grove, Ill: 2000; American Academy of Pediatrics.

Pancreatitis

ETIOLOGY

1. Infection:
   a. Viral: mumps, hepatitis, EB virus, coxsackievirus
   b. *Mycoplasma pneumoniae*
   c. Kawasaki's disease
2. Trauma: blunt, penetrating, or surgical
3. Intoxication:
   a. Diuretics: thiazides, furosemide
   b. Prednisone, oral contraceptive agents
   c. Antibiotics: rifampin, tetracycline, isoniazid
4. Congenital: biliary tract anomalies
5. Structural:
   a. Biliary tract disease
   b. Cholelithiasis
6. Systemic illness:
   a. Systemic lupus erythematosus
   b. Kawasaki's disease
   c. Cystic fibrosis
   d. Diabetes mellitus

DIAGNOSTIC FINDINGS

1. Abdominal pain is the primary complaint, of either insidious or sudden onset. Upper quadrant or epigastric constant or intermittent pain is reported. It may radiate to the back or neck. Relief is obtained in the knee-chest position.
2. Abdominal tenderness and distension are noted, with decreased bowel sounds and ascites. Cullen's (bluish periumbilical discoloration) and Grey Turner's (discoloration of the flank) signs are indicative of pancreatic necrosis and only occur late.
3. Low-grade fever, nausea, vomiting, and lethargy may be present.

Complications

1. Hypotension and shock secondary to third-space losses and intravascular volume depletion
2. Acute respiratory distress syndrome with left-sided pleural effusions and pneumonitis
3. Pancreatic pseudocyst or abscess, usually with delayed onset
4. Disseminated intravascular coagulation

Ancillary Data

1. Electrolyte levels are normal. Glucose level may be increased.
2. Hypocalcemia is a bad prognostic sign.
3. Serum amylase level rises to a peak at 12 to 24 hours and may return to normal in 48 to 72 hours. Lipase level rises early and normalizes less rapidly. A determination that is useful for patients whose serum amylase level is not diagnostic is clearance values calculated from spot urine and serum values:

$$\frac{C_{amylase}}{C_{creatine}} = \frac{\text{Amylase (urine)}}{\text{Amylase (serum)}} \times \frac{\text{Creatinine (serum)}}{\text{Creatinine (urine)}} \times 100$$

This ratio is normally equal to 1% to 4%. A value greater than 6% indicates pancreatitis.

NOTE: Serum amylase value may be elevated in abdominal trauma or infection that does not specifically cause pancreatitis.

4. Liver function values are elevated, particularly the bilirubin level.
5. X-ray films may demonstrate pleural effusions, atelectasis, pneumonitis, and an intestinal ileus or sentinel loop.
6. Prognosis has been studied in adults. Poor prognostic findings upon presentation include a WBC count higher than 16,000 cells/mm^3, serum glucose level higher than 200 mg/dl, serum lactate dehydrogenase (LDH) level higher than 350 U/l, and serum aspartate transaminase (AST) level higher than 250 U/l. At 48 hours, poor prognostic findings include a decrease in hematocrit (Hct) value of more than 10%, an increase in BUN level greater than 5 mg/dl, serum Ca^{++} level lower than 8 mg/dl, base excess higher than 4, PaO_2 less than 60 mm Hg, and fluid sequestration volume greater than 6 liters (adult).

DIFFERENTIAL DIAGNOSIS

1. Infection:
   a. Peritonitis and other causes of surgical abdomen
   b. Pneumonia
2. Trauma: It is essential to differentiate pancreatitis from other abdominal organic involvement. Peritoneal lavage may be necessary. Consider child abuse.

MANAGEMENT

1. Stabilization is of primary importance; initial attention is given to fluid therapy, which usually requires IV replacement of deficits (see Chapter 7). In cases of trauma, it is imperative to be certain that other organs are not involved. Glucose and calcium abnormalities may require intervention.
2. An NG tube attached to suction should be inserted, and the patient put on NPO status until pain has subsided for several days.
3. Analgesia may be used. Meperidine (Demerol), 1 mg/kg/dose q4-6hr IM or IV, is the drug of choice.
4. When the patient can tolerate food, a bland, low-fat diet should be used; pancreatic enzyme supplements are often required. Until that time, IV alimentation is appropriate.
5. Once the patient is stabilized, antacids or cimetidine may be useful.

DISPOSITION

1. Patients must be hospitalized for IV fluids, gastric suction, and monitoring.
2. Long-term follow-up observation is essential because of the delayed onset of pancreatic pseudocyst and abscess.

BIBLIOGRAPHY

Mader TJ, McHugh TP: Acute pancreatitis in children, *Pediatr Emerg Care* 8:157, 1992.

Weizman Z, Durle PR: Acute pancreatitis in childhood, *J Pediatr* 113:24, 1988.

Reye Syndrome

ALERT Vomiting and behavior changes after an acute illness require rapid evaluation and intervention.

Reye's syndrome is an acute, noninflammatory encephalopathy with altered level of consciousness, cerebral edema without perivascular or meningeal inflammation, and fatty metamorphosis of the liver, probably secondary to mitochondrial dysfunction. It is a multisystem disease with a biphasic history marked by an infectious phase followed by an encephalopathic stage. There have been reports of the syndrome in children between 4 months and 14 years old with an average age of 7 years and a peak occurrence between 4 and 11 years. Reye's syndrome often follows a viral infection: influenza B and chickenpox are particularly implicated. Salicylate ingestion may be a predisposing factor. The disease is rare at present.

The term *Reye-like syndrome* has been used to describe a variety of pathologic conditions resulting from defects in urea and fatty acid metabolism, toxicologic injury, and impaired gluconeogenesis.

DIAGNOSTIC FINDINGS

1. A prodrome of respiratory or GI symptoms is consistently present for 2 to 3 days.
2. Vomiting develops and is followed in 24 to 48 hours by an encephalopathic phase with marked behavioral changes, including delirium and combativeness, disorientation, and hallucination. The deteriorating level of consciousness reflects increasing intracranial pressure (ICP). Obtundation and coma may follow, associated with seizures, hyperventilation, and hypothermia.

   Progressive stages have been outlined on the basis of the progression of findings in cephalocaudal evolution of brainstem dysfunction, as follows:

   Stage 0: Alert, wakeful.

   Stage I: Lethargy, follows verbal comments, normal posture, purposeful response to pain, brisk pupillary light reflex, and normal oculocephalic reflex. Vomiting.

   Stage II: Combative or stuporous, inappropriate verbalizing, normal posture, purposeful or nonpurposeful response to pain, sluggish pupillary reaction, and conjugate deviation on doll's eyes maneuver. Hyperventilation.

   Stage III: Comatose, decorticate posture, decorticate response to pain, sluggish but present pupillary reaction, conjugate deviation on doll's eyes maneuver.

   Stage IV: Comatose, decerebrate posture and decerebrate response to pain, dilated fixed pupils, and inconsistent presence or absence of oculocephalic reflex.

   Stage V: Comatose, flaccid, no response to pain, no pupillary response, no oculocephalic reflex, seizures. Respiratory arrest.
3. Hepatomegaly and pancreatitis may be present.
4. In children younger than 1 year, the presentation is often atypical. Vomiting is mild and the predominant findings are apnea, hyperventilation, seizures, hepatomegaly, and hypoglycemia.

Complications

Children in stage IV or V and those progressing rapidly from stage I to stage III have a poor prognosis.

1. Acute respiratory failure
2. Cerebral edema with herniation, reflecting progression of increased ICP (10%)
3. Cardiac dysrhythmia
4. Death (10%)

Ancillary Data

1. Plasma ammonia levels are usually elevated to 1.5 to 3 or greater times the normal values (normal: 40 to 80 μg/dl). Transiently present for 24 to 48 hours after the onset of mental status changes. A level above 300 μg/dl is associated with a poor prognosis.
2. Elevations of serum transaminase value (usually three times normal) and other liver function values, osmolality, and serum amylase value. Normal or slightly elevated bilirubin value. Variable BUN and electrolyte values. Decreased glucose level, particularly in children younger than 4 years.
3. Decreased levels of liver-dependent clotting factor (II, VII, IX, and X), with prolonged PT and partial thromboplastin time (PTT). Fibrinogen level may be decreased. Normal platelets.
4. Arterial blood gas (ABG) analysis, lumbar puncture (assuming no evidence of

increased ICP), blood cultures, and toxicology screen to exclude other potential causes and to monitor the patient.

5. Computed tomography (CT) to exclude intracranial lesions (e.g., abscess) if diagnosis is uncertain. Scan demonstrates cerebral edema.
6. Percutaneous liver biopsy may be useful in patients with an atypical presentation, including infants younger than 1 year in recurrent episodes and familial cases, and in nonepidemic cases without an antecedent infection or vomiting.

DIFFERENTIAL DIAGNOSIS

(see Chapter 15)

1. Infection:
   a. Meningitis/encephalitis (p. 741)
   b. Sepsis
   c. Viral: chickenpox or hepatitis
2. Endocrine/metabolic disorders:
   a. Hypoglycemia (see Chapter 38)
   b. Hypoxia
   c. Amino acid/organic acid inborn errors of metabolism
3. Intoxication: salicylates, acetaminophen, ethanol, lead, camphor (see Table 54-2)
4. Trauma: head
5. Vascular: intracranial hemorrhage

MANAGEMENT

1. General supportive care is crucial in determining the ultimate outcome. Dehydration may be present but should not be fully corrected because of the concurrent cerebral edema. Serum glucose level should be kept between 125 and 175 mg/dl, with a serum osmolality less than 310 mOsm/kg H_2O.
2. Patients with stage I or II Reye's syndrome need frequent monitoring of vital and neurologic signs, IV infusion of 10% to 20% dextrose in water (D10W-D20W), and correction of fluid and electrolyte abnormalities.
3. Patients with stage III through stage V disease need aggressive support and intervention:
   a. Supportive measures:
      (1) Monitoring of venous and arterial pressures; NG tube; and urinary catheter for intake and output measurement.
      (2) Respiratory support, including intubation, mechanical ventilation, and hyperventilation, if indicated.
      (3) IV infusion of D15W at two-thirds maintenance level after cardiovascular stabilization to keep urine output at 1 ml/kg/hr.
      (4) Seizure control: phenytoin (Dilantin), loading dose of 10 to 20 mg/kg/dose and maintenance at 5 mg/kg/24 hr q6hr IV; does not cause sedation; monitor serum drug level.
      (5) Control of temperature.
   b. Metabolic abnormalities: Maintenance of serum glucose level between 125 and 175 mg/dl through the use of glucose and insulin (1 unit of insulin per 5 g of glucose given) infusions.
   c. For coagulation abnormalities:
      (1) Fresh-frozen plasma, 10 ml/kg/dose q12-24hr IV or prn.
      (2) Vitamin K, 1 to 10 mg/dose IV slowly.
      (3) Exchange transfusion rarely indicated.
   d. Intracranial monitoring to measure efficacy of a number of therapeutic modalities. Maintain ICP at 15 to 18 mm Hg or less and cerebral perfusion pressure (CPP) above 50 mm Hg. Measures may be tried individually or concurrently, depending on patient response:
      (1) Mannitol, 0.25 to 0.5 g/kg/dose IV infusion over 20 minutes; may

be repeated q2hr as needed. Monitor osmolality of serum, keeping it below 210 mOsm/kg H_2O.

(2) Hyperventilation to lower $Paco_2$.

(3) Furosemide (Lasix), 1 to 2 mg/kg/dose q4-6hr IV.

(4) Head elevation.

(5) Muscular paralysis: pancuronium (Pavulon), 0.05 to 0.1 mg/kg/dose q1-2hr prn IV. Patient must be intubated with respiratory support.

(6) Pentobarbital (Nembutal), 3 to 20 mg/kg, by IV slowly while blood pressure is monitored. Maintain serum drug level at 25 to 40 (g/dl by maintenance infusion of 1 to 2 mg/kg/hr. Barbiturate coma is maintained for 2 to 3 days while other parameters are monitored if alternative approaches have not been successful (see Chapter 57).

4. Treat complications.

DISPOSITION

All patients must be admitted to an intensive care unit (ICU) capable of intracranial monitoring. Appropriate consultation should be sought.

BIBLIOGRAPHY

Belay ED, Bresee JS, Holman RC et al: Reye's syndrome in the United States from 1981 through 1997, *N Engl J Med* 340:1377, 1999.

Committee on Infectious Diseases (AAP): Aspirin and Reye's syndrome, *Pediatrics* 69:810, 1982.

Hurwitz ES, Barrett MJ, Bregman D et al: Public health service study on Reye's syndrome and medications, *N Engl J Med* 313:849, 1985.

Rogers MF, Schonberger LB, Hurwitz ES et al: National Reye's syndrome surveillance, *Pediatrics* 75:260, 1985.

CONDITIONS REQUIRING SURGERY

Appendicitis

ALERT Severe RLQ pain requires urgent surgical consultation.

DIAGNOSTIC FINDINGS

Clinical symptoms and signs of appendicitis vary according to the severity of inflammation and whether perforation has occurred. The hydration status of the patient may also affect the clinical presentation; most patients are 5% to 10% dehydrated. Patients classically have a low-grade fever and loss of appetite. Symptoms progress to consist of pain followed by vomiting.

1. The crampy abdominal pain is initially periumbilical but gradually shifts to the RLQ over the ensuing 4 to 12 hours. Tenderness is maximal over McBurney's point, which is located 4 to 6 cm from the iliac crest along a line drawn between the iliac crest and the umbilicus. The patient is most comfortable in the supine position with the legs flexed. With rupture of the appendix, there is initial pain relief but subsequent worsening as a result of peritonitis.
2. RLQ guarding and rebound are present. Bowel sounds may be diminished. With perforation, there is less localization, and more generalized peritoneal signs are present.
3. Rectal examination may demonstrate tenderness, greatest on the right.
4. Psoas sign: With the patient in the left lateral decubitus position, pain is elicited by passive extension of the right thigh. Presence of this sign suggests abdominal or pelvic peritoneal inflammation.
5. Obturator sign: With the patient in the supine position, pain is produced by flexion and internal rotation of the right thigh. Presence of this sign suggests pelvic inflammation.

6. In children younger than 2 years, the diagnosis of appendicitis is particularly difficult because of the nonspecific nature of the clinical picture. The morbidity rate is high because about 90% of such patients are not diagnosed until perforation has occurred. About one third of these patients have been seen by a physician 24 to 48 hours before admission:
   a. Vomiting, lethargy or irritability, crying spells, and feeding problems are noted.
   b. Concurrent illness (upper respiratory infection, otitis media, or gastroenteritis) may confuse the diagnostic picture.
   c. The abdomen is diffusely tender, with decrease or absence of bowel sounds, guarding, and tenderness on rectal examination. Patients are febrile, and urinary retention may occur.
   d. Tachypnea with short respiratory excursions may result from diaphragmatic irritation by peritonitis.
7. Mantrel's score may have some value:

Finding	Point Value
Migration of pain to RLQ	1
Anorexia or acetone in urine	1
Nausea/vomiting	1
Tenderness of RLQ	2
Rebound tenderness	1
Elevated temperature	1
Leukocytosis (WBC count >10,000 cells/mm^3)	2
Shift to left of WBC count (>75% neutrophils)	1

A Mantrel score of 7 or higher is highly suspicious for appendicitis; the patient with a score of 5 or 6 should be observed and followed closely; a score of 4 or less signifies a low likelihood of appendicitis. Further study is still needed of this scoring system.

Complications

1. Peritonitis. Perforation is associated with delay in treatment and with younger age.
2. Intraabdominal or pelvic abscess.
3. Ileus or obstruction.
4. Pyelophlebitis.
5. Sepsis and shock.

Ancillary Data

1. WBC count: Above 15,000 cells/mm^3 in about 40% of patients, 93% of whom show a shift to the left (percentage of neutrophils: >50% for 1- to 5-year-old children, >65% for 5- to 10-year-old children, and >75% for 10- to 15-year-old children).
2. C-reactive protein (CRP) measurement may be useful. An increase of 1 mg/dl or more on the second CRP determination after 4 to 12 hours of observation is reliable. A CRP value of more than 6 mg/dl is suggestive.
3. Urinalysis: May demonstrate minimal pyuria secondary to ureteral irritation (UTI must be excluded). Will also assist in assessment of hydration.
4. Chest x-ray film to exclude pneumonia, particularly in the lower lobe.
5. Abdominal x-ray film (three-way view consists of supine and upright abdomen and anteroposterior [AP] chest):
   a. Abnormal gas pattern with decreased gas, air-fluid levels, or diffuse small bowel dilation
   b. Free peritoneal air
   c. Thickening of abdominal wall
   d. Appendolith (about 10% of cases)
   e. Abscess in RLQ
   f. Scoliosis
6. CT is probably the definitive diagnostic tool when performed with rectal contrast agent in patients in whom the history or physical findings are not diagnostic. The results are reproducible and do not depend on the operator.
7. Ultrasonography: Increasingly used to confirm the diagnosis of abscess by experienced clinicians. Studies have demonstrated it to be 89% to 94% specific and

85% to 94% sensitive. It is operator dependent.

8. Barium enema study may on occasion be useful as a diagnostic modality to demonstrate other diseases.
9. Laparoscopy: Indicated for patients with relative contraindications to surgery and equivocal physical findings. Videoscopic surgery is widely used for definitive removal of the appendix.

Differential Diagnosis (Table 76-3)

Children who are misdiagnosed as having appendicitis are more likely to have had pain of more than 2 days' duration and a temperature above 38.3° C and to appear lethargic and irritable. The accuracy of the diagnosis is improved by admitting and observing children in whom examination findings are equivocal.

Management

1. Focus initial management on stabilization of the patient:
   a. IV hydration, initially with 20 ml/kg of D5W 0.9% in normal saline (NS) solution or D5W in lactated Ringer's (LR) solution over 1 hour if there is a fluid deficit (see Chapter 7)
   b. NG tube; NPO status
   c. Oxygen if the patient is in marked distress
   d. Lowering of temperature by cooling blanket or antipyretics
2. Involve surgical consultant early.
3. If any evidence of peritonitis or perforation exists, begin antibiotics:
   a. Ampicillin, 100 to 200 mg/kg/24 hr q4hr IV, *and*
   b. Clindamycin, 30 to 40 mg/kg/24 hr q6hr IV, *and*

TABLE 76-3 Right Lower Quadrant Pain: Diagnostic Considerations

	Infection/ Inflammation	Neoplasm	Congenital
Systemic	Influenza		
Skin	Herpes zoster Cellulitis		
Abdominal wall			Inguinal hernia
Pulmonary	Pneumonia		
Gastrointestinal tract	**Mesenteric adenitis** **Gastroenteritis** (*Salmonella, Shigella, Yersinia*, typhoid) **Appendicitis** Peritonitis Meckel's diverticulum Cholecystitis Duodenal ulcer Hepatitis	Hodgkin's disease Carcinoma	Intussusception Obstruction Meckel's diverticulum
Kidney/ureter	**Pyelonephritis** **Cystitis** Perinephritic abscess	Wilms' tumor	Hydronephrosis
Reproductive tract	**Pelvic inflammatory disease** **Salpingitis** Tuboovarian Pelvic abscess	Endometriosis	Testicular torsion
Spine	Osteomyelitis		

c. Gentamicin, 5.0 to 7.5 mg/kg/24 hr q8hr IV or IM. Some surgeons use cefoxitin (Mefoxin), 80 to 160 mg/kg/24 hr q4-6hr IV.

4. Give analgesia, if necessary, but only after the diagnosis is certain and the decision to operate has been made: meperidine (Demerol), 1 to 2 mg/kg/dose IM (maximum: 50-100 mg/dose)
5. Perform surgery.

Disposition

All patients must be admitted for surgical management.

Patients for whom the diagnosis is uncertain may often benefit from 12 to 24 hours of observation to allow the disease to progress and define itself.

BIBLIOGRAPHY

Balthazar EJ, Rofsky NM, Zucker R: Appendicitis: the impact of computed tomography imaging on negative appendectomy and perforation rates, *Am J Gastroenterol* 93:768, 1998.

Bond GR, Tully SB et al: Use of Mantrel's score in childhood appendicitis: a prospective study of 187 children with abdominal pain, *Ann Emerg Med* 19:1014, 1990.

Chen SC: C-reactive protein in the diagnosis of acute appendicitis, *Am J Emerg Med* 14:101, 1996.

Crady SK, Jones JS, Wyn T et al: Clinical validity of ultrasound in children with suspected appendicitis, *Ann Emerg Med* 22:1125, 1993.

Garcia Pena BM, Taylor GA, Fishman SJ et al: Cost and effectiveness of ultrasonography and limited computed tomography for diagnosis appendicitis in children, *Pediatrics* 106:672, 2000.

Heller RM, Hernanz-Schulman M: Application of new imaging modalities to the evaluation of common pediatric conditions, *J Pediatr* 135:632, 1999.

Northrock SG, Skeach G, Rush JJ: Clinical features of misdiagnosed appendicitis in children, *Ann Emerg Med* 20:45, 1991.

Rao PM, Rhea JT, Novellini RA et al: Effect of computed tomography of the appendix on treatment of patients and use of hospital resources, *N Engl Med* 338:141, 1998.

Vignault F, Filiatrault D, Brandt ML et al: Acute appendicitis in children: evaluation with ultrasound, *Pediatr Radiol* 176:501, 1990.

Zoltie N, Cust MP: Analgesia in the acute abdomen, *Ann R Coll Surg Engl* 68:209, 1986.

Autoimmune	Trauma	Intrapsychic	Vascular	Endocrine/Metabolic
	Black widow spider bite	Functional		Diabetic ketoacidosis Acute prophyria
	Contusion Muscle rupture			
Regional enteritis Ulcerative colitis	**Impacted feces**		Mesenteric infarct	
				Renal calculi
				Mittelschmerz **Dysmenorrhea** Ovarian cyst Threatened abortion Ectopic pregnancy

Hernia, Inguinal (see p. 672)

ALERT Although repair of an inguinal hernia is an elective procedure, bowel incarceration requires urgent surgery.

Inguinal hernias in children represent 37% of all surgical procedures in the pediatric age group. The hernia results from the failure of the processus vaginalis to obliterate in boys and of the canal of Nuck to close in girls. Right-sided (60%) hernias are more common than left-sided (30%) hernias; 10% are bilateral.

A higher incidence of inguinal hernias is associated with increases in peritoneal fluid volume (ventriculoperitoneal shunt, peritoneal dialysis, ascites), abdominal tumors, genitourinary abnormalities (exstrophy of bladder, hypospadias, epispadias), connective tissue disorders, mucopolysaccharides, cystic fibrosis, and intersex syndromes.

DIAGNOSTIC FINDINGS

Parents report a bulge or mass in the groin that enlarges with crying and Valsalva's maneuver. A smooth, firm, sausage-shaped nontender or slightly tender mass can be seen and palpated in the groin. During reduction, there is a gurgling or "swoosh" sound.

The hernia is usually reduced before being seen. A "silk glove" sign may be sought by rubbing the index finger over the spermatic cord at the pubic tubercle; a slippery feel similar to that of two layers of silk rubbing together constitutes presence of this sign.

The herniated bowel may become incarcerated or strangulated, resulting in signs and symptoms of intestinal obstruction. Perforation may also occur.

DIFFERENTIAL DIAGNOSIS

1. Hydrocele is an outpocketing of the peritoneum and lack of complete obliteration of the processus vaginalis. The transillumination finding is positive. A communicating hydrocele changes in size and is associated with an inguinal hernia. Hydroceles usually resolve by 1 year of age (see p. 672).
2. Lymphadenopathy.
3. An undescended or high-riding testicle may retract spontaneously.
4. Urologic problems, including testicular torsion and epididymitis, may occur.

MANAGEMENT

If evidence of intestinal obstruction or perforation exists, immediate intervention is required for stabilization and preparation for surgery.

Patients in whom hernias are easily reduced should be scheduled for semielective surgery. Discharge and close follow-up observation can be arranged after careful instructions have been given about recognition of incarceration or strangulation and the need for immediate intervention.

For incarcerated hernias that do not easily reduce spontaneously, gentle, persistent pressure should be applied. If this does not work, place the patient in Trendelenburg's position with cold compresses over the inguinal area. Sedatives may also be used. Surgical consultation should be initiated for repair. Patients are usually admitted for observation and early surgery.

Strangulated hernias cannot be reduced and need immediate surgical intervention.

BIBLIOGRAPHY

Sparnon AL, Kiely EM, Spitz L: Incarcerated inguinal hernia in infants, *BMJ* 293:376, 1986.

Hirschsprung's Disease

James C. Mitchiner

ALERT Intestinal obstruction in the newborn or infant requires a careful and expeditious evaluation.

Hirschsprung's disease, or congenital megacolon, results from congenital aganglionosis of the distal colon and rectum that leads to failure of effective peristalsis through the aganglionic segment. It is the most common cause of partial intestinal obstruction in early infancy and occasionally manifests in childhood.

DIAGNOSTIC FINDINGS

Neonates may fail to pass meconium in the first 24 hours of life. They also may demonstrate constipation, often not until 2 to 3 weeks of age. Paradoxic diarrhea, caused by mucosal ulcerations in the proximal dilated segment, may develop. Vomiting and failure to thrive may be seen.

Bowel obstruction is usually present, with a distended, tympanitic abdomen, hyperactive or high-pitched bowel sounds, and a history of vomiting. Rectal examination reveals an absence of stool in the ampulla and is often followed by evacuation of gas and liquid stool when the examiner's finger is withdrawn.

Complications

1. Hirschsprung's-associated enterocolitis (HAEC), generally secondary to *Clostridium difficile* infection, with cecal perforation, rectal bleeding, pneumoperitoneum, and pericolic abscess
2. Acute appendicitis
3. Malnutrition
4. Reversible urinary tract obstruction, leading to hydronephrosis, hydroureter, and recurrent UTIs
5. Septicemia, particularly in newborns

Ancillary Data

1. CBC and electrolyte determinations as indicated by clinical condition.
2. Abdominal x-ray film: May show distended, gas-filled proximal segment, or findings may be normal.
3. Barium enema study: Shows a normal diameter in the aganglionic segment associated with a dilated proximal segment tapering at the rectosigmoid. Once the dilated segment is defined, it is not necessary to complete the study; in fact, completing it may be dangerous. A postevacuation film taken 12 to 48 hours later shows residual barium.
4. Rectal biopsy: Ideally performed in the stable patient whose diagnosis is uncertain; often performed when barium enema study results are equivocal. Is performed proximal to the anorectal junction, 2 to 3 cm above the rectal columns. Specimen must be of sufficient depth to include both the mucosal and muscular layers for proper diagnosis. General anesthesia is usually necessary.

   Acetylcholinesterase activity, which is high in Hirschsprung's disease, should be measured in the biopsy material.
5. Manometry demonstrates paradoxic contraction of the internal anal sphincter.

DIFFERENTIAL DIAGNOSIS

1. Congenital disorders:
   a. Colonic or ileal atresia
   b. Hypoplastic left colon syndrome
2. Infection/inflammation: neonatal sepsis, megacolon, necrotizing enterocolitis, ulcerative colitis.
3. Endocrine disorders: hypothyroidism and adrenal insufficiency.
4. Trauma: anal fissure.
5. Intoxication: drug-induced hypomotility (anticholinergics, narcotics).
6. Acquired constipation, which usually occurs after 2 years of age, with associated incontinence, abdominal pain, and obstruction. Stools are usually large in caliber, with larger amounts of stool in the ampulla. Barium enema shows a diffuse megacolon.

   In contrast, Hirschsprung's disease typically manifests in the newborn period with symptoms of failure to thrive and rarely with abdominal pain. The stool is thin and ribbonlike, with decreased frequency and little stool in the ampulla. Barium enema demonstrates a localized constriction with proximal dilation.

MANAGEMENT

1. Intravenous hydration and gastric decompression with an NG tube are essential in the management of acute obstruction.
   a. Fluids: D5W 0.9% NS solution at 20 ml/kg over the first hour, then deficit and maintenance replacement
   b. With evidence of obstruction: intestinal decompression with NG tube
   c. Immediate surgical consultation
2. After stabilization, a barium enema study is indicated if enterocolitis and perforation are not present; if barium enema findings are suggestive, a rectal biopsy should be performed by a pediatric surgeon or gastroenterologist.
3. In general, surgery is the definitive treatment if the biopsy shows no ganglion cells and high acetylcholinesterase (ACE) activity.
   a. Acute surgical therapy typically involves a primary pullthrough procedure. The goal is to place normal ganglion-containing bowel within 1 cm of the anal opening.
   b. In certain cases, a loop colostomy is done to decompress the bowel, and a definitive procedure is performed electively at a later date. The stoma must contain normal bowel.
   c. Laparoscopic pullthrough procedures are being performed more frequently.

BIBLIOGRAPHY

Adzick NS, Nance ML: Pediatric surgery, *N Engl J Med* 342:1651, 2000.

Amiel J, Lyonnet S: Hirschsprung disease, associated syndromes, and genetics: a review, *J Med Genet* 38:729, 2001.

Coran AG, Teitelbaum DH: Recent advances in the management of Hirschsprung's disease, *Am J Surg* 180:382, 2000.

Doig CM: Hirschsprung's disease and mimicking conditions, *Dig Dis* 12:106, 1994.

Foster P, Cowan P, Wrenn EL Jr: Twenty-five years of experience with Hirschsprung's disease, *J Pediatr Surg* 25:531, 1990.

Kays DW: Surgical conditions of the neonatal intestinal tract, *Clin Perinatol* 23:353, 1996.

Sullivan PB: Hirschsprung's disease, *Arch Dis Child* 74:5, 1996.

Swenson O: Hirschsprung's disease: a review, *Pediatrics* 10:914, 2002.

Vinton NE: Gastrointestinal bleeding in infancy and childhood, *Gastrointest Endosc Clin North Am* 23:93, 1994.

Worman S, Ganiats TG: Hirschsprung's disease: a cause of chronic constipation in children, *Am Fam Physician* 51:487, 1995.

Wulkan ML, Georgeson KE: Primary laparoscopic endorectal pull-through for Hirschsprung's disease in infants and children, *Semin Laparosc Surg* 5:9, 1998.

Intussusception

James C. Mitchiner

ALERT Classic signs of abdominal pain, vomiting, and bloody stool with mucus are not always present. Altered mental status may be noted.

Intussusception occurs when a proximal segment of bowel invaginates into the distal bowel, resulting in infarction and gangrene of the inner bowel. It commonly occurs in children younger than 1 year and is usually of the ileocolic type.

A lead point is more commonly found in older children with conditions such as Meckel's diverticulum, polyp, duplication, lymphoma, lymphoid hyperplasia, foreign body, cystic fibrosis, or Henoch-Schönlein purpura, and after surgery.

DIAGNOSTIC FINDINGS

1. Classically, patients have an acute onset of intermittent fits of sudden intense pain with screaming and flexion of the legs.

The episodes occur at 5- to 20-minute intervals. Vomiting, often bilious, commonly occurs, accompanied by passage of blood and mucus ("currant jelly stool") via the rectum. This classic symptom triad is present in less than half of patients. Not all patients have gross or occult blood in the stool.

2. The abdomen is often distended and swollen, with a palpable mass in the right iliac fossa. Peristaltic waves may be visible through the abdominal wall. The rectal and bimanual examinations may reveal bloody stool and a palpable mass.
3. Alteration in mental status may appear, marked by lethargy, behavioral changes, irritability, somnolence, and listlessness. These changes may precede abdominal findings and must be viewed as important symptoms in this condition.

Complications

1. Perforation of bowel with peritonitis
2. Shock and sepsis
3. Recurrent intussusception

Ancillary Data

1. Abdominal x-ray film findings are positive in 35% to 40% of patients:
   - **a.** Decreased bowel gas and fecal material in the right colon
   - **b.** An abdominal mass
   - **c.** The apex of the intussusception outlined by gas
   - **d.** Small bowel distension and air-fluid levels secondary to mechanical obstruction
2. Enema is both diagnostic and therapeutic and is up to 75% successful at achieving reduction:
   - **a.** The success of reduction may partially reflect the duration of the intussusception: In one study, enema was therapeutic in 74% of patients whose symptoms had been present less than 24 hours, compared with 32% in those in whom the intussusception had been present for a longer time. The more distal the intussusception, the less likely the enema can reduce it.
   - **b.** Of patients with intussusception, 97% have no lead point. More than two thirds of the cases with an identifiable lesion in one study were in children older than 2 years.
   - **c.** The procedure is as follows. It should be performed only by an experienced radiologist after surgical consultation:
     - **(1)** A nonlubricated catheter is inserted into the rectum.
     - **(2)** With use of fluoroscopic observation, the barium solution is allowed to flow, filling the rectum by means of gravity.
     - **(3)** The intussusception is identified, and reduction is manifested as free filling of the small intestine proximal to the point of obstruction.
   - **d.** Up to three attempts of 3 minutes each may be tried. Sedation of the patient may be helpful to the success of the procedure. The abdomen should not be palpated or compressed during the study. Hydrostatic studies have also been successful in achieving reduction.
   - **e.** Air-pressure enemas are preferred by some clinicians because of the reduced risk of peritonitis if complications develop.
   - **f.** Contraindications to performing an enema include gangrenous bowel, abdominal free air, peritonitis, and an unstable patient with shock, anemia, or acidosis.
3. Ultrasonography may be useful as a noninvasive screening technique to evaluate intussusception:
   - **a.** Sensitivity is 100%, and specificity approaches 98%.

b. The intussusception typically appears as a "donut" structure, with a hyperechoic core surrounded by a hypoechoic rim of homogeneous thickness.
c. Interpretation is highly operator dependent.

DIFFERENTIAL DIAGNOSIS

(see Chapters 24 and 35)

1. Infection:
   a. Acute gastroenteritis
   b. Appendicitis
2. Infantile colic
3. Intestinal obstruction or peritonitis (e.g., volvulus, postoperative complication, tumor)
4. Incarcerated hernia
5. Testicular torsion

MANAGEMENT

1. Once intussusception is suspected, an IV line should be established, and rehydration initiated. A bolus of D5W 0.9% NS, at 20 ml/kg, should be given over 45 to 60 minutes and should be repeated if there is any evidence of a fluid deficit.
2. Immediate surgical consultation should be obtained.
3. Abdominal x-ray film series should be obtained and, if indicated, a barium enema.
4. If the barium enema is successful at reducing the intussusception, the patient should be hospitalized to observe for recurrence and potential perforation of necrotic bowel.
5. Surgery is indicated immediately if barium enema is unsuccessful or is contraindicated.
   a. If evidence of peritonitis or perforation is present, initiate antibiotic therapy. Treatment options include a triple antibiotic combination—ampicillin, 100 to 200 mg/kg/24 hr q4-6hr IV, clindamycin, 30 to 40 mg/kg/24 hr q6hr IV, and either gentamicin, 5 to 7.5 mg/kg/24 hr q8hr IV, or cefoxitin (Mefoxin), 80 to 160 mg/kg/24 hr q4-6hr IV.
   b. Adults and children older than 4 years commonly need surgery because of the high incidence of diseased lead points.

BIBLIOGRAPHY

Bhisitku DM, Listernick R, Shkolnik A et al: Clinical application of ultrasonography in the diagnosis of intussusception, *J Pediatr* 121:182, 1992.

Daneman A, Alton DJ: Intussusception: issues and controversies in diagnosis and reduction, *Radiol Clin North Am* 34:743, 1996.

DeFiore JW: Intussusception, *Semin Pediatr Surg* 8:214, 1999.

Hickey RW, Sodhi SK, Johnson WR: Two children with lethargy and intussusception, *Ann Emerg Med* 19:390, 1990.

Little KJ, Danzyl DF: Intussusception associated with Henoch-Schönlein purpura, *J Emerg Med* 9:29, 1991.

Losek JD: Intussusception: don't miss the diagnosis, *Pediatr Emerg Care* 9:46, 1993.

Losek JD, Fiete RL: Intussusception and the diagnostic value of testing stool for occult blood, *Am J Emerg Med* 9:1, 1991.

Ong NT, Beasley DW: The leadpoint in intussusception, *J Pediatr Surg* 25:640, 1990.

Stein M, Alton DJ, Daneman A: Pneumatic reduction of intussusception: 5-year experience, *Radiology* 183:681, 1992.

Stephenson CA, Seibert JJ, Strain JD et al: Intussusception: clinical and radiographic factors influencing reducibility, *Pediatr Radiol* 20:57, 1989.

Vinton NE: Gastrointestinal bleeding in infancy and childhood, *Gastroenterol Clin North Am* 23:93, 1994.

Meckel's Diverticulum

James C. Mitchiner

ALERT Meckel's diverticulum must be considered in patients with rectal bleeding or RLQ pain.

Meckel's diverticulum is the most common congenital malformation of the GI tract, resulting from the persistence of the omphalomesenteric duct remnant. Symptomatic diverticula usually contain gastric mucosa and are proximal to the ileocecal valve. Most cases manifest by 2 years of age, a third of which are symptomatic during infancy.

DIAGNOSTIC FINDINGS

1. Although many patients with noninflamed diverticula remain asymptomatic, patients with diverticulitis have crampy, RLQ abdominal pain associated with nausea, vomiting, and anorexia. Symptoms are caused by narrowing of the diverticular mouth as a result of peptic strictures, fecal material, granulomas, foreign bodies, tumors, and so on.
2. Perforation may be present; it is associated with abdominal guarding and rebound, decreased bowel sounds, and fever.
3. Obstruction produces distension with abdominal pain.
4. Lower gastrointestinal hemorrhage may be present in 40% of patients with Meckel's diverticulum. Children have painless rectal bleeding, which may be episodic. The stool blood is usually bright red or dark but rarely tarry. Anemia may be present.

Complications

1. Small bowel obstruction, often from obstruction of the ileum, is the most common complication. Causes include intussusception of the diverticulum into the ileum and volvulus.
2. Massive GI bleeding.
3. Perforation of the diverticulum with peritonitis.
4. Diverticular hernia (Littre's hernia). The diverticulum may manifest as either a femoral or an inguinal hernia.

Ancillary Data

1. WBC count is often elevated and the hematocrit (Hct) value decreased if significant bleeding has occurred.
2. Stool has bright red or dark red blood.
3. Abdominal x-ray examinations are not diagnostic but may demonstrate free air if perforation has occurred or distension and air-fluid levels if obstruction is present.
4. Radionuclide scan, using technetium-99m pertechnetate to identify ectopic gastric mucosa, is diagnostic. False-positive findings are rare, whereas false-negative findings may occur in as many as 30% of cases. In children, technetium scans have a sensitivity of 85% and a specificity of 95%. Diagnostic accuracy may be improved with the addition of pentagastrin, which stimulates metabolism of the ectopic gastric mucosa, and cimetidine, which enhances retention of radionuclide in the mucoid cells.

DIFFERENTIAL DIAGNOSIS

1. Rectal bleeding, most commonly resulting from intestinal polyps, intussusception, volvulus, and anal fissures (see Chapter 35)
2. RLQ pain: appendicitis (p. 658)
3. Small bowel obstruction caused by intussusception or volvulus
4. Other causes of peritonitis

MANAGEMENT

1. Depending on the severity of rectal bleeding and obstruction, patients may need resuscitation and blood products. A NG tube should be inserted for gastric decompression.
2. A rapid evaluation of the patient, including a surgical consultation, is usually required.
   a. Laboratory studies (CBC, electrolyte and glucose measurements, blood typing and cross-match, and urinalysis) should be obtained rapidly.
   b. If the cause of the bleeding is uncertain, a rapid evaluation of the patient should be completed, including abdominal x-ray studies, anoscopy,

technetium scan, and barium enema, depending on likely causes and the patient's clinical status.

3. If evidence of peritonitis or perforation is present, IV antibiotics should be initiated using a triple-antibiotic combination—ampicillin, 100 to 200 mg/kg/24 hr q4-6hr IV, clindamycin, 30 to 40 mg/kg/24 hr q6hr IV, and either gentamicin, 5 to 7.5 mg/kg/24 hr q8hr IV or cefoxitin (Mefoxin), 80 to 160 mg/kg/24 hr q-6hr IV.
4. Laparotomy is the definitive diagnostic and therapeutic procedure. A wedge diverticulectomy, consisting of excision of the diverticulum and a wedge of ileum, should be performed in most symptomatic cases.

DISPOSITION

1. All patients with Meckel's diverticulum should be admitted for evaluation and treatment.
2. A surgical consultation is required.

BIBLIOGRAPHY

Brown CK, Olshaker JS: Meckel's diverticulum, *Am J Emerg Med* 6:157, 1988.

Mackey WC, Direen P: A fifty-year experience with Meckel's diverticulum, *Surg Gynecol Obstet* 156:56, 1983.

Martin JP, Connor PD, Charles K: Meckel's diverticulum, *Am Fam Physician* 6:1037, 2000.

Rossi P, Gourtsoyiannis N, Bezzi M et al: Meckel's diverticulum: imaging diagnosis, *Am J Roentgenol* 144:567, 1996.

Vinton NE: Gastrointestinal bleeding in infancy and childhood, *Gastroenterol Clin North Am* 23:93, 1994.

Pyloric Stenosis

ALERT Pyloric stenosis should be suspected in neonates 3 to 6 weeks old with postprandial, nonbilious vomiting. Projectile vomiting is not always present.

Hypertrophic pyloric stenosis results from hypertrophy and hyperplasia of the circular antral and pyloric musculature, leading to gastric outlet obstruction. Although it has been reported in infants from birth to 5 months, it most commonly occurs at 3 to 4 weeks of life. White boys are more frequently affected, and there is a familial incidence.

DIAGNOSTIC FINDINGS

1. Gradual onset of vomiting between 3 and 4 weeks is common. It progresses to become forceful or projectile, nonbilious emesis. An associated esophagogastritis is present in 20% of children, producing blood-tinged vomitus. The child is hungry and easily refed. Constipation is common.
2. Visible peristaltic waves may be observed traveling from the left upper to the right upper quadrant. These are best visualized postprandially and before emesis.
3. A palpable pyloric "olive" or tumor is present below the liver edge and just lateral to the right rectus abdominis muscle. It is best felt after emesis or when an NG tube has been inserted on low intermittent suction.
4. Dehydration with varying degrees of lethargy may be present, often a hypochloremic alkalosis.
5. Jaundice may be present (8%) as a result of glucuronyl transferase deficiency. It clears after surgery.
6. Administration of erythromycin (or other macrolide) to the mother or infant is a risk factor, especially to infants during the first 2 weeks of life.
7. Pyloric stenosis may be associated with absence of a mandibular frenulum (normal midline extending from the vestibular mucosa of the lower lip to the gingival mucosa of the lower jaw).

Complications

1. Dehydration with metabolic alkalosis, hypokalemia and, in rare cases, shock
2. Esophagitis, gastritis, or gastric ulceration, with upper GI hemorrhage or perforation
3. Failure to thrive and secondary neurologic sequelae

Ancillary Data

1. Electrolyte, BUN, and glucose determinations to evaluate hydration and nutrition. Bilirubin evaluation if patient has jaundice. CBC to exclude infection.
2. X-ray films:
   a. Abdominal plain film demonstrates gastric dilation.
   b. Barium swallow study is indicated if suspected diagnosis is unconfirmed by physical examination. The study shows a "string" or "beak" sign (fine elongated pyloric canal) and delayed gastric emptying. Rarely is pyloric obstruction complete.
   c. Abdominal ultrasonography provides reliable confirmation on the basis of the anatomy of the pylorus.

DIFFERENTIAL DIAGNOSIS

(see Chapter 44)

1. Infection/inflammation:
   a. Gastroenteritis or sepsis
   b. Esophagitis or gastritis
2. Endocrine disorders: adrenal insufficiency (adrenogenital syndrome)
3. Congenital disorders: hiatal hernia, intestinal obstruction, atresia, malrotation
4. Chalasia or poor feeding technique

MANAGEMENT

1. Once the diagnosis is considered, an IV line should be inserted, and fluid deficits corrected. Initially give D5W 0.9% NS at 20 ml/kg IV over 30 to 60 minutes, and then compute deficit and maintenance replacements. Aggressive management of the inevitable hypokalemia is essential in correcting the electrolyte imbalance and alkalosis.
2. An NG tube should be inserted and connected to intermittent low suction.
3. Surgical consultation should be obtained early in the evaluation. Some surgeons are comfortable performing a pyloromyotomy in symptomatic patients with a palpable pyloric mass without further evaluation.
4. Surgery is indicated once the fluid and electrolyte status is stable:
   a. In rare cases, conservative medical management has been attempted, but it results in prolonged hospitalization and significant morbidity.
   b. Pyloromyotomy is performed and is associated with low morbidity and mortality.

DISPOSITION

All patients must be hospitalized and treated surgically.

BIBLIOGRAPHY

Breaux CW, Georgeson KE, Royal SA et al: Changing patterns in the diagnosis of hypertrophic pyloric stenosis, *Pediatrics* 81:213, 1988.

Mahon BE, Rosenman MB, Kleinman MB: Maternal and infant use of erythromycin and other macrolide antibiotics as risk factors for infantile hypertrophic pyloric stenosis, *J Pediatr* 13:380, 2001.

Volvulus

ALERT Acute onset of abdominal pain and obstruction in the child older than 1 year requires evaluation for volvulus.

Volvulus is a closed-loop obstruction with massive distension resulting from the twisting of a section of intestine on its own axis. Although uncommon in children, the rare cases that are reported occur in the first few days of life and in children between 2 and 14 years of age.

The condition may result from congenital malrotation, the presence of a long and freely mobile mesentery, Meckel's diverticulum, or surgical adhesions. Volvulus may occur without malrotation. Sigmoid volvulus is most often seen, although gastric (along axis joining lesser and greater curvatures), midgut, and transverse colon volvulus have been reported.

DIAGNOSTIC FINDINGS

1. Sudden onset of crampy abdominal pain, often greater in the lower quadrants, is common. In rare cases, patients have progressive or intermittent pain over several days or weeks, associated with sporadic twisting. Pain increases with worsening distension.
2. Marked intestinal obstruction is present with sigmoid volvulus, the severity reflecting the competency of the ileocecal valve. Tenderness is present, but guarding and peritoneal signs appear only if complications of peritonitis develop.
3. The rectum is empty of stool. Bloody stool is uncommon.
4. Anorexia and vomiting commonly occur.

Complications

1. Perforation with peritonitis
2. Dehydration

Ancillary Data

1. CBC and electrolyte measurements
2. X-ray films:
   a. Abdominal films show dilated, gas-filled loops with colonic distension. No gas is present in the rectum.
   b. Barium enema study (very carefully performed) demonstrates, in sigmoid volvulus, that the sigmoid colon has a circular pattern and that barium stops at the junction of the sigmoid and left colon.

DIFFERENTIAL DIAGNOSIS

1. Congenital disorders:
   a. Intussusception (usually occurs in children younger than 1 year)
   b. Hirschsprung's disease
2. Inflammatory disorders:
   a. Colitis with megacolon
   b. Peritonitis
3. Uremia

MANAGEMENT

1. Initial stabilization should provide for oxygen, replacement of fluid deficits, and surgical consultation.
2. If peritonitis is present, if it develops, or if reduction is not achieved, immediate surgical repair is necessary. Triple-antibiotic therapy should be initiated—ampicillin, 100 to 200 mg/kg/24 hr q4hr IV, clindamycin, 30 to 40 mg/kg/24 hr q6hr, and gentamicin, 5 to 7.5 mg/kg/24 hr q8hr IV or IM.
3. The necessity for surgical repair on a semielective basis of a sigmoid volvulus in a child whose volvulus has been hydrostatically reduced is controversial. Children, unlike adults, have a lower risk of recurrence.

BIBLIOGRAPHY

Leonidas JC, Magio N, Soberman N et al: Midget volvulus in infants: diagnosis with ultrasound, *Radiology* 179:491, 1991.

Seashore JH, Touloukian RJ: Midget volvulus: an ever-present threat, *Arch Pediatric Adolesc Med* 148:43, 1994.

77 Genitourinary Diseases

Also See Chapter 64 (Genitourinary Tract) and 85 (Renal Disorders)

Epididymitis

ALERT Testicular torsion must be excluded in patients with testicular pain.

ETIOLOGY: INFECTION

1. Infection:
   a. Commonly caused by *Neisseria gonorrhoeae* and *Chlamydia trachomatis*
   b. Uncommon organisms, especially important in younger age group; coliform and *Pseudomonas* bacteria
   c. Virus
2. Trauma
3. Chemical: reflux of sterile urine into ejaculatory duct
4. Systemic disease: Kawasaki's disease, Henoch-Schönlein purpura, sarcoid
5. Idiopathic

DIAGNOSTIC FINDINGS

1. Usually, there is a gradual onset of scrotal and groin pain with edema.
2. Initially, the epididymis is tender and swollen, with a soft, normal testicle. This evolves to diffuse tenderness and edema of the epididymis and testicle, often involving the scrotal wall as well.
3. The patient may have a history of trauma, lifting, or heavy exercise.
4. Dysuria, frequency of urination, and urethral discharge may be present.

Ancillary Data

1. White blood cell (WBC) count may be elevated.
2. Urinalysis and urine culture.
3. Gram stain and culture of urethral discharge.
4. Children younger than 2 years and older patients with reflux should undergo urologic investigation.

DIFFERENTIAL DIAGNOSIS

See p. 674.

MANAGEMENT

The most important part of the management is to be certain of the diagnosis. If there is any question that a testicular torsion exists, immediate urologic consultation should be obtained.

1. For epididymitis, institute scrotal support, bed rest, and analgesia.
2. Start antibiotics (dose for boys weighing more than 45 kg or 100 lb):
   a. Give amoxicillin, 3 g PO once, and probenecid, 1 g PO once, or ceftriaxone, 250 mg IM once. Follow (for boys older than 8 years) with tetracycline, 500 mg q6hr PO, or doxycycline, 100 mg q12hr PO, for 10 days.
3. Children younger than 9 years should receive erythromycin, 50 mg/kg/24 hr q6hr PO.
4. If a specific organism is identified, alter antibiotics as appropriate.

DISPOSITION

Patients may be sent home with supportive care and antibiotics.

BIBLIOGRAPHY

Likitnukul S, McCracken AH, Nelson JD et al: Epididymitis in children and adolescents, *Am J Dis Child* 141:41, 1987.

Turek PJ, Ewalt DH, Snyder HM 3rd, Duckett JW: Normal epididymal anatomy in boys, *J Urol* 151:726, 1994.

Hernias and Hydroceles

HERNIAS (see p. 662)

Hernias result from persistence of the processus vaginalis.

Diagnostic Findings

Patients usually have intermittent, localized swelling in the groin or labia, sometimes accompanied by irritability, pain, abdominal tenderness, or limp.

1. Incarcerated hernias occur when the intestine becomes trapped in the sac, usually before 3 years of age.
2. Strangulated bowel has a compromised blood supply, leading to necrosis. It is tender and swollen, and the overlying skin is usually edematous with a red or violaceous color. It is rare in pediatric patients for the hernia to strangulate. However, in girls the ovary or uterus may become incarcerated, preventing easy reduction.
3. Intestinal obstruction may occur.

Management

1. Uncomplicated hernias may undergo elective surgical repair.
2. Incarcerated hernias can usually be reduced manually, after sedation, with gentle, prolonged pressure and elevation of the foot of the bed. The patient should be hospitalized for observation and then urgent repair 12 to 24 hours after edema has resolved.
3. Strangulated hernias need immediate surgical intervention.

HYDROCELES

Hydroceles occur with closure of the processus vaginalis at the abdominal end and fluid accumulation in the sac.

Diagnostic Findings

1. The testicle appears large, surrounded by a fluid-filled sac. This condition usually resolves by 6 months of age. The sac is transilluminated on examination with a light.
2. If the size of the sac (or amount of fluid) changes from day to day, it is considered to communicate and is associated with a hernia.
3. A varicocele may exist; it feels to palpation like a collection of "worms."

Management

1. Noncommunicating hydroceles resolve by 6 months of age.
2. Communicating hydroceles or those that are still present at 12 months of age require surgical intervention for repair of the associated hernia.
3. Hydroceles in adolescents should be explored surgically because of the potential for underlying neoplasm.

BIBLIOGRAPHY

Skoog SJ, Roberts KP, Goldstein M et al: The adolescent varicocele: what's new with an old problem in young patients? *Radiation* 100:112, 1997.

Penile Disorders

See also Chapter 64.

PHIMOSIS

Phimosis is a narrowing of the foreskin with an inability to retract the prepuce over the glans because of poor hygiene or chronic infection. Normally, retraction of the prepuce is possible by 4 years of age. If obstruction to urinary flow occurs, early circumcision (or dorsal slit) may be necessary.

PARAPHIMOSIS

Paraphimosis occurs when the foreskin retracts and is caught proximal to the coronal sulcus with subsequent swelling and venous congestion, potentially compromising the vascular supply to the glans. It usually occurs with manipulation, masturbation, intercourse, or irritation.

After sedation, an ice and water mixture (usually in a rubber glove) is placed over the foreskin and glans for 3 to 4 minutes. With gentle, continuous, circumferential pressure on the glans for 5 minutes, the foreskin usually slips over. If the foreskin does not slip easily, the shaft of the penis should be held between the thumb and fingers of one hand (after 5 to 10 minutes of squeezing to reduce swelling), and the glans pushed down into the prepuce with a slow, steady pressure with the examiner's free thumb. Alternatively, the shaft may be held in both hands with the thumb on the glans and the foreskin pulled forward over the glans in a slow, steady motion. A dorsal slit with later circumcision is rarely indicated.

In newborns with a Plastibell circumcision, the ring may slip behind the glans onto the shaft of the penis and cannot be slipped forward. In such event, an attempt should be made to reduce the swelling with cold compresses and steady continuous circumferential pressure. The ring also can be cut off.

BALANITIS

Balanitis is a chronic irritation and inflammation of the foreskin and glans, usually a result of poor hygiene. The foreskin is red and swollen with a collection of smegma. There is often a concurrent diaper dermatitis.

Hot baths and local care are usually sufficient for treatment.

COMPLICATIONS OF CIRCUMCISION

Newborn male circumcision is a reflection of cultural, religious, and family beliefs. Some advocate circumcision because of data that the incidence of penile cancer and urinary tract infections (UTIs), as well as other penile disorders discussed earlier, may be lower after circumcision.

Intraoperative complications include hemorrhage, localized and systemic infection, Fournier's syndrome, necrotizing fasciitis, and meatal problems (stenosis or ulcers). Hemorrhage is rare and is usually controlled with pressure or application of silver nitrate. The Plastibell clamp may restrict venous return or may be retained beyond 10 days, in which case it should be removed.

Other nonacute problems may cause skin excess, asymmetry, or redundancy; concealed penis; skin bridges or chordae; and meatal abnormalities.

BIBLIOGRAPHY

Baskin LS, Canning DA, Snyder HM et al: Treating complications of circumcision, *Pediatr Emerg Care* 12:62, 1996.

Testicular Torsion

ALERT Acute onset of testicular pain and tenderness requires immediate urologic consultation.

ETIOLOGY

1. Congenital: A freely mobile testis suspended on a long mesorchium ("bell clapper") is usually present bilaterally.
2. Trauma: Scrotal trauma or exercise may precede the torsion, but torsion can occur at rest or may awaken the patient from sleep.

DIAGNOSTIC FINDINGS

Intermittent or constant testicular pain, which is sudden and intense in onset, occurs. Rarely, it may be gradual in onset with progression of severity. The testicle is tender, rides high, and is often horizontal. Scrotal edema is present. The contralateral testis often has a horizontal axis. Nausea and vomiting often accompany the testicular pain.

The peak incidence is in 3-year-old children, and it is uncommon after the age of 30 years.

Complications

Testicular necrosis will occur within 6 to 8 hours of torsion.

Ancillary Data

1. Doppler examination of the testicle demonstrates decreased pulsatile flow in the affected testicle. Normally, flow is equal in both testicles. This is the preferred approach to evaluation.
2. Technetium nuclear scan shows decreased perfusion and is 90% sensitive and specific for testicular torsion but should not delay surgery inordinately. It is less accurate in children younger than 10 years.

DIFFERENTIAL DIAGNOSIS

Diagnostic considerations must be rapidly excluded in evaluating the patient with testicular pain. Table 77–1 summarizes significant findings.

For *acute scrotal swelling,* a broader list of entities should be considered. *Painful* swelling with a tender testicle may be caused by testicular torsion, trauma with a hematocele, epididymitis, or orchitis. A nontender testicle and painful swelling may be secondary to an incarcerated hernia or torsion of the appendix testicle. In cases of *painless* swelling with an enlarged testicle, a testicular tumor or antenatal testicular torsion must be considered. If the testis is normal, underlying abnormality may include a hydrocele, an incarcerated hernia, Henoch-Schönlein purpura, or generalized edema, or the swelling may be idiopathic.

TABLE 77-1 Testicular Pain: Diagnostic Considerations

Condition	Diagnostic Findings	Ancillary Data
TESTICULAR TORSION	Sudden onset; may follow trauma or occur during sleep or vehicle ride; nausea, vomiting Physical examination: tender testicle with horizontal lie; abdominal or flank pain; palpable cord twist Peak incidence 13 years of age; uncommon in those older than 30 years of age	Urine: normal Technetium scan: decreased activity Doppler examination: decreased flow
TRAUMA	Sudden onset with history of trauma Physical examination: pain and swelling of testicle; hematoma may be present; findings reflect injury	Urine: normal Technetium scan: variable Doppler examination: variable
EPIDIDYMITIS	Usually gradual onset; uncommon in boys before puberty; groin pain; may be associated with trauma, lifting, exercise; recent instrumentation Physical examination: tender epididymis present early with a soft normal testicle, whereas later, diffuse tenderness of epididymis and testicle is noted; febrile; prostatic tenderness	Urine: pyuria, bacteriuria Technetium scan: increased activity Dopper examination: normal or increased flow
TUMOR	Gradual onset unless hemorrhage Physical examination: hard, irregular, and usually painless testicle	Urine: normal Technetium scan: normal Doppler examination: normal

A *varicocele* is present when there is abnormal tortuosity and dilatation of the pampiniform venous plexus secondary to valvular incompetence of spermatic veins. It most commonly appears in adolescence, being on the left in 90% of cases. It may decrease fertility. Surgical repair may reverse testicular growth arrest.

MANAGEMENT

1. Testicular torsion is a urologic emergency. If there is any question about the diagnosis, immediate consultation is required. Doppler and nuclear scanning should be performed.
2. Surgical detorsion is indicated immediately. If this procedure is unavailable, local detorsion by outward twisting (toward the outer thigh) may be cautiously attempted. Edema usually precludes local detorsion from being successful. This procedure may be monitored by Doppler examination, to verify return of blood flow.
3. Analgesia is useful after the diagnosis is certain and the decision has been made to operate.

DISPOSITION

All patients need immediate hospitalization for surgical detorsion and bilateral fixation. Necrosis usually results if torsion has existed for several hours and the cord is twisted three to four complete turns. Various degrees of atrophy have been reported after detorsion.

The salvage rate is 70% if the torsion has existed for 8 to 12 hours, but 80% to 90% with torsion for less than 8 hours. For torsion longer than 12 hours, the salvage rate is 20%.

BIBLIOGRAPHY

Herzog LW, Alvarez SR: The frequency of foreskin problems in uncircumcised children, *Am J Dis Child* 140:254, 1986.

May DC, Lesh P, Lewis S et al: Evaluation of acute scrotum pain with testicular scanning, *Ann Emerg Med* 14:696, 1985.

Nussinovitch M, Greenbaum E, Amir J et al: Prevalence of adolescent varicocele, *Arch Pediatr Adolesc Med* 155:855, 2001.

Petrack MM, Hafeez W: Testicular torsion versus epididymitis: a diagnostic challenge, *Pediatr Emerg Care* 8:347, 1992.

Schul MW, Keating MA: The acute pediatric scrotum, *J Emerg Med* 12:565, 1993.

78 Gynecologic Disorders

Also See Chapter 43 (Vaginal Bleeding)

Gynecologic Examination

The gynecologic examination of the prepubescent patient requires patience, sensitivity, and a modified approach. It is crucial to provide a careful explanation and move slowly while constantly reassuring the patient and parents. These measures usually preclude the necessity to examine the patient under anesthesia. The most shy children are often those 11 to 13 years old, who are just experiencing puberty.

Younger girls are best examined in the presence of their mothers. Examination of the external genitalia by inspection and palpation can usually be accomplished while the child is on the mother's lap. If appropriate, having the child assist the examiner by separating the labia may reassure her. The examiner should simultaneously depress the perineum. Particular attention should be focused on observation for trauma, foreign bodies, lacerations, discharges, vesicles, ulcers, and adenopathy. Labial adhesions are common in young children, usually secondary to irritation or inflammation. They may spontaneously separate by 12 months, but this process may be facilitated by topical application of conjugated estrogens (Premarin) cream nightly for 2 weeks.

Next, the child should be placed in the knee-chest position with her buttocks held up in the air and apart by an assistant. The girl is asked to lie on her abdomen with her bottom up and to let her stomach and back sag. Instrumentation is rarely necessary; the short vagina of the prepubertal girl allows enough visualization to rule out foreign bodies and other lesions. Samples of secretions, discharges, and seminal fluid for culture, cell cytology, or forensic examination may be obtained by using a moistened cotton-tipped applicator or an eyedropper. A small vaginoscope or small nasal speculum should be used if direct visualization is necessary.

All discharges should be evaluated both for *Candida (Monilia)* and *Trichomonas* organisms, with a wet saline and potassium hydroxide (KOH) preparation. Samples to test for trichomoniasis, bacterial vaginosis, and candidiasis can be collected with a cotton swab inserted into the vagina without a speculum. Gram stain and culture of all discharges on a minimum of Thayer-Martin or Transgrow medium should also be done.

Examination for sexual abuse or rape involves a very careful physical examination and social evaluation with specific attention to the "chain of evidence" (see Chapter 25).

Palpation may be required to establish abdominal tenderness and the position of the cervix and to exclude foreign bodies or other masses. A bimanual rectoabdominal or one-finger vaginal examination may be performed with the child on her back.

In the pubescent female, a careful examination should be made, with detailed explanations to maximize the patient's cooperation. The procedures should parallel those for a woman. A straightforward, noncondescending approach to the patient is crucial.

As a component of the examination, sexual maturity should be evaluated. Tanner stage I represents the prepubertal level; stage II, the early pubertal level; stages III and IV, intermediate levels of genital changes during puberty; and stage V, the adult level.

Menstrual Problems

DYSMENORRHEA

Dysmenorrhea commonly has pain associated with menstruation, which is functional in more than 95% of patients. It may result from an increased secretion of prostaglandins causing contractility of the myometrium during a period of falling progesterone levels. Emotional problems or sexual maladjustment may rarely be contributory. Infrequently, endometriosis (rare in children), chronic pelvic inflammatory disease (PID), or anomalies of the müllerian ducts or genitourinary tract may be present as a cause of dysmenorrhea. There is a high correlation with dysmenorrhea in the mother. As many as 29% of girls 12 to 17 years old have pain severe enough to interfere with normal activity; 14% of girls miss an average of 12 to 15 days of school per year because of cramps.

Diagnostic Findings

Crampy abdominal pain in the lower to middle abdomen with radiation to the back and thighs is commonly associated with the menses, often beginning 6 to 18 months after menarche. The discomfort normally commences within 1 to 4 hours of the menstruation, continues for up to 24 hours, and may vary in severity from month to month. In rare cases, the pain begins before bleeding and continues for several days. Nausea, vomiting, and diarrhea may be noted. Emotional problems should be suspected if the pain occurs at menarche or begins with anticipation of menses. Patients may be anxious and irritable, with edema and weight gain or a sense of bloating. Patients also may be fatigued and depressed.

Premenstrual syndrome (PMS), a distinct luteal-phase disorder, starts 7 to 10 days before menses and consists of weight gain, fatigue, headache, pelvic pain, and emotional lability. It is uncommon in adolescents, usually occurring in women in their late 20s and 30s.

With functional dysmenorrhea, physical examination is usually normal. A pelvic examination is indicated to exclude organic causes.

MANAGEMENT

1. Appropriately treat organic causes.
2. If dysmenorrhea is functional, reassurance is of primary importance. Hot baths, heating pads, and relaxation may be used. Mild analgesics may be helpful. Aspirin is particularly useful because it is also a prostaglandin inhibitor and should be tried first, but it may increase bleeding.
3. If further intervention is appropriate, have the patient use a prostaglandin inhibitor on the first day of menses and for 2 to 3 days longer as necessary for pain control. It may be more effective for some patients to begin medication a day before onset of menstruation. Several options exist:
   a. Naproxen (Naprosyn), 375 to 500 mg initially, followed by 250 to 375 mg q8-12hr PO (maximum: 1250 mg/24 hr).
   b. Ibuprofen (Motrin), 400 mg q6hr PO (maximum: 1200 mg/24 hr). Many find an initial dose of 800 mg to be useful. Available as an over-the-counter medication.
4. If discomfort continues to be significant, oral contraceptives may be tried for 3 to 6 months. If the patient is sexually active, oral contraceptives (if there are no contraindications) are particularly useful.
5. Contraindications to the use of oral contraceptives include the following:
   a. Pregnancy
   b. History of thromboembolic disease

c. History of cerebrovascular accident (CVA) or myocardial ischemia
d. History of neoplasm
e. Hepatic dysfunction
f. Hypertension
6. Arrange follow-up visits every 2 to 3 months to provide reassurance and to monitor the clinical response.

PREMENSTRUAL EDEMA

Edema, bloating, and irritability may precede the onset of menstruation. Management includes mild salt restriction; for severe edema, some clinicians suggest initiating diuretic therapy 3 to 4 days before the onset of menses and continuing it for a total of 5 to 7 days. Hydrochlorothiazide (HydroDIURIL), 25 mg/24 hr PO, is appropriate.

MITTELSCHMERZ

Mittelschmerz is thought to be caused by ovulatory bleeding into the peritoneal cavity. It is typically dull and aching, occurring midcycle and predominantly in one lower quadrant. It sometimes lasts 6 to 8 hours but may be severe and cramping, lasting for several days. Distinguishing it from pain caused by appendicitis, torsion or rupture of an ovarian cyst, ectopic pregnancy, and so forth, may be difficult.

1. Physical findings are usually normal.
2. Therapy includes reassurance, mild analgesia, and local application of heat.

DYSFUNCTIONAL UTERINE BLEEDING (HYPERMENORRHEA OR MENORRHAGIA)

Dysfunctional uterine bleeding is related to unopposed estrogen during anovulatory cycles resulting in hyperplasia of the endometrium from continuous estrogenic stimulation. It is often associated with irregular menses and results when flow is frequent (often less than 21 days between episodes), heavy (more than 80 ml in volume), and prolonged (more than 7 days in duration). It is usually painless. The condition may result from dietary changes, stress, and diabetes mellitus as well as from a number of endocrine conditions (hypothyroidism or hyperthyroidism, ovarian tumor, or adrenal insufficiency). Other causes of vaginal bleeding (see Chapter 43) must be excluded before treatment. The hematocrit (Hct) level should be measured to assess the severity of bleeding, as well as routine and orthostatic vital signs.

Management

Management depends on the significance of the bleeding.

1. *Minimal bleeding* in a patient with a hemoglobin (Hb) level higher than 12 g/dl and with little discomfort may be treated with reassurance and follow-up observation. Consider nonsteroidal anti-inflammatory agents (naproxen), iron supplementation, and cyclic oral contraceptives.
2. *Moderate bleeding* associated with a Hb level lower than 12 g/dl and no orthostatic changes often needs pharmacologic intervention:
   a. Medroxyprogesterone (Provera), 10 mg/24 hr PO for 5 days.
      (1) This is the most common approach, and bleeding usually stops in 3 to 5 days in response.
      (2) If bleeding persists with subsequent menses, the patient takes 10 mg/24 hr for 5 days at the beginning of expected menstruation for three cycles, at which time normal cycles should resume.
   b. A combination of estrogen and synthetic progestin given in 21-day cycles separated by 7 days without therapy usually regulates the menstrual cycle. Active bleeding may be controlled by administration of up to four tablets at the time of the emergency department (ED) visit, followed by a tapering dose over the next few days down to one tablet per day during a 21-day cycle.

3. *Severe bleeding* requires hospitalization, treatment of anemia (often, Hb less than 7 g/dl), and high-dose conjugated estrogens such as Premarin, 40 mg/dose q4hr IV for up to 24 hours (maximum: 6 doses), until bleeding stops. Circulatory resuscitation may be required.
   a. Once bleeding has stopped, a high estrogen-progestin oral preparation is begun: Ortho-Novum 5 mg or equivalent; 2 tablets are given initially, followed by 1 tablet QID PO and gradually tapered over 1 month. The patient is placed on a cycle of Ortho-Novum, 2 mg, or equivalent for 2 to 3 months.
   b. Gynecologic consultation is suggested.

Iron-deficiency anemia in menstruating adolescents often can be prevented by treatment with supplemental iron and vitamin C (enhances oral iron absorption) and by monitoring response.

Pelvic Inflammatory Disease (also see Vulvovaginitis and Vaginal Discharge—p. 682)

Pelvic inflammatory disease encompasses a spectrum of illnesses that are seen with growing frequency in adolescents. Asymptomatic or uncomplicated genital infections may involve only the urethra, vagina, or cervix, but they may become disseminated, resulting in generalized PID.

Although PID is normally considered a sexually transmitted disease, and pelvic disease occurs almost exclusively in sexually active women, nonsexual transmission is possible but rare, particularly in children. Factors contributing to sensitivity include foreign bodies such as an intrauterine device (IUD), instrumentation and other trauma, pregnancy, and menstruation. Most cases of gonococcal disease occur within 7 days of the onset of menses.

ETIOLOGY: INFECTION

1. *Neisseria gonorrhoeae*
2. Nongonococcal (often mixed) infection
3. *Chlamydia trachomatis* (most common of nongonococcal causes)
4. Anaerobes: *Bacteroides*, *Peptostreptococcus*, and *Peptococcus* organisms
5. Aerobes: *Escherichia coli*, *Proteus* organisms, *Gardnerella vaginalis*
6. *Mycoplasma hominis* or *Ureaplasma urealyticum*

DIAGNOSTIC FINDINGS

Endometritis, Salpingitis, Parametritis, or Peritonitis

Complicated PID may be divided into acute, subacute, and chronic categories on the basis of onset of symptoms, severity of findings, and number of previous episodes. In general, *N. gonorrhoeae* infection produces more severe symptoms, has a more acute onset, and is usually associated with the menstrual cycle, whereas *Chlamydia* infection is more commonly associated with an insidious course of pelvic pain. However, this differentiation is not reliable for the individual patient. A constellation of findings assists the clinician.

Acute PID

1. Patients usually have high fever. Vital signs reflect the severity of abdominal inflammation, which may consist of endometritis, salpingitis, parametritis, or peritonitis.
2. Abdominal pain is continuous, usually bilateral, and most severe in the lower quadrants. Only 10% of patients have unilateral pain, the presence of which should prompt consideration of ectopic pregnancy, appendicitis, cyst disease, or urinary origin. Peritonitis with rebound, guarding, and decreased bowel sounds may be present. Liver tenderness may result from perihepatitis (Fitz-Hugh–Curtis syndrome).
3. Cervical and adnexal tenderness is present and increases with movement. Uterine bleeding and vaginal discharge may be noted.

4. The minimum clinical criteria to make the diagnosis of PID are as follows:
   a. All three of the following:
      (1) Lower abdominal tenderness
      (2) Cervical motion tenderness
      (3) Adnexal tenderness

   NOTE: Other causes of signs and symptoms should be excluded.
   b. Additional criteria increase the specificity of diagnosing PID:
      (1) Oral temperature above 38.3° C
      (2) Abnormal cervical or vaginal discharge
      (3) Elevated erythrocyte sedimentation rate (ESR)
      (4) Elevated C-reactive protein (CRP)
      (5) Laboratory determination of cervical infection with *N. gonorrhoeae* or *C. trachomatis*
   c. A definitive diagnosis is made from the following:
      (1) Histopathologic evidence of endometritis on endometrial biopsy
      (2) Transvaginal or abdominal ultrasonography showing tuboovarian abscess (TOA) consistent with fallopian tube abnormality
      (3) Laparoscopic demonstration of abnormalities consistent with PID

Subacute PID

1. Patients often have low-grade fever and few systemic signs.
2. Moderate abdominal, cervical, and adnexal tenderness are present.

Chronic PID. Patients have recurrent episodes of abdominal pain, backaches, vaginal discharge, dysmenorrhea, and menorrhagia.

Complications

1. Infection/inflammation:
   a. Peritonitis
   b. TOA; 85% of adolescents have adnexal enlargement or TOA
   c. Endometriosis
   d. Salpingitis
   e. Perihepatitis (Fitz-Hugh–Curtis syndrome)
   f. Recurrent PID
2. Endocrine disorders:
   a. Infertility. After first episode in 10% to 12% of cases; after second episode, 23% to 35%; after third episode, 50% to 75%
   b. Ectopic pregnancy (risk increased in subsequent pregnancies)
3. Chronic pelvic pain

Ancillary Data

1. White blood cell (WBC) count and ESR often are elevated. Hematocrit value may be decreased with extensive bleeding. An elevated ESR (higher than 15 mm/hr) is seen 75% of the time. WBC count is elevated in about 60% of patients.
2. Culdocentesis or laparoscopy is useful for patients with acute abdominal pain and potential pelvic disorders. Purulent cul-de-sac fluid may be present in either ruptured appendicitis or extensive PID. Unclotted blood suggests adnexal cyst rupture or ectopic pregnancy. A clear aspirate containing serous fluid occurs with PID, ruptured ovarian cyst, and other entities that cause a peritoneal reaction.
3. Bacterial culture and Gram stain:
   a. Gram staining of a cervical culture for *N. gonorrhoeae* can be useful. A positive result is defined as presence of gram-negative diplococci in close association with polymorphonuclear (PMN) leukocytes; an equivocal result is presence of only extracellular organisms or atypical intracellular gram-negative diplococci.

      Finding *N. gonorrhoeae* identifies a patient at high risk for PID, but the correlation with the infecting organism of an upper tract infection is not sufficient to serve as a basis for therapy.

Gram staining of urethral discharge is reliable in males.

b. Culture on Thayer-Martin (or Transgrow) medium and, if the infection is complicated, anaerobic cultures.

c. Antigen, nucleic acid amplification, and genetic assays are often more sensitive and specific.

d. Cultures may be useful when results of antigen or genetic assays are negative and the suspicion of infection is high. Cultures should be done if there is a suspicion of child abuse.

4. *Chlamydia* endocervical swab screening is reliable and easily available. Clear as much mucus as possible off the cervix before obtaining the specimen to prevent a false-negative result. Detection of chlamydial antigen or a nucleic acid amplification method such as PCR or ligase chain reaction (LCR) is more sensitive than culture and more specific and sensitive than DNA probe, direct fluorescent antibody (DFA), and enzyme immunoassays (EIA).
5. Ultrasonography to define masses, adnexal enlargement, or TOA, exclude ectopic pregnancy, or localize IUD, if indicated.
6. Pregnancy test, if indicated.
7. Serologic test for syphilis.

DIFFERENTIAL DIAGNOSIS

1. Infection/inflammation:
   a. Urethritis
   b. Urinary tract infection (p. 833)
   c. Appendicitis, diverticulosis (p. 658)
   d. Peritonitis
   e. Gastroenteritis
   f. Mesenteric lymphadenitis
   g. Pancreatitis
   h. Inflammatory bowel disease
   i. Endometriosis
2. Endocrine disorders:
   a. Ovarian cyst, torsion, tumor
   b. Ectopic pregnancy (p. 689)
   c. Spontaneous abortion
   d. Diabetic ketoacidosis

MANAGEMENT

Prescribed doses in the following section are for adolescents (weight more than 45 kg or 100 lb) and adults who are not pregnant.

Support consists of parenteral fluids, analgesics, insertion of a nasogastric (NG) tube (if ileus is present), and bed rest, as indicated, in the hospital.

1. Cefoxitin, 2 g IV q6hr (or cefotetan, 2 g q12hr IV or equivalent); *plus* doxycycline, 100 mg q12hr IV or PO, for at least 48 hours after clinical improvement followed by doxycycline, 100 mg q12hr PO for 10 to 14 days. This regimen provides optimal coverage for *N. gonorrhoeae* and *C. trachomatis*.
2. Clindamycin, 900 mg (15-40 mg/kg/24 hr) IV q8hr; *plus* gentamicin load, 2 mg/kg/dose IV, followed by maintenance of 1.5 mg/kg/dose q8hr IV; *plus* doxycycline, 100 mg q12hr IV or PO, continued for at least 48 hours after clinical improvement; followed by doxycycline, 100 mg q12hr PO, for 10 to 14 days, or clindamycin, 600 mg q8hr PO for 14 days. This approach is preferred when a predominantly facultative or anaerobic infection is probable (i.e., IUD-related). When pyogenic complications are suspected from the findings of anaerobes or gram-negative organisms, consider the addition of clindamycin, 450 mg q6hr PO.
3. If doxycycline is contraindicated or not tolerated, an alternative is erythromycin, 40 mg/kg/24 hr q6hr PO, for prolonged therapy as well.
4. When a patient does not require hospitalization, an ambulatory regimen may be considered:
   - Ofloxacin, 400 mg BID PO for 14 days in patients older than 18 years of age, *plus* metronidazole 500 mg BID PO for

14 days; *or* Cefoxitin, 2 g IM, with concurrent probenecid, 1 g once orally, or ceftriaxone, 250 mg IM once; *plus* doxycycline, 100 mg BID PO for 14 days.

5. Culture should be repeated in 4 to 7 days, and screening at 4 to 6 weeks after completion of treatment.
6. Children weighing less than 45 kg should be treated with ceftriaxone, 100 mg/kg/24 hr q12hr IV or IM, *and* erythromycin, 40 mg/kg/24 hr q6hr IV.

DISPOSITION

Hospitalization is indicated under the following circumstances:

1. Uncertain diagnosis requiring further evaluation
2. Possibility of surgical emergency such as appendicitis, ectopic pregnancy, or peritonitis
3. Moderate to severe disease with fever, nausea, vomiting, peritonitis, and leukocytosis
4. Suspicion of a pelvic mass, TOA, or other abscess
5. Pregnancy
6. Immunodeficiency
7. Poor compliance or inability to take oral medications
8. Failure of response to outpatient therapy
9. Recurrent episodes consistent with chronic PID
10. Any consideration of sexual abuse

Many clinicians recommend that all patients with PID, particularly younger women, be hospitalized to reduce complications, maximize long-term fertility, and emphasize the potential severity of the disease. Indwelling IUDs are commonly removed. A single episode of tubal infection results in tubal closure in 14% of affected women, and the rate of ectopic pregnancies is five times greater than in women without a pelvic infection.

Vulvovaginitis and Vaginal Discharge (see also Pelvic Inflammatory Disease—p. 679)

Vulvovaginitis and vaginal discharges are common problems of prepubertal and pubescent females, although the common causes vary with age.

A careful history should focus on the presence of accompanying pruritus and odor and should define the quality, duration, and volume of the discharge. Other illnesses (diabetes, infections) should be excluded, medications identified (e.g., contraceptives, deodorant sprays, douches, antibiotics), and menstrual history, sexual activity, previous infections, and symptoms in sexual partners clarified. Vaginal discharge associated with cervical motion or adnexal tenderness is usually associated with PID (p. 679).

PREPUBESCENT FEMALE

Nonspecific Causes

Poor hygiene or an allergic reaction is usually the cause of vulvovaginitis or vaginal discharge in a prepubescent girl. Cultures show a variety of organisms, most of which are normal flora. Substances responsible for allergic responses in younger children include bubble bath and, in adolescents and adults, sanitary napkins, chemical douches, and deodorant and contraceptive sprays.

Diagnostic Findings. The discharge is thin and mucoid, and the introitus is painful, erythematous, and swollen. Patients may have a positive history of contact with an irritant. Dysuria may occur.

Management

1. Improved perineal hygiene with particular attention to ensure that the child wipes from front to back after bowel movements
2. Frequent changes of white cotton underpants
3. Avoidance of bubble baths and other irritating substances

4. Sitz baths: may be useful 2 to 4 times/day; the area should be washed with a very mild soap and allowed to air dry
5. For severe cases: 1% hydrocortisone cream for 2 to 3 days
6. If there is no resolution in 2 to 3 weeks: systemic ampicillin (or amoxicillin), 250 to 500 mg q6hr PO, for 10 days

Foreign Body

Articles commonly found in the vagina include paper products, vegetable matter, and, in older patients, forgotten tampons. The discharge is blood tinged and foul smelling. Physical examination should detect the foreign body, which often can be palpated on rectal examination.

Pinworms (p. 593)

Vulvovaginitis is secondary to irritation and itching of the perineum.

Physiologic Leukorrhea

A clear, sticky, nonirritating discharge may develop at the onset of puberty secondary to estrogen stimulation and irritation; it ceases once menarche occurs.

It is common for baby girls to have a thin vaginal discharge in the first few days of life. This discharge may become bloody at 5 to 10 days because of withdrawal of maternal estrogens.

Infection

The infectious causes specified for the pubescent female may cause vulvovaginitis in the younger child. Such infections should be diagnosed and treated with weight-specific doses of drugs as described in the discussion of the postpubescent female.

Nonsexual transmission of sexually transmitted disease is uncommon in prepubescent females beyond the neonatal period. In general, sexual abuse should be considered, particularly in the presence of gonorrhea, *Chlamydia trachomatis, Trichomonas vaginalis,* and condyloma acuminatum.

Although uncommon, *Shigella* organisms can cause a chronic, purulent, blood-tinged discharge that is foul smelling. There may be no associated diarrhea. *E. coli* and group A streptococci have also been associated with vulvovaginitis.

POSTPUBESCENT FEMALES

Causes of vulvovaginitis and vaginal discharge specified for the prepubescent female also occur after puberty, although the infectious agents discussed here are more common.

Gonorrhea and Chlamydia

Although *N. gonorrhoeae* may cause vaginitis in prepubescent girls, it is more often associated with cervicitis and salpingitis in the pubescent female (p. 679). *C. trachomatis* infection is common.

Diagnostic Findings

1. Patients with gonorrhea have a vaginal (urethral in males) discharge that is yellow-green and purulent or mucopurulent. However, 60% to 80% of females (and 10% of males) are asymptomatic. Infection is most likely to occur in proximity to menses. Symptomatic patients have discharge, dysuria, frequency, variable cervical tenderness, and proctitis:
   a. Cervicitis in postpubertal females is marked by purulent discharge, dysuria, and dyspareunia. The cervix is hyperemic and tender on touch but not on movement.
   b. Urethritis occurs in males and, rarely, in females. It is associated with purulent discharge and dysuria.
2. Complications:
   a. PID (p. 679).
   b. Disseminated gonorrhea, often associated with polyarthritis or polytenosynovitis. Endocarditis and meningitis are rare.
   c. Polyarthritis, most commonly the wrist, ankle, or knee (see Chapter 27).
   d. Monoarticular arthritis.

3. Ancillary data (p. 680):
   a. Swab or aspirate of vaginal discharge (and also of rectum and pharynx, when appropriate) is cultured on Thayer-Martin, Transgrow, or similar medium. Urethral or cervical discharge may reveal intracellular gram-negative diplococci on Gram staining. Rectal cultures should be performed in females (and males if appropriate) because rectal culture result is positive in 5% of cases in which cervical culture findings are negative.
   b. Detection of chlamydial or neisserial antigen with nucleic acid amplification (see p. 680). Endocervical or urethral specimens are generally required.
   c. Syphilis serologic tests should be obtained (Venereal Disease Research Laboratory [VDRL] test or equivalent).
   d. Other studies that may be considered are tests for pregnancy, human immunodeficiency virus (HIV) antibody, and hepatitis B, and urinalysis.

Management. Most clinicians believe that despite the isolated nature of an infection, concurrent treatment for *N. gonorrhoeae* and *C. trachomatis* is required. Treatment should be given as follows:

1. For uncomplicated vulvovaginitis, urethritis, epididymitis, proctitis, or pharyngitis in prepuberal children weighing less than 45 kg or 100 lb:
   a. Erythromycin, 40 mg/kg/24 hr (maximum: 2 g/24 hr) q6hr PO for 7 days; *or*
   b. Azithromycin, 10-20 mg/kg (maximum: 1 g) PO.
2. For uncomplicated endocervicitis, urethritis, epididymitis, proctitis, or pharyngitis in children older than 8 years and in nonpregnant adults weighing more than 45 kg or 100 lb:
   a. Doxycycline, 100 mg q12hr PO for 7 days; *or*
   b. Azithromycin, 1 g PO as a single dose
3. For disseminated gonococcal infections such as arthritis and dermatitis syndrome:
   a. Ceftriaxone, 50 mg/kg/24 hr (maximum: 1 g/24 hr) q24hr IV/IM for 7 days, *plus* doxycycline or azithromycin (for children younger than 8 years or pregnant women, use erythromycin)
4. For conjunctivitis:
   a. Ceftriaxone, 50 mg/kg (maximum: 1 g) IM.
5. For pharyngeal gonococcal infections: ceftriaxone, 125 mg IM. An alternative for use in adolescents and adults is ciprofloxacin.
6. Patients who are potentially incubating syphilis (seronegative, without clinical signs) may be cured by regimens that include ceftriaxone and a 7-day regimen of doxycycline or erythromycin.
7. Follow-up culture specimens from the infected site should be obtained 4 to 7 days after treatment. Positive culture findings are often caused by new exposures and require retreatment.

Disposition. Patients who have evidence of peritoneal signs or sepsis (arthritis, liver tenderness) should be hospitalized. Others may generally be followed at home. If outpatient management has failed or compliance is unlikely, close follow-up and frequent contacts may be required.

Candida albicans (Monilia)

C. albicans is an oval-budding fungus. Patients predisposed to infection with the fungus include patients with diabetes, patients who have recently taken antibiotics or used oral contraceptives, and patients who are pregnant or use nylon undergarments.

Diagnostic Findings

1. The discharge, which is thick and white and resembles cottage cheese, often appears 1 week before menses. There often is associated dysuria, intense pruritus, and dyspareunia. The vulva is red and

edematous, with excoriations secondary to the intense itching.

2. Examination of a slide prepared by placing 1 drop of KOH (10%) on a small amount of discharge and applying a coverglass will reveal branching filaments, yeastlike budding hyphae, or both.

Management

1. Sitz baths may provide symptomatic relief.
2. Topical treatment may consists of any of the following:
   a. Miconazole (Monistat): 1 applicatorful before bed for 7 to 14 days. Also available as miconazole, 200-mg suppository (Monistat 3), that requires only 3 days of therapy.
   b. Clotrimazole (Gyne-Lotrimin), 100-mg vaginal tablet or 1% cream, before bed for 7 days.
   c. Nystatin cream or suppository (Mycostatin or Nilstat): two applications per day until symptoms are relieved; then before bed for a total of 10 days.
   d. Ketoconazole (Nizoral), 200 mg q12hr PO, for 5 days in adults. Longer treatment may be required.
3. Discontinue the use of oral antibiotics or contraceptives, if possible.

Trichomonas vaginalis

Diagnostic Findings

1. Discharge is thin, frothy, malodorous, and yellow-green. Commonly, signs and symptoms are itching, erythema, pain, and burning of the vulvovaginal area, with cystitis or urethritis. The cervix typically has red, punctate hemorrhages. In rare cases (10%), patients have abdominal pain.
2. A wet mount examination, with saline, of the cervical discharge shows motile, flagellated organisms, slightly larger than a leukocyte. Direct immunofluorescence with monoclonal antibodies may hold promise for rapid detection.

Management

1. Sitz bath or wet compresses for symptomatic relief
2. Metronidazole (Flagyl), 2 g as a single dose PO. The sexual partner should be treated with metronidazole, 2 g PO as a single dose.
   a. Younger children may receive 15 mg/kg/24 hr, divided into three doses orally for 7 days, or 500 mg BID PO for 7 days, or 40 mg/kg (maximum: 2 g) as a single dose PO.
   b. Patients must not drink alcohol during the course of therapy and for 48 hours after. Do not prescribe metronidazole to a pregnant woman.
3. The patient's sexual partner should be treated concurrently, even if asymptomatic.

Bacterial Vaginosis (*Gardnerella vaginalis*)

Diagnostic Findings

1. Discharge is gray or clear, with a fishy smell. Gram staining shows multiple organisms and PMN leukocytes. Pruritus and burning may be present.
2. Microscopic examination demonstrates epithelial cells coated with small refractile bacteria ("clue cells"). PMN leukocytes are common. Mixing the discharge with 10% KOH liberates a fishy, amine-like odor.

Management. Systemic treatment is most effective. Topical treatment can be used for symptomatic relief only.

1. Systemic treatment:
   a. Metronidazole (Flagyl), 1 g/24 hr q12hr PO for 7 to 10 days (children: 35 mg/kg/24 hr) or 2 g PO as single dose, with second dose in 48 hours; *or*
   b. Clindamycin, 600 mg/24 hr q12hr PO for 7 days.
2. Topical treatment:
   a. Metronidazole gel, 0.25%, 5 g intravaginally BID for 5 days.

b. Clindamycin cream, 2%, 5 g intravaginally at bedtime for 7 days.

3. Treatment of the sexual partner does not influence relapse or recurrence rates.

Herpes Simplex, Type 2

Although both types 1 and 2 can cause infections of the vagina, vulva, and cervix, type 2 is the more common.

Diagnostic Findings

1. Grouped vesicles progress to ulcers in the perineal area, associated with bilateral tender inguinal nodes, pain, burning, and itching. Systemic illness may be present. Each episode of infection is usually self-limited but may last for a prolonged period with recurrence. It is particularly important to determine whether the patient is pregnant because of the risk to the fetus.
2. Wright or Giemsa staining of a vesicle shows giant multinucleated cells and inclusion bodies.

Management

1. Sitz baths or wet compresses
2. Analgesics, if necessary
3. For acute infection:
   a. *Oral* therapy shortens the symptomatic period by reducing the number of new lesions and duration of pain, dysuria, and constitutional symptoms while shortening the shedding of virus. This efficacy has been documented in primary herpes when treatment is initiated early (within 6 days of onset) in the *first episode:*
      - Acyclovir, 400 mg TID for 7 to 10 days or 300 mg 5 times per day for 7 to 10 days; *or*
      - Famciclovir, 250 mg TID PO for 7 to 10 days; *or*
      - Valaciclovir, 1 g BID PO for 7 to 10 days

   b. Topical 5% ointment is less effective in reducing symptoms but may be used every 6 hours for 7 days
4. For recurrent infection, therapy may be useful:
   - Acyclovir, 800 mg BID PO for 5 days or 400 mg TID PO for 5 days or 200 mg 5 times per day for 5 days; *or*
   - Famciclovir, 125 mg BID PO for 5 days; *or*
   - Valaciclovir, 500 mg BID PO for 5 days
5. Severe disease may be treated with acyclovir, 5 to 10 mg/kg q8hr IV for 5 to 7 days or until clinical resolution is noted

BIBLIOGRAPHY

American Academy of Pediatrics: *Report of the Committee of Infectious Diseases*, ed 25, Elk Grove, Ill, 2000, American Academy of Pediatrics.

Corey L, Spear PG: Infections with herpes simplex viruses, *N Engl J Med* 314:686, 1986.

Emans SJ, Goldstein DP: *Pediatric and adolescent gynecology*, ed 3, Boston, 1990, Little, Brown.

Fleming DT, McQuillan GM, Johnson RE et al: Herpes simplex virus type 2 in the United States, 1976 to 1994, *N Engl J Med* 337:1105, 1997.

Friedland LR, Kulick RM, Biro FM: Cost effectiveness decision analysis of intramuscular ceftriaxone versus cefixime in adolescents with gonococcal cervicitis, *Ann Emerg Med* 27:299, 1996.

Gevelber MA, Biro FM: Adolescence and sexually transmitted disease, *Pediatr Clin No Amer* 46:747, 1999.

Magid D, Douglas JM, Schwartz JS: Doxycycline compared with genital *Chlamydia trachomatous* infection: an incremental cost effective analysis, *Ann Intern Med* 124:389, 1996.

Martin DH, Mroczkowski TF, Dalu ZA et al: A controlled trial of single dose azithromycin for the treatment of chlamydial urethritis and cervicitis, *N Engl J Med* 327:921, 1992.

Sirnick A, Melzer-Lange M: Gynecologic and obstetric disorders. In Barkin RM, editor: *Pediatric emergency medicine: concepts and clinical practice*, ed 2, St Louis, 1997, Mosby.

Complications of Pregnancy

Lynne M. Yancey and Benjamin Honigman

The diagnosis of pregnancy is made on the basis of clinical presentation, a positive urine or serum pregnancy test result, and ultrasonography. Pregnancy causes secondary amenorrhea.

Women also have breast fullness and tenderness, darkening of the areola, enlargement of the nipples, and protrusion of Montgomery glands. Fatigue, lassitude, nausea, and vomiting are commonly present early in pregnancy. Urinary frequency may be reported. About 6 weeks after the last menses, early changes, such as softening of the uterine isthmus and cervix (Hegar's sign) and violaceous coloration of the vulva, vagina, and cervix (Chadwick's sign), become evident. These changes progress over the course of pregnancy as a result of hypertrophy of the uterus and its venous plexus.

The physiology of pregnancy forms the basis for pregnancy testing. About 14 days before the next expected menstruation, ovulation is triggered by a surge of luteinizing hormone (LH). Nine days later (1 to 2 days after implantation), human chorionic gonadotropin (hCG) becomes detectable. The hCG maintains the corpus luteum of pregnancy, supporting the secretion of estrogen and progesterone.

The hCG is a sialoglycoprotein with alpha and beta subunits. The beta subunits are immunologically specific. The serum hCG level doubles every 2 to 3 days in early pregnancy, so by the expected day of menstruation, the hCG level is approximately 50 mIU/ml. By 6 weeks' gestation (2 weeks after the first missed period), the level is approximately 3000 mIU/ml, later peaking at 8 to 12 weeks with a level of 20,000 to 100,000 mIU/ml. During the third trimester, the hCG level may decline.

A number of pregnancy tests are available to the clinician. Older bioassays have been replaced by immunoassays with varying sensitivities:

1. Enzyme-linked or solid-phase immunoassays of urine or serum are simple, can be performed within minutes, and are sensitive to an hCG level of 25 to 50 mIU/ml. They can detect pregnancy within 7 to 10 days of conception and are the preferred pregnancy tests for routine testing.
2. Home pregnancy urine tests routinely use hemagglutination inhibition (HAI) or latex agglutination inhibition (LAI) techniques. They can detect hCG at a sensitivity of 150 to 4000 mIU/ml (3 to 6 weeks' gestation). Errors occur from not using a concentrated first morning urine, excessive liquid intake, proteinuria, hematuria, and ingestion of psychotropic drugs.
3. Quantitative hCG levels can help in assessing fetal viability but not location. Because hCG levels double every 2 to 3 days in early pregnancy, serial quantitative measurements can be used to establish normal embryonic growth. Ectopic and aborted pregnancies are usually characterized by plateau or decline of hCG level, although in 15% to 20% of ectopic pregnancies, increases in hCG may be normal. An abnormally high level may be associated with multiple gestations or molar pregnancy.
4. The hCG levels disappear completely 2 to 3 weeks after spontaneous or induced pregnancy loss.
5. Progesterone has also been used to determine the viability of an early pregnancy; however, because of cost, lack of availability, and overlap of serum progesterone values in normal and abnormal pregnancies, these measurements are rarely used in the ED. Progesterone values of 15 mg/ml or less are rarely associated with a viable fetus.
6. Location and viability of early pregnancy are best determined with ultrasonography. Correlation of hCG levels with ultrasonographic findings is useful to guide the clinician in associated management decisions:
   a. Transabdominal ultrasonography can identify an intrauterine pregnancy at 6 weeks' gestational age (hCG levels approximately 6000-6500 mIU/ml).
   b. Transvaginal ultrasonography can detect an intrauterine sac at 4 to 5 weeks (approximately 1500-2000 mIU/ml).

The emergency physician most commonly encounters one of a number of complications of pregnancy that must be considered in the differential diagnosis of presenting complaints. Patients with any of these complications must undergo monitoring of vital signs and hematocrit determination.

ABORTION

ALERT Always consider ectopic pregnancy in a pregnant patient who has pain or bleeding. For any type of abortion, first assess hemodynamic stability and begin volume resuscitation with crystalloid or blood if indicated. Check the patient's Rh type. Patients with Rh-negative blood may need Rho (D antigen) immune globulin (RhoGAM).

Threatened Abortion

Diagnostic Findings

1. Vaginal bleeding during the first trimester of pregnancy; pain may be present.
2. Enlarged and nontender uterus, appropriate for dates. The cervix is closed.
3. Inevitable abortion: the os is open but gestational tissue has not yet passed.
4. If the initial hCG level is within normal range, there is a 79% chance of a favorable outcome.

Management

1. Reassurance and education: 30% to 40% of patients with threatened abortion carry their pregnancies to term. Sexual intercourse, use of tampons, and douching should be avoided because of the increased risk of uterine infection if the os becomes open. There is no contraindication to moderate daily activities. The patient should be aware that any blood pooled in the vagina during rest will become apparent when she stands, giving the impression of profuse bleeding. She should also be reassured that no minor trauma, physical activity, or use of over-the-counter medication has caused her to miscarry. Most nonviable pregnancies can be shown to have been nonviable 1 to 2 weeks before any symptoms develop; therefore, there is nothing she can do or could have done to prevent miscarriage at this early gestational age.
2. For Rh incompatibility in the setting of threatened abortion at less than 12 weeks' gestation, treatment with RhoGAM is controversial, but a dose of 50 μg IM can be offered to the patient. For gestational age of more than 12 weeks, RhoGAM is recommended at a dose of 300 μg.

   NOTE: The patient with an open os eventually aborts her fetus and should be under continuing observation. An outpatient dilation and curettage (D & C) may be indicated in patients in whom the os is open (inevitable abortion).

Incomplete Abortion

Diagnostic Findings

1. First-trimester bleeding is accompanied by cramps and cervical dilation.
2. Enlarged, mildly tender uterus. The cervix admits a ring forceps beyond the internal os without resistance. Do not attempt to introduce forceps if the uterus is large enough to be felt by abdominal examination.
3. Products of conception may be visible in the os.
4. Bleeding may be profuse.

Management

1. Remove any material from the cervical os. Doing so should reduce bleeding.
2. Consult a gynecologist for ongoing management. In the stable patient who has passed what appear to be complete products of conception, expectant management may be appropriate. The os should close and bleeding should slow within 1 to 2 hours.
3. For patients with heavy or ongoing bleeding, place oxytocin (Pitocin), 20 units, in

1000 ml of 5% dextrose in water (D5W), and infuse over 1 to 2 hours. D & C may be indicated.
4. For Rh incompatibility, administer RhoGAM. Normally, Hct and blood type determinations should be obtained.

Complete Abortion

Diagnostic Findings

1. Complete expulsion of products of conception during the first trimester.
2. Small, firm, and nontender uterus. The cervix admits a ring forceps beyond the internal os. Products of conception are in the vagina or have previously been expelled.
3. Hct with complete blood count (CBC) and blood type and hold; Rh determination.
4. There is a 50% decrease in hCG level every 12 to 48 hours; usually less than 5 mIU/ml after 3 to 7 days.

Management

1. Gynecologic consultation. D & C may be indicated in some cases.
2. RhoGAM for Rh incompatibility.
3. Offer resources for counseling and support. Reassure the patient that there is nothing she did to cause the miscarriage, and that grief is normal even when the pregnancy was unplanned.

Missed Abortion (Anembryonic Gestation or Fetal Death)

Diagnostic Findings

1. A nonviable pregnancy that has been retained in the uterus without spontaneous passage. Begins as a threatened or incomplete abortion, followed by decrease in bleeding to a brownish discharge. The symptoms of pregnancy diminish.
2. Small uterus for gestational date, and os will variably admit ring forceps.
3. Hct determination with CBC and blood type and hold; Rh determination.

Management

1. If gestational age is 12 weeks or less: D & C.
2. If gestation is more than 12 weeks: oxytocin drip (see earlier discussion) and hematologic monitoring for hypofibrinogenemia and disseminated intravascular coagulation (DIC).
3. With Rh incompatibility, administration of RhoGAM.

ECTOPIC PREGNANCY

ALERT Amenorrhea, abdominal pain, and vaginal bleeding accompanying symptoms of pregnancy must be rapidly investigated. No specific constellation of signs and symptoms has been identified that can consistently confirm or exclude an ectopic pregnancy (EP); therefore, any pregnant patient with abdominal pain or vaginal bleeding should be assumed to have an ectopic pregnancy until proven otherwise. EPs are normally (95%) tubal. Less than 3% are cornual, ovarian, or abdominal. Predisposing factors include PID, previous EP or tubal surgery, use of an IUD, endometriosis, and a history of infertility. The incidence is greatest in women 35 to 44 years old and lowest in those 15 to 24 years old, although rates in this latter age group are rising.

Diagnostic Findings

Ruptured Ectopic Pregnancy. Abdominal pain is invariably present. Sudden onset of pain associated with vaginal spotting in a pregnant female is very suggestive of a ruptured ectopic pregnancy. The pain may be described as sharp, dull, or aching, and it may be continuous or intermittent, reflecting episodes of intraperitoneal bleeding. Shoulder and back pain suggest peritonitis.

1. Rebound tenderness is present, and in rare cases, a bluish ecchymotic area around the umbilicus (Cullen's sign) may develop if there has been a rupture.
2. The cervix is usually tender and the cul-de-sac full. Adnexal tenderness is present

and, variably, a mass. The uterus is smaller than expected for gestational age.

3. Initial amenorrhea followed by vaginal bleeding can range from spotting to heavy flow; 15% to 30% of patients have a normal menstrual history; 15% experience EP rupture before they miss a period, whereas 50% have abnormal bleeding before any pain.
4. Patients often experience vomiting and nausea (morning sickness), amenorrhea, and, in rare cases, breast engorgement and other suggestions of pregnancy.
5. Patients often demonstrate hypotension, tachycardia, and dyspnea.

Unruptured Ectopic Pregnancy. Unruptured EP is difficult to diagnose because abdominal pain may be the only symptom. A pelvic mass is present in only 10% of patients. Thus, women of childbearing age with abdominal pain should undergo a pregnancy test.

Complications

1. DIC (p. 694)
2. Fertility problems and recurrent ectopic pregnancies
3. Death from hemorrhagic shock

Ancillary Data

1. Hct measurement with CBC and blood type and cross-match.
2. Pregnancy test: The test used should reflect the number of days since the last menses. Although the hCG level is usually lower in ectopic pregnancy than in a viable intrauterine pregnancy, there is significant overlap between the two. In addition, hCG level does not allow distinction between an ectopic pregnancy and an intrauterine pregnancy that is nonviable. In selected cases, serial quantitative hCG determinations may be useful (see "Management").
3. Ultrasonography: A valuable diagnostic aid that should be performed immediately in all pregnant patients with vaginal bleeding or abdominal pain. Findings can be correlated with quantitative hCG levels to aid in assessing risk of ectopic pregnancy. In patients with a β-hCG level of at least 1500 to 2000 mIU/ml, transvaginal ultrasonography can identify an intrauterine sac in patients with a viable intrauterine pregnancy. Absence of an intrauterine sac in this setting should raise concern for an ectopic pregnancy. Transabdominal ultrasonography can identify an intrauterine pregnancy at a β-hCG level of 6000 to 6500 mIU/l. The presence of an intrauterine pregnancy makes the diagnosis of ectopic pregnancy highly unlikely. Most heterotopic pregnancies (simultaneous intrauterine and extrauterine gestations) occur in patients undergoing fertility treatment with embryonic transfer procedures.
4. Culdocentesis: A diagnostic test that may be useful if ultrasonography is not available, if there is a question of infection, or to differentiate abdominal from pelvic disorders before surgery for an acute abdomen. The aspirate results are categorized as follows:
   a. Normal: straw-colored fluid
   b. Dry: nondiagnostic, requiring a repeat tap or other diagnostic procedure (may occur with ectopic pregnancy before rupture)
   c. Positive diagnosis: bloody (nonclotting) aspirate with an Hct greater than 15%. This finding indicates the presence of intraperitoneal blood, although it does not identify the source of bleeding.
5. Laparoscopy: Useful, particularly if available on an emergency basis, to make a definitive diagnosis and initiate treatment.

Differential Diagnosis

In cases of pelvic pain with a positive pregnancy test result, EP, intrauterine pregnancy, and spontaneous or threatened abortion must be considered.

Pelvic pain with a negative pregnancy test result may be caused by an EP (in 5% of symptomatic EPs, hCG level is less than 50 mIU/ml). Other diagnostic possibilities are mittelschmerz, dysmenorrhea, PID, appendicitis, neoplasm, adnexal torsion, endometriosis, fibroids, adhesions, and pelvic congestion.

Management

1. For the unstable patient, intravenous (IV) crystalloid, blood, military antishock trousers (MAST) suit (use is controversial), NG tube, and urinary catheterization for treatment and monitoring should be initiated. Such a patient will likely need immediate surgery.
2. Diagnostic evaluation should include ultrasonography, culdocentesis, or laparoscopy.
3. If diagnosis is confirmed, salpingectomy (either open or laparoscopic) has classically been undertaken to remove the ectopic pregnancy and to ligate the tube. More recently, laparoscopic salpingostomy with preservation of the tube has become the surgical treatment of choice in young nulliparous females, for whom preservation of fertility is a high priority.
4. Methotrexate therapy has become an accepted alternative for selected patients who meet criteria for nonsurgical treatment. Although these criteria may vary from institution to institution, they include size, volume, and specific location of the gestational mass, hCG levels, progesterone levels, the presence or absence of fetal cardiac activity, and the presence or absence of intraperitoneal blood. Most methotrexate protocols involve a single IM dose with close outpatient follow-up and repeat dose(s) as indicated.
5. If the diagnosis of ectopic pregnancy is suspected but cannot be confirmed on initial evaluation, close follow-up is mandatory.
   a. For the stable patient with a clinically benign presentation in whom no intrauterine pregnancy is visualized on transvaginal ultrasonography, most practitioners recommend outpatient follow-up and repeat of hCG measurement in 24 to 48 hours.
   b. For patients in whom the initial hCG level was less than 1500 mIU/ml, transvaginal ultrasonography should be repeated if the hCG level exceeds 3000 mIU/ml.
   c. For patients without reliable outpatient follow-up or in whom clinical suspicion is high, hospitalization is usually indicated.
6. Patients with Rh incompatibility should be given RhoGAM.

ABRUPTIO PLACENTAE AND PLACENTA PREVIA

ALERT Third-trimester vaginal bleeding requires urgent evaluation.

Abruptio placentae is the premature separation of a normally implanted placenta; it has peak incidence between 20 to 29 weeks and again at 38 weeks. It complicates 1% to 5% of cases of minor abdominal blunt trauma in women with last-trimester pregnancy who experience such an injury. Other predisposing factors are maternal hypertension, increasing age or parity, smoking, cocaine use, prior abruption, and underlying bleeding disorders.

Placenta previa occurs when the attachment of a placenta is located over or near the internal os. Its classification as total or partial is dynamic because of the changing location of the placenta with the progression of pregnancy. Predisposing factors include high parity, history of prior cesarean section, and smoking.

Diagnostic Findings

Abruptio Placentae. Patients classically have vaginal bleeding and abdominal pain.

The extent of pain reflects the extent of disruption of the myometrial fibers and intravasation of blood at the site of disruption. The combination of placental separation and uterine spasm can lead to reduced placental perfusion and fetal distress or death. Vaginal bleeding is variably present and may be concealed. The uterus is uniformly tender on abdominal examination. Because placenta previa is part of the differential diagnosis, the cervix should be examined only under specific circumstances and then with extreme caution (see later).

Hypotension may be present. The decrease in blood pressure is often disproportionate to the amount of hemorrhage because of the concealed nature of the blood loss.

Placenta Previa. Vaginal bleeding is the prominent sign, varying from repeated episodes to massive hemorrhage. The initial bleeding episode is classically minimal; in the second episode, bleeding may be profuse. The bleeding is usually painless and bright red. Digital or instrument examination of the cervix should never be performed because it could precipitate catastrophic bleeding in placenta previa. Cervical examination with a sterile speculum should be undertaken only by an obstetrician who is prepared to perform immediate cesarean section.

Hypotension is present, reflecting the amount of blood loss.

Complications

1. DIC (p. 694) in abruptio placentae (rare in placenta previa)
2. Acute tubular necrosis (p. 828)
3. Fetal death

Ancillary Data

1. Hct is decreased. Blood specimen for typing and cross-match should be sent to the laboratory.
2. Fibrinogen level is reduced in the presence of thrombocytopenia and coagulation abnormalities.
3. Ultrasonography localizes the placenta and is appropriate for the stable patient.

Differential Diagnosis

1. Trauma: laceration or other perineal injury
2. Endocrine or coagulation disorders
3. Complications of pregnancy, including uterine rupture or marginal sinus bleeding, premature labor, and abortion

Management

1. Stabilization should include administration of IV fluids and blood, placement of an NG tube, and urinary catheterization. DIC should be treated if present. Initial laboratory evaluations may include hematocrit measurement, blood type and crossmatch, and a DIC screen.
2. Fetal heart tones and status should be monitored continuously.
3. Consult with an obstetrician immediately. Consider transfer after stabilization if no obstetrical services are available. The pelvic examination of the patient should be performed only in the obstetric or operating suite, where double setup precautions are available and an immediate cesarean section can be performed. If the mother and fetus are stable, an ultrasonographic image may be useful in the initial assessment. The decision about vaginal delivery of the fetus is best made by the obstetric and pediatric consultants involved in the examination. Cesarean section is usually indicated if there is any evidence of fetal distress. Support personnel must be available to assist in the management of the unstable or potentially unstable patient.
4. With a diagnosis of placenta previa, an attempt to stop labor should be made with a β-adrenergic agent such as terbutaline (0.25 mg).
5. RhoGAM should be administered in cases of RH incompatibility.

BIBLIOGRAPHY

ACOG Practice Bulletin: medical management of tubal pregnancy, *Int J Gynecol Obstet* 65:97, 1999.

ACOG Practice Bulletin: prevention of RhD alloimmunization, *Int J Gynecol Obstet* 66:63, 1999.

Abbot J, Emmans LS, Lowenstein SR: Ectopic pregnancy: ten common pitfalls in diagnosis, *Am J Emerg Med* 8:515, 1990.

American Academy of Pediatrics Committee on Adolescence: Adolescent pregnancy, *Pediatrics* 83:132, 1989.

Buster JE, Heard MJ: Current issues in medical management of ectopic pregnancy, *Curr Opin Obstet Gynecol* 12:525, 2000.

Creinin MD, Schwartz JL, Guido RS et al: Early pregnancy failure—current management concepts, *Obstet Gynecol Surv* 56:05, 2001.

Cunningham FG, Gant NF, Leveno KG et al: *Williams obstetrics*, ed 2, New York, 2001, McGraw-Hill.

Dart RG: Role of pelvic ultrasonography in evaluation of symptomatic first-trimester pregnancy, *Ann Emerg Med* 33:310, 1999.

Dart RG, Kaplan B, Cox C: Transvaginal ultrasound in patients with low β-human chorionic gonadotropin values: how often is the study diagnostic? *Ann Emerg Med* 30:135, 1997.

Dart RG, Kaplan B, Varaklis K: Predictive value of history and physical examination in patients with suspected ectopic pregnancy, *Ann Emerg Med* 33:283, 1999.

Durham B, Lane B, Burbridge L et al: Pelvic ultrasound performed by emergency physicians for the detection of ectopic pregnancy in complicated first-trimester pregnancy, *Ann Emerg Med* 29:338, 1997.

Gale CL, Stovall TG, Muran D: Tubal pregnancy in adolescence, *J Adolesc Health Care* 11:485, 1990.

Houry D, Abbott JT: Acute complications of pregnancy. In Marx JA et al, editors: *Rosen's Emergency medicine: concepts and clinical practice*, ed 2, St Louis, 2002, Mosby.

Kaplan BC, Dart RO, Moskos M et al: Ectopic pregnancy: prospective study with improved diagnostic accuracy, *Ann Emerg Med* 28:10, 1996.

Lipscomb GH, McCord ML, Stovall TG et al: Predictors of success of methotrexate treatment in women with tubal ectopic pregnancies, *N Engl J Med* 341:1974, 1999.

Lipscomb GH, Stovall TG, Ling FW: Nonsurgical treatment of ectopic pregnancy, *N Engl J Med* 343:1325, 2000.

Olshaker JS: Emergency department pregnancy testing, *J Emerg Med* 14:59, 1996.

79 Hematologic Disorders

Disseminated Intravascular Coagulation

Disseminated intravascular coagulation (DIC) is an acquired coagulopathy that may occur in a variety of clinical settings in which the clotting mechanism is triggered. It results in the deposition of thrombi within the microcirculation, consumption of coagulation factors (I, II, V, VIII) and platelets, and, ultimately, bleeding. The severity and clinical significance of DIC varies greatly among patients.

ETIOLOGY

The following are common triggers of DIC:

1. Infection:
   a. Bacterial:
      (1) Gram-negative sepsis
      (2) Meningococcemia (p. 729)
      (3) Gram-positive sepsis: *Streptococcus pneumoniae* and *Staphylococcus aureus*
   b. Viral:
      (1) Herpes simplex
      (2) Measles
      (3) Chickenpox
      (4) Cytomegalovirus
      (5) Influenza
   c. Rocky Mountain spotted fever
2. Shock (see Chapter 5)
3. Respiratory distress syndrome and asphyxia
4. Trauma:
   a. Burns (see Chapter 46)
   b. Multiple trauma (see Chapter 56)
   c. Snake bites (p. 315)
   d. Heat stroke (see Chapter 50)
   e. Head injury
5. Complications of pregnancy (p. 686)
6. Neoplasms
7. Necrotizing enterocolitis
8. Hemangioma
9. Intravascular hemolysis:
   a. Incompatible blood transfusion
   b. Autoimmune hemolytic anemia

DIAGNOSTIC FINDINGS

The primary determinant of the clinical presentation is the triggering condition. In addition to the signs and symptoms related to that disease, a number of specific findings may be present with DIC.

1. Simultaneous evidence of diffuse bleeding and thrombosis, including petechiae, purpura, peripheral cyanosis, ischemic necrosis of the skin and subcutaneous tissues, hematuria, and melena
2. Prolonged bleeding from venipuncture and other sites of injury

Complications

1. Organ damage as a result of bleeding and infarction. May include gastrointestinal (GI) hemorrhage, hematuria, central nervous system (CNS) bleeding first appearing as mental status changes, apnea, seizures, and coma
2. Purpura fulminans: occurs as patchy hemorrhagic infarction of the skin and subcutaneous tissue
3. Complications of the precipitating event
4. Death from hemorrhage

Ancillary Data

1. Complete blood count (CBC) and peripheral blood smear:

a. Evidence of hemolysis with fragmented RBCs resulting from microangiopathy.
b. Anemia may occur as a result of bleeding or hemolysis.
c. Thrombocytopenia is usually present.

2. Coagulation studies: Typical findings include the following:
   a. Prolongation of the partial thromboplastin time (PTT) as a result of decrease in consumable clotting factors (fibrinogen, II, V, VIII).
   b. Elevation of fibrin split (degradation) products.
   c. Elevation of fibrin monomer.
   d. Once the consumption of coagulation factors has ceased, values normalize (fibrinogen and factor VIII in 24 to 48 hours; platelet count in 7 to 14 days).

DIFFERENTIAL DIAGNOSIS

1. Bleeding (see Chapter 29)
2. Precipitating conditions

MANAGEMENT

Initial attention must be directed to stabilizing the patient and treating the underlying condition triggering DIC. If this precipitating event can be quickly reversed (e.g., shock, hypoxia, endotoxin release), further therapy is often unnecessary.

1. Administer fresh whole blood or packed red blood cells (RBCs) if there is significant hemorrhage.
2. Replacement of depleted coagulation factors is usually necessary with active or impending bleeding:
   a. Fresh-frozen plasma (FFP): fibrinogen (I) and other clotting factors (II, V, and VIII):
      (1) Usually deficient if hypoxia or acidosis is present.
      (2) Administration of 10 to 15 ml/kg/dose IV repeated as indicated by follow-up coagulation studies.
   b. Cryoprecipitate: fibrinogen (I) and factor VIII: Indicated only if there is no response to FFP, the fibrinogen value is less than 100 mg/dl, and the PTT remains very prolonged. Does not correct deficiencies of other coagulation factors:
      (1) For infants: 1 bag cryoprecipitate per 3 kg of body weight; for older children: 1 bag cryoprecipitate per 5 kg.
      (2) Generally raises fibrinogen value above 100 mg/dl, a level sufficient to promote hemostasis.
   c. Platelet concentrate: platelets plus aged plasma:
      (1) Platelet level usually deficient if DIC was triggered by infection.
      (2) Administration of 1 platelet pack per 5 to 6 kg of body weight or, for infants, 10 ml/kg should increase platelet count by 50,000 to 100,000 cells/mm^3.
   d. Vitamin K: for infants, 1 to 2 mg/dose IV slowly; for children and adults, 5 to 10 mg/dose IV.
3. Heparin: Indicated in the presence of widespread thrombosis or active bleeding that cannot be controlled by replacement of clotting factors and platelets coupled with aggressive treatment of the triggering disorder. In this setting, the intent of heparin therapy is to block further consumption of clotting factors. It is not recommended until other therapies have failed. Heparin should be used early in the course of DIC associated with meningococcemia because of the frequent occurrence of fulminant thrombosis and tissue necrosis in this setting.
   - Heparin is administered preferentially by continuous IV infusion:
     a. Load with 50 units/kg IV.
     b. Give continuous drip of 10 to 15 units/kg/hr IV.

c. With purpura fulminans, give higher dosage if necessary: 20 to 25 units/kg/hr IV.
d. If bolus infusion approach is used, give four times the hourly dose q4hr IV.

- Replacement therapy with FFP and platelet concentrate should be continued after the initiation of heparin therapy to minimize bleeding risk.
- The efficacy of heparin therapy is monitored through measurement of the fibrinogen level and, later, the platelet count and watching for increase and return to normal.

e. Unresponsive DIC in neonates: Exchange transfusion may occasionally be indicated for those who show no response to normal medical management.

DISPOSITION

1. Patients must be admitted to an intensive care unit (ICU) for treatment of the underlying disease as well as the DIC.
2. Critical care is required, with involvement of a hematologist and of those with expertise in the management of the underlying pathologic condition.

Hemophilia

Rochelle A. Yanofsky

ALERT Minor pain often signifies deep muscle or joint bleeding requiring factor replacement. Any head trauma requires urgent intervention.

Hemophilia A (classic hemophilia) and hemophilia B (Christmas disease) are inherited as X-linked recessive conditions. However, as many as one third of cases are caused by recent genetic mutations, resulting in a family history negative for bleeding problems.

Hemophilia A and B are clinically indistinguishable. The diagnosis of both diseases is made on the basis of coagulation factor assays. Hemophilia A is characterized by a deficiency of factor VIII coagulant activity (with a normal level of von Willebrand factor); hemophilia B is characterized by a deficiency of factor IX. The normal range for factor VIII coagulant activity at all ages, and for factor IX activity after age 6 months, is 0.5 to 1.5 U/ml (or 50% to 150%).

Patients are classified as having severe (factor VIII or IX coagulant level less than 0.01 U/ml [<1%]), moderate (factor VIII or IX coagulant level 0.01 to 0.05 U/ml [1% to 5%]), or mild (factor VIII or IX coagulant level low but higher than 0.05 U/ml [>5%]) disease. Patients with severe hemophilia bleed spontaneously; those with moderate hemophilia bleed with mild trauma; and those with mild hemophilia bleed with major trauma. Bleeding is usually deep-seated and delayed.

Type 2N von Willebrand's disease may be confused with hemophilia A. The former disorder is autosomal recessive and is characterized by a shortened half-life of factor VIII coagulant activity caused by defective binding of that moiety to von Willebrand factor. Measurements of factor VIII–von Willebrand factor binding are needed to establish the diagnosis; this disorder cannot be distinguished from hemophilia A from standard coagulation factor assays.

The rare factor IX Leiden variant of hemophilia B is thought to be caused by a mutation at the androgen-sensitive promoter region of the gene. Patients with this variant of hemophilia B have severe hemophilia until age 15 years, after which their factor IX levels gradually rise, sometimes to levels as high as 0.50 U/ml (50%).

DIAGNOSTIC FINDINGS

Bleeding commonly occurs in muscles or joints, either spontaneously or as a result of minor trauma. A local tingling sensation and pain are often the first signs of bleeding. Hemophilia should be suspected in any male who bleeds excessively after trauma or who has bled into joints or muscles. Common sites for bleeding include the following:

1. Musculoskeletal:
   a. Joints most commonly involved are the elbow, knee, and ankle. Tenderness, swelling, and limitation of range of motion may be present in the involved joint, but these are later findings. Septic arthritis may occur but is uncommon.
   b. Muscle bleeding in the forearm flexor group or the gastrocnemius muscle may cause a compartment syndrome.
   c. Signs of bleeding into the iliopsoas muscle include lower quadrant abdominal pain and tenderness (may simulate appendicitis), pain in the groin or back, and limp. Compression of the femoral nerve may cause anterior thigh pain as well as paresthesia, hypesthesia, weakness of the quadriceps muscle, and even permanent paralysis of the thigh flexors. The hip is held in flexion. Range of hip movement is full if the hip is kept flexed. The psoas sign is present. Significant blood loss may occur.
2. Subcutaneous hematomas ("raised" bruises).
3. Intracranial: Bleeding may be subdural, subarachnoid, intraventricular, cerebellar, or cerebral. Without provocation, or after seemingly minor head trauma, patients may experience headache, vomiting, altered mental status, or seizures. With severe bleeding, signs of increased intracranial pressure may develop (see Chapter 57).
4. Spinal cord hematomas: May cause paralysis, weakness, back pain, and asymmetric neurologic findings.
5. Upper or lower GI bleeding: May be associated with hematemesis, melena, abdominal tenderness and distension, and shock. Intussusception is rare. Intraperitoneal or retroperitoneal hemorrhage may be present.
6. Retropharyngeal hematomas: May produce dyspnea, dysphagia, and potential GI or respiratory obstruction.
7. Mild hematuria is common.

Complications

1. DIC and thromboembolism have been reported with the repetitive use of large doses of low-purity factor IX (prothrombin complex) concentrates as well as with activated prothrombin complex concentrates, particularly with the concomitant use of antifibrinolytic agents (ε-aminocaproic acid [EACA] or tranexamic acid), or in the presence of liver dysfunction or other factors that would increase the risk of thrombosis.
2. Either hepatitis B or, more commonly, hepatitis C may develop secondary to plasma-derived factor replacement therapy. All patients with hemophilia who are seronegative for hepatitis B should be immunized with recombinant hepatitis B vaccine. Hepatitis A virus and parvovirus may be transmitted in plasma-derived factor concentrates, despite the current viral attenuation processes used. In addition to the hepatitis B vaccine, it is probably worthwhile to administer the hepatitis A vaccine to patients who have tested negative for immunoglobulin (Ig) G antibodies to hepatitis A and who are likely to receive plasma-derived coagulation products.
3. Human immunodeficiency virus 1 (HIV-1). Plasma-derived factor VIII and factor IX concentrates in current use have been subjected to various methods of viral attenuation and appear to be safe in terms of transmission of HIV, HTLV, hepatitis B, and hepatitis C. Acquired immunodeficiency syndrome (AIDS) has been documented in individuals with hemophilia who previously received blood products contaminated with HIV-1. Evidence of immune dysfunction (AIDS-related

complex, or ARC) is seen more commonly than full-blown AIDS in patients with hemophilia who demonstrate HIV seropositivity. Hepatosplenomegaly, lymphadenopathy, lymphopenia, high levels of IgG, thrombocytopenia, and Coombs' test positivity may be part of ARC.

4. Death may result from intracranial hemorrhage, underlining the necessity of rapid intervention in patients with (even minimal) head trauma
5. Repeated hemorrhages can occur into a "target" joint. The ensuing persistent inflammation and hyperemia can result in a chronic joint effusion (chronic synovitis), as well as progressive degeneration of joint bone and cartilage (hemophilic arthropathy). Primary or secondary prophylaxis with factor concentrate is sometimes used to minimize these problems.
6. Muscle wasting and contractures may develop as a result of bleeding into muscles or joints. A cyst may develop within muscle as a result of a previous intramuscular hematoma. A pseudotumor may develop as a result of an intraosseous or subperiosteal hematoma and may require surgical excision in addition to factor replacement therapy and local measures. Possible complications of pseudotumors are spontaneous rupture, fistula formation, nerve or vessel entrapment, and fracture of the adjacent bone.
7. A factor VIII (hemophilia A) or factor IX (hemophilia B) IgG inhibitor may develop (in about 20% to 33% of individuals with moderate or severe hemophilia A, and in 1% to 4% of individuals with hemophilia B, usually during childhood), making the treatment of bleeding episodes more difficult. A bleeding episode that does not respond to the usual dose of factor replacement therapy should prompt investigations for an inhibitor. In addition, patients with hemophilia should be screened for the development of an inhibitor at least yearly as well as before undergoing elective surgery.

Ancillary Data

1. CBC with hematocrit (Hct) determination, if significant bleeding has occurred.
2. The CBC and differential count, platelet count, prothrombin time (PT), and thrombin time are normal, unless other diseases coexist. The bleeding time is usually normal but is not routinely measured as part of the workup for hemophilia. The PTT is prolonged. However, the severity of PTT prolongation varies according to the sensitivity of the reagent used and the severity of the deficiency. On occasion, the PTT may be normal in individuals with mild hemophilia. Assays for factors VIII and IX define the deficiency and are useful in the initial evaluation (see Table 29-2):
   a. PTT is prolonged. Specific factor level is low.
   b. Factor replacement therapy for major bleeding episodes and perioperative management of hemostasis are guided by coagulation factor assay results.
   c. Urinalysis: Mild hematuria is common. Severe or persistent hematuria requires evaluation and factor replacement therapy.
3. Skeletal x-ray films are helpful in a search for degenerative joint changes or fractures; they are not used to assess acute hemarthroses. If symptoms of a retropharyngeal hematoma develop, a soft tissue lateral neck view defines the extent of swelling.
4. Computed tomography (CT) of the brain should be considered in any patient with hemophilia and head trauma, even if neurologic symptoms and signs are minimal to absent. Evolving neurologic deficits require

immediate factor replacement and, often, neurosurgical intervention.

5. Contrast studies of the genitourinary (GU) and GI tracts are indicated for evaluation of serious bleeding from those sites.
6. Ultrasonography and CT are useful in defining the extent of a hematoma; they are particularly helpful for evaluating bleeding in retroperitoneal sites.
7. Aspiration of involved joints is indicated only if the cause is uncertain and infection is suspected. Factor replacement must be given prior to joint aspiration (Tables 79-1 and 79-2). Hematologic consultation should be obtained before the procedure.

DIFFERENTIAL DIAGNOSIS

See Chapter 29.

MANAGEMENT

1. Stabilization of the patient requires intravenous (IV) fluids or blood for major hemorrhages. Airway management, if obstruction is present, must receive first priority.
2. Factor replacement should be initiated immediately as outlined in Tables 79-1 and 79-2: "Factor first" (i.e., treat first and investigate later). Use vials of factor concentrate that are as close as possible to the desired dose of factor concentrate. In general (except possibly in small infants), do not waste factor concentrate. Use whole vials. Round dose up to the nearest vial.
   a. One unit (U) of factor VIII or IX equals the activity of factor contained in 1 ml of plasma.
   b. One unit of factor VIII per kg of body weight raises the patient's plasma level by approximately 0.02 U/ml (2%). The plasma half-disappearance time for factor VIII is about 12 hours.
   c. One unit of factor IX per kg of body weight raises the patient's plasma level by approximately 0.01 U/ml (1%). The yield is lower than this with recombinant factor IX concentrates (see Table 79-2). The plasma half-disappearance time for factor IX is about 24 hours.
   d. Available products for the treatment of bleeding episodes in hemophilia A include plasma-derived factor concentrates as well as recombinant factor VIII concentrates (Box 79-1). Recombinant factor VIII concentrates are the safest factor VIII products available with respect to viral transmission and are currently considered the factor concentrates of choice for individuals with hemophilia A. Cryoprecipitate is now rarely used in developed countries because of (among other things) the lack of viral inactivation processes for this product.
   e. Available alternatives for treatment of bleeding episodes in hemophilia B include plasma-derived factor IX concentrates of high and low purity, as well as recombinant factor IX concentrate (Box 79-2). Recombinant factor IX concentrates are the safest factor IX products available with respect to viral transmission and are currently considered the factor concentrates of choice for individuals with hemophilia B. Prothrombin complex concentrates are now rarely used to treat hemophilia B in developed countries because of the variable factor content, as well as the risk for DIC and thrombotic problems associated with the use of prothrombin complex concentrates.
   f. All plasma-derived factor concentrates are now subjected to various methods of viral inactivation. Lower-purity plasma-derived factor concentrates may be immunosuppressive, particularly in individuals who are

TABLE 79-1 Hemophilia A: Recommended Dosages of Factor VIII

Actual or Potential Site of Bleeding	Initial Dose* (factor VIII U/kg)	Subsequent Doses* (factor VIII U/kg)	Comments
Life-threatening situations†	50	25 q12hr (or by continuous IV Infusion as advised by local hemophilia center)	Significant blood loss may occur with retroperitoneal bleeding. Factor dosing is guided by factor assays.
Central nervous system hemorrhage			
Major trauma			
Tongue or neck bleeding with potential airway obstruction			
GI bleeding			
Retroperitoneal bleeding (including Iliopsoas bleeding)			
Intraocular bleeding†	50	25 q12hr or as advised by local hemophilia center	Threat to vision. Suspect if there has been an injury around the eye. Formal ophthalmologic examination is required.
Fracture†	50		Factor replacement first. Then x-ray and cast.
Head trauma (no evidence of CNS bleeding)†	50		Close follow-up observation for 14 days.
Surgery preoperative and postoperative care†	50	25 q12hr (or by continuous IV infusion as advised by local hemophilia center)	Evaluation for inhibitor before elective surgery. Perioperative and postoperative plans must be in place preoperatively.
Before spinal tap or other invasive procedure†	50		

Joint or superficial muscles	25-50	25 q12-24hr prn	Several doses may be necessary. Rest, immobilization of involved muscles, or joint therapy and physiotherapy may be needed. Calf/forearm bleeding is limb threatening (compartment syndrome). Use lower end of dose range for early/mild bleeding and higher doses for more severe/late bleeding.
Hematuria (persistent or severe)	40-50	30-40 q24hr	Increase fluid intake. Rest. Prednisone (1-2 mg/kg/day) is sometimes given for 3-7 days. Look for cause. Antifibrinolytic agents are contraindicated.
Mouth bleeding or in preparation for dental work (tooth extraction or deep nerve block)	25-50	25 q12-24hr prn	Use of antifibrinolytic agent for 5-7 days will reduce the need for ongoing factor replacement. Soft diet.
Subcutaneous hematoma (enlarging)	20-25	Rarely needed	
Minor lacerations of skin: before suture placement and removal	25-50		
Before IM injections	15-25		Avoid IM injections if possible. Use subcutaneous route for routine immunizations. If IM injection is required, give it with a small-bore (25-gauge) needle and apply firm pressure to the needle site for 10 minutes after the injection. Some comprehensive hemophilia centers do not routinely give factor replacement before an immunization.

* In individuals who have mild hemophilia A, DDAVP (desmopressin) is the treatment of choice rather than factor VIII concentrates for mild bleeding episodes.
† These cases should be treated in consultation with patient's comprehensive hemophilia center.

TABLE 79-2 Hemophilia B: Recommended Dosages of Factor IX

Actual or Potential Site of Bleeding	Initial Dose* (Factor IX U/kg)	Subsequent Doses* (Factor IX U/kg)	Comments
Life-threatening situations[†] Central nervous system hemorrhage Major trauma Tongue or neck bleeding with potential airway obstruction GI bleeding Retroperitoneal bleeding (including Iliopsoas bleeding)	100	50 q24hr (or by continuous IV Infusion as advised by local hemophilia center)	Significant blood loss may occur with retroperitoneal bleeding. Factor dosing is guided by factor assays.
Intraocular bleeding[†]	100	50 q24hr (or as advised by local hemophilia center)	Threat to vision. Suspect if there has been an injury around the eye. Formal ophthalmologic examination required.
Fracture[†]	100		Factor replacement first. Then x-ray and cast.
Head trauma (no evidence of CNS bleeding[†]	100		Close follow-up observation for 14 days.
Surgery: preoperative and postoperative care[†]	100	50 q24hr (or by continuous IV infusion as advised by local hemophilia center)	Evaluate for inhibitor before elective surgery. Perioperative and postoperative plans must be in place preoperatively.
Before spinal tap or other invasive procedures[†]	100		

Joint or superficial muscles	30-60	30-40 q24hr prn	Several doses may be necessary. Rest, immobilization of involved muscle or joint, and physiotherapy may be needed. Calf/forearm bleeding is limb threatening (compartment syndrome). Use lower end of dose range for early/mild bleeding and higher doses for more severe/late bleeding.
Hematuria (persistent or severe)	80-100	40-50 q24hr	Increase fluid intake. Rest. Prednisone (1-2 mg/kg/day) is sometimes given. Look for cause. Antifibrinolytic agents are contraindicated.
Mouth bleeding or in preparation for dental work (tooth extraction or deep nerve block)	50	30-40 q24hr prn	Use of antifibrinolytic agent for 5-7 days will reduce the need for ongoing factor replacement but is relatively contraindicated when low purity or activated factor IX (prothrombin complex) concentrates are given. Soft diet.
Subcutaneous hematoma (enlarging)	25-30	Rarely needed	
Minor lacerations of skin: before suture placement and removal	40-80		
Before IM injections	25-40		Avoid IM injections if possible. Use subcutaneous route for routine immunizations. If IM injection is required, give it with a small-bore (25-gauge) needle and apply firm pressure to the needle site for 10 minutes after the injection. Some comprehensive hemophilia centers do not routinely give factor replacement before an immunization.

* Doses of factor IX specified in the table are for plasma-derived factor IX concentrates. The dose of recombinant factor IX required is substantially higher because of its lower recovery, particularly in children. Recommended dosing for recombinant factor IX is as follows: For children younger than 15 years, multiply above doses by 1.4. For patients older than 15 years, multiply above doses by 1.2.

† These cases should be treated in consultation with the patient's comprehensive hemophilia center.

Box 79-1

FACTOR TREATMENT PRODUCTS (AND MANUFACTURERS) AVAILABLE IN NORTH AMERICA FOR HEMOPHILIA A IN PATIENTS WITHOUT INHIBITORS OR WITH LOW-TITER/LOW-RESPONDING INHIBITORS

RECOMBINANT FACTOR VIII CONCENTRATES

Product of choice (all of the products that are currently commercially available use human or bovine protein in the culture medium. Clinical trials are in progress evaluating recombinant factor VIII products that do not contain any animal protein):

- Bioclate (Baxter)
- Helixate FS (Bayer)
- Kogenate FS (Bayer)
- Recombinate (Baxter)
- ReFacto (Wyeth)

PLASMA-DERIVED POOLED CONCENTRATES

All are purified and virally inactivated.

- Alphanate SD (Alpha)
- Hemofil M (Baxter)
- Humate-P (Aventis Behring): used primarily to treat von Willebrand's disease
- Koāte-DVI (Bayer)
- Monarc M (Baxter)
- Monoclate P (Aventis Behring)

PLASMA-DERIVED

No viral inactivation.

- Cryoprecipitate: rarely used now in developed countries because of (among other things) the lack of a viral inactivation process for this product

infected with HIV-1. Most children with hemophilia are treated with very high purity or recombinant factor concentrates to minimize this risk as well as to reduce the risk of viral transmission. The more purified (and recombinant) products are considerably more expensive.

3. DDAVP increases the factor VIII coagulant level to about two to three times the baseline value in patients with mild hemophilia A. However, considerable interpatient variation in response is seen. DDAVP may be given to patients with mild hemophilia A to treat mild bleeding episodes or to prepare them for minor surgery, as long as they have previously demonstrated an adequate rise in factor VIII coagulant level after receiving DDAVP.
   a. DDAVP is usually given intravenously but can also be given subcutaneously or intranasally. The dosage of DDAVP for intravenous or subcutaneous use is 0.3 μg/kg/dose (or 10 μg/m^2/dose, whichever is less) to a maximum of 20 μg/dose; for IV use, it is mixed with 50 ml of normal saline and infused over 20 to 30 minutes. The 15 μg/ml concentration of DDAVP should be used for subcutaneous injection.
   b. The dose of DDAVP nasal spray (Stimate) is 150 μg for individuals weighing less than 50 kg and 300 μg (i.e., 150 μg in each nostril) for

Box 79-2

FACTOR TREATMENT PRODUCTS (AND MANUFACTURERS) AVAILABLE IN NORTH AMERICA FOR HEMOPHILIA B IN PATIENTS WITHOUT INHIBITORS OR WITH LOW-TITER/LOW-RESPONDING INHIBITORS

RECOMBINANT FACTOR IX CONCENTRATES

Do not contain any human or animal protein. Product of choice. Note lower yield with recombinant factor IX concentrates (see text).

Benefix (Wyeth)

PURIFIED POOLED PLASMA-DERIVED FACTOR IX CONCENTRATES

All are virally inactivated.

AlphaNine SD (Alpha)
Immunine (Immuno)
Mononine (Aventis Behring)

LOW-PURITY POOLED PROTHROMBIN COMPLEX CONCENTRATES

All are virally inactivated. They contain factors II, IX, and X as well as small amounts of factor VII. Rarely used to treat hemophilia B in the industrialized world because of variable factor content and risk for thrombosis and DIC.

Bebulin VH (Baxter)
Konyne 80 (Bayer)
Profilnine SD (Alpha)
Proplex T (Baxter)
Prothromplex-TIM4 (Immuno)

individuals weighing less than 50 kg. The effect of intravenous DDAVP peaks 30 to 60 minutes after the drug is given; the effect of subcutaneous DDAVP peaks at 60 minutes; the effect of intranasal DDAVP peaks about 60 to 90 minutes after DDAVP is administered.

c. DDAVP should not be administered more often than every 24 hours. It should not be used for more than 2 or 3 consecutive days without evaluation of response (factor levels), because tachyphylaxis (diminishing effectiveness) may occur when DDAVP is given more often than every 48 hours. DDAVP has a potent antidiuretic effect. In patients receiving IV fluids, care must be taken to avoid overhydration for 24 hours after the drug is given. Any IV fluids administered within 24 hours after DDAVP is given should contain the equivalent of normal saline (NS) (e.g., lactated Ringer's solution [LR] or 5% dextrose in water [D5W] 0.9% NS). See product monograph for other precautions and a list of other possible adverse effects.

4. A maxim in the management of bleeding episodes is, "If in doubt, treat" with factor replacement therapy. Considerable controversy exists regarding the dosage of factor replacement therapy required to treat bleeding episodes. However, all agree that higher doses of factor replacement and longer duration of therapy are required to treat potentially life-threatening bleeding episodes and severe hemarthrosis.
5. Postoperatively, or for management of serious bleeding episodes, the total daily

dose of factor VIII (or IX) can be given by continuous IV infusion after an initial bolus dose. The continuous infusion method is superior to the intermittent bolus method in that the former achieves a constant therapeutic factor level and uses less factor concentrate than would be required by intermittent bolus dosing.

6. Secondary prophylaxis (with the infusion of factor VIII concentrate three times per week or of factor IX concentrate twice a week) is given to patients in whom a "target" joint is developing. Despite clinical improvement with secondary prophylaxis, many patients still have radiologic evidence of hemophilic arthropathy.
7. Studies show that primary prophylaxis (with factor VIII concentrate three times per week or factor IX concentrate twice a week, starting at age 1 to 3 years) is effective in preventing joint bleeding and joint damage. (The aim of primary prophylaxis is to keep the factor VIII or IX level above 1% at all times).
8. Antifibrinolytic agents (EACA and tranexamic acid) are available in IV, oral, and topical forms and are useful adjuncts in the prevention or treatment of bleeding from the mouth, nose, or GI tract. The dosage of systemic EACA (Amicar) is 50 to 100 mg/kg/dose (maximum: 6 g/dose) q6-8hr IV or PO. The dosage of systemic tranexamic acid is 25 mg/kg/dose PO (maximum: 1.5 g/dose) q6-8hr or 10 mg/kg/dose IV (maximum: 1 g/dose) q8hr. Systemic antifibrinolytic therapy is usually administered for 5 to 7 days or until healing occurs. Antifibrinolytic drugs are contraindicated in the presence of hematuria and are not usually given in conjunction with the lower-purity or activated prothrombin complex concentrates because of concern about the risk of thrombosis.
9. Prednisone, 1 to 2 mg/kg/24 hr, is sometimes used as an adjunct in the treatment of hematuria or chronic synovitis resulting from recurrent hemarthroses.
10. Patients with moderate or severe hemophilia A or B may develop an inhibitor that is an IgG antibody to the transfused clotting factor. The inhibitor may be detected either during routine screening or because of failure of bleeding episodes to resolve with appropriate factor replacement therapy. The inhibitor titer is measured in Bethesda units.
11. The treatment of bleeding episodes in patients with inhibitors is challenging and individualized. A hematologist should be consulted for advice on managing every bleeding episode in a hemophilia patient with an inhibitor as soon as the patient arrives. Treatment decisions are made on the basis of the severity of the bleeding, the inhibitor level, and the inhibitor response to transfused factor (i.e., a patient with hemophilia A who is a "high responder" has a marked rise in inhibitor level about 5 to 10 days after factor VIII is given, whereas the level of inhibitor does not rise significantly in a "low responder" who is given factor VIII concentrate).
    a. In patients with hemophilia A or B who have a low inhibitor titer and are low responders, bleeding episodes are usually treated with higher doses of factor concentrate. More frequent dosing or continuous factor infusion may be required to achieve hemostatic factor levels.
    b. In patients with hemophilia A or B who have a high titer inhibitor or are high responders, bleeding episodes are treated with recombinant factor VIIa, low-purity or activated prothrombin complex concentrates, or porcine factor VIII (for hemophilia A patients) (Box 79-3). Recombinant

Box 79-3

TREATMENT OPTIONS AVAILABLE IN NORTH AMERICA FOR HEMOPHILIA A OR B IN PATIENTS WITH HIGH-TITER OR HIGH-RESPONDING INHIBITORS

RECOMBINANT FACTOR VIIa

Niastase (Novo Nordisk): dose is 90 μg/kg IV every 2-3 hours

ACTIVATED PROTHROMBIN COMPLEX CONCENTRATES

Also referred to as AICC products (anti-inhibitor coagulant complex concentrates): 75-100 U/kg repeated once or twice every 8-12 hours if needed. (All are virally inactivated. Note risk for thrombosis and DIC associated with the use of these products.) Risk for allergic reaction in some hemophilia B patients who have inhibitors.

Autoplex T (Baxter)

FEIBA VH (Baxter, Immuno)

LOW-PURITY POOLED PROTHROMBIN COMPLEX CONCENTRATES

See list of prothrombin complex concentrates and risks associated with use in Box 79-2. Also risk for allergic reaction in some patients with hemophilia B who have inhibitors. Dose is 100 U/kg.

PORCINE FACTOR VIII

Hyate C (Ipsen): For patients with hemophilia A only. Initial dose is 100-150 U/kg. May be used if antibody to human factor VIII does not strongly react with porcine factor VIII. Propensity to cause anamnestic rise in antibody titer to both porcine and human factor VIII. May cause thrombocytopenia. Risk of transmission of porcine parvovirus with this product. Occasional recipients have allergic reactions.

PLASMAPHERESIS

factor VIIa is the safest product with respect to viral transmission. Some patients with hemophilia B who have inhibitors may exhibit an allergic or anaphylactic reaction to any product that contains factor IX.

c. Occasionally, the temporary removal of antibody by plasmapheresis can allow the short-term use of specific factor replacement for life-threatening or limb-threatening hemorrhage.

d. On a long-term basis, induction of immune tolerance may be attempted and is often successful. It involves the administration of large doses of factor VIII concentrate (or factor IX concentrate for hemophilia B), on a daily or alternate-day basis, sometimes in conjunction with a short course of steroids, cyclophosphamide, or IV immunoglobulin. The inhibitor level often falls with this therapy, although it may take several months. Once the inhibitor has been eradicated (which may take years), factor replacement is administered every 2 to 3 days to prevent the reappearance of the inhibitor.

12. Other considerations in the management of all patients with hemophilia include the following:

a. Listen to the patient and family. They are usually very knowledgeable about hemophilia.

b. If in doubt about appropriate management, or if consideration is being given to withholding factor replacement therapy, discuss the approach with a hematologist or the local hemophilia treatment center.

c. Treat the patient's veins with care. Use the smallest-gauge needle possible.

After venipuncture, apply pressure to the site for at least 5 minutes to prevent hematoma formation. No jugular or femoral vein sticks should be performed except in life-saving situations. Caution is advised if antecubital veins are used.

13. Aspirin-containing medications are contraindicated. Nonsteroidal antiinflammatory drugs (NSAIDs) should be avoided.
14. Intramuscular (IM) injections should be avoided if possible. Note that most routine immunizations can be given subcutaneously (preferred route, rather than intramuscular). See Tables 79-1 and 79-2 for factor replacement guidelines and suggested local measures for IM injections.
15. Immobilization of affected areas and rest for 24 to 72 hours should be used for acute muscle and joint bleeding. Analgesia is often required. Rehabilitation with physiotherapy may be required.
16. Hematology consultation should be sought for acute management and ongoing comprehensive care. Contact information for local comprehensive hemophilia centers can be obtained from the following sources:
    - The National Hemophilia Foundation; telephone 1-800-424-2634; Web site: www.hemophilia.org
    - The Canadian Hemophilia Society; telephone: 1-800-668-2686; Web site: www.hemophilia.ca
    - The World Federation of Hemophilia (for information about hemophilia centers anywhere in the world); Web site: www.wfh.org
17. Immediate surgical consultation should be sought for anterior compartment syndrome, intracranial bleeding, or spinal cord compression.
18. Methods for carrier detection and prenatal diagnosis are now available.

DISPOSITION

1. Most patients can be treated and discharged. Admission is required in the following circumstances:
    a. Head trauma, acute onset of headache, or spinal cord hematoma
    b. Retropharyngeal hematoma
    c. Muscle bleeding with impending or actual compartment syndrome
    d. GI bleeding
    e. Retroperitoneal or severe iliopsoas bleeding
    f. Poor patient compliance
2. Immediate consultation with a hematologist should be obtained under the following circumstances:
    a. Before any surgical or invasive procedure
    b. Intracranial, retropharyngeal, or GI bleeding
    c. Bleeding in patients with inhibitors
3. Other consultants should be involved for specific indications.
4. All patients should be monitored in a comprehensive hemophilia clinic.
5. Early treatment of joint and muscle bleeding, coupled with an aggressive physical therapy program, helps prevent prolonged disability. Home transfusion programs can expedite early intervention.

BIBLIOGRAPHY

Andrew M, Paes B, Johnston M: Development of the hemostatic system in the neonate and young infant, *Am J Pediatr Hematol Oncol* 12:95, 1990.

DiMichele D: Hemophilia: a new approach to an old disease, *Hematol/Oncol Clin North Amer* 12:1315, 1998.

Eyster ME, Gill FM, Blatt PM et al: Central nervous system bleeding in hemophiliacs, *Blood* 51:1179, 1978.

Jadhav M: Anaphylaxis in patients with hemophilia, *Thromb Haemost* 26:205, 2000.

Kulkarni R: Therapeutic choices for patients with hemophilia and high-titer inhibitors, *Am J Hematology* 67:240, 2001.

Morgan LM, Kissoon N, deVebber BL: Experience with the hemophiliac child in a pediatric emergency department, *J Emerg Med* 11:519, 1993.

Silverman R, Kwiatkowski T, Bernstein S et al: Safety of lumbar puncture in patients with hemophilia, *Ann Emerg Med* 22:1739, 1993.

Idiopathic Thrombocytopenic Purpura

Idiopathic thrombocytopenic purpura (ITP) results from increased destruction of platelets that occurs on an autoimmune basis. It is associated with a spectrum of viral illnesses, including measles, rubella, mumps, chickenpox, infectious mononucleosis, and the common cold. Most cases of childhood ITP are self-limited, with 70% to 90% resolving within 6 months.

DIAGNOSTIC FINDINGS

1. An antecedent viral illness is reported in 50% of cases.
2. Symptomatic thrombocytopenia with abrupt onset of petechiae, purpura, and spontaneous bleeding of the skin and mucous membranes. Epistaxis and hemorrhage of the buccal mucosa are common. Bleeding usually responds to pressure.

Complications

1. Intracranial hemorrhage: Occurs in approximately 1% of patients, usually within the first 2 to 4 weeks. May be life threatening. Patients with headache or altered level of consciousness need emergency care.
2. GI bleeding.
3. Massive hematuria.
4. Chronic ITP: Thrombocytopenia of more than 6 months' duration. Most common in girls older than 10 years. Patients have a greater likelihood of associated autoimmune, collagen vascular, or malignant disease.

Ancillary Data

1. CBC, blood smear, and platelet count. Normal platelet count is 150,000 to 400,000 platelets/mm^3; in patients with ITP, it is usually less than 100,000 platelets/mm^3 at the time of presentation. If the count falls to less than 20,000 platelets/mm^3, the patient is at risk of major hemorrhage.
2. Bone marrow puncture and analysis should be performed early in the evaluation to confirm the diagnosis in patients with fewer than 50,000 platelets/mm^3 or when bone marrow disease is suspected. A normal or increased number of megakaryocytes is present in an otherwise normal aspirate or biopsy specimen. Some hematologists recommend a bone marrow examination only in patients with an atypical presentation.

DIFFERENTIAL DIAGNOSIS (PARTIAL)

Thrombocytopenia

1. Increased destruction of platelets:
   a. Consumption:
      (1) Microangiopathic state: hemolytic-uremic syndrome (HUS), DIC, local ischemic disease (necrotizing enterocolitis [NEC])
      (2) Prosthetic heart valves
      (3) Hyaline membrane disease (HMD)
   b. Autoimmune: systemic lupus erythematosus (SLE), Evans's syndrome
2. Sequestration/maldistribution: splenomegaly or hypothermia.
3. Decreased production of platelets:
   a. Marrow infiltration: leukemia, lymphoma, storage disease, or solid tumor
   b. Marrow dysfunction:
      (1) Congenital: Wiskott-Aldrich syndrome, etc.
      (2) Infection: viral
      (3) Drugs
         (a) Cytotoxic drugs
         (b) Anticonvulsants: phenytoin, carbamazepine, valproate
         (c) Antibiotics: sulfonamides, chloramphenicol, rifampin, trimethoprim with sulfamethoxazole

Platelet Dysfunction (Normal Count)

1. Congenital: von Willebrand's disease.
2. Drugs: aspirin, antihistamines, antibiotics (carbenicillin), NSAIDs.
3. Uremia.

Purpura and Petechiae without Thrombocytopenia or Platelet Dysfunction

Purpura and petechiae without thrombocytopenia or platelet dysfunction include vasculitides such as Henoch-Schönlein purpura (HSP) and SLE and connective tissue disorders such as Ehlers-Danlos syndrome.

MANAGEMENT

Once the diagnosis is confirmed by bone marrow testing, expectant observation is indicated for several days, with close monitoring for developing CNS signs and symptoms. Because the antibodies responsible for ITP react with both patient and donor platelets, platelet transfusions are generally of little help in management. ITP is usually self-limited, with 80% of patients recovering spontaneously within 6 months.

Steroid Therapy

If the platelet count is less than 10,000 to 20,000 platelets/mm^3 or if there are extensive bleeding manifestations, most authorities recommend starting steroid therapy:

- Prednisone, 2 mg/kg/24 hr (maximum: 60 mg/24 hr) q8hr PO for 2 to 3 weeks; then tapering at 5- to 7-day intervals

Steroids raise the platelet count by blocking reticuloendothelial consumption of antibody-coated platelets. They may also lessen the fragility of capillary membranes, further decreasing bleeding.

The effects of steroid therapy are usually apparent by 48 to 72 hours, and more than 50% of children with ITP show a response. However, the effect is transient and may last only as long as therapy is continued. Some clinicians suggest that if there is no initial response to steroids or the platelet count falls when therapy is discontinued, a 4-week course of steroids should be repeated a month after the first course was discontinued, with monitoring of the patient during that interval. This measure should be taken after consultation.

Emergent Intervention

For the patient with ITP and severe GI bleeding, epistaxis, hematuria, headache, or intracranial hemorrhage, emergent intervention is essential:

1. RBC transfusion for hypotension and anemia should be initiated.
2. Steroids are administered: hydrocortisone (Solu-Cortef), 4 to 5 mg/kg/dose q6hr IV, followed by prednisone, 2 mg/kg/24 hr PO q8hr. Others have suggested the use of methylprednisolone (Solu-Medrol), 30 mg/kg/24 hr PO for 7 days. Steroids may have an effect in 48 to 72 hours.
3. Hematuria may respond to a push of fluids.
4. Emergency splenectomy is usually necessary. Risk of infection is higher after surgery.
5. IV infusions of gamma globulin (1 g/kg/dose IV over 4 to 8 hours up to three doses or 0.5 g/kg/dose each day for 5 days) may be indicated in patients in whom a rapid rise in platelet count is needed (surgery, trauma, or life-threatening mucosal or internal hemorrhages).
6. Platelet transfusions may be used for massive bleeding unresponsive to pressure. Adolescents and adults need 5 to 10 units, depending on their size, the age of platelet packs, and the response. The half-life of transfused platelets is very short and usually fails to provide prolonged hemostasis.

Chronic ITP

A sequential therapeutic plan is needed for chronic ITP:

1. Steroids: prednisone, as previously described.

2. If no improvement: splenectomy. The patient whose platelet count does not improve with splenectomy should be evaluated for an accessory spleen by means of a blood smear examination for Howell-Jolly bodies and a spleen scan.
3. Immunosuppressive drugs such as vincristine and cyclophosphamide and IV immunoglobulins have been tried with some success.

DISPOSITION

1. Patients with platelet counts lower than 50,000 platelets/mm^3 should be admitted for initial evaluation, monitoring, education, and treatment. A hematologist should be involved to perform a bone marrow examination and to assist in management. Asymptomatic patients with higher platelet counts may be monitored as outpatients after evaluation.
2. If no complications develop, the patient may be discharged after 3 days, with close follow-up to ensure that thrombocytopenia resolves and no complications develop. Activity should be restricted, and close follow-up evaluation ensured.

Parental Education

1. Watch for bleeding or any evidence of CNS abnormality.
2. Contact sports, as well as high-risk endeavors (e.g., skiing, diving), should be avoided.
3. The child should wear seat belts when traveling in a motor vehicle.
4. Young children (less than 4 years old) can be fitted with padded helmets to decrease the risk of head trauma.
5. Aspirin and other drugs that inhibit platelet function should be avoided. The child should use a soft toothbrush and a stool softener, and activity should be limited.

BIBLIOGRAPHY

Albayrak D, Islek I, Kalayei AG et al: Acute immune thrombocytopenia: a comparison study of very high oral doses of methylprednisolone and intravenously administered immune globulin, *J Pediatr* 125:1004, 1994.

Halperin DS, Doyle JJ: Is bone marrow examination justified in idiopathic thrombocytopenia purpura? *Am J Dis Child* 142:508, 1988.

Oncologic Presentations

Julie D. Zimbelman and Thomas J. Smith

Cancer is an important cause of death in children and can occur at any age. Specific presentations may complicate the primary disease process. In as many as 7% of patients with cancer, the initial diagnosis is made in the emergency department (ED). Leukemia most commonly manifests as pallor and weakness in addition to hepatosplenomegaly, petechiae or ecchymoses, fever, tachycardia, bone pain, or cytopenias. Children with CNS tumors frequently present with headache, vomiting, or balance problems. Children with non-CNS solid tumors typically have symptoms related to the location of the neoplasm. Oncologic emergencies are associated with an undiagnosed neoplasm, a new presentation of an existing cancer, recurrent disease, or therapy-induced toxicities. An oncologist should be consulted in all of these situations.

FEVER AND NEUTROPENIA

Infection, inflammation, transfusion, medications, and tumor necrosis may cause fever in children with cancer. Children with neutropenia (fewer than 500 polymorphonuclear [PMN] leukocytes per mm^3) and a fever need immediate evaluation. Common bacterial pathogens are *S. pneumoniae*, *Streptococcus* species, *S. aureus*, *Klebsiella*, *Enterococcus*, *Escherichia coli*, and *Pseudomonas*. Fungal infections and *Pneumocystis carinii* may also be noted. Viral infections such as adenovirus and cytomegalovirus can be life threatening in severely immunocompromised children, such as those who have received bone marrow transplants. Varicella is also life threatening in children undergoing chemotherapy.

After evaluation, expectant management is essential with a combination of intravenous broad-spectrum antibiotics. Immunosuppressed patients in whom herpes simplex or varicella infection is suspected or develops should receive acyclovir. The oncologist should be notified immediately.

SUPERIOR VENA CAVA SYNDROME/SUPERIOR MEDIASTINAL SYNDROME

Compression, infiltration, or thrombosis surrounding the superior vena cava may cause this syndrome, which usually results from tumors of the mediastinum such as lymphoma and mediastinal adenopathy. Patients have venous hypertension within the area drained by the superior vena cava. Tracheal compression can occur with superior vena cava syndrome. Intravascular thrombosis can occur. Periorbital, conjunctival, and facial swelling is present. Progression may lead to thoracic and neck vein distension, facial edema, tachypnea, wheezing, stridor, plethora of the face, edema of the upper extremities, and cyanosis. Shortness of breath, stridor, cough, dyspnea, orthopnea, and chest pain may be reported. In addition, anxiety, confusion, somnolence, headache, visual changes, and syncope may occur. Tumor lysis syndrome is a risk.

Chest x-ray usually demonstrates a mass with or without a pleural or pericardial effusion. Chest CT (prone), echocardiogram, and pulmonary function studies can further define the effect of the mass and aid in evaluating the risk with anesthesia, which is significant.

Sedation and overhydration should be avoided. The head is generally elevated, and the patient carefully monitored. Steroids and irradiation may be needed emergently.

ACUTE TUMOR LYSIS SYNDROME

Tumor lysis syndrome is most commonly seen in rapidly growing tumors as well as tumors that are very sensitive to chemotherapy. Burkitt's lymphoma and hyperleukocytosis are commonly associated with tumor lysis syndrome.

Lysis occurs 1 to 5 days after initiation of chemotherapy but can be present before beginning of treatment (spontaneous tumor lysis). Patients may experience renal failure, dysrhythmias, and neuromuscular symptoms as a result of the metabolic abnormalities. Uric acid, potassium, and phosphorus values may be elevated. Hyperuricemia may produce nephropathy, nephrolithiasis, and, ultimately, renal failure. Hypocalcemia is not uncommon.

Allopurinol or rasburicase administration, phosphate binders, hydration, and alkalinization of urine are necessary. Urine output, blood pressure, weight, and levels of electrolytes, creatinine, uric acid, phosphorus, and calcium must be followed closely. Alkalinization of the urine pH to 6.5 to 7.5 with sodium bicarbonate ($NaHCO_3$) IV is indicated, unless the phosphorus value is elevated. Treatment for hyperuricemia is with allopurinol or rasburicase, fluids, and alkalinization of the urine. Dialysis is sometimes necessary.

OTHER METABOLIC DISTURBANCES

Hypercalcemia may occur in patients with cancer, usually secondary to paraneoplastic syndromes. It may be associated with tumors of the breast, ovary, lung, kidney, and thyroid. Ensuing complications and cardiac tamponade may develop. Neurologic findings may be acute or chronic, usually as a result of direct involvement of the CNS. Treatment depends on severity but can include IV hydration, furosemide (Lasix), biphosphonates, and other medications. Dialysis is sometimes indicated. Close monitoring of electrolytes is imperative.

Hypokalemia and SIADH may be seen secondary to the primary disease or therapies.

HYPERLEUKOCYTOSIS

Hyperleukocytosis is defined as a total white blood cell (WBC) count greater than

100,000 cells/mm^3. Hyperleukocytosis increases blood viscosity and may cause sludging in the microcirculation, resulting in end-organ damage, respiratory failure, CNS changes, and hemorrhage. The mortality from CNS hemorrhage in patients with acute myelogenous leukemia and a WBC count greater than 300,000/mm^3 is near 60%. Concomitant coagulopathies associated with some myeloid leukemias raise the risks of bleeding. Evaluation for hypoxia, acidosis, tachypnea, blurred vision, headache, lethargy, confusion, and chest pain are imperative. Examination should include evaluation for papilledema.

Management of hyperleukocytosis consists of transfusing platelets to keep the level higher than 20,000 platelets/mm^3 and avoiding other nonessential transfusions (do not raise hemoglobin level above 8 to 10 g/dl) because of the risk of increasing blood viscosity. Further, correct underlying coagulopathy that may be present, and manage the metabolic abnormalities (see preceding discussion of tumor lysis syndrome). Begin hydration, alkalinization, and allopurinol or rasburicase. WBC apheresis is sometimes necessary.

NEUROLOGIC EMERGENCIES

Compression of the spinal cord, changes in mental status, seizures, and stroke may occur in patients with cancer at any time as a result of the tumor or the associated therapies.

Cord compression is usually associated with back pain. A thorough neurologic examination is essential. If deficits are noted or if back pain is persistent despite normal neurologic findings, magnetic resonance imaging (MRI) of the entire spine is necessary. Prompt diagnosis and intervention can prevent severe neurologic morbidity. Dexamethasone, irradiation, and spinal cord decompression can all be therapeutic. Not all tumors are radioresponsive. Neurosurgical evaluation is necessary in all patients with spinal cord compression.

Mental status changes and seizures can occur secondary to many things, including metastatic disease, primary CNS tumor, infection, hemorrhage, and metabolic abnormalities. Chemotherapeutic agents can also have neurologic sequelae. A thorough evaluation for increases in intracranial pressure and glucose and electrolyte levels, liver and kidney abnormalities, and DIC is needed. CT of the head may be indicated. Management is dictated by the abnormalities found. If infection is being considered, broad-spectrum parenteral antibiotics should be given.

Strokes can result from spread of the tumor, infection, hemorrhage, or thrombosis. Chemotherapy and disease-related coagulopathies can lead to stroke. Radiation therapy can result in strokes occurring months or years after therapy. Assessment includes CT or MRI (potentially magnetic resonance angiography or venography) of the head, CBC, DIC screen, and antithrombin III determination. A lumbar puncture may be required. Anticoagulation, steroids, and mannitol may be indicated.

ABDOMINAL EMERGENCIES

Abdominal emergencies may arise secondary to inflammation, mechanical obstruction, hemorrhage, or perforation in patients with cancer. Appendicitis, typhlitis, and hemorrhagic pancreatitis can occur in such patients and require prompt recognition. The physical findings may be subtle in a patient with neutropenia.

Typhlitis is a necrotizing colitis of the cecum that occurs in patients with neutropenia. Initial assessment includes thorough examination, CBC, electrolytes, blood cultures, DIC screen, plain three-view x-ray films of the abdomen, CT scan of the abdomen, and a surgical consultation. Medical management, consisting of bowel rest, IV fluids, broad-spectrum antibiotics (including coverage for anaerobic organisms and double coverage for gram-negative bacteria), and supportive care, is the mainstay of therapy. Vasopressors may be required. Surgical intervention is indicated if free air is present or hypotension persists despite aggressive medical management.

Hemorrhagic pancreatitis may occur in patients undergoing asparaginase therapy. Serum amylase and lipase levels should be measured in patients with abdominal pain and vomiting who have received prior asparaginase. Management consists of measurements of electrolyte levels, serum amylase and lipase levels, ultrasonography or CT of the abdomen, bowel rest, nasogastric decompression of the bowel, antibiotics, and IV fluids. Surgical intervention may be needed.

Hemorrhage from ulcerations may occur, especially in patients undergoing high-dose steroid therapy and those with increased intracranial pressure or prior high-dose irradiation. Medical management with histamine$_2$ blockers, antacids, lavage, correction of thrombocytopenia, and coagulopathies is needed. Surgical intervention may be indicated.

BIBLIOGRAPHY

Bachman BT, Barkin RM, Brennan SA et al: Hematologic and oncologic disorders. In Barkin RM, editor: *Pediatric emergency medicine: concepts and clinical practice,* ed 2, St Louis, 1997, Mosby.

Jaffe D, Fleisher G, Grosflam J: Detection of cancer in the pediatric emergency department, *Pediatr Emerg Care* 1:11, 1985.

Pizzo PA, Rubin M, Freifeld A et al: The child with cancer and infection. I: empiric therapy for fever and neutropenia and preventive strategies, *J Pediatr* 119:679, 1991.

Albano E, Ablin A: Oncologic emergencies. In Ablin AR, editor: *Supportive care of children with cancer*, Baltimore, 1997, Johns Hopkins University Press.

Pizzo PA, Poplack DG: *Principles and practice of pediatric oncology,* ed 3, Philadelphia, Lippincott-Raven, 1997.

Sickle Cell Disease

Thomas J. Smith and Julie D. Zimbelman

Sickle cell anemia (SS disease) is an inherited disorder of hemoglobin synthesis, resulting from a single amino acid substitution (valine for glutamate) in the beta subunit of the hemoglobin molecule. Homozygotes for the sickle gene produce a predominance of sickle hemoglobin and experience symptomatic SS anemia. SS disease occurs in approximately 1 in 500 African Americans and may occasionally be seen in other racial groups from the Mediterranean region, the Middle East, and India.

Sickle hemoglobin C (SC) disease and sickle-β-thalassemia are less common variants with similar but less severe clinical manifestations. Heterozygotes (AS) for the sickle gene produce both sickle (S) and normal adult (A) hemoglobin and remain asymptomatic carriers of the sickle trait except under conditions of severe hypoxia (including tourniquet surgery). These carriers are not anemic, and their blood smears do not contain sickle cells. Newborn screening for sickle cell disease, when combined with extensive follow-up and education, significantly reduces patient mortality.

Screening for sickle cell disease is now mandatory in all states. Identification of SS disease at birth enhances early recognition of sepsis and splenic sequestration, use of prophylactic penicillin and appropriate vaccines, and referrals to sickle cell centers.

DIAGNOSTIC FINDINGS (Table 79-3)

The clinical course of SS disease is a chronic illness punctuated by acute episodes ("crises") that threaten the life or comfort of the patient.

Anemia Crises

Sickling of erythrocytes results in chronic hemolytic anemia. Any process that further decreases the circulating RBC mass may produce a profound level of anemia.

Aplastic Crisis. Impairment of RBC production in the bone marrow may cause exacerbation of the chronic hemolytic anemia. Profound anemia may lead to high-output congestive heart failure (CHF). Hematocrit value and reticulocyte count are reduced in comparison with baseline values. Impairment of erythropoiesis can be related to infection or folic acid deficiency. Recent evidence suggests that

TABLE 79-3 Sickle Cell Disease: Clinical Manifestations

Crisis	Category	Symptoms and Signs	Evaluation	Management
Anemia	Aplastic	Fatigue, exercise intolerance, pallor, tachycardia, worsening anemia, low reticulocyte count	CBC, reticulocytes, bilirubin	Hospitalize, support intravascular volume, transfuse to replace RBCs to slightly above baseline value
	Hyperhemolytic	As above, except high reticulocyte count, worsening icterus, increased bilirubin	As above	As above
	Splenic sequestration	Signs of anemia with splenomegaly (usually marked)	As above	As above; splenectomy may be necessary if recurrent problem
Vasoocclusive	Musculoskeletal	Pain, warmth, swelling, often in extremities (dactylitis)	CBC, reticulocytes (x-ray films of little help)	Control pain, hydrate
	Gastrointestinal	Pain, no peritoneal signs	CBC, reticulocytes, liver function tests; consider abdominal ultrasound for cholelithiasis	Control pain, hydrate
	Neurologic	Headache, focal neurologic findings, paralysis, seizures	CBC, reticulocytes, MRI of head without contrast agent	Hospitalize, hydrate, hematology consult, consider immediate RBC pheresis
	Priapism	Prolonged painful erection	CBC, reticulocytes	Control pain, hydrate, urology consultation; consider RBC transfusion or pheresis; avoid local heat or cold
Chest syndrome	Pulmonary	Chest pain, fever, tachypnea, hypoxia, focal pulmonary findings	CBC, reticulocytes, blood culture, pulse oximetry, ABG, chest x-ray ($\dot{V}/\dot{Q}$ scan of little help)	Hospitalize, hydrate, oxygen, antibiotics, hematology consult; may require RBC transfusion or pheresis if progressive
Infection	Fever	Fever with or without focal signs	CBC, reticulocytes, blood, and other appropriate cultures or x-ray films	Immediate antibiotics, may need hospitalization
	Pneumonia	See "Chest Syndrome"		See "Chest Syndrome"
	Osteomyelitis	Focal pain, warmth, swelling, fever; difficult to distinguish acutely from vasoocclusive crisis	CBC, reticulocytes, blood culture, plain film of site	Control pain, hydrate, consider aspiration; antibiotics only if diagnosis is clear

human parvovirus B19 infection is the predominant cause of aplastic crises in SS disease.

Hyperhemolytic Crisis. Acceleration of the already rapid rate of RBC destruction may occasionally cause worsening of the underlying anemia. Episodes may be related to concurrent glucose-6-phosphate dehydrogenase (G6PD) deficiency or infection.

Splenic Sequestration Crisis. A young child with SS disease may suddenly pool a large portion of the peripheral blood volume in the spleen. This results in massive splenomegaly, severe anemia, and hypovolemic shock, which evolve over a period of hours to days. This crisis occurs most commonly between 4 months and 6 years of age, before autoinfarction of the spleen. It may be precipitated by infection.

Vasoocclusive Crises

Gelation of the abnormal hemoglobin within erythrocytes causes them to sickle, making them less deformable and leading to recurrent thromboses of the microvasculature. Local ischemia and tissue infarction result. Sickling is enhanced by dehydration, stasis, hypoxemia, acidosis, and hypertonicity. Bones, pulmonary parenchyma, abdominal viscera, and the CNS are the sites most often affected by the vasoocclusive process.

Musculoskeletal System

1. Bone pain, particularly of the extremities.
2. Dactylitis (hand-and-foot syndrome): symmetric, nonpitting edema of the hands and feet, accompanied by warmth and tenderness. Most common in children younger than 4 years. Often, dactylitis may be the first manifestation of SS disease, alerting the clinician to evaluate the patient for this underlying disorder.
3. Aseptic necrosis of bone, particularly of the femoral or humeral head.
4. Leg ulcers.

Gastrointestinal Tract

1. Abdominal pain that is caused by a crisis is usually without peritoneal signs or decreased bowel sounds. In addition, the patient often has experienced this pain previously, without a fever or an increase in the baseline WBC count or band count.
2. Autosplenectomy by 5 years of age in those with SS disease.
3. Cholelithiasis caused by chronic hemolysis is increasingly prevalent after 10 years of age. Cholelithiasis may cause acute or insidious right upper quadrant pain and jaundice.
4. Hepatomegaly: A mild degree of enlargement is usually present, but it may progress because of one of the following:
   a. Acute hepatic sludging/right upper quadrant syndrome. Sickling may obstruct blood flow within the liver, leading to noncolicky right upper quadrant pain, progressive hepatomegaly, malaise, and jaundice.
   b. Viral hepatitis usually secondary to prior blood transfusions.
   c. Hepatic sequestration after infarction of the spleen.

Central Nervous System. Thrombotic or hemorrhagic stroke occurs in about 8% of patients with SS disease. Patients may have severe headache, nuchal rigidity, focal neurologic findings, seizures, coma, or xanthochromic cerebrospinal fluid (CSF).

Priapism. Painful erections, caused by obstruction of the venous drainage of the corpus cavernosum, can be either "stuttering" (multiple short episodes) or prolonged (for more than 24 hours).

Acute Chest Syndrome

Patients initially have chest pain, dyspnea, infiltrate, fever, leukocytosis, and rub or effusion. Often, pulmonary infarction cannot be differentiated from pneumonia. Infarction usually occurs in children older than 12 years and may be associated with a painful crisis; infection is a more common trigger in younger children. The chest x-ray film is often clear initially with a positive findings on ventilation-perfusion ($\dot{V}/\dot{Q}$) scan. Lower lobe involvement is common.

Infection

1. Functional asplenia leads to higher risk of serious bacterial infection. Sepsis, meningitis, pneumonia, and osteomyelitis occur with greater frequency and severity. Common causative organisms are listed in Table 79-4.
2. It is important to compare the WBC count with baseline value. Patients with SS disease often have a high baseline WBC count as a result of a hyperactive bone marrow.
3. The likelihood of bacterial infection is increased when the count of nonsegmented neutrophils (bands) in the CBC is more than 1000 cells/mm^3.
4. Children with SC or sickle-β-thalassemia have a lower (but still high) risk of sepsis than those with SS disease.

Other Diagnostic Findings

1. Impaired growth and delayed puberty are common.
2. CHF (see Chapter 16).
3. Psychosocial problems.
4. Retinopathy resulting from vasoocclusive phenomena. Marked by dilated and tortuous retinal vessels, microaneurysms, neovascularization, and retinal hemorrhage.
5. Premature births and spontaneous abortions are common during pregnancy.
6. Irreversible renal hyposthenuria is present in all patients by 5 years of age.
7. Hematuria may occur in both SS disease and sickle trait. Risk of urinary tract infections is increased.

Ancillary Data

1. CBC and reticulocyte count are both abnormal. Baseline values for an individual patient are particularly important in the evaluation of acute problems (Table 79-5). Patients with sickle cell trait generally have no anemia or sickle cells on smear.
2. Hemoglobin electrophoresis confirms the diagnosis in coordination with the newborn metabolic screen. Early diagnosis allows initiation of preventative measures before the onset of signs or symptoms at 2 to 4 months. Solubility tests (e.g., Sickledex) are poor screening tests because they are insensitive during the newborn period; they do not distinguish between sickle cell disease and trait and fail to detect other hemoglobinopathies.

TABLE 79-4 Sickle Cell Disease: Infections

Infection	Common Organisms	Initial Antibiotic Therapy*
Fever/presumed sepsis or meningitis	*S. pneumoniae* *H. influenzae*	Cefotaxime, 150 mg/kg/24 hr (adult: 6 g/24 hr) q6-8hr IV, or ceftriaxone, 100 mg/kg/24 hr (adult: 4 g/24 hr) q12hr IV Add vancomycin, 30-45 mg/kg/24 hr (adult: 2 g/24 hr) q8-12hr IV for severe illness
Acute chest syndrome	*S. pneumoniae* *H. influenzae* *M. pneumoniae*	Cefotaxime or ceftriaxone as above; also, erythromycin, 40 mg/kg/24 hr q6hr PO; add vancomycin for severe illness
Osteomyelitis	*Salmonella* *S. aureus* *S. pneumoniae*	Cefotaxime or ceftriaxone as above and nafcillin, 100 mg/kg/24 hr q4hr IV, and gentamicin, 5-7.5 mg/kg/24 hr q8hr IV

* In critically ill children, more broad-spectrum antibiotics may be initiated. Therapy should be altered when culture and sensitivity data are available.

3. Unconjugated (indirect) bilirubin value is elevated (range: 1.5 to 4.0 mg/dl) because of chronic hemolysis. Other liver function test (LFT) results are normal unless there is supervening hepatobiliary disease (e.g., hepatitis, cholelithiasis, hepatic sludging).
4. Pulse oximetry and arterial blood gas (ABG) analysis are helpful in the evaluation of pneumonia, pulmonary infarction, acute chest syndrome, CHF, and metabolic acidosis. Knowledge of baseline pulse oximetry values is helpful.
5. Cultures: blood, urine, bone, CSF as indicated. Blood cultures are imperative with any febrile episode.
6. Urinalysis: hematuria common. Specific gravity is not accurate in reflecting dehydration.
7. X-ray studies.
   a. Chest x-ray film: acute chest syndrome, infarction, infection, CHF. This study is especially indicated in children who are febrile as well as those with cough, chest pain, or physical findings that suggest chest problems.
   b. Abdominal x-ray or ultrasonography: cholelithiasis.
   c. Bone x-ray study: infarction, infection, aseptic necrosis. X-ray films usually cannot distinguish acute infarction from infection.
   d. Magnetic resonance imaging (MRI): stroke.
8. Electrocardiogram (ECG): biventricular hypertrophy is common. Cor pulmonale may result from recurrent pulmonary infarcts.
9. Family studies: CBC with indices and reticulocyte count, blood smear, and hemoglobin electrophoresis in parents and siblings may help clarify the patient's diagnosis.

MANAGEMENT

Fluids

1. Maintain euvolemia. More fluids are necessary only if patient is hypotensive or dehydrated or insensible losses are increased.
2. Administer 1 to 1¼ times maintenance fluids IV or PO during vasoocclusive crisis.
3. Monitor patient for dehydration, fluid overload, and high-output CHF. In splenic sequestration crisis, emergent fluid resuscitation with isotonic crystalloid, colloid, or blood is necessary to treat potential vascular collapse.

Blood Products

1. Restore circulating RBC during aplastic or hyperhemolytic crises by administering packed RBCs, 5 to 10 ml/kg over 3 to 4 hours.

   If more rapid replacement of sickle erythrocytes is required (e.g., stroke, acute chest syndrome, priapism), if CHF is present, or if there is concern about

TABLE 79-5 Sickle Cell Disease: Hematologic Values

	Normal (AA) Average	Sickle Cell Disease (SS) Average (Range)
Hematocrit (%)	36	22 (17–29)
Hemoglobin (g/dl)	12	7.5 (5.5–9.5)
Reticulocytes (%)	1.5	12 (5–30)
WBC count (per mm^3)	7500	20,000 (12,000–35,000)
Peripheral smear	Normal	Sickle cell present

Modified from Pearson HA, Diamond LK: In Smith CA, editor: *The critically ill child*, Philadelphia, 1985, WB Saunders.
NOTE: Patients with sickle cell trait have normal values and RBC morphology.

augmenting sickling with greater blood viscosity after transfusion, partial-exchange transfusion or RBC pheresis can be used.

2. Reduction of cells containing sickle hemoglobin to 30% or less of the total circulating RBCs effectively prevents further sickling. This can be accomplished with a long-term transfusion program by which transfusions are given every 3 to 4 weeks. Adequacy of transfusion therapy can be assessed through the use of the sodium metabisulfite sickling test or quantitative hemoglobin electrophoresis.

Oxygen

Hypoxia precipitates sickling and should be corrected when present, particularly in pulmonary disease, stroke, severe anemia, and CHF. Oxygen should be used to keep pulse oximetry value at 92% or higher. Excessive oxygen may suppress reticulocyte count and exacerbate anemia.

Analgesia

A variety of agents may be selected from:

- Codeine, 4 mg/kg/24 hr q4-6hr PO.
- Ketorolac (Toradol): Children older than 2 years, 0.5 to 1 mg/kg/dose q6hr IV; adults, 30 to 60 mg initially followed by 15 to 30 mg q6hr IV up to daily maximum of 150 mg. First parenteral NSAID. Not to be used for longer than 48 hours.
- Morphine, 0.1 to 0.2 mg/kg/dose q2-4hr IV. Maximum dose: 10 mg/dose. May need continuous infusion.

  NOTE: Prolonged use of meperidine (Demerol) should be avoided because of risk of seizures.
- Hydromorphone (Dilaudid), 1 to 4 mg/dose q4-6hr PO (or IV). Not recommended for children younger than 10 years.

A useful analgesic routine for inpatient management of severe pain may include the following; in most cases, prn analgesia orders are not appropriate:

1. First 24 hours: morphine sulfate, 0.05 to 0.1 mg/kg/dose (maximum: 10 mg/dose) q2hr IV on a schedule. Monitoring is required. May be supplemented with ibuprofen or acetaminophen q4hr PO. Alternatively, ketorolac, 0.5 to 1.0 mg/kg/dose IV q6hr on schedule (maximum duration: 5 days) supplemented with morphine sulfate for breakthrough pain.
2. After 24 to 48 hours or when acute pain has diminished: Taper parenteral dose by 20% daily but do not change interval. When half of the starting parenteral dose is achieved, switch to oral analgesics every 4 hours and then slowly decrease interval to a prn basis.
3. Obviously, any regimen needs to be individualized.

Antibiotics

Antibiotics (see Table 79-4) should be given urgently if the patient has a fever. Antibiotic administration should not be delayed for the sake of IV access or x-rays.

1. Culture specimens should be obtained before treatment is initiated and should determine the ultimate choice of antibiotic.
2. An identifiable source of the fever still requires parenteral, broad-spectrum antibiotics.
3. A bacterial infection is more likely if there are more than 1000 neutrophil bands per mm^3 of blood but should be considered in all febrile patients.
4. The route of administration of antibiotics and the necessity of hospitalizing the patient are determined by the level of toxicity and the nature of systemic involvement. Prophylactic penicillin initiated by 4 months of age has been shown to reduce infection-related morbidity and mortality rates in children younger than 5 years.
5. For chest syndrome or bone pain, it may be impossible to distinguish between infection and infarction. Chest syndrome should always be treated with appropriate antibiotics. In the child with bone

pain, it may be prudent to treat with hydration and analgesia and to institute antibiotic therapy only if symptoms persist 2 to 3 days (if no fever).

Surgery

1. If surgery is required, a hematologist should be consulted.
2. Cholecystectomy: symptomatic cholelithiasis
3. Splenectomy: recurrent splenic sequestration crises
4. Arthroplasty: aseptic necrosis of femoral or humeral head

Transfusion Therapy

Long-term transfusion therapy is 90% effective in preventing recurrent strokes after an episode of actual cerebrovascular accident (CVA). Therapy must be continued indefinitely. Long-term transfusions may also be needed for recurrent chest syndrome or priapism.

DISPOSITION

1. Hospitalization is indicated for patients with splenic sequestration crisis, aplastic crisis with severe anemia, stroke, acute chest syndrome, suspected bacterial infection, severe or prolonged priapism, or severe vasoocclusive pain crisis for which parenteral analgesia or IV hydration is required. It is important not to prolong ambulatory management of such patients in the ED. Patients showing no response in the first 2 hours with appropriate pain medication and hydration should usually be admitted.
2. Hydroxyurea. Hydroxyurea therapy significantly decreased the severity of anemia and frequency of vasoocclusive crisis in some children with SS disease. Nevertheless, it is a potent chemotherapeutic agent whose long-term toxicity is unknown and should be used by hematologists with expertise in chemotherapy.
3. Bone marrow transplantation. An allogeneic bone marrow transplant from an HLA-identical sibling can change the patient's hemoglobin electrophoresis pattern to that of the donor and eliminate sickle-related symptoms. The main problems are predicting the clinical severity of SS disease for any given child, finding a matched sibling donor, and the side effects of bone marrow transplant.
4. Long-term follow-up is essential. Health maintenance considerations should include the following:
   - **a.** Prophylactic penicillin. Consideration should be given to stopping this prophylaxis at age 5 years, although the issue is still under study.
   - **b.** Pneumococcal, *Haemophilus influenzae*, meningococcal, and hepatitis B vaccines.
   - **c.** Folic acid therapy (1 mg/day PO).
   - **d.** Long-term transfusion therapy.
   - **e.** Genetic counseling.
   - **f.** Ophthalmologic examination for sickle retinopathy.
   - **g.** Routine cardiac and pulmonary screening.
   - **h.** Yearly evaluation for blood-borne infections.
   - **i.** Yearly ultrasonography for gallstones after age 13.
   - **j.** Psychosocial counseling.
   - **k.** Coordination of patient care and services through a comprehensive hemoglobinopathy program.

BIBLIOGRAPHY

American Academy of Pediatrics, Section of Hematology/Oncology: Health supervision for children with sickle cell disease, *Pediatrics* 109:326, 2002.

Buchanan GR, Glader BE: Leukocyte counts in children with sickle cell disease, *Am J Dis Child* 132:398, 1978.

Charache S, Lubin B, Reid CD: *Management and therapy of sickle cell disease*, US Department of Health and Human Services, NIH Publication No. 91-2117, 1991.

DiMichele D: Hemophilia 1996: a new approach to an old disease, *Pediatr Clin North Am* 43:709, 1996.

Falletta JM, Woods GM, Verter JI et al: Discontinuing penicillin prophylaxis in children with sickle cell anemia, *J Pediatr* 127:685, 1995.

Galloway SJ, Harwood-Nuss AL: Sickle cell anemia: a review, *J Emerg Med* 6:213, 1988.

Gaston MH, Verter JJ, Woods G et al: Prophylaxis with oral penicillin in children with sickle cell anemia, *N Engl J Med* 314:1593, 1986.

Mills ML: Life-threatening complications of sickle cell disease in children, *JAMA* 254:1487, 1985.

Pollack CV, Sanders DY, Severance HW: Emergency department analgesia without narcotics for adults with acute sickle cell pain crisis: case reports and review of crisis management, *J Emerg Med* 9:445, 1991.

Poncz M, Kane E, Gill FM: Acute chest syndrome in sickle cell disease: etiology and clinical correlates, *J Pediatr* 107:861, 1985.

Scott J, Hillary CA, Brown ER et al: Hydroxyurea therapy in children severely affected with sickle cell disease, *J Pediatr* 128:820, 1996.

Vermulen C, Counu F: Bone marrow transplantation for sickle cell disease: the European experience, *Am J Pediatr Hematol Oncol* 16:18, 1994.

Vichinsky E, Hurst D, Eaules A et al: Newborn screening for sickle cell disease: effect on mortality, *Pediatrics* 81:749, 1998.

80 Infectious Disorders

Also See Chapter 34 (Fever in Children)

Acquired Immunodeficiency Syndrome

Children contract acquired immunodeficiency syndrome (AIDS) from their mothers during the perinatal period or through contaminated blood or blood products. The former mode of transmission accounts for 90% of new cases in the United States. Sexual activity is a rare mode of transmission in children but is obviously a major concern in adolescents and adults.

Human T-lymphotropic virus type III (HTLV-III), called human immunodeficiency virus (HIV), is etiologic. It is tropic for helper T (CD4) lymphocytes and macrophages, causing cell dysfunction, immune deficiencies, and death. Human retrovirus, of which HIV is one, uses enzyme reverse transcriptase to copy deoxyribonucleic acid (DNA) from the viral ribonucleic acid (RNA). The DNA is incorporated into human cellular DNA, where it can remain latent for months or years.

DIAGNOSTIC FINDINGS

Maternal HIV infections may be suspected if there is clinical evidence of infection or immunodeficiency. Intravenous drug abuse, sexual promiscuity, and residence in an area of high HIV prevalence also increase the risk. Perinatal transmission occurs in 25% to 40% of offspring of infected women. Breast milk has been implicated in the transmission of HIV infection. *Infants* may be small for gestational age or may fail to thrive; problems develop by 3 to 6 months of age.

Older children have hepatosplenomegaly, lymphadenopathy, salivary gland enlargement, recurrent or persistent infections, and high immunoglobulin G (IgG) levels in association with AIDS-related complex (ARC), which ultimately progresses to AIDS. Chronic interstitial pneumonia *(Pneumocystis carinii)* as well as other opportunistic infections may develop. Hemoptysis is associated with pneumococcal pneumonia and tuberculosis. Otitis media, sinus infections, hepatitis, hepatosplenomegaly, failure to thrive, nephropathy, cardiomyopathy, malignancy, immune thrombocytopenia purpura, and chronic diarrhea are noted. Neurologic deficits include developmental delay, generalized weakness with pyramidal signs, loss of milestones, and chronic or progressive encephalopathy with ataxia and seizures.

Common opportunistic infections in children include the following:

1. *P. carinii* pneumonitis
2. *Candida* esophagitis
3. Disseminated cytomegalovirus
4. Cryptosporidiosis associated with watery diarrhea
5. *Mycobacterium avium-intracellulare*
6. Chronic herpes simplex virus
7. *Cryptococcus*
8. *Toxoplasma gondii,* which causes central nervous system (CNS) mass

Ancillary Data

1. Screening studies include HIV antibody testing by enzyme-linked immunosorbent assay (ELISA). If the result is positive, the assay should be repeated, and if the second result is positive, the results should be confirmed by Western

blot assay to minimize false-positive results. If possible, obtain DNA polymerase chain reaction (PCR) and P24 antigen tests. If the study findings are initially negative after a specific exposure, a second screening may be warranted in 1 month. Informed consent to obtain these studies is sometimes appropriate.

2. Immune evaluation:
   a. Complete blood count (CBC) and differential count
   b. T cell: delayed hypersensitivity skin test, complete T-cell subset evaluation, and mitogen and antibody stimulated lymphocyte blastogenesis
   c. B cell: quantitative immunoglobulins, preimmunization and postimmunization antibody levels, and B-cell enumeration
3. Other evaluations include tests of liver and renal function, chest x-ray examination, and lumbar puncture, usually in consultation with a center commonly caring for patients with AIDS.
   a. In patients with fever, CBC and differential, blood culture, chest x-ray examination, and other studies should generally be done to exclude specific infections. A more extensive evaluation is indicated for recurrent or unexplained fever.

MANAGEMENT

No definitive treatment exists for AIDS. Supportive care is essential and parallels that for immunocompromised individuals, as outlined in Chapter 79. Referral for ongoing care is essential to ensure appropriate evaluation, continuity, and access to evolving protocols.

1. Opportunistic infections must be recognized and treated aggressively.
2. The antiviral agents zidovudine (ZVT) and didanosine (DDI) are approved for use in HIV-infected children. ZVT administered during pregnancy of a woman with HIV infection may reduce vertical transmission. Newer regimens, perhaps combined with cesarean section, may be prophylactic.
3. Provide psychologic support.
4. Use universal precautions.
5. The National AIDS Hotline may be useful (800-342-AIDS).

BIBLIOGRAPHY

American Academy of Pediatrics Task Force on Pediatric AIDS: Guidelines for human immunodeficiency virus (HIV) infection in children and their foster families, *Pediatrics* 89:681, 1992.

Centers for Disease Control and Prevention: Guidelines: revised guidelines for prophylaxis against *Pneumocystis carinii* pneumonia for children infected with or permanently exposed to human immunodeficiency virus, *MMWR* 44(RR-4), 1995.

Krasinski K: Antiretroviral therapy in children, *Acta Paediatr* 400(suppl 1):63, 1994.

Luzuriaga K, Bryan Y, Krogstad P et al: Combination treatment with zidovudine, didanosine, and nevirapine in infants with HIV type I infection, *N Engl J Med* 336:1343, 1997.

Rogers M, Caldwell M, Qwinn M et al: Epidemiology of pediatric human immunodeficiency virus infection in the United States, *Acta Paediatr* 400(suppl 1):5, 1995.

Botulism

Botulism results from the ingestion of preformed toxins (e.g., canned vegetables), ingestion of spores (infant botulism: honey), or spore contamination of open wounds. *Clostridium botulinum* produces a neurotoxin that blocks the presynaptic release of acetylcholine. The incubation period of foodborne infection is 12 to 36 hours (range 6 hours to 8 days), whereas it is 4 to 14 days with wound infections. Infant botulism has an incubation period of 3 to 30 days.

DIAGNOSTIC FINDINGS

1. A symmetric descending paralysis is noted, with weakness and equal deep tendon reflexes (DTRs):
   a. Pupils are fixed and dilated with oculomotor paralysis, blurred vision, diplopia, ptosis, and photophobia.

b. Slurred speech, dysphagia, and sore throat are reported.
c. Nausea, vomiting, vertigo, dry mouth, constipation, and urinary retention occur.
d. Dyspnea and rales are commonly noted. In rare cases, secondary bacterial infection and total respiratory failure occur as a result of paralysis.

2. The sensorium and sensory findings are normal.
3. If a wound is present, it may suppurate with gas formation.

Ancillary Data

1. *C. botulinum* toxin assay, if available
2. Lumbar puncture (LP) may show increased protein in cerebrospinal fluid (CSF)
3. Chest x-ray film and arterial blood gas (ABG) analysis as indicated

DIFFERENTIAL DIAGNOSIS

Botulism should be distinguished from intoxication (see Chapter 54) caused by heavy metals or organophosphates (p. 351).

MANAGEMENT

1. Initially, focus on airway management as well as other aspects of cholinergic blockage. Place a nasogastric (NG) tube and urinary catheter. All patients need intensive monitoring. In one study of 57 children with infant botulism, 77% were intubated and required mechanical ventilation.
2. Irrigate and debride all wounds.
3. Administer human-derived botulinum antitoxin or equine botulinum antitoxin, the latter after testing for hypersensitivity to equine sera. Trivalent ABE antitoxin is available from the Centers for Disease Control and Prevention (CDC) (daytime phone: 404-639-3670; nighttime/weekend/holiday phone: 404-639-2888) or a state health department.
4. Give antitoxin to individuals exposed to the source by ingestion.
5. Botulism may be prevented by boiling all foods adequately (more than 10 minutes). Children younger than 1 year should not eat honey.

BIBLIOGRAPHY

Burmingham M, Walter F, Mecham C et al: Wound botulism, *Ann Emerg Med* 24:1184, 1994.

Long SS, Gajewski JL, Brown LW et al: Clinical laboratory and environmental features of infant botulism in Southeastern Pennsylvania, *Pediatrics* 75:935, 1985.

Shriener MS, Field E, Ruddy R: Infant botulism: a review of 12 years' experience at the Children's Hospital of Philadelphia, *Pediatrics* 87:159, 1991.

Diphtheria

Corynebacterium diphtheriae, a club-shaped, gram-positive, pleomorphic bacillus, produces an exotoxin that accounts for much of the systemic disease of diphtheria and its complications. The incubation period is 2 to 5 days.

DIAGNOSTIC FINDINGS

Four distinct clinical presentations have been described:

1. Pharyngeal-tonsillar: sore throat, fever, vomiting, swallowing difficulty, and malaise associated with a gray, closely adherent pseudomembrane. It may progress to respiratory obstruction.
2. Laryngeal: less common. Initially occurs with hoarseness, loss of voice, and may extend into the pharynx.
3. Nasal: serosanguineous nasal discharge that may persist for weeks.
4. Cutaneous: sharply demarcated ulcer with membranous base. Common in the tropics.

Complications

Complications are primarily the result of the effects of exotoxin on organs beyond the respiratory tract.

1. Cardiac: myocarditis, endocarditis (p. 567), dysrhythmias (atrioventricular [AV]

block, left bundle branch block) (see Chapter 6)
2. Respiratory obstruction and failure
3. Palatal and oculomotor palsy and peripheral polyneuritis (see Chapter 41)
4. Death, usually from respiratory or cardiac complications

Ancillary Data

1. Cultures (Loeffler's medium and tellurite agar) and Gram staining
2. CBC (variable, platelets decreased)
3. Cardiac enzymes, electrocardiogram (ECG), and ABG analysis as needed

DIFFERENTIAL DIAGNOSIS

See p. 614.

MANAGEMENT

1. Initially focus on stabilization of the airway and treatment of cardiac dysfunction.
2. Give a tetanus and diphtheria toxoid (Td) booster to exposed, immunized, asymptomatic contacts. Give erythromycin (as described later) to asymptomatic, unimmunized individuals for 7 days, and begin immunization schedule as outlined in Appendix B-7.
3. Corticosteroids have no proven beneficial role in preventing ECG changes or neuritis.

Antitoxin

1. Sensitivity may be determined by diluting 0.5 ml serum in 10 ml saline or 5% dextrose in water (D5W). Give this slowly. Observe for 30 minutes; if no reactions, serum diluted 1:20 may be given at a rate of 1 ml/min.
2. If the membrane is pharyngeal or laryngeal and of less than 48 hours' duration, give 20,000 to 40,000 units of antitoxin; for nasopharyngeal lesions, 40,000 to 60,000 units; and for extensive disease of 3 days or more in duration, 80,000 to 100,000 units.
3. With cutaneous disease, some clinicians recommend 20,000 to 40,000 units of antitoxin to prevent progression to toxic sequelae.
4. CDC may be a source of antitoxin (daytime phone: 404-639-3670; nighttime/weekend/holiday phone: 404-639-2888).

Antibiotics

Antibiotics are required to eradicate the organism and prevent spread; they are not a substitute for antitoxin:

- Aqueous penicillin G, 100,000 to 150,000 U/kg/24 hr q4-6hr IV, for 7 to 10 days; *or* procaine penicillin G, 25,000 to 50,000 U/kg/24 hr q12hr IM, for 14 days

Parenteral erythromycin is an alternative.

Once parenteral therapy is no longer required, a 10-day course of oral penicillin (or, for a patient allergic to penicillin, erythromycin) is begun:

- Penicillin V, 25,000 to 50,000 units (15 to 30 mg)/kg/24 hr q6hr PO; *or*
- Erythromycin, 30 to 50 mg/kg/24 hr q6hr PO.

Asymptomatic, previously immunized close contacts should receive a booster immunization if they have not received a booster dose of diphtheria toxoid within 5 years.

Asymptomatic close contacts who have not been immunized or whose immunization status is unknown should receive prophylaxis (erythromycin, 40 to 50 mg/kg/24 hr for 7 days, or benzathine penicillin G, 600,000 to 1,200,000 units IM).

Culture specimens should be collected from all close contacts.

DISPOSITION

Patients should be hospitalized for close observation and respiratory isolation. Carriers need antibiotics and immunization.

Parental Education

Active immunization should be encouraged.

BIBLIOGRAPHY

Report of the Committee on Infectious Disease, Elk Grove, Ill, American Academy of Pediatrics, 1997.

Thisyakorn USA, Wongvarich J, Kumpeng V: Failure of corticosteroid therapy to prevent diphtheritic myocarditis or neuritis, *Pediatr Infect Dis* 3:126, 1984.

Kawasaki's Disease

Adam Z. Barkin, MD

Kawasaki's disease (KD) is a multisystem disease primarily affecting children younger than 5 years during the late winter and early spring. The disease is rare in infants younger than 3 months with a peak at the ages of 1 to 2 years. The disease was formerly known as mucocutaneous lymph node syndrome. Although it is generally self-limited, coronary artery vasculitis can result in significant morbidity. The etiology for Kawasaki's disease is thought to be infectious, but an agent has not been isolated.

DIAGNOSTIC FINDINGS

The disease is triphasic in clinical presentation. An *acute* phase lasts for 1 to 2 weeks and consists of fever and the appearance of four of five diagnostic criteria. The *subacute* phase begins with resolution of fever, rash, and lymphadenopathy, and lasts until approximately 4 weeks from onset of illness. This phase is notable for thrombocytosis, desquamation, and the highest risk of sudden cardiac death. The *convalescence* phase lasts 6 to 8 weeks and is notable for an absence of clinical signs, normalization of the erythrocyte sedimentation rate (ESR), and an ongoing high risk of death.

The diagnostic criteria for Kawasaki's disease are fever greater than 38.5° C (usually 38.5° to 40.0° C) for at least 5 days plus four of the following five criteria.

1. Discrete, bilateral nonexudative conjunctival injection that usually appears within 2 days of the onset of fever and sometimes lasts 1 to 2 weeks.
2. Mouth changes, which appear 1 to 3 days after onset of fever and may last 1 to 2 weeks:
   a. Erythema, fissuring, and crusting of lips
   b. Diffuse, oropharyngeal erythema
   c. Strawberry tongue
3. Peripheral changes, most of which begin 3 to 5 days after onset of fever and last 1 to 2 weeks:
   a. Induration of the hands and feet, with possible edema
   b. Erythema of the palms and soles
   c. Desquamation of the tips of the fingers and toes 2 to 3 weeks after the onset of illness
   d. Transverse nail grooves are common during convalescence
4. Erythematous, polymorphous rash concurrent with the fever and spreading from the extremities to the trunk. May be pruritic. The rash usually disappears within 1 week but may be followed by desquamation of the distal extremities, particularly the tips of the fingers and toes.
5. Cervical lymphadenopathy with one node larger than 1.5 cm.

Other possible findings are:

1. Cardiovascular: coronary artery disease (see discussion of complications)
2. Gastrointestinal: vomiting, diarrhea, abdominal pain, hydrops of the gallbladder, obstructive jaundice, pancreatitis
3. Hematologic: leukocytosis, normocytic anemia, elevated ESR, elevated C-reactive protein value, thrombocytopenia or thrombocytosis
4. Genitourinary: urethritis, proteinuria, pyuria
5. Respiratory: pneumonia, cough
6. Musculoskeletal: arthralgia, arthritis
7. Neurologic: meningismus, cerebrospinal fluid (CSF) pleocytosis, irritability, photophobia, uveitis, iritis

Complications

Kawasaki's disease is a vasculitis most severe in medium-sized arteries, including coronary arteries. This vasculitis results in aneurysm formation, coronary artery disease, and the potential for thrombosis and myocardial infarction. Twenty percent to 25% of untreated patients have coronary abnormalities, including aneurysms and diffuse dilatation. Children younger than 1 year and older than 5 years at onset of disease are at greatest risk. The condition may be asymptomatic but accounts for a mortality rate of 1% to 2%. The risk is greatest during the subacute and convalescent phases, 70% of all deaths occurring 15 to 45 days after the onset of fever.

Congestive heart failure (CHF) is commonly observed, accompanied by carditis with complications such as dysrhythmias, pericarditis, mitral insufficiency, myocardial ischemia, and myocardial infarction.

Ancillary Data

1. White blood cell (WBC) count is frequently elevated with bandemia in the acute phase.
2. Normocytic anemia.
3. Thrombocytosis, usually in the second to third week of illness, often as high as 1 million cells/mm^3. Thrombocytopenia if associated with severe coronary disease or myocardial infarction.
4. ESR is elevated from the first week to 4 to 6 weeks.
5. Elevated C-reactive protein value.
6. Sterile pyuria and proteinuria may be present.
7. Increased serum transaminases and bilirubin values.
8. Aseptic meningitis with CSF pleocytosis may be present.
9. ECG is not diagnostic. Echocardiography or arteriography is often needed to define the extent of coronary artery disease. The most common coronary artery involvement is simple dilation.
10. Results of blood, urine, CSF, and throat culture are negative.

DIFFERENTIAL DIAGNOSIS

Differentiating Kawasaki's disease from other entities is important for both acute care and long-term follow-up (Table 80-1). The patient with this disorder is unlikely to have discrete intraoral lesions, exudative conjunctivitis, or generalized lymphadenopathy.

1. Infection:
   a. Viral: adenovirus, enterovirus, measles, Epstein-Barr virus, rubella
   b. Bacteria: scarlatiniform rash (group A streptococci and *S. aureus*), staphylococcal or streptococcal scalded skin syndrome, toxic shock syndrome
   c. Rickettsial: Rocky Mountain spotted fever
   d. Erythema multiforme: hypersensitivity reaction precipitated by drugs (penicillin, sulfonamides, anticonvulsants), infection (herpes simplex, virus, *Mycoplasma pneumoniae*), malignancies. Stevens-Johnson syndrome is severe form
2. Drug reaction: Stevens-Johnson syndrome, erythema multiforme, sulfonamides
3. Autoimmune: juvenile rheumatoid arthritis (JRA), systemic lupus erythematosus (SLE)

MANAGEMENT

1. Initial stabilization with focus on airway, breathing, and cardiovascular stability.
2. Supportive care is essential; attention is given to fluids, antipyretic agents, and treatment of CHF, if present (see Chapter 16).
3. Intravenous immune gamma globulin (IVIG), 2 g/kg over 10 to 12 hours. Treatment within the first 10 days of illness reduces the rate of cardiac sequelae from 20% to 25% to 2% to 4%. Retreatment may be necessary in 10% of children

TABLE 80-1 Erythroderma: Diagnostic Considerations

Condition	Etiology	Diagnostic Findings
Scarlatiniform rash (p. 291)	Group A streptococcus *S. aureus*	Diffuse erythroderma, prominent flexion creases; fingertip desquamation; pharyngitis; strawberry tongue
Scalded skin syndrome	*S. aureus* phage group 2	Painful erythroderma with bullae and presence of Nikolsky's sign with shedding superficial layers; generally starts on face, neck, axillae, groin; mucous membranes not involved; toxic; may have fluid loss
Toxic epidermal necrolysis (p. 589)	Drugs (penicillin, sulfas, anticonvulsants, NSAIDS); may be part of continuum of erythema multiforme	Tender, erythema of skin and mucosa followed by cutaneous and mucosal blistering, desquamation; Nikolsky's sign present with shedding of entire epidermis; primarily adults; mortality 2° fluid loss, infection
Erythema multiforme (p. 589)	Hypersensitivity, drugs; infection (herpes simplex, other viruses, *Mycoplasma pneumoniae*); malignancy	Erythematous macules or papules progressing to "iris" or "target" lesions (erythematous plaques with dusky center, bright red border); mucous membranes in 25% of patients; usually extremity; may last 2-3 weeks
Stevens-Johnson Syndrome (p. 590)	Severe erythema multiforme with ≥ 2 mucosal surfaces involved	Bullous mucocutaneous lesions that erode; multiple mucosal surfaces; toxic; fever, myalgia, arthralgias; fluid loss, ocular (corneal ulceration), renal involvement
Kawasaki's disease (p. 726)	Unknown	Polymorphous erythroderma; desquamation of tips of fingers and toes; fever; conjunctival injection; red fissured lips; lymphadenopathy
Toxic shock syndrome (p. 736)	*S. aureus* Rarely, group A streptococcus	Diffuse erythroderma; desquamation, especially of palms and soles; fever; shock; multisystem involvement
Leptospirosis	*Leptospira*	Erythematous, macular, papular, petechial, or purpuric rash; fever, conjunctivitis, pharyngitis, lymphadenopathy; multisystem (renal, liver, central nervous system) involvement

whose fever is persistent (lasting longer than 48 to 72 hours) or recrudescent.

4. Aspirin, 80 to 100 mg/kg/day PO q6hr through day 14, when fever has resolved; then aspirin, 3 to 5 mg/kg/day PO qd. Monitoring of salicylate levels is not essential, except in nonresponsive cases, because of decreased absorption and increased clearance. In patients without coronary artery abnormalities, this lower dose is maintained for 6 to 8 weeks or until the platelet count and ESR are normal.
5. A cardiologist should be involved in the management to ensure immediate assessment and long-term follow-up observation. Recommendations for echocardiography include a baseline study during the acute phase with follow-up studies at 2 to 3 weeks and 6 to 8 weeks.
6. Treatment of myocardial infarctions as in adults.
7. Steroids are not indicated and may actually raise the incidence of aneurysms.

DISPOSITION

1. All patients should be hospitalized early in the course of disease for initial stabilization and treatment as well as to ensure adequate and rapid assessment to exclude other diagnostic possibilities.
2. Patients need follow-up for several years after their illness, with particular attention to coronary artery disease; 50% of aneurysms occur within 1 to 2 years of initial diagnosis.

BIBLIOGRAPHY

Akagi T, Rose V, Benson LN et al: Outcome of coronary artery aneurysms after Kawasaki disease, *J Pediatr* 121:689, 1992.

Burns JC: Kawasaki disease, *Adv Pediatr* 48:157, 2001.

Nakamura Y, Fujita Y, Nagai M et al: Cardiac sequelae of Kawasaki disease in Japan: statistical analysis, *Pediatrics* 88:1144, 1991.

Newburger JW: Kawasaki disease, *Curr Treat Options Cardiovasc Med* 2:227, 2000.

Rowley AH, Shulman ST: Kawasaki syndrome, *Pediatr Clin North Am* 2:313, 1999.

Tse SML, Silverman ED, McCrindle BW et al: Early treatment with intravenous immunoglobulins in patients with Kawasaki disease, *J Pediatr* 140:450, 2002.

Williams RV, Minich LL, Tani LY: Pharmacological therapy for patients with Kawasaki disease, *Paediatr Drugs* 3:649, 2001.

Meningococcemia

Neisseria meningitidis is a gram-negative diplococcus responsible for a spectrum of clinical infections. Meningococcemia is life threatening and presents a diagnostic dilemma. In rare cases, *Haemophilus influenzae* infection can produce a comparable clinical picture.

DIAGNOSTIC FINDINGS

1. The onset varies, ranging from insidious to fulminant. The insidious form is particularly difficult to suspect until a skin eruption is present.
2. Patients have fever, malaise, headache, weakness, lethargy, vomiting, and arthralgia as well as signs and symptoms of complicating conditions. Extremity pain or refusal to walk is often associated with invasive disease.
3. Two patterns of skin eruptions are noted:
   a. Pink maculopapular and generalized petechial rash, including palms and soles
   b. Purpuric and ecchymotic (often in a centrifugal distribution), which is associated with a very high mortality
4. Unfavorable prognostic factors include the following:
   a. Presence of petechiae for less than 12 hours before hospitalization
   b. Shock
   c. Absence of meningitis (fewer than 20 WBCs/mm^3 of CSF)
   d. WBC count normal or low (less than 10,000 cells/mm^3)
   e. ESR normal or low (less than 10 mm/hr)
5. Survival is usually determined in the first 12 hours after treatment has begun.

Complications

1. Meningitis or meningoencephalitis (see Chapter 81)
2. Pericarditis (p. 574)
3. Cervicitis
4. Disseminated intravascular coagulation (DIC) (p. 694), Waterhouse-Friderichsen syndrome
5. Hypotension (see Chapter 5), cardiac collapse, and death

Ancillary Data

1. WBC and platelet counts, bleeding screens
2. Cultures of blood, CSF, nasopharynx, and other involved organs
3. Skin scraping of the purpuric lesion may yield a positive culture.

DIFFERENTIAL DIAGNOSIS

(see Table 42-2)

One study of children with fever and petechiae demonstrated that 20% had bacterial infections. Of the infections, 50% were caused by *N. meningitidis*, 30% by *H. influenzae*, and the remainder by a variety of agents.

MANAGEMENT

Patients with meningococcemia need immediate resuscitation (fluids, ventilation and airway support, and pressor agents, if necessary), supportive care, and treatment of complications.

Antibiotics

- Penicillin, 250,000 U/kg/24 hr q4hr IV (maximum: 20 million U/24 hr), for 7 to 10 days

Chloramphenicol for allergic patients; cefotaxime or ceftriaxone may also be considered.

Treatment of Contacts

Contacts are people who have slept or eaten in the same household as the patient with the index case and hospital personnel who have had intimate respiratory contact with the patient, such as would occur with mouth-to-mouth resuscitation. Contacts should be clinically monitored.

Rifampin

1. Children: 10 mg/kg q12hr PO for 2 days
   - To administer to children, a liquid formulation can be prepared. Mixing the powder in vehicles such as applesauce can result in irregular absorption.
2. Adults: 600 mg q12hr PO for 2 days

DISPOSITION

1. All patients with systemic disease must be admitted to an intensive care unit (ICU) with provision for respiratory isolation.
2. Contacts need treatment and should notify the primary physician if fever, headache, stiff neck, or malaise develops. A vaccine is available for administration to high-risk groups; epidemic control may also be an indication.

BIBLIOGRAPHY

Berg S, Trollfors B, Alestig K et al: Incidence, serogroups, and case-fatality of invasive meningococcal infections in a Swedish region 1975-1989, *Scand J Infect Dis* 24:333, 1992.

Olivareis R, Bouyer J, Hubert B: Risk factors for death in meningococcal disease, *Pathol Biol* 41:164, 1993.

Mononucleosis, Infectious

An acute viral illness caused by Epstein-Barr (EB) virus, infectious mononucleosis most frequently occurs in adolescents and young adults.

DIAGNOSTIC FINDINGS

1. Although the severity varies, most patients have a prodrome of 3 to 5 days with malaise, anorexia, nausea, and vomiting.
2. Patients rapidly experience high fevers, pharyngitis, lymphadenopathy, particularly cervical, and splenomegaly. Lymph nodes are usually symmetric, firm, discrete, and mildly to moderately tender.
3. The symptoms may persist for weeks, particularly those associated with the prodrome.

4. Young children may have fever, diarrhea, pharyngitis, otitis media, pneumonia, lymphadenopathy, hepatomegaly, and splenomegaly.
5. An erythematous, maculopapular rash may develop, commonly with the use of ampicillin. It is most prominent on the trunk and proximal extremities.

Complications

Complications are more commonly noted in adolescents than in young adults.

1. Upper airway obstruction from marked tonsillar hypertrophy.
2. Splenic rupture, often preceded by abdominal pain secondary to splenomegaly. Risk is greatest between 14 and 28 days of illness.
3. Hepatitis (p. 649).
4. Autoimmune hemolytic anemia, leukopenia, and thrombocytopenia.
5. Encephalitis or Landry-Guillain-Barré syndrome (see Chapter 41). Oculomotor paralysis.
6. Pericarditis (p. 574).
7. Glomerulonephritis.
8. Orchitis.

Ancillary Data

1. WBC count is elevated, with a marked predominance of lymphocytes, 50% to 90% of which are atypical.
2. Thrombocytopenia.
3. Monospot test. Heterophil antibody test is rarely indicated. Results of both tests are usually negative in children younger than 5 years (EB virus titer may be needed). In adolescents and adults, positive test result is found during the second week of illness.

   Serologic diagnosis can be achieved by measurement of antibody to viral capsid antigen (VCA), which rises above 1:160 during acute infection.
4. Throat culture for identifying group A streptococci, which may be concurrently present; 15% to 18% of patients with infectious mononucleosis have group A streptococci.
5. Liver function tests should be performed in patients with right upper quadrant (RUQ) tenderness.
6. ECG and ABG analysis rarely indicated.

DIFFERENTIAL DIAGNOSIS

1. Infection:
   a. Pharyngitis: group A streptococci, diphtheria, or viral
   b. Toxoplasmosis
   c. Infectious hepatitis
   d. Meningoencephalitis, viral
2. Neoplasm: leukemia or lymphoma

MANAGEMENT

1. Support and symptomatic care are required:
   a. Establishment of an airway if obstructed
   b. Bed rest, fluids, and antipyretics
2. Steroids may be indicated for patients with complications of severe disease (e.g., severe hemolytic anemia, airway obstruction from tonsillar hypertrophy, thrombocytopenia): hydrocortisone (Solu-Cortef), 4 to 5 mg/kg/dose q6hr IV, or prednisone, 1 to 2 mg/kg/24 hr q6hr PO, for 7 days followed by tapering of dosage over 2 weeks.

DISPOSITION

Patients with significant symptoms and complications must be hospitalized. Others may be sent home if hydration, observation, and support will be adequate.

Pertussis (Whooping Cough)

Pertussis (whooping cough) is caused by *Bordetella pertussis* and occurs in all age groups, although its greatest morbidity is in children younger than 1 year. The incidence peaks in late summer and early fall. The incubation period is 7 to 10 days.

DIAGNOSTIC FINDINGS

Three stages categorize the progression of pertussis in children.

1. Catarrhal: minor respiratory complaints of fever, rhinorrhea, and conjunctivitis lasting up to 2 weeks.
2. Paroxysmal: severe cough associated with hypoxia, unremitting paroxysms, and vomiting. As many as 40 episodes/day may occur, and this period may last for 2 to 4 weeks. In rare cases, the cough is associated with apnea.
3. Convalescent: residual cough.

The infant with pertussis often has only a paroxysmal cough and rhinorrhea. Stages are indistinct. Adults often have only rhinorrhea, sore throat, and persistent cough.

Pertussis should be suspected in children younger than 18 months with persistent respiratory illness and vomiting who are poorly immunized. Partially immunized children have less severe disease.

Complications

1. Pneumonia caused by secondary infection
2. Crepitus from subcutaneous or mediastinal emphysema
3. Pneumothorax
4. Seizures and encephalitis
5. Hypoxia
6. Apnea

Ancillary Data

1. WBC count: markedly increased with a tremendous shift to the right (lymphocytosis)
2. Chest x-ray study: peribronchial thickening, infiltrates, and "shaggy" heart border
3. Culture: nasopharyngeal or cough specimen plated on Bordet-Gengou medium
4. Fluorescent antibody (FA) stain of nasopharyngeal swab (a rapid diagnostic technique)

DIFFERENTIAL DIAGNOSIS

Pertussis should be differentiated from other causes of pneumonia (p. 811).

MANAGEMENT

1. Of primary importance is pulmonary support, consisting of oxygen, postural drainage, and, rarely, intubation with sedation. Patients with severe paroxysms should be monitored to ensure that hypoxia and bradycardia are treated.
2. Antibiotic therapy decreases the contagiousness of the patient: erythromycin, 30 to 50 mg/kg/24 hr (adult: 250 mg/dose) q6hr PO (if possible), for 7 to 14 days. It may also shorten the symptomatic course if given early in the catarrhal phase. Additional antibiotics should be given if there is evidence of superinfection.
3. Patients should be isolated. Those exposed may be treated with erythromycin, as already described, for 10 days.
4. Pertussis immune globulin is not effective.
5. Corticosteroids and albuterol may reduce paroxysms of coughing. Further studies are required (p. 790).

DISPOSITION

1. Patients who are younger than 1 year or have any complication should be hospitalized for careful monitoring and pulmonary support.
2. Older children in the catarrhal phase or experiencing only minor paroxysms may be discharged.

Parental Education

1. Importance of active immunization in disease prevention (see Appendix B-7).
2. Prophylaxis and isolation of household and other close contacts of pertussis cases should be considered, as follows:
   a. All household or other close contacts younger than 1 year (regardless of diphtheria-tetanus-pertussis [DTP] immunization status) should receive

14 days of oral erythromycin, 40 mg/kg/24 hr q6hr PO.

b. All household or other close contacts 1 to 7 years old who have received fewer than 4 doses of DTP or whose last dose of DTP was more than 3 years ago should receive 14 days of oral erythromycin, and many recommend a DTP immunization. Alternative agents:
- Zithromax, 10 mg/kg (max: 500 mg) on the first day; then 5 mg/kg (max: 250 mg) days 2 to 5; *or*
- Clarithromycin (Biaxin) 7.5 mg/kg (max: 500 mg) BID PO for 7 days

c. Asymptomatic household or other close contacts need not be excluded from school or work if they are taking antibiotics or their DTP immunization is up to date (4 doses of DTP, the last within 3 years).

d. Persons with a positive laboratory test result for pertussis should be excluded from school or work until they have taken antibiotics for 14 days, although 7 days may be adequate.

e. Adults and children with early symptoms who are household contacts should be excluded from school or work until they have completed 5 days of antibiotic therapy.

f. All household contacts 7 years or older should receive antibiotics if their last DTP was given 3 years ago or longer.

3. If the patient has been discharged, the parent should call the physician immediately if any of the following occurs:

a. Breathing difficulty recurs or worsens.
b. Skin or lips turn blue.
c. Restlessness or sleeplessness develops.
d. Fluid intake decreases.
e. Medicines are not tolerated.

BIBLIOGRAPHY

Halperin SA, Bartoluss R, Langley JM et al: Seven days of erythromycin estolate is as effective as fourteen days for the treatment of *Bordetella pertussis* infection, *Pediatrics* 100:65, 1997.

Yaari E, Yafe-Zimerman Y, Schwartz SB et al: Clinical manifestations of *Bordetella pertussis* infection in immunized children and young adults, *Chest* 115:1254, 1999.

Rabies

Although rare, rabies in humans is a fatal viral disease resulting from skin or mucous membrane contact with an infected animal. The incubation is 10 days to several months after the initial exposure, the duration reflecting the site and severity of the wound. The primary goal must be prevention.

DIAGNOSTIC FINDINGS

Initially, hypoesthesia or paresthesia is noted at the site of injury. Progression of symptoms, including hydrophobia, apprehension, and hyperexcitability associated with a clear sensorium, is rapid. Seizures, delirium, and lethargy are noted in the period before death in 5 to 7 days. Cardiovascular, respiratory, and CNS instability may be noted in the interim.

Ancillary Data

Rabies virus may be isolated from the saliva or brain of infected individuals. Examination of the biting animal's brain with fluorescent antibody testing or Negri body identification, confirmed by viral isolation, provides additional verification.

MANAGEMENT

Although the mortality rate is extremely high, there have been several cases of survival with intense, supportive care.

Prevention of Rabies

Risk Factors

1. Bites and wounds inflicted by animals must be individually considered with regard to the risk of rabies. Skunks, foxes, coyotes, raccoons, wild dogs and cats, and bats are most commonly infected.

Rodents (mice, rats, squirrels, chipmunks), rabbits, and hares are not normally considered to be risks.

2. The circumstances of the biting incident must be considered. Unprovoked attacks are more likely than provoked attacks to indicate that the animal was rabid.
3. The type of exposure is a factor. Rabies is transmitted by the introduction of virus into open cuts or wounds in skin or via mucous membranes:
   a. Bite: any penetration of the skin by teeth
   b. Nonbite: scratches, abrasions, open wounds, or mucous membrane contaminated with saliva
4. Epizootic conditions of rabies in the area should be considered.

Management of the Biting Animal

1. A healthy domestic dog or cat should be confined and observed for 10 days. If any suggestive signs develop, the animal should be killed, and the head removed and shipped under refrigeration to the designated health department, provided that there is risk of rabies in the area. A stray or wild dog or cat should be killed and its brain examined.
2. A wild animal that has bitten or scratched a person should be killed and its brain examined.

Local Treatment of the Wound

1. Immediate and thorough washing and debridement are appropriate.
2. Tetanus prophylaxis should be given, if indicated.

Immunization (Table 80-2)

Antirabies immunization after exposure should include both passively administered antibody and vaccine unless the patient has been immunized before exposure.

1. Read the instructions for administration carefully on inserts for products. If immune globulin or vaccine is unavailable, call the CDC (daytime phone: 404-639-3670; nighttime/weekend/holiday phone: 404-639-2888).
2. Human rabies immune globulin (HRIG) is supplied in 2- and 10-ml (150 IU/ml) vials. It should be administered at a dose of 20 IU/kg. If anatomically feasible, approximately half the dose is used to infiltrate the wound and the remainder is given IM.
3. Human diploid cell rabies vaccine (HDCV) (Imovax Rabies) is administered IM in five 1-ml doses; the first dose is administered at the time of exposure, followed by the remaining doses at 3, 7, 14, and 28 days. Rabies vaccine absorbed (RVA) is another option.
4. Preexposure HDCV (Imovax Rabies) may be administered to at-risk individuals. In adults, give 1 ml IM in 3 doses at 0, 7, and 28 days with a booster every 2 years. May also be given 0.1 ml intradermally according to the same schedule. If the antibody titer is 1:5 or above, the booster may be omitted, and the patient monitored. RVA may also be used.

BIBLIOGRAPHY

Centers for Disease Control: Human rabies prevention, US–1999, *MMWR* 48:1, 1999.

Tetanus

Tetanus results from puncture or other wounds with the introduction of *Clostridium tetani*, which produces a neurotoxin. Severe skeletal muscle hypertonicity occurs. The incubation period ranges from 3 days to 3 weeks (average: 8 days). Generally, the shorter the incubation period, the more severe the clinical presentation.

DIAGNOSTIC FINDINGS

1. A wound is present in 80% of patients.
2. The onset of symptoms is marked by increased tone of the skeletal

TABLE 80-2 Rabies Postexposure Prophylaxis Guide

Species of Animal	Condition of Animal at Time of Attack	Treatment of Exposed Human*
DOMESTIC		
Dog, cat, ferret	Healthy and available for 10 days of observation	None†
	Rapid or suspected rabid; unknown	HRIG and HDCV; consult public health officer†
WILD		
Skunk, bat, fox, coyote, raccoon, bobcat, and other carnivores	Regard as rabid unless proved negative by laboratory test or geographic area is known to be free of rabies‡	HRIG and HDCV
OTHER		
Livestock, rodents; lagomorphs (rabbits, hares)	Consider individually. Squirrels, hamsters, guinea pigs, gerbils,chipmunks, rats, mice, rabbits, and hares are almost never considered to be rabid.	

Adapted from American Academy of Pediatrics: *Report of the committee on infectious diseases,* Elk Grove, Ill, 2000. These recommendations are only a guide. They should be applied in conjunction with information about the animal species involved, the circumstances of the exposure, the vaccination status of the animal, and the presence of rabies in the region.

HRIG, Human rabies immune globulin; *HDCV,* human diploid cell rabies vaccine.

* All bites and wounds should immediately be thoroughly cleansed with soap and water. If antirabies treatment is indicated, both HRIG and HDCV should be given as soon as possible, regardless of the interval from exposure.

† During the usual holding period of 10 days, begin treatment with HRIG and HDCV at the first sign of rabies in the animal. The symptomatic animal should be killed immediately and examined.

‡ The animal should be killed and tested as soon as possible. Holding for observation is not recommended. Discontinue treatment if test findings are negative.

muscles that initially involves the jaw and neck. This becomes generalized over the next 24 to 48 hours, with spasms increasing in frequency and intensity.

   a. Trismus: inability to open the mouth because of spasms of the masseter muscles
   b. Risus sardonicus: peculiar, sustained facial distortion
   c. Opisthotonic posturing from spasms of neck and back
   d. Boardlike abdomen
   e. Stiff and extended extremities

3. A low-grade fever, headache, tachycardia, and anxiety are often present. The sensorium is totally normal.
4. Tetanus neonatorum occurs in the first 3 to 10 days of life; it is marked by muscle rigidity, particularly of the jaw and neck, difficulty swallowing, and irritability.

Complications

1. Respiratory: laryngospasm, pneumonia, pulmonary edema, and respiratory failure
2. Compression or subluxation injuries of the vertebrae

Ancillary Data

1. WBC count: variably increased
2. LP and CSF analysis: normal
3. ABG analysis: indicated if there is respiratory compromise

TABLE 80-3 Schedule for Td Toxoid and TIG at Time of Exposure

	CLEAN, MINOR WOUNDS		ALL OTHER WOUNDS*	
History of Tetanus Immunizations	**Td**	**TIG**	**Td**	**TIG**
Uncertain or less than 3 doses	Yes	No	Yes	Yes
3 or more doses‡	No†§	No	No†‖	No

Adapted from American Academy of Pediatrics: *Report of the committee on infectious diseases*, Elk Grove, Ill, 2000.
Td, Tetanus diphtheria; *TIG*, tetanus immune globulin.
* Including but not limited to, contaminated wounds as well as puncture wounds, avulsions, and wounds resulting from missiles, crushing, burns, and frostbite.
† If only 3 doses of fluid toxoid have been previously received, a fourth dose of absorbed toxoid should be given.
‡ Single dose of 3000 to 6000 units IM.
§ Unless >10 yr have elapsed since the last dose.
‖ Unless >5 yr have elapsed since the last dose.

4. Vertebral x-ray films: for patients with pain and severe opisthotonic posturing

DIFFERENTIAL DIAGNOSIS

1. Trauma: head and neck
2. Infection: dental abscess, peritonsillar abscess
3. Intoxication: phenothiazines, strychnine
4. Endocrine/metabolic: hypocalcemia (tetany)
5. Intrapsychic: hysteria, conversion reaction

MANAGEMENT

At Time of Exposure

1. Tetanus and diphtheria (Td) toxoid and tetanus immune globulin (TIG) are indicated (see schedule in Table 80-3 and Appendix B-7). DT (pediatric) may be used for children less than 6 years of age.
2. The wound must be cleansed and debrided.

Treatment of Acute Disease

1. The patient must have immediate evaluation and support of the airway with oxygen and active intervention, when indicated.
2. Muscle spasms and associated pain must be controlled with the following:
   - Diazepam (Valium), 0.1 to 0.3 mg/kg/dose q4-8hr IV or 0.1 to 0.8 mg/kg/24 hr q6-8hr PO; minimize external stimuli
3. Tetanus immune globulin antitoxin should be administered, 3000 to 6000 units IM, with a portion infiltrated around the wound.
4. An antibiotic should be given: penicillin G, 100,000 U/kg/24 hr q4hr IV for 10 to 14 days.

Prevention

Active immunization (see Appendix B-7) is recommended.

DISPOSITION

1. All patients with tetanus must be admitted to an ICU.
2. Patients with tetanus exposure may be discharged after appropriate immunologic therapy.

BIBLIOGRAPHY

Richardson J, Knight A: The management and prevention of tetanus, *J Emerg Med* 11:737, 1993.

Toxic Shock Syndrome

Toxic shock syndrome (TSS) primarily affects menstruating young women; however, nonmenstruating women, men, and premenarcheal girls have also had the syndrome, usually in association with a definable site of infection.

ETIOLOGY: INFECTION

1. Although the pathophysiology remains unclear, a toxic shock syndrome toxin-1 (TSST-1), elaborated by coagulase-positive *S. aureus* (phage group I), is absorbed through the vaginal mucosa, causing systemic signs and symptoms.
2. There is a temporal relationship between tampon use, menstruation, and the onset of the syndrome.

DIAGNOSTIC FINDINGS

The onset of the illness is often preceded by a prodromal illness lasting less than 12 hours and consisting of high fever, profuse diarrhea, and vomiting. Patients typically seek medical care 12 to 18 hours after prodromal illness, usually because of dizziness or confusion.

Clinically, a diagnosis of TSS can be made only if the following features are present:

1. Fever >38.9° C
2. Rash (diffuse, blanching macular, erythematous, nonpruritic); erythroderma
3. Desquamation 1 to 2 weeks after the onset of illness, particularly on the palms and soles
4. Hypotension (systolic blood pressure 90 mm Hg for adults or less than 5% by age for children or orthostatic changes), usually with hypovolemia
5. Involvement of three or more of the following organ systems:
   - **a.** Gastrointestinal: vomiting or diarrhea, usually at the onset of illness
   - **b.** Muscular: severe myalgia
   - **c.** Mucous membrane: vaginal, oropharyngeal, or conjunctival hyperemia
   - **d.** Renal: blood urea nitrogen (BUN) or creatinine level at least twice normal or more than 5 WBCs per high-power field (HPF) on urine examination with no urinary tract infection (UTI)
   - **e.** Hepatic: bilirubin, serum glutamic oxaloacetic transaminase (SGOT), or serum glutamic pyruvic transaminase (SGPT) level at least twice normal
   - **f.** Hematologic: platelet count 100,000 cells/mm^3 or lower
   - **g.** CNS: disorientation or alteration in consciousness without focal signs
6. Negative results on the following tests, if obtained: serologic tests for Rocky Mountain spotted fever, leptospirosis, or measles, and cultures of blood, throat, and CSF.

   NOTE: Blood culture may grow *S. aureus* (variable).

Patients often have a 2-day prodrome, composed of fever, vomiting, diarrhea, and myalgia. Sore throat is a prominent complaint.

Group A streptococcal sepsis is similar to toxic shock syndrome; it is mediated by a pyrogenic exotoxin A elaborated by the streptococcus. Clinically, in addition to the primary infection, erythroderma, hypotension, DIC, renal dysfunction, hypoalbuminemia, hypocalcemia, and respiratory failure develop over several days. The onset of illness is often preceded by pain at the site of the skin lesion; local necrosis may occur. Patients may also have fever, chills, myalgia, diarrhea, and subsequent desquamation.

Complications

1. Cardiovascular collapse and shock with myocardial failure.
2. Adult respiratory distress syndrome with pulmonary edema. More common in children younger than 10 years.
3. Coagulopathy with DIC is usually mild.
4. Recurrence. Usually mild, not meeting all criteria.

Ancillary Data

1. Hematologic: increased WBC count with shift to left, thrombocytopenia, and variable coagulation study results.

2. Chemistry: electrolyte, BUN, creatinine, and calcium levels may be abnormal. Elevations of liver function values and serum bilirubin are common.
3. Urinalysis: proteinuria and pyuria.
4. Cultures: vaginal culture for *S. aureus*. Blood, throat, and CSF culture results vary. Group A streptococcus should be sought as well.
5. Chest x-ray study and ABG analysis in a patient with respiratory distress.

DIFFERENTIAL DIAGNOSIS

See Table 80-1.

MANAGEMENT

General supportive care is essential because of the multisystem involvement of the disease and the progressive nature of organ involvement.

1. Fluids for hypotension and abnormal loss from vomiting and diarrhea. Often very large volumes of fluids are required, with two to five times normal maintenance fluids being necessary. Fluids should not be restricted or diuretics administered unless an adequate filling pressure can be maintained.
2. Pressor agents may be required for significant hypotension unresponsive to fluid therapy: dopamine, 5 to 15 μg/kg/min IV constant infusion, often in combination with other pressors after volume deficits have been replaced. Echocardiography and Swan-Ganz catheter monitoring are indicated if myocardial failure is noted.
3. Ventilatory support with positive end-expiratory pressure (PEEP), particularly in the presence of adult respiratory distress syndrome (ARDS) with pulmonary edema.
4. If incriminated, removal of tampon and irrigation of vagina. Aggressive drainage of sites of staphylococcal infection must be achieved. Abscesses and empyemas always need surgical drainage.
5. Antibiotics should be initiated, although their role is unclear. They decrease the incidence of recurrence but do not clearly alter the course of the illness. The patient is given:
   - Nafcillin, 100 to 200 mg/kg/24 hr (adult: 1 g/dose) q4hr IV (or equivalent β-lactamase–resistant penicillin), for at least 7 days; *or*
   - Cephalosporin: cephalothin (Keflin), 75 to 150 mg/kg/24 hr (adult: 1 g/dose) q4hr IV
6. Corticosteroid therapy reduces the severity of illness and duration of fever if initiated within 2 to 3 days of illness: methylprednisolone (Solu-Medrol), 10 to 20 mg/kg/24 hr IV.
7. Calcium supplementation is usually required.
8. Renal dialysis may be needed if renal failure develops.
9. Patients with group A streptococcal sepsis, in addition to the support noted, must be given penicillin, 100,000 U/kg/24 hr q4hr IV.

DISPOSITION

Hospitalization is needed for all patients with definite TSS because of the progression of findings. Admission to an ICU is usually indicated.

Upon discharge, long-term monitoring for renal and neuromuscular sequelae is essential.

BIBLIOGRAPHY

Bergovac J, Marton E, Lisic M et al: Group A beta-hemolytic streptococcal toxic shock-like syndrome, *Pediatr Infect Dis J* 9:369, 1990.

Resnick S: Toxic shock syndrome recent developments in pathogenesis, *J Pediatr* 116:321, 1990.

Todd JK, Ressman M, Caston SA et al: Corticosteroid therapy for patients with toxic-shock syndrome, *JAMA* 252:3399, 1984.

Tuberculosis

The resurgence in the United States of tuberculosis caused by *Mycobacterium tuberculosis* has been well documented to be caused by coinfection in patients with HIV as well as the decline in access to rapid diagnosis and treatment and increasing immigration from high-prevalence countries. The disease results from the inhalation of aerosol droplets produced by individuals with infectious pulmonary tuberculosis. Children rarely transmit the disease because of insufficient inoculum in their respiratory tracts.

DIAGNOSTIC FINDINGS

The period from exposure to positive result of a tuberculin skin test is usually 2 to 10 weeks. Most infections resolve without disease. Manifestations occur in the first 6 to 11 months, causing either pulmonary or extrapulmonary findings. Extrapulmonary disease consists of miliary tuberculosis, meningitis, and lymphadenitis, and renal, bone, and joint involvement.

Most patients are identified through routine skin testing or chest x-ray films.

Ancillary Data

1. Tuberculin Mantoux skin test (5 units): A positive test result is defined as induration 15 mm or larger in healthy patients and 5 mm or larger in a patient with HIV infection, documented exposure, or radiographic evidence of disease. Induration of 10 mm or more is a positive result in patients from high-incidence or medically underserved areas as well as those from long-term care facilities. Additional consideration should be given to IV drug users and those who have diabetes, immunosuppression from steroid or other therapy, and end-stage renal disease.
2. Culture specimens should be obtained for isolation and identification of antibiotic sensitivity patterns. Gastric aspirate is often helpful, especially in children younger than 1 year.
3. Chest x-ray films should be obtained in all patients with positive culture or skin test results.

MANAGEMENT

1. Patients with a positive skin test result should be started on preventive therapy with isoniazid (INH), 10 mg/kg/24 hr for 9 months.
2. Uncomplicated pulmonary disease is treated with a 6-month course of therapy:
   a. For the first 2 months: INH, 10 mg/kg/24 hr; rifampin, 10 to 15 mg/kg/24 hr; and pyrazinamide, 20 to 30 mg/kg/24 hr for the first 2 months.
   b. For remaining 4 months: twice-weekly INH, 20 to 40 mg/kg/dose, and rifampin, 10 to 20 mg/kg/24 hr.
3. Tuberculous meningitis, miliary disease, or bone or joint infection requires prolonged therapy and infectious disease consultation.

BIBLIOGRAPHY

Barnes PF, Bloch AB, Davidson PT et al: Tuberculosis in patients with human immunodeficiency infection, *N Engl J Med* 324:1644, 1991.

Committee on Infectious Disease: *Report of the Committee*, Elk Grove, Ill, 2000, American Academy of Pediatrics.

Hoge CW, Schwartz KB, Talkington DF et al: The changing epidemiology of invasive group A streptococcal infections and the emergence of streptococcal shock-like syndrome: a retrospective population-based study, *JAMA* 269:384, 1993.

Huebner R, Schein M, Bass J: The tuberculin test, *Adv Pediatr Infect Dis* 8:23, 1993.

Jacobs R, Eisenach K: Childhood tuberculosis, *Adv Pediatr Infect Dis* 8:23, 1993.

Snider JDE, Roper WL: The new tuberculosis, *N Engl J Med* 326:703, 1992.

Starke JR, Jacobs RF, Jereb J: Resurgence of tuberculosis in children, *J Pediatr* 120:839, 1992.

81 Neurologic Disorders

Also See Chapters 15 (Coma), 21 (Status Epilepticus), 23 (Syncope), 28 (Ataxia), 36 (Headache), 39 (Irritability), 41 (Paralysis and Hemiplegia), 57 (Head Trauma), and 61 (Spine and Spinal Cord Trauma)

Breath-Holding Spells

Breath-holding spells may result after prolonged crying, producing cyanosis and, ultimately, loss of consciousness. They have a median age at onset of 6 to 12 months and may continue until 4 years of age. Fifteen percent of cases occur in children younger than 6 months. A family history is present in 34% of children.

DIAGNOSTIC FINDINGS

1. Vigorous crying is precipitated by a fall or injury or by anger. The child subsequently becomes cyanotic, unconscious, and limp. The episodes are self-limited, lasting less than 1 minute.
2. Some evidence of disturbance at home or in the maternal-child interaction may be evident. Youth of parents, maternal depression, or difficulty in setting limits can usually be detected.

Complications

Tonic-clonic seizures may be noted as a result of cerebral hypoxia in less than 15% of children with breath-holding spells.

DIFFERENTIAL DIAGNOSIS

It is usually easy to differentiate breath-holding spells from a seizure. Patients with seizures lose consciousness and then become cyanotic; the reverse is true with breath-holding spells, which rarely occur at night. It is important to note that cerebral anoxia may cause brief seizures with breath-holding spells.

MANAGEMENT

1. Reassurance and calmness of the parents must be emphasized. The episodes are self-limited. Behavior patterns that initiate breath-holding spells and secondary gain from that behavior must be reduced.
2. Anticonvulsants are not indicated. The focus must be on behavior modification and family support.

Parental Education

1. Minimize the events or factors that trigger the spells.
2. Attempt to be firm and consistent in management of behavior problems.
3. Call the physician if the nature, duration, or frequency of the breath-holding spells changes.

BIBLIOGRAPHY

DiMario FJ: Breath-holding spells in childhood, *Am J Dis Child* 146:125, 1992.

DiMario FJ: Prospective study of children with cyanotic and pallid breath-holding spells, *Pediatrics* 107:265, 2001.

Gordon N: Breath-holding spells, *Dev Med Child Neurol* 29:805, 1987.

Mattie-Luksic M, Javornisky G, DiMario FJ: Assessment of stress in mothers of children with severe breath-holding spells, *Pediatrics* 106:1, 2000.

Meningitis

ALERT Infections elsewhere do not exclude the presence of meningitis. The younger the child with meningitis, the less specific the presenting signs and symptoms. In unstable patients with suspected meningitis, immediate attention to the ABCs (airway, breathing, circulation) and empiric treatment (after specimens have been obtained for blood studies including culture) with antibiotics may be needed.

ETIOLOGY: INFECTION

1. Bacterial:
   a. The child's age is the predominant determinant of the common bacterial causes:

Age Group	Predominant Organism
<2 mo	*Escherichia coli*, group B streptococci *(S. agalactiae), Listeria monocytogenes, Haemophilus influenzae, Neisseria meningitidis, Streptococcus pneumoniae*
2 mo to 9 yr	*S. pneumoniae, H. influenzae, N. meningitidis*
>9 yr	*N. meningitidis, S. pneumoniae*

   The incidence of *H. influenzae* meningitis has dramatically declined since the introduction of routine immunization.

   b. Ventriculoperitoneal (VP) shunt: 25% of patients with VP shunts have infections associated with alterations in the shunt, usually caused by *Staphylococcus epidermidis* and, less commonly, *Staphylococcus aureus.* Less common organisms may be gram negative *(E. coli, Klebsiella pneumoniae, Pseudomonas aeruginosa*) or anaerobic *(Propionibacterium acnes).*
2. Viral: most commonly enteroviral (Table 81-1).
3. Fungal and *Mycobacterium tuberculosis:* uncommon, but should be considered if endemic or patient is immunocompromised.

DIAGNOSTIC FINDINGS: BACTERIAL MENINGITIS

1. In younger children, the initial presentation is nonspecific, consisting of fever, hypothermia, dehydration, bulging fontanelle, lethargy, irritability, anorexia, vomiting, seizures, respiratory distress, or cyanosis (Table 81-2). Children younger than 12 months are commonly toxic in appearance with impaired mental status. The diagnosis may therefore be difficult to confirm clinically; lumbar puncture (LP) with analysis of cerebrospinal fluid (CSF) remains the definitive test.
2. Older patients may have the symptoms listed in item 1 as well as the more classic findings such as nuchal rigidity, Kernig's sign (pain on extension of legs), Brudzinski's sign (flexion of the neck produces flexion at knees and hips), and headaches. Meningeal signs are present in 87% of children older than 12 months. Otitis media is often present.
3. Historically, the progression of illness, associated symptoms, exposures, and underlying health problems are important.
4. Partially treated children with bacterial meningitis less commonly have a temperature above 38.3° C and altered mental status. Immunization to prevent *H. influenzae* disease has reduced the incidence of associated meningitis. Similarly, immunization may be able to reduce the incidence of meningitis caused by *S. pneumoniae.*
5. The distinction between a simple febrile seizure and a seizure-complicating meningitis is difficult to make in younger children and often requires an LP (p. 763). In one study, 23% of patients with *S. pneumoniae* meningitis had seizures.
6. Patients with a VP or other shunt may have a somewhat different presentation in association with a low-grade ventriculitis, including headache, nausea, minimal fever, and malaise.

TABLE 81-1 Viral Meningoencephalitis

Agent	Epidemiology	Clinical Manifestations
ENTEROVIRUS	Epidemic, with summer and fall peak incidence; all ages affected, particularly <12 yr	Most common; usually mild; rash often present; rarely with focal findings or sequelae
MUMPS	Epidemic, occurring year-round with increase in spring; all ages affected, particularly 2- to 14-year-old children	Mild to moderate meningoencephalitis accompanied by parotitis (>50%); focal findings and sequelae rare
HERPES SIMPLEX	Year-round; most commonly affecting patients <1 yr and >15 yr	Severe and progressive encephalitis; 50%-75% having focal findings; severe motor and mental deficits occur in as many as 75% of survivors; high mortality rate; treatment: acyclovir, support
OTHER		
California equine	Occurs in rural areas with peak incidence in June-Oct; 5- to 9-year-old children most commonly affected	Mild meningoencephalitis with accompanying seizures (50%) and focal findings (15%-40%); long-term behavioral problems (15%-20%)
St. Louis equine	Peaks in July-Oct; adults primarily involved	Commonly asymptomatic in children
Western equine	July-Oct peak incidence; primarily (20%-30%) affects infants	Sudden high fever with focal or generalized seizures, rare focal findings and coma; sequelae occur in >50% of children affected in first year of life

TABLE 81-2 Bacterial Meningitis: Presentation By Age

Diagnostic Findings	<2-3 Mo	2-3 Mo-2 Yr	>2 Yr
Apnea/cyanosis	Common	Rare	Rare
Fever	Common	Common	Common
Hypothermia	Common	Rare	Rare
Altered mental status	Common	Common	Common
Headache	Rare	Rare	Common
Seizures	Early finding	Early finding	Late finding
Ataxia	Rare	Variable	Early finding
Jitteriness	Common	Common	Rare
Vomiting	Common	Common	Variable
Stiff neck	Rare	Late finding	Common
Bulging fontanelle	Common	Common	Closed

a. Components of a VP shunt: The ventricular catheter is passed into the anterior horns of the lateral ventricles through a right occipital or frontal burr hole. The catheter is attached subcutaneously to a reservoir that may be percutaneously tapped to obtain ventricular fluid. This reservoir is attached to a distal catheter containing a pump and one-way valve to regulate pressure and flow in the system. The distal catheter commonly passes into the peritoneum.

b. Assessment of shunt function: The reservoir is pumped; this is normally done easily with a rapid refill of the reservoir in less than 3 seconds. If it cannot be depressed, there is a distal block, whereas if it pumps but does not refill, it is blocked proximally, at the ventricular end. Poor pumping may indicate a relative dysfunction. Pressure may be assessed by percutaneous needle access of the reservoir: High pressure indicates distal obstruction, whereas low pressure suggests proximal obstruction or overdrained ventricles. One third of obstructed shunts are infected.

c. Withdrawing fluid from the shunt for analysis or because of abnormal pumping is usually performed in conjunction with a neurosurgeon. A computed tomography (CT) study and plain radiographs comparing the present status with previous findings may be helpful in the assessment.

7. Aseptic (viral, fungal, mycobacterial) meningoencephalitis usually has a less toxic and acute clinical manifestation. Diagnosis of encephalitis is often made on the basis of clinical evaluation (see Table 81-1).

Complications of Bacterial Meningitis

1. Cerebral edema with potential for increased intracranial pressure (ICP) and herniation. The sickest patients are at greatest risk, particularly after LP. These patients have focal neurologic signs, unresponsiveness, and decerebrate posturing.
2. Septic shock and disseminated intravascular coagulation, particularly with *N. meningitidis* although also in association with all organisms.
3. Bacteremia with associated hematogenous involvement of joints (particularly the hip), pericardium, and myocardium.
4. Inappropriate antidiuretic hormone (ADH) with hyponatremia.
5. Subdural effusion and empyema. Of patients aged 1 to 18 months, 39% have subdural effusions. Associated risk factors are young age, rapid onset of illness, low peripheral white blood cell (WBC) count, and high CSF protein level. Initially, patients with subdural effusions are more likely to have seizures, but on long-term follow-up, they do not have a higher incidence of seizures, hearing loss, neurologic deficits, or developmental delay. Specific therapy may not be required, but consultation is indicated.
6. Anemia, especially with *H. influenzae.*
7. Of patients with meningococcal or pneumococcal meningitis, 90% are afebrile by the sixth day, in contrast to only 72% of those with *H. influenzae* as the etiologic agent. Conditions associated with persistent fever are untreated disease, subdural effusion, nosocomial infection, phlebitis, and drug fever.

   The widespread use of dexamethasone (Decadron) in patients with bacterial meningitis has altered this pattern, particularly in children with *H. influenzae* disease. These children may have a relatively low temperature early in the illness with an elevated temperature becoming evident once steroids are stopped on day 4.
8. Neurologic findings, both transient and persistent, may include deficits in cranial nerves (particularly CN VI), hearing, vision, and retardation as well as later behavioral problems. Follow-up evaluation of children with bacterial meningitis in one study noted that 14% had persistent deficits (10% sensorineural hearing loss and 4% multiple neurologic problems) 1 year after the illness; 7% had one or more late seizures not associated with fever. A study of patients with *S. pneumoniae* meningitis suggested a morbidity of

20% to 30% and a case-fatality rate lower than 10%.

9. Children with viral aseptic meningitis often are not toxic and do not have meningeal signs.

Ancillary Data

Lumbar Puncture (see Appendix A-4)

1. CSF is the basis for evaluation of the patient with clinical signs of meningitis. Analysis of the fluid is essential (Table 81-3). Meningitis may exist in the absence of a CSF pleocytosis.
2. Partial treatment with antibiotics before LP rarely alters the CSF enough to interfere with an appropriate interpretation. The blood culture, Gram stain of CSF, and latex agglutination testing are useful in identifying the causative organisms in patients receiving antibiotics before the LP is performed.

LP results after pretreatment with third-generation cephalosporins are as follows:

- Meningococcal meningitis: one-third sterile within 1 hour and all sterile by 2 hours
- Pneumococcal meningitis: negative cultures usually noted by 4 hours; positive culture results were present in the setting of decreased susceptibility

TABLE 81-3 Cerebrospinal Fluid Analysis

	NORMAL				
	Preterm*	**Term**	**>6 Mo**	**Bacterial**	**Viral**
Cell count (WBC/mm^3)†					
Mean	9	8	0	>500	<500
Range	0-25	0-22	0-4		
Predominant cell type	Lymph	Lymph	Lymph	80% PMN leukocytes	PMN leukocytes initially, may be lymphocytes later
Glucose (mg/dl)					
Mean	50	52	>40	<40	>40
Range	24-63	34-119			
Protein (mg/dl)					
Mean	115	90	<40	>100	<100
Range	65-150	20-170			
CSF/blood glucose (%)					
Mean	74	81	50	<40	>40
Range	55-150	44-248	40-60		
Gram stain	Negative	Negative	Negative	Positive‡§	Negative
Bacterial culture	Negative	Negative	Negative	Positive‡§	Negative

Modified from Sarff LD, Platt LH, McCracken GH Jr: *J Pediatr* 88:473, 1976; Portnoy JM, Olson LC: *Pediatrics* 75:484, 1985; and Rodriguez AF, Kaplan SC, Mason ED: *J Pediatr* 116:971, 1990.

* Infants <1000 g have a mean cell count of 4 ± 3 WBC/mm^3 (range 0-14 cells/mm^3). The mean protein level is 150 ± 56 mg/dl (range 95-370 mg/dl) and glucose of 61 ± 34 mg/dl (range 29-217 mg/dl). Infants 1001-1500 g have a mean cell count of 6 ± 9 WBC/mm^3 (range 0-44 cells/mm^3). The mean protein level is 132 ± 43 mg/dl (range 5-227 mg/dl) and glucose of 59 ± 21 (range 31-109 mg/dl).

† Total WBC/mm^3 by age in the normal child can be further delineated as follows (mean ± 2 SD): <6 wk: 3.7 ± 6.8; 6 wk-3 mo: 2.9 ± 5.7; 3 mo-6 mo: 1.9 ± 4.0; 6-12 mo: 2.6 ± 4.9; >12 mo: 1.9 ± 5.4

‡ If Gram stain finding is negative, a methylene blue stain may distinguish intracellular bacteria from nuclear material.

§ Of partially treated patients 85% will have a positive Gram stain result and >95% have positive culture findings. Counterimmunoelectrophoresis (CIE) may be helpful if the culture result is negative.

3. Although conflicting evidence exists regarding the potential risk of seeding the meninges with bacteria when performing an LP in the bacteremic patient, this consideration should not delay obtaining CSF in patients who are clinically at risk of having meningitis. The occurrence of meningitis after bacteremia is related to the organism causing the bacteremia rather than to whether the patient underwent an LP.
4. If it is difficult to distinguish bacterial from viral meningitis on the basis of the initial CSF results, an enteroviral polymerase chain reaction (PCR) test may be useful.

   Approximately 57% of children with aseptic meningitis during enteroviral season have a predominance of polymorphonuclear (PMN) leukocytes. In many patients, the second LP specimen still shows a predominance of PMN leukocytes even when collected more than 5.8 hours after the first LP and more than 48 hours after the onset of signs and symptoms.
5. An LP may appropriately be delayed if the patient is hemodynamically unstable, there is evidence of increased ICP, infection is present in the area to be traversed by the needle, or the procedure cannot logistically be performed. A blood culture specimen should be obtained before antibiotic therapy is started; antibiotic therapy should not be delayed.

   LP should be performed only cautiously, if at all, in the patient with suspected papilledema, neurologic findings, unresponsiveness, decerebrate posturing, or increased ICP or in patients who are uncooperative. Consultation and CT scan are usually indicated before an LP is performed.
6. In patients with bacterial meningitis, a second LP may be done at 36 to 48 hours, and a third 10 days after initiation of therapy if the clinical response has been slow or the therapy inadequate. Otherwise, repeat LPs are rarely required.
7. Bloody spinal taps create a diagnostic dilemma:
   a. Hemorrhage into the subarachnoid space caused by bleeding results in equal numbers of red blood cells (RBCs) in the first and last samples of fluid. The fluid should be xanthochromic after centrifugation.
   b. Although the appraisal may be inexact and fraught with errors, the number of leukocytes in spinal fluid obtained after a traumatic tap may be estimated as follows:
      (1) 1000 RBCs/mm^3 contribute 1 or 2 WBCs/mm^3.
      (2) Number of WBCs introduced per mm^3:

$$\frac{(\text{Peripheral WBCs}) \times (\text{RBCs in CSF})}{\text{Peripheral RBC count}}$$

      (3) The result is then compared with the actual number of WBCs counted in the CSF.
      (4) 1000 RBCs/mm^3 in the CSF raises the protein level by about 1.5 mg/dl.
8. Cultures for tuberculosis or fungi may be done, if indicated.
9. Determinations of CSF lactic acid and lactate dehydrogenase (LDH) have not proved to be of value.
10. A ratio of immature to mature neutrophils greater than 0.12:1 is associated with, and is more sensitive for, the presence of bacterial meningitis than total peripheral WBC count. However, it is not sensitive enough to diagnose or exclude meningitis without an LP.
11. Approximately 90% of children with VP shunts in whom the CSF WBC count is higher than 100 cells/mm^3 are infected.

The leukocyte count in the malfunctioning shunt is 18 WBCs/mm^3, in contrast to an average of 156 WBCs/mm^3 in an infected shunt. The CSF glucose level is usually normal, and the organisms are usually less virulent.

12. The infant's airway should never be compromised during LP. This precaution is particularly important in small infants who are held tightly, which could potentially cause suffocation or impaired central venous return.

Blood Cultures. Blood cultures may provide bacteriologic confirmation of the infecting organism and should always be obtained. A blood culture is positive in nearly 100% of patients with *S. pneumoniae* or *H. influenzae* meningitis, if pretreated children are excluded.

Cultures of Infected Sites. Aspirates of purpuric lesions, joints, and abscesses or middle ear infections should be obtained.

Counterimmunoelectrophoresis. Rapid bacteriologic diagnosis may be possible through the detection of antisera against capsular antigen to *H. influenzae* type B, *S. pneumoniae, N. meningitidis,* and group B streptococcus. This method is useful in children who have previously received antibiotics. The limited sensitivity and specificity restrict the usefulness of bacterial antigen detection tests (BADTs) as routine evaluations. An enteroviral PCR analysis may be useful if aseptic meningitis is suspected.

Other Studies

1. A specimen for blood glucose measurement should be obtained before LP is performed.
2. WBC and platelet counts. The peripheral WBC count may be noted to increase after the LP.
3. Electrolyte determinations. Should initially be performed every 1 to 2 days to monitor for inappropriate ADH.
4. PCR analysis may be useful in achieving an early diagnosis of herpes and enterovirus.

Chest X-Ray Film. A film should be taken if there are associated respiratory symptoms.

CT Scan. CT is indicated if the patient has focal neurologic signs or seizures or clinical evidence of an intracranial mass effect. It is also appropriate if the patient had preceding trauma.

Normal CT findings do not guarantee the safety of an LP in a patient with meningitis.

Subdural Taps. A subdural tap should be performed if there is evidence of increasing head circumference, expanding and bulging anterior fontanel, or continuing fever with poor clinical response (see Appendix A-6).

DIFFERENTIAL DIAGNOSIS
(see Chapters 15, 34, and 39)

Differential diagnostic considerations in the patient with a stiff neck are meningitis, adenitis, osteomyelitis, trauma with secondary fracture, hematoma, or muscle injury, tumor, hysteria, torticollis, and oculogyric crisis from drugs such as phenothiazines (p. 393).

Infection

Because of the nonspecific signs and symptoms of meningitis, particularly in younger children, it is often difficult, without an LP, to distinguish this disease from a number of other infections, for instance:

1. Pneumonia
2. Acute gastroenteritis with dehydration, particularly if caused by *Shigella* organisms
3. Acute illness associated with a febrile seizure
4. Less common: brain abscess, subdural empyema, and acute obstruction of a VP shunt

Vascular Disorder

Subarachnoid bleeding or a cerebrovascular accident may develop acutely and may be associated with a systemic infection.

Intoxication

The stress of an acute infection may lead some individuals to overdoses, purposeful or accidental. Infection changes the kinetics of drugs such as theophylline.

Trauma

Head trauma producing a subdural or epidural hematoma may be difficult to distinguish from meningitis, sometimes necessitating a CT scan before LP. Heat stroke may cause fever, dehydration, meningism, and marked changes in mentation.

MANAGEMENT

1. Initial management must focus on stabilizing the patient. Intravenous access should be established after ensuring adequate airway and ventilation. Assessment of vital signs with concomitant evaluation for hypoxia, dehydration, increased ICP, acidosis, electrolyte abnormalities, and disseminated intravascular coagulation (DIC), when appropriate, must be rapidly done.
2. LP should be performed and the CSF should be rapidly analyzed.

Bacterial Meningitis

Immediate intervention is required for bacterial meningitis.

Antibiotics. Parental administration of antibiotics should be initiated, with selection of agent based on the Gram stain response, the patient's age, immunologic status, and allergy history, and any underlying disease as guides. The agent should be altered if needed once culture and sensitivity data are available. *S. pneumoniae* resistant to penicillin is becoming a more important pathogen. Although *H. influenzae* is less common because of widespread immunization, the organism may be resistant to ampicillin, chloramphenicol, or both (Table 81-4).

Cerebral Edema. An uncommon complication, cerebral edema may develop with focal neurologic signs or evidence of herniation.

1. If the patient is intubated, hyperventilate control $PaCO_2$ (p. 424).
2. Give mannitol (20% solution), 0.5 to 1.0 g/kg/dose q4-6hr.
3. Give diuretic: furosemide (Lasix), 1 mg/kg/dose q4-6hr IV.

NOTE: In most patients who have symptomatic increased ICP and who need aggressive treatment as just described, an intracranial monitor should be placed by a neurosurgeon. Prognosis is improved if the cerebral perfusion pressure (CPP = difference between ICP and blood pressure [BP]) is greater than 30 mm Hg.

Seizures. Seizures should be treated with diazepam (Valium), 0.2 to 0.3 mg/kg/dose q5-10min IV (maximum: 10 mg), or lorazepam (Ativan), 0.05 to 0.15 mg/kg/dose IV. Phenobarbital or phenytoin should be initiated for maintenance therapy (see Chapter 21). Prophylactic anticonvulsants are generally not indicated.

Physical Examination. A complete physical examination, including head circumference measurement, should be performed daily. Particular attention should be given daily to secondary complications such as septic arthritis and subdural effusion.

Fluid Therapy. Fluid therapy should be conservative, reflecting hydration and vital signs. After stabilization, fluids should be continued at 80% to 100% of maintenance requirements. Serum sodium level should be monitored; if serum sodium level is decreased, spot urine and serum sodium and potassium measurements should be performed and osmolality should be determined. If hyponatremia as a result of inappropriate ADH secretion occurs, fluid should be further restricted.

Steroids. Administration of steroids during the treatment of bacterial meningitis in children older than 6 weeks of age may reduce the incidence of subsequent hearing loss. Although steroids are often routinely used in bacterial meningitis, the exact benefit is under continuing study and results are somewhat conflicting. The initial studies were done with *H. influenzae type B* meningitis; current evidence does not clearly support its use with other pathogens, partially

TABLE 81-4 Bacterial Meningitis: Antibiotic Treatment

Cause	Treatment
Patient <6 wk old	
Unknown cause*	Ampicillin, 100-200 mg/kg/24 hr q4-6hr IV, and cefotaxime (or equivalent), 100-150 mg/kg/24 hr q8-12hr IV; or ampicillin, as above, and gentamicin, 5-7.5 mg/kg/24 hr q8-12hr IV (or tobramycin, 4-6 mg/kg/24 hr q8-12hr IV); if *S. pneumoniae* suspected by Gram stain or antigen testing, add vancomycin (30 mg/kg/24 hr q12hr IV)
E. coli	Cefotaxime, as above; treat 21 days or longer
Group B streptococci (*S. agalactiae)*	Penicillin G, 150,000-250,000 units/kg/24 hr q4-6hr IV, and gentamicin, as above; treat 14 days or longer
L. monocytogenes	Ampicillin, as above; treat 14-21 days or longer
Patient 6 wk-18 yr old	
Unknown cause†	Cefotaxime, 200 mg/kg/24 hr q6-8hr IV (or ceftriaxone, 100 mg/kg/24 hr q12hr IV or equivalent)
H. influenzae	Cefotaxime, 200 mg/kg/24 hr q6-8hr IV (or ceftriaxone, 100 mg/kg/24 hr q12hr IV, or ceftizoxime 200 mg/kg/24 hr q8hr IV) or equivalent
S. pneumoniae	Vancomycin, 30-45 mg/kg/24 hr q6hr IV, and ceftriaxone, 100 mg/kg/24 hr q12hr IV, pending sensitivities for 10-14 days,
N. meningitidis	Penicillin G, 250,000 units/kg/24 hr q4hr IV; treat 7-10 days‡

Duration of therapy in uncomplicated cases in children <2 mo of age is generally 14-21 days or longer. Older children may generally be treated for 7-10 days, depending on the response to therapy and the pathogen. Patients with complicated cases require longer duration.

* In preterm, low-birth-weight infant <1 mo, vancomycin (30 mg/kg/24 hr q12hr IV) and ceftazidime (100-150 mg/kg/24 hr q8hr IV) may be used because of risk of *S. aureus* and gram-negative bacilli.

† If *S. pneumoniae* is suspected, vancomycin and cefotaxime/ceftriaxone should be initiated until pathogen is identified and sensitivities completed.

‡ Adult: 10 million-20 million units/24 hr q4hr IV.

because of limited studies. Dosage is dexamethasone, 0.6 mg/kg/24 hr q6hr IV, for first 4 days or 16 doses of therapy. The optimum time for starting dexamethasone is either before or concomitant with the first dose of parenteral antibiotics.

Steroids produce a more rapid improvement in the opening CSF pressure and CPP. They decrease meningeal inflammation and concentration of cytokines. They may also reduce the temperature during the first few days of therapy.

Disposition. All patients with bacterial meningitis must be hospitalized. Those with high-risk features (younger than 1 year or demonstrate shock, coma, seizures, petechiae for less than 12 hours, low CSF glucose level, or very high CSF protein level) should be monitored very closely, often in an intensive care unit (ICU).

If the patient is seen initially in a setting without facilities to perform LP and has signs and symptoms highly suggestive of bacterial meningitis, blood culture specimens should be obtained and parenteral antibiotics (IV preferably) administered before transport.

Coma, shock, respiratory distress, or a low CSF WBC count (<1000 cells/mm^3) at the time of admission are associated with a poor prognosis in patients with *S. pneumoniae* meningitis. Worse sequelae in those with bacterial meningitis are associated with duration of symptoms of more than 48 hours, prehospital seizure activity, presence of peripheral vasoconstriction, CSF WBC count less than 1000 cells/mm^3, and an admission body temperature of 38° C or less.

Twenty-five percent of school-aged survivors of bacterial meningitis have sequelae.

Chemoprophylaxis is indicated in the following situations:

1. Individuals who have had intimate contact with a patient who has meningitis caused by *N. meningitidis* should receive prophylaxis: rifampin, 10 mg/kg/dose q12hr PO for 4 doses (adult: 600 mg/dose q12hr PO for 4 doses; children <1 month, 5 mg/kg/dose q12hr PO for 4 doses).
2. Prophylaxis for exposure to other systemic disease—especially meningitis caused by *H. influenzae*—is controversial but guidelines have been developed:
   a. Prophylaxis is recommended for all members of a household with children younger than 4 years who have systemic *H. influenzae* type B disease.
   b. Prophylaxis in daycare settings is indicated if they resemble households such as those with children younger than 2 years in which contact is 25 hours per week or more. It is also used if two or more cases of invasive disease occurred in attendees within 60 days.
   c. Dosage of rifampin is 20 mg/kg/dose (maximum: 600 mg/dose) q24hr PO for 4 doses. Some clinicians recommend reducing the dosage to 10 mg/kg/dose for infants younger than 1 month; the efficacy is uncertain.
   d. Exposed children who have a febrile illness should receive prompt medical evaluation, and treatment should be initiated if indicated.
3. Rifampin can be administered to children by having a liquid preparation formulated. Do not give to patients with liver disease or pregnant females.
4. Parents should be warned of the increased risk for secondary *H. influenzae* meningitis in children younger than 1 year.
5. In epidemic *Neisseria* meningitis, immunization of potential contacts is indicated.

With good clinical response, patients may be discharged within 24 hours after completion of antibiotic therapy. They should be monitored closely, with particular attention to potential neurologic deficits and hearing loss.

All children who have experienced bacterial meningitis should undergo audiologic evaluation. Children younger than 2 years should have routine immunization to *H. influenzae* because the disease does not provide long-term immunologic protection.

Viral Meningitis or Meningoencephalitis (see Table 81-1)

The patient with viral meningitis or meningoencephalitis needs supportive therapy:

1. If there is any concern about the reliability of the diagnosis, a second LP should demonstrate a marked decrease in the percentage of PMN leukocytes in 6 to 8 hours after the first LP in untreated patients.
2. Most patients with viral meningitis should be hospitalized initially to ensure adequate fluid intake and pain management and to allow monitoring for deterioration. If herpes is considered, acyclovir may be initiated. Complications require aggressive management. After an initial assessment and stabilization period, patients may be discharged with close follow-up observation.
3. Although a definitive treatment for viral meningitis is unavailable, patients should be monitored closely on a long-term basis because of associated neurologic and learning deficits that may develop in subsequent months. Poor outcomes appear to be associated with young age, impaired consciousness, and abnormal oculocephalic responses.

BIBLIOGRAPHY

American Academy of Pediatrics, Committee on Infectious Diseases: Therapy for children with invasive pneumococcal infection, *Pediatrics* 99:289, 1997.

Arditi M, Mason EO, Bradley JS et al: Three year multi-center surveillance of pneumococcal meningitis in children:

clinical characteristics and outcome related to penicillin susceptibility and dexamethasone, *Pediatrics* 102:1087, 1998.

Blisitkul DM, Hogan AE, Tanz RR: The role of bacterial antigen detection tests in the diagnosis of bacterial meningitis, *Pediatr Emerg Care* 10:67, 1994.

Coant PN, Kornberg AE, Duffy LC et al: Blood culture results as determinants in the organisms identification of bacterial meningitis, *Pediatr Emerg Care* 8:200, 1992.

Geiman BJ, Smith AL: Dexamethasone and bacterial meningitis: a meta analysis of randomized controlled trials, *West J Med* 157:27, 1992.

Grimwood K, Anderson VA, Bond L et al: Adverse outcomes of bacterial meningitis in school-age survivors, *Pediatrics* 95:646, 1995.

Jafari HS, McCracken OH: Dexamethasone therapy in bacterial meningitis, *Pediatr Ann* 23:82, 1994.

Kaaresen P, Flaegstad T: Prognostic factors in childhood bacterial meningitis, *Acta Paediatr* 84:873, 1995.

Kanegaye JT, Soliemanzedah P, Bradley JS: Lumbar puncture in pediatric bacterial meningitis: defining the time interval for recovery of cerebrospinal fluid pathogens after parenteral antibiotic treatment, *Pediatrics* 108:1169, 2001.

Key CB, Rothrock SC, Falk JL: Cerebrospinal fluid shunt complications: an emergency medicine perspective, *Pediatr Emerg Care* 11:265, 1995.

Kornelisse RE: Prognosis of pneumococcal meningitis, *Clin Infect Dis* 21:1390, 1995.

Lembo RM, Rubin DH, Krowchuk DP et al: Peripheral white blood cell counts and bacterial meningitis: implications regarding diagnostic efficacy in febrile children, *Pediatr Emerg Care* 7:4, 1991.

Naradzay JFX, Browne BJ, Rolnick MA et al: Cerebral ventricular shunts, *J Emerg Med* 17:311, 1999.

Negrini B, Kelleher KJ, Wald ER: Cerebrospinal fluid findings in aseptic versus bacterial meningitis, *Pediatrics* 105:316, 2000.

Quagliarella VJ, Scheld WM: Treatment of bacterial meningitis, *N Engl J Med* 336:708, 1997.

Rodriquez AF, Kaplan SL, Mason EO: Cerebrospinal fluid values in the very low birth weight infant, *J Pediatr* 116:971, 1990.

Rorabaugh ML, Berlin LE, Heldrich F et al: Aseptic meningitis in infants younger than two years of age: acute illness and neurologic complications, *Pediatrics* 92:206, 1993.

Rothrock SG, Green SM, Wren J et al: Pediatric bacterial meningitis: is prior antibiotic therapy associated with an altered clinical presentation? *Ann Emerg Med* 21:146, 1992.

Schaad UB, Wedgewood-Krucke J, Tschaeppoelee H: Reversible ceftriaxone-associated biliary pseudolithiasis in children, *Lancet* 2:1411, 1988.

Schlesinger Y, Sawyer MH, Storch GA: Enteroviral meningitis in infancy, potential role for polymerase chain reaction in pain management, *Pediatrics* 94:157, 1994.

Schoendorf KC, Adams WO, Kiely JL et al: National trends in *Haemophilus influenzae* meningitis mortality and hospitalization among children, 1980-1991, *Pediatrics* 93:663, 1994.

Snedeker JB, Kaplan SL, Dodge P et al: Subdural effusion and its relationship with neurologic sequelae of bacterial meningitis in infancy: a prospective study, *Pediatrics* 86:163, 1990.

Taylor HG, Mills EL, Ciampi A et al: The sequelae of *Haemophilus influenzae* meningitis in school-age children, *N Engl J Med* 323:1657, 1990.

Unhanand M, Mustafa MM, McCracken GH et al: Gram-negative enteric bacillary meningitis: a twenty-one-year experience, *J Pediatr* 122:15, 1993.

Wald ER, Kaplan SL, Mason EQ et al: Dexamethasone therapy for children with bacterial meningitis, *Pediatrics* 95:21, 1995.

Walsh-Kelly C, Nelson DB, Smith DS et al: Clinical patterns of bacterial versus aseptic meningitis in childhood, *Ann Emerg Med* 21:910, 1992.

Migraine Headache

Migraines are recurrent headaches with initial intracranial vasoconstriction followed by extracranial vasodilation, producing a throbbing pain, that may occur in any age group. A positive family history commonly is present (50%). There is a 3:1 prevalence in women. The headache is often precipitated by stress and may first develop during puberty. It is episodic and has a variable frequency.

DIAGNOSTIC FINDINGS

1. The classic headaches are unilateral but may be bilateral with a throbbing or pulsatile quality and aura:
   - **a.** They are commonly preceded by an aura, which may be visual (stars, spots, or circles), sensory (hyperesthesia), or motor (weakness) and are accompanied by abdominal pain, nausea, vomiting, anorexia, vertigo, ataxia, and syncope. A symptom-free period after the aura is usually less than 60 minutes long.
   - **b.** Headaches subsequently become recurrent.

c. Onset may be associated with exertion, stress, or coughing.

2. Common migraines may be generalized, without an aura—more common in younger children:
   a. Generalized malaise, dizziness, photophobia, nausea, and vomiting are prominent.
   b. Aggravated by walking or routine activities.
3. Less commonly, specific migraine complexes may be present.
   a. *Ophthalmoplegic* migraines cause unilateral eye pain with limitation of extraocular movement involving cranial nerves III, IV, and VI.
   b. *Basilar* migraines involve the basilar artery, producing headaches, vertigo, ataxia, cranial nerve palsy, blindness, syncope, acute confusion without neurologic findings, cyclic vomiting, recurrent abdominal pain, and paroxysmal disequilibrium. Progressive mental status deterioration may be noted.
   c. *Hemiplegic* migraines primarily cause transient motor deficits.
4. Migraines are often relieved by rest.

Ancillary Data

1. Electroencephalogram (EEG) may show slowing but is not diagnostically or therapeutically useful.
2. Tests to exclude other causes of headaches or specific presenting neurologic findings: Diagnostic studies, minimally including a CT scan, should normally be obtained in children younger than 6 years, those with large head circumference, and those who exhibit new neurologic signs or persistent or unusual headache, do not return to a normal state of health, or experience either increasing frequency or severity of headaches or personality changes.

DIFFERENTIAL DIAGNOSIS

See Chapter 36.

MANAGEMENT

1. Initial management must attempt to relieve pain. Many cases respond to mild analgesia such as acetaminophen or acetaminophen with codeine. Relief usually is achieved with sleep. Oxygen may be helpful.
2. Nonpharmacologic therapy should focus on trigger factors. Reducing stress and exertion and avoiding certain foods and oral contraceptives reduce the incidence rate. Biofeedback, relaxation therapy, psychotherapy, and hypnotherapy may be useful.
3. Once the diagnosis is established, abortive treatment of the acute episode is best achieved if medication is initiated early in the course.
   a. If mild analgesics (acetaminophen, ibuprofen, naproxen) provide inadequate relief, aspirin, phenacetin, and caffeine combinations (Fiorinal or Fenbutal) should be initiated:
      - In children younger than 5 years of age, ½ tablet; in those 5 to 12 years, 1 tablet; repeat 1 hour later if no relief is obtained. Older children receive 1 to 2 tablets.
   b. In the postpubertal child with classic migraine, Midrin (isometheptene mucate, 65 mg, dichloralphenazone, 100 mg, and acetaminophen, 325 mg) given at the onset of pain with an additional tablet 1 hour later may be useful.
   c. Sumatriptan (Imitrex) (adult: 6 mg SC or 100 mg PO; SC dose may be repeated in 1 hour if there is no response to initial SC dose; suggested pediatric dose is 0.6 mg/kg SC). The onset of response is rapid with 70% recovering within 1 hr; 35% of patients have a recurrence during the

subsequent 24 hours. There is limited experience with this agent in children. Sumatriptan is also available as a nasal spray.

d. If the patient arrives with a severe attack that has been going on for some time, chlorpromazine (Thorazine), 12.5 mg q20min IM up to a total adult dose of 37.5 mg, is helpful. Ketorolac (Toradol) is a parenteral nonsteroidal antiinflammatory agent given in children older than 2 years at a dosage of 1 mg/kg/dose q6hr IM; adults are initially normally given 30 to 60 mg/dose, followed by 15 to 30 mg/dose q6hr. This latter agent is as effective as meperidine and hydroxyzine in some studies.

e. Severe migraines may be treated with one of a number of regimens that have been used in adolescents and adults:

(1) *Initial dose:*
- Dihydroergotamine (DHE), 1 mg IM, *plus* hydroxyzine, 0.7 mg/kg IM; *or*
- Meperidine, 1.5 mg/kg IM, *plus* hydroxyzine, 0.7 mg/kg IM

(2) *If there is no resolution after 60 minutes, second doses may be considered:*
- Dihydroergotamine, 1 mg IM, *plus* hydroxyzine, 0.35 mg/kg IM; *or*
- Meperidine 0.75 mg/kg IM, *plus* hydroxyzine, 0.35 mg/kg IM

f. If relief from a severe migraine is not easily achieved, ergotamine preparations may be used in subsequent attacks. Ergotamine (1 mg with 100 mg caffeine) tablets should be used at the onset of pain, and the dose should be repeated every 30 minutes up to 3 doses per headache in children younger than 12 years or up to no more than 6 doses per headache in older patients. Suppositories are available if the patient is vomiting (one suppository per headache for children younger than 12 years; no more than two suppositories per headache for older patients). Caffeine potentiates the ergotamine by increasing absorption, but it may prevent sleep.

g. Metoclopramide (Reglan), in a dose of 10 mg IV, has been found useful in adults.

h. Dexamethasone has been used.

4. Long-term prophylactic management of disabling migraines in adolescents and adults may include one of a number of agents. Control is often achieved through the use of a variety of agents that are attempted on an empiric basis:

a. Propranolol, 2 mg/kg/24 hr q8hr PO. Side effects include bradycardia, nausea, fatigue, hypotension, hypoglycemia, and depression. The agent is contraindicated in patients with asthma, congestive heart failure, or depression. Metoprolol (2 to 6 mg/kg/24 hr for adults) is recommended as a β-blocker in patients with asthma.

b. Phenytoin (Dilantin), 3 to 5 mg/kg/24 hr q12-24hr PO. Side effects include drowsiness, impairment of learning, idiosyncratic hypersensitivity, and gingival hypertrophy.

c. Amitriptyline (Elavil), 0.2 to 0.5 mg/kg/dose given at night, especially to older children with depressive characteristics. Side effects include dry mouth, dizziness, fatigue, and urinary retention.

d. Cyproheptadine (Periactin), 0.2 to 0.4 mg/kg/24 hr q6-8hr PO (maximum: 32 mg/24 hr), is an antihistamine that may cause weight gain and sedation.

e. Calcium channel blockers may be effective as well. Verapamil, 4 to 10 mg/kg/24 hr (240 to 480 mg/24 hr) TID PO, may be used.

DISPOSITION

1. Most patients with migraine can be sent home with appropriate short-term and long-term medications and close follow-up observation.
2. Hospitalization is indicated only for severe pain.

BIBLIOGRAPHY

Bell R, Montoya D, Shuaib A et al: A comparative trial of three agents in the treatment of acute migraine headache, *Ann Emerg Med* 19:1079, 1990.

Bulloch B, Tenenbein M: Emergency department management of pediatric migraine, *Pediatr Emerg Care* 16:196, 2000.

Carleton SC, Shesser RF, Pietrzak MP et al: Double blind multi-center trial to compare the efficacy of intramuscular dihydroergotamine plus hydroxyzine versus intramuscular meperidine plus hydroxyzine for the emergency department treatment of acute migraine headache, *Ann Emerg Med* 32:129, 1998.

Cooper PJ, Bawden HN, Camfield PR et al: Anxiety and life events in childhood migraine, *Pediatrics* 79:999, 1987.

Duarte C, Dunaway F, Turner L et al: Ketorolac versus meperidine and hydroxyzine in the treatment of acute migraine headache: a randomized prospective double blind trial, *Ann Emerg Med* 21:1116, 1992.

Ellis GL, Delaney J, De Hart DA et al: The efficacy of metoclopramide in the treatment of migraine headache, *Ann Emerg Med* 22:191, 1993.

Igarashi M, May WN, Golden GS: Pharmacologic treatment of childhood migraine, *J Pediatr* 120:653, 1992.

Larkin GL, Prescott JE: A randomized, double-blind comparative study of the efficacy of ketorolac tromethamine versus meperidine in the treatment of severe migraine, *Ann Emerg Med* 21:919, 1992.

Olesen J: Understanding the biologic basis of migraine, *N Engl J Med* 331:1713, 1994.

Subcutaneous sumatriptan international study group: Treatment of migraine attacks with sumatriptan, *N Engl J Med* 325:316, 1991.

Welch KMA: Drug therapy of migraine, *N Engl J Med* 329:1476, 1993.

Pseudotumor Cerebri

Benign intracranial hypertension or pseudotumor cerebri occurs when there is increased ICP in the absence of a local, space-occupying lesion or there is acute brain swelling accompanying an identifiable infectious or inflammatory process.

ETIOLOGY

Although the pathogenesis is unknown, pseudotumor cerebri is associated with a host of clinical entities:

1. Infection: upper respiratory tract (URI) infection, acute otitis media (AOM), roseola infantum, sinusitis
2. Allergy
3. Deficiency: anemia, including iron deficiency, leukemia, vitamin A deficiency, overdose
4. Endocrine/metabolic disorders: steroid medication, oral contraceptive pills, uremia, hyperthyroidism, hypothyroidism, Addison's disease, galactosemia
5. Trauma: minimal head trauma
6. Vascular disorder: congenital or acquired heart disease
7. Intoxication: tetracycline, steroids, oral contraceptives, vitamin A
8. Idiopathic disorder

DIAGNOSTIC FINDINGS

1. Younger children may have only a bulging fontanelle with some irritability or listlessness.
2. Older children have headache, nausea, vomiting, and dizziness. Eye examination may demonstrate papilledema, sixth nerve palsy, diplopia, blurred vision, and enlarged blind spot.
3. The level of consciousness is relatively normal, given the signs of increased ICP.

Ancillary Data

1. LP: normal with the exception of increased pressure
2. CT scan: may be indicated to exclude mass lesion

DIFFERENTIAL DIAGNOSIS

1. Infection:
   a. Meningitis or encephalitis: LP for evaluation
   b. Brain abscess: CT scan and subsequent LP

2. Optic neuritis: slit-lamp examination
3. Trauma (subdural effusion or hemorrhage): subdural tap or CT scan
4. Neoplasm: CT scan (may be diagnostic)

MANAGEMENT

Although pseudotumor cerebri is a benign entity with an excellent prognosis, it is a diagnosis of exclusion, and other entities such as meningitis in the febrile child must be considered. Once the diagnosis is confirmed, treatment of the underlying disease is appropriate.

Adjunctive therapy, implemented in conjunction with a neurologist, may include the following:

1. Acetazolamide (Diamox), 5 mg/kg/dose (maximum: 250 to 375 mg/dose) q24-48hr PO; or
2. Serial LPs.

Uncontrolled, increased ICP and papilledema may result in visual loss. The patient should therefore be followed by an ophthalmologist with testing of visual fields if possible.

BIBLIOGRAPHY

Amacher AL, Spence JD: Spectrum of benign intracranial hypertension in children and adolescents, *Child Nerv Syst* 1:81, 1985.

Lessell S: Pediatric pseudo tumor cerebri (idiopathic intracranial hypertension), *Surg Ophthalmol* 37:155, 1992.

Seizures

ALERT If ongoing seizures are occurring, refer to status epilepticus (see Chapter 21). Underlying conditions must be sought and managed.

A seizure or convulsion is a paroxysmal disturbance in nerve cells resulting in abnormalities in motor, sensory, autonomic, or psychic function. (See febrile seizures, p. 763.)

ETIOLOGY (Box 81-1 and Table 81-5)

The most common causes of acute onset of seizures in children, which often occur because the threshold for seizure is lowered, are infection, trauma, poor compliance, intoxications, and idiopathic disorders. Epilepsy accounts for most chronic seizure disorders.

Box 81-1

SEIZURES: CAUSE BY AGE AT ONSET*

FIRST DAY OF LIFE

Hypoxia
Drugs
Trauma
Infection
Hyperglycemia
Hypoglycemia
Pyridoxine deficiency

DAY 2-3 OF LIFE

Infection
Drug withdrawal
Hypoglycemia
Hypocalcemia
Developmental malformation
Intracranial hemorrhage
Inborn error of metabolism
Hypo/hypernatremia

DAY 4-6 MO

Infection
Hypocalcemia
Hyperphosphatemia
Hyponatremia
Developmental malformation
Drug withdrawal
Inborn error of metabolism

6 MO-3 YR

Febrile seizures
Birth injury
Infection
Toxin
Trauma
Metabolic disorder
Cerebral degenerative disease

>3 YR

Idiopathic
Infection
Trauma
Cerebral degenerative disease

* Differential considerations must be individualized.

TABLE 81-5 Seizures: Diagnostic Considerations

Condition	Diagnostic Findings	Comments
EPILEPSY	Variable seizure types as described in this chapter	Multiple causes, including idiopathic
INFECTION		
Febrile (p. 763)	Fever; grand mal seizure; variable focal seizure; self-limited; peak: 5 mo-5 yr; high association with *Shigella*; LP normal	Must distinguish from meningitis
Meningitis (p. 741)	Fever, stiff neck, headache, Kernig's and Brudzinski's signs; in young child, dehydration, bulging fontanel, lethargy, irritability, vomiting, cyanosis; LP diagnostic	May be viral or bacterial
Encephalitis (p. 743)	Headache, fever, vomiting, irritability, listlessness, stupor, variable focal neurologic signs; LP may be diagnostic or equivocal	Epidemiology important; usually viral
Intracranial abscess	Insidious onset; fever; variable focal neurologic findings; CT scan diagnostic	
S/P DTP immunization	History of immunization, fever; seizure within 48 hr	May have permanent sequelae
Misc: pertussis, rabies, tetanus, syphilis	Disease-specific signs and symptoms	
Subacute bacterial endocarditis (p. 567)	Fever; usually insidious; focal neurologic findings; splenomegaly; embolic phenomenon; variable heart disease; positive blood culture results	
TRAUMA (Chapter 57)		
Concussion	History of trauma, variable abnormal neurologic findings; focal or grand mal seizure within 24 hr; CT findings variably WNL	May be recurrent; close neurologic monitoring; may not require anti-convulsants
Acute		Immediate neurosurgical intervention
Subdural	Variable focal neurologic signs; change in mental status; progression with increased intracranial pressure; positive CT findings	
Epidural	Lucid period after trauma; eventual lapse into coma with herniation	Immediate neurosurgical intervention
CONGENITAL (Chapters 10 and 11)		
Birth asphyxia	History of perinatal injury; neurologic abnormality; premature; low Apgar score	Infection, placental insufficiency, difficult birth
Neurocutaneous syndrome	Pathognomonic skin findings; variably abnormal neurologic findings, family history; CT scan may be useful	

Continued

TABLE 81-5 Seizures: Diagnostic Considerations—cont'd

Condition	Diagnostic Findings	Comments
INTRAPSYCHIC		
Breath-holding (p. 740)	Precipitated by crying, anger, injury, and cyanosis, followed by loss of consciousness, may be opisthotonic; seizures rare and self-limited	Peak: 6 mo-4 yr; cyanosis precedes loss of consciousness; in seizures consciousness is lost first; usually maternal-infant problems
Hyperventilation		
Hysteria		
ENDOCRINE/METABOLIC		
Hypoglycemia (Chapter 38)	Sweating, pallor, syncope, vasovagal reaction; newborn: irritability, apnea, cyanosis, listlessness, poor feeding	Definition varies with age; glucose level: newborn <2500 g, (<20 mg/dl); term newborn, (<30 mg/dl); older infant and child, (<40 mg/dl)
Hyponatremia (Chapter 8)	Listlessness, variable stupor; associated condition (e.g., dehydration, head trauma, inappropriate ADH, Addison's disease, water intoxication); usually temp <36.5°C	
Hypernatremia (Chapter 8)	Listlessness or irritability; associated condition (dehydration)	Rarely causes seizures unless rehydration is rapid
Hypocalcemia	Muscle cramps, pain, Chvostek's, Trousseau's sign, variable increased intracranial pressure, headache	Common in premature, parathyroid deficiency
Hypomagnesemia	Tetany, tremor, irritability	Difficult to determine true body deficit
Kernicterus (Chapter 11)	Jaundice, developmental delay	Rare at present
Inborn errors		
Phenylketonuria (PKU)	Neurologically abnormal; developmental delay; variable acidosis; need urine and blood screen	
Amino and organic acidemia		
Uremia (p. 828)	Signs and symptoms of renal failure	

INTOXICATION (Chapter 54)		
Aspirin Amphetamine Anticholinergics (e.g., tricyclic, antidepressants, phenothiazine) Theophylline Carbon monoxide PCP, cocaine Propoxyphene Lead Drug withdrawal (e.g., alcohol, anticonvulsants)	Signs and symptoms of associated drug intoxication or withdrawal	See Chapters 54 and 55 for complete listing
DEGENERATIVE/DEFICIENCY		
Pyridoxine deficiency or dependence	Mental retardation, anemia, diarrhea	Responds well to pyridoxine, (5-10 mg IV/IM), then 0.3-0.5 mg/24 hr
Tay-Sachs disease	Blindness, spastic, floppiness, cherry-red spot	Eastern European background
Juvenile Huntington's chorea	Rigidity, dementia	
Metachromatic leukodystrophy	Incoordination, upper and lower neurologic signs	
Other CNS diseases	Variable	
NEOPLASM	Often focal neurologic findings	Glioma, most common; supratentorial lesions more likely to cause seizure
VASCULAR (Chapter 18)		
Dysrhythmia	Irregular pulse, sudden event, abnormal ECG (e.g., long QT, block)	
Intracranial hematoma Cerebral Extradural Subarachnoid	Acute-onset headache, neurologic findings; variable increased intracranial pressure	Associated with AV malformation, bleeding disorder (e.g., hemophilia), heart disease, sickle cell, trauma
Hypertensive encephalopathy (Chapter 18)	High blood pressure; vomiting, hyperpyrexia, ataxia, coma; facial paralysis	May be secondary to stroke
Embolism	Focal neurologic findings	Predisposing factors: heart disease, peripheral embolism
Transient ischemic attack/infarct	Variable neurologic finding, dependent on site; fever; broad deficits; altered sensation	Differentiate from Todd's paralysis

By age of onset, specific causes are most common (see Box 81-1).

Classification

1. *Partial seizures*:
   a. *Partial simple seizure* (consciousness retained): Patient may have motor (jacksonian), somatosensory (metallic, headache), autonomic (flushing, sweating), or psychiatric (déjà vu) symptoms.
   b. *Partial complex seizure* (consciousness impaired): Simple partial seizures at onset progress to impaired consciousness, or consciousness is impaired at onset of seizure. Previously called "psychomotor seizures." An aura that includes automatisms, alteration of perception, and hallucinations may occur before alteration of consciousness develops.
   c. Partial seizures that secondarily generalize
2. *Generalized seizures* (involves both sides of brain):
   a. Nonconvulsive:
      (1) *Absence seizures:* Characterized by brief lapses in awareness, sometimes accompanied by minor motor manifestations (staring, rhythmic eye blinking, head dropping) without postictal period. Previously called "petit mal."
      (2) Atypical absence seizures.
   b. Convulsive:
      (1) *Myoclonic seizures:* Brief contractions that occur unilaterally or bilaterally.
      (2) *Clonic, tonic, tonic-clonic seizures: Tonic* movements reflect sustained muscle contracting resulting in limb and trunk rigidity. *Clonic* movements are rhythmic jerking and flexor spasms of the extremities.
      (3) *Atonic seizures*: Abrupt loss of muscle tone that causes the child to collapse or drop.

DIAGNOSTIC FINDINGS

Patients usually have a history of seizures, but if ongoing seizures are present, evaluation and management as described in Chapter 21 should be implemented.

1. The initial assessment must determine the characteristics of the seizure, defining its focality or generalized nature, and frequency, associated sensory and autonomic functions, and behavioral changes. Predisposing factors, such as fever, intoxications, perinatal asphyxia, trauma, and preexisting abnormalities in growth and development, require definition.
2. A complete neurologic examination is essential, differentiating long-standing from acute changes. Evidence of asymmetry of findings, increased ICP, or infection must be carefully assessed.

Ancillary Data

Evaluation must reflect the nature of the seizure and potential causes.

Blood Studies. A glucose determination should be performed on all patients:

1. Initially, screening with reagent strips (Dextrostix or Chemstrip).
2. Measurements of electrolyte, Ca^{++}, Mg^{++}, and PO_4^{--} levels as indicated. Laboratory studies have the highest yield in patients with active seizures or body temperature lower than 36.5° C and in patients younger than 1 month.

Hematology. For febrile patients, a complete blood count (CBC) and urinalysis should be performed.

Lumbar Puncture. An LP should be performed in febrile patients, if indicated (p. 848). Evaluation of the CSF must include Gram stain (and methylene blue stain), culture, cell count, and glucose and protein measurements.

Seizures can cause some elevation of cell counts but generally less than 20 $WBCs/mm^3$ or 9 $neutrophils/mm^3$.

Cultures. In addition to a CSF culture and Gram stain in the febrile child, cultures of blood and urine should be obtained. Cultures of other specimens should be done as indicated.

X-Ray Films

1. A CT scan has a very low yield in generalized seizures without focal findings in the pediatric age group and is usually not required. It may be useful in cases with preceding head trauma or abnormal neurologic status.

   The CT findings in a patient with an acute seizure are usually normal if none of the following is present: malignancy, neurocutaneous disorder, recent closed head injury, recent CSF shunt revision, age younger than 6 months old, seizure of more than 15 minutes' duration, and recent onset of focal neurologic deficit.
2. A skull radiograph is indicated when there is evidence of trauma preceding the seizure and when a CT scan is not readily available.
3. Magnetic resonance imaging (MRI) may be useful for recurrent or progressive findings.

Drug Levels

1. Evaluation for possibility of drug ingestion (see Chapter 54).
2. Anticonvulsant medication levels should be measured if the patient is receiving long-term therapy. Subtherapeutic levels are a very common cause of seizures.

Subdural Tap (see Appendix A-6). A subdural tap may be indicated in the young child who has associated trauma or infection, particularly if the fontanel is full and the child is deteriorating. If the child is stable, a CT scan may be diagnostic. A subdural tap is usually performed in consultation with a neurosurgeon.

Electroencephalogram. An EEG is indicated to assess electrical seizure activity. The period of greatest yield (finding epileptiform abnormalities as a seizure focus) is immediately after the seizure, and the yield declines with time. Nonspecific background changes may persist for 1 to 6 weeks after any type of seizure, including febrile or hypoxic breath-holding.

DIFFERENTIAL DIAGNOSIS

See Table 81-5 and Box 81-2.

MANAGEMENT

1. Initial treatment of the patient with ongoing seizure activity (see Chapter 21) must include oxygen, dextrose, and anticonvulsants.
2. In the absence of active seizure activity, efforts should be focused on rapidly determining possible causes and instituting specific treatment.

Box 81-2

CLINICAL ENTITIES SIMULATING SEIZURES

INFANT
Jitteriness
Apnea
Micturitional shivering
Tremor
Dysrhythmia

CHILD
Breath-holding spell
Micturitional/cough syncope
Night tremor/terrors
Migraine
Tics
Dysrhythmia

ADOLESCENT
Vasomotor syncope
Micturitional/cough syncope
Hyperventilation
Pseudoseizures
Orthostatic hypotension
Hysteria

a. Metabolic derangements need specific therapy to correct the abnormality.
b. For seizures after trauma, immediate neurosurgical consultation and CT scan are required if the patient remains neurologically impaired.
c. Infectious causes require antibiotic therapy and supportive care.

3. If no cause is determined, consider anticonvulsants after consultation with a neurologist. At present, some controversy exists regarding the advisability of treating the first tonic-clonic seizure; many clinicians prefer to wait until subsequent seizures occur, when a more definite diagnosis of epilepsy can be made. If medication is begun, loading is required (Table 81-6 and Box 81-3). Monotherapy is effective in about half the patients. Of those children whose seizures are not controlled by the first anticonvulsant, 42% have complete remission if their therapy is switched to a different anticonvulsant.
   a. If the patient is taking medication, increase anticonvulsant dosage if the level is found to be subtherapeutic.
   b. If poor compliance is the basis for the low levels, reload the patient (in full or part, depending on the level) and give instructions about the importance of taking medications. Close follow-up observation with monitoring of the levels is necessary.
   c. Anticonvulsants usually are continued for at least 2 years after the last seizures. They may be stopped at that time, provided that the child has been doing well.
   d. Erythromycin may decrease the metabolism of phenytoin and carbamazepine, requiring a reduction in anticonvulsant dose.
   e. Generic carbamazepine and primidone may have different bioavailability than brand agents.
4. Newborns require slightly different management (see Chapter 11).
5. A Glasgow Coma Scale score (p. 419) of 3 to 8 appears to be somewhat predictive of posttraumatic seizure. Prophylactic phenytoin may be indicated in consultation with a neurosurgeon.

DISPOSITION

1. Patients with first seizures of unknown cause are often admitted to the hospital for evaluation and control and as a response to parental anxiety.
2. After a period of observation, patients with chronic seizure disorders who are taking subtherapeutic doses or who need alteration in the therapeutic regimen can be discharged once the drugs are changed and follow-up evaluations have been arranged.
3. Patients with febrile seizures do not need to be hospitalized if no underlying life-threatening infection is detected, as described in the next section of the chapter.
4. All patients with seizure disorders need close follow-up of clinical status and therapeutic response. Periodic assessment of serum anticonvulsant levels is indicated. Patients with complex recurrent

Box 81-3
SUGGESTED ANTICONVULSANTS ALTERNATIVES BY SEIZURE TYPE

Partial seizures: CBZ, FBM, GBP, PHT, PRM, VPA
Generalized seizures
- Absence: ETX, VPA
- Tonic-clonic: CBZ, FBM, PB, PHT, PRM, VPA
- Myoclonic: BZD, FBM, VPA
- Atonic: BZD, FMB, VPA

Anticonvulsants listed alphabetically.
See Table 81-6 for drug identification and dosage.
BZD, Benzodiazapines.

TABLE 81-6 Common Anticonvulsants

Drug/Availability	Primary Indication	Maintenance Dosage and PO Frequency	Loading Dose* (mg/kg)	Serum Half-life (hr)	Serum Therapeutic Range (μg/ml)
Carbamazepine (Tegretol) Susp: 100 mg/5 ml Tab: 100 (chew), 200 mg	Generalized tonic-clonic, partial seizures	10-40 mg/kg/24 hr (adult: 800-1600 mg/24 hr) BID		11-22	4-14
Clonazepam (Klonopin) Tab: 0.5, 1, 2 mg	Absence seizures, secondary for complex partial and tonic seizures	0.05-0.2 mg/kg/24 hr (adult: 1.5-2.0 mg/24 hr) BID		24-36	0.10-0.80
Diazepam (Valium) Vial: 5 mg/ml	Status epilepticus	NA	0.2-0.3 IV (<1 mg/min) 0.5 PR		
Ethosuximide (Zarontin) Syr: 250 mg/5 ml Cap: 250 mg	Absence seizures	20-40 mg/kg/24 hr (adult: 750-1750 mg/24 hr) QD or BID		24-42	40-100
Felbamate (Felbatol) Susp: 600 mg/5 ml Tab: 400-600 mg	Partial seizures, generalized tonic-clonic	15-45 mg/kg/24 hr (adult: 1200-3600 mg/24 hr) TID or QID		14-20	30-80
Gabapentin (Neurontin) Cap: 100, 300, 400 mg	Adjunctive drug for partial seizures Secondary drug for generalized tonic-clonic (>12 yr)	15-30 mg/kg/24 hr (adult: 900-2400 mg/24 hr) TID		4-8	Unknown
Lamotrigine (Lamictal) Tab: 25, 100, 150, 200 mg	Generalized seizures, partial seizures, refractory absence seizures	3-5 mg/kg/24 hr QD (14 days), then BID (adult: 100-500 mg/24 hr) (no concurrent valproic acid)		12-48 (mean: 25)	2-4
Lorazepam (Ativan) Vial: 2, 4 mg/ml	Status epilepticus	NA	0.05-0.10 IV	16	
Phenobarbital Elixir: 15, 20 mg/5 ml Tab: 15, 30, 60, 100 mg Vial: 65, 130 mg	Generalized tonic-clonic, partial seizures	2-6 mg/kg/24 hr (adult: 100-300 mg/24 hr) BID or QHS	15-20 IV (<1 mg/kg/min) IM erratically absorbed	48-72	15-35 (may be higher)

Continued

TABLE 81-6 Common Anticonvulsants—cont'd

Drug/Availability	Primary Indication	Maintenance Dosage and PO Frequency	Loading Dose* (mg/kg)	Serum Half-life (hr)	Serum Therapeutic Range (μg/ml)
Phenytoin (Dilantin) Susp: 125/5 ml Tabs (chew): 50 mg Cap: 30, 100 mg Amp: 50 mg/ml Amp (fosphenytoin—Cerebyx): 50 mg/ml equivalent	Generalized tonic-clonic, partial seizures	5-10 mg/kg/24 hr (adult: 200-400 mg/24 hr) BID	10-20 IV; or IM, use fosphenytoin	6-30	10-20
Primidone (Mysoline) Susp: 250 mg/5 ml Tab: 50, 250 mg	Generalized tonic-clonic, partial seizures	10-25 mg/kg/24 hr (adult: 750-1250 mg/24 hr) TID or BID		6-12	6-12 (or phenobarbital level)
Valproic acid (Depakene)† Syr: 250 mg/5 ml Cap: 250 mg Vial: 100 mg/ml (Depacon)	Generalized tonic-clonic	15-60 mg/kg/24 hr (adult: 1000-3000 mg/24 hr) TID or BID	Adult: 500-1000 mg IV followed by 500 mg q12hr (<20 mg/min)‡	6-18	50-100
Vigabatrin (Sabril)	Partial seizures	40-80 mg/kg/24 hr (adult: 1500-3000 mg/24 hr)		5-17	Unknown

* When no specific loading dose specified, oral administration after several doses will achieve therapeutic range.
† May cause carnitine deficiency.
‡ IV dose administered over 60 minutes (<20 mg/min) for less than 14 days. Limited pediatric experience.

seizures should routinely be referred to a neurologist.

5. The majority of patients with epilepsy in childhood are free of seizures by adulthood although they are at increased risk for social and educational problems.

Parental Education

1. Give all medications as prescribed.
2. If a seizure does occur, institute seizure precautions to protect the child from self-injury. Maintain the airway.
3. Close follow-up observation is very important. Please keep all health care appointments.
4. Call your physician if either of the following occurs:
   a. There is any change in the pattern or frequency of seizures.
   b. The child shows behavior changes or has problems with medication.

BIBLIOGRAPHY

Abramowicz M, editor: Drugs for epilepsy, *Med Lett Drug Ther* 37:37, 1995.

Callagham N, Garrett A, Goggin T: Withdrawal of anticonvulsant drugs in patients free of seizures for two years, *N Engl J Med* 318:942, 1988.

Camfield PR, Camfield CS, Gordon K et al: If a first antiepileptic drug fails to control a child's epilepsy, what are the chances of success with the next drug? *J Pediatr* 131:821, 1997.

Chamberlain J, Altieri M, Futterman C et al: Seizures in children, *Pediatr Emerg Care* 13:92, 1997.

Hirtz D, Ashwal S, Berg A et al: Practice parameters: evaluating a first nonfebrile seizure in children: report of the quality standards subcomittee of the American Academy of Neurology, the Child Neurology Society, and the American Epilepsy Society, *Neurology* 55:616, 2000.

Laxer K: Guidelines for treating epilepsy in the age of felbamate, vigabatrin, lamotrigine, and gabapentin, *West J Med* 161:309, 1994.

Lewis RJ, Yee L, Inkelis SH et al: Clinical predictors of post-traumatic seizures in children with head trauma, *Ann Emerg Med* 22:1114, 1993.

Pellock JM: Managing pediatric epilepsy syndromes with new antiepileptic drugs, *Pediatrics* 104:1106, 1999.

Rider LG, Thapa PB, Del Beccaro MA et al: Cerebrospinal fluid analysis in children with seizures, *Pediatr Emerg Care* 11:336, 1995.

Scarfone RJ, Pond K, Thompson K et al: Utility of laboratory testing for infants with seizures, *Pediatr Emerg Care* 16:309, 2001.

Scheuer ML, Pedley TA: The evaluation and treatment of seizures, *N Engl J Med* 323:1468, 1990.

Shinnar S, Berg AT, Moshe SL et al: Risk of seizure recurrence following a first unprovoked seizure, *Pediatrics* 85:1076, 1990.

Sillanpaa M, Jalava M, Kaleva Q et al: Long-term prognosis of seizures with onset of childhood, *N Engl J Med* 338:1715, 1998.

Vining EPG: Pediatric seizures, *Emerg Med Clin North Am* 12:973, 1994.

Warden CR, Brownstein DR, Del Beccaro MA: Predictors of abnormal findings of computed tomography of the head in pediatric patients presenting with seizures, *Ann Emerg Med* 29:518, 1997.

Febrile Seizures

ALERT Meningitis must be considered as a potential cause in the febrile child who has seizures.

Febrile seizures are generalized seizures occurring in children with febrile illnesses that do not specifically involve the central nervous system (CNS). They occur in 2% to 5% of children between 5 months and 5 years of age, with the peak incidence between 8 and 20 months.

ETIOLOGY: INFECTION

1. URIs are commonly present, representing more than 70% of underlying infections. Pharyngitis, otitis media, and pneumonitis are most common.
2. Gastroenteritis, urinary tract infections, measles, and immunization such as diphtheria-tetanus-pertussis (DTP) are less common.
3. Roseola (exanthema subitum) is associated with a high fever, often complicated by a seizure before the onset of the rash.
4. *Shigella* organisms produce high fevers and a neurotoxin. Seizures are common.
5. Meningitis occurs in about 2% of children with fevers and seizures.

DIAGNOSTIC FINDINGS

1. Typically, there is a preceding infectious illness and high fever (usually >39° C). Patients have signs and symptoms of the underlying systemic infection. Of obvious importance is exclusion of meningitis; in patients having lethargy, fever, headache, vomiting, etc. (p. 741).
2. Seizures are generalized tonic-clonic episodes lasting less than 15 minutes. The seizures are classified as complex when an episode lasts more than 15 minutes, is focal, or is followed by transient or persistent neurologic abnormalities.
3. Behavior and state of alertness are altered:
   a. Children are postictal.
   b. The underlying illness produces irritability, lethargy, and other changes in mental status.
4. Aggressive antipyretic therapy early in the management facilitates evaluation.

Complications

Febrile seizures are usually self-limited, although they may be recurrent or complex, resulting in hypoxia and self-injury.

Ancillary Data

Lumbar Puncture. LP is a useful part of the evaluation of the patient, particularly for a patient with a first febrile seizure (see Appendix A-4). LP should generally be performed in the patient:

1. Who is younger than 1 year.
2. Who is younger than 2 years and has a temperature of 41.1° C or more.
3. Who remains irritable or lethargic or demonstrates other abnormal behavior after aggressive antipyretic therapy.
4. For whom there is any question of the reliability of the examination, the caretaker, or follow-up.

Other factors worthy of consideration are a prior physician visit within 48 hours, generalized seizure in the emergency department (ED), and focal seizure.

Evaluation of the CSF should include Gram stain, culture, cell count, and protein and glucose determinations. Prior antibiotic management may complicate the interpretation of the assessment.

Blood Glucose. Serum glucose should be measured immediately, either by quantitative methods or with a reagent strip (Dextrostix or Chemstrip).

CBC with Differential Count. CBC and differential count are usually unreliable because of the demargination resulting from catecholamine release.

Electrolytes and Blood Urea Nitrogen. Determination of electrolyte and blood urea nitrogen values is indicated if there is a preceding problem with intake or output. Ca^{++} and PO_4^{--} determinations are not indicated in previously normal children except for neonates.

Other Studies. Skull roentgenograms or CT scan is obtained if there is associated trauma. An EEG usually is not obtained, because it has little or no prognostic value, although transient abnormalities may be noted.

DIFFERENTIAL DIAGNOSIS
(see Table 81-5)

1. Infection:
   a. CNS infection, including that caused by bacterial, viral, fungal or mycobacterial agents. LP is required for differentiation.
   b. Postinfectious encephalitis.
   c. Brain abscess with fever, seizures, and variable CSF findings.
   d. Immunization, particularly DTP.
2. Intoxication:
   a. Hydrocarbon ingestion with aspiration pneumonitis, fever, and seizures.
   b. Salicylate overdose.
3. Intrapsychic problem. Breath-holding spells may occur during intercurrent febrile illness.

MANAGEMENT (see Chapter 21)

1. Patients with acute seizures need intervention with oxygen, suction, and maneuvers to minimize self-injury. Rarely is active airway management required. Establish venous access for drug administration. Only rarely is a patient having seizures by the time of arrival at the ED. For a patient still having a seizure, give dextrose, 0.5 to 1.0 g/kg/dose (2 to 4 ml 25% dextrose in water (D25W) per kg per dose) IV.
2. Administer anticonvulsants (see Table 81-6) if patient continues to have active seizures after airway and breathing are stabilized:
   - **a.** Diazepam (Valium): 0.2 to 0.3 mg/kg/dose IV given over 2 to 3 minutes at a rate not to exceed 1 mg/min. May be repeated every 5 to 10 minutes if seizures continue (maximum total dose: 10 mg). Used to stop seizures.
   - **b.** Lorazepam (Ativan): 0.05 to 0.15 mg/kg/dose IV over 1 to 3 minutes. Repeat doses are rarely beneficial (maximum total dose in adult: 5 mg).
   - **c.** Phenobarbital: 15 to 20 mg/kg/dose IV (25 to 50 mg/min or 1 mg/kg/min IV) or IM (erratic absorption), given as loading dose as an alternative, followed by maintenance. May be used as maintenance drug (3 to 5 mg/kg/24 hr IV, PO) as well as in the management of the patient with acute seizures.
   - **d.** Phenytoin (Dilantin): 10 to 20 mg/kg/dose IV infusion (concentration of ≤6.7 mg/ml in saline solution, not water; not to exceed 40 mg/min or 0.5 mg/kg/min). Maximum loading dose: 1250 mg total dose. Maintenance dose of 5 mg/kg/24 hr IV or PO. Fosphenytoin (Cerebyx) is a preparation that may be administered more rapidly IV without complications. It may also be given IM.
   - **e.** Erythromycin may decrease metabolism of phenytoin, requiring a reduction in the anticonvulsant dose.
3. Patients who are not having active seizures need rapid evaluation and antipyretic therapy. Questioning should be focused on potential infectious sources, history of seizures, neurologic deficits, developmental problems, family history, medications, precipitating events, and preceding illness.
   - Antipyretic therapy should include acetaminophen, 10 to 15 mg/kg/dose q4-6hr PO, and tepid water sponging. Ibuprofen, 10 mg/kg/dose q6hr PO, may also be useful. Aspirin may also be used if neither chickenpox nor influenza-like illness is present.
4. Obtain laboratory data, including an LP, as appropriate.
5. Treat underlying infections as appropriate.
6. Long-term anticonvulsants reduce, but do not eliminate, recurrent febrile seizures. Consider phenobarbital (5 mg/kg/24 hr q12-24hr PO after a loading dose) in the following circumstances (see Table 81-6):
   - **a.** Patient with two or more of the following risk factors:
     - **(1)** Abnormal neurologic or developmental history before the seizures
     - **(2)** Complex seizure: seizure that lasts more than 15 minutes, is focal, or is followed by transient or persistent neurologic abnormalities
     - **(3)** Positive family history for afebrile seizures in a first-degree relative
   - **b.** Child younger than 12 months at the time of the first seizure.
   - **c.** Child in whom there was only a brief interval (1 hour) between the onset of fever and the initial seizure.

     NOTE: If anticonvulsants are initiated, they are continued for 2 years if the patient remains seizure free, although this decision must be

individualized. Intermittent use of anticonvulsant agents is of no value.
- Family anxiety and other social factors may modify the decision to initiate anticonvulsant therapy.
- Learning disorders and hyperactivity may be associated with the use of phenobarbital.

Anticonvulsants should be initiated only for appropriate reasons. Most children do not need medication.

DISPOSITION

1. Patients with simple febrile seizures may be discharged after appropriate fever control has been achieved. Underlying infections must also be treated.
2. Patients who need phenobarbital therapy may similarly be discharged with close follow-up observation and neurologic consultation after a loading dose has been given and maintenance therapy has been initiated. Phenobarbital therapy is normally prescribed for 2 years when deemed appropriate, with dosage adjustments to accommodate growth. Intermittent phenobarbital is of no value.
3. Approximately 40% of children with a simple febrile seizure have a recurrence, half of which occur within 6 months of the first episode.
4. Recurrent febrile seizures are also related to a fever less than 1 hour before (44%) as well as to a lower body temperature at the time of the seizure.

Parental Education

Parental counseling is essential to provide reassurance. A number of issues must be discussed with the parents:

1. Benign nature of febrile seizures in healthy children. Reassuring points include the high incidence (2% to 5%), the only slightly higher incidence of epilepsy in children identified as being at high risk, the low frequency of recurrences, and the rare incidence of death or sequelae.
2. Home treatment, which must include first aid to protect the airway and minimize self-injury. Fever control must be reviewed.
3. The risks and benefits of anticonvulsant therapy. It may reduce recurrences, but it has adverse effects.
4. The parent should call the physician after the initial evaluation if any of the following occurs:
   a. Fever continues more than 36 hours; behavioral changes develop; severe vomiting, headache, nonblanching rash, or stiff neck develops; or another seizure occurs.
   b. The child is taking medication and becomes lethargic, hyperactive, or irritable or has a rash from phenobarbital. Sedation early in the course of treatment is common.

BIBLIOGRAPHY

American Academy of Pediatrics: Practice parameters: the neurodiagnostic evaluation of the child with a first simple febrile seizure, *Pediatrics* 97:169, 1996.

Anderson AB, Desisto MJ, Marshall PC et al: Duration of fever prior to onset of a simple febrile seizure: a predictor of significant illness and neurologic course, *Pediatr Emerg Care* 5:12, 1989.

Berg AT, Shinnar S, Darefsy AS et al: Predictors of recurrent febrile seizures, *Arch Pediatr Adolesc Med* 151:371, 1997.

Berg AT, Shinnar S, Hauser WA: A prospective study of recurrent febrile seizures, *N Engl J Med* 327:1122, 1992.

Bettis DB, Ater SB: Febrile seizures: emergency department diagnosis and treatment, *J Emerg Med* 2:341, 1985.

Depiero AD, Teach SJ: Febrile seizures, *Pediatr Emerg Care* 17:384, 2001.

Duffner PK, Baumann RJ: A synopsis of the AAP practice parameters on the evaluation and treatment of children with febrile seizures, *Pediatr Rev* 20:285, 1999.

82 Orthopedic Disorders

Also See Chapters 27 (Arthralgia and Joint Pain), 40 (Limp), and 66 through 70 (Orthopedic Injuries)

Septic Arthritis

ALERT Immediate drainage and antibiotics are indicated if the joint is to be salvaged.

Septic arthritis is an infection of the synovial membrane and joint space resulting from either hematogenous spread or direct inoculation.

Predisposing factors include systemic bacterial infections, gonorrhea, and impaired immunologic status.

ETIOLOGY: INFECTION

1. *Staphylococcus aureus:* represents 20% to 30% of isolates and is often preceded by trauma
2. *Haemophilus influenzae*
   - **a.** Most common in children younger than 5 years but found in older children; less common with widespread immunization
   - **b.** Often associated with infections elsewhere (meningitis)
3. Streptococci: group A, group B, anaerobic, *Streptococcus viridans*
4. *Streptococcus pneumoniae*
5. *Neisseria gonorrhoeae*: primarily knee, wrist, and hand
6. Uncommon
   - **a.** Gram-negative enteric: neonates and immunosuppressed patients
   - **b.** *Pseudomonas* organisms: neonates, immunosuppressed persons; persons with puncture wounds

DIAGNOSTIC FINDINGS

1. Patients inconsistently have systemic illness with fever, anorexia, and listlessness.
2. Local findings include pain and tenosynovitis, particularly with gonorrhea. The joints are tender, with warmth, swelling, effusion, and limitation of movement (see Chapter 40). It is primarily a monoarticular disease, involving the large, weight-bearing joints of the knee, hip, shoulder, wrist, and elbow. The patient may have concurrent osteomyelitis.
3. In one series of *H. influenzae* septic arthritis, 35% had associated otitis media and 30% had meningitis.

Complications

Complications of septic arthritis involve damage to growth plate and joint cartilage, leading to poor growth and a stiff or destroyed joint.

Ancillary Data

1. White blood cell (WBC) count variable; erythrocyte sedimentation rate (ESR) is usually elevated and normalizes with recovery.
2. Blood cultures: positive results in 50% of cases of nongonococcal disease and 20% of gonococcal infections.
3. Cultures of the cervix, rectum, and pharynx if gonorrhea is suspected: positive results in 80% of patients with gonococcal disease.

4. Arthrocentesis and analysis of the synovial fluid, including glucose content, cell count and differential, Gram stain, and culture (Table 82-1 and Appendix A-2). Culture results may be negative in gonococcal arthritis.
5. X-ray films: plain films of joint:
   a. Early changes consist of joint fluid with capsular distension. If a film is difficult to interpret, comparison views may help.
   b. Bony demineralization and subsequent cartilaginous and bony destruction may develop; however, radiographs may be normal and therefore are not sensitive enough to be used as a screen.
6. Nuclear scan:
   a. Indicated when joint tap is contraindicated (overlying infection, small joints, axial skeleton involved).
   b. Technetium (Tc 99m) scan: positive result within 24 hours of symptoms and may remain positive. Three-phase study may be helpful in differentiating septic arthritis from osteomyelitis (see p. 769).
   c. Gallium (Ga 67) scan: result positive within 24 to 48 hours of symptoms but reverts to normal with adequate treatment.

DIFFERENTIAL DIAGNOSIS

There is significant overlap of ESR findings, temperature, and WBC count in children with septic arthritis and transient synovitis of the hip.

See Chapter 27.

MANAGEMENT

1. Initial management must exclude other conditions in the differential diagnosis. Delay in treatment of septic arthritis exposes the patient to permanent joint damage.
2. Once septic arthritis is considered, the joint should be aspirated and the fluid analyzed (see Table 82-1).
3. The joint should be immobilized and physical therapy initiated once recovery is partially achieved.

Antibiotics

Initial antibiotics are selected on the basis of the Gram stain result of the fluid obtained from the arthrocentesis and on the patient's drug allergies. Once final culture results and

TABLE 82-1 Common Synovial Fluid Findings

Category	Etiology	Appearance	Leukocytes (cells/mm^3)	Percentage of Neutrophils $\left[\frac{\text{synovial}}{\text{blood}}\right]$	Percentage of Glucose	Mucin* Clot
Normal		Clear	<100	25	>50	Good
Bacterial	Septic arthritis	Turbid, purulent	>50,000	>75	<50	Poor
Inflammatory	Juvenile rheumatoid arthritis Rheumatic fever Mycobacterial, viral, and fungal arthritis	Clear or turbid	500-75,000	50	>50	Poor
Traumatic		Clear or bloody	<5,000†	<50	>50	Good

* For mucin clot: add 4 ml of water to 1 ml of synovial fluid supernatant. Mix in 2 drops of 5% glacial acetic acid. If normal, a tight rope of mucin will form. If infection or inflammation is present, clot will flake and shred.

† May have red blood cells.

sensitivity data are available, the antibiotic agents may be altered.

For known organisms, the following agents and dosages are recommended:

S. aureus: Nafcillin, 100 to 200 mg/kg/24 hr q4hr IV, or an equivalent semisynthetic penicillin

H. influenzae: Cefotaxime, 150 mg/kg/24 hr q6-8hr IV; *or* ceftriaxone, 75 mg/kg/24 hr q12hr IV; *or* ceftizoxime, 150 mg/kg/24 hr q8hr IV

S. pneumoniae: Penicillin G, 100,000 U/kg/24 hr q4hr IV

N. gonorrhoeae: Penicillin G, as above

For unknown organisms, the following agents are recommended:

All patients: Nafcillin

Neonates: Add gentamicin, 5.0 to 7.5 mg/kg/24 hr q8-12hr IV or IM

Infants (≤5 yr): Add cefotaxime or ceftriaxone

1. Clinical trials have substantiated the value of third-generation cephalosporins in the treatment of joint infections.
2. Traditionally, parenteral antibiotics are continued for a minimum of 2 weeks (gonococci, streptococci, and *Haemophilus* organisms) to 3 weeks (staphylococci, gram-negative enteric organisms, and *Pseudomonas* organisms). Some investigators have used oral medications after 1 week of parenteral drugs associated with resolution of signs and symptoms while carefully monitoring clinical response. Serum drug levels, which must have a bactericidal level of at least a dilution of 1:8, may be monitored in patients who show slow response or require antibiotics to achieve moderate levels. May also be used to monitor compliance.

Joint Drainage

1. Initially, needle aspiration of the joint is attempted to relieve pressure and decompress the joint, unless surgical drainage is more appropriate. Aspiration also allows specimens to be obtained for evaluation.
2. Surgical drainage is indicated in the following situations, although some clinicians prefer to drain joints in other circumstances as well:
   - **a.** The hip, elbow, ankle, or shoulder is involved.
   - **b.** Thick, purulent material is obtained.
   - **c.** Adhesions are present, or inadequate decompression is achieved after 2 to 3 days of repeated needle aspiration.
   - **d.** Response to therapy is poor after 36 to 48 hours of antibiotics.
   - **e.** Long delay in the initiation of treatment has occurred.

DISPOSITION

All patients must be hospitalized. Immediate orthopedic consultation should be obtained. The outcome is better in patients who are hospitalized and treated within 5 days of onset of symptoms.

BIBLIOGRAPHY

Barton LL, Dunkle LM, Habib FH: Septic arthritis in children, *Am J Dis Child* 145:898, 1987.

Del Beccaro MA, Champoux AN, Bochers T, Mendelman PM: Septic arthritis versus transient synovitis of the hip: the value of screening laboratory tests, *Ann Emerg Med* 21:1418, 1992.

Volberg FM, Sumner TE, Abramson JS et al: Unreliability of radiographic diagnosis of septic hip in children, *Pediatrics* 73:118, 1984.

Osteomyelitis

ALERT Acute onset of limp or local tenderness, warmth, or erythema requires a careful evaluation. A prolonged course of antibiotics is indicated.

Acute osteomyelitis is an infection of bone, occurring most commonly by hematogenous spread but also in association with direct inoculation that is secondary to open fractures, penetrating wounds, or surgical procedures.

The metaphysis of a long bone, particularly the femur or tibia, is most commonly involved.

Factors predisposing an individual to osteomyelitis include trauma, systemic bacterial disease, drug abuse, sickle cell disease, and impaired immunologic status.

ETIOLOGY: INFECTION

1. *S. aureus:* accounts for 60% to 90% of isolates
2. *H. influenzae:* most common in children younger than 3 years although incidence is decreasing
3. *Pseudomonas* organisms: common in drug abusers and with osteomyelitis caused by penetrating injury of the foot, usually through a rubber-soled shoe in older children
4. Other organisms associated with infection:
   a. Streptococcal species: group A and B (in neonates usually B)
   b. *Staphylococcus epidermidis*
   c. *Salmonella* organisms: usually in patients with sickle cell disease
   d. Gram-negative enteric organisms: usually in newborns
   e. Mycobacteria
   f. Fungal: usually in immunocompromised patients

DIAGNOSTIC FINDINGS

1. The clinical findings are extremely variable, and the physician should be suspicious for osteomyelitis. Most patients have a fever and occasionally report a predisposing factor. Systemic disease may be present.
2. Patients may have a limp (see Chapter 40) and limitation of movement or merely a history of favoring the extremity.
3. Inconsistent local systems are tenderness, warmth, erythema, and pain over the involved site.
4. Children younger than 1 year have little systemic toxicity.

Complications

1. Septic arthritis (p. 767). More common in infants.
2. Growth disturbance of the limb if there is disruption of the epiphyseal growth plate.
3. Chronic osteomyelitis with persistent infection, often a result of inadequate treatment.

Ancillary Data

1. WBC count: often elevated, although most patients have counts between 5000 and 15,000 cells/mm^3.
2. ESR and C-reactive protein (CRP) value: commonly elevated; provides a useful parameter to assess the adequacy of treatment because it normalizes with resolution of inflammation. The CRP value normalizes earlier than the ESR, and its normalization correlates with a good outcome.
3. Blood cultures: results positive in more than 50% of patients.
4. X-ray film: plain film of extremity.
   a. Soft tissue findings develop 3 to 4 days after the onset of symptoms:
      (1) Swelling of deep soft tissues next to metaphysis with displacement of fat lines
      (2) Obliteration of lucent planes between muscles
      (3) Subcutaneous edema
   b. Bony changes are noted 7 to 10 days after symptomatic onset:
      (1) Periosteal elevation
      (2) Lytic lesions
      (3) Sclerosis with new bone formation
5. Nuclear bone scan with Tc 99m:
   a. Initial scan and delayed study (4-8 hr) may be useful. Taking films 24 hours after initial infusion may improve specificity. Three-phase scan may show (1) increased flow on radionuclide angiogram, (2) increased activity on blood pool images, and (3) focal increased bone activity on delayed images. Cellulitis appears as increased

activity on blood pool images but as normal soft tissue activity on delayed images.

b. Nuclear bone scan findings often become abnormal 1 to 2 days after onset of symptoms with increased uptake in area of inflammation.

c. Results may be falsely negative in up to 25% of cases, particularly in newborns and children younger than 1 year.

d. Uptake of radionuclide is locally increased in osteomyelitis, septic arthritis, cellulitis, trauma, and neoplastic disease.

6. Aspiration of involved bone (usually performed by orthopedist): provides definitive identification and sensitivity of etiologic organism.
- Gram stain of aspirate may provide initial etiologic information.

7. Serum bactericidal titers may be useful in monitoring therapeutic regimens. However, the high serum levels achieved with many oral antibiotics decrease the importance of this measure.

DIFFERENTIAL DIAGNOSIS

1. Infection:
  a. Septic arthritis (p. 767)
  b. Cellulitis (p. 582)

2. Trauma:
  a. Local soft tissue injury
  b. Fracture

3. Neoplasm: Ewing's tumor

MANAGEMENT

1. The key to appropriate management is early identification of the patient with osteomyelitis.

2. Culture specimens should be obtained before therapy is initiated.

3. Aspiration of the lesions by an orthopedist is indicated. Many clinicians recommend drainage and curettage if pus is obtained on aspiration. Open drainage also is indicated if there is poor response in the first 36 to 48 hours after initiation of antibiotic therapy.

4. Immobilization of the involved extremity may minimize pain in the initial treatment stages (i.e., evaluation and stabilization).

Antibiotics

1. Give nafcillin (or other semisynthetic penicillin: methicillin or oxacillin), 100 to 200 mg/kg/24 hr q4hr IV (assuming no allergy). Alternative regimens include cefazolin or cephalothin, 100 mg/kg/24 hr q4-6hr IV.

2. Administer additional antibiotics if an organism other than *S. aureus* is suspected.

  a. In a child younger than 5 years, consider adding cefuroxime, 150 mg/kg/24 hr q6-8hr IV, to cover for *H. influenzae.*

  b. If the patient has sickle cell disease or is a neonate, a *Salmonella* organism or gram-negative enteric may be etiologic:
  - Give ampicillin, 200 mg/kg/24 hr q4hr IV, and gentamicin, 5.0 to 7.5 mg/kg/24 hr q8-12hr IV or IM. Prolonged therapy is indicated.

  c. With a puncture wound of the foot through a rubber-soled shoe or if the patient is a drug abuser and routine management is not adequate, a *Pseudomonas* organism should be considered and treated with the following:
    (1) Surgical drainage, as needed.
    (2) Carbenicillin, 400 to 600 mg/kg/24 hr q4hr IV, and gentamicin, as already described; *or* ceftazidime (Fortaz), 100 to 150 mg/kg/24 hr q8hr IV.

3. In the routine care of osteomyelitis caused by *S. aureus*, patients are normally treated parenterally for 5 to 7 days, assuming that local inflammation decreases and the ESR normalizes.

4. After the initial course of parenteral therapy and resolution of signs and symptoms, patients may be switched to oral therapy for 3 to 6 weeks. Studies suggest that with a good therapeutic response, the total treatment period may be reduced to as short as 3 weeks. The influence of shorter regimens on the rate of recurrence is still under investigation.

- Dicloxacillin, 75 to 100 mg/kg/24 hr q6hr PO; *or*
- If the patient is allergic to penicillin: cephalexin, 50 to 100 mg/kg/24 hr q6hr PO, *or* clindamycin, 15 to 25 mg/kg/24 hr q6hr PO

5. Antibiotics may be modified by the results of Gram stain, culture, and sensitivity testing.
6. During the phase of oral therapy, patients are often hospitalized to ensure continuing compliance.
7. Throughout the course of treatment, serum bactericidal levels or serum antibiotic levels, if monitored, should achieve a bactericidal titer at a dilution of 1:8 or greater.

DISPOSITION

1. All patients should be hospitalized for therapy.
2. An orthopedic consultation should be obtained. Infectious disease consultants may also be useful in the evaluation and long-term management of the patient, particularly if an unusual organism is suspected or identified.

BIBLIOGRAPHY

Chisholm CD, Schlesser JF: Plantar puncture wounds: controversies and treatment recommendations, *Ann Emerg Med* 18:1352, 1989.

Faden H, Grossi M: Acute osteomyelitis in children, *Am J Dis Child* 145:65, 1991.

Jacobs NM: Pneumococcal osteomyelitis and arthritis in children, *Am J Dis Child* 145:70, 1991.

Mustafa MM, Saez-Llorens X, McCracken GH et al: Acute hematogenous pelvic osteomyelitis in infants and children, *Pediatr Infect Dis J* 9:416, 1990.

Peltola H, Unkila-Kallio L, Kallio MLT et al: Simplified treatment of acute staphylococcal osteomyelitis of childhood, *Pediatrics* 99:846, 1997.

Unkila-Kallio L: Serum C-reactive protein, erythrocyte sedimentation rate, and white blood cell count in acute hematogenous osteomyelitis of children, *Pediatrics* 93:59, 1994.

83 Psychiatric Disorders

Management Principles

The psychiatric examination of children and their families requires, above all else, sensitivity and a belief in one's own intuition. Data in the psychiatric evaluation may be "hard"—for example, an admission by the patient that he or she is suicidal or homicidal—but may also be "soft." At times the only clue to an adolescent's violent inclination may be an uneasiness or anxiety on the part of the evaluator. Such feelings in the examiner, termed *countertransference,* can be used with great acumen to diagnose a variety of psychiatric ailments. If used appropriately, such data complement the more objective data obtained in a history.

The evaluator also must be willing to ask probing and difficult questions. Objectivity in the history taking maximizes the chances that the patient will respond honestly and candidly. The examiner who is in a hurry or does not want to hear about certain aspects of the patient's behavior subtly encourages a patient not to discuss his or her depression, suicidal ideation, or sexual perversions, for example. The examiner who is calm and maintains an empathic stance with patients will be amazed at how many describe really pressing psychiatric problems. The humbling statistic that nearly 50% of all patients who commit suicide have seen a physician sometime in the previous months speaks to such patients' desire to talk about problems and receive help, and, sadly, to physicians' frequent lack of responsiveness.

The approach to the preadolescent patient is usually different from that to the adolescent. Initially, it is often appropriate to see the child's parents first and gather as much history from them as possible. Then the child can be seen, usually alone, unless he or she is too upset about being separated from the parents. The evaluator should first ask about the child's understanding of the evaluation. Clarifying that no shots will be given and that confidentiality will be maintained (unless information about the child being in danger emerges) can help loosen up a child. Even a 3-year-old child can communicate. Toys and drawings (which may reveal unconscious problems) should be saved for last. Particular attention should be paid to how the child relates to the examiner (oblivious? clinging?), to the child's activity level, and to how he or she relates to the parents. The question "How do you [does he or she] get along with friends?" posed to child and parents is the best single screening question for major psychologic disorder. If the child is isolated or has major interactive problems, a significant psychopathologic condition can be expected. If not, the child is usually in reasonable shape.

In contrast, the adolescent should always be seen first and alone. The typical adolescent bristles at the idea that the evaluator is the parents' agent and thus must understand that the examiner is there to help him or her. This can be achieved through honesty and *objectivity* (regardless of personal morals and values). Teenagers can usually see through any falseness in the evaluator, who (1) should try to leave his or her own adolescence in the waiting room and avoid the use of adolescent language that is not natural and (2) should not encumber the patient with personal feelings about such issues as marijuana, sex, and high school. Particular attention should be paid to such concerns as emancipation from the family,* peer pressure, and heterosexual and homosexual exposure. These are the issues that dominate adolescent development and that lie at the root of an adolescent's psychiatric problems.

Conversion Reactions

Classic conversion reactions are rare, but conversion components of true physical illness may exist and may occur concomitantly with other serious psychopathologic conditions. The *initial* approach to a patient with a possible conversion disorder should be *both* medical and psychiatric. Conversion reaction is not a diagnosis of exclusion. Conversely, even when no physical cause is found to explain the loss of functioning, medical care should not be abandoned, because a large percentage of cases of conversion reaction are subsequently found to have an organic disease as the cause.

DIAGNOSTIC FINDINGS

1. Loss of physical functioning, suggesting a physical disorder.
2. Psychologic factors as part of the symptoms.

   NOTE: Many investigators believe it is possible to have simultaneous true organic abnormality and a conversion component.
3. Symptoms that are not conscious or voluntary. The loss of functioning is usually in the voluntary nervous system, rarely autonomic.
4. Symptoms that defy anatomic explanation usually have some symbolic significance that may reduce anxiety; they may manifest at times of stress.
5. Associated findings:
   - **a.** "La belle indifference" is probably of no value in verifying the diagnosis.
   - **b.** Some symbolism may be involved in the development of the symptom (e.g., paralyzed arm prevents patient from hitting wife). The patient may try to emulate a relative's symptoms.
   - **c.** A history of somatic symptoms is often present.
   - **d.** Previous central nervous system (CNS) abnormality or trauma increases the risk for conversion disorder.
   - **e.** Secondary gain is often present (i.e., the sick role is gratifying to the patient).

DIFFERENTIAL DIAGNOSIS

Conversion reactions should be differentiated from true organic disorders. Psychiatric disorders that must be excluded include the following:

1. Hypochondriasis: an unrealistic interpretation of normal body signs
2. Malingering: a conscious attempt to get attention through *voluntarily* feigned symptoms
3. Munchausen's syndrome: an unconscious attempt to gain attention through voluntarily feigned symptoms
4. Depression: may occur with somatic symptoms in the absence of other signs of depression

MANAGEMENT

1. Conversion symptoms are often transient and disappear on their own. The patient may need to be hospitalized until the symptoms partially resolve.
2. Psychotherapy is indicated in refractory cases.
3. The patient may retrench and worsen if an attempt is made (especially initially) to prove that the symptoms are emotional.
4. Any other underlying psychopathologic condition (e.g., schizophrenia) should be treated.

* For the adolescent runaway, two resources may be useful: Runaway Hotline (800-231-6946) and National Runaway Switchboard (800-621-4000).

5. The prognosis is good, especially with acute onset, short duration of the symptom, adequate premorbid personality, and minimal secondary gain from the symptom. It is crucial to focus on the reduction of stress.

Acute Psychoses

In the patient with acute psychosis, immediate attention must be paid to the level of self-destructiveness and potential for violence. If any doubt exists, the patient should be legally and physically restrained (e.g., with hospital guards) until these questions can be answered. Although psychiatrists disagree about subtypes of psychoses in childhood, several categories have emerged as distinct diagnostic entities that should be familiar to anyone involved in caring for pediatric emergencies. A child with an acute psychosis often seems "off" or detached. Accurate diagnosis and disposition are paramount because many such children, when they arrive at an ED, have come from isolated, suspicious families who rarely frequent hospitals.

INFANTILE AUTISM

Etiology

1. Unproven former theories of autism that involve "refrigerator parents" and abnormal child-rearing have been discarded in favor of a more dynamic cause potentially involving multiple organic disorders that lead to challenging parenting issues and abnormal interpersonal interactions.
2. The illness is probably evenly distributed among socioeconomic groups.

Diagnostic Findings

1. Age at onset is usually less than 30 months
2. Highly unusual responses to environment (need for sameness, stereotypes), with poor social relations
3. Gross deficits in language development; abnormal speech patterns (echolalia, pronoun reversals)
4. Absence of delusions or hallucinations
5. Commonly associated findings:
   a. Congenital blindness
   b. Retardation (70% of patients have an intelligence quotient [IQ] below 70)
   c. Grand mal seizures before adolescence
6. Pockets of normal or even precocious development (e.g., unusual memory or ability to calculate quickly)
7. Abnormal auditory-evoked responses

Differential Diagnosis

1. Mental retardation: Usually with uniform lags in development in all spheres (e.g., motor, social, language). Mentally retarded children ordinarily demonstrate some social relatedness.
2. Diffuse CNS disease (cytomegalovirus, phenylketonuria, hepatic encephalopathy).
3. Deafness: Audiogram helps differentiate.

Management

1. Multifaceted management (behavioral, structured educational program, psychotherapy) is indicated. Hospitalization should always be considered.
2. Neuroleptics may help symptoms of agitation, anxiety, and destructiveness. For example, thioridazine [Mellaril], at a starting dosage of 0.5 to 1 mg/kg/24 hr q8-12hr PO (adult: 25 mg q8-12hr PO). Dosage is then titrated to the response.

The prognosis is very guarded, being best for children with a high IQ and good language development.

SCHIZOPHRENIA

Etiology

There are multiple causative theories for schizophrenia, ranging from abnormal family patterns to a faulty neurotransmitter mechanism (dopamine hypothesis). Schizophrenia has a strong familial predilection.

Diagnostic Findings

1. Usual onset in late adolescence but may occur in earlier childhood
2. Lengthy prodrome of at least 6 months, during which patients exhibit gradual withdrawal from previous relationships and functioning
3. Delusions
4. Hallucinations (usually auditory)
5. Abnormal content of speech (loosening of associations)
6. Altered affect, which often is inappropriate to the content of speech (e.g., laughing while describing the death of a relative) but not predominantly euphoric or depressed
7. Associated findings:
   a. Catatonia with either excitement or motoric rigidity
   b. Excitation can be life threatening; poor impulse control or paranoia can make patients with schizophrenia very dangerous

Differential Diagnosis

1. Other nonorganic psychoses (manic-depression, which shows a predominant mood problem).
2. Organic psychoses: Patient usually has faulty cognition, which can be demonstrated with tests of memory (remembering three unrelated objects at 3 minutes) and orientation (to person, place, and time; disorientation to time is the first to be affected). Causes are multiple but, in the pediatric population, most commonly are ingestions (e.g., hallucinogens).
3. Reactive psychoses (also called schizophreniform psychoses): More acute and short-lived.
4. Acute grief reaction.

Management

The patient should be hospitalized for protection.

Neuroleptics. Neuroleptic agents should usually be administered after 1 to 2 days of hospitalization to see how well the patient responds to a safe environment, unless the patient is agitated, combative, or in need of seclusion:

- Thiothixene (Navane), 10 to 30 mg/24 hr, *or* thioridazine (Mellaril), 200 to 800 mg/24 hr PO, reflecting the patient's age, size, and response to therapy.

Side effects are important and must be considered (p. 393):

1. Acute dystonias, especially with high-potency neuroleptics (e.g., haloperidol [Haldol]): Treat with an anticholinergic agent (e.g., benztropine [Cogentin], 1-2 mg PO or IM q12hr).
2. Parkinsonian side effects: Treat with an anticholinergic agent (Cogentin as in 1).
3. Akathisia (motor restlessness): Difficult to treat and often requires adjustment in neuroleptic dosage.
4. Anticholinergic signs and symptoms, especially with low-potency neuroleptics (e.g., chlorpromazine, thioridazine [Mellaril]).
5. Tardive dyskinesias: Incidence increases with duration of treatment. May be "unmasked" when dosage of neuroleptic is lowered. No effective treatment at this time.
6. Rash, cholestatic jaundice.

Other Considerations

1. Electroconvulsive therapy only if all else fails or if patient is in serious danger (e.g., agitatedly catatonic or acutely suicidal)
2. Family and individual psychotherapy
3. Discharge planning and follow-up: crucial in preventing relapse
4. Prognosis: guarded

ORGANIC PSYCHOSES
Diagnostic Findings

1. Evidence of an organic cause: ingestion (hallucinogens, cocaine, amphetamines, over-the-counter anticholinergics);

systemic illness; endocrine disorder (adrenal, thyroid); renal, cardiac, or liver failure; sensory deprivation (intensive care unit [ICU] "psychosis")
2. Cognitive impairment (memory and disorientation)
3. Predominantly visual hallucinations (if any) versus auditory hallucinations in schizophrenia

Management

1. Treatment of underlying disorder
2. Occasionally, seclusion, restraint, or neuroleptics (neuroleptics have sedative and anticholinergic properties and may be contraindicated)

MANIC-DEPRESSIVE PSYCHOSIS

Diagnostic Findings

Manic-depressive psychosis is rare in childhood and principally involves the following:

1. Increased motor activity
2. Flight of ideas
3. Euphoric or dysphoric mood change
4. Associated findings: spending binges, decreased need for sleep, grandiosity, delusions, hallucinations, increased sexual activity

Differential Diagnosis

Adolescents who have taken stimulants or phencyclidine (PCP) or who have sustained brain damage may have some of these findings.

Management

Patients should be hospitalized and given some combination of neuroleptic and lithium treatment.

DEPRESSION

Diagnostic Findings

Children may demonstrate signs and symptoms of depression, which must be recognized and treated. Typically, patients have a variable appetite and some weight loss because of poor intake; other patients gain weight as a result of increased appetite. Insomnia or hypersomnia is common, with a loss of interest and pleasure in usual activities. Depressed individuals have thoughts of worthlessness and self-reproach and suicidal ideation.

Management

Of primary importance is recognizing the depressed state of the patient and making referral for both short-term evaluation and long-term therapy. The urgency of such counseling must reflect the severity of the depression and ensure that there is no immediate danger to the patient from self-injury.

Psychophysiologic Presentations

A psychophysiologic illness has three components; the patient must (1) have an underlying biologic or genetic disposition for a disease, (2) have a characteristic personality style, and (3) be in a stressful situation. Peptic ulcer disease and thyrotoxicosis are examples of such illnesses. Various illnesses are considered psychosomatic in that psychologic factors are seen as contributing to the actual disease process, but personality profiles and biologic markers and processes have yet to be delineated. The symptoms are often used to avoid undesirable activities, as in school phobias. The following are perhaps the most common presentations:

1. Rumination: An infant regurgitates and may have low weight, and symptoms worsen during separation from the mother.
2. Cyclic vomiting: In response to a subtle stress, a child vomits for several days and then is well for days to weeks. Usually starts around 5 years of age and ends in early adolescence.
3. Abdominal pain: Abdominal pain may result from a variety of physical conditions but also may be caused by a psychophysiologic illness (peptic ulcer,

ulcerative colitis) or, possibly, anorexia nervosa. When no cause is found, abdominal pain may be a conversion symptom.

4. Headache: A very common symptom, headache is usually transient in anxiety states but may be disabling when it is secondary to repressed anger, sexual wishes, etc.
5. Anorexia nervosa: Nonorganic extreme weight loss in the preadolescent or adolescent female, anorexia nervosa is initially associated with voluntary dieting and a preoccupation with obesity that does not diminish with weight loss. The patient has amenorrhea, withdrawal, depression, and an intense interest in physical activity that may lead to bradycardia and hypotension.
6. Bulimia nervosa: Binge eating is followed by purging, usually occurring twice weekly for at least 3 months. The weight is usually in the normal range. The patient's self-evaluation is overly dependent on weight and body shape. Patients are usually ambivalent about treatment, preferring to hide their behaviors.

Differential considerations for anorexia nervosa and bulimia nervosa include hypopituitarism, ovarian dysfunction, malabsorption, and malignancy. Behavioral modification with positive reinforcement is the basis for management to create a weight gain. The patient must be allowed to gain autonomy, effectiveness, and self-esteem. Hospitalization is often needed initially for both psychiatric and medical therapy.

School phobia or school refusal may manifest as one or more of the preceding problems. It is most common with the initial entrance into school, with a change of school, or at the beginning of the school year. Anxiety and separation anxiety may be present. After organic disease has been excluded, this disorder is best treated with insistence that the child attend school, along with provision of reassurance and encouragement of peer relationships.

Suicide Attempts

The incidence of suicide and suicide attempts in childhood is rising. Any seemingly innocent ingestion or accident should raise the question of a suicide attempt. Furthermore, any child who appears depressed should be asked about suicidal ideation, because suicide occurs most often in depressed individuals. Studies of suicidal people reveal that the risk of attempting or reattempting suicide is usually limited to a short crisis period. Therefore, safeguarding the patient with hospitalization or well-established supports is paramount in suicide management.

DIAGNOSTIC FINDINGS

Evaluation of the patient who has attempted or is threatening suicide should include the following:

1. Try to discover the precipitant. Usually a loss or reminder of a loss (anniversary reaction) is causative, but sometimes a simple event such as an argument with parents can trigger an attempt.
2. Assess risk factors:
   a. Girls attempt suicide more often than boys, but boys are more successful.
   b. A chronic illness in the patient raises the risk.
   c. A family history of suicide is often found.
   d. A personal history of previous suicide attempt is an ominous sign.
   e. An intoxicated patient is at greater risk. Substance abuse is a risk factor.
   f. Depression in the patient increases the risk.
   g. Estrangement from a loved one is also a risk factor.
   h. A personality with any of the following characteristics increases risk: hopeless, hostile, impulsive, perfectionism, poor social skills.

3. Carefully evaluate the present illness and suicidal behavior:
   a. How lethal was the method of suicide (gun or hanging versus ingestion of a few Valium)? Always ask about suicidal intent and plan.
   b. Was suicide attempted in complete isolation, or had the patient considered that he or she might be found before dying?
   c. Does any suicide note or afterthought explain a motivation?
   d. Is the patient depressed or schizophrenic or taking drugs?
   e. Would he or she try again if discharged?

The four factors found to be most useful in detecting suicide risk are current suicidal behavior, past suicidal ideation, past self-destructive behaviors, and current stressors.

Common pitfalls in evaluation are the following:

1. No one asks the patient about suicidal ideation or plan. Plan: Ask the patient directly.
2. On recovering from an overdose, the patient disappears. Plan: Always have patients guarded or in a locked unit until their freedom would not jeopardize them.
3. The physician or staff treats the patient roughly or unempathetically. Plan: Treat suicidal behavior medically, *not* judgmentally.

MANAGEMENT

1. Treat the medical or surgical sequelae of the suicide attempt.
2. Protect the patient with hospitalization or a sheltered environment if necessary.
3. Always include a psychiatrist in management. Ideally, this is done at the initial encounter to maximize insight into the precipitating event and to initiate discussion.
4. Try to shore up family and other sources of emotional support.
5. Remove all sources of potential self-injury if the patient is to return home.
6. Treat the underlying psychiatric illness:
   a. Depression—antidepressants, psychotherapy. Warning: Remember that the lethal dose ratio of tricyclic antidepressants is very low; dispense with caution.
   b. Schizophrenia—neuroleptics and hospitalization are usually needed.
   c. Intoxication or ingestion—perform serial suicide evaluations and mental status examinations until parameters return to baseline. Reevaluation is performed when the patient is sober.
7. At discharge, carefully evaluate your alliance with the patient (i.e., will he or she call you if needed and before the next attempt?).

Posttraumatic Stress Disorder

Anxiety may be associated with a known external traumatic event. The significance of the event relates to the level of exposure, appraisal of threat, and the personal impact. The two most likely stressors are a serious threat to the child's, a family member's, or a close friend's life and witnessing injury or death as a result of an accident or physical violence. Stressors resulting in posttraumatic stress disorder in children include the following:

- Kidnapping and a hostage situation
- Exposure to violence, including terrorism, gang violence, sniper attacks, and war atrocities
- Sexual or physical abuse
- Severe accidental injury, including burns and hit-and-run accidents
- Life-threatening illnesses and life-endangering medical procedures
- Train, airplane, ship, and auto accidents
- Major disasters

DIAGNOSTIC FINDINGS

Clinically, children actually respond to stress in a fashion parallel to the adult response. Several behavioral patterns may be noted in the months after a specific event. The phenomenon is often reexperienced through dreams, repetitive planning, or distress at traumatic reminders. Children may try to regulate their emotions or behavior by avoiding specific thoughts, feelings, or situations associated with the trauma. Interest in usual activities may be reduced. Isolation and memory disturbances are common. Patients may exhibit state of greater arousal, with sleep disturbances, irritability, and hypervigilance.

MANAGEMENT

The presence of this problem must first be recognized, and the child supported and counseled. This step is essential for all those involved in the initial stabilization and long-term management of the child. The focus must be on assisting in the recognition of traumatic reminders that elicit anxiety as well as helping children anticipate and understand the nature of the initial event. Family functioning strongly influences the child's reaction and recovery. The goals must be to restore a sense of personal security, to validate and explain responses, and to anticipate reminders. The school can also play a useful role.

Acute Grief Reaction

A sudden loss of a family member or friend from sudden infant death syndrome (SIDS), accidental death, or suicide or the loss of a job may result in a classic picture of grief and mourning. The behavior often follows a typical pattern over a period of weeks to months, from shock and denial or anger, through bargaining, depression (powerlessness over the event), and acceptance. Optimally, the patient or parent can constructively deal with the loss and its consequences.

Some patients experience a depressive mood disorder accompanied by sadness, insomnia, anorexia, agitation, and impaired concentration. Obviously, support is required. When findings persist beyond 2 months, suicidal ideation exists, or the patient is hallucinating or debilitated, formal intervention is appropriate.

Substance Abuse

Substance abuse is a major problem in the adolescent population. It is a significant risk factor in suicide and other psychiatric disorders. Substance abuse may result from, may exacerbate, or may uncover an associated psychiatric disorder. It should be considered in any patient who has psychiatric complaints or symptoms, and toxicologic screening as outlined in Chapter 54 may be required.

BIBLIOGRAPHY

Barnett TM: Psychiatric and behavioral disorders. In Barkin RM, editor: *Pediatric emergency medicine: concepts and clinical practice,* ed 2, St Louis, 1997, Mosby.

Frame DS, Kercher EE: Acute psychosis: functional versus organic, *Emerg Med Clin North Am* 9:123, 1991.

Hotowitz LM, Wang PS, Koocher GP et al: Detecting suicide risk in a pediatric emergency department: development of a brief screening tool, *Pediatrics* 107:1133, 2001.

Jari S, White M, Rosenberg LA et al: Munchausen syndrome by proxy, *Int Psych Med* 22:343, 1992.

Maisami M, Freeman JM: Conversion reactions in children as body language: a combined child psychiatry/neurology team approach to the management of functional neurologic disorders in children, *Pediatrics* 80:46, 1987.

Pynoos RS: Post-traumatic stress disorder in children and adolescents. In Garfunkul BD, Carlson GA, Waller ED, editors: *Psychiatric disorders in children and adolescents,* Philadelphia, 1990, WB Saunders.

Schecker N: Childhood conversion reactions in the emergency department: general and specific features, *Pediatr Emerg Care* 6:46, 1990.

Terr LC: Childhood traumas: an outline and overview, *Am J Psychiatry* 148:10, 1991.

Tueth MJ: Predicting suicide in the ED, *Am J Emerg Med* 14:434, 1996.

84 Pulmonary Disorders

Also See Chapters 13 (Apnea), 17 (Cyanosis), 20 (Respiratory Distress), 31 (Cough), and 62 (Thoracic Trauma)

Asthma

ALERT Not all wheezing is caused by asthma. The patient with asthma in severe respiratory distress may not wheeze. Oximetry and assessment of ventilation are essential for all patients. All patients with distress, tachypnea, or hypoxemia should receive oxygen.

Bronchoconstriction results from intrinsic mechanisms related to autonomic dysfunction or extrinsic sensitizing agents. A number of factors precipitate airway reactivity leading to hypoxia (Fig. 84-1).

An increase in intracellular cyclic adenosine 3′-5′ monophosphate (cAMP) resulting from the promotion of its biosynthesis (β-adrenergic agents) or inhibition of its degradation (theophylline) produces bronchodilation. Activation of the β-adrenergic receptors on airway smooth muscle leads to the activation of adenylate cyclase as well as an increase in the intracellular concentration of cAMP. This increase activates protein kinase A, which inhibits the phosphorylation of myosin and lowers intracellular ionic calcium concentrations, resulting in relaxation of the smooth muscle of the airways.

A rise in cyclic guanosine monophosphate (cGMP), produced by parasympathetic stimulation by cholinergic receptors, causes bronchoconstriction. Parasympathetic agents such as atropine antagonize the action of acetylcholine, inhibiting the release of cGMP. The decrease in vagal tone and relaxation promotes bronchodilation.

ETIOLOGY: PRECIPITATING AND AGGRAVATING FACTORS

1. Infection: associated with viral origin in 19% to 42% of cases
2. Allergic or irritant:
   a. Environmental: pollen, mold, animal dander
   b. Occupational chemicals or allergens: chlorine, ammonia
   c. Irritants: smoke, pollutants, gases, aerosols
   d. A family history of asthma or parental smoking contributes to airway responsiveness at an early age
   e. Environmental changes: moving to new home, vacation, etc.
   f. Food and additives
3. Exercise
4. Intrapsychic: emotional stress, phobias
5. Intoxication: bronchoconstrictors (propranolol, β-blockers, aspirin, nonsteroidal antiinflammatory drugs)

DIAGNOSTIC FINDINGS

In management of the patient after initial stabilization of the airway and breathing, it is essential to focus on the acute episode as well as previous experiences and management of reactive airway disease. Medications (type, dose, and time of last dose), duration of acute symptoms, associated illness, history of aspiration, and exposure must be determined. In addition to specific issues related to pulmonary

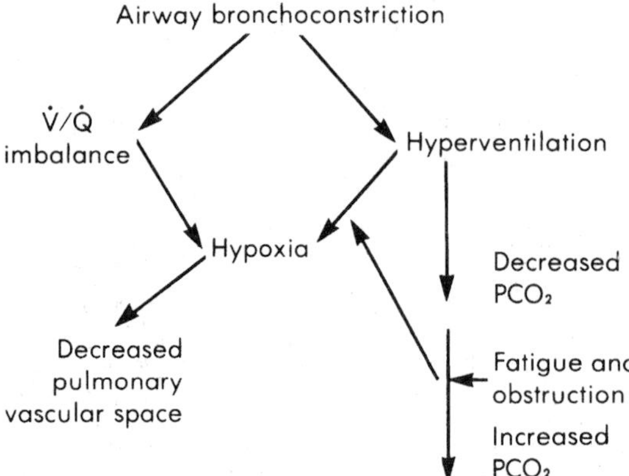

Fig. 84-1 Physiologic effect of bronchoconstriction.

disease, it is important to estimate fluid intake and determine the pattern of response to previous episodes and medication.

History

1. Symptoms: cough, wheezing, chest tightness, sputum production, associated rhinitis, sinusitis, nasal polyposis, and atopic dermatitis. Pattern of symptoms in terms of seasonality, episodic versus continuous, onset, duration, frequency, and progression.
2. Precipitating and aggravating factors.
3. Pattern of disease related to age of onset and diagnosis, progression, previous evaluation, response to treatment, and ongoing management and evaluation. Prior hospitalizations and ventilatory support should be assessed because they affect disposition and prognosis.
4. Profile of typical exacerbation, including prodromal signs and symptoms, temporal progression, management, and outcome.
5. Family history of allergy and asthma.
6. Medical history of patient, focusing on other allergic manifestations, gastrointestinal disturbances, reactions to foods and drugs, croup, reflux, passive exposure to smoking, pneumonia, and early injury to lungs or airway associated with bronchopulmonary dysplasia (BPD), intubation, or congenital abnormalities.
7. Effect of disease on patient and family. Limitations of activities should be specifically assessed so that attention may be directed toward normalization of pulmonary function at follow-up on an outpatient basis.
8. Living environment, focusing on type of home and heating/cooling, humidifier, carpeting, pets, and exposure to smoke. Environmental smoke exposure is an important risk factor for recurrence of asthma.
9. Assessment of family's and patient's perception of illness.

Physical Examination

1. Labored respirations with retractions, nasal flaring, tachypnea, and tachycardia are present. Pulsus paradoxus may be present and, when combined with the degree of retractions, correlates with value of forced expiratory volume at 1 second (FEV_1). These are good indications of the severity of airway obstruction.
   a. Diffuse inspiratory and expiratory wheezing is noted with a prolonged expiratory phase. The patient with respiratory distress and without wheezing may not be moving enough air to generate air movement and may have a silent chest. This patient has severe disease.
   b. Rales and rhonchi may be present.
   c. Pulsus paradoxus may accompany severe asthma, pericardial tamponade, and pneumothorax. Its presence is determined by having the patient breathe quietly while the examiner lowers the blood pressure cuff toward the systolic level. The pressure when the first sound is heard is noted. The pressure is further dropped until sounds can be heard throughout the respiratory cycle. A difference of

10 mm Hg or greater indicates the presence of pulsus paradoxus.

2. Patients may have cyanosis (usually confirmed by oximetry or arterial blood gas [ABG] values), diminished blood pressure, and fever as late findings.
3. Diaphoresis, agitation, somnolence, or confusion may result from hypoxia, hypercapnia, exhaustion, or drug intoxication, and the patient needs emergent intervention because of impending respiratory failure.
4. Status asthmaticus is present when a patient has moderate to severe obstruction and fails to respond significantly to β_2-agonist agents administered in the initial treatment regimen.
5. Chronic cough may occasionally be the only presentation for ongoing mild reactive airway disease. The chest may sound clear, but wheezing can be induced by having the patient exercise. The condition requires a therapeutic trial of oral or inhaled bronchodilators.

Complications

1. Pneumothorax or pneumomediastinum.
2. Pneumonia.
3. Respiratory failure with $Pa{O_2}$ less than 50 mm Hg and $Pa{CO_2}$ greater than 50 mm Hg at room air, sea level. These parameters may be useful, as is the pattern of progression of disease. Patients often have significant retractions, decrease or absence of breath sounds, impairment of mental status and agitation, decreased response to pain, and labored speech.
4. Dehydration.
5. Inappropriate antidiuretic hormone (ADH) secretion.
6. Theophylline overdose (p. 398).
7. Death resulting from respiratory failure with cardiac decompensation or dysrhythmias.

Ancillary Data

1. Oxygen saturation has important prognostic and therapeutic usefulness; oximetry may be more predictive of the need for admission than pulmonary function tests (PFTs). Furthermore, clinical assessment of hypoxemia does not correlate well with oximetry values. Patients with a low initial oxygen saturation, even if they show response to nebulized albuterol, have been shown to be at high risk and require aggressive management and admission. An increase in oxygen saturation in response to nebulization therapy in the emergency department (ED) does not necessarily mean a good outcome and may be transient. Furthermore, many children actually have a decreased oxygen saturation after nebulization therapy because of greater ventilation-perfusion mismatch caused by diffuse mucous plugging, emphasizing the importance of reevaluating oxygen saturation after intervention.
2. ABG measurements are recommended in children with relatively severe disease and those who have clinically impaired ventilation. Oximetry should not be viewed as a substitute for ABG values in severely ill children because it does not assess ventilation.
3. PFTs are useful in monitoring asthmatic patients and provide important prognostic information for an acute episode:
   a. The peak expiratory flow (PEF) rate and the FEV_1 have proved useful in helping to assess the extent of airflow obstruction and severity. The technique, however, is not sufficient to enable one to make a diagnosis or fully evaluate physiologic impairment because it is effort dependent and measures only large-airway function. Furthermore, each patient must establish a "personal best" when he or she is well, with which measurements

may be compared to assess the deterioration during an acute illness or to monitor long-term management (Table 84-1). PEF is particularly helpful for monitoring the patient over time on an outpatient basis with a peak flow meter. A PEF level of 50% to 80% of personal best signals caution, whereas a PEF level less than 50% suggests a medical alert. A level in the lower part of the 50% to 80% range should warrant greater concern.

TABLE 84-1 Predicted Average Peak Expiratory Flow (liters/minute) for Normal Children and Adolescents (Males and Females)

Height (inches)	Peak Expiratory Flow (L/min)
43	147
44	160
45	173
46	187
47	200
48	214
49	227
50	240
51	254
52	267
53	280
54	293
55	307
56	320
57	334
58	347
59	360
60	373
61	387
62	400
63	413
64	427
65	440
66	454
67	467

From National Asthma Education Program: *Guidelines for the diagnosis and management of asthma*, Besthesda, Md, 1991; National Institutes of Health, US Department of Health and Human Services, Publication 91-3042/3042A.

b. PFTs can measure a patient's response; the lack of improvement may reflect variable effort or worsening clinical condition.

c. Evaluation of patients with a nonspecific symptom such as cough or shortness of breath on exertion may require PFTs for assessment of the contribution of bronchoconstriction associated with "cough-variant asthma."

4. A variety of parameters are useful for estimating the severity of an acute exacerbation (Table 84-2).

5. A chest x-ray film classically demonstrates hyperinflation and, in rare cases, an infiltrate. Children whose respiratory distress is increasing or who do not show the expected response to conventional therapy should be studied to exclude an associated process that requires specific therapy or to eliminate other causes of wheezing. Any patient with signs suggestive of an air leak or foreign body aspiration should undergo x-ray studies. These are rarely indicated in children who show good response to initial therapy.

The distinction between infiltrate and atelectasis may be difficult to make, because both appear as opacification on a chest x-ray film:

	Infiltrate	Atelectasis
Diaphragm	Normal	Elevated
Mediastinal shift	None	Toward lesion
Air bronchogram	Common	Variable

6. Serum theophylline level is crucial in managing patients with an acute episode who are taking "therapeutic" doses of theophylline. Therapeutic levels are in the range of 10 to 20 μg/ml. Rapid assays of serum theophylline levels facilitate this process.

7. Complete blood count (CBC) may be useful in children who have been febrile. Optimally, it should be obtained before administration of β-adrenergic agents.

TABLE 84-2 Estimating Severity of Asthma Exacerbations*

	Mild	Moderate	Severe	Respiratory Arrest Imminent
SYMPTOMS				
Breathless	While walking	While talking (infant—softer, shorter cry; difficulty feeding)	While at rest (infant—stops feeding)	
	Can lie down	Prefers sitting	Sits upright	
Talks in	Sentences	Phrases	Words	
Alertness	May be agitated	Usually agitated	Usually agitated	Drowsy or confused
SIGNS				
Respiratory rate (breaths/min)	Increased	Increased	Often > 30	
	Guide to rates of breathing in awake children:			
	Age	*Normal Rate*		
	<2 mo	<60		
	2-12 mo	<50		
	1-5 yr	<40		
	6-8 yr	<30		
Use of accessory muscles; suprasternal retractions	Usually not	Commonly	Usually	Paradoxical thoracoabdominal movement
Wheeze	Moderate, often only end expiratory	Loud; throughout exhalation	Usually loud; throughout inhalation and exhalation	Absence of wheeze
Pulse (beats/min)	<100	100-120	>120	Bradycardia
	Guide to normal pulse rates in children:			
	Age	*Normal Rate*		
	2-12 mo	<160		
	1-2 yr	<120		
	2-8 yr	<110		
Pulsus paradoxus	Absent <10 mm Hg	May be present; 10-25 mm Hg	Often present; >25 mm Hg (adult), 20-40 mm Hg (child)	Absence suggests respiratory muscle fatigue

Continued

TABLE 84-2 Estimating Severity of Asthma Exacerbations*—cont'd

	Mild	Moderate	Severe	Respiratory Arrest Imminent
FUNCTIONAL ASSESSMENT				
PEF (% predicted or % personal best)	80%	Approximately 50%-80%	<50% predicted/ personal best or response lasts <2 hr	
Pa_{O_2} (on room air)	Normal (test not usually necessary)	>60 mm Hg (test not usually necessary)	<60 mm Hg: possible cyanosis	
and/or				
P_{CO_2}	<42 mm Hg (test not usually necessary)	<42 mm Hg (test not usually necessary)	≥42 mm Hg: possible respiratory failure	
Sa_{O_2} (on room air) at sea level	>95%	91%-95%	<91%	
	Hypercapnia (hypoventilation) develops more readily in young children than in adults and adolescents.			

From the National Asthma Education and Prevention Program: *Guidelines for the diagnosis and management of asthma*, Bethesda, Md, 1997, National Institutes of Health, National Heart, Lung and Blood Institute, NIH Publication 97-4051A.

* Notes: The presence of several parameters, but not necessarily all, indicates the general classification of the exacerbation. Many of these parameters have not been systematically studied, so they serve only as general guides.

8. Electrolytes should be monitored periodically in the severely ill patient who is hospitalized to exclude inappropriate ADH secretion. Hypokalemia has been associated with prolonged use of albuterol.

DIFFERENTIAL DIAGNOSIS

(see Chapter 20)

The differential diagnostic considerations in the child with wheezing vary with the age of the child. In the *infant*, bronchiolitis, asthma, foreign body aspiration, gastroesophageal reflux, cystic fibrosis, cardiac disease, congenital and structural abnormalities (e.g., tracheoesophageal fistula, vascular ring), and upper airway congestion or obstruction must be excluded. *Older children* may have asthma, foreign body aspiration, pneumonia, or mediastinal tumors or lymph nodes. Cystic fibrosis and other chronic lung diseases should also be considered after infancy. Other diagnostic entities include the following:

1. Infection/inflammation:
   a. Pneumonia (p. 811)
   b. Bronchiolitis (p. 797)
   c. Aspiration
2. Trauma (see Chapter 62):
   a. Pneumothorax (may be spontaneous)
   b. Foreign body (p. 808)
3. Vascular disorder:
   a. Compression of trachea by vascular anomaly
   b. Pulmonary edema (see Chapter 19)
   c. Pulmonary embolism (p. 578)
   d. Congestive heart failure (CHF) (see Chapter 16)
4. Vocal cord dysfunction may mimic asthma. It is due to an adduction of the true and false vocal cords throughout the respiratory cycle and is often a response to stress or anxiety paralleling a conversion reaction.
5. Congenital disease:
   a. Cystic fibrosis
   b. Tracheoesophageal fistula or tracheal anomaly
6. Hyperventilation.
7. Intoxication: metabolic acidosis (may cause tachypnea) (p. 365), toxic inhalation.
8. Neoplasm: mediastinal or pulmonary.

MANAGEMENT

The patient is often the best indicator of both the severity of the attack and the most effective therapeutic regimen. If the history or physical examination suggests that asthma is not the most likely cause, an appropriate evaluation (e.g., inspiratory and forced expiratory x-ray film, cardiac examination, fluoroscopy, bronchoscopy) should be initiated after stabilization of the patient's respiratory status. ED and hospital management are outlined in Fig. 84-2.

1. When appropriate, stabilize airway, ventilation, and blood pressure, and correct acid-base abnormalities.
2. Administer humidified oxygen by nasal cannula or facemask at 3 to 6 L/min (30% to 40%) to all patients with significant wheezing. Once the patient is stabilized, titrate the oxygen down as appropriate. Utilizing a nasal cannula reduces claustrophobia and allows the child to drink easily without interruption of oxygen administration but may not provide adequate oxygen supplementation.
3. Cardiac monitoring is important during administration of adrenergic agents particularly in patients with moderate or severe disease (status asthmaticus).
4. Initiate continuous oximetry monitoring early, and preferably obtain the first reading before oxygen is initiated.
5. Patients with severe asthma who are in respiratory failure, patients with persistent hypoxemia and hypercarbia with maximal therapy, and patients with fatigue or no response to aggressive bronchodilation may need intubation. Fortunately, this intervention is rarely needed.

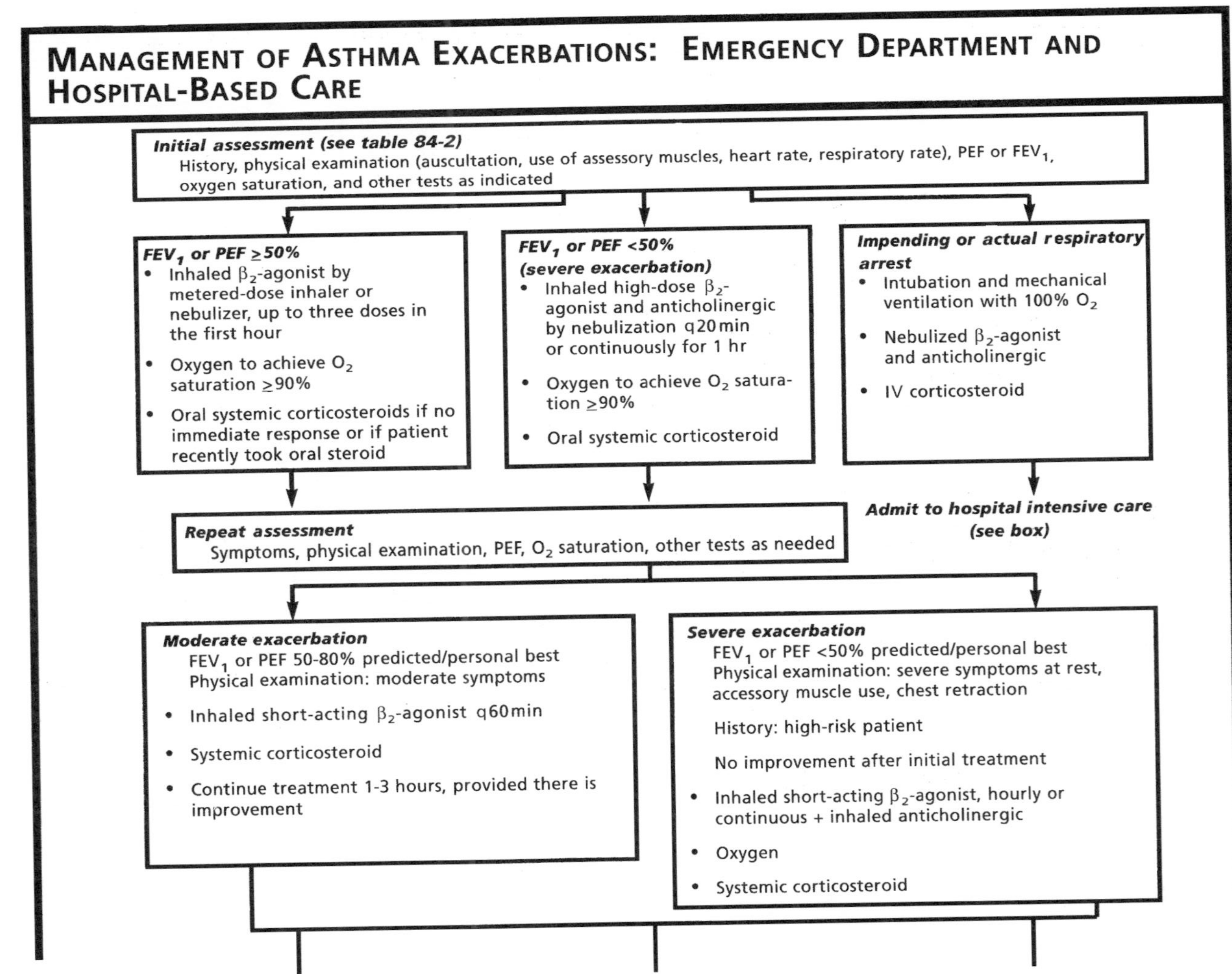
MANAGEMENT OF ASTHMA EXACERBATIONS: EMERGENCY DEPARTMENT AND HOSPITAL-BASED CARE
Initial assessment (see table 84-2)
History, physical examination (auscultation, use of assessory muscles, heart rate, respiratory rate), PEF or FEV_1, oxygen saturation, and other tests as indicated
FEV_1 or PEF ≥50%
• Inhaled β_2-agonist by metered-dose inhaler or nebulizer, up to three doses in the first hour
• Oxygen to achieve O_2 saturation ≥90%
• Oral systemic corticosteroids if no immediate response or if patient recently took oral steroid
FEV_1 or PEF <50% (severe exacerbation)
• Inhaled high-dose β_2-agonist and anticholinergic by nebulization q20min or continuously for 1 hr
• Oxygen to achieve O_2 saturation ≥90%
• Oral systemic corticosteroid
Impending or actual respiratory arrest
• Intubation and mechanical ventilation with 100% O_2
• Nebulized β_2-agonist and anticholinergic
• IV corticosteroid
Admit to hospital intensive care (see box)
Repeat assessment
Symptoms, physical examination, PEF, O_2 saturation, other tests as needed
Moderate exacerbation
FEV_1 or PEF 50-80% predicted/personal best
Physical examination: moderate symptoms
• Inhaled short-acting β_2-agonist q60min
• Systemic corticosteroid
• Continue treatment 1-3 hours, provided there is improvement
Severe exacerbation
FEV_1 or PEF <50% predicted/personal best
Physical examination: severe symptoms at rest, accessory muscle use, chest retraction
History: high-risk patient
No improvement after initial treatment
• Inhaled short-acting β_2-agonist, hourly or continuous + inhaled anticholinergic
• Oxygen
• Systemic corticosteroid

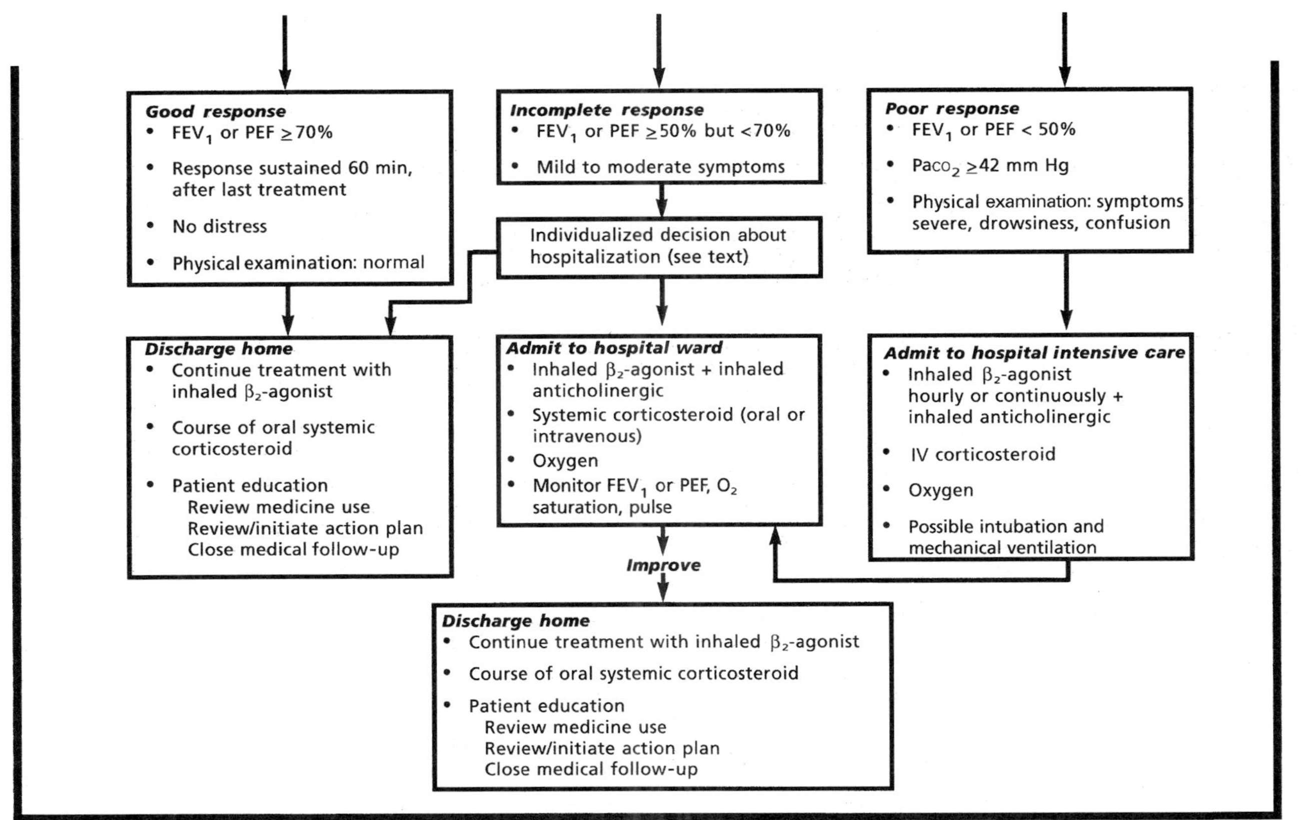

Fig. 84-2 Management of asthma exacerbations: emergency department and hospital-based care.

(From National Asthma Education and Prevention Program: *Guidelines for the diagnosis and management of asthma*, Bethesda, Md, 1997, National Institute of Health, National Heart, Lung, and Blood Institute, NIH Publication 97-4051A.)

Adrenergic Agents

Initially, a rapid-acting β-agonist bronchodilator is administered by inhalation. In general, during the initial stabilization, nebulized agents may be given every 20 minutes or, with severe disease, continuously. Nebulized agents may be continued on an ongoing basis, the frequency reflecting the duration of effect, the clinical response, and the severity of illness.

Nebulized inhalation administration is generally more effective than parenteral therapy and is the ideal route for administration of β-agonist agents. The optimal deposition of drug particles in the lower respiratory tract is achieved by using an oxygen/air flow of 6 to 7 L/min, diluted in a volume of 3.5 to 4.5 ml.

Metered-dose inhalers (MDIs) are available for many agents, including albuterol, terbutaline, steroids, and ipratropium. Such devices may routinely be used in children 6 years and older and with a spacer device in those older than 3 years. A spacer-and-mask device for use with an MDI is available for children and has been found to be equally effective to the nebulizer when used appropriately, even in acutely ill children. The MDI is not usually employed in patients who are developmentally unable to use a T-piece (children <5 years) or patients with altered consciousness.

Albuterol and terbutaline are relatively pure β_2 agents, producing relatively few cardiac side effects. Their wide therapeutic indices allow for safe administration of doses often exceeding traditional recommendations, with careful monitoring. During stabilization, most agents may be given two or three times as tolerated clinically to provide rapid bronchodilation. Often, a combination of a β agonist and ipratropium is most effective; in the severely ill child, the correct agents must be determined empirically or by prior experience in managing the specific child.

1. Albuterol (0.5% solution or 5 mg/ml) (Proventil, Ventolin): 0.03 ml (0.15 mg)/kg/dose up to a maximum of 1.0 ml (5.0 mg)/dose diluted in 2 ml of 0.9% NS administered q2-4hr by nebulization. Many clinicians recommend an initial trial dose of 0.5 ml (2.5 mg). Higher dosages, up to 0.30 mg/kg, have been shown to be safe and to result in greater pulmonary improvement. Treatments may be given more often as tolerated and clinically appropriate, especially in the early assessment and stabilization period. Continuous albuterol may be efficacious and logistically easier in the management of the seriously ill child. Generally, continuous albuterol administration should not exceed 10 to 15 mg/hour.
   - **a.** Peak of onset is 30 to 60 minutes, with a duration of 4 to 6 hours.
   - **b.** Elevations of CPK-MB (isoenzyme of creatine phosphokinase containing M and B subunits) have been noted with prolonged, aggressive, continuous use, emphasizing the importance of ongoing cardiac monitoring in specific patients.
   - **c.** Levalbuterol (Xopenex), a single isomer of albuterol, may be useful during acute management or for ongoing outpatient treatment after stabilization. Less frequent dosing may be possible than with albuterol.
2. Nebulized racemic epinephrine probably has no specific advantage in the management of asthma when compared with albuterol.

Parenteral agents have limited usefulness because of the greater efficacy of inhaled agents, the associated side effects (headache and tachycardia), and the pain of injection. Parenteral administration may have a role in the uncooperative, severely ill patient or when inhalation therapy is logistically impractical (e.g., equipment, cooperation). Intravenous (IV) agents may ultimately have a role in the child who is "in extremis."

1. Epinephrine (Adrenalin) (1:1,000):0.01 ml (0.01 mg)/kg/dose to a maximum of 0.35 ml/dose given SC q20min up to a total of

three administrations if tolerated and the heart rate is less than 180 beats/min. Peak onset is 15 to 30 minutes, with a duration up to 2 hours. Efficacy is less than that of inhaled agents. Significant α- and β-agonist side effects limit usefulness.

If this agent is used with a good response, some clinicians have historically elected to administer Sus-Phrine (1:200), 0.005 ml/kg/dose (maximum: 0.15 ml/dose) SC, to achieve a longer duration of efficacy. The single-vial ampule should be used to ensure consistency of dosage.

2. Terbutaline (0.1% solution) (Brethine): 0.01 ml/kg/dose to a maximum of 0.25 mg (0.25 ml)/dose SC q20min up to a total of three administrations if tolerated. Peak of onset is 30 minutes, and the duration is 3 to 4 hours. This is a good parenteral agent because of the reduced side effects, although the inhaled route is preferred.
3. Albuterol is available outside the United States as an IV preparation. The initial loading dose is 1 μg/kg/min for 10 minutes followed by a continuous infusion of 0.2 μg/kg/min. The dose can be increased by 0.1 μg/kg q15min on the basis of the patient's response. The adult dose is 200 μg over 10 minutes IV followed by a continuous infusion of 3 to 12 μg/min. Studies also suggest that a single IV infusion of salbutamol (15 μg/kg) given in the ED to children who show no response to initial nebulization therapy may produce a rapid response. Further data are required before this agent is accessible.

Status asthmaticus exists when the initial response to 2 to 3 doses of β-adrenergic agents is poor. Hypoxia, acidosis, and hypotension must be rapidly corrected, and other causes of wheezing considered. The lack of improvement is often caused by airway obstruction from a prolonged inflammatory process, suggesting that steroid therapy may be useful in such patients.

Oral agents may be used in mild disease or ongoing, long-term treatment, although their efficacy is limited and they are not widely recommended. Albuterol (2 mg/5 ml) is used in a dosage of 0.1 to 0.15 mg/kg/dose q6-8hr PO up to a maximum of 4 mg/dose. It is also available in 2- and 4-mg tablets. Peak of onset is 1 to 2 hours, and duration is 4 to 6 hours.

For long-term β-agonist therapy, many products are available. Advair Diskus, a combination product of inhaled corticosteroids (fluticasone) and long-acting β_2 agonist (salmeterol) used BID, is useful in children older than 12 years. This combination may be more effective than higher doses of inhaled corticosteroids. Budesonide inhalation suspension may be more effective than nebulized cromolyn sodium in children with persistent asthma. The Foradil Aerolizer, consisting of a long-acting β_2 agonist (formoterol), is approved for maintenance therapy in patients older than 5 years. Leukotriene receptor antagonists (see p. 794) are widely used as well.

Alternative agents include fenoterol (0.5% solution): children younger than 2 years, 0.1 ml/dose; children 2 to 9 years, 0.2 ml/dose; children older than 9 years, 0.3 ml/dose.

Anticholinergic Agents

1. Ipratropium (Atrovent): derivative of atropine with less cardiac effect; administered as an inhaled agent. Ipratropium (Atrovent) is available for nebulization in a 0.02% solution. The 500-μg unit dose is diluted in 2.2 ml for a total volume of 2.5 ml. Pediatric dosage is generally considered to be 250 μg/dose QID (one-half the adult dose). It is also available for MDI administration. The adult MDI dose is two inhalations (36 μg) QID. Safety and dosage studies in children show the agents to be beneficial in combination with a β agonist with fewer side effects than atropine. Peak of onset is 1 to 2 hours, and duration is 3 to 4 hours.

NOTE: Ipratropium has a beneficial effect with albuterol in patients with only a moderate response to albuterol. It may not have as significant an additive effect when used with levalbuterol. Ipratropium has not been demonstrated to improve clinical status in children with bronchiolitis.

2. Atropine: 0.02 mg/kg/dose up to a maximum of 2 mg/dose in 2 ml of 0.9% normal saline (NS) administered by nebulization q4-6hr or as tolerated.

Steroids

1. All patients with moderate or severe asthma (status asthmaticus) should receive a minimum of 3 to 4 days of steroid therapy. Administer methylprednisolone (Solu-Medrol), 1 to 2 mg/kg/dose q6hr IV. This therapy shortens the length of hypoxia and hospitalization. Oral corticosteroids, when tolerated, are equally effective.
2. In children who are minimally to moderately ill and who have a good response to β-agonist agents, steroids may be initiated to facilitate recovery; they are often given orally or by MDI. Patients who show only a partial response or initial response and then return for additional therapy may also benefit from steroids. The effectiveness of inhaled steroids has been shown to depend on the time of intervention: the earlier the better.

   In children with recurrent asthma, the severity of the attack may be reduced if steroids are administered in combination with albuterol at the first signs of upper respiratory tract infection and before any sign of wheezing. This therapy is often initiated by parents who have been given specific guidelines. Begin prednisone or prednisolone, 1 to 2 mg/kg/24 hr q6-12hr PO, for 3 to 7 days. A liquid concentrated steroid preparation is prednisolone (Prelone or Orapred, the latter having a more palatable taste), 15 mg/5ml. Some prefer crushed prednisone tablets mixed with applesauce, yogurt, etc. Dexamethasone, 0.6 mg/kg/day given orally for 2 days, is equivalent to 5 days of oral prednisone.
3. In patients who have taken steroids within 12 months (including those taking steroids administered by inhalation) or who have a history of respiratory failure associated with asthma, steroid therapy should be initiated early for an acute exacerbation.

   If more than four bursts of steroid therapy have been given in 1 year, a brief course of glucocorticoids should be initiated for stress such as surgery.
4. Patients with severe asthma, particularly those with severe exacerbations, may benefit from long-term steroid therapy. Systemic steroids (prednisone, 1 to 2 mg/kg/24 hr q6-12hr PO) are commonly used initially for long-term therapy. Many patients needing 20 mg/day or less of prednisone may be changed to inhalation administration with maintenance of good respiratory function and reduction of adverse reactions. Beclomethasone (Vanceril, Beclovent) is provided in an MDI delivering 42 μg/puff. Children 6 to 12 years use 1 to 2 puffs q6-8hr (maximum: 10 puffs/24 hr), whereas older children and adults use 2 puffs q6-8hr (maximum: 20 puffs/24 hr). MDIs are now available that use hydrofluoroalkane (HFA) as the propellant.

   Second-generation inhaled steroids (triamcinolone [Azmacort] and flunisolide [Aerobid]) have fairly short half-lives, whereas third-generation agents (fluticasone [Flovent]) are usually effective in once-a-day or twice-a-day doses. The maintenance dose is 400 to 500 μg/day. Use of a spacer or rinsing the mouth after inhalation reduces side effects such as oral thrush. The risk of systemic side effects with long-term use, including growth delay, cataracts, adrenal suppression, and immunosuppression, is undefined.

Cromolyn

Cromolyn (Intal) bullets (each 20 mg): Adult dosage is 20 mg/dose; infant and neonatal dosage is 10 to 20 mg/dose. It may be given three to four times per day and has been used during acute management, although its efficacy in this role has not been documented. Cromolyn is often used in conjunction with β-agonist agents, in patients with exercise- or cold-induced problems, and with other components of long-term therapy to reduce wheezing after an acute exacerbation.

Theophylline

Theophylline is rarely utilized because it has not been shown to benefit patients in the hospital setting more than administration of nebulized albuterol and steroids.

Parenteral, oral, and rectal preparations are available. All require appropriate loading before the patient is started on maintenance therapy.

If the patient is taking theophylline at the time of the encounter, the amount and time of the last dose and the duration of therapy must be established so that the need for a loading dose can be determined. A serum theophylline measurement is usually required in acutely ill patients.

1. If the patient is taking a subtherapeutic dose, half the loading dose may be given pending determination of the theophylline level.
2. Therapeutic serum theophylline level is 10 to 20 μg/ml. 1 mg/kg of theophylline raises the theophylline concentration by about 2 μg/ml.
3. The dosage of theophylline must be adjusted to reflect changes in clearance. Alter the dosage as indicated for the following conditions:

	Increase Maintenance Dose for (Clearance Increased):	Decrease Maintenance Dose for (Clearance Decreased):
Drugs	Phenobarbital, phenytoin (Dilantin), rifampin, carbamazepine, marijuana	Cimetidine, erythromycin, oral contraceptives
Diet	High-protein, low-carbohydrate, charcoal-broiled meat	
Illness		Viral infection, fever, CHF, abnormal liver/renal function
Other:	Smokers, hyperthyroidism, cystic fibrosis	Infants <3 mo, pregnancy (esp. third trimester)

4. Dosage determination is made on the basis of lean body weight and must reflect serum theophylline levels. Aminophylline is about 85% theophylline.
5. The half-life of IV theophylline in children is approximately 2.5 hours; in adults it is 4.6 hours.
6. Theophylline toxicity results in tachycardia, dysrhythmias, irritability, and seizures as well as nausea, vomiting, and abdominal pain (p. 398). Attention and achievement problems are usually associated with preexisting problems. It is imperative to ascertain that gastrointestinal symptoms are not evidence of toxicity

Parenteral Therapy. On rare occasions and usually after consultation, patients with unresponsive severe obstructive disease may try theophylline. A loading dose is normally given over 20 minutes, followed by an IV infusion of maintenance theophylline. The maintenance infusion may be mixed with aminophylline,

100 mg in 100 ml 0.9% NS (1 mg/ml of aminophylline or 0.85 mg/ml of theophylline).

The following doses of aminophylline (theophylline) are for patients who have not previously received theophylline products:

Age Group	Loading Dose* (mg/kg)	Maintenance Dose* (mg/kg/hr)
1-6 mo	6-7 (5-6)	0.5 (0.4)†
6-12 mo	6-7 (5-6)	1.0 (0.85)†
1-9 yr	6-7 (5-6)	1.5 (1.2)
10-16 yr	6-7 (5-6)	1.2 (1.0)

* Aminophylline dose (theophylline dose).

† Lower doses may be required because of the variability of pharmacokinetics. Very close monitoring of theophylline levels is required, usually within 6 to 12 hours of loading and then periodically.

Other Agents

1. *Magnesium sulfate* ($MgSO_4$) has been studied in the management of severe asthma (PEF at 25% to 30% at presentation, lack of response to initial therapy, and failure of PEF to improve beyond 60% after an hour of therapy) with some success. At a dosage of 25 mg/kg/dose (some recommend a dose as high as 40 mg/kg/dose) over 20 minutes (adult: 1.2 to 2 g/dose) in 100 ml of 0.9% NS, this agent has generally been found to be effective in patients older than 6 years whose asthma is unresponsive to adrenergic and anticholinergic agents.
2. Sedation has certainly been necessary as appropriate but only if ventilation is ensured. *Ketamine* is particularly useful because it is also a bronchodilator. It has been administered in relatively low dosages (to reduce incidence of dysphonic reactions), with a loading dose of 0.1 mg/kg followed by an infusion of 0.5 mg/kg/hr.
3. *Leukotriene-receptor antagonists* have been noted to have a beneficial effect, serving as a complement to other agents for long-term management. Zafirlukast (Accolate; 20-mg tablets) and zileuton (Zyflo; 20-mg tablets) are currently available for adults, and extensive studies in children are ongoing.

   Montelukast (Singulair) has been approved for children 6 to 14 years of age in a dose of 5 mg/day taken in the evening. Once-daily therapy has been recommended for children with mild persistent asthma and exercise-induced asthma. It may be used in combination with inhaled steroids.
4. *Nitric oxide* is a potent pulmonary vasculator that, when delivered continuously by ventilator, may be beneficial.

DISPOSITION

1. Patients with moderate or severe asthma in status asthmaticus need immediate hospitalization and continuation of the therapy initiated in the ED. Although parameters indicating admission are not well defined, risk factors include the following:
   - **a.** Presence of symptoms for more than 24 hours.
   - **b.** Marked retractions, hypoxia, or hypercapnia.
   - **c.** Respiratory obstructions (PEF ≤50% of expected).
   - **d.** Poor response to initial β-agonist agent (PEF ≤40% of expected). Failure of response to initial ED management is a firm indication for admission.
   - **e.** History of hospitalization or respiratory failure, especially with previous admission to an intensive care unit (ICU).
   - **f.** Multiple-drug therapy; long-term or intermittent use of steroids.
   - **g.** Concurrent infection.
   - **h.** Progressive fatigue.
   - **i.** Multiple visits for same episode.
2. A low oxygen saturation on admission to the ED (≤90% to 93% at sea level) has been associated with a consistent need for hospitalization.

3. The patient who has mild disease that clears may be discharged after appropriate loading and with adequate oral therapy. A more aggressive and perhaps more effective approach is to use home nebulizer machines in younger children and MDIs in older ones, with albuterol as the drug of choice. Steroids may be used in some children. Frequent telephone communications and health care visits are necessary.
4. Good follow-up (including monitoring of clinical response and frequency of exacerbations) is essential for all patients with asthma. Often psychiatric intervention is required because of the emotional component of asthma in many children.

Parental Education

1. Give all doses of the medication(s).
2. Push clear liquids. Warm fluids are particularly helpful.
3. Try to keep your child calm.
4. Try to identify substances that precipitate attacks, and avoid them. Passive smoking may exacerbate wheezing.
5. Many patients experience reactive airway disease in response to an infection. Such children should have bronchodilator therapy (asthma medicine) at the first sign of a cough or respiratory infection if they do not use such therapy every day.
   - Initiate inhalation treatments at the first sign of respiratory infection, with albuterol administered by nebulizer or MDI.
   - Some clinicians may begin steroids at home in children with recurrent problems.
6. The correct use of a nebulizer or MDI with spacer requires appropriate training and explanation before discharge from the hospital. Please ask questions and be certain that you understand the equipment and its use.
7. Call your physician immediately if any of the following occurs:
   a. Breathing difficulty recurs or worsens, color changes, restlessness develops, or fluid intake decreases, or if the child has difficulty speaking because of respiratory distress.
   b. Nausea, vomiting, or irritability develops because of the theophylline medicine, or the child is unable to take medication.
   c. Cough or wheezing persists or fever or chest pain develops.

BIBLIOGRAPHY

Abulhosn RS, Morray BH, Llewellyn C et al: Passive smoke exposure impairs recovery after hospitalization, *Arch Pediatr Adolesc Med* 151:135, 1997.

Alario AJ, Lewander WJ, Dennhey P et al: The relationship between oxygen saturation and clinical assessment of acutely wheezing infants and children, *Pediatr Emerg Care* 11:331, 1995.

Amirav I, Newhouse MT: Metered-dose inhaler accessory devices in acute asthma, *Arch Pediatr Adolesc Med* 151:876, 1997.

Barnett PU, Caputo GL, Baskin M et al: Intravenous versus oral corticosteroids in the management of acute asthma in children, *Ann Emerg Med* 29:212, 1997.

Besbes-Ouanes, Nouira S, Elastrous E et al: Continuous versus intermittent nebulization of salbutamol in acute severe asthma: a randomized controlled trial, *Ann Emerg Med* 36:198, 2000.

Bisgaard H: Leukotriene modifiers in pediatric asthma management, *Pediatrics* 107:381, 2001.

Browne GJ, Penna AS, Phung X et al: Randomized trial of intravenous salbutamol in early management of acute severe asthma in children, *Lancet* 349:301, 1997.

Ciarallo L, Brousseau D, Reinert S: Higher-dose intravenous magnesium therapy for children with moderate to severe acute asthma, *Arch Pediatr Adolesc Med* 154:979, 2000.

Craig VC, Bigos D, Brill RJ: Efficacy and safety of continuous albuterol nebulization in children with severe status asthmaticus, *Pediatr Emerg Care* 12:1, 1996.

Cram EF, Weirs KB, Fagan MJ: Pediatric asthma care in US emergency departments, *Arch Pediatr Adolesc Med* 149:893, 1995.

Craven P, Kercsmur CM, Myers TR et al: Ipratropium plus nebulized albuterol for treatment of hospitalized children with acute asthma, *J Pediatr* 138:51, 2000.

DiGiulio GA, Kercsmar CM, Krug SE et al: Hospital treatment of asthma: lack of benefit from theophylline given in addition to nebulized albuterol and intravenously administered corticosteroids, *J Pediatr* 122:464, 1993.

Emerman CL, Cydulka RK, Crain EF et al: Prospective multicenter study of relapse after treatment for acute asthma among children presenting to the emergency department, *J Pediatr* 138:318, 2001.

Emond SD, Camargo CA, Nowak RM: 1997 national asthma education and prevention guidelines: a practical summary for emergency physicians, *Ann Emerg Med* 31:579, 1998.

Geelhoed GC, Landau LI, LeSouef PN: Evaluation of Sao_2 as a predictor of outcome in 280 children presenting with acute asthma, *Ann Emerg Med* 23:1236, 1994.

Granit CC, Duggan AK, DeAngelis C: Independent parental administration of prednisone in acute asthma: a double blind placebo controlled crossover study, *Pediatrics* 96:224, 1995.

Hickey RW, Gochman RF, Chande V et al: Albuterol delivered via metered-dose inhaler with spacer for outpatient treatment of young children with wheezing, *Arch Pediatr Adolesc Med* 148:189, 1994.

Howton JC, Rose J, Duffy S et al: Randomized double blind placebo-controlled trial of intravenous ketamine in acute asthma, *Ann Emerg Med* 27:170, 1996.

Jagoda A, Shepherd SM, Spevitz A et al: Refractory asthma: part I: epidemiology, pathophysiology pharmacology and intervention; part II: airway interventions and management, *Ann Emerg Med* 29:275, 1997.

Karem E, Levison H, Schuh S et al: Efficacy of albuterol administered by nebulizer versus spacer device in children with acute asthma, *J Pediatr* 123:313, 1993.

Keogh KA, MacArthur C, Parkin PC et al: Prediction of hospitalization in children with acute asthma, *J Pediatr* 139:223, 2001.

Kudukis TM, Manthous CA, Schmidt GA et al: Inhaled helium oxygen revisited: effect of inhaled helium oxygen during the treatment of status asthmaticus in children, *J Pediatr* 130:217, 1997.

Landwehr UP, Wood RP, Blager FB et al: Vocal cord dysfunction mimicking exercise-induced bronchospasm in adolescents, *Pediatrics* 98:971, 1996.

Lara M, Rosenbaum S, Rachelefsky G et al: Improving childhood asthma outcomes in the United States: a blueprint for policy action, *Pediatrics* 109:919, 2002.

Leflein JG, Szefler SJ, Murphy KR et al: Nebulized budesonide inhalation suspension compared with cromolyn sodium nebulizer solution for asthma in younger children: results of a randomized outcomes trial, *Pediatrics* 109:866, 2002.

Leversha AM, Campanella SG, Aickin RP et al: Cost and effectiveness of spacer versus nebulizer in young children with moderate and severe acute asthma, *J Pediatr* 136:497, 2000.

Maneker AJ, Perack EM, Krug SE: Contribution of routine pulse oximetry to evaluation and management of patients with respiratory illness in a pediatric emergency department, *Ann Emerg Med* 25:36, 1995.

Mower WR, Sachs C, Nicklin EL et al: Pulse oximetry as a fifth pediatric vital sign, *Pediatrics* 99:681, 1997.

Nakagawa TA, Johnston SJ, Falkos SA et al: Life-threatening status asthmaticus treated with inhaled nitric oxide, *J Pediatr* 137:119, 2000.

Nelson HS, Bensch G, Plaskow WW et al: Improved bronchodilation with levalbuterol compared with racemic albuterol in patients with asthma, *J Allergy Clin Immunol* 102:943, 1998.

Pabon H, Monem G, al Kissoon N: Safety and efficacy of magnesium sulfate infusions in children with status asthmaticus, *Pediatr Emerg Care* 10:200, 1994.

Parks DP, Ahrens RC, Humphries T et al: Chronic cough in childhood: approach to diagnosis and treatment, *J Pediatr* 115:S856, 1989.

Plint AC, Osmond MH, Klassen TP: The efficacy of nebulized racemic epinephrine in children with acute asthma. A randomized, double-blind trial, *Acad Emerg Med* 7:1097, 2000.

Poirier MP, Pancioli AM, DiGuilio GA: Vocal cord dysfunction presenting as acute asthma in a pediatric patient, *Pediatr Emerg Care* 12:213, 1996.

Qureshi F, Pestian J, Davis P et al: Effect of nebulized ipratropium on the hospitalization rates of children with asthma, *N Engl J Med* 339:1030, 1998.

Qureshi F, Zaritsky A, Lakkis H: Efficacy of nebulized ipratropium in severely asthmatic children, *Ann Emerg Med* 29:205, 1997.

Qureshi F, Zaritsky A, Poirier MP: Comparative efficacy of oral dexamethasone versus oral prednisone in acute pediatric asthma, *J Pediatr* 139:20, 2001.

Reijonen T, Korppi M, Kuikka U et al: Antiinflammatory therapy reduces wheezing after bronchodilator, *Arch Pediatr Adolesc Med* 150:512, 1996.

Rowe BH, Bretzlaff JA, Bourdon C et al: Intravenous magnesium sulfate treatment for acute asthma in the emergency department: a systematic review of the literature, *Ann Emerg Med* 36:181, 2000.

Scarfone RJ, Capraro GA, Zorc JJ et al: Demonstrated use of metered dose inhalers and peak flow meters by children and adolescents with acute asthma exacerbations, *Arch Pediatr Adolesc Med* 156:378, 2002.

Scarfone RJ, Loiselle JM, Joffe MD et al: A randomized trial of magnesium in the emergency department treatment of children with asthma, *Ann Emerg Med* 36:572, 2000.

Schuh S, Johnson DW, Callahan S et al: Efficacy of frequent nebulized ipratropium bromide added to frequent high-dose albuterol therapy in severe childhood asthma, *J Pediatr* 126:639, 1995.

Schuh S, Parkin F, Rojan A et al: High versus low dose frequently administered nebulized albuterol in children with severe acute asthma, *Pediatrics* 83:513, 1989.

Wright AL, Holberg C, Martinez FD et al: Relationship of parental smoking to wheezing and non-wheezing lower respiratory tract illnesses in infancy, *J Pediatr* 118:207, 1991.

Young S, LeSouef PN, Geelhoed GC et al: The influence of family history of asthma and parental smoking on airway responsiveness in early infancy, *N Engl J Med* 324:1168, 1991.

Bronchiolitis

ALERT Patients with marked tachypnea, retractions, cyanosis, or decreased air exchange need immediate attention and hospitalization. Hydration status and oxygenation must be assessed.

Bronchiolitis is an acute lower respiratory infection that produces inflammatory obstruction of the small airways and reactive airway disease. It commonly occurs in children younger than 2 years, with the highest incidence in those younger than 6 months. The relationship of bronchiolitis to asthma and later reactive airway disease is unclear at present. In contrast to asthma, which primarily has bronchoconstriction with secondary inflammation, bronchiolitis is primarily an inflammatory process with a bronchoconstrictive component that is variably present.

Children at greatest risk of significant complications are preterm infants (<32 weeks' gestational age), those younger than 6 months, and those with underlying cardiac, pulmonary, or immunologic problems. Smoking by parents or other household members raises a child's risk for development of bronchiolitis.

ETIOLOGY

Viral infection caused by respiratory syncytial virus (RSV) accounts for 90% of isolates in cases of bronchiolitis. Parainfluenza, adenovirus, and influenza are less common.

DIAGNOSTIC FINDINGS

1. Most patients have a respiratory tract infection that is followed by the onset of marked tachypnea (often >60 breaths/min) and diffuse wheezing.
   a. Most children appear well and are attentive, alert, and in no distress despite the tachypnea.
   b. Many have an accompanying otitis media, often bacterial, and viral pneumonia.
2. Patients with respiratory distress have marked retractions, nasal flaring, and cyanosis. With the progression of inflammation, air movement may decrease, with disappearance of audible wheezing. Vital signs may be altered.
3. Restless and apprehensive behavior may appear if hypoxia or fatigue is present.

Complications

1. Apnea is most commonly found in children younger than 6 months who were born prematurely.
2. Dehydration may be exacerbated by the abnormal insensible losses from the rapid respiratory rate. Intake may be decreased because of the greater respiratory effort. During acute respiratory illness, feeding is less effective as a result of poorer coordination of breathing and swallowing.
3. Bacterial pneumonia may result from secondary infection. Serious bacterial infections are rare in previously well children.
4. Pneumothorax may occur with severe obstructive disease.
5. Residual parenchymal and airway disease may result from any acute episode of bronchiolitis, causing long-term abnormalities in pulmonary function. The relationship to asthma and later pulmonary and allergic disorders is uncertain.
6. Atrial tachycardia.
7. Bronchiolitis fibrosa obliterans results from progressive fibrotic reaction, which obliterates the bronchioles.
8. Death in 1% to 2% of patients is secondary to respiratory failure.

Ancillary Data

1. ABG analysis or oximetry is useful in assessing hypoxia and hypercapnia when the clinical findings are not conclusive. Continuous oximetry is often indicated, supplemented by an ABG analysis if there is concern about ventilation or growing fatigue.
2. Chest x-ray films demonstrate hyperinflation, often in association with a diffuse, patchy infiltrate. These films are not required routinely. A pulmonary consolidation or atelectasis enhances a child's risk of requiring prolonged hospitalization.
3. Fluorescent antibody (FA) testing for RSV, performed on nasal washings, is rapid and diagnostically important. A parallel test may be done for pertussis if that infection is a consideration.
4. Eosinophilia during bronchiolitis is associated with subsequent wheezing after the episode of bronchiolitis.

DIFFERENTIAL DIAGNOSIS

(see Chapter 20)

The most common considerations are asthma, pneumonia, and foreign bodies.

1. Asthma usually occurs in children older than 1 year (children with asthma generally experience more respiratory distress). Asthma is caused primarily by bronchoconstrictive disease, whereas bronchiolitis is primarily an inflammatory process.
2. Pneumonia may produce wheezing and asymmetric breath sounds. A chest x-ray film may be useful. Viral pneumonia often accompanies bronchiolitis.
3. Foreign bodies may be excluded by a negative history and normal inspiratory and expiratory films.
4. Other entities that should be excluded are CHF, cystic fibrosis, vascular ring, neoplasm, and toxic or smoke inhalation.

MANAGEMENT

1. The initial assessment should determine whether acute stabilization is required. Oxygen, airway intervention, and fluids may be initiated.
2. A trial of β-agonists is worthwhile, particularly in the child with any degree of respiratory distress or tachypnea. Studies variably demonstrate clinical improvement after β-agonists; mortality is not altered. One of a number of nebulized agents may be used to determine efficacy in a specific child (p. 790). The treatment should usually be administered with a mask and nebulizer machine. Up to two or three consecutive treatments of one of the following agents may be indicated:
   a. Albuterol (0.5% solution) (Proventil, Ventolin): 0.03 ml (0.15 mg)/kg/dose diluted in 2 ml of 0.9% NS administered q2-4hr. Many clinicians recommend an initial trial dose of 0.5 ml (2.5 mg). Treatments may be given more often as tolerated and clinically appropriate, especially in the early assessment and stabilization. The concentration is 5 mg/ml.
   b. Racemic epinephrine (2.25% solution): 0.1 ml/kg diluted in 2 ml of 0.9% NS may be more effective than albuterol in some children.
   c. L-Epinephrine (1:1000 solution): 2.5 ml via nebulizer in 2 ml of 0.9% NS.
   d. Terbutaline (0.1% solution for parenteral administration) (Brethine): 0.03 mg (0.03 ml)/kg/dose in 2 ml 0.9% NS administered q4hr or more often as tolerated, especially during early stabilization. Peak of onset is 30 minutes, and duration is 3 to 4 hours. Rarely used.
3. The efficacy of steroid therapy in bronchiolitis is somewhat controversial. Limited studies have demonstrated the clinical improvement of patients after

administration of dexamethasone, 1 mg/kg/dose PO early in the course of the illness.

4. Ipratropium (Atrovent) has no proven benefit.
5. The patient must be evaluated for signs of respiratory distress:
   a. The patient who has a respiratory rate of more than 60 breaths/min or any evidence of hypoxia, hypercapnia, fatigue, or progression should be hospitalized for humidified oxygen therapy, fluid therapy, and monitoring.
   b. If respiratory failure is present or imminent (Pao_2 less than 50 mm Hg and $Paco_2$ greater than 50 mm Hg), the patient should be in an ICU, and active airway intervention initiated. Continuous positive airway pressure (CPAP) should be instituted for rising respiratory rate or pulse, decreased responsiveness, decreasing Pao_2, or increasing $Paco_2$. Oxygen at 30% to 40% with 5 cm H_2O pressure may be used. Mechanical ventilation with intubation is necessary if CPAP fails or apneic spells are frequent.
6. Aerosolized ribavirin may speed up improvement of illness in children with severe RSV lower respiratory tract disease, usually after documentation of the virus. Such intervention may be considered for severe disease in the patient with an underlying cardiopulmonary abnormality or immunocompromise. Special precautions are required for children who need mechanical ventilation.
7. Palivizumab, a humanized mouse monoclonal antibody given intramuscularly (IM), may reduce the risk of hospitalization when used prophylactically in high-risk children such as those younger than 2 years of age who have chronic lung disease and in whom pulmonary intervention was required in the prior 6 months. Infants without chronic lung disease who were born at 32 weeks' gestation or earlier may benefit as well. Children born between 32 and 35 weeks' gestation should be considered for this therapy if specific additional risk factors are present. Those with immunodeficiencies may also benefit. Palivizumab is administered in a dose of 15 mg/kg IM once a month during the RSV season.

DISPOSITION

The most serious risk factors are apnea, hypoxia on admission, radiopaque consolidation, atelectasis, congenital heart disease, prematurity, and immune suppression.

1. Patients should be hospitalized if they show any evidence of apnea, lethargy, or dehydration, or if they have unreliable caretakers, live a long distance from a health care facility, or are premature.
2. Factors associated with more severe illness include the following:
   a. "Ill" or "toxic" appearance
   b. Oxygen saturation less than 95% at sea level (the single best objective predictor)
   c. Gestational age less than 34 weeks
   d. Respiratory rate greater than 70 breaths/min
   e. Atelectasis indicated by chest x-ray study
   f. Age less than 3 months
3. Patients without respiratory distress, abnormal oximetry, or other modifying factors may be discharged with close follow-up observation.

Parental Education

1. Give all prescribed medications.
2. Push clear liquids. Do not worry about giving solid foods.
3. Humidified air may decrease congestion.
4. Ambulatory patients may take several weeks to return to baseline.
5. Call your physician if any of the following occurs:
   a. Breathing effort or retractions increase.

b. Cyanosis or apnea is noted.
c. Fluid intake decreases.
d. Fever, toxicity, or fatigue increases.

BIBLIOGRAPHY

Andrade MA, Hoberman A, Glustein J et al: Acute otitis media in children with bronchiolitis, *Pediatrics* 101:617, 1998.

Bulow SM, Nir M, Levin E et al: Prednisolone treatment of respiratory syncytial virus infection: a randomized controlled trial of 147 infants, *Pediatrics* 104:e77, 1999.

Donnerstein RL, Berg RA, Shebab Z et al: Complex atrial tachycardia and respiratory syncytial virus infections in infants, *J Pediatr* 125:23, 1994.

Ehlenfield DR, Cameron K, Welliver RC: Eosinophilia at the time of respiratory syncytial virus bronchiolitis predicts childhood reactive airway disease, *Pediatrics* 105:79, 2000.

Flores G, Horwitz RI: Efficacy of β_2-agonists in bronchiolitis: a reappraisal and meta-analysis, *Pediatrics* 100:233, 1997.

Gadomski AM, Lichenstein R, Horton L et al: Efficacy of albuterol in the management of bronchiolitis, *Pediatrics* 93:907, 1994.

Garrison MM, Christakis DA, Harvey E et al: Systemic corticosteroids in infant bronchiolitis: a metaanalysis, *Pediatrics* 105:849, 2000.

Kellner JD, Ohlsson A, Gadomsici AM et al: Efficacy of bronchodilator therapy in bronchiolitis: a metaanalysis, *Arch Pediatr Adolesc Med* 150:1166, 1996.

Klassen TP, Rowe PC, Sutcliffe T et al: Randomized trial of salbutamol in acute bronchiolitis, *J Pediatr* 118:807, 1991.

Kuppermann N, Bank DE, Walton EA et al: Risks of bacteremia and urinary tract infections in young febrile children with bronchiolitis, *Arch Pediatr Adolesc Med* 151:1207, 1997.

Menon K, Sutcliffe T, Klassen TP: A randomized trial comparing the efficacy of epinephrine with salbutamol in the treatment of acute bronchiolitis, *J Pediatr* 126:1004, 1995.

Navas L, Wang E, Carvalho VD et al: Improved outcome of respiratory syncytial virus infection in a high-risk hospitalized population of Canadian children, *J Pediatr* 121:348, 1992.

Parcell K, Fergie J: Concurrent serious bacterial infections in 2396 infants and children hospitalized with respiratory syncytial virus lower respiratory tract infection, *Arch Pediatr Adolesc Med* 156:322, 2002.

Pearlstein PH, Koagal UR, Bolling C et al: Evaluation of an evidence-based guideline for bronchiolitis, *Pediatrics* 104:1334, 1999.

Prober CG, Sullender WM: Advances in prevention of respiratory syncytial virus infection, *J Pediatr* 135:546, 1999.

Rodriquez WJ, Gruber WC, Welliver RC et al: Respiratory syncytial virus (RSV) immune globulin intravenous therapy for RSV lower respiratory tract infection in infants and young children at high risk for severe RSV infections, *Pediatrics* 99:454, 1997.

Roosevelt G, Sheehan K, Grupp-Phelan J et al: Dexamethasone in bronchiolitis: a randomised controlled trial, *Lancet* 348:292, 1996.

Sanchez I, DeKoster J, Powell RE et al: Effect of racemic epinephrine and salbutamol on clinical score and pulmonary mechanics in infants with bronchiolitis, *J Pediatr* 122:145, 1993.

Schuh S, Canny G, Reisman JJ et al: Nebulized albuterol in acute bronchiolitis, *J Pediatr* 117:633, 1990.

Schuh S, Coates AL, Binnie R et al: Efficacy of oral dexamethasone in outpatients with acute bronchiolitis, *J Pediatr* 140:27, 2002.

Schuh S, Johnson D, Callahan S et al: Efficacy of frequent nebulized ipratropium bromide added to frequent high-dose albuterol in severe childhood asthma, *J Pediatr* 126:639, 1995.

Schweich PJ, Hurt TL, Walkley EI et al: The use of nebulized albuterol in wheezing infants, *Pediatr Emerg Care* 8:184, 1992.

Swingler GH, Hussey GD, Zwarenstein M: Duration of illness in ambulatory children diagnosed with bronchiolitis, *Arch Pediatr Adolesc Med* 154:997, 2000.

VanWoensel JB, Simpen JL, Sprikkelman AB et al: Long-term effect of prednisone in acute phase of bronchiolitis caused by respiratory syncytial virus, *Pediatr Pulm* 30:92, 2000.

Wang EEL, Law BJ, Stephens D et al: Pediatric investigator's collaborative network on infections in Canada: prospective study of risk factors and outcome in patients hospitalized with respiratory syncytial viral lower respiratory tract infection, *J Pediatr* 126:212, 1995.

Croup and Epiglottitis

ALERT Ensure adequate airway. Differentiate croup from epiglottitis.

Any patient with epiglottitis must be intubated. Always consider tracheitis, foreign body, and allergic croup in the differential diagnosis. A clinician skilled in airway management must accompany the patient until diagnosis and stabilization are complete.

Infections of the supraglottic area result in swelling of the laryngeal and epiglottic structures and may additionally involve the trachea, as in croup (laryngotracheobronchitis).

ETIOLOGY

1. Infection:
   a. Croup is viral, and the agents include parainfluenza, RSV, and influenza.
   b. Epiglottitis is caused by *Haemophilus influenzae*; in rare cases, other bacteria may be causative. The incidence has decreased with the widespread use of *H. influenzae* vaccine. The condition is becoming increasingly prevalent in adults. A parallel presentation has been noted to occur with infection by group A streptococcus.
2. Allergy: Allergic croup is a rapid supraglottic swelling resulting from exposure to a precipitating or sensitizing agent.

DIAGNOSTIC FINDINGS (Table 84-3)

1. Respiratory failure may occur with both croup and epiglottitis; may be accompanied by pulmonary edema.
2. With spasmodic or allergic croup, there is a rapid onset of croup syndrome after exposure to a precipitating factor and without the preceding viral respiratory infection seen with infectious croup.
3. Other conditions resulting in upper airway obstruction and dyspnea must be considered in the history and physical examination.
4. Extraepiglottic foci commonly are associated with epiglottitis. Pneumonia, lymphadenitis, and otitis media are most common. Pulmonary edema occurs, not uncommonly, after relief of the obstruction.

DIFFERENTIAL DIAGNOSIS (see Chapter 20)

Stridor indicates that some degree of upper airway obstruction exists. Inspiratory stridor usually indicates a supraglottic lesion, whereas

TABLE 84-3 Comparison of Croup and Epiglottitis

	Croup	Epiglottitis
Age	6 mo-3 yr	Any age (peak: 2-5 yr)
Seasonal occurrence	Fall/winter	Any
Worst time of day	Night/early AM	Throughout day
Etiology	Viral	*H. influenzae*
Clinical signs/symptoms:		
Onset	Insidious	Rapid
Preceding URI	Yes	Rare
Fever	<39.5° C	High
Toxic	No	Yes
Sore throat	Variable	Yes
Voice	Hoarse	Muffled
Drooling	None	Yes
Dysphagia	None	Yes
Cough	"Barking seal"	None
Preferred position	Variable	Prefers sitting
Stridor	Inspiratory/expiratory	Inspiratory
Epiglottis	WNL	"Cherry red"
Ancillary data:		
WBC	WNL	High
Blood culture	Negative	Positive
ABG	Variable	Variable
X-ray, lateral neck (Fig. 84-4)	WNL	Enlarged epiglottis

expiratory stridor usually emanates from a lower airway involvement. Common entities to consider include the following:

1. Supraglottic (extrathoracic):
   a. Viral infection.
   b. Bacterial infection: group A streptococcus, *Staphylococcus aureus,* anaerobes of the mouth *(Peptococcus, Bacteroides), Corynebacterium diphtheriae.* Retropharyngeal abscess (p. 617) and peritonsillar abscess (p. 612) must be considered.
   c. Epiglottitis: *H. influenzae.* Group A streptococcus is being reported more commonly at present.
   d. Noninfectious: foreign body, trauma, caustic ingestion, neoplasm, angioneurotic edema.
   e. **Uvulitis** may be caused by a number of entities, including *H. influenzae* and group A streptococcus. It may result from allergic exposures, angioneurotic edema, and caustic ingestions. Fever, dysphagia, and drooling are common.
2. Infraglottic or subglottic (laryngitis, laryngotracheitis, laryngotracheobronchitis):
   a. Viral: parainfluenza, influenza A and B, measles, adenovirus, RSV.
   b. *Mycoplasma pneumoniae.*
   c. Of bacterial infections, which are usually secondary, the most important entity is **bacterial tracheitis**. This is secondary to superinfection of damaged trachea from an antecedent viral infection or instrumentation. It is commonly caused by *S. aureus, Streptococcus pneumoniae, Moraxella catarrhalis,* or *H. influenzae,* with accumulation of pus in the trachea causing a thick plug and ultimately leading to obstruction. It often is associated with pneumonia and appears clinically as a crouplike syndrome with toxicity and rapid progression. Active airway intervention is often required, combined with aggressive pulmonary drainage and toilet and appropriate antibiotics for potential pathogens.

MANAGEMENT (Fig. 84-3)

1. The patient with upper airway obstruction from croup or epiglottitis requires urgent attention:
   a. Ensure adequate airway
   b. Differentiate croup from epiglottitis
   c. Provide ongoing management and airway stabilization
2. Respiratory failure caused by upper airway obstruction may occur. Airway intervention is indicated if hypoxia (PaO_2 less than 50 mm Hg with supplemental O_2) or hypercapnia ($PaCO_2$ greater than 50 mm Hg) is present, if the patient demonstrates evidence of fatigue, or if there is progressive anxiety or severe obstruction. Patients with epiglottitis (see later discussion) usually need intubation on a prophylactic basis. Intubation should be performed with extreme care and maximal support, commonly under controlled conditions in the operating room with equipment and personnel mobilized (see Fig. 84-3). Often a smaller tube is used to minimize the risk of subglottic stenosis. The tube should be well immobilized. There may be some consideration of bacterial tracheitis in children with severe disease before direct visualization and diagnosis, particularly in those with croup who need intubation.
3. After evaluation for respiratory failure, the epiglottis should be visualized to determine its configuration, size, and color. The epiglottis in the child is somewhat easier to see because it is at the level of C2-C3 rather than at the C5-C6 level as found in adults.
   a. If there is evidence of obstruction or the clinical signs and symptoms are consistent with epiglottitis, visualization is optimally done in the operating room with clinicians experienced

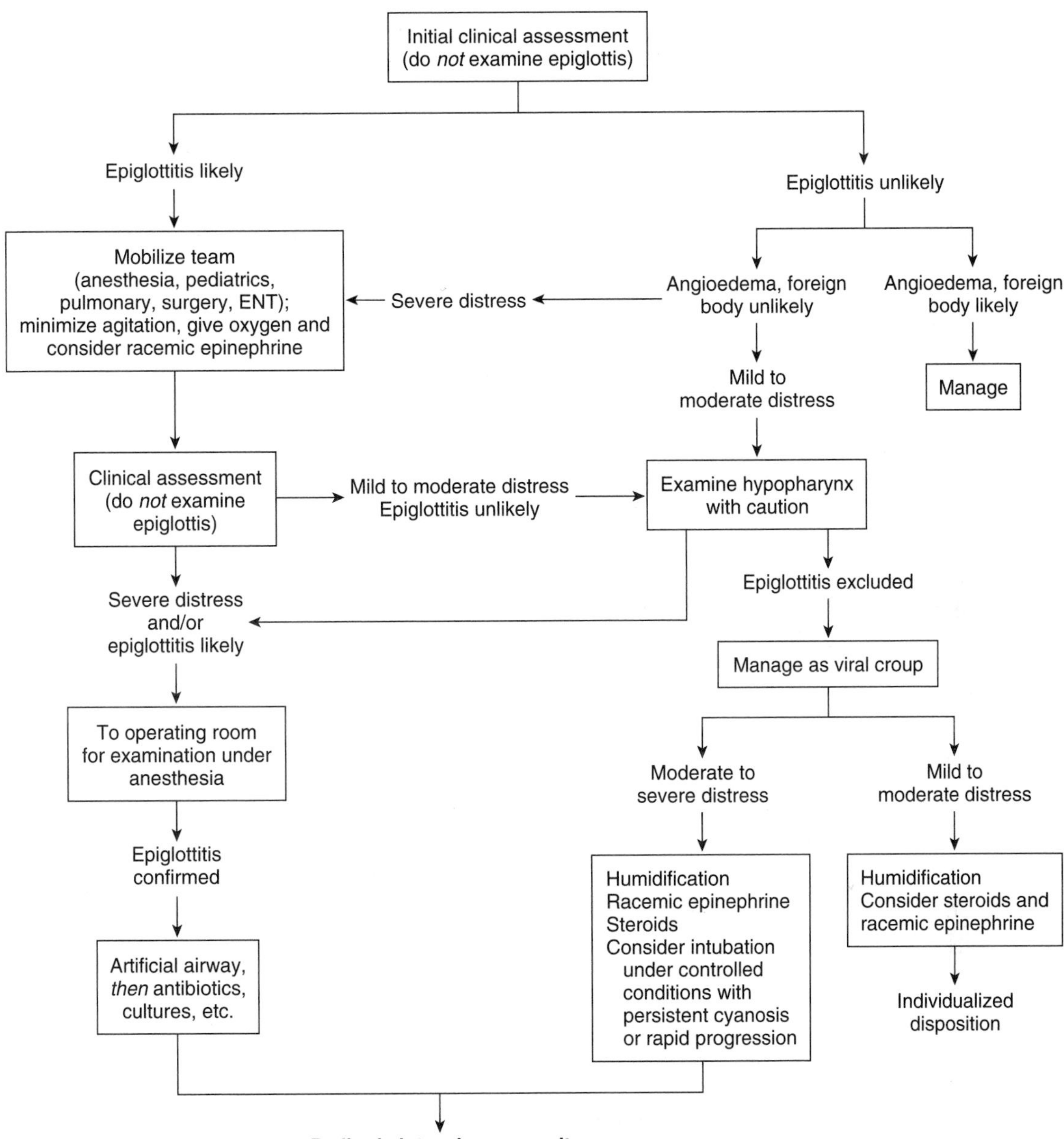

Fig. 84-3 Optimal assessment and management of upper airway obstruction caused by epiglottitis or severe croup. Care must be individualized to reflect resources and logistic issues within a given institution and family.

in surgical airway management (anesthesiologist, otolaryngologist, and surgeon) present. Patients should be preoxygenated and initially allowed to sit in the most comfortable position. Children are usually more comfortable sitting; a supine position may lead to acute obstruction. Minimize agitation. At the time of visualization, the patient care team must be prepared to intubate the child if obstruction occurs or epiglottitis is diagnosed (see Fig. 84-3).

b. Some clinicians prefer to use a lateral neck x-ray film before visualization because of the potential risk of exacerbating the disease if the posterior pharynx is further inflamed. This approach may be useful if the child is not in severe respiratory distress and there is no evidence of obstruction, but direct controlled visualization is usually more desirable. A clinician capable of intubating the patient must accompany the patient at all times. Use of a portable x-ray machine should be considered. Classic findings for croup on lateral radiograph include ballooning of the hypopharynx with narrowing of the cervical trachea on inspiration and ballooning of the cervical trachea on expiration (Fig. 84-4). The ratio of the aryepiglottic width to the body of the third cervical vertebra is a useful parameter. A ratio of 0.35 or more is 100% specific and 90% sensitive for epiglottitis. Lateral neck radiographs in patients with epiglottitis may not be diagnostic in many patients. The rate of false-negative results must be considered in the radiographic evaluation of such patients.

Epiglottitis (see Fig. 84-3)

Immediate intervention is required. Initially, 100% oxygen should be given. The patient who already has obstruction may be ventilated by bag-and-mask positive pressure with a 100% oxygen bag. The patient should be intubated with an endotracheal or nasotracheal tube one to two sizes smaller than would normally be indicated. Topical 4% cocaine or topical epinephrine may be useful, as may atropine (0.01 to 0.02 mg/kg IV), the latter decreasing the vagal response. After intubation, most patients are allowed to breath spontaneously with 4 to 6 mm Hg of CPAP and 40% FiO_2 (humidified). The CPAP helps stabilize the lungs after relief of the obstruction.

1. If time and clinical status permit, the optimal place to perform intubation (and visualize the epiglottis) is in the operating room with appropriate relaxation and with the assistance of an anesthesiologist and others experienced in airway management.
2. An otolaryngologist or surgeon should be available to assist if the airway must be established surgically.
3. If personnel resources are limited, intubation, if necessary, can usually be achieved by a clinician skilled in pediatric airway management. The older child can often be intubated in the position of greatest comfort (usually sitting up and leaning forward). In such cases, clinicians have been successful with blind intubation; the intubator is positioned behind the child (usually sitting on a stretcher with the child). To be successful, this approach usually requires that the child (older than 6 years) be able to tolerate a 6-mm tube.
4. After intubation, patients are monitored in an ICU. Blood cultures and other studies may be performed, and antibiotic therapy initiated. Patients usually remain intubated for 36 ± 14 (1 SD) hour.
5. Children should be reevaluated after 24 hours and then every 12 hours thereafter. The clinical course may be used to

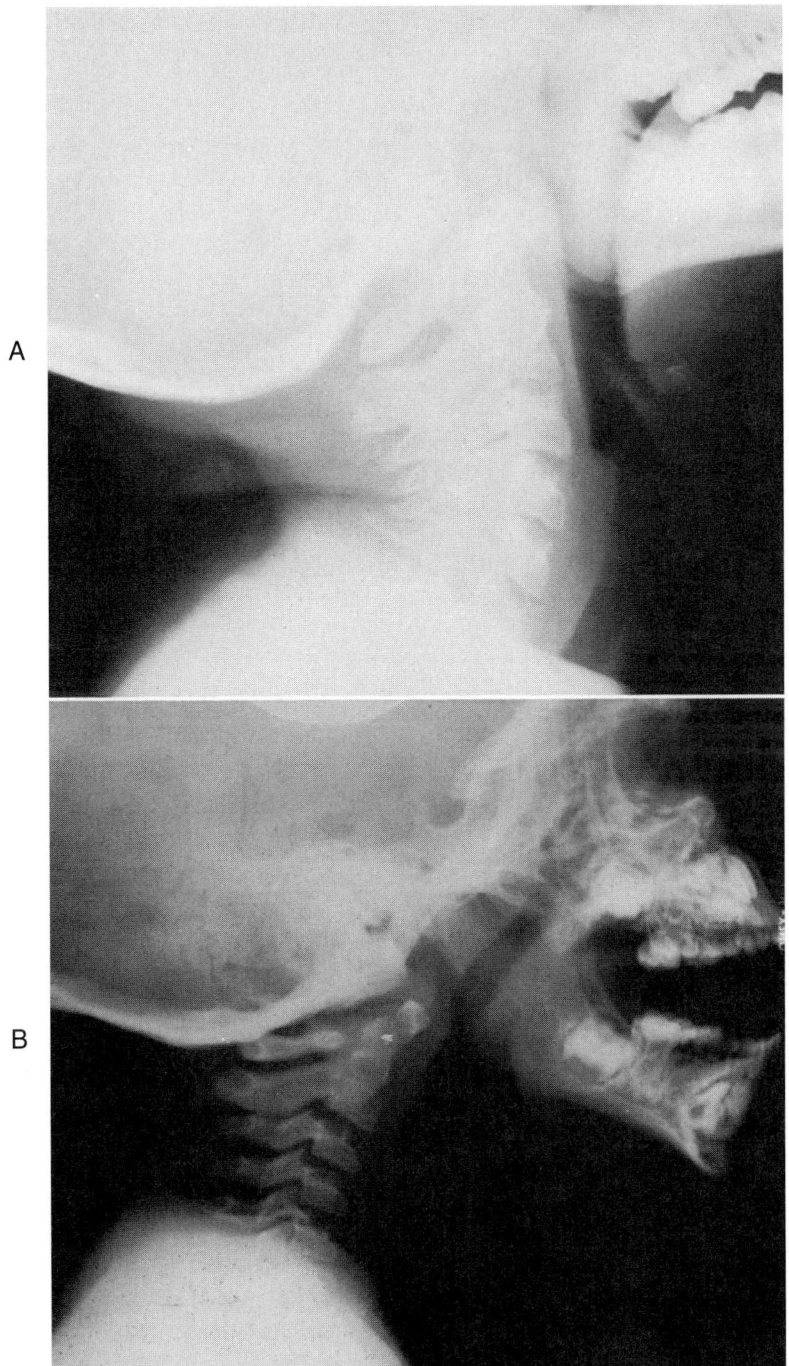

Fig. 84-4 Soft tissue lateral neck films. **A,** Normal. **B,** Markedly swollen epiglottis. Patients with epiglottitis have narrow valleculae and a thick mass of tissue ("thumb" sign) extending from the valleculae to the arytenoids.

(Courtesy of S.Z. Barkin, Denver, Colo.)

determine the timing of elective extubation and may include the following:

a. Mild to moderate respiratory distress followed by improvement in edema and erythema of the epiglottis.

b. Moderate to severe respiratory distress followed by improvement in edema and erythema demonstrated by two successive laryngoscopic examinations.

c. Very severe respiratory distress followed by near-normal epiglottis and aryepiglottic folds.

Intravenous Line. After airway stabilization, an IV line should be started if it has not already been established. Fluid status should be assessed, and maintenance and deficit therapy (if any) initiated.

Antibiotics. Antibiotics should be given parenterally for at least 5 days (at which time they may be changed to oral therapy for a total course of 10 days), with any of the following agents:

- Cefotaxime, 50 to 150 mg/kg/24 hr q6-8hr IV
- Ceftriaxone, 50 to 75 mg/kg/24 hr q12hr IV
- Cefuroxime, 100 mg/kg/24 hr q6-8hr IV

Antibiotic agent may be altered to reflect sensitivity results from blood culture specimens obtained before antibiotic therapy was started.

Disposition

1. All patients with epiglottitis must be admitted to an ICU on an emergency basis for airway management and monitoring. If transport is necessary, it should be performed by an ambulance equipped for airway intervention, ventilatory support, and resuscitation. Trained personnel and an experienced physician should accompany the patient. *Transport without means to control the airway and ventilate the patient is inappropriate.* Ongoing involvement by an anesthesiologist, otolaryngologist, and critical care physician is helpful.
2. Patients can be extubated under controlled conditions after an average of 36 hours if clinical response indicates, and they can usually be discharged 4 to 6 days after admission.

Croup

If the epiglottis is normal and other entities within the differential diagnosis have been excluded, treatment for croup should be initiated, according to whether the patient has stridor when at rest.

Absence of Stridor at Rest. Humidified air is the mainstay of therapy and may be achieved with a variety of cool-air vaporizers. Warm-air humidifiers may be used, but they have the potential disadvantage of possibly causing burns.

Parents should watch for changes in breathing patterns. Stridor often worsens in the early morning hours.

Disposition. The patient who has croup without stridor at rest may be sent home if parents can observe the child, administer fluids, and provide humidified air. Presence or absence of access to a phone and transportation in case the child deteriorates may serve to modify the disposition.

Parental education

1. Keep room air humidified, preferably with a cool-mist humidifier.
2. Push clear liquids.
3. Control fever to make the child more comfortable.
4. If the child awakens with stridor, take him or her outside for 5 minutes. If the stridor persists, bring the child to the hospital.
5. Call your physician immediately if any of the following occurs:
   - **a.** The stridor worsens
   - **b.** The child has more difficulty breathing
   - **c.** The child turns blue or begins drooling
   - **d.** The child becomes agitated or listless
   - **e.** Intake is poor
   - **f.** The croup does not improve in 4 to 5 days

Stridor at Rest

1. Patients with croup and stridor at rest should be observed for a long period or

hospitalized. Humidified air remains the mainstay of therapy and may be achieved with a vaporized room or a mist tent. The latter has the disadvantage of decreasing patient visibility.

2. Racemic epinephrine is useful for patients with stridor at rest and respiratory distress:
   a. Racemic epinephrine is administered after dilution of the solution (2.25%) (child weighing less than 20 kg: 0.25 ml in 2.5 ml saline solution; child weighing 20 to 40 kg: 0.5 ml in 2.5 ml saline solution; child weighing more than 40 kg: 0.75 ml in 2.5 ml saline solution), which is given by nebulizer with or without intermittent positive-pressure breathing (IPPB) up to every 2 hours for increasing stridor at rest.
   b. The therapeutic effect lasts up to 4 hours, and the patient's clinical status often returns to the pretreatment level. However, this rebound may be avoided by initiating steroids at the time of administration of racemic epinephrine.
   c. Racemic epinephrine also has a bronchodilator effect.
   d. L-Epinephrine is an alternative to racemic epinephrine, containing the active isomer and producing therapeutic equivalency. L-Epinephrine (1:1000 solution), 2.5 to 5.0 ml nebulized in 2 ml 0.9% NS.
3. Steroids reduce the severity of disease and shorten the stay in the ED. They are indicated for patients who need racemic epinephrine because of stridor at rest and respiratory distress. Many clinicians use steroid therapy for less severe cases as well.
   a. Dexamethasone (Decadron), 0.6 mg/kg/dose IV, IM, or PO, is given for 1 to 4 doses q12-24hr. There is no clinical difference between oral and IM formulations. Lower doses, 0.15 mg/kg/dose and 0.3 mg/kg/dose, are probably similar. Nebulized steroids are inconsistently equivalent.
   b. Early administration of steroids avoids rebound from racemic epinephrine.
4. Hydration must be maintained by oral or parenteral therapy. Antipyretics are often useful.
5. Oxygen without intubation rarely is indicated because hypoxia is usually an indication for airway intervention. Oxygen, when administered, should be given only in an ICU, where intensive monitoring and observation are possible. On occasion, intubation is required because of respiratory failure.
6. Heliox (helium-oxygen mixture for respiratory distress), when available, has been used to decrease the work of breathing in patients with an incomplete response to epinephrine. A trial may be considered.

Disposition. Most patients with stridor at rest should be observed in a unit that provides close supervision and access to airway intervention in case it is necessary. In many patients, the stridor resolves rapidly after treatment with racemic epinephrine and dexamethasone. If the patient is relatively asymptomatic 3 to 4 hours after the last nebulization treatment and there is good follow-up observation, early discharge may be contemplated with the assurance of careful monitoring.

Spasmodic or Allergic Croup. Spasmodic or allergic croup has a rapid onset and is usually treated very effectively with nebulized racemic epinephrine, 0.25 to 0.5 ml (adult: 0.75 ml) diluted in 2.5 ml of saline. Patients show dramatic response but may need additional treatments in the ensuing 24 hours.

Patients with allergic croup should be hospitalized for observation, administration of humidified air, and additional racemic epinephrine treatments.

BIBLIOGRAPHY

Aquino V, Terndrup TE: Uvulitis in three children: etiology and respiratory distress, *Pediatr Emerg Care* 8:206, 1992.

Bernstein T, Brilli R, Jacobs D: Is bacterial tracheitis changing? a 14-month experience in the pediatric intensive care unit, *Clin Infect Dis* 27:458, 1998.
Birtto J, Habibi P, Walters S et al: Systemic complications associated with bacterial tracheitis, *Arch Dis Child* 74:249, 1996.
Cruz MN, Stewart G, Rosenberg N: Use of dexamethasone in the outpatient management of acute laryngotracheitis, *Pediatrics* 96:220, 1995.
Donaldson JO, Maltby CC: Bacterial tracheitis in children, *J Otolaryngol* 18:101, 1989.
Geelhoed GC: Sixteen years of croup in a Western Australia teaching hospital: effects of routine steroid treatment, *Ann Emerg Med* 28:621, 1996.
Husby S, Agertoft L, Mortensen S et al: Treatment of croup with nebulized steroids (budesonide), *Arch Dis Child* 68:353, 1993.
Johnson DW, Schuh S, Karen G et al: Outpatient treatment of croup with nebulized dexamethasone, *Arch Pediatr Adolesc Med* 150:349, 1996.
Kelley PB, Simon JE: Racemic epinephrine use in croup and disposition, *Am J Emerg Med* 10:181, 1992.
Kunkel NC, Baker MD: Use of racemic epinephrine, dexamethasone and mist in the outpatient management of croup, *Pediatr Emerg Care* 12:156, 1996.
Ledwith CA, Shea LH, Mauro RD: Safety and efficacy of nebulized racemic epinephrine in conjunction with oral dexamethasone and mist in the outpatient treatment of croup, *Ann Emerg Med* 25:331, 1992.
Luria JW, Gonzalez-del-Rey JA, DiGiulio GA et al: Effectiveness of oral or nebulized dexamethasone for children with mild croup, *Arch Pediatr Adolesc Med* 155:1340, 2001.
Mauro RD, Poole SR, Lockhart CH: Differentiation of epiglottitis from laryngotracheitis in children with stridor, *Am J Dis Child* 142:679, 1988.
Ritticier KK, Ledwith CA: Outpatient treatment of moderate croup with dexamethasone: intramuscular versus oral dosing, *Pediatrics* 106:1344, 2000.
Rothrock SG, Pignatiello GA, Howard RM: Radiologic diagnosis of epiglottitis: objective criteria for all ages, *Ann Emerg Med* 19:978, 1990.
Rowe PC, Klassen TP: Corticosteroids for croup, *Arch Pediatr Adolesc Med* 150:344, 1991.
Stroud RH, Friedman NR: An update on inflammatory disorders of the pediatric airway: epiglottitis, croup and tracheitis, *Am J Otolaryngol* 22:268, 2001.
Super DM, Cartelli NA, Brooks LJ et al: A prospective randomized double-blind study to evaluate the effect of dexamethasone in acute laryngotracheitis, *J Pediatr* 115:323, 1989.
Valdepena HG, Wald ER, Rose E et al: Epiglottitis and *Haemophilus influenzae* immunization: the Pittsburgh experience, *Pediatrics* 96:424, 1995.
Waisman Y, Klein BL, Boenning DH et al: Prospective randomized double-blind study comparing L-epinephrine and racemic epinephrine aerosols in the treatment of laryngotracheitis (croup), *Pediatrics* 89:302, 1992.
Weber JE, Chudnofsky CR, Younger JG et al: A randomized comparison of helium-oxygen mixture (Heliox) and racemic epinephrine for the treatment of moderate to severe croup, *Pediatrics* 107:e96, 2001.

Foreign Body in Airway

ALERT The patient with a laryngotracheal foreign body needs immediate airway stabilization, by either removal of the material or surgical intervention. Foreign bodies may cause wheezing.

The clinical presentation of a child with an airway foreign body reflects the acuteness and location of the obstruction. Laryngotracheal foreign bodies typically cause an acute obstruction, whereas bronchial foreign bodies produce a more subacute course. Bronchial obstruction may result from a variety of mechanisms:

1. Check valve, in which air is inhaled but not expelled leading to emphysema
2. Stop valve, which allows no inhaled air to pass, resulting in distal atelectasis
3. Ball valve, in which the foreign body is dislodged during expiration but becomes reimpacted on inspiration, resulting in atelectasis
4. Bypass valve, which produces a partial obstruction to inflow and outflow with decreased aeration on the affected side

Food and vegetable matter (nuts, seeds, grapes, raisins, hard candy, sausage-shaped meat such as hot dogs, raw carrots) are most commonly aspirated by children. Objects usually measure 32 mm or less; round objects are more likely to plug the airway completely. The age range of highest risk is from birth to 48 months; the peak age group is between 1 and 2 years (see Chapter 20).

DIAGNOSTIC FINDINGS

1. Although a history of aspiration is useful, the absence of a positive history does not exclude a foreign body and is often not reported.

2. Acute airway obstruction resulting from material in the laryngotracheal area causes acute, life-threatening respiratory distress. Cyanosis, apnea, stridor, wheezing, cough, and dysphonia may be present. Facial petechiae may appear as a result of increased intrathoracic pressure.
3. Subacute obstruction occurs with bronchial foreign bodies and, rarely, partial obstruction of the laryngotracheal segment. Patients demonstrate air trapping, wheezing, cyanosis, a muffled voice, and cough. Atelectasis is commonly present. At least one component of the triad consisting of wheezing, coughing, and decreased breath sounds is not present in 61% of patients who have obstruction.

Complications

1. Specific pulmonary complications include atelectasis, pneumonia, erosion through the trachea and bronchus, and abscess.
2. Respiratory arrest occurs with any delay in clearing of an acute obstruction. Attempts to remove bronchial foreign bodies may produce total obstruction.
3. Dysrhythmias and other complications of hypoxia may develop, including a full cardiac arrest.
4. Pulmonary edema occasionally results from obstruction and increased intrathoracic pressure.

Ancillary Data

Relief of the obstruction should not be delayed by a wait for the results of ancillary testing. Immediate intervention may be necessary. However, if obstruction is only partial, a number of ancillary diagnostic tests may be useful in defining the location of the foreign body and for consideration of other diagnostic entities:

1. Oximetry and ABG analysis to determine ventilatory status if compromised.
2. Chest x-ray films, both inspiratory and expiratory, to determine whether a bronchial foreign body is likely to be present. It is often important to distinguish whether the foreign body is in the trachea or esophagus. Foreign bodies lie in the plane of least resistance. Flat foreign bodies, such as coins in the esophagus, lie in the frontal plane, appearing as a full circle on the posteroanterior (PA) view, whereas those in the trachea rest in the sagittal plane and appear end-on on the PA chest x-ray film and flat on a lateral view.

   Radiopacity is a relative quality rather than an absolute property. In one study, tracheobronchial tree findings indicated obstruction in 66% of cases, atelectasis in 13%, radiopaque foreign body in 11%, and pneumonia in 5%; in 5% of patients, the findings were normal.
3. Soft tissue lateral neck.
4. Laryngoscopy may be both diagnostic and therapeutic. Magill forceps or a Kelly clamp can be used to remove the foreign body with direct visualization of the laryngotracheal area.
5. Fluoroscopy may be useful. Tracheal foreign bodies may have paradoxic movement.
6. Bronchoscopy is the definitive therapy but is also useful as a diagnostic tool. The procedure is rapidly and safely performed with fiberoptic equipment used by an experienced physician.

DIFFERENTIAL DIAGNOSIS

See Chapter 20.

MANAGEMENT

1. The initial stabilization of the patient with a foreign body involves attention to the airway and simultaneous management of shock, respiratory or cardiac arrest, and the complications of hypoxia the patient has experienced. Concurrent with immediate resuscitation, other differential diagnostic considerations must be evaluated.

2. Efforts should be initiated on the first contact to relieve airway obstruction according to the guidelines of the American Heart Association. Attempts to clear the airway followed by back blows and manual thrusts should be regarded as an essential part of prehospital care and will, ultimately, determine the patient's prognosis.
3. If the child has acute obstruction and is obviously in respiratory distress, immediate intervention is required:
   a. If the infant is younger than 12 months, the rapid increase in pressure resulting from five back blows may expel or loosen a foreign body, which often lodges high in the trachea or throat. If the material is not expelled, five manual chest thrusts should be performed immediately to provide a more sustained increase in pressure and air flow. Repeat as indicated.
   b. In older children, five manual abdominal (Heimlich) thrusts constitute the primary technique. Repeat as indicated. The chest wall compliance in older children reduces the efficacy of chest thrusts, which therefore cannot be recommended.
   c. Blind probing of the airway to dislodge a foreign body is discouraged. The airway may be opened by the jaw thrust maneuver. If a foreign body is seen, it can be removed with the fingers or available instruments (Magill forceps or Kelly clamp).
   d. The preceding recommendations are made on the basis of the best available information, which suggests that a combination of maneuvers may be more effective than any single method, especially in the infant. These methods are under constant reevaluation.
4. If the preceding procedures are not rapidly successful, an attempt may be made to remove the foreign body with laryngoscopy and Magill forceps or Kelly clamp.
5. Bronchoscopy is the definitive therapy and must be performed rapidly in all patients who have unrelieved respiratory obstruction or in whom a bronchial foreign body has been present for more than 24 hours.
6. If these procedures are not available or immediately successful at relieving the obstruction, surgical intervention by cricothyroidotomy may be appropriate.
7. Postural drainage in an ICU, in combination with inhaled bronchodilators, may be useful in removing nonvegetable matter foreign bodies that have been present in the tracheobronchial tract for less than 24 hours and that are not causing respiratory distress. Bronchoscopy may, of course, be used instead.

DISPOSITION

1. Patients who have experienced significant hypoxia or any other complications of an upper airway foreign body should be hospitalized for monitoring if definitive therapy has been rendered either before arrival at the hospital or in the ED.
2. Patients with ongoing obstruction need emergent airway stabilization and critical care facilities.
3. The patient who has experienced a very transient episode of obstruction or choking and is free of distress or signs and symptoms referable to the incident may be monitored closely as an ambulatory patient.

Parental Education

Small, hard foods such as nuts, seeds, raisins, hard candy, sausage-shaped meat, and raw carrots should not be given to small children unless cut into very small pieces. Parents should be taught the techniques of back blow and manual chest thrust for infants and abdominal thrust for older children.

BIBLIOGRAPHY

Imaizuma H, Kaneko M, Nara S et al: Definitive diagnosis and location of peanuts in the airway using magnetic resonance imaging techniques, *Ann Emerg Med* 23:1379, 1994.

Puhakka H, Svedstrom E, Kero P et al: Tracheobronchial foreign body, *Am J Dis Child* 143:543, 1989.

Svedstrom E, Puhakka H, Kero P: How accurate is chest radiography in the diagnosis of tracheobronchial foreign body in children? *Pediatr Radiol* 19:520, 1989.

Schlass MD, Pham-Dang H, Rosales JK: Foreign bodies in the tracheo-bronchial tree: a retrospective study of 217 cases, *J Otolaryngol* 12:212, 1983.

Pneumonia

Pneumonia is an acute infection of the lung parenchyma manifesting as an interstitial process that involves either the alveolar walls or the alveoli.

ETIOLOGY AND DIAGNOSTIC FINDINGS: INFECTION

1. Respiratory findings (Table 84-4) and tachypnea are often associated with pneumonia. The risk of pneumonia increases with age-specific respiratory rates:

Age	Respiratory Rate (breaths/min)
<6 mo	>59
6-11 mo	>52
1-2 yr	>42

   A combination of grunting and an oxygen saturation value of 93% or less suggests the presence of findings consistent with pneumonia on chest x-ray film.

2. Bacterial infection (Table 84-5).
   a. Common organisms: *Streptococcus pneumoniae, H. influenzae,* group A streptococci, and *Staphylococcus aureus.* With *S. pneumoniae,* sputum is often rust colored. The relative frequency of complicated disease in hospitalized children with pneumococcal pneumonia is increasing.
   b. Unusual organisms:
      (1) Pertussis: catarrhal stage followed by staccato, paroxysmal cough (p. 731).

TABLE 84-4 Differentiating Features of Pneumonia

	Bacterial	Viral	*Mycoplasma*
Age	Any	<5 yr	5-15 yr
Season	Any	Epidemic	Any
Onset	Rapid	Gradual	Gradual
Toxicity	Severe	Mild/moderate	Mild
Fever	High	Moderate	Low
Chills	Common	Rare	Rare
Tachypnea	Moderate/severe	Mild/moderate	Mild/moderate
Cough	Productive, variable	Dry, variable	Dry, prominent
Myalgia/headache	None	Common	Headache, pharyngitis
Auscultation	↓ breath sounds, rales, rhonchi	Rare wheezes, rare rales	Very rare rales
Pleural effusion	Common	Very rare	Rare
Segmental consolidation	Common	Rare	Variable
Chest x-ray	Lobar consolidation	Interstitial, delayed resolution	Interstitial (more than physical findings would indicate)
White blood cell count (cells/mm^3)	>10,000	Normal	Normal
Diagnostic procedures	Positive blood culture result; rarely, lung tap or thoracentesis	Viral culture, serologic evaluation	Cold agglutinin, complement fixation
Primary antibiotics	See Table 84-6	None	Erythromycin

(2) *Pseudomonas aeruginosa:* usually in debilitated or immunocompromised patients, especially those with cystic fibrosis. May involve pulmonary tract, ear, sinus, or meninges. Sputum is commonly green.

(3) *Klebsiella pneumoniae:* usually in infants, alcoholics, or immunocompromised patients. Explosive pulmonary symptoms with gastroenteritis and neurologic findings. Chest x-ray film shows bulging fissures. Sputum has current-jelly appearance.

(4) Anaerobes such as *Peptostreptococcus* organisms, often as secondary infection or abscess with feculent sputum.

3. Viral infections: RSV and parainfluenza predominant in children younger than 2 years; influenza A and B in older children; also adenovirus, measles, and chickenpox.
4. *Mycoplasma pneumoniae:* common in children older than 5 years.
5. *Chlamydia trachomatis:*
   a. Tachypnea, staccato cough, conjunctivitis, rarely toxic; fairly common in the second to sixth weeks of life.
   b. Chest x-ray film: hyperexpansion; CBC shows eosinophilia.
6. *Mycobacterium tuberculosis:*
   a. History of exposure; fever, anorexia, cough.
   b. Chest x-ray film with hilar adenopathy and apical findings; sputum and gastric aspirates may be helpful. Purified protein derivative (PPD) skin test of patient and family should be performed.
7. Parasitic infection: *Pneumocystis carinii:*
   a. Fever, tachypnea, cough, dyspnea, cyanosis; occurs in immunosuppressed or malnourished patients.
   b. Chest x-ray film: diffuse interstitial pneumonitis; ABG analysis shows hypoxia, usually greater than would be indicated by chest x-ray study; lung aspirate or biopsy with methenamine-silver nitrate stain.

TABLE 84-5 Bacterial Pneumonias: Diagnostic Findings

	Streptococcus pneumoniae	*Haemophilus influenzae**	Group A Streptococci	*Staphylococcus aureus*
Age	≤4 yr	≤8 yr	>10 yr	<1 yr
Onset	Rapid	Gradual	Gradual	Rapid
Diagnostic features	Infant: poor feeding, cough, irritable Child: fever, cough, toxic, abdominal pain	Fever, cough, toxic, otitis media (variable)	Fever, tachypnea, chill, pleuritic pain, hemoptysis	High fever, respiratory distress, nausea, vomiting
Complications	Bacteremia Empyema Effusion	Bacteremia Meningitis Empyema Lung abscess Bronchiectasis	Empyema (serosanguineous)	Pneumatocele Empyema Pneumothorax Pyopneumothorax
Chest x-ray film	Lobar consolidation, patchy bronchopneumonia	Unilateral lobar consolidation	Infiltrate	Segmental, lobar infiltrate

* Decreasing incidence with widespread immunizations.

8. Fungal infection:
   a. Coccidioidomycosis:
      (1) Fever, pleuritis, productive cough with weight loss, anorexia, myalgias, headache, and rash
      (2) Chest x-ray study: pneumonia (interstitial), effusions, granuloma, cavitation
      (3) Skin test and complement-fixation test
   b. Histoplasmosis:
      (1) Pulmonary cavitation, hemoptysis, variable hepatosplenomegaly, variable weight loss, lymphadenopathy
      (2) Chest x-ray film: pulmonary calcification; CBC shows anemia
9. Rickettsial infection: Q fever.
   a. Fever, chest pain, headache, sore throat, chills, and respiratory symptoms; self-limited disease lasts 3 weeks.
   b. Complement fixation test.

Ancillary Data

Laboratory studies must be individualized for the specific patient and the presenting clinical complex.

1. Chest x-ray films: PA and lateral views. In the absence of respiratory signs in children younger than 8 weeks, abnormalities are unusual.
   a. Children with the following factors commonly do not have pneumonia: illness in summer months, absence of cough, dyspnea, respiratory distress (grunting, flaring, retracting), respiratory rate less than 60 breaths/min, absence of rales or decreased breath sounds, presence of normal color, or white blood cell (WBC) count less than 19,000 cells/mm^3.
   b. An empiric chest radiograph may be indicated in children with a temperature of 39° C or higher and a WBC count of 20,000 cells/mm^3 or higher without an alternative source of the infection. Nearly 20% of such children were noted to have an occult pneumonia in one study.
   c. Inspiratory and expiratory views may be useful in excluding a foreign body if in doubt.
   d. Lateral decubitus views can define an effusion.
2. CBC with differential count.
3. ABG analysis: For all patients with significant cyanosis, apnea, dyspnea, or respiratory distress. Oximetry may be useful if child has good ventilation.
4. Blood cultures: Positive result in 10% to 20% of all patients with bacterial pneumonias; 2.1% of patients with pneumonia seen in the ED have positive culture results. Blood cultures should be obtained for patients needing hospitalization (e.g., toxic, respiratory distress).
5. Counterimmunoelectrophoresis (CIE) may be useful in hospitalized patients with negative culture results.
6. Cold agglutinin measurement. Positive correlation between cold agglutinin titer of at least 1:64 and presence of *M. pneumoniae.* The procedure is performed as follows:
   (1) Place 4 drops of whole blood in small purple top tube (EDTA), which is then placed on ice bath for at least 30 seconds.
   (2) Roll the tube on its side and observe for coarse flocculation.

Pulmonary Cultures. Invasive procedures are indicated for patients with severe toxicity and life-threatening infection, for those showing no response to appropriate antibiotic therapy, and for those who are immunosuppressed. Consultation is usually appropriate.

Nasopharyngeal (NP) or throat cultures are of no value except for pertussis (NP swab) and viral cultures.

1. Sputum: usually difficult to obtain in children and is contaminated with mouth flora. Results reliable only in a

patient with productive cough and if a single organism is recovered.

2. Tracheal suctioning by direct laryngoscopy: fairly reliable but patient may have upper airway contamination.
3. Transtracheal aspiration: difficult to perform in children and usually should be avoided. Absolute contraindication is a bleeding diathesis or an uncooperative, young child.
4. Bronchoscopy with direct aspiration and brush-border biopsy. Excellent approach yielding direct visualization with aspiration of good culture material. Requires equipment and experience, which are rarely available emergently.
5. Direct needle aspiration of the lung (useful in critically ill and immunocompromised children):
   a. Unless the infiltrate is in the upper lobes, the patient is placed in a sitting position and is told to take a deep breath and hold in expiration if old enough to cooperate. A needle (18- to 20-gauge, 1 to 1½ in) is inserted rapidly under negative pressure, along the top of the rib, with an attached syringe containing nonbacteriostatic saline solution. Patient must be hospitalized for observation after the procedure.
   b. Aspirate is an excellent specimen for Gram staining and culture.
   c. Contraindications include hyperexpansion with air trapping, pneumothorax, bleeding diathesis, pulmonary hypertension, uncontrolled coughing or seizures, poor cooperation, and lack of a facility to observe the patient after the procedure.

Thoracentesis (see Appendix A-8). Thoracentesis is indicated for the removal of pleural fluid for either diagnostic or therapeutic purposes.

1. Patient is kept in an upright position, and the site for thoracentesis is defined with the use of x-ray film and physical examination.
2. A needle (18- to 20-gauge) with a 20-ml syringe is attached to a three-way stopcock. With the use of negative pressure, the needle is passed along the top of the ribs, and fluid is withdrawn. The amount removed should reflect the extent of respiratory distress and the amount required for diagnosis. Patient must be hospitalized for observation after the procedure.

Evaluation of the fluid should include Gram stain and culture, cell count and differential, and measurements of protein, lactate dehydrogenase (LDH), and glucose levels.

DIFFERENTIAL DIAGNOSIS

(see Chapter 20)

1. Allergy: asthma (p. 781)
2. Trauma:
   a. Foreign body (p. 808)
   b. Drowning (see Chapter 47)
3. Atelectasis
4. Vascular disease:
   a. CHF and pulmonary edema (see Chapters 16 and 19)
   b. Pulmonary embolism (p. 578)
5. Intoxication: hydrocarbon (p. 385)
6. Recurrent aspiration (gastroesophageal reflux, vascular ring, pharyngeal incoordination, H type tracheoesophageal fistula)
7. Congenital absence of lung, hemangioma, etc.
8. Neoplasm: primary or metastatic

MANAGEMENT

1. Most patients with pneumonia have only mild disease and do not need immediate stabilization or airway support. However, if respiratory distress is present, stabilization of the airway is of the highest priority:
   a. Initiate oxygen, optimally with humidification, if respiratory distress is present.

b. Intubation may be indicated if respiratory failure (Pa_{O_2} less than 50 mm Hg and Pa_{CO_2} greater than 50 mm Hg) is present.

2. ABG analysis is indicated for a moderately ill patient.
3. Suctioning and postural drainage are useful adjunctive measures.
4. Initiate antibiotic therapy for all cases of pneumonia in which bacteria or mycoplasma is the suspected pathogen (Table 84-6):
   a. If appropriate, obtain culture specimens (blood and rarely lung tap) before initiating therapy.
   b. Viral infections do not require antibiotics, although if the patient is toxic or having respiratory distress, antibiotics are indicated until culture results are available.
   c. Most patients may be treated with oral medications and as outpatients.
   d. The initial choice of antibiotic must reflect common causes for the patient's age, allergies, signs and symptoms, and known bacterial sensitivity patterns.
   e. Antibiotic therapy failures commonly occur with infection by resistant organisms (particularly *H. influenzae*), viral infections, or poor compliance.
   f. Infection with organisms such as *Mycobacterium tuberculosis* and *P. carinii* need alternative therapy.
5. Bronchodilators are indicated if wheezing or reactive airway disease is present (p. 790).
6. Special considerations must be recognized in the management of the newborn (see Chapter 11).

DISPOSITION

Hospitalization is rarely necessary but is indicated for any of the following circumstances:

1. Significant toxicity with high fever, dyspnea, apnea, cyanosis, or fatigue
2. Any evidence of potential respiratory failure or progression

TABLE 84-6 Antibiotic Therapy for Bacterial Pneumonia

		ANTIBIOTIC THERAPY	
Age Group	**Major Causes**	**PO**	**IV**
<2 mo*	*E. coli* Group B streptococci *S. aureus* *C. trachomatis*	Rarely given	Ampicillin, 100-200 mg/kg/24 hr q6-12hr, **and** gentamicin, 5-7.5 mg/kg/24 hr q8-12hr
2 mo-8 yr	Virus *S. pneumoniae*† *H. influenzae* *S. aureus* (rare)	Amoxicillin, 30-50 mg/kg/24 hr q8hr, **or** Augmentin **or** cefaclor	Ampicillin, 200 mg/kg/24 hr q4hr, **or** ceftriaxone, 50 to 100 mg/kg/24 hr q12hr IV‡ **If poor response, add** nafcillin (or equiv), 100 mg/kg/24 hr q4hr
≥9 yr	Virus *S. pneumoniae*† *Mycoplasma* *S. aureus* (rare) Group A streptococci (rare) *H. influenzae* (rare)	Erythromycin, 30-50 mg/kg/24 hr q6hr	Ampicillin, 200 mg/kg/24 hr q4hr, **or** ceftriaxone, 50-100 mg/kg/24 hr q12hr IV; if poor response, consider erythromycin (PO) or nafcillin

* If *C. trachomatis* is suspected, **add** erythromycin, 30-50 mg/kg/24 hr q6hr PO.
† If *S. pneumoniae* is suspected and child is toxic, initially add vancomycin, 40 mg/kg/24 hr q6hr IV.
‡ Alternatives are cefuroxime, 100 mg/kg/24 hr q6-8hr IV, and cefotaxime, 50-150 mg/kg/24 hr q6hr IV.

3. Patient younger than 2 or 3 months
4. Immunocompromised host as a result of underlying disorder (e.g., leukemia), drugs (steroids or other immunosuppressive agents), or sickle cell disease
5. Acute deterioration and distress in a patient with cystic fibrosis or other chronic pulmonary disease; the aims of hospitalization are infection control and institution of aggressive pulmonary toilet
6. Presence of pleural effusion or after lung aspiration or thoracentesis
7. Unreliable home environment or questionable compliance

Most patients may be discharged with appropriate medications:

1. Close follow-up must be ensured so that the patient's condition may be assessed after 24 and 48 hours to determine that resolution has occurred.
2. A second chest x-ray film should be obtained 4 to 6 weeks after the initial diagnosis in patients who have segmental or lobar infiltrates.

Parental Education

1. Give medication for entire course of treatment
2. Call the primary care physician or bring your child to his or her office in 24 hours for assessment of the response to treatment
3. Perform postural drainage, if suggested
4. Call your physician if any of the following occurs:
   a. Your child is having more difficulty breathing or has a high fever, more rapid breathing, increased retractions, cyanosis, or apnea
   b. Your child has trouble taking medications or fluids
   c. Your child is not afebrile and much improved in 48 hours.

BIBLIOGRAPHY

Bachur R, Perry H, Harper MB: Occult pneumonia: empiric chest radiographs in febrile children with leukocytosis, *Ann Emerg Med* 33:166, 1999.

Courtoy I, Lande AE, Turner RB: Accuracy of radiographic differentiation of bacterial from nonbacterial pneumonia, *Pediatrics* 28:261, 1989.

Hickey RW, Bowman MJ, Smith GA: Utility of blood cultures in pediatric patients found to have pneumonia in the emergency department, *Ann Emerg Med* 27:721, 1996.

Inselman LA: Tuberculosis in children: an unsettling forecast, *Contemp Pediatr* 7:10, 1990.

Losek JO, Kishaba RG, Berens RJ et al: Indications for chest roentgenograms in the febrile young infant, *Pediatr Emerg Care* 5:149, 1989.

Mhabee-Gittens EM, Dowd MD, Beck JA et al: Clinical factors associated with focal infiltrates in wheezing infants and toddlers, *Clin Pediatr (Phila)* 39:387, 2000.

Tan TQ, Mason EO, Wald ER et al: Clinical characteristics of children with complicated pneumonia caused by *Streptococcus pneumoniae*, *Pediatrics* 110:1, 2002.

Taylor J, Del Beccaro M, Done S et al: Establishing clinically relevant standards for tachypnea in febrile children younger than 2 years, *Arch Pediatr Adolesc Med* 149:283, 1995.

85 RENAL DISORDERS

Also See Chapters 37 (Hematuria and Proteinuria) and 64 (Genitourinary Trauma)

MARK A. HOSTETLER and JOSEPH T. FLYNN

Acute Glomerulonephritis

Although glomerulonephritis is a histopathologic diagnosis, *acute glomerulonephritis* is commonly used to refer to the clinical presentation of gross hematuria, edema, and hypertension. It occurs after an immunologic trigger that causes inflammation and proliferation of glomerular tissue, most commonly as a sequela of group A β-hemolytic streptococcal infection involving either the pharynx or the skin. Infections with other bacteria, *Mycoplasma*, and certain viruses may produce a similar picture. The pathogenesis is poorly understood but probably results from the deposition of circulating immune complexes in the kidney.

The disease most commonly occurs in older school-age children and adolescents.

Although the disease is self-limited with careful clinical management, strict attention must be given to the initial evaluation, differential diagnosis, and recognition of complications.

DIAGNOSTIC FINDINGS

1. Usually a streptococcal infection or exposure occurs 1 to 2 weeks (mean, 10 days) before the onset of glomerulonephritis. An interval less than 4 days is associated with an exacerbation of preexisting disease rather than an initial attack.
2. Patients commonly have hematuria (90%), fluid retention and edema (100%), hypertension (60% to 70%), and oliguria (80%). Fever, malaise, and abdominal pain are frequently reported.

Complications

1. Circulatory congestion is sometimes noted, with dyspnea, cough, pallor, and pulmonary edema.
2. Hypertensive encephalopathy with confusion, headaches, somnolence, and seizures may develop.
3. Anuria and renal failure occur in 2% of patients.

Ancillary Data

1. Urinalysis (UA):
   a. Hematuria may be microscopic or gross. Erythrocyte casts are present in up to 80% of affected children.
   b. Leukocyturia and hyaline and granular casts are common.
   c. Proteinuria is usually less than 2 g/m^2/24 hr.
   d. Urinary concentrating ability is preserved.
2. Fractional excretion of sodium (p. 830) may be reduced.
3. Antistreptococcal antibodies are present. An antistreptolysin O (ASO) measurement is most commonly ordered but is less specific than anti-DNAse B measurement. The Streptozyme slide test screens

for five different antistreptococcal antibodies, values of which are almost always elevated.

4. Levels of total serum complement, and specifically of C3, are depressed in 90% to 100% of patients during the first 2 weeks of illness, returning to normal within 6 to 8 weeks. Persistently low levels suggest the presence of a chronic renal disease.
5. Immunoglobulin (Ig) G values are elevated, often in association with rheumatoid factor titers greater than 1:32.
6. Anemia may be present, possibly because of dilution. Thrombocytopenia is reported, and fibrinogen, factor VIII, and plasma activity values may be acutely elevated.
7. Blood urea nitrogen (BUN) is elevated disproportionately to the serum creatinine. Hyponatremia and hyperkalemia may be present, specifically related to the degree of oliguria.
8. Chest x-ray film may show cardiomegaly and pulmonary congestion.

DIFFERENTIAL DIAGNOSIS

(see Chapter 37)

The diagnosis of poststreptococcal acute glomerulonephritis is established from the acute onset of edema, hypertension, and gross or microscopic hematuria with erythrocyte casts and proteinuria. Evidence of an antecedent streptococcal infection, decreased complement, and spontaneous improvement in the renal disease and its complications further support the diagnosis. Other diagnoses should be considered when the clinical syndrome is aberrant, the renal failure is severe, the individual's age does not fall within the predicted range, or resolution is prolonged. Other common causes of nonstreptococcal glomerulonephritis in children are IgA nephropathy, membranoproliferative glomerulonephritis, Henoch-Schönlein purpura, systemic lupus erythematosus, and idiopathic rapidly progressive glomerulonephritis.

MANAGEMENT

Hypertension (see Chapter 18)

1. Acute management may involve a number of agents that may be used individually or in combination, as follows:
   a. Diazoxide, 1 to 3 mg/kg/dose q6hr IV (potent vasodilator)
   b. Furosemide (Lasix), 1 to 2 mg/kg/dose IV (diuretic)
   c. Labetalol, 0.4 to 1.0 mg/kg/dose q4-6hr IV
2. Maintenance, ongoing therapy involves the following agents, to be used individually or in combination:
   a. Propranolol, 1 mg/kg/dose q6-8hr PO
   b. Hydralazine, 1 to 3 mg/kg/24 hr q6hr PO
   c. Isradipine, 0.05 to 0.2 mg/kg/dose q 8 hr PO

Fluid Overload

1. Fluid and sodium are restricted to minimize fluid retention.
2. Diuretics may be required.

DISPOSITION

1. All patients who have evidence of uncontrolled hypertension, congestive heart failure (CHF), or severe azotemia should be hospitalized. Children without any of these problems can be monitored at home provided that close follow-up is available, including frequent blood pressure measurements.
2. Referral to a nephrologist is recommended.

BIBLIOGRAPHY

Herthelius M, Berg U: Renal function during and after childhood acute poststreptococcal glomerulonephritis, *Pediatr Nephrol* 13:907, 1999.

Hricik DE, Chung-Park M, Sedor JR: Glomerulonephritis, *N Engl J Med* 229:888, 1998.

O'Meara YM, Brady HR: Lipoxins, leukocyte recruitment and the resolution phase of acute glomerulonephritis, *Kidney Int Supl* 58:S56, 1997.

Popovic-Rolovic M, Kostic M, Antic-Peco A et al: Medium and long term prognosis of patients with acute poststreptococcal glomerulonephritis, *Nephron* 58:393, 1991.
Simckes AM, Spitzer A: Poststreptococcal acute glomerulonephritis, *Pediatr Rev* 16:278, 1995.
Travis LB, Kalia A: Acute nephritic syndrome. In Postlewaite RJ, editor: *Clinical paediatric nephrology*, Oxford, 1994, Butterworth-Heinemann.

Hemolytic-Uremic Syndrome

Hemolytic-uremic syndrome (HUS) consists of the classic triad renal failure, microangiopathic hemolytic anemia, and thrombocytopenia. HUS most often follows an episode of bloody diarrhea but has also been reported in association with a respiratory infection. It is primarily a disease of young children and usually occurs in those younger than 5 years. Predisposing factors include exposure to contaminated meat or to other children with gastroenteritis in daycare centers. There is some seasonal variability, with peaks in the late summer and early fall. HUS has also been reported after exposure to certain medications, including oral contraceptive pills (OCPs) and cyclosporine. In addition, there is an atypical familial pattern without known predisposing factors.

HUS results from localized intravascular coagulation and endothelial injury within the kidney. Clinical evidence of thrombotic microangiopathy is usually limited to the kidneys but may also be seen in extrarenal organs, including the colon, brain, and pancreas. Platelet aggregation results in consumptive thrombocytopenia. The vascular endothelial cell injury produces swelling and detachment from the basement membrane with accumulation of a fluffy material. The prostacyclin-thromboxane (coagulation/anticoagulation) equilibrium is disturbed.

ETIOLOGY

1. Bacteria: Verotoxin-producing *Escherichia coli* serotype 0157:H7 is the most common organism involved. Evidence of *E. coli* 0157:H7 infection has been found in 72% of patients affected. Other bacteria that have been implicated in HUS are *Shigella, Salmonella,* and group A streptococci.
2. Virus: coxsackievirus, influenza, and respiratory syncytial virus (RSV).
3. Drugs: OCPs, cyclosporine.

DIAGNOSTIC FINDINGS

1. Patients with typical HUS have a history of gastroenteritis with vomiting, bloody diarrhea, and crampy abdominal pain for up to 2 weeks before the onset of HUS. Absence of a gastrointestinal (GI) prodrome is associated with a poor prognosis.
2. The spectrum of clinical disease is highly variable, ranging from mild elevation of BUN without anemia to acute renal failure with marked anemia and thrombocytopenia. Approximately two thirds of patients experience at least some degree of oliguria. In patients with anuria for more than 8 days, or oliguria more than 15 days, chronic disease often develops.
3. Patients may have marked hypertension, pallor, petechiae and easy bruising, hepatosplenomegaly, and edema. Hypertension occurs in as many as 50% of patients.
4. Central nervous system (CNS) findings, which occur relatively often, include irritability and lethargy and in some cases progress to coma, seizures, and hemiparesis.

Complications

1. Renal failure, rarely progressing to end-stage renal disease in children with typical HUS. However, some renal abnormality may be found on long-term follow-up in up to 30% to 50% of all patients with HUS.
2. High-output cardiac failure may occur because of volume overload. Rarely, myocarditis is seen.

3. Bowel perforation or necrosis.
4. Insulin-dependent diabetes mellitus, secondary to pancreatic involvement.
5. Seizures occur in 40% of cases, especially in patients with hyponatremia or severe azotemia. Other CNS findings are drowsiness, personality changes, focal weakness, cerebral infarction, and coma.
6. Atypical HUS is marked by recurrences, often without prodrome.
7. Mortality may be as high as 15%.

Ancillary Data

1. Assessment of renal function (p. 830).
   a. Electrolytes (elevated K^+ level and acidosis may be present), BUN, creatinine, calcium (often low), and phosphorus levels (usually elevated).
   b. UA demonstrating hematuria and proteinuria.
   c. In dehydration, the BUN value is often elevated and should decrease by 50% after 24 hours of appropriate rehydration. If BUN value does not fall, HUS should be considered.
2. Hematologic findings:
   a. Anemia is usually present. Peripheral smear reveals microangiopathic hemolytic anemia with burr cells and fragments.
   b. The white blood cell (WBC) count is usually elevated. A polymorphonuclear leukocyte count greater than 15,000 cells/mm^3 is associated with severe manifestations.
   c. Thrombocytopenia: platelets usually less than 50,000 cells/mm^3.
   d. Results of coagulation studies are normal. Presence of fibrin split products and evidence of disseminated intravascular coagulation (DIC) are rare.
3. Arterial blood gas (ABG) analysis may be helpful for evaluation of acidosis and hypoxemia.
4. Bacterial and viral cultures, when appropriate, including stool for *E. coli* serotyping.

DIFFERENTIAL DIAGNOSIS

1. Vascular lesions are similar in HUS and thrombotic thrombocytopenic purpura (TTP). Whereas renal failure is the hallmark of HUS, TTP is more commonly associated with CNS involvement.
2. DIC, which is differentiated by the presence of fibrin split products and grossly abnormal coagulation study results.
3. Inflammation and infection:
   a. Acutely dehydrated patients with acute tubular necrosis. Anemia and thrombocytopenia should be less pronounced or absent.
   b. Ulcerative colitis may be accompanied by bloody diarrhea and anemia with a chronic pattern.
   c. Surgical abdomen secondary to infection, perforation, or necrosis.
4. Trauma may be associated with hematuria and anemia and, occasionally, thrombocytopenia.
5. Other causes of acquired hemolytic anemia (p. 212).

MANAGEMENT

1. Treatment is supportive. The initial management, after the diagnosis is established, should involve careful assessment and treatment of the volume status of the patient. Many patients have volume overload associated with electrolyte abnormalities, hypertension, and high-output cardiac failure.
2. Acute renal failure may necessitate the treatment of hypertension, volume overload, hyperkalemia, acidosis, hypocalcemia, hyperphosphatemia, and other metabolic abnormalities. Consultation with a nephrologist should be obtained. If routine medical management is ineffective, dialysis may be necessary in the

patient who has hypervolemia with oliguria or anuria, more than 24 hours of anuria, unresponsive electrolyte abnormalities, or life-threatening hyperkalemia and in whom more conservative management is contraindicated.

3. Red blood cell (RBC) transfusions are indicated if the hematocrit (Hct) value is less than 15% or the hemoglobin (Hgb) level is less than 5 to 6 g/ml at any time, less than 20% in the presence of continuing decline, or if the patient is symptomatic (e.g., hypoxemic, gallop rhythm, or high output failure). Initially, it is important to transfuse only a small amount of blood slowly (5 ml/kg over 4 hours) to minimize volume overload. Blood pressure may rise dramatically concomitant with or after the transfusion. If the patient is hyperkalemic, transfusion should be delayed until after dialysis.
4. Platelet transfusions are usually not recommended. Platelets have a shortened survival time, and transfused platelets may contribute to platelet plugging in the renal microvasculature. Platelet counts less than 10,000 cells/mm^3 associated with spontaneous bleeding are uncommon. Platelet transfusions may be considered in children with active bleeding and platelet counts consistently less than 20,000 cells/mm^3, or in patients with counts less than 50,000 cells/mm^3 who are about to undergo invasive procedures. In such cases, 1 unit of platelets may be transfused for every 10 kg of body weight.
5. Seizures are controlled with lorazepam (Ativan), 0.1 mg/kg/dose IV, or diazepam (Valium), 0.2 mg/kg/dose IV, repeated every 5 to 10 minutes as required. Phenobarbital or phenytoin should be initiated for maintenance therapy (see Chapter 21). Prophylactic loading with phenytoin, 10 to 20 mg/kg/dose IV administered at a rate of 0.5 mg/kg/min, may be considered in patients with neuromuscular irritability (e.g., muscular twitching). Fosphenytoin permits more rapid or IM administration.
6. Azotemia should be closely monitored. Protein intake should be restricted to limit azotemia. Adequate calories are provided in the form of carbohydrates and fat to enable anabolism. The indications and route of dialysis are somewhat controversial, but dialysis is usually initiated in the presence of complicating clinical signs, such as hyperkalemia and encephalopathy.
7. Multiple investigational therapies have been attempted, including heparin, antiplatelet agents (aspirin or dipyridamole), fibrinolytic agents (urokinase), plasmapheresis, diuretic infusions, prostacyclin infusions, and intravenous IgG infusions. Results have been suboptimal. Plasma exchange may be helpful if severe neurologic involvement is present. Consultation with a nephrologist is recommended.

DISPOSITION

1. Patients with HUS should be hospitalized, and a nephrology consultation obtained.
2. In rare cases, patients may be discharged home if they show no clinical evidence of disease (normal blood pressure [BP], CNS status, and volume) and only minimal laboratory abnormalities (mildly hemolytic smear and normal Hgb and Hct values, platelet count, and BUN and creatinine levels). In such cases, however, the underlying diagnosis would have to be questioned. If the patient is discharged, he or she must have close outpatient follow-up.
3. Given that siblings may get HUS, it is important that other household members also be monitored.
4. Long-term follow-up (for up to 10 years) is indicated because of the possibility of delayed onset of renal failure and hypertension.

BIBLIOGRAPHY

Bell BP, Griffin PM, Lozano P et al: Predictors of hemolytic uremic syndrome in children during a large outbreak of *Escherichia coli* O157:H7 infections, *Pediatrics* 100:E12, 1997.

Brandt JR, Fouser LS, Watkins SL et al: *E. coli* 0157:H7-associated hemolytic-uremic syndrome after ingestion of contaminated hamburgers, *J Pediatr* 125:519, 1994.

Fitzpatrick MM, Walters MDS, Trompeter RS et al: Atypical (non-diarrhea-associated) hemolytic uremic syndrome in childhood, *J Pediatr* 122:532, 1993.

Gordjani N, Sutor AH, Zimmerhackl LB: Hemolytic uremic syndromes in childhood, *Semin Thromb Hemost* 23:281, 1997.

Gravitz A, Rosmini F, Capioli A et al: Haemolytic-uraemic syndrome in childhood: surveillance and case control studies in Italy, *Pediatr Nephrol* 8:705, 1994.

Hahn JS, Havens PC, Higgins JJ et al: Neurologic complications of hemolytic uremic syndrome, *J Child Neurol* 4:108, 1989.

Kelles A, Van Dyck M, Proesman W: Childhood haemolytic uraemic syndrome: long-term outcome and prognostic features, *Eur J Pediatr* 153:38, 1994.

Matsumae T, Takebayashi S, Naito S: The clinico-pathological characteristics and outcome in hemolytic uremic syndrome of adults, *Clin Nephrol* 45:153, 1996.

Niaudet P, Gagnadoux MF, Broyer M: Hemolytic uremic syndrome: hereditary forms and forms associated with hereditary diseases, *Adv Nephrol Necker Hosp* 30:261, 2000.

Remuzzi G: Hemolytic uremic syndrome: past and present, *Am J Kidney Dis* 36:54, 2000.

Rowe PC, Orrbine E, Ogborn M et al: Epidemic *E. coli* 0157:H7 gastroenteritis and hemolytic-uremic syndrome in a Canadian Inuit community: intestinal illness in family members as a risk factor, *J Pediatr* 124:21, 1994.

Schulman SL, Kaplan BS: Management of patients with hemolytic uremic syndrome demonstrating severe azotemia but not uremia, *Pediatr Nephrol* 10:671, 1996.

Siegler RL, Milligan MK, Burningham TH et al: Long-term outcome and prognostic indicators in the hemolytic uremic syndrome, *J Pediatr* 118:195, 1991.

Henoch-Schönlein Purpura

Henoch-Schönlein purpura (HSP) is an acute vasculitis of unknown etiology. It is thought to be an IgA-mediated autoimmune response to a variety of causes, including group A streptococcus, *Mycoplasma pneumoniae,* and viral (e.g., varicella, Epstein-Barr [EB] virus) infections; drugs (penicillin, tetracycline, aspirin, sulfonamides, and erythromycin); and allergens (insect bites, chocolate, milk, and wheat). Antigen-antibody complexes form and deposit throughout the body and activate pathways leading to necrotizing vasculitis. HSP most commonly occurs in the winter months, and a male predominance has been noted.

Multisystem involvement occurs primarily in children 2 to 11 years old. Progression of renal disease occurs more commonly in older children and adults (children: 5%; adults: 15%). Children younger than 3 months may have only skin manifestations without GI or renal involvement.

DIAGNOSTIC FINDINGS

1. Skin lesions are pathognomonic and usually begin on the gravity-dependent areas of the legs and buttocks and the extensor surfaces of the arms. They begin as erythematous, maculopapular lesions that blanch and progress to become petechial and purpuric, at which time they are often palpable. They may be discrete, confluent, clustered, or individual. The entire body may be involved, although the lower extremities usually demonstrate the greatest eruption. A rash is the presenting symptom in 50% of patients and lasts an average of 3 weeks. It may recur in 40% of patients within 6 weeks, often without systemic signs.
2. Colicky abdominal pain with diarrhea, often bloody, is commonly present. Approximately 60% to 85% of patients have abdominal pain. Melena or hematemesis may also be noted. Intussusception (ileo-ileal) or perforation must be considered.
3. Nephritis associated with hematuria, proteinuria, and other nephrosis may develop. Renal involvement occurs in 50% of patients, may begin after other symptoms, and requires ongoing follow-up observation. Microscopic hematuria is most common and carries a

benign long-term prognosis. A "nephritic-nephrotic" presentation portends a poor long-term prognosis.

4. Migratory polyarthritis, often transient, may be present, with the greatest frequency in the ankles, knees, and, less commonly, the wrists. It may occur in up to 75% of patients. Effusions are not typical.
5. Other findings are soft tissue edema (scalp, ear, face, and dorsum of hands and feet), testicular pain, and parotitis.

COMPLICATIONS

1. Renal involvement is the primary source of long-term sequelae. Severe renal involvement may progress to chronic renal failure.
2. Intussusception and abdominal distension.
3. CNS presentations include mental status change, hemiparesis, seizures, and intracranial hemorrhage.

Ancillary Data

1. Complete blood count (CBC) often reveals an elevated WBC count with a variable left shift. Anemia may be present. Coagulation study results and platelet count are usually normal.
2. Erythrocyte sedimentation rate (ESR) is often elevated, but the finding is nonspecific.
3. UA reflects the extent of renal involvement, with hematuria, proteinuria, leukocytosis, and cylindruria. If results are abnormal, other assessments of renal function are indicated (basic metabolic profile).
4. Throat cultures may be indicated to rule out group A streptococcus.
5. Blood cultures should be performed if bacteremia is a diagnostic consideration (i.e., fever or elevated WBC count) (see discussion of differential diagnosis).
6. Serum complement level is usually normal.
7. Barium enema study may be indicated to exclude intussusception (ileo-ileal) if there is severe abdominal pain.
8. If indicated, renal biopsy may be performed after the acute phase of the illness. Mesangial IgA deposition is classically seen.
9. Skin biopsy specimens of the purpuric lesions, examination of which would demonstrate IgA deposition, are rarely necessary.

DIFFERENTIAL DIAGNOSIS

1. HSP is most often a diagnosis of exclusion. Patients are unusually well-appearing despite a prominent rash that is often purpuric. Infections, particularly those associated with petechial and purpuric eruption (e.g., meningococcemia, Rocky Mountain spotted fever) must be excluded (see Table 42-1).
2. Thrombocytopenic purpura (platelet count should differentiate).
3. Nonthrombocytopenic purpura: Ehlers-Danlos syndrome, scurvy, massive steroid therapy, vasculitis.
4. Glomerulonephritis.
5. Other GI or intraabdominal abnormality (intussusception, trauma, appendicitis).

MANAGEMENT

1. Assess and stabilize airway, breathing, and circulation. If there is evidence of GI hemorrhage or hypovolemia, initiate fluid resuscitation.
2. In cases of significant abdominal pain:
   a. Exclude the possibility of an acute abdomen.
   b. Evaluation for intussusception in patient with severe abdominal pain.
   c. Corticosteroids (prednisone, 1 to 2 mg/kg/24 hr q12hr PO for 1 week) may be useful for significant GI pain (once an acute abdomen is excluded) or polyarthritis. Steroids may also play a beneficial role in soft tissue

and joint swelling and in preventing the progression of renal manifestations.

3. Manage complications of renal disease if there is abnormal function. If acute renal failure or nephrosis is present, consult a nephrologist. Specific attention must be given to the control of blood pressure and intake and output.
4. Exclusion of other life-threatening conditions (most notably meningococcemia).

DISPOSITION

Most patients can be managed successfully as outpatients. Admission may be indicated for patients with severe dehydration, renal involvement, or abdominal pain.

BIBLIOGRAPHY

Blanco R, Martinez-Taboada VM, Rodriguez-Valverde V et al: Henoch-Schönlein purpura in adulthood and childhood: two different expressions of the same syndrome, *Arthritis Rheum* 40:859-64, 1997.

Lanzkowsky S, Lanzkowsky L, Lanzkowsky P: Henoch-Schönlein purpura, *Pediatr Rev* 13:130-7, 1992.

Mollica F, LiVolti S, Garozzo R et al: Effectiveness of early prednisone treatment in preventing the development of nephropathy in anaphylactoid purpura, *Eur J Pediatr* 151:140, 1992.

Robson W, Leung A: Henoch-Schönlein purpura, *Adv Pediatr* 41:163, 1994.

Rostoker G et al: High-dose immunoglobulin therapy for severe IgA nephropathy and Henoch-Schönlein purpura, *Ann Intern Med* 120:476, 1994.

Szer IS: Henoch-Schönlein purpura: when and how to treat, *J Rheumatol* 23:1661-5, 1996.

Nephrotic Syndrome

Nephrotic syndrome is characterized by pronounced proteinuria and occurs as a result of increased glomerular permeability. Most commonly affecting children younger than 6 years of age, the disorder is marked by massive proteinuria, edema, hypoalbuminemia, and hyperlipidemia.

ETIOLOGY

1. Primary renal disorders:
   a. Minimal change disease is the most common form of nephrotic syndrome in children, and its prevalence is inversely proportional to the age at onset
   b. Focal segmental glomerulosclerosis is a heterogeneous condition, affecting 7% to 10% of all children with nephrotic syndrome
   c. Membranoproliferative glomerulonephritis may be associated with a nephritic pattern and is more common in older children and adolescents
   d. Membranous glomerulonephritis is rare in children younger than 10 years and is seen mostly in adolescents
2. Intoxication: heroin, mercury, probenecid, silver
3. Allergic hypersensitivity reactions:
   a. Poison ivy or oak, pollens
   b. Bee sting
   c. Snake venom
4. Infection:
   a. Bacterial
   b. Viral: hepatitis B, cytomegalovirus, EB virus
   c. Protozoa: malaria, toxoplasmosis
5. Neoplasm: Hodgkin's disease, Wilms' tumor, etc.
6. Autoimmune disorders: systemic lupus erythematosus
7. Metabolic disorder: diabetes mellitus
8. Cardiac disorders: congenital heart disease and CHF, pericarditis
9. Vasculitis: Henoch-Schönlein purpura, Wegener's granulomatosis

DIAGNOSTIC FINDINGS

1. Patients may report a recent upper respiratory infection or flulike symptoms before the development of edema; however, the significance of this association is unknown.

2. Patients commonly have generalized peripheral edema that may be associated with ascites and hepatomegaly.
3. BP may be decreased if intravascular volume is depleted, or it may be increased because of renal impairment. Approximately 20% to 30% of patients with minimal change disease have hypertension. Hypertension may be exacerbated by steroid therapy.
4. Respiratory and cardiovascular status will reflect the extent of edema. Pleural effusion, pericardial effusion, pulmonary edema, and CHF may be present.
5. Patients with nephrotic syndrome may be relatively immunosuppressed. Appropriate culture specimens should be obtained in all febrile children, and empiric antibiotic therapy started.

Complications

1. Infection: Patients are at increased risk of peritonitis and are susceptible to systemic infection. Septicemia, cellulitis, peritonitis, and pneumonitis are most commonly caused by *Streptococcus pneumoniae.* They may also be caused by gram-negative organisms such as *E. coli,* or other gram-positive organisms such as *Staphylococcus aureus.*
2. Renal failure related to intravascular volume depletion.
3. Thromboembolism: Patients have hypercoagulation because of urinary losses of protein S, protein C, and antithrombin III. Renal venous thrombosis, although relatively uncommon in children, may occur and may lead to renal failure.
4. Long-term effects of hypercholesterolemia, especially in patients who show no response to steroids.
5. Complications of drug therapy: Corticosteroids are associated with a number of unwanted side effects, including excessive weight gain, behavioral changes, alterations in growth, hyperglycemia, osteoporosis, and immune suppression. Other, less commonly used agents also carry significant morbidity (e.g., diuretics, other immunosuppressive agents).

Ancillary Data

1. UA invariably reveals marked proteinuria. Hematuria varies according to the type of nephrotic syndrome. Of those with minimal change disease, microscopic hematuria occurs in 20% to 30%, and macroscopic hematuria in 3% to 4% (see Chapter 37).
2. WBC count may be elevated, even in the absence of infection. Because infection often exacerbates nephrotic syndrome, evidence should be sought.
3. Electrolytes, BUN, creatinine, calcium, and phosphorus measurements. BUN and creatinine values may be normal at the onset of nephrotic syndrome, and can become elevated in 25% of children with minimal change disease. Factitious hyponatremia (related to hyperlipidemia) is common.
4. Triglyceride and cholesterol determinations. Levels of plasma cholesterol carriers (low-density lipoprotein [LDL] and very-low-density lipoprotein [VLDL]) are increased. Lipid elevations result from increased synthesis as well as a defect in catabolism of phospholipid.
5. Hypoalbuminemia.
6. Spot urine protein-creatinine ratio greater than 1.0. A 24-hour urine collection is usually not routinely necessary. By definition, the protein level in a 24-hour urine collection is greater than 40 $mg/m^2/hr$.
7. Further tests to identify the underlying cause include serum complement (C3) measurement, ASO titer or Streptozyme test, antinuclear antibody (ANA) test, hepatitis studies (B and C), and human immunodeficiency virus (HIV) test (Fig. 85-1).

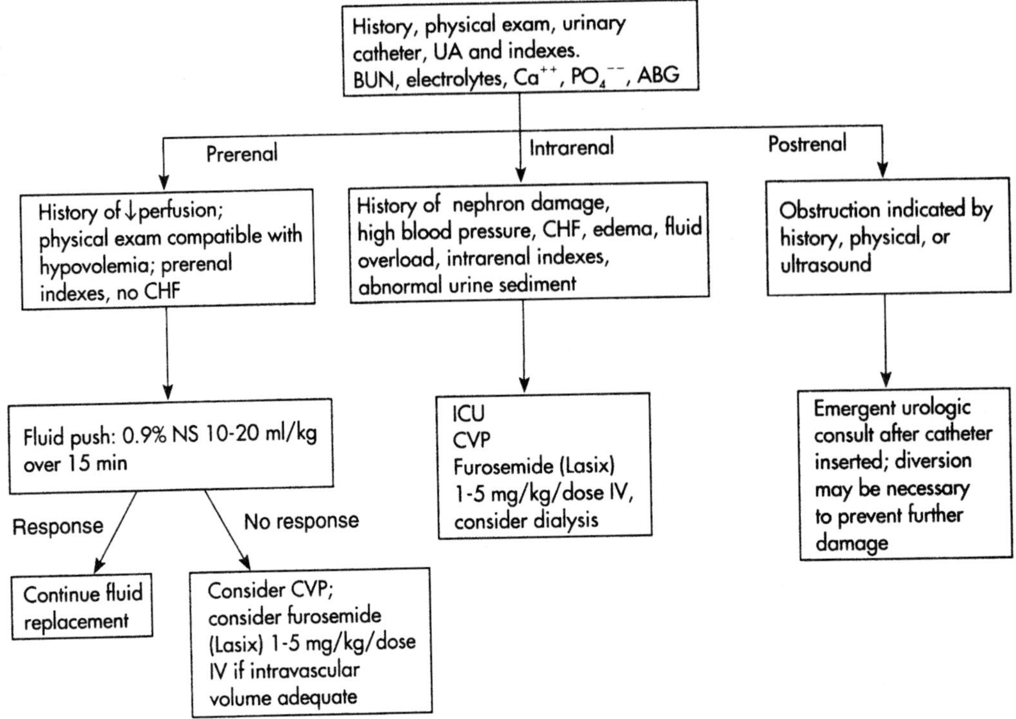

Fig. 85-1 Acute renal failure: initial assessment and treatment.

8. No routine imaging studies are indicated. Renal ultrasonography may reveal slightly enlarged kidneys with normal or increased echogenicity.
9. Renal biopsy is needed for the following poor prognostic indicators:
   a. Patient older than 10 years
   b. Decreased complement value, positive ANA test result
   c. No response to steroid therapy
   d. Coexistence of significant hematuria, hypertension, or azotemia

DIFFERENTIAL DIAGNOSIS
(see Chapter 37)

Diagnostic considerations in evaluating the patient with generalized edema include the following:

1. Renal: nephrotic syndrome, glomerulonephritis, renal failure
2. Cardiovascular: CHF, vasculitis, acute thrombosis
3. Endocrine/metabolic: hypothyroidism, starvation
4. Hematologic: hemolytic disease of the newborn
5. GI: cirrhosis, protein-losing enteritis, cystic fibrosis, lymphangitis
6. Iatrogenic: drugs (steroids, diuretics), water overload

MANAGEMENT

1. Corticosteroids are the mainstay of treatment, usually starting with prednisone, 2 mg/kg/dose (maximum: 80 mg/day) divided BID for 4 to 6 weeks. Then a maintenance dose, of 1.5 mg/kg/dose every other morning, is used for 4 to 6 weeks longer. Ninety percent of cases of minimal change disease respond to

corticosteroids. Of the cases that do respond, 73% do so within 14 days, and 94% within 28 days. Limited response to initial steroid therapy is generally predictive of a poor outcome.

a. If remission occurs (defined as clearing of proteinuria and return of serum albumin to normal) and the patient has a relapse, begin prednisone again. A short course of high-dose daily steroids is continued until the patient is free of proteinuria for 3 days, followed by a maintenance-tapering course of alternate-day steroids for 4 to 6 weeks. Some cases are steroid dependent, relapsing as steroid dosage is tapered.
b. After four relapses in less than 1 year, or if the disease is steroid dependent, cytotoxic agents may be considered. Either cyclophosphamide, 2 mg/kg/24 hr for 12 weeks, or chlorambucil, 0.2 mg/kg/24 hr for 12 weeks, is given in conjunction with prednisone, 1.0 to 1.5 mg/kg QOD. Consultation with a pediatric nephrologist should be obtained before cytotoxic agents are given.
c. Patients whose disease is steroid resistant (defined as failure to enter remission after more than 8 weeks of steroid therapy) are unlikely to have minimal change disease and should be referred to a pediatric nephrologist for a renal biopsy. Drugs that may be useful in such patients include cyclosporine A, "pulse" IV Solu-Medrol (with or without cytotoxic agents), tacrolimus, and angiotensin-converting enzyme (ACE) inhibitors.
d. Teenagers with nephrotic syndrome are less likely to be steroid sensitive than younger children, and early referral to a pediatric nephrologist should be considered.

2. Initiate sodium restriction (2-3 g/day) to minimize edema formation. A high-protein diet is not indicated and may even increase urinary protein losses.
3. Loop diuretics such as furosemide, 1 to 2 mg/kg/day, may be helpful to decrease edema in cases of mild hypertension. These agents should be used with caution, however, because further sodium and fluid losses may be associated with hypovolemia. Hypertension is rarely observed in patients with minimal change disease and, when present, is often difficult to manage.
4. Treatment of severe fluid overload (anasarca):
   a. Albumin: 25% albumin infusion, 2 g/kg/day IV, over 24 hours.
   b. Furosemide: 6 to 8 hours after albumin infusion is begun. Furosemide, 1 mg/kg/dose IV, q8-12hr.
   c. Observe carefully for complications of albumin infusion, including hypertension and pulmonary edema.
5. Some clinicians recommend prophylactic low-dose amoxicillin (children weighing less than 20 kg, 125 mg BID; children weighing more than 20 kg, 250 mg) to reduce the risk of infection from encapsulated organisms.
6. Low-dose aspirin is recommended by some authorities to reduce the risk of thromboembolism, especially in teenagers and in steroid-resistant cases.

DISPOSITION

1. Most children with uncomplicated nephrotic syndrome can be managed as outpatients
   a. Patients' parents should perform daily urine protein analysis by dipstick and keep a log of results
   b. Close follow-up should be arranged with the primary care practitioner
2. Admission to the hospital may be indicated for:
   a. Anuria, severe oliguria, or significant azotemia

b. Severe, symptomatic hypertension
c. Massive edema (anasarca)
d. Peritonitis or other severe infection
e. Thrombosis

3. Antibiotic coverage should be provided as indicated

BIBLIOGRAPHY

Bagga A, Hari P, Srivastava RN: Prolonged versus standard prednisolone therapy for initial episode of nephrotic syndrome, *Pediatr Nephrol* 13:824, 1999.

Eddy AA, Schnaper HW: The nephrotic syndrome: from the simple to the complex, *Semin Nephrol* 18:304, 1998.

Hogg RJ, Portman RJ, Milliner D et al: Evaluation and management of proteinuria and nephrotic syndrome in children: recommendations from a pediatric nephrology panel established at the National Kidney Foundation conference on proteinuria, albuminuria, risk, assessment, detection, and elimination (PARADE), *Pediatrics* 105:1242, 2000.

Sakarcan A, Timmons C, Seikaly M: Reversible idiopathic acute renal failure in children with primary nephrotic syndrome, *J Pediatr* 125:723, 1994.

Tarshish P, Tobin JN, Bernstein J: Prognostic significance of the early course of minimal change nephrotic syndrome: report of the International Study of Kidney Diseases in Children, *J Am Soc Nephrol* 8:769, 1997.

Warshaw BL: Nephrotic syndrome in children, *Pediatr Ann* 23:495, 1994.

Acute Renal Failure

Acute renal failure (ARF) is defined as a sudden decrease in glomerular filtration rate (GFR), accompanied by accumulation of nitrogenous wastes, that occurs over a short period (hours to days). ARF may occur in response to three types of injury: prerenal (decreased perfusion of the kidney), intrarenal (damage to the kidney tissue itself), or postrenal (obstruction of the urinary tract). In addition to treating the complications of ARF, it is imperative to determine, if possible, the underlying cause.

ETIOLOGY

ARF may occur as a result of a wide variety of causes (Table 85-1).

DIAGNOSTIC FINDINGS (Table 85-2)

1. The history can provide some important clues regarding the potential cause of the renal failure:
   a. Patients with prerenal failure have a history of decreased perfusion of the kidney. This may include dehydration from vomiting, diarrhea, diabetic ketoacidosis, decreased intravascular volume as a result of nephrotic syndrome, burns, or shock resulting from hemorrhage, sepsis, cardiac failure, or anaphylaxis. The most common causes of ARF in children are prerenal.
   b. Intrarenal failure results from direct intrinsic nephron damage occurring in glomerulonephritis (hematuria, proteinuria, edema, and hypertension), in HUS (anemia, uremia, and thrombocytopenia), with nephrotoxins (aminoglycosides, radiocontrast material), in autoimmune diseases (systemic lupus erythematosus, sarcoidosis, lymphoma), with massive crush injuries, with vascular catastrophes (renal thrombosis or embolic phenomena), in overwhelming infection, or in DIC.
   c. Postrenal failure results from obstruction and is commonly seen in genitourinary (GU) malformations (posterior urethral valves, ureteropelvic junction obstruction) or in the presence of stone disease or abdominal masses. If the onset is acute, the failure may be accompanied by abdominal and flank pain.
2. Physical findings can reflect underlying renal and fluid abnormalities:
   a. Hypovolemia (tachycardia, hypotension or orthostatic changes).
   b. Volume overload (increased blood pressure, edema, CHF).
   c. Obstruction (increased kidney size or large bladder).

TABLE 85-1 Common Causes of Acute Renal Failure

Prerenal (Decreased Perfusion of an Intact Nephron)*	Intrarenal (Damage of the Actual Nephron)	Postrenal (Downstream Obstruction with Initially Intact Nephron)*
Shock: hypovolemic	Primary glomerular disease	Posterior urethral valves
Dehydration	Acute poststreptococcal nephritis	Ureteropelvic junction (if bilateral)
Hemorrhagic	Membranoproliferative glomerulonephritis	Stones (bilateral)
Diabetic ketoacidosis	Rapidly progressive glomerulonephritis	Crystals
Burn	Systemic disease	Sulfonamides
Shock: distributive	Henoch-Schönlein purpura	Uric acid
Septic	Hemolytic-uremic syndrome	Retroperitoneal fibrosis or tumor
Anaphylactic	Vasculitides	Trauma to collecting system
Shock: cardiogenic	Bacterial endocarditis	Ureterocele
Nephrotic syndrome with intravascular volume depletion from decreased oncotic pressure	Systemic lupus erythematosus	Acquired urethral obstruction
	Nephrotoxins	Abscess
	Antibiotics (aminoglycoside, methicillin)	Constipation
	Metals (gold, lead)	
	Antihypertensives (captopril)	
	Anticonvulsant (phenytoin)	
	Rhabdomyolysis (pigment damage to nephron)	
	Radiocontrast materials	
	Nonsteroidal antiinflammatory drugs (e.g., indomethacin, ibuprofen)	
	Organic solvent (carbon tetrachloride, methanol, toluene)	
	Vascular	
	Renal vein thrombosis	
	Renal artery thrombosis or embolism	
	Acute tubular necrosis (caused by prolonged decreased perfusion)	

* Prolonged obstruction or uncorrected hypoperfusion eventually leads to irreversible nephron damage.

   d. Abdominal or flank mass.
   e. Signs of systemic infection or autoimmune disease.
3. Patients may be oliguric (urine output less than 1 ml/kg/hr) or nonoliguric with a volume inappropriate to maintain hemostasis. Azotemia (increase in plasma concentration of nitrogenous waste products, i.e., BUN and creatinine) is present.

Complications

1. Fluid overload with CHF.
2. Hypertension caused by fluid overload or inappropriate renin production.
3. Azotemia with elevated potassium, BUN, and creatinine values.
4. Hyperkalemia resulting in dysrhythmias and myocardial dysfunction.

TABLE 85-2 Differential Diagnosis of Acute Renal Failure

Prerenal	Intrarenal	Postrenal
Ultrasound: normal	Ultrasound: can have increased renal density or slight swelling	Ultrasonography: dilated bladder or kidney
Serum BUN-to-creatinine ratio >15:1		History and examination may be diagnostic
Urine Na^+ <15 mEq/L	Urine Na^+ >20 mEq/L	Indexes not helpful
Urine osmolality >500 mOsm/kg H_2O	Urine osmolality <350 mOsm/kg H_2O	
Urine-to-plasma creatinine ratio >40:1	Urine-to-plasma creatinine ratio <20:1 (often <5:1)	
Fractional excretion of Na^+ <1 (<2.5 in neonates)	Fractional excretion of Na^+ > 2 (>2.5 in neonates)	
Urine sediment benign	Urine sediment "active" (casts, RBCs, WBCs, tubular cells)	Urine sediment benign

$$\text{Fractional excretion of Na}^+ = \frac{\text{Urine Na}^+ \text{ (mEq/L)}}{\text{Plasma Na}^+ \text{ (mEq/L)}} \times \frac{\text{Plasma creatinine (mg/dl)}}{\text{Urine creatinine (mg/dl)}}$$

5. Hypocalcemia and hyperphosphatemia, leading to cardiac dysrhythmias, tetany, and altered mental status.
6. Acidosis from diminished H^+ secretion by the kidney.
7. Altered level of consciousness, seizures, and coma from metabolic derangements (e.g., elevations of BUN and potassium and decrease of Ca^{++}), cerebral edema, and hypertension.
8. Bleeding resulting from platelet dysfunction associated with uremia.
9. Anemia resulting from decreased erythropoietin production by the kidney.
10. Infections are particularly common in patients with ARF.

Ancillary Data

1. Measurements of electrolytes, Ca^{++}, PO_4^{--}, BUN, and creatinine, CBC, and platelet count
2. UA with microscopic examination of urinary sediment
3. Urine sodium, creatinine, potassium, and osmolality determinations
4. Renal ultrasonography, including Doppler assessment of arterial and venous flow
5. Chest x-ray film (helpful in assessing volume status)
6. Electrocardiogram (ECG) and cardiac monitor
7. Computed tomography (CT) may be helpful for evaluating abdominal masses

DIFFERENTIAL DIAGNOSIS

Combining data from history, physical examination, and serum, urine, and radiologic studies is the best method of determining whether the failure is prerenal, intrarenal, or postrenal (see Table 85-2).

MANAGEMENT

Initial stabilization must focus on determining the cause and classification of the ARF to permit appropriate therapeutic intervention. The initial approach is outlined in Fig. 85-1. Intake and output must be closely monitored. A urinary catheter may be necessary. Monitoring of central venous pressure (CVP) is helpful in cases of abnormal volume status.

Fluid Balance

Furosemide. Furosemide (Lasix) is a potent diuretic, and its administration should be considered if the intravascular volume is adequate or overloaded according to CVP measurements.

1. Give 2 to 4 mg/kg/dose (higher dosages may be used if the creatinine is elevated).
2. If there is no response after two doses at maximum amount, no further doses should be given because of potential nephrotoxicity and ototoxicity.
3. Do not give if evidence of obstruction is present.
4. A good response to diuretics is the formation of 6 to 10 ml/kg of urine over the subsequent 1 to 3 hours.
5. If patient shows response to the initial dose of furosemide, consider starting a continuous infusion at 0.25 to 1.0 mg/kg/hr.

Administration of Fluids. In a patient who clearly has a prerenal form of ARF (because of dehydration, hemorrhage, etc.), fluid boluses should be administered to restore intravascular volume. This may help prevent the renal failure from progressing.

If the patient remains oliguric or anuric, fluids should be restricted to keep the patient euvolemic. Replace insensible losses with dextrose in water (estimated as one third of maintenance fluid requirements), urine losses with 0.45% normal saline (NS), and other fluid losses (vomitus, diarrhea) with lactated Ringer's solution (LR) or 0.45% NS. Intake and output fluids should be closely monitored, and electrolyte balance should be assessed periodically.

Caloric requirements and protein intake must be considered. In general, protein intake should be limited to slow the rise of BUN, and adequate calories should be given in the form of carbohydrates and fat to ensure an anabolic, rather than catabolic, state.

Dopamine. Low-dose infusion of dopamine (5 µg/kg/min) IV may increase renal blood flow and potentiate sodium excretion. However, recent data have not demonstrated a beneficial effect.

Dialysis. Rapid referral for dialysis is mandatory for patients with severe fluid overload or metabolic derangement and no response to the conservative measures already listed.

Hypertension (see Chapter 18)

Hypertension may be caused by fluid overload or high renin secretion. Any child with acute hypertension and a diastolic pressure greater than the 99th percentile for age should be treated. In the acute phase, parenteral administration of antihypertensive agents allows for titration of dosage to desired effect and minimizes the risk of aspiration in event of seizure or encephalopathy. In general, only a mild reduction in pressure is needed in an acute situation, perhaps down to the 90th to 95th percentile of blood pressure level for age.

Parenteral Therapy. Parenteral therapy should be given sequentially, with observation for a response:

1. Furosemide (Lasix), 1 mg/kg/dose q6hr IV, facilitates action of vasodilators by volume contraction. Will be helpful only in patients who have urine output.
2. Diazoxide (Hyperstat), 1 to 3 mg/kg/dose by rapid infusion; may be repeated q30-60min. It is a vasodilator, and fluid infusion reverses severe hypotension. Magnitude and duration of effect are unpredictable.
3. Nitroprusside (Nipride) may be used instead of diazoxide: Begin at 0.1 to 1 µg/kg/min IV infusion. This agent is a potent vasodilator, so its use requires constant monitoring. Nitroprusside provides the most exact method of controlling malignant hypertension because of its very short half-life. Buildup of thiocyanate (produced by breakdown of nitroprusside) limits the time that nitroprusside can be used to 48 to 72 hours.
4. Hydralazine may be used if a slower-acting, longer-duration vasodilator is preferred in place of diazoxide or nitroprusside: 0.1 to

0.2 mg (rarely up to 0.5 mg)/kg/dose q4-6hr IV or IM. Use in combination with diazoxide to potentiate effect.

5. Another good option is labetalol, 0.4 to 1.0 mg/kg/dose, which may be repeated up to a total of 3.0 mg/kg over first hour of treatment. Labetalol can also be given by constant infusion at a dose of 0.25 to 3.0 mg/kg/hr. Its use is contraindicated in patients with asthma.
6. Nicardipine is an IV calcium channel blocking agent that has been used in severe hypertension in both children and adults. It is given as a constant infusion at 1 to 3 μg/kg/min. Unlike nitroprusside, it can be given for prolonged periods.

The choice of medication depends on the urgency of treatment, a knowledge of the agents, and the availability of monitoring equipment. Vasodilators may eventually cause compensatory tachycardia, requiring the addition of a β-blocker such as propranolol (Inderal), 1 mg/kg/24 hr q6hr PO.

Hyperkalemia

Hyperkalemia results in excess membrane excitability and cardiac dysrhythmias. Potassium levels greater than 6.5 mEq/L are associated with ECG changes consisting of peaked T waves and widened QRS complex. Cardiac toxicity is enhanced by hypocalcemia, hyponatremia, or acidosis.

Treatment

1. Calcium is cardioprotective:
   a. Calcium chloride 10%, 20 (0.2 ml) mg/kg/dose (maximum 5 ml or 500 mg/dose), or calcium gluconate, 100 mg (1 ml)/kg/dose IV. Calcium chloride may cause bradycardia and should be given slowly over 5 to 10 minutes. It can also cause severe tissue necrosis if it extravasates.
   b. Calcium changes the cell's action potential and stabilizes the membrane, protecting the heart from dysrhythmias.
   c. Effects last approximately 30 minutes, and the dose may be repeated up to four times if necessary.
2. $NaHCO_3$ (moves K^+ intracellularly):
   a. $NaHCO_3$, 1 to 2 mEq/kg/dose IV.
   b. Useful in emergent situations as well as in combination with Kayexalate (see later). May be repeated every 2 to 4 hours or as required by pH.
   c. Exchanges H^+ for K^+, thereby moving potassium intracellularly and normalizing membrane potential.
3. Glucose and insulin (moves K^+ intracellularly):
   a. Glucose, 0.5 to 1.0 g/kg (2-4ml/kg D50W), followed by 1 unit of insulin for every 4 g of glucose infused, IV.
   b. May be repeated in 10 to 30 minutes.
   c. Monitor serum glucose with reagent strips (Dextrostix, Accu-Chek) carefully. The effect lasts 1 to 3 hours.
4. Kayexalate (ion exchange resin in GI tract):
   a. Kayexalate, 1 g/kg/dose mixed with 70% sorbitol PO (may use a nasogastric [NG] tube or administer per rectum [PR]).
   b. For newborns, give 1 g/kg/dose, with Kayexalate dissolved in 10% dextrose in water to make 25% solution.
   c. May be repeated every 4 to 6 hours.
   d. Useful in combination with $NaHCO_3$ for K^+ level less than 6.5 mEq/L.
   e. May cause hypocalcemia, hypomagnesemia, gastric irritation, and diarrhea.
5. Albuterol:
   a. Albuterol by continuous nebulization will lower serum K^+ by shifting it intracellularly and is readily available.
   b. Onset of effect is rapid, occurring within minutes, and will last 2 to 4 hours. Doses can be repeated until definitive treatment is available. The major adverse effect is tachycardia.

c. Albuterol is useful as an adjunctive measure, but administration of Kayexalate or dialysis is still required for definitive elimination of potassium.

Metabolic Acidosis

Give $NaHCO_3$, 1 to 2 mEq/kg/dose q6hr IV push, or as indicated by ABG values, exercising care to avoid fluid and sodium overload. If severe acidosis and fluid overload are present, rapid dialysis is required.

Hyponatremia

Hyponatremia is usually the result of excess free water. Water intake should be restricted to insensible loss plus replacement of losses as detailed previously.

Hyperphosphatemia

Calcium carbonate, calcium acetate, and aluminum hydroxide act to bind dietary phosphorus. Aluminum is potentially toxic, however, and should be used only for short-term therapy.

Dialysis (Peritoneal Dialysis or Hemodialysis)

Indications for dialysis are as follows:

1. Fluid overload refractory to medical management with CHF or hypertension
2. Severe hyperkalemia
3. Severe hyponatremia or hypernatremia
4. Unresponsive metabolic acidosis, particularly with fluid overload
5. BUN value higher than 80 to 100 mg/dl (although not an absolute indication)
6. Uremia producing alteration in consciousness or seizures

Technology has made dialysis possible for even the smallest infant. In the intensive care unit (ICU) setting, newer continuous renal replacement therapies (hemofiltration, hemodiafiltration) may be preferable because of the ability to give large volumes of parenteral nutrition and other fluids.

Other Considerations

Intravenous pyelograms and CT scans with IV contrast agents should not be performed in a patient with ARF because of the risk of nephrotoxicity from the dye. Ultrasonography and nuclear renal scans are preferable for initial evaluation.

DISPOSITION

All patients with ARF need hospitalization and consultation with a nephrologist.

BIBLIOGRAPHY

Alkhunaizi AM, Schrier RW: Management of acute renal failure: new perspectives, *Am J Kidney Dis* 28:315-28, 1996.

Druml W: Prognosis of acute renal failure, *Nephron* 53:8, 1996.

Flynn JT: Causes, management approaches, and outcome of acute renal failure in children, *Curr Opin Pediatr* 10:184, 1998.

Groshong T: Hypertensive crisis in children, *Pediatr Ann* 25:368, 1996.

Klahr S, Miller SB: Acute oliguria, *N Engl J Med* 338:671, 1998.

McClure RJ, Prasad VK, Brocklebank JT: Treatment of hyperkalemia using intravenous and nebulised salbutamol, *Arch Dis Child* 70:126, 1994.

Moghal NE, Brocklebank JT, Meadow SR: A review of acute renal failure in children: incidence, etiology and outcome, *Clin Nephrol* 49:91, 1998.

Peter JR, Steinhardt GF: Acute urinary retention in children, *Pediatr Emerg Care* 9:205, 1993.

San A, Selcuk Y, Tonbul Z, Soypacaci Z: Etiology and prognosis in 438 patients with acute renal failure, *Ren Fail* 118:593, 1996.

Thadhani R, Pascual M, Bonventre JV: Acute renal failure, *N Engl J Med* 334:1448, 1996.

Weiner ID, Wingo CS: Hyperkalemia: a potential silent killer, *J Am Soc Nephrol* 9:1535, 1998.

Urinary Tract Infection

Suzanne Z. Barkin

ALERT Symptoms often are nonspecific. Appropriate cultures, treatment, and follow-up observation are required.

Urinary tract infections (UTIs) range from being asymptomatic to causing systemic disease associated with pyelonephritis. Long-term sequelae include hypertension and chronic renal failure in some children with recurrent infections and vesicoureteral reflux.

ETIOLOGY: INFECTION

Bacteria causing most infections are normal rectal and perineal flora, including *E. coli* (90%), *Klebsiella* organisms, enteric streptococci, and, rarely, *S. aureus* or *Staphylococcus epidermidis*. Organisms gain entry into the GU tract by hematogenous spread in infants, whereas vesicoureteral reflux is the major risk factor in older children.

Uncommonly, viral, fungal, and mycobacterial agents are causative.

DIAGNOSTIC FINDINGS

Symptoms in younger children are often nonspecific. The diagnosis in this age group is particularly important because it may indicate the presence of vesicoureteral reflux or another anatomic abnormality that may predispose the child to recurrent infections. In addition, the risk of renal scarring is greatest in children younger than 1 year.

1. Neonates may have fever or hypothermia, irritability, poor feeding, failure to thrive, jaundice, sepsis, or cyanosis. In one study, a UTI was found in 7.5% of asymptomatic, afebrile infants with jaundice who were younger than 8 weeks. These infants were more likely to have onset of jaundice after 8 days of age.
2. Infants may experience vomiting, diarrhea, fever, irritability, and poor feeding.
3. Older children have the more classic signs and symptoms: fever, abdominal, suprapubic, back or costovertebral (CVA) pain, vomiting, enuresis, and urinary frequency, dysuria, and urgency.

Systemic toxicity accompanied by high temperatures, chills, and variably, CVA pain often accompanies upper urinary tract disease and pyelonephritis.

Historically, it is important to ascertain whether the patient has had previous episodes of infection. The physical examination should determine whether evidence of genitourinary malformations, hypertension, or poor growth exists.

Predisposing factors include poor perineal hygiene, the short urethra of females, infrequent voiding, and sexual activity. Circumcision may reduce the male's risk of UTI. Females have a higher incidence; the prevalence of UTIs in girls aged 2 months to 2 years is twice that of boys. Males with UTI have a higher incidence of anatomic abnormality. The risk of recurrence is greatest in the first month after a UTI and increases with repeated infections.

Complications

1. Chronic renal failure resulting from recurrent pyelonephritis or reflux nephropathy.
   a. Incidence of scarring is greatest in children younger than 1 year but can still be seen in older children.
   b. Scarring can be prevented by early detection and treatment of infection as well as detection of vesicoureteral reflux.
2. Bacteremia or sepsis. In infants up to 3 months of age, UTI is associated with a 30% incidence of sepsis.
3. Perinephric abscess.
4. Urolithiasis is uncommon but may follow infection. Findings include abdominal or flank pain, recurrent or persistent pyuria, and gross hematuria.

Ancillary Data

Urine Culture. Urine culture is the basis for making the diagnosis, and the quality of the specimen is an important determinant of the results. In asymptomatic or minimally ill patients in whom antibiotic therapy may be delayed until culture results are available, a clean-catch midstream specimen (CCMS) may be obtained after careful cleansing of the perineum and urethra. In patients who are toxic, specimens should be obtained by suprapubic aspiration (see Appendix A-7) or a straight catheterization, particularly in infants. In younger children, the catheterization may be done by using a 5-Fr sterile feeding tube. The first 5 ml of urine is discarded, and the remainder is sent for culture. Bag urine, which has a 70% contamination rate, is not satisfactory for adequate diagnosis.

1. The specimen must be plated for culture within 30 minutes or placed in a refrigerator. If not, the colony count may be elevated and is not reliable.
2. The interpretation of the culture result varies with the method of collection (Table 85-3). Cultures with uninterpretable results must be repeated after a reliable method has been used to collect another specimen. False-negative results may occur from dilution (e.g., specimen that is not the first morning void), improper culture medium, recent antimicrobial therapy, infection by fastidious organisms, bacteriostatic agent in urine, or complete obstruction of a ureter.

Urinalysis. UA is a useful diagnostic tool but its results are not definitive. They may be normal in infants with UTI. Dilute urine specimens can be particularly misleading.

1. Pyuria (the finding of more than 5 WBCs per high-power field [HPF]) is present in more than half of patients with UTI. It is often not present in neonates with UTIs.

TABLE 85-3 Culture Criteria for Diagnosis of UTI

	PROBABILITY OF INFECTION (BASED ON CFU/ML*)		
Collection-Method	Unlikely	Possible†	Likely
Suprapubic	0		Any
Catheterization	$<10^3$	10^3-10^4	$\geq 10^4$
CCMS	$<10^3$	10^4-10^5	$\geq 10^5$

CCMS, Clean-catch midstream; *CFU*, colony-forming units.
* Pure culture (single organisms).
† Patient symptomatic or if dilute urine sample.

2. Causes of pyuria besides UTI include chemical (bubble bath), physical (masturbation), or other types of irritation, dehydration, renal tuberculosis, trauma, acute glomerulonephritis, respiratory infections, appendicitis, other abdominal and pelvic infections, gastroenteritis, and administration of oral polio vaccine.
3. The presence of leukocyte esterase correlates with the presence of pyuria, which is often but not always present with UTI.
4. A positive nitrite test result implies that bacteria capable of fixing the nitrate normally found in urine have been present in the urine. A first morning urine is the optimal specimen.
5. Gram staining of urinary sediment is more reliable than dipstick methods of diagnosis and may be superior to the traditional UA. Identification of any organisms on Gram stain is particularly useful in predicting a UTI in children younger than 60 days with fever.

X-Ray Films. X-ray films are only rarely indicated on an emergent basis unless the patient is severely toxic or has evidence of obstruction. Children in whom radiologic evaluation is required after UTI include the following:

1. Infants younger than 3 months
2. Boys (increased likelihood of anomaly)
3. Clinical signs and symptoms consistent with pyelonephritis
4. Clinical evidence of renal disease (e.g., high blood pressure, BUN value, or creatinine level)
5. After the second documented lower tract UTI in girls; some authorities recommend that these patients should be studied after the first infection

The optimal approach to evaluation remains controversial. Ultrasonography should be performed in most settings after the first infection to evaluate renal size, evidence of hydronephrosis, and bladder abnormalities. In girls older than 3 months, evaluation may be delayed until a second documented infection occurs. The fluoroscopic voiding cystourethrogram (VCUG) is also an important screening test in children. It shows whether vesicoureteral reflux is present and if so, its severity (graded I to V) while permitting visualization of the urethra, with its potentially correctable lesions. Many clinicians are substituting a nuclear cystogram for a fluoroscopic VCUG in girls.

In the acute setting, normal renal ultrasonographic findings do not exclude the diagnosis of pyelonephritis. The most sensitive test for demonstration of renal parenchymal involvement is the nuclear DMSA renal scan.

Intravenous pyelograms (IVPs) are performed less commonly because the nuclear DMSA renal scan is a more sensitive indicator of renal scarring. The optimal use of DMSA scans, however, has yet to be determined.

Blood Cultures. Blood cultures are indicated in the febrile, toxic patient with a UTI.

Blood Creatinine and Urea Nitrogen Determinations. Blood creatinine and BUN should be measured in patients with evidence of pyelonephritis, recurrent infections, or hypertension.

DIFFERENTIAL DIAGNOSIS

1. Trauma: Chemical (bubble bath) or physical (masturbation or perineal injury) irritation, foreign body, and sexual abuse may cause discomfort.
2. Infection:
   - **a.** Viral, mycobacterial, and fungal agents may cause similar symptoms with associated pyuria. Culture techniques must be specific for these organisms.
   - **b.** Vaginitis may cause irritation with comparable symptoms. Vulvovaginitis is a common cause of dysuria, especially in school-aged girls.
   - **c.** Pinworms may cause perineal pain resulting from both inflammation and itching.
   - **d.** Urethritis caused by *Neisseria gonorrhoeae* or *Chlamydia trachomatis* is often associated with a discharge. It may cause dysuria, suprapubic discomfort, and, in the male, prostatic or rectal tenderness.
   - **e.** Appendicitis.
3. Nephrolithiasis.

MANAGEMENT

1. When UTI is suspected, an appropriate urine culture should be obtained. Suprapubic or catheterized specimens are indicated for moderately ill patients. A CCMS specimen for the minimally ill individual may be considered in patients who are not going to be treated until culture results are available; if results are abnormal, the culture should be repeated.
2. UA should be performed. If results are normal, urine should be sent for culture. If pyuria or bacteriuria is found, or the nitrite/leukocyte esterase is abnormal, the specimen should also be sent for culture, and the appropriate medication initiated. Urine sediment can also undergo Gram stain to assist in the diagnosis.
3. A lower urinary tract infection (cystitis) commonly has the associated urinary symptoms of urgency, frequency, and dysuria. Appropriate management is to push fluids initially and to treat with antibiotics for a minimum of 10 days:
   - Amoxicillin, 30-50 mg/kg/24 hr q8hr PO; *or*
   - Trimethoprim (TMP) with sulfamethoxazole (SMZ), 8 mg TMP and 40 mg SMZ/kg/24 hr q12hr PO; *or*
   - Cephalexin (Keflex), 25 to 100 mg/kg/24 hr q6hr PO; *or*
   - Nitrofurantoin (Macrodantin), 5 to 7 mg/kg/24 hr q6hr PO.
     - **a.** Final choice of antibiotics should reflect sensitivity and clinical response.
     - **b.** Duration of therapy should be 7 to 10 days, except in adolescent girls

with uncomplicated cystitis, in whom shorter regimens (1 to 3 days) may be adequate.

4. Pyelonephritis has associated systemic toxicity (temperature, chills, CVA tenderness) and must be treated with antibiotics that have broader coverage. Until culture and sensitivity testing results are available (24 to 48 hours), a combination of one of the drugs noted previously for lower tract infection with gentamicin or tobramycin, 5.0 to 7.5 mg/kg/24 hr q8-12hr IM or IV, should be given. For the patient with only moderate toxicity who is to be monitored as an outpatient, administration of gentamicin, 2.0 to 2.5 mg/kg/dose (maximum: 80 mg/dose), or ceftriaxone, 50 mg/kg/dose (maximum: 2.0 g/dose) IM once, in combination with continuing oral therapy, provides sufficient treatment until results of culture and sensitivity testing are known in 24 to 48 hours, although some clinicians suggest that oral therapy alone may be adequate. Cefixime (Suprax), 8 mg/kg/24 hr q12hr PO, is an excellent broad-spectrum antibiotic that may be useful in this setting. Patients who must be hospitalized should be treated with standard parenteral daily doses.
5. If urinary dysuria, urgency, or frequency is a predominant symptom, temporary relief can be obtained with phenazopyridine (Pyridium), a urinary tract analgesic, at 12 mg/kg/24 hr orally in three doses q8hr up to 200 mg/dose for 1 to 3 days. It turns the urine orange.
6. Follow-up evaluation in 48 hours should be ensured to determine that the patient is clinically improved and that the etiologic organism is sensitive to the medication. If there is any question, a second specimen for UA and culture should be obtained. Medication may have to be altered.
7. The patient should return in 14 days for another UA and culture after completing the 10-day course of antibiotics. Close follow-up observation over the next year is appropriate because of the higher risk of recurrence. The greater the number of previous episodes, the more likely the infection will recur. In the first year, the chance of recurrence is as high as 50%.

DISPOSITION

1. Patients who are toxic, younger than 3 months, pregnant, or immunocompromised; who are unable to maintain hydration or retain medications; or who have debilitating systemic disease should generally be hospitalized. In addition, those with previous renal disease associated with impaired function, obstruction, foreign bodies (catheter), or stones should be hospitalized. Other criteria that should be considered are the likelihood of resistant organisms, failure of previous outpatient therapy, previous pyelonephritis within 30 days, and the reliability of the patient.
2. Most patients may be monitored at home with appropriate antibiotic therapy. Compliance must be ensured, and follow-up evaluation in 1 to 2 days arranged.
3. High-risk patients should be evaluated radiologically (Table 85-4):
   a. If vesicoureteral reflux is present, the patient is typically kept on prophylactic antibiotic therapy (TMP/SMZ, 2 mg/kg/day of TMP given QHS) and a follow-up cystogram is obtained in 12 to 18 months. A urologist should usually be involved in the follow-up.
   b. Patients with recurrent UTI despite prophylaxis or with high-grade vesicoureteral reflux should be referred to a pediatric urologist.
4. If signs of renal damage are present (creatinine elevation, proteinuria, or hypertension), the patient should be referred to a pediatric nephrologist.

TABLE 85-4 Radiologic Evaluation of Children with Urinary Tract Infections

Age	Clinical Setting	IMAGING EVALUATION	
		Ultrasound	Voiding Cystourethrogram
Infant <3 mo	Any infection	Within 2-3 days	Within 1-2 wk
Girls 3 mo-adolescence	Afebrile cystitis	As above	After second episode
	Febrile infection	As above	After first episode up to age 6 yr
	Any infection	As above	Within 1-2 wk
Boys 3 mo-adolescence			
Adolescent girls	Cystitis	After second or third episode within 12-18 mo	If ultrasonogram abnormal or if voiding dysfunction present

Adapted from Hellerstein S: *Pediatr Clin North Am* 42:1433, 1995.

Parental Education

1. Give all of the medication. Call your physician if your child does not tolerate the medication.
2. A urine culture has been ordered. In 2 days you should contact your care provider to discuss whether the child is taking the correct medicine and feeling better.
3. Two weeks after your initial visit, your care giver will want to see the child again for another culture. Periodic checks will be made over the next year.
4. To help prevent repeat infections, particularly in girls, try the following:
   a. Teach your daughter to wipe correctly from front to back.
   b. Do not use bubble baths or let the soap float around in the bath.
   c. Treat constipation with mineral oil or a stool softener.
   d. Encourage frequent urination.
5. Call your physician if any of the following occurs:
   a. Fever or pain with urination is not gone in 48 hours after antibiotics have been started.
   b. The child feels worse or does not tolerate the medication.

BIBLIOGRAPHY

Benador D, Benador N, Slosaan DO et al: Cortical scintigraphy in the evaluation of renal parenchymal changes in children with pyelonephritis, *J Pediatr* 124:17, 1994.

Choi H, Snyder HM, Duckett JW: Urolithiasis in childhood: current management, *J Pediatr Surg* 22:158, 1987.

Dayan PS, Bennett J, Best R et al: Test characteristics of urine gram stain in infants ≤60 days of age with fever, *Pediatr Emerg Care* 18:12, 2002.

Dick PT, Feldman W: Routine diagnostic imaging for childhood urinary tract infection: a systematic overview, *J Pediatr* 128:15, 1996.

Garcia FJ, Nager AL: Jaundice as an early diagnostic sign of urinary tract infection in infancy, *Pediatrics* 109:846, 2002.

Hellerstein S: Urinary tract infections, *Pediatr Clin North Am* 42:1433, 1995.

Hoberman A, Chao HP, Keller DM et al: Prevalence of urinary tract infection in febrile infants, *J Pediatr* 123:17, 1993.

Hoberman A, Wald ER, Hickey RJ et al: Oral versus initial intravenous therapy for urinary tract infections in young febrile children, *Pediatrics* 104:79, 1999.

Lockhart GR, Lewander WJ, Cimini DM: Use of urinary gram stain for detection of urinary tract infection in infants, *Ann Emerg Med* 25:31, 1995.

Lohr JA: The foreskin and urinary tract infections, *J Pediatr* 114:502, 1989.

Mahant S, To T, Friedman J: Timing of voiding cystourethrogram in the investigation of urinary tract infections in children, *J Pediatr* 139:568, 2000.

Majad M, Rushton HG: Renal cortical scintigraphy in the diagnosis of acute pyelonephritis, *Semin Nucl Med* 22:98, 1992.

Pollack CV, Pollack ES, Andrew ME: Suprapubic bladder aspiration versus urethral catheterization in ill infants: success, efficiency and complication rates, *Ann Emerg Med* 23:224, 1994.

Smeilie JM, Jodal U, Lax H: Outcome of 10 years of severe vesicoureteral reflux managed medically, *J Pediatr* 139:656, 2001.

A Procedures

Several procedures are unique to the pediatric patient. Others are rarely performed and require some familiarity with the crucial landmarks. The descriptions included in this section are meant not to be inclusive but to serve as reminders of important aspects of techniques to those individuals who have had experience performing them in a supervised setting that included direct observation and instruction. This section is not intended to be a training manual for practitioners who do not have previous experience in invasive procedures. Informed consent should be obtained from a parent or guardian after appropriate discussion when appropriate but should not delay lifesaving procedures in unstable patients.

Preparing a child for a procedure may facilitate the process and must be related to the child's age, developmental status, and ability to understand. Initially, determine what the parents know about the procedure and what they have told the child. Encourage the child to ask questions while presenting information in small amounts. Describe the procedure in terms of what the child will feel, taste, see, or smell, while making the child as comfortable as possible. Appeal to older toddlers (2 to 4 years), who desire to please, by encouraging them to help, assist with the Band-Aid, or make choices when appropriate.

Appendix A-1: Arterial Punctures

Arterial punctures are used routinely to obtain heparinized blood for arterial blood gas (ABG) determinations. Most laboratories can make the determination with less than 1 ml of heparinized blood. A tuberculin syringe is filled with heparin that is then squirted out, allowing a small amount to remain in the hub. A 25-gauge needle is used in newborns and infants. The site is identified and prepared before puncture. After withdrawal of the needle, pressure should be applied to the site for at least 5 minutes.

1. The radial artery is the preferred site because of its stability and lack of an accompanying vein. It is entered tangentially (Fig. A-1).
2. The posterior tibial artery, located between the medial malleolus and the Achilles tendon.
3. The femoral artery should be used only in life-threatening situations. A useful mnemonic is NAVL (nerve, artery, vein, lymph node).

Appendix A-2: Arthrocentesis

Arthrocentesis is essential in excluding infection in a joint that is acutely swollen or painful or that has limited range of motion.

SITE AND POSITION

Knee

The patient is placed on the back with the knee fully extended. The needle (18-gauge) is passed laterally or medially beneath the midpoint of the patella so that it enters the knee joint midway between the patella and the patellar grove of the femur.

Ankle

The ankle is approached either medially or laterally, reflecting the area of maximal swelling. For those with lateral swelling, the foot is

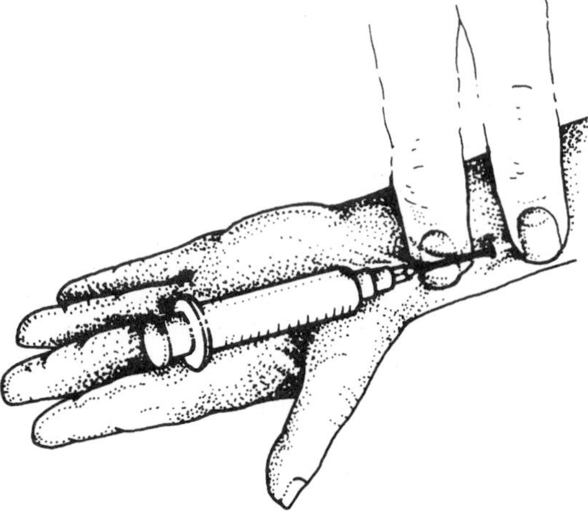

Fig. A-1 Localization of radial artery for puncture.

placed in neutral position, and a 20- to 22-gauge needle is inserted horizontally 1 cm both medial and inferior to the tip of the lateral malleolus. Medial swelling also requires the foot to be in a neutral position, and the 20- to 22-gauge needle is directed horizontally just above and lateral to the medial malleolus, medial to the extensor hallucis longus tendon.

Elbow

Lateral aspiration is done by positioning the elbow joint at a 90-degree angle. The needle (20- to 22-gauge) is inserted perpendicularly, below the lateral epicondyle and above the olecranon process.

Hip

Arthrocentesis of the hip is usually performed by an orthopedic consultant.

PROCEDURE

Aseptic technique is essential. The area should be shaved (if necessary), and the skin prepared with a povidone-iodine (Betadine) scrub, followed by cleansing with an alcohol scrub. The procedure is not routinely done in the presence of overlying cellulitis or a coagulation disorder.

Anesthetic agents (1% to 2% lidocaine) are infiltrated into the skin with a 23- to 25-gauge needle. A new bottle of anesthetic agent should be used to ensure sterility.

A large 18-gauge needle normally should be attached to a 5- to 10-ml syringe for aspiration of large joints (20- to 22-gauge for smaller joints). If large amounts of fluid are anticipated, the syringe may be connected to a stopcock, and a larger syringe attached once free flow is established. Negative pressure is usually maintained.

COMPLICATIONS

Bleeding within the joint or in the subperiosteum may occur, as may infection. Strict aseptic technique must be maintained.

FLUID ANALYSIS (see Table 82-1)

Fluid obtained by arthrocentesis should always be analyzed completely. This analysis should include the following:

1. Cell count
2. Gram stain and culture, for both aerobic and anaerobic organisms
3. Protein and glucose measurements
4. Examination for crystals (monosodium urate or calcium pyrophosphate dihydrate)
5. Mucin clot test

Appendix A-3: Venous Infusion

Obtaining venous access in the pediatric patient requires familiarity with potential sites and techniques as well as expertise and patience. The choice of technique may require modification because of the nature of the injury or illness and the patient's condition, size, and fluid requirements.

PERIPHERAL VEIN PERCUTANEOUS PUNCTURE

Site

Peripherally, the preferred sites are the antecubital vein, veins on the dorsa of the hand and foot, and, in the child younger than 2 years, the scalp. The external jugular (p. 843) or femoral vein also may be used.

Position

1. The patient is immobilized to the extent necessary. For smaller children a papoose board may be useful.
2. Extremities require careful immobilization with tape (Fig. A-3, *A*). Hands may be better positioned if a small amount of cotton or gauze is placed under the wrist when using veins on the dorsum of the hand.

Preparation

1. Cleanse the area to be entered.
2. Shave the area if necessary (e.g., the head).

Tourniquet

1. Apply a tourniquet proximal to the point of venous access.
2. On the head, a rubber band may serve as the tourniquet. Place a small amount of tape at one point on the rubber band to facilitate removal of the rubber band (Fig. A-3, *B*).

Needles and Cannulas. The choice is made on the basis of personal preference.

1. *Scalp vein needle.* May be used in all areas except for veins overlying joints. The inherent problem is the lack of true stability of the needle after it is inserted.
   a. Before inserting the needle, flush with saline solution, leaving the syringe attached until the skin is punctured. Once the skin is entered, remove the syringe to permit a flashback to appear on entering the vein.
   b. Insert the needle tangentially through the skin approximately 1 cm distal to the point of vein entry. Grasp the needle by the winged tabs. Advance the needle gently until the vein is entered and a flashback is visible. Unless the vein is large, do not thread the needle further.

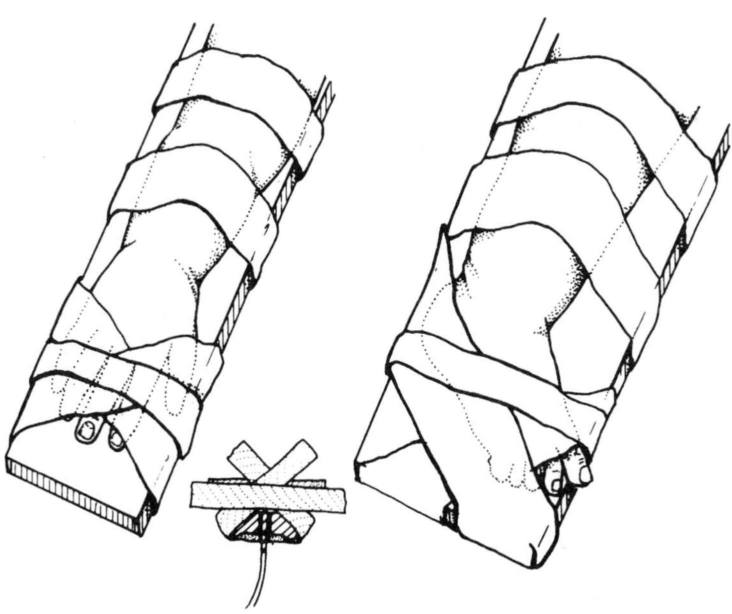

Fig. A-3 **A,** Immobilization of extremity for percutaneous venous puncture. Scalp vein needle taping.

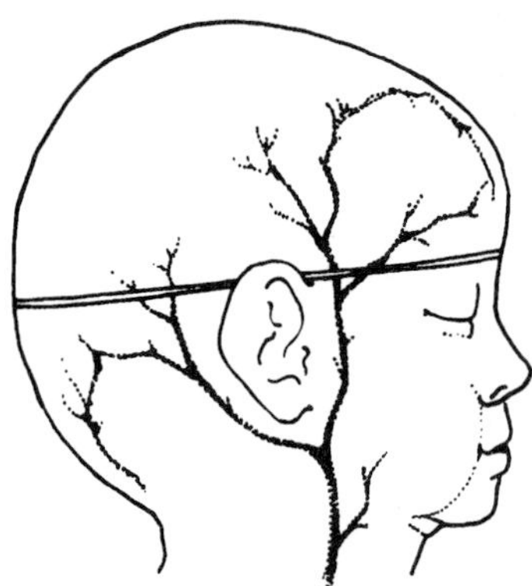

Fig. A-3 B, Location of scalp veins. Rubber band used for tourniquet.

   c. Place a 1-cm-wide tape over the needle at the point of entry to provide initial stabilization, and loop a second piece around the winged tabs.
   d. Intermittently flush the needle to ensure patency and position.
   e. Tape the needle carefully to minimize movement. Placement of a half medicine cup with the edges taped over the point of insertion and needle provides additional protection.
2. *Over-the-needle catheter.* Inserted according to manufacturer's directions. Remember that once a flashback is noted in the over-the-needle catheter, the needle should be inserted 1 to 3 mm more to ensure that it is well into the vein before an attempt is made to advance the catheter.

Intravenous Infusion. An intravenous (IV) infusion set should be attached after the patient is stabilized. In children younger than 5 years, there should always be a volume-limiting device such as a Buretrol in line to prevent excessive fluid administration.

VENOUS CUTDOWN

Site

The greater saphenous vein is located anterior to the medial malleolus and medial to the anterior tibial tendon.

Position

The foot is immobilized with careful visualization of the malleolus.

Procedure

1. After cleansing, draping, and infiltrating locally with 1% lidocaine, apply a tourniquet.
2. Make a 1-cm transverse incision perpendicular to the vein, usually one fingerbreadth above and one fingerbreadth anterior to the medial malleolus.
3. Bluntly dissect down to the tibia in the direction parallel to the vein, and identify the vein. Free the vein, and place two 3-0 Vicryl or silk sutures loosely around it:
   a. The distal suture is ligated to control venous return.
   b. The proximal suture is tied after the venous catheter has been placed. At this time it is left loose.
4. Some clinicians have recommended a more rapid approach:
   a. An incision from the posterior border of the malleolus is extended anteriorly to the "shin" or the anterior border of the tibia.
   b. A curved, closed hemostat pointing downward is scraped along the tibia from the anterior to the posterior aspect of the incision.
   c. All tissue is picked up and the hemostat is turned upward and opened.
   d. The saphenous vein is identified.
5. Another approach involves identification and isolation of the vein and subsequent cannulation using a guidewire technique.

Catheterization

1. Select the appropriate size catheter. Using the proximal suture for traction, make a small flap incision in the anterior third of the vein with a No. 11 scalpel blade. The vein can also be cannulated by direct puncture, which does not require ligation.

2. Insert the catheter with traction from the proximal tie while elevating the vein flap. Remove the tourniquet and ensure that there is free flow.
3. Secure the catheter by tightening the proximal tie. Flush the vein with 1 to 2 ml of 1% lidocaine to overcome venous spasm, if necessary. Begin the IV infusion.

Closure

1. Close the wound with 4-0 Vicryl or Dexon sutures (some prefer silk or nylon), and further secure the catheter with extensive taping.
2. Cover with sterile dressing.

EXTERNAL JUGULAR VEIN

Site

The external jugular vein is easily accessible in children whose necks are not unduly short or obese. The vein courses from the angle of the mandible to the middle of the clavicle over the sternocleidomastoid muscle. The vein may be used for venipuncture as well as to establish peripheral or central venous access.

Position

The child is restrained in a supine position on a firm table. The head is rotated to the side away from the procedure and held off the edge of the table with the shoulders firmly touching the table (Fig. A-3, *C*).

Although the vein may be visible without additional measures, distension may be increased by placing the child in modified Trendelenburg's position, by having the child cry, or by occluding the vein with a finger on the clavicle.

Catheterization

After the area is prepared and draped, the catheter is inserted.

1. If peripheral access is desired, the largest catheter that is easily inserted should be used.

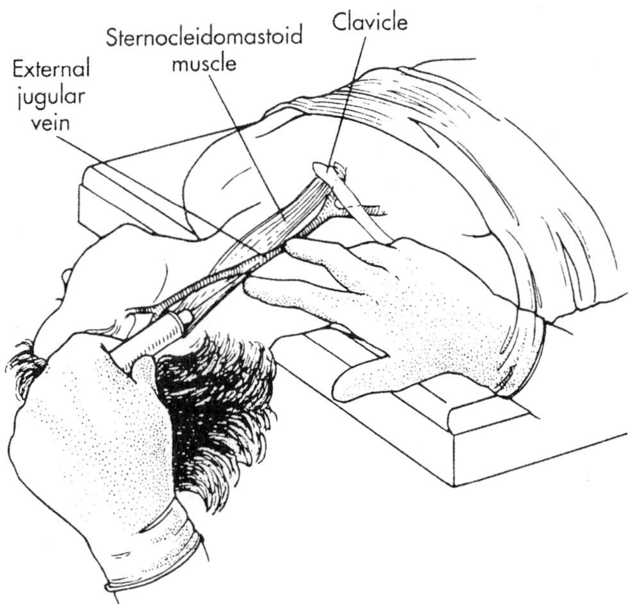

Fig. A-3 **C,** Percutaneous external jugular vein puncture.

(From Barkin RM: *Pediatric emergency medicine*, ed 2, St Louis, 1997, Mosby.)

2. If central access is desired, a guide-wire technique normally is used, as described on p. 845.
3. The IV infusion is attached, and the catheter secured.

INTRAOSSEOUS (IO) INFUSIONS

Bone marrow infusion provides a route to venous access when conventional routes are unavailable. The intramedullary vessels are supported by bone architecture and therefore accessible in children because the tibial marrow is still actively producing red blood cells. The data would suggest that the IO approach may be used in most age groups. This allows access into the sinusoids and ultimately the large medullary venous channels (Fig. A-3, *D*).

The technique is useful in life-threatening conditions requiring immediate venous access on a temporary basis for infusion of crystalloids and drugs. Besides fluids, numerous pharmacologic agents, including diazepam, inotropic agents, sodium bicarbonate, lidocaine, antibiotics, and insulin, have been administered without complications. The safety of infusion of hypertonic and strongly alkaline solutions has not been fully established on a long-term basis.

Bone marrow aspirate may be useful for laboratory studies such as blood culture and electrolyte determinations.

Position

The patient is immobilized in the supine position. It is often useful to position a small sandbag under the leg, immediately behind the operative site. Restrain the leg.

Needle

Special intraosseous needles are available and are the optimal devices because of ease of use and the band that facilitates immobilization. Other options are an 18- to 20-gauge spinal needle with stylet or a small 15- to 18-gauge bone marrow trephine needle.

Procedure (Fig. A-3, *E*)

1. Strict aseptic technique must be maintained.
2. Local infiltration with lidocaine is desirable but is often precluded by the emergent nature of the procedure and the depressed sensorium of the patient.
3. The needle is inserted perpendicular to the skin or at a 45- to 60-degree angle away from the epiphyseal plate. The proximal tibia or distal femur is preferred. If the tibia is used, a site two to three fingerbreadths below the tibial tuberosity is selected. A screwing motion is used to push the needle through the cortex.
4. The needle is in the marrow when there is a lack of resistance after the needle passes through the cortex and stands upright

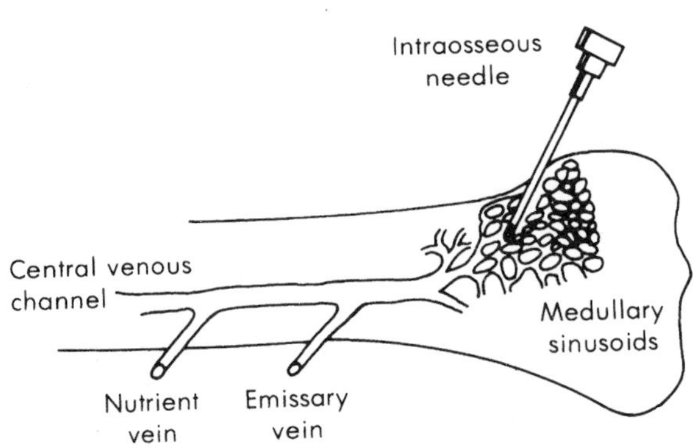

Fig. A-3 **D**, Venous drainage from marrow of long bone with intramedullary needle in place.

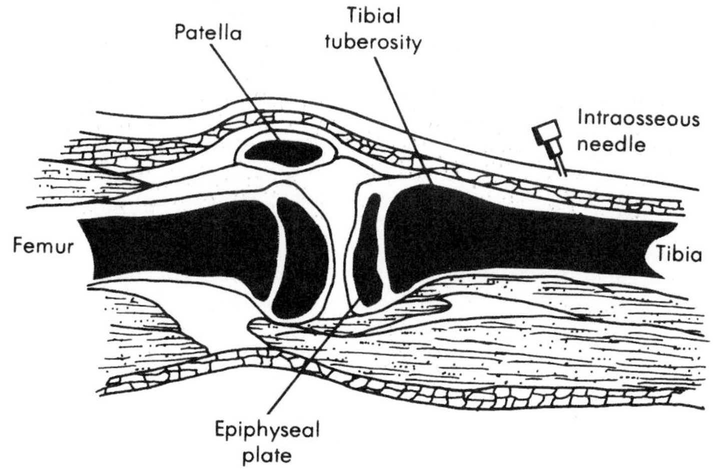

Fig. A-3 **E,** Intraosseous insertion of needle.

without support. Bone marrow is aspirated by the syringe, and the infusion flows smoothly. Once the needle is inserted, a member of the team should be assigned to protect the IO site.

Complications

The procedure is meant as a temporizing measure and should be replaced once stable access is achieved. Complications may include the following:

1. Osteomyelitis or abscess, usually from prolonged insertion.
2. Leakage around the needle, with compartment syndrome. If the needle comes out, it is difficult to insert in the same leg because of the leakage problem from a second puncture.
3. Potential injury to the bone marrow cavity.
4. Fat and bone marrow emboli.
5. Tibial fracture.
6. No impairment of bone growth has been observed.

CENTRAL VENOUS ACCESS

Obtaining central venous access involves the subclavian or internal jugular veins. The femoral vein also may be used and is preferred by many. Central venous access provides venous access as well as measurement of central venous pressure.

Position

The patient is immobilized in Trendelenburg's position (15 to 20 degrees) if condition permits, head turned away from the site of puncture.

Site and Needle

The site is cleansed with povidone-iodine (Betadine), infiltrated with 1% lidocaine, and draped if time permits.

Needles, catheters, and guidewires are available as disposable kits from a variety of companies and are generally complete with catheters, guidewires, and needles. (Fig. A-3, *A*, and A-3, *B*, and Table A-3, A).

Internal Jugular Vein. The vein runs posterior to the sternocleidomastoid muscle between its two heads and behind the anterior portion of the clavicular head as it courses to meet the subclavian vein just above the medial end of the clavicle.

For the central or middle approach:

1. Landmarks are the triangle created by the sternal and clavicular heads of the sternocleidomastoid muscle and the clavicle at

TABLE A-3, A Approximate Conversion of French Size to Gauge to mm

French Size	Gauge	mm
1	29	0.33
2	23/22	0.66
3	20/19	1.00
4	18/17	1.35
5	16/15	1.68
6	15/14	2.00

the base. The internal jugular vein is just behind the medial border of the clavicular head. The carotid artery is just medial to it.

2. The needle is inserted at the apex of the triangle at a 45-degree angle and aimed caudal and toward the ipsilateral nipple. The needle is inserted only 1 to 2 cm, and blood should be free-flowing. If the vein is not entered, the needle is withdrawn and redirected slightly more laterally (Fig. A-3, *F*).
3. Once the vein is entered, the needle is left in place while the attached syringe is removed. The guidewire is then inserted through the needle.
4. The needle is then removed over the guidewire. A small cut is made at the point of skin entry, and the catheter is inserted according to the manufacturer's directions.

Subclavian Vein. The vein crosses over the first rib and passes in front of the anterior scalene muscle and continues behind the medial third of the clavicle, where it unites with the internal jugular vein to form the innominate vein.

1. Estimate the length of the catheter needed by measuring from the site of insertion to the sternomanubrial angle.
2. Insert the needle infraclavicularly at the juncture of the middle and medial thirds of the clavicle parallel to the frontal plane. Direct it medially and slightly cephalad behind the clavicle toward the sternal notch.

   NOTE: It is often useful to place a finger in the suprasternal notch for reference (Fig. A-3, *G*).
3. Insert the needle with the bevel upward. Once the lumen of the vessel is entered, rotate it so that the bevel is directed caudally.
4. Attach the needle to a syringe and insert under negative pressure until a free flow of blood back into the syringe is achieved. The syringe is then removed and a thumb placed over the needle hub to prevent air embolization.
5. A supraclavicular approach is preferred by some clinicians. The site of insertion is the angle and junction formed by the lateral border of the sternocleidomastoid muscle and the clavicle. The needle is inserted behind the sternocleidomastoid

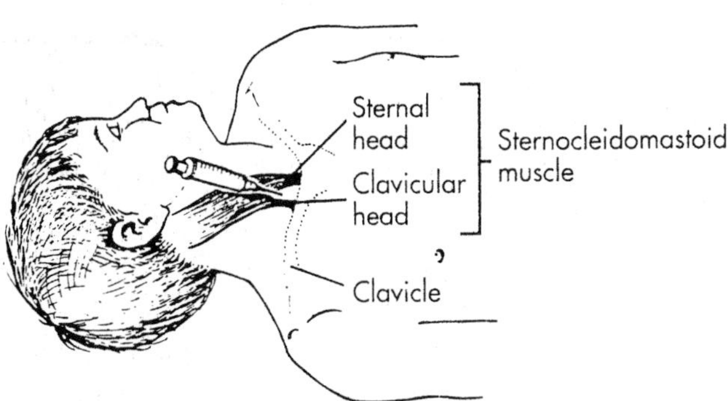

Fig. A-3 **F,** Percutaneous internal jugular vein insertion.

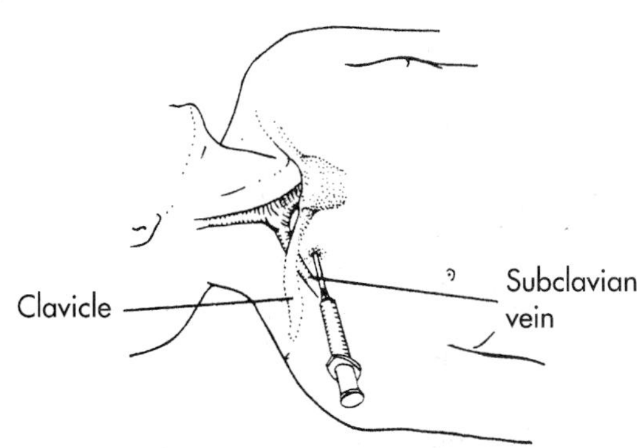

Fig. A-3 G, Subclavian vein puncture.

muscle and clavicle at an angle bisecting the angle formed by the landmarks and directed toward the contralateral nipple. The needle is advanced with the barrel of the syringe 5 to 10 degrees below the horizontal plane. The vein is entered 0.5 to 4.0 cm of depth. If unsuccessful, elevate the syringe 5 degrees above the horizontal plane.

Femoral Vein. The femoral vein may be cannulated by locating the femoral pulse and inserting a needle 2 cm distal to the inguinal ligament and 0.5 cm medial. The remainder of the approach using a guidewire is similar to other routes.

The Cannula

The *cannula* type determines the next step.

1. If the *catheter-through-the needle* technique is used, the catheter is slipped through the needle the appropriate distance and the needle is slid off the cannula once the cannula is in place. The catheter is never withdrawn through the needle because of the risk of shearing it.
2. If a *guidewire* is used, a wire guide is inserted through the needle and the needle is withdrawn. The dilator and overlying catheter are then fed over the wire and, once the catheter is in place, the wire and dilator are removed.

Procedure

1. The IV infusion is attached with an inline manometer to measure central venous pressure (CVP).
2. The catheter is secured with a suture through the skin and wrapped around the catheter. A sterile dressing is applied.
3. CVP is determined.

Cautions

1. A bright-red blood return indicates that an artery has been punctured. Remove the needle and apply pressure for a minimum of 10 minutes.
2. If unable to advance the catheter, remove the needle and catheter together. Never withdraw the cannula through the needle.
3. The right side usually is preferred, because the dome of the lung is lower on the right, it is a more direct path to the right atrium, and there is a smaller thoracic duct on the right.
   a. If there is pulmonary injury, such as a pneumothorax or major pulmonary contusion and a central line is to be placed for monitoring, place the central catheter on the side of the injury.
   b. If there is potential vascular injury to the subclavian, internal jugular, or innominate veins, place the catheter on the other side.
4. After insertion, chest x-ray films (anteroposterior [AP] or posteroanterior [PA] and lateral) should be obtained to define placement as well as to exclude immediate complications.

   NOTE: Many believe that the external jugular is the safest approach, followed by the internal jugular technique.

Complications

Complications include pneumothorax, hemothorax, hydrothorax, air or catheter embolization, and brachial plexus injury. Preparations always should be made to treat them. Cervical hematomas are common, and although bleeding is usually trivial, it can occlude the airway. A common error, if a pneumothorax occurs, is to try to reverse it with too small an intrathoracic catheter. A thoracostomy should be performed with underwater drainage and, at times, additional suction.

UMBILICAL ARTERY AND VEIN

Access via the umbilical artery and vein is useful in the newborn (see Chapter 9).

Appendix A-4: Lumbar Puncture

Lumbar punctures (LPs) are commonly performed to exclude central nervous system (CNS) infection. It is important to exclude potential increased intracranial pressure on the basis of history and physical examination before performing the LP. If there is any question, computed tomography (CT) should be obtained before the LP.

POSITION

The patient's position is crucial. The patient should be placed at the edge of a firm examination table and maintained in a position with the neck flexed and the knee drawn upward (fetal position). The key to performing an LP is to properly position the child (Fig. A-4).

1. The shoulders and back of the patient should be perpendicular to the table.
2. An alternative position for the small infant is to have the patient sitting, flexing the thighs up to the abdomen. This is recommended only if the holder and clinician are experienced with this approach.
3. In the preterm infant, the optimal position is either the lateral recumbent one with the hips flexed and partial neck extension or the upright position. Full flexion of the neck may cause hypoventilation.

PROCEDURE

1. The patient's back is cleansed with a surgical solution—using povidone-iodine (Betadine)—and then draped. Steri-drapes are particularly useful, because they are adherent and do not obscure the landmarks.
2. Meticulous sterile technique is used.
3. Local anesthetic is used for children above 5 years of age who will cooperate more easily if the pain is minimized.

Site

The puncture is at the intersection of the line joining the superior portion of the iliac crest

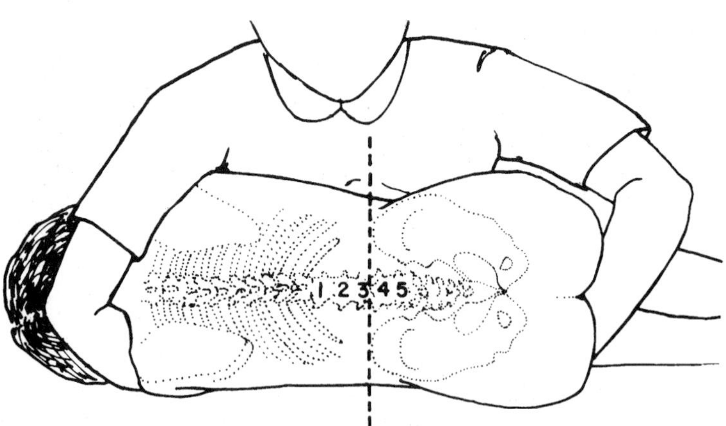

Fig. A-4 Position for lumbar puncture.

with the spine. This point is the spinous process of L4. The needle is optimally inserted at L3-L4 but may be inserted one space above or below.

Spinal Needle

This is a 22-gauge, 1-inch needle for children younger than 5 years; a longer needle is used in older children and adults.

Insertion

The needle is inserted into the designated spot with the stylet in place.

1. The needle should be inserted perpendicular to the back and aimed toward the umbilicus.
2. In the younger child it is advisable to puncture the skin and allow the child to calm down and then to reassess the position before proceeding.
3. Lumbar puncture in younger children does not demonstrate the increasing resistance and "pop" noted in older children. It is advisable to frequently remove the stylet and examine the needle hub for fluid as the needle with stylet is advanced.

Manometry

This can be performed in cooperative children older than 5 years when it is important. A three-way stopcock and manometer are attached to the spinal needle, and the pressure determined. Normal relaxed pressure is 5 to 15 cm H_2O.

Fluid Analysis (see Table 81-3)

Analysis of the cerebrospinal fluid (CSF) must be done expeditiously.

1. Tube No. 1: culture and Gram stain. If Gram stain result is negative: methylene blue. Cultures beyond routine bacterial ones should be specified.
2. Tube No. 2: protein and glucose measurements. (Serum glucose level should be obtained before performing the LP.)
3. Tube No. 3: cell count. If bloody, it may be desirable to compare tube No. 1 and tube No. 3 cell counts to determine whether the tap was traumatic.
4. A fourth tube may be collected for additional studies such as viral cultures.
5. The CSF pressure can be estimated (cm H_2O) by counting the number of drops in a specified counting period (seconds). Child must be relaxed and not crying.

Needle (gauge)	Length (in)	Counting Period (sec)
22	1.5	21
22	3.5	39
20	3.5	12

6. Analysis is outlined in detail in Table 81-3, p. 744.

COMPLICATIONS

1. Cardiac respiratory arrest may result from the child being held too tightly, with subsequent respiratory arrest and impaired venous return. Children must be observed closely to prevent this problem.
2. Infection may occur as a result of introduction of pathogens during the procedure. Controversy exists as to the risk of performing an LP in the child with bacteremia. The risk is not substantiated, and this question should not serve to inhibit clinicians from performing necessary studies.
3. Herniation through the foramen magnum may occur because of antecedent increased intracranial pressure. If increased pressure is noted at the time of the procedures, only a small amount of fluid should be withdrawn, and the needle quickly removed. The patient obviously needs immediate evaluation and treatment. Optimally an LP is avoided in such patients.
4. Headaches are more common in adults.
5. Intraspinal dermoids are avoided by using only needles with stylets.
6. Penetration of a nerve causes pain. In this case the needle is withdrawn and redirected.

7. Spinal cord hematoma occurs, particularly in patients with thrombocytopenia or coagulation defects.

Appendix A-5: Pericardiocentesis

Fluid collection in the pericardial sac, whether it results from effusion, infection, or hemorrhage, may be removed in the acute situation for both diagnostic and therapeutic reasons by pericardiocentesis. An ultrasonogram or echocardiogram may be an important diagnostic tool in the stable patient to establish the presence of an effusion. After this life-saving procedure, definitive surgical care is immediately indicated.

POSITION

The patient is supine, leaning backward at a 45-degree angle, supported by the bed or pillows (reverse Trendelenburg position).

SITE

The left subxiphoid is used, with the needle aimed cephalad and backward toward the tip of the left scapula (Fig. A-5). Some clinicians recommend aiming the needle toward the right scapula.

NEEDLE

An 18- or 20-gauge metal spinal needle (3-inch) is attached to a three-way stopcock and 20-ml syringe. One end of an alligator clip is attached to the needle's base and the other end to the V lead on an electrocardiogram (ECG). (Limb leads should be attached as usual.)

PROCEDURE

1. After preparation, cleansing, and draping of the patient, the needle is inserted slowly under negative pressure through the puncture site, penetrating the diaphragm. As the pericardium is entered, there is a distinct "pop." A current of injury with ST-T wave changes will be noted if the epicardium is entered, and the needle should be withdrawn slightly.
2. Aspiration is performed. As little as 2 ml may be temporarily effective at relieving tamponade and improving cardiac output.
3. Vital signs should be monitored throughout the procedure.

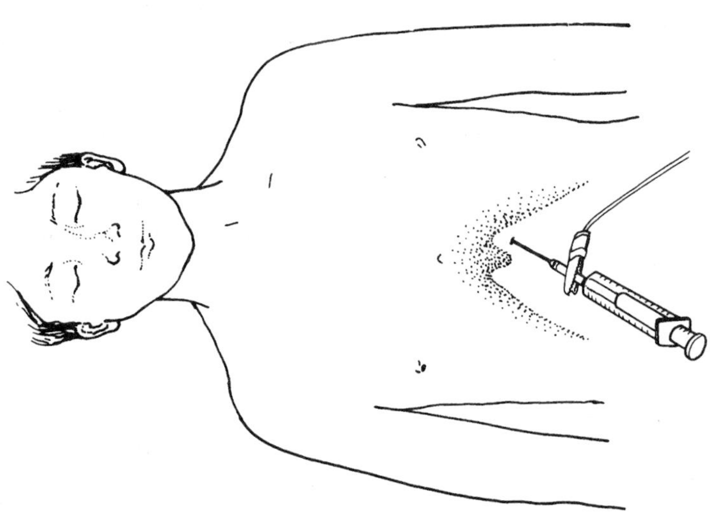

Fig. A-5 Position of needle for pericardiocentesis.

4. Ultrasonography may facilitate this procedure.

COMPLICATIONS

1. Pneumothorax.
2. Coronary artery injury or myocardial laceration.
3. Dysrhythmias.
4. Bleeding. In the stable patient, prothrombin time (PT), partial thromboplastin time (PTT), and platelet count may be obtained before the procedure.

Appendix A-6: Subdural Tap

The subdural space is a noncommunicating space between the dura mater and the arachnoid membrane. Although a CT scan can delineate the presence of fluid in the subdural space, the tap is performed to define the nature of the collection—hematoma, effusion, or empyema. This is commonly done in conjunction with a neurosurgeon.

SITE

The *puncture site* is the lateral corner of the anterior fontanelle or farther lateral along the suture. Optimally, this is at least 5 cm from the midline or 1 to 2 cm lateral to the edge of the anterior fontanelle, which is generally "open" until 12 months of age (Fig. A-6).

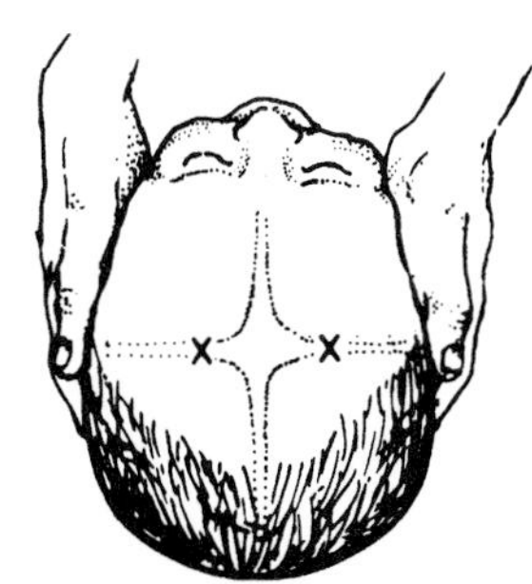

Fig. A-6 Puncture site for subdural tap.

POSITION

The patient is in the supine position with the head at the edge of an examining table. An assistant should immobilize the patient with the help of a papoose board, other device, or sedation.

NEEDLE

A *subdural needle* (short bevel) is used. If one is unavailable, a short spinal needle with a short bevel may be substituted. It is often advisable with this needle to place a hemostat on the needle at the point of entry to prevent excessive penetration.

PROCEDURE

1. The anterior two thirds of the scalp are shaved and surgically scrubbed with povidone-iodine solution (Betadine). Meticulous surgical technique is essential. The needle is inserted slowly at a right angle to the skin surface with total finger control. It is advanced slowly with the stylet in place until there is a sudden decrease in resistance, usually associated with a "pop," representing penetration of the dura.
2. The stylet is removed, and up to 15 to 20 ml of fluid is allowed to drain by gravity, avoiding aspiration. Normally, there are only a few drops in this space. Sometimes none is obtained.
3. In most cases, the procedure is repeated on the other side.
4. If excessive fluid is present or reaccumulates, repeat taps may be necessary over a period of time. A neurosurgeon should be consulted.

ANALYSIS OF THE FLUID

This analysis should parallel the studies performed on specimens obtained by LP: culture, Gram stain, glucose and protein measurements, and cell count (p. 744). A subdural effusion is usually associated with grossly xanthochromic or bloody fluid.

COMPLICATIONS

1. Infection resulting from introduction of pathogens during the procedure.
2. Bleeding from small vessels (lateral position of puncture site should be maintained to avoid superior sagittal sinus).
3. Removal of more than 20 ml/tap can produce CNS sequelae. If more than 20 ml is present, a neurosurgeon should be consulted.
4. Injury to the cerebral cortex if needle is inserted too deeply.

Appendix A-7: Suprapubic Aspiration

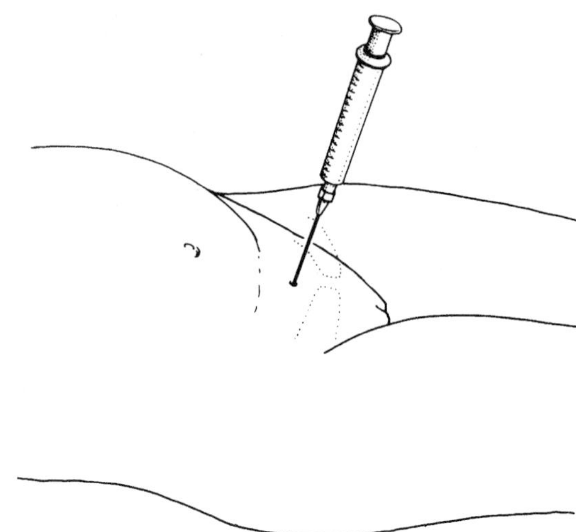

Fig. A-7 Suprapubic aspiration.

Suprapubic aspiration is a relatively safe method of obtaining urine from the newborn and infants younger than 2 years because the distended bladder in this age group is primarily intraabdominal.

The infant's bladder must be full. Determining that the diaper has been dry for 45 minutes is good evidence of a full bladder. Dehydration reduces the success. Ultrasonographic confirmation of a full bladder may be helpful.

POSITION

The patient is restrained in the supine position.

SITE

The site is 2 cm (a fingerbreadth) above the symphysis.

PROCEDURE

1. Cleanse the suprapubic area as for surgery with povidone-iodine (Betadine).
2. Identify the pubic bone without contaminating the area of puncture.
3. Insert a 1-inch, 22-gauge needle attached to a 5-ml syringe at midline, angling the needle 10 to 20 degrees cephalad and advancing it through the skin under negative pressure at all times (Fig. A-7).

Entry into the bladder is indicated by return of urine. If no urine is obtained:

1. Angle the needle perpendicular to the frontal plane and try once more.
2. Avoid excessive probing or manipulation of the needle.
3. If no urine is obtained, try again in 15 minutes, or use a different technique, such as catheterization (an infant can be catheterized with a 3.5- or 5.0-Fr feeding tube).

COMPLICATIONS

Complications include gross hematuria (some hematuria usually will follow the procedure), anterior abdominal wall abscess, and bowel puncture. Peritonitis is uncommon.

Appendix A-8: Thoracentesis

Thoracentesis is indicated to remove pleural fluid for diagnostic or therapeutic reasons or in the emergency treatment of a pneumothorax pending placement of a chest tube.

POSITION

For posterior or posterolateral approaches to fluid removal, the patient sits in a flexed position, leaning forward against a bed stand or chair back. A small infant may be held in the "burping" position.

1. If the patient is too ill to sit, the procedure may be performed with the patient lying on the involved side on a firm surface with a portion of the lateral chest wall extending over the edge of the bed. An alternative for gaining access to the lateral chest wall is for the patient to lie across two beds or examination tables with the involved side down.
2. If a pneumothorax is to be decompressed, the patient should be lying supine.

SITE

The site of puncture depends on the location of the pleural fluid. If a pneumothorax is being decompressed before placement of a chest tube (see Fig. A-9), venting is done at the second or third intercostal space at the midclavicular line.

NEEDLE

An 18- or 19-gauge needle with a short bevel attached to a three-way stopcock and 10-ml syringe is used. If fluid is expected, plastic tubing is attached to the sidearm of the stopcock to facilitate removal of fluids.

Flexible cannulas over needle also are useful and may replace the needle. They decrease the risk of lung puncture and are particularly valuable for emergency intervention.

PROCEDURE

1. The area is prepared and draped, and 1% lidocaine is infiltrated locally.
2. With sterile technique, the needle or catheter-over-needle is inserted, passing over the superior edge of the rib under negative pressure, and advanced slowly. There is a sudden decrease in resistance once the pleural space is reached. A hemostat should be placed on the needle at the skin to prevent further penetration once the pleural space is entered.
3. Fluid is aspirated, the volume reflecting cardiopulmonary status and the therapeutic goals of the procedures.

ANALYSIS OF THE FLUID

Analysis should include a culture, Gram stain, protein, glucose, and lactose dehydrogenase (LDH) measurements, cell count, and a check for chyle (see later).

The distinction between transudate and exudate may be useful in differentiating the causes of pleural effusion. Transudates usually are associated with congestive heart failure, cirrhosis, nephrotic syndrome, acute glomerulonephritis, myxedema, and peritoneal dialysis. Exudates with protein content higher than 3 g/dl occur

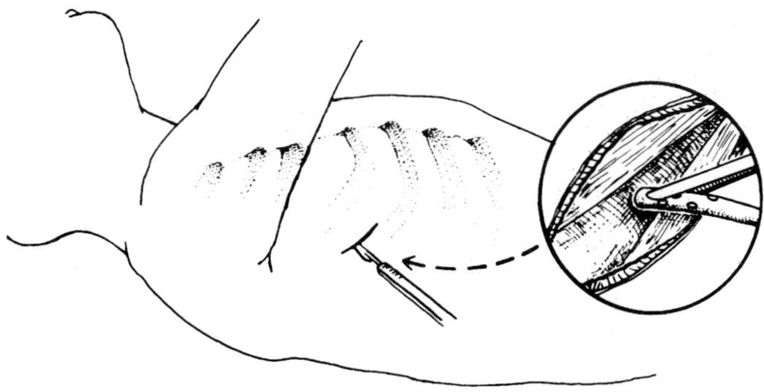

Fig. A-9 Placement of chest tube.

(Modified from Rosen P, Sternbach G: *Atlas of emergency medicine*, Baltimore, 1983, Williams and Wilkins. Reproduced by permission of the author.)

	Transudate	Exudate
Etiology	CHF, cirrhosis	Infection: bacterial, mycobacterial; infarction, neoplasm, pancreatitis
Protein	<3.0 g/dl (PF/S <0.5)	>3.0 g/dl (PF/S >0.5)
LDH	Low (<200 IU/L) (PF/S <0.6)	High (>200 IU/L) (PF/S >0.6)
Glucose	Same as blood	Variable (infection: low)
RBC	<10,000/mm^3	Variable (if >100,000/mm^3; consider infarction, trauma, neoplasm)
WBC	<1000/mm^3	>1000/mm^3 (infection)

PF, Pleural fluid; *S,* serum.

with pulmonary infarction, neoplasms, infection (viral or bacterial such as *Staphylococcus aureus, Haemophilus influenzae,* or streptococcus; tuberculosis; fungus; or parasites), collagen vascular disease, subphrenic abscess, trauma, and lymphatic abnormalities.

COMPLICATIONS

Complications include introduction of infection, pneumothorax, hemothorax, or pulmonary laceration. Hospitalize the patient for observation after the procedure.

Appendix A-9: Thoracostomy

Chest tubes are used for the treatment of pneumothorax or hemothorax, often before a definitive radiologic diagnosis is made (see Chapter 62). Management in newborns is discussed in Chapter 11.

INDICATIONS

1. Tension pneumothorax.
2. Traumatic moderate to large pneumothorax. A small (<10% simple) pneumothorax in a symptom-free patient (with no increase on repeat x-ray film) may be observed in the hospital if general anesthesia or mechanical ventilation is not required for other injuries.
3. Any pneumothorax with respiratory symptoms.
4. Enlarging pneumothorax after initial conservative therapy.
5. Pneumothorax in a patient who needs mechanical ventilation or general anesthesia.
6. Associated hemothorax.
7. Bilateral pneumothorax.

POSITION

The patient is supine with appropriate immobilization.

SITE

The site for insertion is at the fourth or fifth intercostal space in the midaxillary line.

TUBE SIZE

The tube should be the largest one that can be inserted. This is particularly important if a hemothorax is present.

1. The following are estimates of appropriate size:

Patient Age	Tube Size (French)
Newborn	8 to 12
Infant	14 to 20
Child	20 to 28
Adolescent	28 to 42

2. The length of the tube should be approximated before insertion. All holes in the tube must be within the pleural cavity.
3. A Seldinger technique (tube-over-wire) may be an alternative to the traditional chest tube insertion.

PROCEDURE

1. The area is prepared, draped, and locally infiltrated with 1% lidocaine down to the rib and along the subcutaneous tissue to be tunneled.
2. The skin is incised with a scalpel parallel to the long axis of the rib. The incision should be adequate to permit manipulation of the tube (3 to 5 cm).
3. The area is bluntly dissected down to the rib with a clamp or scissors. If tunneling is desired, the dissection is continued across the intercostal space above the incision site and over the next rib. A clamp is then curved over the superior edge of the rib, dividing the intercostal muscles down to the parietal pleura, which is penetrated. The opening is enlarged by blunt dissection.
4. In older infants and children, a finger is inserted to ensure that there are no adhesions of the lung and that the tube will be inserted into the chest and not subdiaphragmatically.
5. The thoracostomy tube is grasped at the tip by a curved clamp and advanced through the tunnel and intercostal space into the chest. It is directed posteriorly and apically. The interspace is entered superior to the rib to avoid injuring the neurovascular bundle (Fig. A-9). All holes must be within the pleural cavity.
6. The tube is attached to an underwater seal. If there is a continuous air leak or an associated hemothorax, additional pleural suction may be needed up to 15 to 25 cm H_2O.
7. The tube is sutured in place and dressed with a sterile covering, often including a petrolatum-soaked gauze as an air seal.
8. A chest x-ray film should be obtained after the procedure.

COMPLICATIONS

1. Inserting the tube too low, causing penetration of the diaphragm and injury to the liver or spleen
2. Injury to the neurovascular bundle, causing persistent hemorrhage
3. Injury to the underlying lung
4. Air leak if the tube is not placed far enough to include all the holes in the pleural cavity, causing extensive subcutaneous emphysema and failure to reexpand the collapsed lung
5. Empyema

BIBLIOGRAPHY

Ahmed MY, Silver P, Wimroff L et al: The needle-wire-dilator technique for insertion of chest tubes in pediatric patients, *Pediatr Emerg Care* 11:252, 1995.

Ellis RW, Strauss LC, Wiley JM et al: A simple method of estimating cerebrospinal fluid pressure during lumbar puncture, *Pediatrics* 89:895, 1992.

Fiser BH: Intraosseous infusion, *N Engl J Med* 322:1579, 1990.

Fiser RT, Walker WM, Seibert JJ et al: Tibia length following intraosseous infusion: a prospective radiographic analysis, *Pediatr Emerg Care* 13:186, 1997.

Glaeser PW, Hellmich JR, Szewczuga D et al: Five-year experience in prehospital intraosseous infusions in children and adults, *Ann Emerg Med* 22:1119, 1993.

Orlowski JP, Julius CJ, Petras RE et al: The safety of intraosseous infusion: risks of fat and bone marrow emboli to the lungs, *Ann Emerg Med* 18:1062, 1989.

Orlowski JP, Parembka DT, Gallagher JM et al: The bone marrow as a source of laboratory studies, *Ann Emerg Med* 18:1348, 1989.

Orlowski JP, Parembka DT, Gallagher JM et al: Companion study of intraosseous infusions of emergency drugs, *Am J Dis Child* 144:112, 1990.

Pollack CV, Pollack ES, Andrew ME: Suprapubic bladder aspiration vs. urethral catheterization in all infants: success, efficiency and complication rates, *Ann Emerg Med* 23:225, 1994.

Proter FL, Miller JP, Cole FS et al: A controlled clinical trial of local anesthesia for lumbar puncture in newborns, *Pediatrics* 88:663, 1991.

Shockley LW, Butzier DJ: A modified well-guided technique for venous cutdown access, *Ann Emerg Med* 19:393, 1990.

B Reference Standards

Appendix B-1: Growth Curves

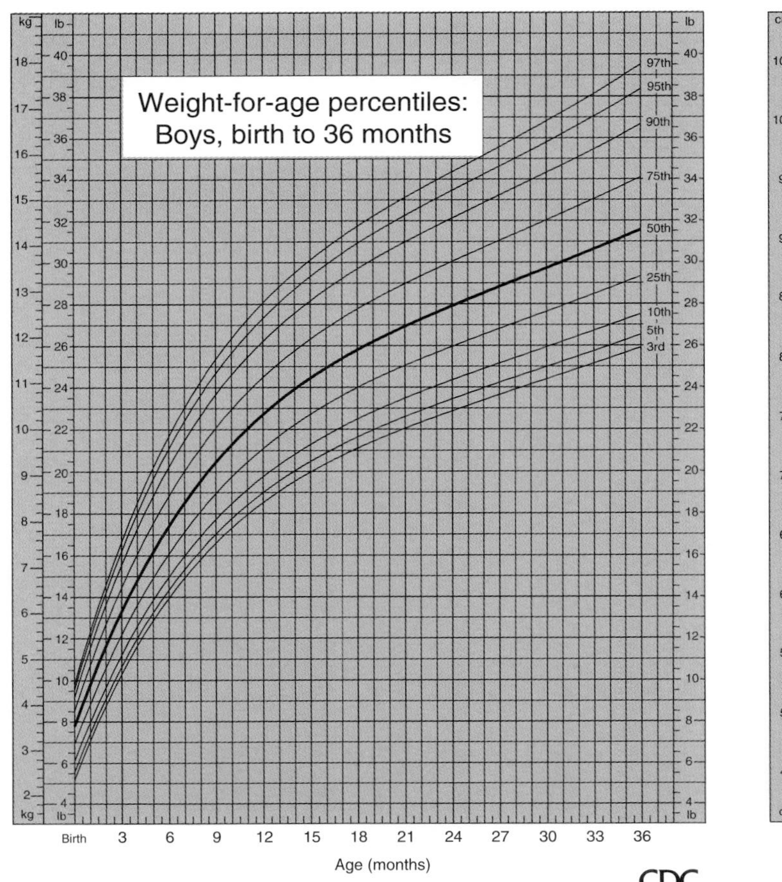

Fig. B-1 **A,** Weight-for-age percentiles: boys, birth to 36 months.

(Developed by the National Center for Health Statistics in collaboration with the National Center for Chronic Disease Prevention and Health Promotion [2000].)

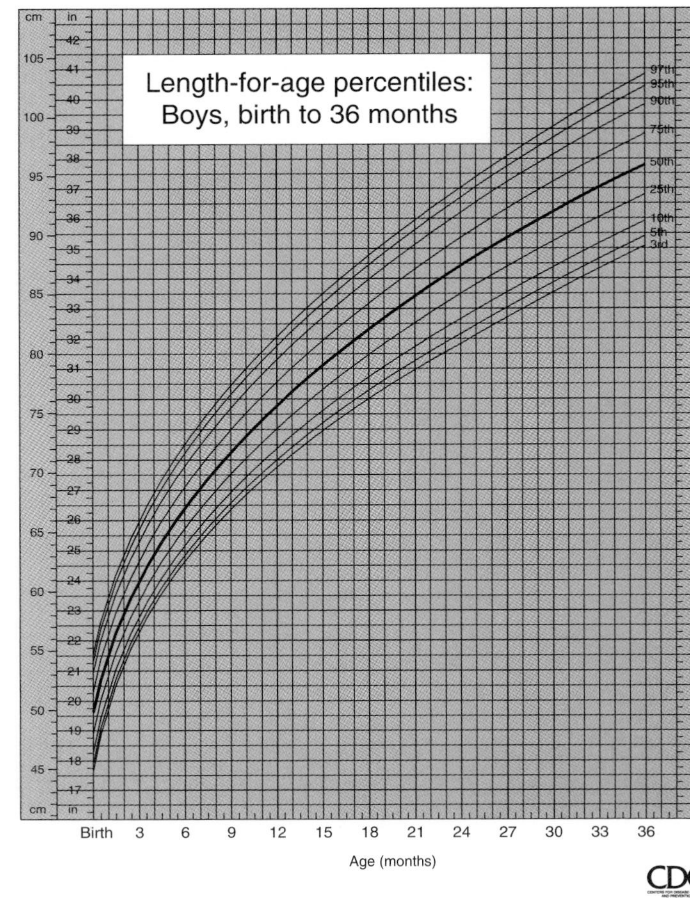

Fig. B-1 **B,** Length-for-age percentiles: boys, birth to 36 months.

(Developed by the National Center for Health Statistics in collaboration with the National Center for Chronic Disease Prevention and Health Promotion [2000].)

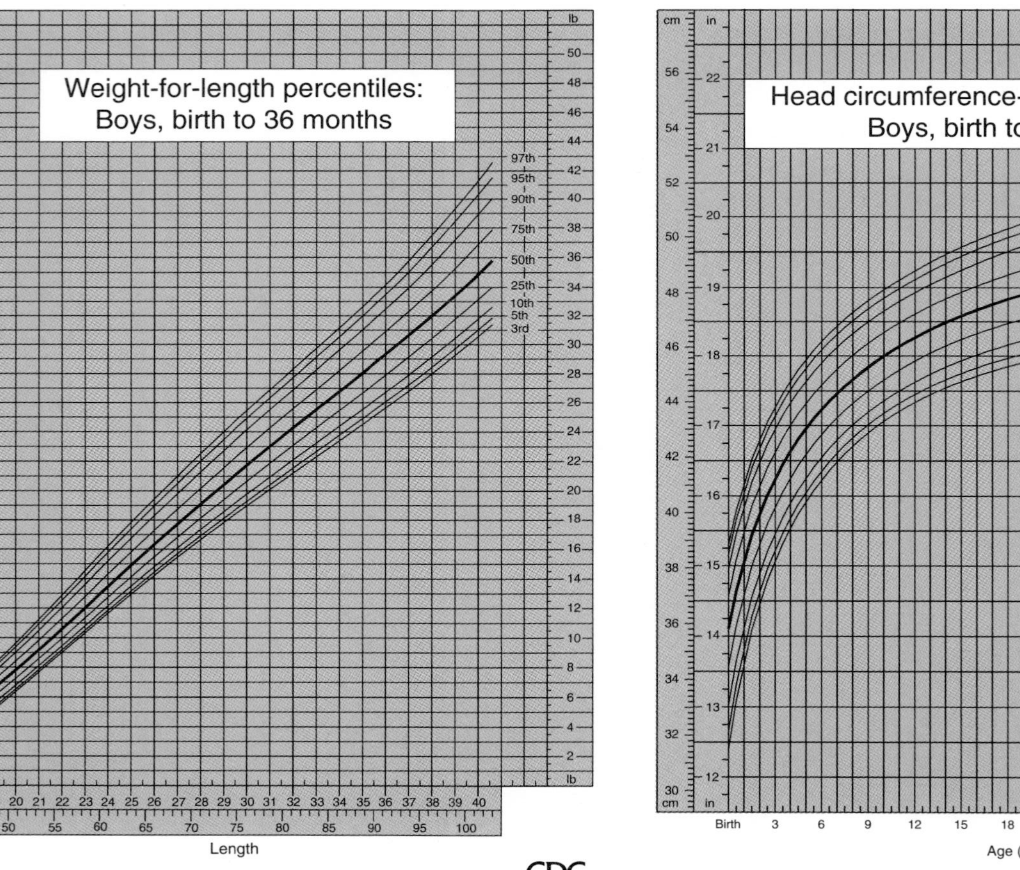

Fig. B-1 **C,** Weight-for-length percentiles: boys, birth to 36 months.

(Developed by the National Center for Health Statistics in collaboration with the National Center for Chronic Disease Prevention and Health Promotion [2000].)

Fig. B-1 **D,** Head circumference-for-age percentiles: boys, birth to 36 months.

(Developed by the National Center for Health Statistics in collaboration with the National Center for Chronic Disease Prevention and Health Promotion [2000].)

Fig. B-1 E, Weight-for-age percentiles: girls, birth to 36 months.

(Developed by the National Center for Health Statistics in collaboration with the National Center for Chronic Disease Prevention and Health Promotion [2000].)

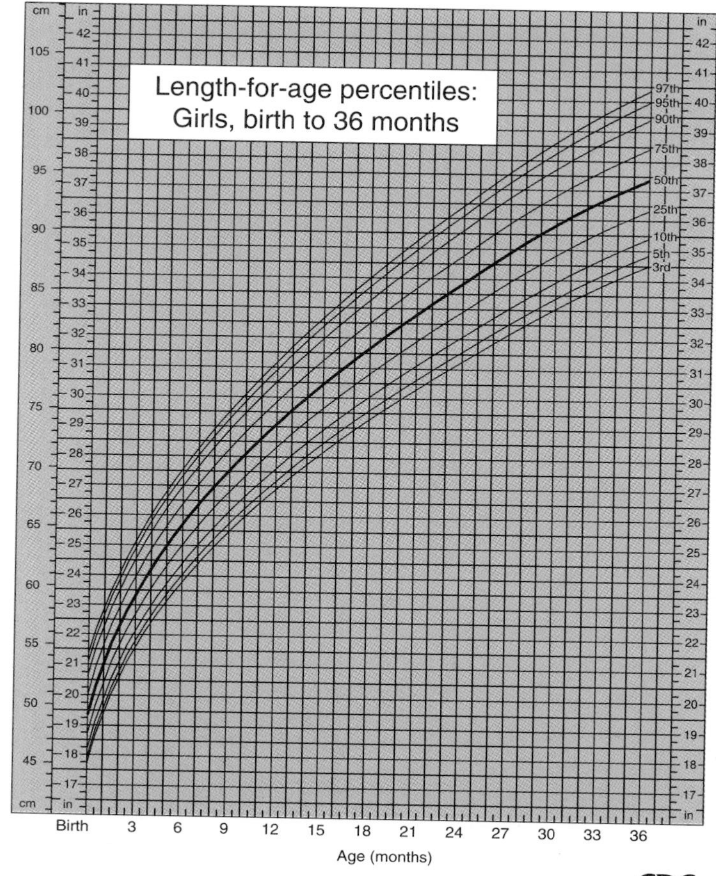

Fig. B-1 F, Length-for-age percentiles: girls, birth to 36 months.

(Developed by the National Center for Health Statistics in collaboration with the National Center for Chronic Disease Prevention and Health Promotion [2000].)

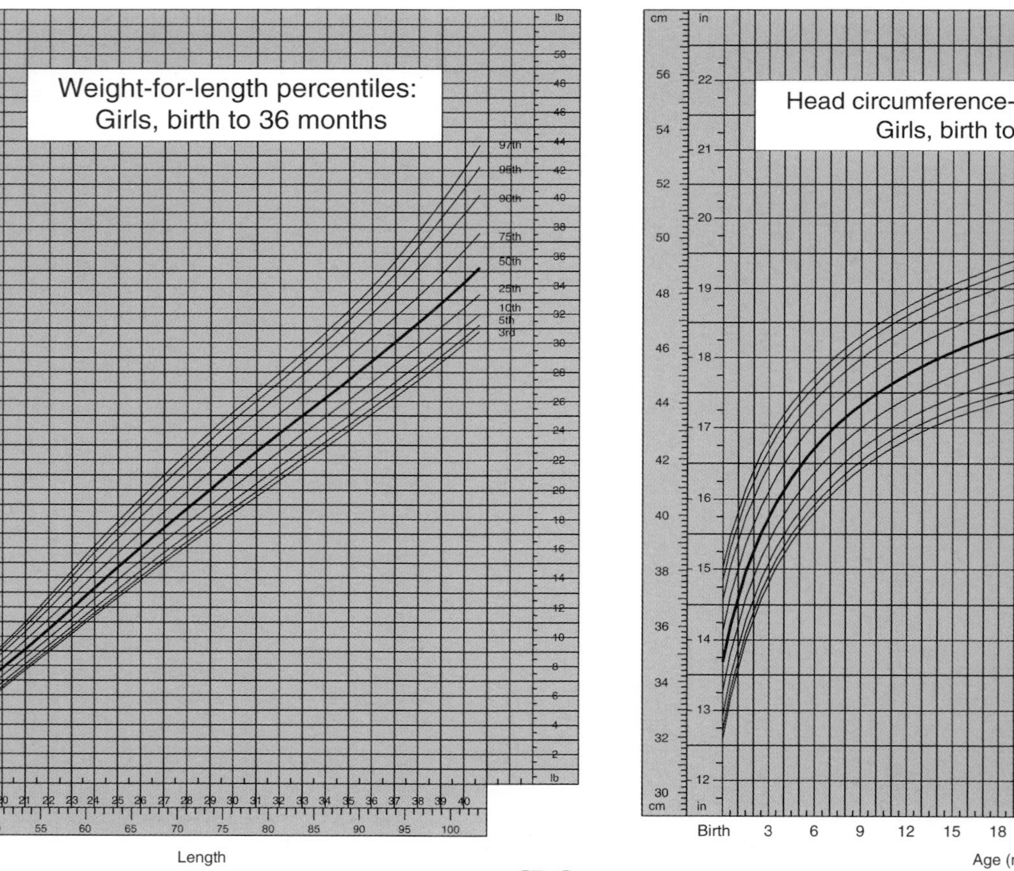

Fig. B-1 **G,** Weight-for-length percentiles: girls, birth to 36 months.

(Developed by the National Center for Health Statistics in collaboration with the National Center for Chronic Disease Prevention and Health Promotion [2000].)

Fig. B-1 **H,** Head circumference-for-age percentiles: girls, birth to 36 months.

(Developed by the National Center for Health Statistics in collaboration with the National Center for Chronic Disease Prevention and Health Promotion [2000].)

Weight-for-age percentiles: Boys, 2 to 20 years

Fig. B-1 I, Weight-for-age percentiles: boys, 2 to 20 years.

(Developed by the National Center for Health Statistics in collaboration with the National Center for Chronic Disease Prevention and Health Promotion [2000].)

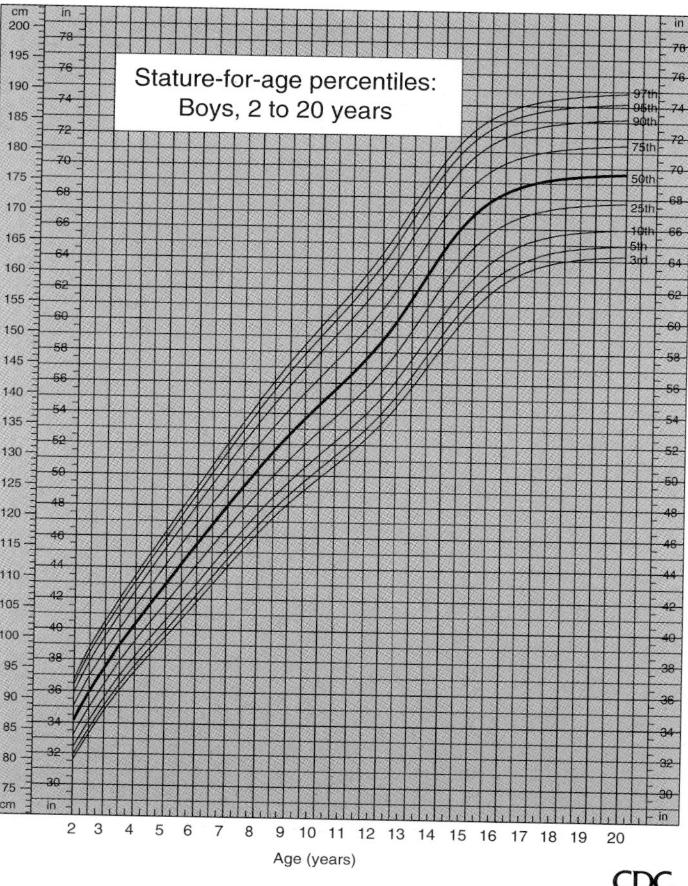

Fig. B-1 J, Stature-for-age percentiles: boys, 2 to 20 years.

(Developed by the National Center for Health Statistics in collaboration with the National Center for Chronic Disease Prevention and Health Promotion [2000].)

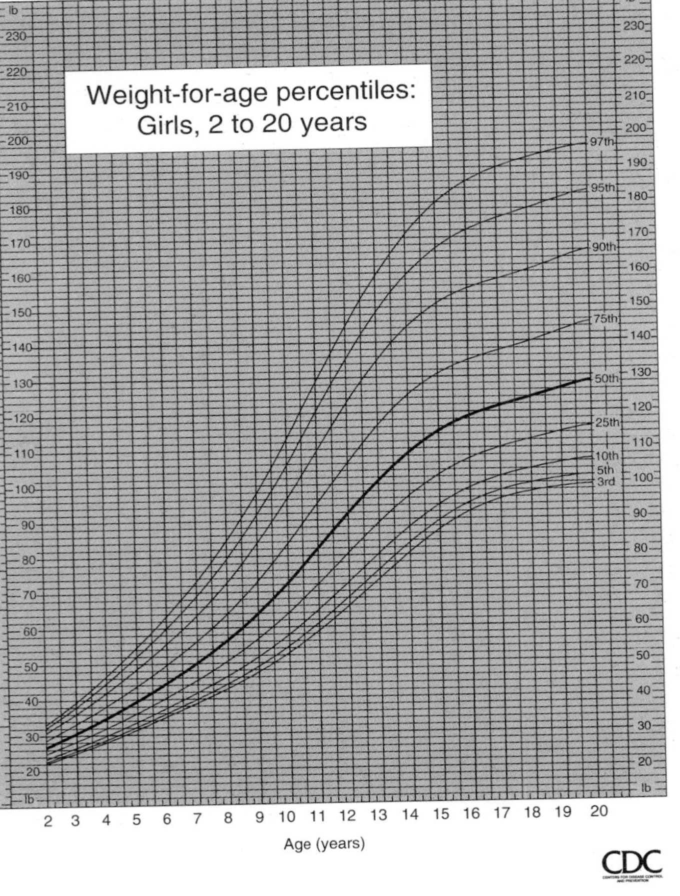

Fig. B-1 **K,** Weight-for-age percentiles: girls, 2 to 20 years.

(Developed by the National Center for Health Statistics in collaboration with the National Center for Chronic Disease Prevention and Health Promotion [2000].)

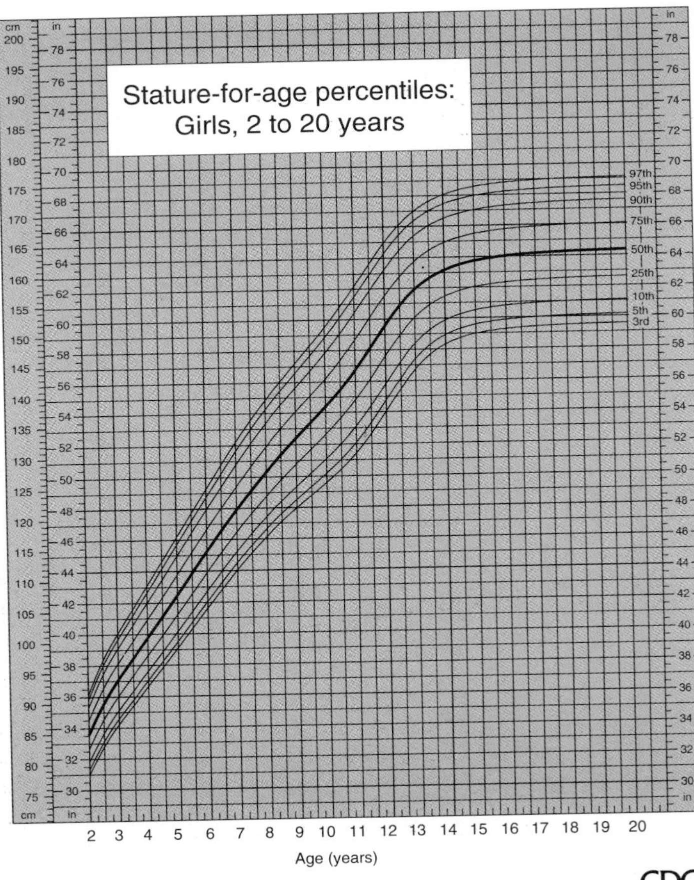

Fig. B-1 **L,** Stature-for-age percentiles: girls, 2 to 20 years.

(Developed by the National Center for Health Statistics in collaboration with the National Center for Chronic Disease Prevention and Health Promotion [2000].)

Appendix B-2: Vital Signs and Ancillary Ventilatory Support

Age	Weight (kg)	Heart Rate (average/min)	Respiratory Rate	BLOOD PRESSURE		ET TUBE		Suction Catheter (Fr)	Chest Tube (Fr)	Laryngoscopy Blade
				Systolic	Diastolic*	ID† (mm)	Length (cm)			
Premature	1	145	>40	42 ± 10	21 ± 8	2.5	10	6	8-10	0 st
Newborn	1-2	135		50 ± 10	28 ± 8	3.0	11	6-8	10-12	1 st
Newborn	2-3	125		60 ± 10	37 ± 8	3.5	12	8		
1 mo	4	120	38 ± 10	80 ± 16	46 ± 16	3.5	13			
6 mo	7	130		89 ± 29	60 ± 10	3.5-4.0	14			
1 yr	10	125	39 ± 11	96 ± 30	66 ± 15	4.0-4.5	15	8-10	16-20	1 st
2-3 yr	12-14	115	28 ± 4	99 ± 25	64 ± 25	4.5	16	10	20-24	
4-5 yr	16-18	100	27 ± 6	99 ± 20	65 ± 20	5.0-5.5	17		20-28	2
6-8 yr	20-26	100	24 ± 6	See figures on pp. 864-865		5.5-6.0	18			
10-12 yr	32-42	75	21 ± 4			5.5-7.0	20	12	28-32	2-3
>14 yr	>50	70	20 ± 4			7.5-8.5	24		32-42	3

* Point of muffling (Nadas).

† Variability of 0.5 mm is common. Estimate: $\frac{16 + \text{age(yr)}}{4}$

95TH PERCENTILE OF SYSTOLIC AND DIASTOLIC BLOOD PRESSURE BY HEIGHT AND AGE, BOYS

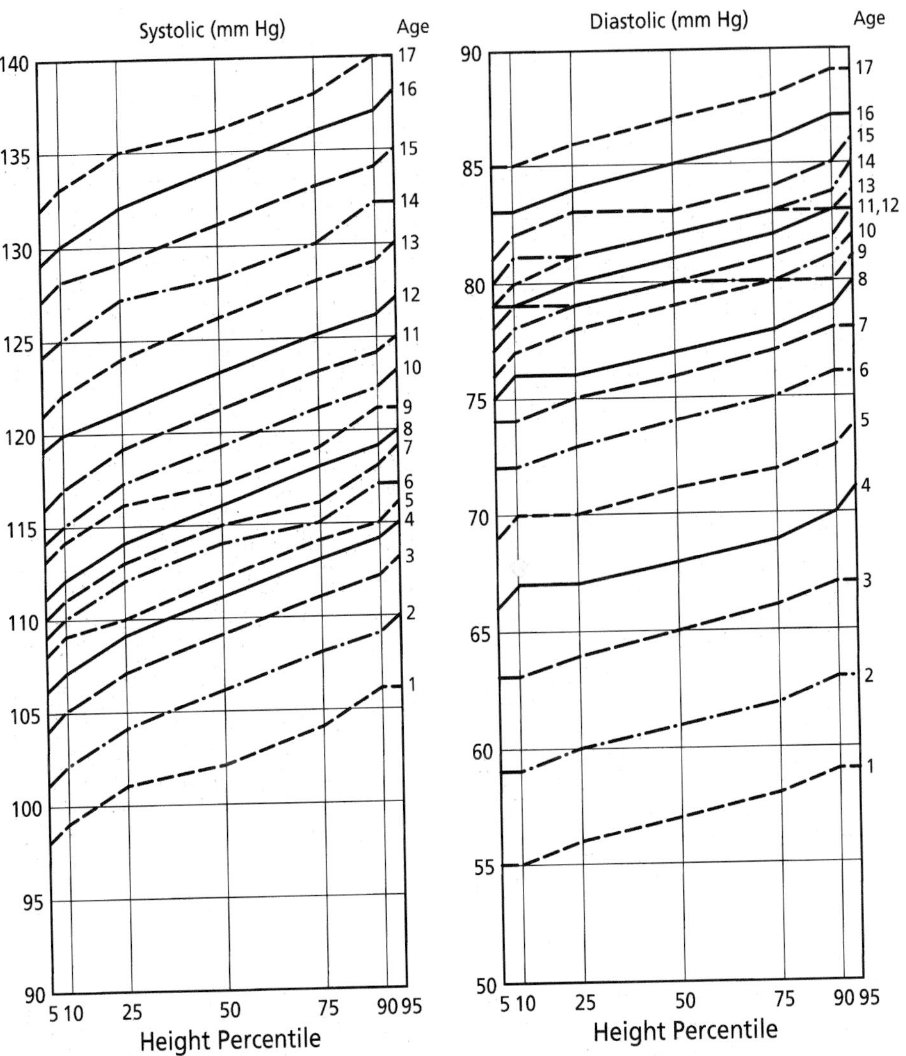

Fig. B-2 95th percentile of systolic and diastolic blood pressure by height and age, boys.

(From *Update on the task force report (1997) on high blood pressure control in children and adolescents: a working group report from the National High Blood Pressure Education Program.* National Institutes of Public Health, National Heart, Lung, and Blood Institute, NIH Publication No. 96-3790, 1996.)

95TH PERCENTILE OF SYSTOLIC AND DIASTOLIC BLOOD PRESSURE BY HEIGHT AND AGE, GIRLS

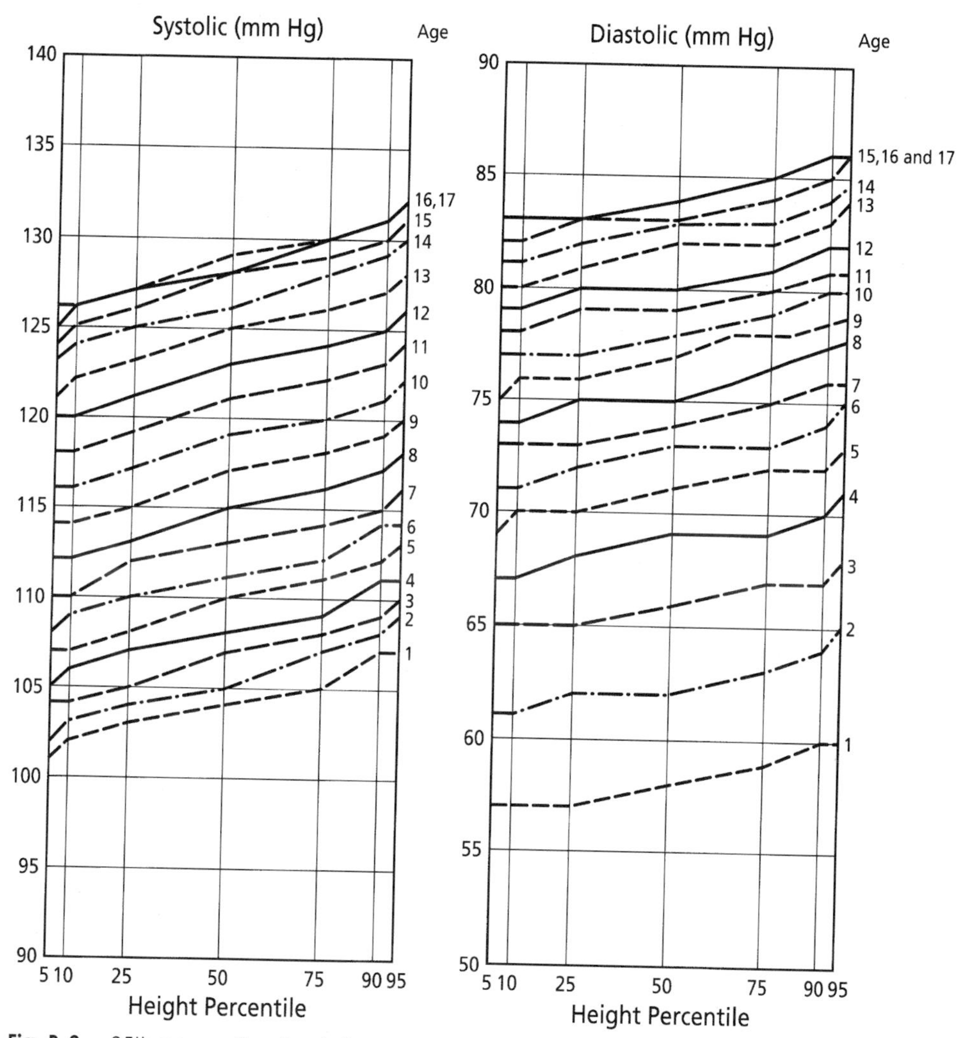

Fig. B-3 95th percentile of systolic and diastolic blood pressure by height and age, girls.

(From *Update on the task force report (1997) on high blood pressure control in children and adolescents: a working group report from the National High Blood Pressure Education Program.* National Institutes of Public Health, National Heart, Lung, and Blood Institute, NIH Publication No. 96-3790, 1996.)

Appendix B-3: Electrocardiographic Criteria

Age	Heart Rate (/min)	QRS Axis (degrees)	PR Interval (sec)	QRS Duration* (sec)
0–1 mo	100–180 (120)†	+75 to +180 (+120)	0.08–0.12 (0.10)	0.04–0.08 (0.06)
2–3 mo	110–180 (120)	+35 to +135 (+100)	0.08–0.12 (0.10)	0.04–0.08 (0.06)
4–12 mo	100–180 (150)	+30 to +135 (+60)	0.09–0.13 (0.12)	0.04–0.08 (0.06)
1–3 yr	100–180 (130)	0 to +110 (+60)	0.10–0.14 (0.12)	0.04–0.08 (0.06)
4–5 yr	60–150 (100)	0 to +110 (+60)	0.11–0.15 (0.13)	0.05–0.09 (0.07)
6–8 yr	60–130 (100)	−15 to +110 (+60)	0.12–0.16 (0.14)	0.05–0.09 (0.07)
9–11 yr	50–110 (80)	−15 to +110 (+60)	0.12–0.17 (0.14)	0.05–0.09 (0.07)
12–16 yr	50–100 (75)	−15 to +110 (+60)	0.12–0.17 (0.15)	0.05–0.09 (0.07)
>16 yr	50–90 (70)	−15 to +110 (+60)	0.12–0.20 (0.15)	0.05–0.10 (0.08)

QT INTERVAL‡

Rate/Min	R-R Interval (sec)	Q-T Interval (sec)
40	1.5	0.38-0.50 (0.45)†
50	1.2	0.36-0.48 (0.43)
60	1.0	0.34-0.46 (0.41)
70	0.86	0.32-0.43 (0.37)
80	0.75	0.29-0.40 (0.35)
90	0.67	0.27-0.37 (0.33)
100	0.60	0.26-0.35 (0.30)
120	0.50	0.24-0.32 (0.28)
150	0.40	0.21-0.28 (0.25)
180	0.33	0.19-0.27 (0.23)
200	0.30	0.18-0.25 (0.22)

T-WAVE ORIENTATION

Age	V_1, V_2	aVF	I, V_5, V_6
0-5 days	Variable	Upright	Upright
6 days-2 yr	Inverted	Upright	Upright
3 yr-adolescent	Inverted	Upright	Upright
Adult	Upright	Upright	Upright

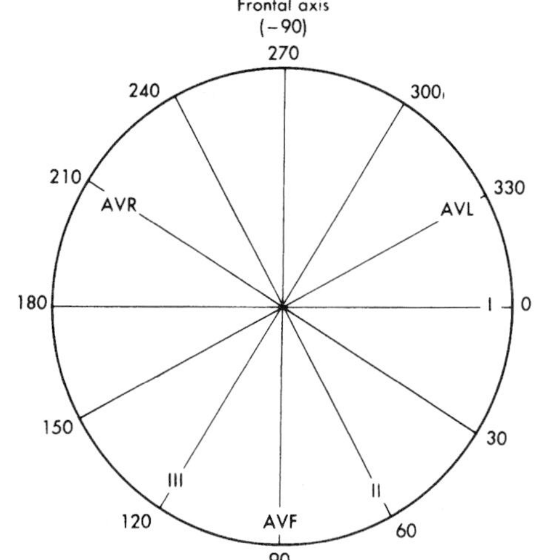

* If QRS duration is normal, add R + R′ and compare total (R + R′) with standards; R/S undefined because S can be equal to 0.

† Minimum-maximum (mean).

‡ $QT_c, \dfrac{\text{measured Q-T interval (sec)}}{\sqrt{\text{R-R interval (sec)}}}$

QT_c should not exceed 0.45 in child <6 mo, 0.44 in children or 0.425 in adolescents/adults.

Adapted from Garson A, Jr, Gillette PC, McNamara DG: *A guide to cardiac dysrhythmias in children,* New York, 1980, Grune & Stratton, Inc; Guntheroth WGS: *Pediatric electrocardiography,* Philadelphia, 1965, WB Saunders.

LEAD V_1			LEAD V_6			
R-Wave Amplitude (mm)	S-Wave Amplitude (mm)	R/S Ratio	R-wave Amplitude (mm)	S-Wave Amplitude (mm)	R/S Ratio	Age
4-25 (15)	0-20(10)	0.5 to ∞ (1.5)	1-21 (6)	0-12 (4)	0.1 to ∞ (2)	0-1 mo
2-20 (11)	1-18 (7)	0.3 to 10.0 (1.5)	3-20 (10)	0-6 (2)	1.5 to ∞ (4)	2-3 mo
3-20 (10)	1-16 (8)	0.3 to 4.0 (1.2)	4-20 (13)	0-4 (2)	2.0 to ∞ (6)	4-12 mo
1-18 (9)	1-27 (13)	0.5 to 1.5 (0.8)	3-24 (12)	0-4 (2)	3.0 to ∞ (20)	1-3 yr
1-18 (7)	1-30 (14)	0.1 to 1.5 (0.7)	4-24 (13)	0-4 (1)	2.0 to ∞ (20)	4-5 yr
1-18 (7)	1-30 (14)	0.1 to 1.5 (0.7)	4-24 (13)	0-4 (1)	2.0 to ∞ (20)	6-8 yr
1-16 (6)	1-26 (16)	0.1 to 1.0 (0.5)	4-24 (14)	0-4 (1)	4.0 to ∞ (20)	9-11 yr
1-16 (5)	1-23 (14)	0 to 1.0 (0.3)	4-22 (14)	0-5 (1)	2.0 to ∞ (9)	12-16 yr
1-14 (3)	1-23 (10)	0 to 1.0 (0.3)	4-21 (10)	0-6 (1)	2.0 to ∞ (9)	>16 yr

Chamber Enlargement ("Hypertrophy")

Right ventricular
1. RV1 >20 mm (>25 mm under 1 mo)
2. SV6 >6 mm (>12 mm under 1 mo)
3. Abnormal R/S ratio (VI >2 after 6 mo)
4. Upright TV3R, RV1 after 5 days
5. QR pattern in V3R, V1

Left ventricular
1. RV6 >25 mm (>21 mm under 1 yr)
2. SV1 >30 mm (>20 mm under 1 yr)
3. RV6 + SV1 >60 mm (use V_5 if RV5 >RV6)
4. Abnormal R/S ratio
5. SV1 >2 × RV5

Combined
1. RVH and SV1 or RV6 exceed mean for age
2. LVH and RV1 or SV6 exceed mean for age

Right atrial
1. Peak P valve >3 mm (<6 mo), >2.5 mm (≥6 mo)

Left atrial
1. PII >0.09 sec
2. PV1 late negative deflection >0.04 sec and >1 mm

MAXIMAL P-R INTERVAL (SEC)

Rate/Min	<1 Mo	1 Mo-1 Yr	1-3 Yr	3-8 Yr	8-12 Yr	Adult
<60					0.18	0.21
60-80				0.17	0.17	0.21
80-100	0.12			0.16	0.16	0.20
100-120	0.12		0.16	0.16	0.15	0.19
120-140	0.11	0.14	0.14	0.15	0.15	0.18
140-160	0.11	0.13	0.14	0.14		0.17
>160	0.11	0.11				

Appendix B-4: Normal Laboratory Values*

DETERMINATION FOR

(S) = Serum
(B) = Whole blood
(P) = Plasma

ACID-BASE MEASUREMENTS (B)

pH: 7.38-7.42
$Pa{O_2}$: 65-76 mm Hg
$Pa{CO_2}$: 36-38 mm Hg
Base excess: -2 to +2 mEq/L

ACID PHOSPHATASE (S, P)

Newborns: 7.4-19.4 IU/L
2-13 yr: 6.4-15.2 IU/L
Adult males: 0.5-11 IU/L
Adult females: 0.2-9.5 IU/L

ALANINE AMINOTRANSFERASE (SGPT) (S)

Newborns (1-3 days): 1-25 IU/L
Adult males: 7-46 IU/L
Adult females: 4-35 IU/L

ALKALINE PHOSPHATASE (S)

Age	IU/L
Newborn (1-3 days)	95-368
2-24 mo	115-460
2-7 yr	115-460
8-9 yr	115-345
10-11 yr	115-437
12-13 yr	92-403
14-15 yr	78-446
16-18 yr	35-331
Adults	39-137

AMMONIA (P)

Newborns: 9-150 μg/dl (53-88 μmol/L); higher in premature and jaundiced infants
Thereafter: 0-60 μg/dl (0-35 μmol/L) when blood is drawn correctly

* Values may vary with laboratory, technique, determination, underlying conditions, etc.

AMYLASE (S)

Neonates: undetectable
2-12 mo: levels increase to adult levels
Adults: 28-108 IU/L

ASPARTATE AMINOTRANSFERASE (SGOT) (S)

Newborns (1-3 days): 16-74 IU/L
Adult males: 8-46 IU/L
Adult females: 7-34 IU/L

BICARBONATE (P)

18-25 mEq/L

BILIRUBIN (S)

After 1 mo
Conjugated: 0-0.3 mg/dl
Unconjugated: 0.1-0.7 mg/dl

BLEEDING TIME

1-3 min

CALCIUM (S)

Premature infants: 3.5-4.5 mEq/L
Full-term infants: 4-5 mEq/L
Infants and thereafter: 4.4-5.3 mEq/L

CARBOXYHEMOGLOBIN (B)

<5% of total hemoglobin

CATION-ANION GAP (S, P)

8-12 mEq/L

CHLORIDE (S, P)

96-116 mmol/L

CHOLESTEROL (S, P)

Full-term newborns: 45-167 mg/dl
3 days-1 yr: 69-174 mg/dl
2-14 yr: 120-205 mg/dl
14-19 yr: 120-210 mg/dl
20-29 yr: 120-240 mg/dl
30-39 yr: 140-270 mg/dl
40-49 yr: 150-310 mg/dl
50-59 yr: 160-330 mg/dl

CHOLINESTERASE (S)

2.5-5 μmol/min/ml of serum (pseudocholinesterase)
2.3-4 μmol/min/ml of red cells

COMPLEMENT (S)

C3: 96-195 mg/dl
C4: 15-20 mg/dl

CREATININE (S, P)

Values in mg/dl

Age	Males	Females
Newborns (1-3 days)	0.2-1.0	0.2-1.0
1-3 yr	0.2-0.7	0.2-0.6
4-10 yr	0.2-0.9	0.2-0.8
11-17 yr	0.3-1.2	0.3-1.1
<18 yr	0.5-1.3	0.3-1.1

CREATININE CLEARANCE†

Newborns (1 day): 5-50 ml/min/1.73 m^2 (mean, 18 ml/min/1.73 m^2)
Newborns (6 days): 15-90 ml/min/1.73 m^2 (mean, 36 ml/min/1.73 m^2)
Infants (1 mo): 65 ml/min/1.73 m^2
Infants (2 to 12 mo): 85 ml/min/1.73 m^2
Adult males: 85-125 ml/min/1.73 m^2
Adult females: 75-115 ml/min/1.73 m^2

GLUCOSE (S, P) (see Chapter 38)

Premature infants: 20-80 mg/dl
Full-term infants: 30-100 mg/dl
Children and adults (fasting): 60-105 mg/dl

γ-GLUTAMYL TRANSPEPTIDASE (S)

0-1 mo: 12-27 IU/L
1-2 mo: 9-159 IU/L
2-4 mo: 7-98 IU/L
4-7 mo: 5-45 IU/L
7-15 mo: 3-30 IU/L
Adult males: 9-69 IU/L
Adult females: 3-33 IU/L

GLYCOHEMOGLOBIN (HEMOGLOBIN A_{IC}) (B)

Normal: 6.3%-8.2% of total hemoglobin
Well-controlled diabetic patients ordinarily have levels <10%

HEMATOCRIT (B) (see p. 213)

At birth: 44%-64%
14-90 days: 35%-49%
6 mo-1 yr: 30%-40%
4-10 yr: 31%-43%

HEMOGLOBIN ELECTROPHORESIS (B)

A_1 hemoglobin: 96%-98.5% of total hemoglobin
A_2 hemoglobin: 1.5%-4% of total hemoglobin

FETAL HEMOGLOBIN

At birth: 50%-85% of total hemoglobin
At 1 yr: <15% of total hemoglobin
1-2 yr: up to 5% of total hemoglobin
>2 yr: <2% of total hemoglobin

IMMUNOGLOBINS (S)

Age	IgG (mg/dl)	IgA (mg/dl)	IgM (mg/dl)
2 wk-3 mo	299-852	3-66	15-149
3-6 mo	142-988	4-90	18-118
6-12 mo	418-1142	14-95	43-223
1-6 yr	356-1381	13-209	37-239
6-12 yr	625-1598	29-384	50-278
>12 yr	660-1548	81-252	45-256

IRON (S, P)

Newborns: 20-157 μg/dl
6 wks-3 yr: 20-115 μg/dl
3-9 yr: 20-141 μg/dl
9-14 yr: 21-151 μg/dl
14-16 yr: 20-181 μg/dl
Adults: 44-196 μg/dl

IRON-BINDING CAPACITY (S, P)

Newborns: 59-175 μg/dl
Children and adults: 275-458 μg/dl

LACTATE DEHYDROGENASE (LDH) (S, P)

Newborns (1-3 days): 40-348 IU/L
1 mo-5 yr: 150-360 IU/L
5-12 yr: 130-300 IU/L
12-16 yr: 130-280 IU/L
Adult males: 70-178 IU/L
Adult females: 42-166 IU/L

LACTATE DEHYDROGENASE ISOENZYMES (S)

LDH_1 (heart): 24%-34%
LDH_2 (heart, red cells): 35%-45%
LDH_3 (muscle): 15%-25%
LDH_4 (liver [trace], muscle): 4%-10%
LDH_5 (liver, muscle): 1%-9%

MAGNESIUM (S, P)

Newborns: 1.5-2.3 mEq/L
Adults: 1.4-2 mEq/L

PARTIAL THROMBOPLASTIN TIME (PTT) (P)

Children: 42-54 seconds (varies with control)

PHOSPHORUS, INORGANIC (S, P)

Full-term infants:
  At birth: 5-7.8 mg/dl
  3 days: 5.8-9 mg/dl
  6-12 days: 4.9-8.9 mg/dl
1-10 yr: 3.6-6.2 mg/dl
Adults: 3.1-5.1 mg/dl

PROTEIN (S)

POTASSIUM (S, P)

Premature infants: 4.5-7.2 mEq/L
Full-term infants: 3.7-5.2 mEq/L
Children and adults: 3.5-5.8 mEq/L

PROTHROMBIN TIME (P)

Children: 11-15 seconds (varies with control)

SEDIMENTATION RATE (ESR) (MICRO) (B)

<2 yr: 1-5 mm/h
>2 yr: 1-8 mm/h

SODIUM (S, P)

Children and adults: 135-148 mEq/L

UREA NITROGEN, BLOOD (BUN) (S, P)

<2 yr: 5-15 mg/dl
>2 yr: 10-20 mg/dl

PROTEIN TABLE FOR Appendix B-4

Age	Total Protein (gm/dl)	Albumin (gm/dl)	α_1 Globulin (gm/dl)	α_2 Globulin (gm/dl)	β Globulin (gm/dl)	Gamma Globulin (gm/dl)
Birth	4.6-7.0	3.2-4.8	0.1-0.3	0.2-0.3	0.3-0.6	0.6-1.2
3 mo	4.5-6.5	3.2-4.8	0.1-0.3	0.3-0.7	0.3-0.7	0.2-0.7
>1 yr	5.4-8.0	3.7-5.7	0.1-0.3	0.4-1.1	0.4-1.0	0.2-1.3

† Creatinine clearance (ml/min/1.73 m²) = $\frac{UV}{P} \times \frac{1.73}{SA}$

P, U, Plasma or urinary concentration of creatinine (mg/dl); *V,* volume of urine divided by number of minutes in collection period (24 hr = 1440 min); *SA,* surface area (m²).

Appendix B-5: Conversions, Estimates, and Nomograms

TEMPERATURE

To convert Celsius to Fahrenheit: (9/5 × temperature) + 32
To convert Fahrenheit to Celsius: (temperature − 32) × 5/9

Celsius	Fahrenheit	Celsius	Fahrenheit
34.2	93.6	38.6	101.4
34.6	94.3	39.0	102.2
35.0	95.0	39.4	102.9
35.4	95.7	39.8	103.6
35.8	96.4	40.2	104.3
36.2	97.1	40.6	105.1
36.6	97.8	41.0	105.8
37.0	98.6	41.4	106.5
37.4	99.3	41.8	107.2
37.8	100.0	42.2	108.0
38.2	100.7	42.6	108.7

WEIGHT

To change pounds to grams: multiply by 454
To change kilograms to pounds: multiply by 2.2

If patient weighs ≤10 lb, the following are used, with the intermediate value in pounds and ounces added to determine the final conversion:

10 lb	4.53 kg	110 lb	49.89 kg
20 lb	9.07 kg	120 lb	54.43 kg
30 lb	13.60 kg	130 lb	58.96 kg
40 lb	18.14 kg	140 lb	63.50 kg
50 lb	22.68 kg	150 lb	68.04 kg
60 lb	27.21 kg	160 lb	72.57 kg
70 lb	31.75 kg	170 lb	77.11 kg
80 lb	36.28 kg	180 lb	81.64 kg
90 lb	40.82 kg	190 lb	86.18 kg
100 lb	45.36 kg	200 lb	90.72 kg

Growth Patterns

Birth weight (avg): 3.3 kg (7 lb 5 oz)
A newborn loses up to 10% of birth weight initially but should be up to birth weight again by 10 days
An infant gains 30 g (1 oz)/day for the first 1-2 mo
5 mo: birth weight should be doubled
12 mo: birth weight should be tripled
2 yr: birth weight should be quadrupled

Estimates of Weight

4 to 8-year-old: 6 × Age + 12 = Weight (lb)
8 to 12-year-old: 7 × Age + 5 = Weight (lb)

Weight conversion table (pounds and ounces to grams)

Ounces	0 lb	1 lb	2 lb	3 lb	4 lb	5 lb	6 lb	7 lb	8 lb	9 lb
0		454	907	1361	1814	2268	2722	3175	3629	4082
1	28	482	936	1389	1843	2296	2750	3204	3657	4111
2	57	510	964	1418	1871	2325	2778	3232	3686	4139
3	85	539	992	1446	1899	2353	2807	3260	3714	4168
4	113	567	1020	1474	1928	2382	2835	3289	3742	4196
5	142	595	1049	1503	1956	2410	2863	3317	3771	4224
6	170	624	1077	1531	1984	2438	2892	3345	3799	4253
7	198	652	1106	1559	2013	2467	2920	3374	3827	4281
8	227	680	1134	1588	2041	2495	2948	3402	3855	4309
9	255	709	1162	1616	2070	2523	2977	3430	3884	4338
10	284	737	1191	1644	2098	2552	3005	3459	3912	4366
11	312	765	1219	1673	2126	2580	3034	3487	3940	4394
12	340	794	1247	1701	2155	2608	3062	3516	3969	4423
13	369	822	1276	1729	2183	2637	3090	3544	3997	4451
14	397	850	1304	1758	2211	2665	3119	3572	4026	4479
15	425	879	1332	1786	2240	2693	3147	3601	4054	4508

LENGTH

To convert inches to centimeters: multiply by 2.54

To convert centimeters to inches: multiply by 0.394

Growth Patterns

Birth length (avg): 50 cm (20 in)

12 mo: birth length should be doubled

HEAD CIRCUMFERENCE

Growth Patterns

Birth head circumference (avg): 35 cm (14 in)

12 mo head circumference (avg): 47 cm (19 in)

Head circumference: grows 1 cm/mo during first 9 mo

BLOOD PRESSURE (ESTIMATE)

Systolic BP (mm Hg) = 2 × Age (yr) + 80

Diastolic BP (mm Hg) = $\frac{2}{3}$ systolic

OTHER CONVERSION FACTORS

To Convert	To	Multiply By
1 mm Hg	psi	0.0193
1 cm H_2O	mm Hg	0.735
1 mm Hg	cm H_2O	1.259
1 cm	inch	0.3937
1 inch	cm	2.541
1 kg	pound	2.204
1 pound	kg	0.4536
1 French size	mm	0.33

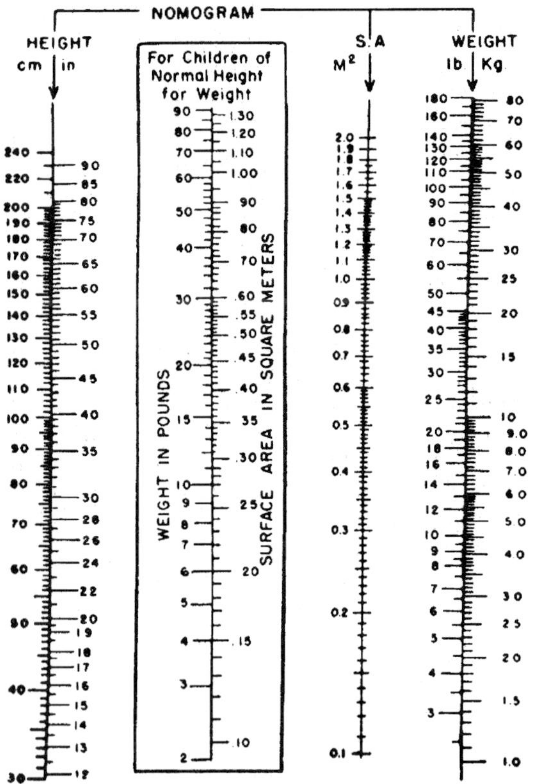

Fig. B-6 Nomogram for estimation of surface area. The surface area is indicated where a straight line that connects the height and weight levels intersects the surface area column; or the patient is roughly of average size, from the weight alone *(enclosed area)*.

(Modified from data of E Boyd by CD West.)

Appendix B-6: Denver Developmental Screening Test

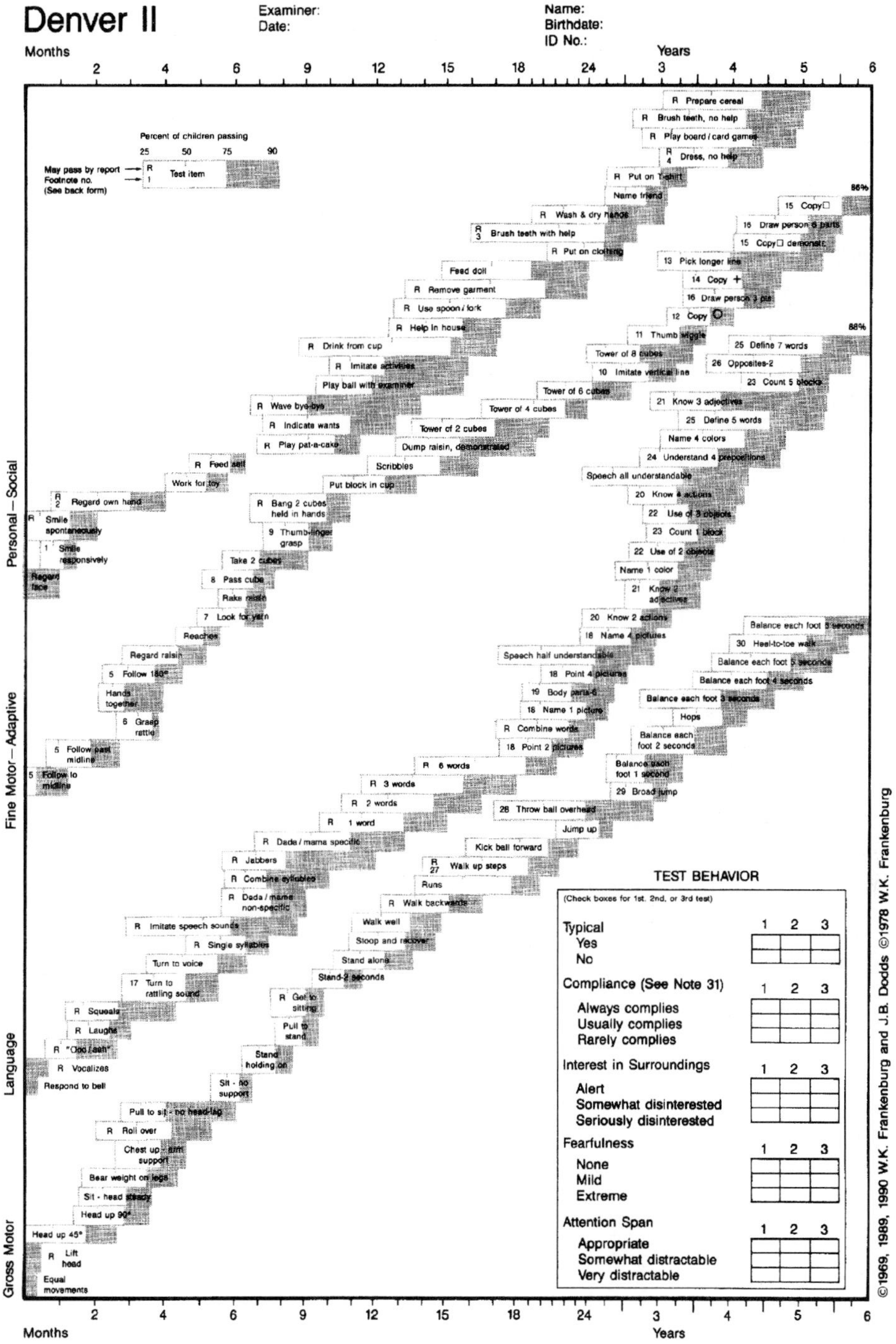

Fig. B-7 (Reproduced with permission from Frankenburg WK, Dodds J, Archer P et al: *Pediatrics* 89:93, Figure 2, copyright 1992.)

Appendix B-7: Recommended Childhood Immunization Schedule: United States

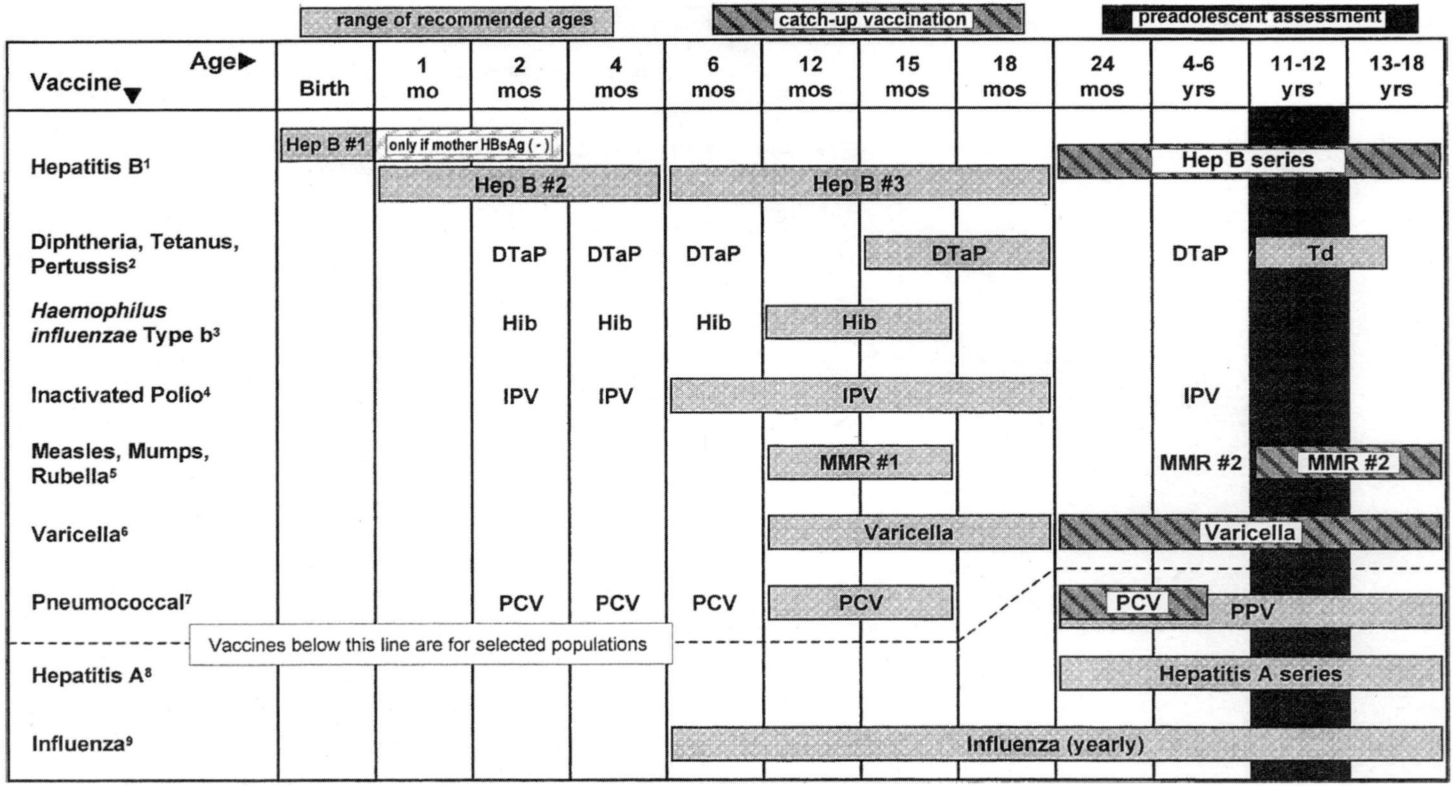

range of recommended ages | catch-up vaccination | preadolescent assessment

Vaccine ▼ / Age ►	Birth	1 mo	2 mos	4 mos	6 mos	12 mos	15 mos	18 mos	24 mos	4-6 yrs	11-12 yrs	13-18 yrs
Hepatitis B[1]	Hep B #1	only if mother HBsAg (-)								Hep B series		
		Hep B #2			Hep B #3							
Diphtheria, Tetanus, Pertussis[2]			DTaP	DTaP	DTaP		DTaP			DTaP	Td	
Haemophilus influenzae Type b[3]			Hib	Hib	Hib	Hib						
Inactivated Polio[4]			IPV	IPV		IPV				IPV		
Measles, Mumps, Rubella[5]						MMR #1				MMR #2	MMR #2	
Varicella[6]							Varicella				Varicella	
Pneumococcal[7]			PCV	PCV	PCV	PCV			PCV		PPV	
Vaccines below this line are for selected populations												
Hepatitis A[8]											Hepatitis A series	
Influenza[9]								Influenza (yearly)				

Approved by the Advisory Committee on Immunization Practices (www.cdc.gov/nip/acip), the American Academy of Pediatrics (www.aap.org), and the American Academy of Family Physicians (www.aafp.org).

This schedule indicates the recommended ages for routine administration of currently licensed childhood vaccines for children through age 18 years. Any dose not given at the recommended age should be given at any subsequent visit when indicated and feasible. [hatched box] Indicates age groups that warrant special effort to administer those vaccines not previously given. Additional vaccines may be licensed and recommended during the year. Licensed combination vaccines may be used whenever any components of the combination are indicated and the vaccine's other components are not contraindicated. Providers should consult the manufacturers' package inserts for detailed recommendations. For additional information about vaccines, vaccine supply, and contraindications for immunization, please visit the National Immunization Program Website at *www.cdc.gov/nip* or call the National Immunization Hotline at 800-232-2522 (English) or 800-232-0233 (Spanish).

1. **Hepatitis B vaccine (Hep B).** All infants should receive the first dose of hepatitis B vaccine soon after birth and before hospital discharge; the first dose may also be given by age 2 months if the infant's mother is HBsAg-negative. Only monovalent hepatitis B vaccine can be used for the birth dose. Monovalent or combination vaccine containing Hep B may be used to complete the series; four doses of vaccine may be administered if combination vaccine is used. The second dose should be given at least 4 weeks after the first dose, except for Hib-containing vaccine which cannot be administered before age 6 weeks. The third dose should be given at least 16 weeks after the first dose and at least 8 weeks after the second dose. The last dose in the vaccination series (third or fourth dose) should not be administered before age 6 months.
<u>Infants born to HBsAg-positive mothers</u> should receive hepatitis B vaccine and 0.5 mL hepatitis B immune globulin (HBIG) within 12 hours of birth at separate sites. The second dose is recommended at age 1-2 months and the vaccination series should be completed (third or fourth dose) at age 6 months.
<u>Infants born to mothers whose HBsAg status is unknown</u> should receive the first dose of the hepatitis B vaccine series within 12 hours of birth. Maternal blood should be drawn at the time of delivery to determine the mother's HBsAg status; if the HBsAg test is positive, the infant should receive HBIG as soon as possible (no later than age 1 week).

2. **Diphtheria and tetanus toxoids and acellular pertussis vaccine (DTaP).** The fourth dose of DTaP may be administered as early as age 12 months, provided 6 months have elapsed since the third dose and the child is unlikely to return at age 15–18 months. **Tetanus and diphtheria toxoids (Td)** is recommended at age 11–12 years if at least 5 years have elapsed since the last dose of tetanus and diphtheria toxoid-containing vaccine. Subsequent routine Td boosters are recommended every 10 years.

3. ***Haemophilus influenzae* type b (Hib) conjugate vaccine.** Three Hib conjugate vaccines are licensed for infant use. If PRP-OMP (PedvaxHib® or ComVax® [Merck]) is administered at ages 2 and 4 months, a dose at age 6 months is not required. DTaP/Hib combination products should not be used for primary immunization in infants at ages 2, 4 or 6 months, but can be used as boosters following any Hib vaccine.

4. **Inactivated polio vaccine (IPV).** An all-IPV schedule is recommended for routine childhood polio vaccination in the United States. All children should receive four doses of IPV at ages 2 months, 4 months, 6–18 months, and 4–6 years.

5. **Measles, mumps, and rubella vaccine (MMR).** The second dose of MMR is recommended routinely at age 4–6 years but may be administered during any visit, provided at least 4 weeks have elapsed since the first dose and that both doses are administered beginning at or after age 12 months. Those who have not previously received the second dose should complete the schedule by the 11–12 year old visit.

6. **Varicella vaccine.** Varicella vaccine is recommended at any visit at or after age 12 months for susceptible children, i.e., those who lack a reliable history of chickenpox. Susceptible persons aged ≥13 years should receive two doses, given at least 4 weeks apart.

7. **Pneumococcal vaccine.** The heptavalent pneumococcal conjugate vaccine (PCV) is recommended for all children age 2–23 months. It is also recommended for certain children age 24–59 months. **Pneumococcal polysaccharide vaccine (PPV)** is recommended in addition to PCV for certain high-risk groups. See MMWR 2000;49(RR-9);1–35.

8. **Hepatitis A vaccine.** Hepatitis A vaccine is recommended for use in selected states and regions, and for certain high-risk groups; consult your local public health authority. See MMWR 1999;48(RR-12);1–37.

9. **Influenza vaccine.** Influenza vaccine is recommended annually for children age ≥6 months with certain risk factors (including but not limited to asthma, cardiac disease, sickle cell disease, HIV, diabetes; see MMWR 2001;50(RR-4);1–44), and can be administered to all others wishing to obtain immunity. Children aged ≤12 years should receive vaccine in a dosage appropriate for their age (0.25 mL if age 6–35 months or 0.5 mL if aged ≥3 years). Children aged ≤8 years who are receiving influenza vaccine for the first time should receive two doses separated by at least 4 weeks.

10. **A combination vaccine,** diphtheria and tetanus toxoids, acellular pertussis adsorbed, hepatitis B (recombinant), and inactivated poliovirus (Pediarix) may be used for primary immunization beginning at 2 months of age and administered IM (0.5 ml) at 6 to 8 week intervals.

ADDITIONAL NOTES

Precautions and Contraindications

Minor Illness or Fever. Although immunizations are generally reserved for healthy patients, minor illness and fever are not contraindications to administration of immunization. Deferring administration may lead to unimmunized status. However, if the fever or other manifestations suggest a moderate or serious illness, deferral of an immunization is appropriate.

Immunocompromise. Immunocompromised children need special consideration, whether the condition is a congenital immunodeficiency, human immunodeficiency virus (HIV) infection, malignancy, or receipt of immunosuppressive therapy.

Egg Allergy

Children with egg allergy, even those with severe hypersensitivity, are at low risk of anaphylactic reactions to measles and mumps vaccine, singly or in combination; skin testing result does not predict an allergic reaction. When vaccine is administered, it should be given as one injection, and the child should be observed for 90 minutes with immediate availability of emergency equipment.

Influenza Vaccine (Inactivated)

Recommended in high-risk patients older than 6 months of age including those with renal, metabolic, cardiac, or pulmonary disease as well as immunocompromised hosts. The recommendations are reassessed *annually*, but in general, children 6 to 35 months old receive 0.25 ml (split virus) twice given 4 weeks apart; children 3 to 12 years old receive 0.5 ml (split virus) twice; and children older than 12 years should be given 0.5 ml (whole or split virus) once. Healthy children age 6 to 23 months are encouraged to receive the vaccine because of their increased risk for influenza-related hospitalization.

Pneumococcal Vaccine

Recommended for children older than 2 years who are at risk of severe pneumococcal infection. Indications are sickle cell disease; functional or anatomic asplenia; nephrotic syndrome, chronic renal failure; conditions associated with immunosuppression, such as organ transplantation, drug therapy, and cytoreduction therapy; HIV infection; and cerebrospinal fluid (CSF) leaks.

Prematurity

The appropriate age for initiating most immunizations in the prematurely born infant is the usual recommended chronologic age. Vaccine doses should not be reduced for preterm infants. Studies are in progress.

Lapsed Immunizations

A lapse in the immunization schedule dose does not require reinstituting the entire series. If a dose of DTaP (or DTP), poliovirus vaccine, Hib, or hepatitis B vaccine is missed, the next immunization should be given as if the usual interval had elapsed.

Adverse Reactions

Before a vaccine is administered, information about previous adverse reactions should be sought. Unexpected events occurring soon after administration of any vaccine should be described in detail and reported to the Vaccine Adverse Events Reporting System (800-338-2382).

Informed Consent

Parents and patients should be informed about the benefits to be derived from vaccines in preventing disease in individuals and the risks of those vaccines. Questions should be encouraged to ensure that they understand the information.

Health care providers should make note in the patient's record of the information that was provided. In addition, the date of administration of the vaccine, the manufacturer and lot of the vaccine, and the name of the provider should be recorded.

BIBLIOGRAPHY

American Academy of Pediatrics: *Report of the committee on infectious diseases,* ed 25, Elk Grove, Ill, 2000, The Academy.

Committee on Infectious Diseases, AAP: Poliomyelitis prevention recommendations for use of inactivated poliovirus vaccine and live oral poliovirus vaccine, *Pediatrics* 99:300, 1997.

Evans G: National childhood vaccine injury act: revision of the vaccine injury table, *Pediatrics* 98:1179, 1996.

Goldstein KP, Kviz FJ, Daum RS: Accuracy of immunization histories provided by adults accompanying preschool children to a pediatric emergency department, *JAMA* 270:2190, 1993.

Lindegren ML, Atkinson WL, Farizo KM et al: Measles vaccination in pediatric emergency departments during a measles outbreak, *JAMA* 270:2185, 1993.

Robinson PE, Gausche M, Gerardi MJ et al: Immunization of the pediatric patient in the emergency department, *Ann Emerg Med* 28:334, 1996.

Rodewald LE, Szilagyi PG, Humiston SG et al: Effect of emergency department immunization rates and subsequent primary care visits, *Arch Pediatr Adolesc Med* 150:1271, 1996.

C Formulary

APPENDIX C-1 Common Medications

Drugs	Dosages	Comments
Acetaminophen (Tylenol, Tempra) Drop: 80 mg/0.8 ml Elix: 160 mg/5 ml Tab: 80 (chew), 160 (junior), 325 mg Supp: 120, 325 mg	10-15 mg/kg/dose q4-6hr PO (adult: 10 gr/dose); (maximum: 3.6 g/24 hr)	May give ibuprofen for synergistic antipyretic effect; also see Codeine Tox: hepatic; overdose (Chapter 55)
Acetazolamide (Diamox) Tab: 125, 250 mg Cap (SR): 500 mg Vial: 500 mg/5 ml	Diuretic: 5 mg/kg/24 hr q6-24hr PO, IV (adult: 250-375 mg/24 hr) Epilepsy: 8-30 mg/kg/24 hr q6-8hr PO, IM, IV (maximum: 1 g/24 hr)	Carbonic anhydrase inhibitor; IM painful; half-life: 4-10 hr; prophylaxis for high-altitude sickness; Table 16-3 Tox: hypokalemia, acidosis (long-term therapy), paresthesias
Acetylcysteine (Mucomyst) Sol'n: 10% (100 mg/ml) 20% (200 mg/ml)	Acetaminophen OD: load 140 mg/kg PO, then 70 mg/kg q4hr PO × 17 doses Nebulizer: 2-20 ml (10%) or 1-10 ml (20%) sol'n q2-6hr	Primary treatment for acetaminophen overdose (Chapter 55); pulmonary mucolytic; IV preparation available (investigational) Tox: mucosal irritant, bronchospasm
Acyclovir (Zovirax) Cap: 200 mg Vial: 500 mg/10 ml Ointment: 5%	Herpes genitalis: 200 mg q4hr (5 doses/24 hr) PO × 5-10 days Herpes neonatorum: 30 mg/kg/24 hr q8hr IV × 10 days Varicella: 80 mg/kg/24 hr q6hr PO × 5 days (maximum: 3200 mg/24 hr)	IV therapy indicated in immunocompromised patient; effective in newborn; modified dose for recurrent episode or suppression; reduce with renal failure Tox: diaphoresis, hematuria, phlebitis (IV)
Adenosine (Adenocard) Vial: 3 mg/ml	0.1-0.2 mg/kg bolus as rapidly as possible; may repeat and double in 2 min if unsuccessful Adult: 6 mg IV as rapid (1-2 min) bolus; repeat 12 mg IV up to 2 times if no response in 2 min	No controlled studies in children but commonly used for paroxysmal supraventricular tachycardia Tox: facial flushing, dyspnea, nausea, metallic taste

Many oral drugs may be given 3-4 times/day with more flexibility than implied by the specific intervals noted. Adult dose provided as guideline for maximum dose. *NB*, Newborns <7 days of age; *Pen*, penicillin; *SR*, sustained release; *Tox*, toxicity of drug.

APPENDIX C-1 Common Medications—cont'd

Drugs	Dosages	Comments
Albumin 25% salt-poor albumin (25 g/dl) 5% with 0.9% NS (5 g/dl)	0.5-1 g/kg/dose IV repeated prn	Salt-poor albumin has 0.6 mEq Na^+/g; caution with hypervolemia, CHF
Albuterol (Proventil, Ventolin) Syr: 2 mg/5 ml Sol'n (inhalation): 0.5%: 5 mg/ml Tab: 2, 4 mg	Inhalation: 0.03 ml (0.15 mg)/kg/dose to maximum of 0.5-1.0 ml/dose diluted in 2 ml 0.9% NS; may repeat q20min × 3 or as needed Oral: 0.1-0.2 mg/kg/dose q6-8hr PO (maximum: 4 mg/dose)	β_2 Agonist with little cardiac effect; higher dosage more effective; available as MDI; single isomer available (levalbuterol)
Allopurinol (Zyloprim) Tab: 100, 300 mg	10 mg/kg/24 hr q6hr PO (<6 yr, 150 mg/24 hr; 6-10 yr: 300 mg/24 hr) (maximum: 600 mg/24 hr)	Titrate to serum uric acid level; reduce dosage with renal failure Tox: rash, hepatic, cataract
Aluminum hydroxide (Amphojel) Tab: 300, 600 mg Susp: 320 mg/5 ml **Maalox** (also magnesium hydroxide) Tab: 200/200, 400/400 mg Susp: 225/200 mg/5 ml	Peptic ulcer: 5-15 ml (adult: 15-45 ml) 1 and 3 hr after meals and before bed PO Prophylaxis GI bleeding; infant: 2-5 ml/dose q1-2hr PO; child: 5-15 ml/dose (adult: 30-60 ml) q1-2hr PO	Should be initiated early for prophylaxis; alternatives include cimetidine
Amantidine (Symmetrel) Syr: 50 mg/5 ml Cap: 100 mg	4.4-8.8 mg/kg/24 hr q12hr PO (>9 yr and adult: 100 mg q12hr PO or 200 mg q24hr PO)	Continue for at least 10 days and longer in unprotected high-risk patient with ongoing exposure to influenza A; only children >1 yr; effective if given early Tox: depression, CHF, psychosis, seizures
Amikacin (Amikin) Vial: 50, 250 mg/ml	15 mg/kg/24 hr q8hr IM, IV slowly over 30 min (maximum: 1.0 g/24 hr) (NB: 15 mg/kg/24 hr q12hr)	Therapeutic peak level: <35 μg/ml: caution in renal failure (reduce dosage) Tox: renal, CN VIII
Aminocaproic acid (Amicar) Syr: 250 mg/ml Tab: 500 mg Vial: 250 mg/ml	Load: 200 mg/kg PO (maximum: 6 g); 100 mg/kg/dose q6hr PO (maximum: 24 g/24 hr) × 5-7 days or until healing occurs Load: 100 mg/kg IV, then 33.3 mg/kg/hr IV up to 30 g/24 hr	Useful for oral bleeding; also available for IV use; Chapter 79 Tox: thrombosis, rash, hypotension Reduce dose with renal disease

Continued

APPENDIX C-1 Common Medications—cont'd

Drugs	Dosages	Comments
Aminophylline	Load: 7.5 mg/kg PO; maintenance: 5 mg/kg/dose q6hr PO Load: 6 mg/kg IV slowly, maintenance: 0.8-1.2 mg/kg/hr IV Neonatal apnea load: 5 mg/kg; then 2-3 mg/kg q12hr PO	85% theophylline: therapeutic level: 10-20 μg/ml; neonatal apnea (Chapter 84) Tox: nausea, vomiting, irritability, seizures, dysrhythmias
Amiodarone (Cardarone) Vial: 50 mg/ml Tab: 200 mg	Load: 5 mg/kg IV (maximum: 15 mg/kg/24 hr) 10 mg/kg/24 hr q12hr PO × 7-10 days, then reduce to 5 mg/kg/24 hr (maximum: 15 mg/kg/24 hr for 2-3 wk) (adult: load with 800-1600 mg/24 hr for 1-3 wk, then 600-800 mg/24 hr × 1 mo, then 200-400 mg/24 hr)	If pulseless VF or VT, administer rapidly; if perfusing tachycardia, give IV over 20-60 min; avoid combination with drugs prolonging QT interval
Amoxicillin (Amoxil, Larotid) Susp: 125, 250 mg/5 ml Cap: 125, 250 mg	30-100 mg (average: 50 mg)/kg/24 hr q8hr PO (adult: 250-500 mg q8hr)	Do not use for *Shigella* Tox: similar to ampicillin but less diarrhea; see Penicillin G
Amoxicillin (AMX)-clavulanic acid (CLA) (Augmentin) Susp: 125 mg AMX/31.25 CLA/5 ml, 250 mg AMX/62.50 CLA/5 ml Tab: 250 mg AMX/125 CLA, 500 mg AMX/125 CLA Tab (chew): 125 mg AMX/31.25 CLA, 250 mg AMX/62.5 CLA	30-50 mg AMX/kg/24 hr q8hr PO (adult: 250-500 mg AMX q8hr PO)	Dosage is based on amount of amoxicillin; 2 tab 250 mg are not equivalent to 500 mg tab; β-lactamase inhibitor Tox: diarrhea, similar to amoxicillin
Amphotericin (Fungizone) Vial: 50 mg	0.6 mg/kg/24 hr IV over 1-4 hours; begin at 0.2 mg/kg/24 hr and increase dosage	May also be given intrathecal; only for severe fungal infection; initial test dose 0.1 mg/kg over 20-60 min Tox: fever, chills, bone marrow suppression
Ampicillin (Omnipen, Polycillin) Susp: 125, 250 mg/5 ml Cap: 250, 500 mg Vial: 250, 500, 1000 mg	50-100 mg/kg/24 hr q6hr PO (adult: 250-500 mg/dose PO); 100-400 mg/kg/24 hr q4-6hr IV (NB: 50-100 mg/kg/24 hr q12hr IV) (adult: 4-12 g/24 hr IV)	Higher parenteral doses with severe infection: 3 mEq Na^+/g Tox: rash (especially with infectious mononucleosis), diarrhea, superinfection; see Penicillin G

Many oral drugs may be given 3-4 times/day with more flexibility than implied by the specific intervals noted. Adult dose provided as guideline for maximum dose. *NB*, Newborns <7 days of age; *Pen*, penicillin; *SR*, sustained release; *Tox*, toxicity of drug.

APPENDIX C-1 Common Medications—cont'd

Drugs	Dosages	Comments
Ampicillin (AMP)/Sulbactam (SUL) (Unasyn) Vial: 1.5, 3 g	Adult: 1 g AMP/0.5 g SUL q6hr IV	Intraabdominal, gynecologic infections; semisynthetic β-lactamase inhibitor Little experience in children <12 yr
Aspirin (salicylate, ASA) Tab: 81 (chew), 325 mg Supp: 65, 130, 195, 325 mg	10-15 mg/kg/dose q4-6hr PO (adult: 10 gr or 650 mg/dose) Rheumatoid: 60-100 mg/kg/24 hr q4-6hr PO (maximum: 3.6 g/24 hr PO)	Synergistic antipyretic effect with acetaminophen; avoid with chickenpox or influenza-like illness Therapeutic level: 15-30 mg/dl Tox: GI irritation, tinnitus, platelet dysfunction; overdose (Chapter 54)
Atenolol (Tenormin) Tab: 50, 100 mg	Hypertension: 1-2 mg/kg/dose q24hr PO (adult: 50 mg q24hr PO up to 100 mg q24hr PO)	Little experience in children; response seen in 1 wk; also available for IV use
Atropine Vial: 0.1, 0.4, 1 mg/ml	0.02 mg/kg/dose IV (minimum: 0.1 mg/dose) (adult: 0.6-1.0 mg/dose; maximum total dose 2 mg) q5min prn; may also be given ET	Infants require higher dose (0.03 mg/kg); organophosphate poisoning (0.05 mg/kg) (Chapter 54) Tox: dysrhythmias, anticholinergic
Azithromycin (Zithromax) Cap: 250 mg Pack: 1 g	Otitis media: 10 mg/kg/24 hr q24hr PO followed by half dose on days 2-5 Pharyngitis: 12 mg/kg/24 hr q24hr PO × 5 days Uncomplicated genital chlamydia: 1 g PO	Pharyngitis relapse high
Beclomethasone (Beclovent, Vanceril) MDI (inhalation: 42 μg/dose)	6-12 yr: 1-2 puffs QID >12 yr: 2 puffs QID	
Benztropine (Cogentin) Tab: 0.5, 1, 2 mg Vial: 1 mg/ml	>3 yr: 0.02-0.05 mg/kg/dose q12-24hr PO, IV Adult: 1-4 mg/dose IV	Pediatric dose not well established
Bethanechol (Urecholine) Tab: 5, 10, 25 mg Vial: 5 mg/ml	0.6 mg/kg/24 hr q8hr PO (adult: 10-30 mg QID PO) 0.15-0.2 mg/kg/24 hr SC (adult: 2.5-5 mg/24 hr)	

Continued

APPENDIX C-1 Common Medications—cont'd

Drugs	Dosages	Comments
Bicarbonate, sodium ($NaHCO_3$) Vial: 8.4% (50 mEq/50 ml) 7.5% (44 mEq/50 ml) 4.2% (0.5 mEq/ml) for newborns	1 mEq/kg/dose q10min IV prn	Monitor ABG: dilute 1:1 with D5W or sterile water; incompatible with calcium, catecholamines Tox: alkalosis, hyperosmolality, hypernatremia
Budesonide (Pulmicort Turbuhaler) 200 μg/metered dose	>6 yr: 1-2 puffs BID Adult: 2 puffs BID	Inhaled steroid for long-term management of asthma
Bumetanide (Bumex) Vial: 0.25 mg/ml Tab: 0.5, 1 mg	Begin with 0.015-0.1 mg/kg/dose q8-12hr IV up to a maximum of 0.3 mg/kg/dose or 10 mg/24 hr	Limited experience in children
Calcium chloride Vial: 10% (100 mg/ml-1.36 mEq Ca^{++}/ml)	20-30 mg/kg/dose IV (slow) (maximum: 500 mg/dose) q10min prn; 250 mg/kg/24 hr q6hr PO (mix 2% soln)	Monitor heart, avoid extravasation; caution in digitalized patient; incompatible with $NaHCO_3$ Tox: bradycardia, hypotension
Calcium gluconate Vial: 10% (100 mg/ml-0.45 mEq Ca^{++}/ml) Tab: 1 g	100 mg/kg dose IV (slow) (maximum: 1 g/dose) q10 min prn; 500 mg/kg/24 hr q6hr PO	See Calcium chloride
Captopril (Capoten) Tab: 12.5, 25, 50, 100 mg	1-6 mg/kg/24 hr q8hr PO (maximum: 450 mg/24 hr) (adult: initial 25 mg q8hr PO)	Table 18-2 Tox: renal, proteinuria, neutropenia, rash
Carbamazepine (Tegretol) Tab: 100 mg (chewable), 200 mg	10-40 mg/kg/24 hr q8-12hr PO (adult: 800-1600 mg/24 hr; begin 100-200 mg/dose q12hr PO with 100 mg/24 hr increments)	Therapeutic level: 4-14 μg/ml: Table 81-6 Tox: hepatic, nystagmus, nausea, aplastic anemia
Carbenicillin (Geopen, Geocillin) Vial: 1, 2, 5, 10 g Tab: 382 mg	400-600 mg/kg/24 hr q4-6hr IV; 30-50 mg/kg/24 hr q6h PO (NB: 200 mg/kg/24 hr q12hr IV) (adult: 40 g/24 hr IV; 2 g/24 hr PO)	Used in combination therapy with aminoglycoside; 5.2-6.5 mEq Na^+/g Tox: platelet dysfunction, rash; adjust dose with renal failure; see Penicillin G

Many oral drugs may be given 3-4 times/day with more flexibility than implied by the specific intervals noted. Adult dose provided as guideline for maximum dose. *NB*, Newborns <7 days of age; *Pen*, penicillin; *SR*, sustained release; *Tox*, toxicity of drug.

APPENDIX C-1 Common Medications—cont'd

Drugs	Dosages	Comments
Cefaclor (Ceclor) Susp: 125, 250 mg/5 ml Cap: 250, 500 mg	20-40 mg/kg/24 hr q8hr PO (adult: 250-500 mg q8hr)	Active against ampicillin-resistant *H. influenzae*; second-generation cephalosporin Tox: renal, diarrhea, vaginitis; cross-reacts with penicillin
Cefadroxil (Duricef) Susp: 125, 250, 500 mg/5 ml Cap: 500 mg Tab: 1 g	30 mg/kg/24 hr q12hr PO (maximum: 2 g/24 hr)	Relatively long half-life; first-generation cephalosporin Tox: diarrhea, pruritus; cross-reacts with penicillin
Cefazolin (Ancef) Vial: 0.25, 0.5, 1 g	25-100 mg/kg/24 hr q6-8hr IM, IV (NB: 40 mg/kg/24 hr q12hr) (adult: 2-12 g/24 hr)	First-generation cephalosporin Tox: renal, hepatic, rash, phlebitis; cross-reacts with penicillin; adjust dosage with renal failure
Cefixime (Suprax) Syr: 100 mg/5 ml Tab: 200, 400 mg	8 mg/kg/24 hr q12-24hr PO (adult: 400 mg/24 hr)	Third-generation cephalosporin
Cefoperazone (Cefobid) Vial: 1, 2 g	100-150 mg/kg/24 hr q8-12hr IV (maximum: 12 g/24 hr) Adult: 2-12 g/24 hr q6-12hr IV slowly, IM	Third-generation cephalosporin; limited experience in children; half-life 2 hr Tox: diarrhea, hypersensitivity
Cefotaxime (Claforan) Vial: 1, 2 g	50-150 mg/kg/24 hr q6-8hr IV, IM (neonatal meningitis: 100-150 mg/kg/24 hr q8-12hr) (adult: 1-2 g q4-6hr up to maximum: 12 g/24 hr)	Third-generation cephalosporin; excellent broad-spectrum coverage; meningitis, UTI, bacteremia, pneumonia, skin infection; half-life 1 hr Tox: hypersensitivity (cross-reacts with penicillin), phlebitis, pain (IM), diarrhea, colitis, renal, hepatic
Cefoxitin (Mefoxin) Vial: 1, 2 g	80-160 mg/kg/24 hr q4-6hr IV (maximum: 12 g/24 hr) PID: adult: 2 g q6hr IV	Second-generation cephalosporin; good anaerobic coverage Tox: pain at site if IM injection, nausea, vomiting; adjust dosage with renal failure

Continued

APPENDIX C-1 Common Medications—cont'd

Drugs	Dosages	Comments
Cefpodoxime (Vantin) Susp: 50, 100 mg/5 ml Tab: 100, 200 mg	10 mg/kg/24 hr q12hr PO (maximum: 800 mg/24 hr)	Second-generation cephalosporin
Cefprozil (Cefzil) Susp: 125, 250 mg/5 ml Tab: 250, 500 mg	15-30 mg/kg/24 hr q12hr PO (maximum: 1000 mg/24 hr)	Second-generation cephalosporin
Ceftazidime (Fortaz) Vial: 0.5, 1, 2 g	100-150 mg/kg/24 hr q8hr IV (adult: 3-6 g/24 hr)	Third-generation cephalosporin; limited CNS data Tox: diarrhea; cross-reacts with penicillin
Ceftizoxime (Cefizox) Vial: 1, 2 g	150-200 mg/kg/24 hr q6-8hr IV (neonatal meningitis: 100-200 mg/kg/24 hr q8-12hr IV) (adult: 6-12 g/24 hr)	Third-generation cephalosporin Tox: diarrhea; cross-reacts with penicillin
Ceftriaxone (Rocephin) Vial: 0.25, 0.5, 1, 2 g	50-100 mg/kg/24 hr q12-24hr IV, IM (adult: 1-2 g/dose q12-24hr IV, IM)	Third-generation cephalosporin; use in children >1 mo; less frequent administration; half-life 5-8 hr; reports of delayed CNS sterilization Tox: diarrhea, abnormal liver function, cholecystitis
Cefuroxime (Zinacef, Ceftin) Vial: 750, 1500 mg Tab: 125, 250, 500 mg	50-240 mg/kg/24 hr q6-8hr IV (adult: 4.5-9.0 g/24 hr q6-8hr IV) 30 mg/kg/24 hr q12hr PO; >12 yr: 250-500 mg q12hr PO	Second-generation cephalosporin; oral formulation; higher dosage IV for meningitis but slower sterilization; useful for *H. influenzae* disease; do not use for neonatal meningitis, sepsis; oral form for nontoxic child with respiratory, skin, or urinary infections; 5 days oral treatment for otitis media
Cephalexin (Keflex) Susp: 125, 250 mg/5 ml Cap: 250, 500 mg	25-50 mg/kg/24 hr q6hr PO (adult: 250-500 mg/dose q6hr)	First-generation cephalosporin Tox: nausea, vomiting, renal, hepatic; cross-reacts with penicillin; adjust dosage with renal failure

Many oral drugs may be given 3-4 times/day with more flexibility than implied by the specific intervals noted. Adult dose provided as guideline for maximum dose. *NB*, Newborns <7 days of age; *Pen*, penicillin; *SR*, sustained release; *Tox*, toxicity of drug.

APPENDIX C-1 Common Medications—cont'd

Drugs	Dosages	Comments
Cephalothin (Keflin) Vial: 1, 2, 4 g	75-125 mg/kg/24 hr q4-6hr IM, IV (NB: 40 mg/kg/24 hr q12hr) (adult: 4-12 g/24 hr)	First-generation cephalosporin Tox: renal, hepatic, phlebitis, neutropenia; cross-reacts with penicillin; adjust dosage with renal failure
Cephradine (Anspor, Velosef) Susp: 125, 250 mg/5 ml Cap: 250, 500 mg Vial: 0.25, 0.5, 1 g	25-50 mg/kg/24 hr q6hr PO; 50-100 mg/kg/24 hr q6hr IM (deep), IV (maximum: 4 g/24 hr)	First-generation cephalosporin Tox: renal, hepatic, nausea, vomiting, neutropenia, vaginitis, phlebitis, cross-reacts with penicillin; adjust dosage with renal failure
Charcoal, activated	1 g/kg or 15-50 g PO (adult: 50-100 g/dose)	First dose may be mixed with 35%-70% sorbitol; may require NG tube for administration
Chloral hydrate (Noctec) Syr: 500 mg/5 ml (also 250 mg/5 ml) Cap: 250, 500 mg	Hypnotic: 50-100 mg/kg/24 hr q6-8hr PO (maximum: 1 g/dose in children; 2 g/dose in adults) Sedative: ½ hypnotic dose	Hypnotic dose often needed for sedation; do not use with renal, hepatic disease; two strengths of syrup
Chloramphenicol (Chloromycetin) Susp: 150 mg/5 ml Cap: 250 mg Vial: 1 g (100 mg/ml)	50-100 mg/kg/24 hr q6hr IV (NB: 25 mg/kg/24 hr q12hr IV) (adult: maximum 2-4 g/24 hr)	Tox: bone marrow suppression (reversible) and aplastic anemia; therapeutic level: 10-25 μg/ml
Chloroquine phosphate (Aralen) Tab: 500 mg (300 mg base)	10 mg base/kg/24 hr q24hr PO	Several forms available; see Appendix C-3
Chlorothiazide (Diuril) Susp: 250 mg/5 ml Tab: 250, 500 mg	10-20 mg/kg/24 hr q12hr PO (NB: 30 mg/kg/24 hr PO) (adult: 500-1000 mg q12-24hr PO)	Table 16-3 Tox: hyponatremia, hypokalemia, alkalosis; reduce dosage with renal failure
Chlorpheniramine (Chlor-Trimeton) Syr: 2 mg/5 ml Tab: 4 mg Tab/cap (SR): 8, 12 mg	0.35 mg/kg/24 hr q6hr PO (adult: 4 mg q4-6hr) Sustained release in children >12 yr: 16-24 mg/kg/24 hr q8-12hr PO	OTC antihistamine Tox: drowsiness, anticholinergic (Chapter 55), hypotension (IM)
Chlorpromazine (Thorazine) Syr: 10 mg/5 ml Tab: 10, 25, 50, 100 mg Cap (SR): 30, 75, 150 mg Supp: 25, 100 mg Vial: 25 mg/ml	0.5 mg/kg/dose q6-8hr PO, IM, IV prn (adult: 25-50 mg/dose) 1.0 mg/kg/dose q6-8hr PR prn (adult: 50-100 mg/dose PR)	Only children >6 mo old Tox: phenothiazine-extrapyramidal, anticholinergic (Chapter 55)

Continued

APPENDIX C-1 Common Medications—cont'd

Drugs	Dosages	Comments
Cimetidine (Tagamet) Susp: 300 mg/5 ml Tab: 200, 300 mg Vial: 150 mg/ml	20-30 mg/kg/24 hr q6hr PO, IV (maximum: 2.4 g/24 hr) (adult: 300 mg/dose q6hr PO)	Tox: diarrhea renal, neutropenia; reduce dosage with renal failure
Ciprofloxacin (Cipro) Tab: 250, 500, 750 mg	Adult: 250-750 mg q12hr PO	Should not be used in children <12 yr (probably causes arthropathy); reduce dosage if impaired renal function
Clarithromycin (Biaxin) Susp: 125, 250 mg/5 ml Tab: 250, 500 mg	15 mg/kg/24 hr q12hr PO Adult: 250-500 mg q12hr PO	Increases theophylline and carbamazepine levels; do not refrigerate oral suspension
Clindamycin (Cleocin) Sol'n, topical: 1% Cap: 75, 150 mg Amp: 300, 600 mg	10-25 mg/kg/24 hr q6hr PO (adult: 600-1800 mg/24 hr PO) 15-40 mg/kg/24 hr q6-8hr IM, IV (NB: 15-20 mg/kg/24 hr q6-8hr IV) (maximum: 4.8 g/ 24 hr IV)	Caution in renal, hepatic disease; topical solution useful for acne Tox: colitis, rash, diarrhea, phlebitis; only for child >1 mo
Clonazepam (Klonopin) Tab: 0.5, 1, 2 mg	0.05-0.2 mg/kg/24 hr q8-12hr PO; start at 0.01 mg/kg/24 hr and add 0.25-0.5 mg/24 hr q3days until control (adult: 1.5-2.0 mg/ 24 hr) (maximum total dose: 20 mg/24 hr)	Therapeutic level: 0.013-0.072 μg/ml; caution in renal disease; titrate dosage slowly every third day; Table 81-6; previously Clonopin Tox: drowsiness, ataxia, personality change
Clonidine (Catapres) Tab: 0.1, 0.2, 0.3 mg	0.005-0.01 mg/kg/24 hr q6hr PO (maximum: 0.9 mg/24 hr) (adult: 0.1 mg q12hr PO initially; increase 0.1-0.2 mg/24 hr up to 2.4 mg/24 hr PO)	May be used acutely in hypertension; widely used for ADHD (initial dose: 0.05 mg/24 hr) Tox: drowsiness, headache, dysrhythmia
Clotrimazole (Gyne-Lotrimin, Mycelex) Tab (vag): 100 mg Cream (vag): 1%	1 tablet or applicatorful vaginally nightly × 7-14 days	Tox: local irritation
Cloxacillin (Tegopen) Sol'n: 125 mg/5 ml Cap: 250, 500 mg	50-100 mg/kg/24 hr q6hr PO (maximum: 4 g/24 hr)	Administer on empty stomach Tox: GI irritant, see Penicillin G

Many oral drugs may be given 3-4 times/day with more flexibility than implied by the specific intervals noted. Adult dose provided as guideline for maximum dose. *NB*, Newborns <7 days of age; *Pen*, penicillin; *SR*, sustained release; *Tox*, toxicity of drug.

APPENDIX C-1 Common Medications—cont'd

Drugs	Dosages	Comments
Codeine Elix: 10 mg/5 ml (with antitussive) Tab: 15, 30, 60 mg Vial: 30, 60 mg/ml	Analgesic: 0.5-1.0 mg/kg/dose q4-6hr PO, IM (adult: 30-60 mg/dose) Antitussive: 1.0 mg/kg/24 hr q4-6hr PO (adult: 10-20 mg/dose)	Also available combined with acetaminophen 120 mg with 12 mg codeine/5 ml and tablets (acetaminophen 300 mg with 7.5 mg codeine [#1], 15 mg codeine [#2], or 30 mg codeine [#3]). Tox: dependence, CNS and respiratory depression (Chapter 55)
Cortisone Tab: 5, 10, 25 mg Vial: 25, 50 mg/ml	Maintenance: 0.25 mg/kg/24 hr q12-24hr IM; 0.50-0.75 mg/kg/24 hr q6-8hr PO	Table 74-2
Cromolyn (Intal) Vial: 20 mg powder/sol'n	20 mg q6-8hr by nebulization	MDI may also be used to administer; for ongoing management of bronchospasm
Cyproheptadine (Periactin) Syr: 2 mg/5 ml Tab: 4 mg	0.25 mg/kg/24 hr q8-12hr PO (adult: 12-16 mg/24 hr)	
Dantrolene (Dantrium) Cap: 25 mg Vial: 20 mg	0.5 mg/kg/dose q12hr PO, then increase to 0.5 mg/kg/dose q6-8hr PO and increase up to maximum of 3 mg/kg/dose	Little information about use in children <5 yr; IV solution for surgical prophylaxis for malignant hyperthermia (1 mg/kg IV; repeat up to total dose of 10 mg/kg)
Deferoxamine (Desferal) Amp: 500 mg	If no shock: 90 mg/kg/dose q8hr IM (adult: 1-2 g/dose × 1; maximum: 6 g/24 hr) If shock: 15 mg/kg/hr IV	Urine turns rose colored if SI >TIBC in iron overdose; Chapter 55 Tox: urticaria, hypotension
Dexamethasone (Decadron) Vial: 4, 24 mg Elix: 0.5 mg/5 ml Tab: 1.5, 4, 6 mg	Croup: 0.25-0.6 mg/kg/dose q6hr IM, IV, PO Meningitis: 0.15 mg/kg/dose q6hr IV × 16 doses	Table 74-2
Dextrose D5W (0.5 g/ml)	0.5-1.0 g (2-4 ml D25W)/kg/dose IV	Dilute D50W 1:1 to prevent hypertonicity; measure glucose

Continued

APPENDIX C-1 Common Medications—cont'd

Drugs	Dosages	Comments
Diazepam (Valium) Tab: 2, 5, 10 mg Vial: 5 mg/ml	Status epilepticus: 0.2-0.3 mg/kg/dose IV (<1 mg/min) q2-5 min prn (maximum total dose: child, 10 mg; adult, 30 mg) Sedation, muscle relaxation: 0.1-0.8 mg/kg/24 hr q6-8hr PO	If used for status epilepticus, must initiate additional drug; may be given as 0.5 mg/kg/dose PR; respiratory depression (Chapter 55); see flumazenil Tox: drowsiness, respiratory depression (increased with second drug)
Diazoxide (Hyperstat) Vial: 15 mg/ml	1-3 mg/kg/dose q4-24hr IV up to 150 mg/dose (fast); repeat in 30 min if no effect; may use intermittent smaller dose	Vasodilator: prompt (3-5 min) response (Table 18-2); also used to treat hyperinsulinemic hypoglycemia
Dicloxacillin (Dynapen) Susp: 62.5 mg/5 ml Cap: 125, 250, 500 mg	25-100 mg/kg/24 hr q6hr PO (adult: 125-500 mg/dose)	Do not use for NB; although optimally given on empty stomach, may have to use open capsule mixed with food Tox: GI irritant, see Penicillin G
Dicyclomine (Bentyl) Syr: 10 mg/5 ml Cap: 10, 20 mg	Children (>6 mo): 5-10 mg/dose q6-8hr PO; adult: 20-40 mg/dose q6-8hr PO	
Digoxin	See Tables 6-4 and 16-2	
Dimercaprol (BAL in oil) Amp: 100 mg/ml	Mild gold or arsenic poisoning: 2.5 mg/kg q6hr IM × 2 days, q8hr × 1 day, then q24hr × 10 days Severe arsenic or gold poisoning: 3 mg/kg q4hr × 2 days, q6hr × 1 day, then q12hr × 10 days Mercury poisoning: 5 mg/kg initially, then 2.5 mg/kg q12-24hr × 10 days Lead encephalopathy: 4 mg/kg/dose q4hr in combination with edetate calcium disodium × 2-7 days; if less severe, 3 mg/kg/dose	

Many oral drugs may be given 3-4 times/day with more flexibility than implied by the specific intervals noted. Adult dose provided as guideline for maximum dose. *NB*, Newborns <7 days of age; *Pen*, penicillin; *SR*, sustained release; *Tox*, toxicity of drug.

APPENDIX C-1 Common Medications—cont'd

Drugs	Dosages	Comments
Diphenhydramine (Benadryl) Elix: 12.5 mg/5 ml Cap: 25, 50 mg Vial: 10, 50 mg/ml	5 mg/kg/24 hr q6hr PO, IM, IV (maximum: 300 mg/24 hr) Anaphylaxis or phenothiazine overdose: 1-2 mg/kg/dose q6hr PO, IM, IV	Antihistamine: OTC Tox: sedation, anticholinergic (Chapter 55); may inhibit breast milk
Diphenoxylate with atropine (Lomotil) Tab: 2.5 mg DPL/0.025 ATP Liq: 2.5 mg DPL/0.025 ATP/5 ml	0.3-0.4 mg DPL/kg/24 hr q6hr PO (adult: 2 tab QID PO)	Not recommended in children <2 yr; use liquid in children <13 yr; reduce dosage or discontinue after control; prevent accidental ingestion
Dobutamine (Dobutrex) Vial: 250 mg	2-20 μg/kg/min IV infusion (maximum: 40 μg/kg/min IV) **Dilute:** 6 mg × weight (kg) in 100 ml D5W. Rate of infusion in μg/kg/min = ml/hr (1 ml/hr delivers 1 μg/kg/min); **or** 250 mg (1 vial) in 500 ml D5W = 500 μg/ml	Table 5-2
Docusate (Colace) Syr: 20 mg/5 ml Cap: 50, 100 mg	3-5 mg/kg/24 hr TID PO; (adult: 60-480 mg/24 hr)	
Dopamine (Intropin) Amp: 40 mg/ml Vial: 80 mg, 160 mg/ml	Low: 2-5 μg/kg/min IV drip Mod: 5-20 μg/kg/min IV drip High: >20 μg/kg/min IV drip **Dilute:** 6 mg × weight (kg) in 100 ml D5W. Rate of infusion in μg/kg/min = ml/hr (1 ml/hr delivers 1 μg/kg/min); **or** 200 mg (1 amp of 5 ml) in 500 ml D5W = 400 μg/ml	Table 5-2
Doxycycline (Vibramycin) Syr/susp: 25, 50 mg/5 ml Cap: 50, 100 mg Vial: 100, 200 mg	5 mg/kg/24 hr q12hr PO or IV slowly over 2-4 hr (adult: 100-200 mg/24 hr)	Do not use in children <9 yr of age Tox: GI irritant, hepatic, photosensitization, superinfection; adjust dosage with renal failure; BR
Droperidol (Inapsine) Vial: 2.5 mg/ml	0.1 mg/kg/dose IM, IV for anesthetic premedication; 0.05 mg/kg/dose q4-6hr prn for nausea, vomiting (adult: 1.25-5 mg/dose IM, IV)	Monitor respirations; minimal pediatric data; associated QT prolongation and torsades de pointes; perform ECG before prescribing; other agents usually preferred

Continued

APPENDIX C-1 Common Medications—cont'd

Drugs	Dosages	Comments
Edrophonium (Tensilon)		
Vial: 10 mg/ml	Test for myasthenia gravis: 0.2 mg/kg/dose and if no response in 1 min, give 1-mg increments up to maximum total dose of 5-10 mg IV (adult test dose: 2 mg) (NB: 1 mg single dose IV)	Have atropine available; may precipitate cholinergic crisis
Epinephrine (Adrenalin)		
Vial (1:1000-1 mg/ml) (1: 10,000-0.1 mg/ml) Sus-Phrine (1:200-5 mg/ml in oil)	Asthma: 0.01 ml (1:1000)/kg/dose (maximum: 0.35 ml/dose) q15-20min SC prn × 3 Asystole: 0.1 ml (1:10,000)/kg/ dose (maximum: 5 ml/dose) IV initially; subsequent dose and initial ET dose is 0.1 mg/kg or 0.1 ml/kg of 1:1000 solution Shock; 0.05-1 μg/kg/min IV infusion **Dilute** (for infusion in shock): 0.6 mg × weight (kg) in 100 ml D5W. Rate of infusion in 0.1 μg/kg/min = ml/hr (1 ml/hr delivers 0.1 μg/kg/min; **or** 1 mg in 500 ml D5W = 2 μg/ml	Inhalation (albuterol, terbutaline) therapy preferred for asthma Use in shock only after isoproterenol and dopamine are ineffective; not effective with acidotic patient; Table 5-2 Tox: tachycardia, dysrhythmia, tremor, hypertension
Epinephrine, racemic		
Soln: 2.25%	0.25-0.75 ml in 2.5 ml of sterile water or saline administered by nebulizer	Rebounds, always observe patient; often given with steroids; some bronchodilator effect
Erythromycin (Pediamycin, E.E.S., Erythrocin, E-Mycin, ERYC) Susp: 200, 400 mg/5 ml Tab: 200 (chew), 250, 400, 500 mg	20-50 mg/kg/24 hr q6hr PO (adult: 250-1000 mg/dose)	Also available as combination: erythromycin 200 mg + sulfisoxazole 600 mg/5 ml (Pediazole) Tox: GI irritant, rash
Ethambutol (Myambutol)		
Tab: 100, 400 mg	Initial TB treatment: 15 mg/kg q24hr PO Retreatment: 25 mg/kg q24hr PO	Multiple drug treatment indicated; monthly eye examination advised

Many oral drugs may be given 3-4 times/day with more flexibility than implied by the specific intervals noted. Adult dose provided as guideline for maximum dose. *NB*, Newborns <7 days of age; *Pen*, penicillin; *SR*, sustained release; *Tox*, toxicity of drug.

APPENDIX C-1 Common Medications—cont'd

Drugs	Dosages	Comments
Ethanol		
100% (1 ml = 790 mg)	Methanol, ethylene glycol overdose: 1 ml/kg over 15 min, then 0.15 ml (125 mg)/kg/hr IV	Maintain ethanol level at ≥100 mg/dl; Table 54-4
Ethosuximide (Zarontin)		
Syr: 250 mg/5 ml Cap: 250 mg	20-40 mg/kg/24 hr q12-24hr PO; begin 250 mg q24hr (3-6 yr old) and increase 250 mg/24 hr at 4- to 7-day interval; maximum: 1.5 g/24 hr	Therapeutic level: 40-100 μg/ml; Table 81-6 Tox: GI irritant, neutropenia, drowsiness, dizziness, headache
Factor VIII, IX		
	Tables 79-2 and 79-3	
Famciclovir (Famvir)		
Tab: 125, 250, 500 mg	Adult: 500 mg/dose q8hr × 7 days	Preferably begin within 12 hr of onset of rash; not studied in children <18 yrs
Famotidine (Pepcid)		
Tab: 20, 40 mg Susp: 40 mg/5 ml Vial: 10 mg/ml	1-2 mg/kg/24 hr q12-24hr IV, PO Adult: 20-40 mg q24hr PO; 20 mg q12hr IV	
Felbamate (Felbatol)	Table 81-6	
Fentanyl (Sublimaze)		
Amp: 50 μg/ml	1-5 μg/kg/dose IV slowly (adult: 50-100 μg/dose)	Narcotic; half-life: 20 min; monitor oxygenation and ventilation
Fexofenadine (Allegra) Cap: 60 mg	6-11 yr: 30 mg q12hr PO Adult: 60 mg q12hr PO	Second-generation H_1-receptor blocker; limited experience in children <12 yr
Fluconazole (Diflucan)		
Susp: 10, 40 mg/ml Tab: 50, 100, 200 mg	*Oral candidiasis*: load: 6 mg/kg PO; then 3 mg/kg/24 hr PO	Usually treat 2-3 weeks
Fludrocortisone (Florinef)		
Tab: 0.1 mg	0.05-0.1 mg/24 hr q24hr PO	
Flumazenil (Romazicon)		
Vial: 0.1 mg/ml	0.01 mg/kg initially, repeating 0.01 mg/kg q1min to a maximum total dose of 1 mg; adult: 0.2 mg IV initially; then 0.3 mg IV and then 0.5 mg if no response up to a cumulative dose of 3 mg	Management of suspected benzodiazepine overdose
Folic acid Tab: 0.1, 0.4, 1 mg	0.2-1.0 mg/24 hr PO (adult: 1-3 mg/24 hr)	
Fosphenytoin (Cerebyx)	See Phenytoin	
Furazolidone (Furoxone)		
Liq: 50 mg/15 ml Tab: 100 mg	*Giardia*: 6 mg/kg/24 hr q6hr PO (adult: 100 mg q6hr)	Do not use in children <1 mo; avoid alcohol; see Table 76-1 Tox: nausea, vomiting, rash

Continued

APPENDIX C-1 Common Medications—cont'd

Drugs	Dosages	Comments
Furosemide (Lasix) Sol'n: 10 mg/ml Tab: 20, 40, 80 mg Amp: 10 mg/ml	1 mg/kg/dose q6-12hr IV initially (may repeat q2hr IV prn); 2 mg/kg/dose q2-12hr PO initially; may increase dosage by 1 mg/kg increments (maximum: 6 mg/kg/dose PO, IM, IV)	Rapid acting; Table 16-3 Tox: hypokalemia, hyponatremia, alkalosis, prerenal azotemia; ototoxicity
Gabapentin (Neurontin)	See Table 81-6	
Gentamicin (Garamycin) Vial: 10, 40 mg/ml	5.0-7.5 mg/kg/24 hr q8hr IM, IV (maximum: 300 mg/24 hr) (NB: 5 mg/kg/24 hr q12hr) (adult: 3-5 mg/kg/24 hr q8hr)	Therapeutic peak level: 6-12 μg/ml; caution in renal failure (adjust dosage); slow IV infusion Tox: renal, VIII nerve
Glucagon Amp: 1 mg (1 unit)/ml	0.03-0.1 mg/kg/dose q20min SC, IM, IV prn (NB: 0.1-0.2 mg/kg/dose q4hr prn) (adult: 0.5-1.0 mg/dose)	Hypoglycemia: not adequate as only glucose support, especially in NB; treatment of propranolol (β-blocker) overdose
Glucose (see Dextrose)		
Griseofulvin Microsize (Grisactin, Grifulvin V) Susp: 125 mg/5 ml Tab/cap: 125, 250, 500 mg Ultramicrosize (Gris-PEG, Fulvicin P/G) Tab: 125, 250, 330 mg	Microsize: 10 mg/kg/24 hr q24hr PO (adult: 500-1000 mg q12-24hr PO) Ultramicrosize: 5 mg/kg/24 hr q24hr PO (adult: 250-500 mg/24 hr q12-24hr PO)	Give with meals; either formulation is adequate; treatment period of 4-6 wk Tox: renal, hepatic, neutropenia, rash, headache
Haloperidol (Haldol) Tab: 1, 2, 5, 10 mg Sol'n: 2 mg/ml Amp: 5 mg/ml, 100 mg/ml (decanoate)	Psychosis: 0.05-0.15 mg/kg/24 hr q8-12hr PO; begin at 0.5 mg/24 hr and increase Nonpsychotic behavior: 0.05-0.075 mg/kg/24 hr q8-12hr PO Adult: initial 0.5-2.0 mg/dose PO (maximum: 5 mg q8-12hr PO)	
Heparin (Liquaemin, Panheprin) Vial: 100, 1000, 5000, 10,000, 20,000, 40,000 units/ml	Load: 50-75 units/kg IV bolus Maint: 10-25 units/kg/hr IV infusion **or** 100 units/kg/dose q4hr IV Adult: load (5,000 units) with maint (20,000-30,000 unit over 24 hr IV continuous infusion **or** 5000-10,000 q4hr)	Titrate to maintain PTT at 2 times control; antidote: protamine Tox: bleeding, allergy rash, wheezing, anaphylaxis

Many oral drugs may be given 3-4 times/day with more flexibility than implied by the specific intervals noted. Adult dose provided as guideline for maximum dose. *NB*, Newborns <7 days of age; *Pen*, penicillin; *SR*, sustained release; *Tox*, toxicity of drug.

APPENDIX C-1 Common Medications—cont'd

Drugs	Dosages	Comments
Hydralazine (Apresoline) Tab: 10, 25, 50, 100 mg Amp: 20 mg/ml	Crisis: 0.1-0.4 mg/kg/dose (1.7-3.5 mg/kg/24 hr) q4-6hr IM, IV prn (adult: 10-40 mg/dose) Maintenance: 0.75-3 mg/kg/24 hr q6-12hr PO (adult: 10-75 mg/dose q6hr PO)	Vasodilator, prompt (10-30 min response if IV) decrease BP; may also be given as 1.5 μg/kg/min IV infusion; limited availability in parenteral form (being reformulated); Table 18-2 Tox: tachycardia, angina, SLE-like syndrome; reduce dosage with renal failure
Hydrochlorothiazide (Esidrix, HydroDiuril) Tab: 25, 50, 100 mg	1-2 mg/kg/24 hr q12hr PO (NB: 2-3 mg/kg/24 hr PO) (adult: 25-100 mg q12-24hr)	Table 16-3 Tox: hyponatremia, hypokalemia, alkalosis; reduce dosage with renal failure
Hydrocortisone (Solu-Cortef) Susp: 10 mg/5 ml Tab: 5, 10, 20 mg Vial: 100, 250, 500, 1000 mg	Maintenance: 0.5 mg/kg/24 hr q8hr PO Asthma: 4-5 mg/kg/dose q6hr IV	Table 74-2
Hydroxyzine (Atarax, Vistaril) Syr/susp: 10, 25 mg/5 ml Tab (Atarax): 10, 25, 50 mg Cap (Vistaril): 25, 50, 100 mg Vial (Vistaril): 25, 50 mg/ml	2 mg/kg/24 hr q6hr PO (adult: 200-400 mg/24 hr q6hr PO) 0.5-1 mg/kg/dose q4-6hr IM prn (adult: 25-100 mg/dose q4-6hr IM prn)	Antihistamine, potentiates meperidine, barbiturates Tox: sedation, anticholinergic (Chapter 55); may inhibit breast milk
Ibuprofen (Motrin) Tab: 300, 400, 600, 800 mg Susp: 100 mg/5 ml Chewable: 50, 100 mg	40 mg/kg/24 hr q6-8hr PO (adult: 1.2 g/24 hr) Adult: 200-400 mg q24hr PO; Maximum: 1.2 g/24 hr PO	Available over the counter. Tox: GI irritant, keratopathy, hematuria, retinopathy, rash
Imipenem (IMP)-**Cilastatin** (CIL) (Primaxin) Vial: 250 mg IMP/250 mg CIL, 500 mg IMP/500 mg CIL	(60 mg IMP + 60 mg CIL)/kg/24 hr q6hr IV (adult: 250-1000 mg IMP + 250-1000 mg CIL/dose) (maximum: 50 mg/kg/24 hr **or** 4 g/24 hr of each agent)	Limited experience in children but has been studied in those >3 mo Tox: phlebitis, diarrhea, renal
Imipramine (Tofranil) Tab: 10, 25, 50 mg	Enuresis: 25-75 mg at bedtime PO	
Immune serum globulin	Exposure to measles <1 yr of age (0.25 ml/kg IM) or immunocompromised (0.5 ml/kg IM); viral hepatitis type A contact within 14 days of exposure (0.02 ml/kg IM); and selected immunodeficiency disease; hepatitis B immune globulin (HBIG) is used with significant exposure to HBsAg-positive blood within 24 hr and 1 mo later (0.06 ml/kg/dose IM)	

Continued

APPENDIX C-1 Common Medications—cont'd

Drugs	Dosages	Comments
Indomethacin (Indocin)		
Cap: 25, 50 mg	1-3 mg/kg/24 hr q6-8hr PO (maximum: 100-200 mg/24 hr)	Not approved in children <14 yr; may be used to close PDA (with CHF) in neonate; 0.1-0.2 mg/kg/dose q12hr up to maximum 0.6 mg/kg IV Tox: nausea, vomiting, headache, corneal opacity
Insulin	Table 74-3	
Iodoquinol	See Appendix C-3	
Ipecac, syrup of	6-12 mo: 10 ml/dose PO 12 mo: 15 ml/dose PO Adult: 30 ml/dose PO Give initial dose and may repeat × 1	Do not use in children <6 mo; push fluids; contraindicated in caustic ingestions and patients who are comatose or having seizures, Chapter 54
Ipratropium (Atrovent)		
MDI (18 μg/dose) Sol'n: (0.02%): 500 μg in 2.5 ml	Adult: 2 inhalation (MDI) puffs QID; solution (500 μg/dose in 2.5 ml) by nebulization q6hr prn in adults; child: administer partial (half) adult dose	Efficacious as MDI or nebulization solution
Iron, elemental (Fe) (Fer-In-Sol, Feosol)		
Drop: 75 mg (15 mg Fe)/0.6 ml Syr: 90 mg (18 mg Fe)/5 ml Tab: 200 mg (40 mg Fe), 325 mg (65 mg Fe)	Therapeutic: 6 mg elemental Fe/kg/24 hr q8hr PO Prophylactic: 1-2 mg elemental Fe/kg/24 hr q8-24hr PO (maximum: 15 mg elemental Fe/24 hr)	Ferrous sulfate is 20% elemental iron (Fe) (Chapter 26) Tox: GI irritant (reduce by giving with food); overdose (Chapter 55)
Isoetharine (Bronkosol, Bronkometer)		
Sol'n: 1% (10 mg/ml) Aerosol	Nebulizer: 0.25-0.5 ml diluted in 2.5 ml saline q4hr prn Aerosol: 1-2 puffs q2-4hr prn	Administer by nebulizer; rarely used Tox: tachycardia, hypertension
Isoniazid (INH)		
Syr: 50 mg/5 ml Tab: 50, 100, 300 mg	10-20 mg/kg/24 hr q12-24hr PO (adult: 300 mg/24 hr)	Supplemental pyridoxine (10 mg/100 mg INH) needed in adolescents, adults Tox: peripheral neuropathy, hepatitis, seizure, acidosis

Many oral drugs may be given 3-4 times/day with more flexibility than implied by the specific intervals noted. Adult dose provided as guideline for maximum dose. *NB*, Newborns <7 days of age; *Pen*, penicillin; *SR*, sustained release; *Tox*, toxicity of drug.

APPENDIX C-1 Common Medications—cont'd

Drugs	Dosages	Comments
Isoproterenol (Isuprel) Amp: 200 μg/ml	Shock: 0.05-1.5 μg/kg/min IV infusion; begin at 0.05 μg/kg/min and increase by 0.1 μg/kg/min increments (maximum: 1.5 μg/kg/min) **Dilute** for infusion in shock: 0.6 mg × weight (kg) in 100 ml D5W; rate of infusion in 0.1 μg/kg/min = ml/hr (1 ml/hr delivers 0.1 μg/kg/min); **or** 200 μg (1 ml) in 200 ml D5W = 1 μg/ml	Table 5-2
Ivermectin	See Appendix C-3	
Kanamycin (Kantrex) Vial: 37.5, 250, 333 mg/ml	15 mg/kg/24 hr q8hr IM, IV (maximum: 1 g/24 hr) (NB: 15 mg/kg/24 hr q12hr)	Therapeutic peak level: 25-30 μg/ml; caution in renal failure (adjust dosage; infusion IV slowly Tox: renal, hearing
Ketamine Vial: 10, 50, 100 mg/ml	1 mg/kg/dose IV (maximum: 100 mg); 5 mg/kg/dose IM (maximum: 50 mg); 5-10 mg/kg PO (maximum: 50 mg)	Administer slowly; half-life 2½ hr, redistribution half-life 10-15 min; monitor
Ketorolac (Toradol) Syringe: 15, 30, 60 mg Tab: 10 mg	1 mg/kg/dose q6hr IM (children >2 yr) Adult: 30-60 mg IM initial, then 15-30 mg q6hr IM (maximum: 120 mg/24 hr); 10-20 mg q6hr PO	Limited experience in children <16 yr; do not give if patient hypovolemic
Labetalol	0.4-1.0 mg/kg/dose IV slow push; repeat up to 3 mg/kg/hr IV (adult: 2 mg/min or 20 mg/dose; titrate 20-80 mg q10min; maximum: 300 mg)	Tox: hypotension; Table 18-2
Lamotrigine (Lamictal)	See Table 81-6	
Levothyroxine (Synthroid) Tab: 25, 50, 100, 200, 300 μg Vial: 500 μg	Infancy: 7-9 μg/kg/24 hr PO; thereafter 100 μg/m^2/24 hr PO (child: 3-5 μg/kg/24 hr PO)	Monitor T_4 and thyroid-stimulating hormone

Continued

APPENDIX C-1 Common Medications—cont'd

Drugs	Dosages	Comments
Lidocaine (Xylocaine) Vial (IV): 10, 20 mg/ml Vial (anesthetic): 10 mg (1%), 20 mg (2%), 40 mg (4%)/ml	Load: 1 mg/kg/dose q5-10min IV prn to maximum of 5 mg/kg Maintenance: 20-50 μg/kg/min IV infusion Adult: load same; maintenance: 2-4 mg/min **Dilute**: 150 mg × weight (kg) in 250 ml D5W; rate of infusion in μg/min = 10 × ml/hr	Antidysrhythmic; may be given ET (dilute 1:1); Table 6-4 Tox: seizures, drowsiness, euphoria, muscle twitching, dysrhythmias, and titrate dosage
Loperamide (Imodium) Cap: 2 mg Liq: 1 mg/5 ml	Children (>2 yr): 0.4-0.8 mg/kg/24 hr q6-12hr PO until diarrhea resolves (adult: 2 mg q8hr PO)	Limited efficacy OTC
Loracarbef (Lorabid) Cap: 200, 400 mg	Adult: 200-400 mg q12hr PO × 7 days	Urinary tract infection in children ≥13 yr
Loratadine (Claritin) Tab: 10 mg Syr: 5 mg/5 ml	10 mg PO QD for up to 2 weeks	Limited trials in children 6-12 yr; may use 5 mg/day in children 2-5 yr; effective seasonal allergic rhinitis; second-generation H_1-receptor blocker
Lorazepam (Ativan) Vial: 2, 4 mg/ml	0.05-0.10 mg/kg/dose IV at rate 2 mg/min (adult: 2.5-10 mg/dose)	May consider repeating × 1 dose in 15-20 min if necessary
Magnesium hydroxide (see aluminum hyroxide) (Maalox)		
Magnesium sulfate Crystal: Epsom salt Vial: 100, 125, 250, 500 mg/ml	Catharsis: 250 mg/kg/dose PO (adult: 20-30 g/dose PO) Hypomagnesemia: 25-50 mg/kg/dose q4-6hr × 3-4 doses IV (adult: 1-4 g/24 hr) Asthma/torsades de pointes: 25-50 mg/kg (maximum 2 g) per dose IV over 10-20 min Anticonvulsant: 20-100 mg/kg/dose q4-6hr IV (adult: 1 g q6hr IV × 4)	Caution in renal failure; follow magnesium and calcium levels; Chapter 54 Tox: hypotension
Mannitol Vial: 20% (200 mg/ml) 25% (250 mg/ml)	Diuretic: 750 mg/kg/dose IV: do not repeat with persistent oliguria (adult: 300 mg/kg/dose) Cerebral edema: 0.25-0.5 g/kg IV slowly over 10-15 min q3-4hr prn (maximum: 1 g/kg/dose IV)	Maintain serum osmolality <320 mOsm/L; may be CNS rebound, intracranial monitor indicated Tox: hypovolemia, volume overload, hyperosmolality
Mebendazole (Vermox) Tab (chew): 100 mg	Pinworm: 100 mg PO, repeat in 1 wk Ascaris, hookworm: 100 mg q12hr PO × 3 days	Not studied in children <2 yr; see Appendix C-3 Tox: diarrhea

Many oral drugs may be given 3-4 times/day with more flexibility than implied by the specific intervals noted. Adult dose provided as guideline for maximum dose. *NB*, Newborns <7 days of age; *Pen*, penicillin; *SR*, sustained release; *Tox*, toxicity of drug.

APPENDIX C-1 Common Medications—cont'd

Drugs	Dosages	Comments
Meperidine (Demerol) Syr: 50 mg/5 ml Tab: 50, 100 mg Vial: 25, 50, 100 mg/ml	1-2 mg/kg/dose q3-4hr PO, IM, IV prn (adult: 50-150 mg/dose) (maximum: 100 mg/dose in children)	75 mg meperidine = 10 mg morphine Also potentiated by hydroxyzine Tox: CNS, respiratory depression, seizure, overdose (Chapter 55)
Metaraminol (Aramine) Vial: 10 mg/ml	0.01 mg/kg/dose IV prn **or** 1-4 μg/kg/min IV infusion	Tox: tachycardia, dysrhythmia, local tissue slough
Methicillin (Staphcillin) Vial: 1, 4, 6 g	100-200 mg/kg/24 hr q4-6hr IM, IV (maximum: 12 g/24 hr) (NB: 50-75 mg/kg/24 hr q8-12hr)	Equivalent to nafcillin, oxacillin Tox: interstitial nephritis (hematuria), bone marrow suppression; see Penicillin G
Methsuximide (Celontin) Cap: 150, 300 mg	Adult: 300 mg/24 hr q24 hr PO × 1 wk; 300 mg/24 hr/wk increments q3wk prn (maximum: 1.2 g/24 hr)	Petit mal seizures Tox: CNS symptoms, behavioral change; use with caution in liver or renal disease
Methyldopa (Aldomet) Tab: 125, 250, 500 mg Vial: 50 mg/ml Susp: 250 mg/5 ml	Crisis: 2.5-5 mg/kg/dose q6-8hr IV (maximum: 20-40 mg/kg/24 hr or 500 mg/dose IV) Chronic: 10 mg/kg/24 hr q6-12hr PO (maximum: 40 mg/kg/24 hr or total dose 2 g/24 hr)	Table 18-2 Tox: somnolence, hemolytic disease, ulcerogenic; reduce dosage with renal failure
Methylene blue Vial: 1% (10 mg/ml)	1-2 mg/kg/dose IV q4hr prn	Use for methemoglobinemia
Methylphenidate (Ritalin) Tab: 5, 10, 20 mg	Initial dose (>6 yr): 5 mg in AM/PM PO; titrate; maximum: 60 mg/24 hr	Toxicity may be increased when combination therapy used; do ECG if using multiple agents for ADHD; sustained-release forms available (Concerta: 18, 36, 54 mg; Ritalin SR: 20 mg; Metaclate CD: 20 mg)
Methylprednisolone (Solu-Medrol) Vial: 40, 125, 500, 1000 mg	Asthma: 1-2 mg/kg/dose q6hr IV	Table 74-2; different preparation for intraarticular route

Continued

APPENDIX C-1 Common Medications—cont'd

Drugs	Dosages	Comments
Metoclopramide (Reglan) Syr: 5 mg/5 ml Tab: 5, 10 mg Vial: 5 mg/ml	0.1 mg/kg/dose q6hr PO, IV Adult: 10-15 mg q6hr PO, IV	For gastroesophageal reflux, nausea, and vomiting; higher dosage (1 mg/kg/dose) may be used IV before chemotherapy to reduce vomiting; extrapyramidal reactions
Metolazone (Zaroxolyn) Tab: 2.5, 5, 10 mg	0.2-0.4 mg/kg/24 hr q12-24hr PO Adult: 2.5-10 mg/24 hr PO	Little experience in children; useful when no response to other diuretics and decreased glomerular filtration rate; Table 16-3 Tox: azotemia, ↓ K^+, hypotension, lethargy, coma
Metronidazole (Flagyl) Tab: 250, 500 mg	*Haemophilus vaginalis* - (*Gardnerella*) vaginitis: 500 mg q8hr PO × 7-10 days *Tricomonas vaginalis*: 15 mg/kg/24 hr q8hr PO × 7 days (adult: 250 mg q8hr × 7 days) *Giardia lamblia*: 15 mg/kg/24 hr q8hr PO × 5 days (adult: 250 mg q8hr × 5 days) Amebiasis: 35-50 mg/kg/24 hr q8hr PO × 10 days (adult: 750 mg q8hr × 10 days)	IV form available for severe anaerobic infections Tox: nausea, diarrhea, neutropenia, urticaria, do not give to pregnant patient
Miconazole (Monistat) Vag cream (2%) Supp: 200 mg (Monistat 3)	*Candida (Monilia)* vaginitis: 1 applicator-full before bed × 7-14 days; supp: 200 mg before bed × 3 days	Systemic form available
Midazolam (Versed) Vial: 1.5 mg/ml	Conscious sedation: 0.05-0.10 mg/kg/dose (maximum: 5 mg) IV; 0.3-0.7 mg/kg PO; 0.4 mg/kg intranasal	Often used in combination with narcotic such as low-dose fentanyl, morphine, meperidine; See Chapter 65
Milrinone (Primacor) Vial: 1 mg/ml	Load: 50-75 μg/kg over 5 min Infusion: 0.5-0.75 μg/kg/min IV	Tox: hypotension, risk of ventricular dysrhythmia
Minoxidil (Loniten) Tab: 2.5, 10 mg	0.2-1.0 mg/kg/24 hr q24hr PO (adult: 10-40 mg q24hr PO) (maximum: 100 mg/24 hr)	Peripheral vasodilator; limited experience in children; increase dose gradually
Morphine Vial: 5, 8, 10, 15 mg/ml	0.1-0.2 mg/kg/dose (maximum: 10-15 mg/dose) q2-4hr IM, IV	Antidote: naloxone (Chapter 55) Tox: CNS, respiratory depression, hypotension

Many oral drugs may be given 3-4 times/day with more flexibility than implied by the specific intervals noted. Adult dose provided as guideline for maximum dose. *NB*, Newborns <7 days of age; *Pen*, penicillin; *SR*, sustained release; *Tox*, toxicity of drug.

APPENDIX C-1 Common Medications—cont'd

Drugs	Dosages	Comments
Mupirocin 2% (Bactroban) Oint: 15 g	Apply small amount TID	May substitute for systemic treatment of impetigo with small lesions
Nafcillin (Unipen) Vial: 0.5, 1, 2g	50-200 mg/kg/24 hr q4-6hr IM, IV (maximum: 12 g/24 hr) (NB: 40 mg/kg/24 hr q 12hr)	Equivalent to methicillin, oxacillin; IM painful; oral form available Tox: allergy, see Penicillin; low renal toxicity
Naloxone (Narcan) Amp: 0.4, 1.0 mg/ml	0.1 mg/kg/dose (minimum: 0.4 mg; maximum: 2.0 mg) IV	Narcotic antagonist; propoxyphene (Darvon) and pentazocine (Talwin) require very large doses to reverse; Chapter 55; may have role in septic shock
Naproxen (Naprosyn) Tab: 250, 375, 500 mg Susp: 125 mg/5 ml	2.5-5 mg/kg/dose q8hr PO (adult: 250-375 mg q8-12hr PO) (maximum: 15 mg/kg or 1250 mg for adult/24 hr) Dysmenorrhea: load 500 mg PO, then 250 mg q8-12hr PO	Nonsteroidal antiinflammatory Tox: GI irritant, vertigo, headache, platelet dysfunction; not approved in children <2 yr
Nifedipine (Procardia) Cap: 10, 20 mg	0.25-0.50 mg/kg q15-30min PO, sublingual, buccal (adult: 10-20 mg/dose)	Negative inotropic effect; contraindicated with intracranial hemorrhage
Nitrite, amyl	Inhale pearl q60-120sec	For cyanide poisoning, follow with sodium nitrite and sodium thiosulfate
Nitrite, sodium (3%)	0.27 ml (8.7 mg)/kg (adult: 10 ml [300 mg]) IV slowly if Hgb 10 g	For cyanide poisoning, precede with amyl nitrite and follow with sodium thiosulfate
Nitrofurantoin (Furadantin, Macrodantin) Susp: 25 mg/5 ml Tab: 50, 100 mg Cap: 25, 50, 100 mg	5-7 mg/kg/24 hr q6hr PO; chronic: 2.5-5 mg/kg/24 hr (adult: 50-100 mg/dose q6hr PO; chronic: 50-100 mg before bed PO)	Do not use for renal disease, G6PD deficiency, child <1 mo, pregnancy Tox: hypersensitivity
Nitroprusside (Nipride) Vial: 50 mg	0.5-10 μg (avg: 3 μg)/kg/min IV infusion **Dilute**: 6 mg × weight (kg) in 100 ml D5W; rate of infusion in μg/kg/min = ml/hr **or** 50 mg (1 vial) in 100 ml of D5W = 500 μg/ml	Precise, rapid (1-2 min) BP control; requires constant monitoring; light sensitive; Tables 5-2 and 18-2 Tox: hypotension, cyanide poisoning (monitor thiocyanate level)

Continued

APPENDIX C-1 Common Medications—cont'd

Drugs	Dosages	Comments
Norepinephrine (Levophed) Vial: 1 mg/ml	0.1-1.0 μg/kg/min IV infusion **Dilute**: 0.6 mg × weight (kg) in 100 ml D5W; rate of infusion in 0.1 μg/kg/in = ml/hr (1 ml/hr delivers 0.1 μg/kg/min); **or** 1 mg (1 ml) in 100 ml of D5W = 10 μg/ml	Table 5-2; titrate dosage to response
Norfloxacin (Noroxin) Tab: 400 mg	Adult: 400 mg q12hr PO	Quinolone antibiotic No pediatric recommendation because of risk of arthropathy
Nystatin (Mycostatin) Cream: 100,000 unit/g Susp: 100,000 unit/ml Tab (vag): 100,000 unit	Thrush: 1 ml in each side of the mouth q4-6hr PO Diaper rash *(Candida)*: apply cream with diaper changes (q2-6hr) Vaginitis: 1 tab in vagina before bed × 10 days	Continue oral and topical therapy for 2-3 days after clearing
Ondansetron (Zofran) Tab: 4, 8 mg	4-11 yr: 4 mg q8hr PO; >11 yr: 8 mg q8hr PO; IV: 0.1-0.15 mg/kg infused over 30 min; may repeat in 4-8 hr	Antiemetic for cancer chemotherapy or postoperative nausea, vomiting
Oseltamivir (Tamiflu) Susp: 60 mg/5 ml Cap: 75 mg	<15 kg: 30 mg BID PO; >15-23 kg: 45 mg BID PO: >23-40 kg: 60 mg BID PO; >40 kg: 75 mg BID PO	Begin within 2 days of onset of symptoms of influenza; children >1 yr; 5-day course
Oxacillin (Prostaphin) Sol'n: 250 mg/5 ml Cap: 250, 500 mg Vial: 0.5, 1, 2, 4 g	50-100 mg/kg/24 hr q6r PO (adult: 500-1000 mg q6hr PO); 50-200 mg/kg/24 hr q4-6hr IM, IV (maximum: 8 g/24 hr) (NB: 25-50 mg/kg/24 hr q8-12hr IM, IV)	Equivalent to methicillin, nafcillin; oral form optimally given on empty stomach Tox: see Penicillin G
Pancuronium (Pavulon) Vial: 1, 2 mg/ml	Load: 0.04-0.1 mg/kg/dose IV (intubation: 0.06-0.1 mg/kg/dose IV) (NB: 0.02 mg/kg/dose IV) Maintenance: 0.01-0.02 mg/kg/dose q20-40min IV prn (NB: adjust on basis of loading dose)	Peak effect in 2-3 min; duration 40-60 min; must be able to support respirations
Paraldehyde (Paral) Soln: 1 g/ml Amp: 1 g/ml	Sedative: 0.15 ml (150 mg)/kg/dose PO, IM Anticonvulsant: 0.3 ml (300 mg)/kg/dose q4-6hr PR prn (maximum: 5 ml) (NB: 0.1-0.2 ml [100-200 mg]/kg/dose diluted in 0.9% NS q4-6hr PR prn; 0.15 ml/kg/dose q4-6hr IM, IV pm)	For PR, dissolve 1:2 in cottonseed, olive, or mineral oil; for IM, give deep; do not give if hepatic or pulmonary disease is present Tox: IV (pulmonary edema, CHF), IM (sterile abscess), PR (proctitis), respiratory depression

Many oral drugs may be given 3-4 times/day with more flexibility than implied by the specific intervals noted. Adult dose provided as guideline for maximum dose. *NB*, Newborns <7 days of age; *Pen*, penicillin; *SR*, sustained release; *Tox*, toxicity of drug.

APPENDIX C-1 Common Medications—cont'd

Drugs	Dosages	Comments
Penicillin G (sodium or potassium salt) Susp: 125, 250 mg/5 ml Tab: 125, 250, 500 mg Vial: 1, 5, 20 million units	25-50 mg (40,000-80,000 units)/kg/24 hr q6hr PO (adult: 300,000-1.2 million units/24 hr PO); 50,000-250,000 units/kg/24 hr q4hr IM, IV (NB: 50,000-150,000 units/kg/24 hr q8-12hr IM, IV)	1 mg = 1600 units; salt content (1 million units contains 1.68 mEq Na^+ or K^+); PO erratically absorbed, give on empty stomach Tox: allergy (anaphylaxis, rash, uticaria), superinfection *(Candida)* hemolytic anemia, interstitial nephritis; adjust dosage with renal failure
Penicillin G benzathine and Penicillin G procaine (Bicillin C-R 900/300) 900,000 units benz and 300,000 units proc/2 ml	*Weight (lb)* — *Benzathine pen G (Bicillin L-A)* <30 — 300,000 units 31-60 — 600,000 units 61-90 — 900,000 units >90 — 1,200,000 units	*Benzathine/procaine pen G (Bicillin C-R 900/300)* 300,000:100,000 units 600,000:200,000 units 900,000:300,000 units Not available
Penicillin V (Pen-Vee K, V-Cillin K) Susp: 125 mg (200,000 units), 250 mg (400,000 units)/5 ml Tab: 125, 250, 500 mg	25-50 mg (40,000-80,000 units)/kg/24 hr q6hr PO (adult: 250-500 mg q6hr PO)	More resistant to destruction by gastric acid Tox: see Penicillin G
Pentamidine (Pentam) Vial: 300 mg	4 mg/kg/24 hr q24hr IM	May be given IV slowly
Pentobarbital (Nembutal) Elix: 20 mg/5 ml Cap: 30, 50, 100 mg Supp: 30, 60, 120, 200 mg Vial: 50 mg/ml	Sedation: 6 mg/kg/24 hr q8hr PO, PR, IM, IV (adult: 30 mg q6-8hr) Cerebral edema: load: 3-5 mg/kg slow IV; maintenance: 1-2 mg/kg/hr IV	Short-acting barbiturate; treatment of increased intracranial pressure must include monitor Pentobarbital to maintain intracranial pressure <15 mm Hg and barbiturate level 25-40 μg/ml; support respirations, monitor BP Tox: CNS excitement, respiratory depression, hypotension (Chapter 55)
Phenazopyridine (Pyridium) Tab: 100, 200 mg	6-12 yr of age: 100 mg q8hr PO (adult: 200 mg q8hr PO) × 1-3 days	Use until dysuria gone and diagnosis made; urine color orange/red; avoid with G6PD deficiency Tox: hemolytic anemia, methemoglobinemia

Continued

APPENDIX C-1 Common Medications—cont'd

Drugs	Dosages	Comments
Phenobarbital (Luminal) Elix: 20 mg/5 ml Tab: 8, 15, 30, 60, 90, 100 mg Vial: 65, 130 mg/ml	Seizures: load: 15-20 mg/kg PO, IM (erratic absorption), IV (<1 mg/kg/min); with status epilepticus and no response in 20-30 min, repeat 10 mg/kg IV (adult: 100 mg/dose IV q20min prn × 3) Maintenance: 2-6 mg/kg/24 hr q12-24hr PO (adult: 100-300 mg/24 hr PO) Sedation: 2-3 mg/kg/dose PO q8hr prn	May be used as first-line drug in status epilepticus (IV) or after seizures controlled by diazepam (Valium); Chapters 21 and 81 Therapeutic level: 15-35 μg/ml Tox: drowsiness, irritability, learning problems, CNS and respiratory depression with high dosages (Chapter 55) Reduce dosage with renal failure
Phentolamine (Regitine) Vial: 5 mg/ml	0.05-0.1 mg/kg/dose q1-4hr IV (adult: 2.5-5 mg/dose IV)	Specific for pheochromocytoma and MAO-induced hypertension; rapid onset; dose, especially PO, must be individualized; may be given as continuous infusion Tox: dysrhythmia, hypotension
Phenytoin (Dilantin, diphenylhydantoin) Susp: 125 mg/5 ml Tab: (chew): 50 mg Cap: 30, 100 mg Amp: 50 mg/ml Amp: (fosphenytoin [Cerebyx]): 50 mg/ml equivalent	Seizures: load: 10-20 mg/kg PO, IV (<0.5 mg/kg/min unless using fosphenytoin); maintenance: 5-10 mg/kg/24 hr q12-24 hr PO (adult: 200-400 mg/24 hr PO) Dysrhythmia load: 5 mg/kg IV (<0.5 mg/kg/min) (adult: 100 mg/dose q5min prn up to 1 g IV); maintenance: 6 mg/kg/24 hr q12hr PO (adult: 300 mg/24 hr PO)	Therapeutic level: 10-20 μg/ml: good for digoxin- and cyclic antidepressant–induced dysrhythmias; fosphenytoin has reduced toxicity and may be given IM; Chapters 21 and 81 Tox: nystagmus, ataxia, hypotension, gingival hyperplasia, SLE-like syndrome, hirsutism
Physostigmine (Antilirium) Vial: 1 mg/ml	Child: 0.02 mg/kg/dose up to 0.5 mg/dose IV (over 3 min) q10min prn (maximum total dose: 2 mg) Adult: 1-2 mg IV (over 3 min) q10min prn (maximum total dose: 4 mg in 30 min)	Anticholinesterase; use in life-threatening anticholinergic overdose (Chapter 55) Tox: neurologic, dysrhythmias

Many oral drugs may be given 3-4 times/day with more flexibility than implied by the specific intervals noted. Adult dose provided as guideline for maximum dose. *NB*, Newborns <7 days of age; *Pen*, penicillin; *SR*, sustained release; *Tox*, toxicity of drug.

APPENDIX C-1 Common Medications—cont'd

Drugs	Dosages	Comments
Piperacillin (Pipracil) Vial: 2, 3, 4 g	200-300 mg/kg/24 hr q4-6hr IV (maximum: 24 g/24 hr) (NB: 100 mg/kg/dose q12 hr IV)	Good *Pseudomonas* coverage Tox: neurologic, GI
Polystyrene sodium sulfonate (Kayexalate) Powder: 450 g	1 g/kg/dose q6hr PO or q2-6hr PR (adult: 15 g PO or 30-60 g PR q6hr)	1 level tsp = 3.5 g; 4.1 mEq Na^+/g: exchanges 1 mEq K^+ for 1 g resin, which delivers 1 mEq Na^+ for each 1 mEq K^+ removed; mix 30%-70% suspension in D10W, 1% methylcellulose, or 10% sorbitol Tox: electrolyte problems, constipation
Pralidoxime (Protopam, 2-PAM) Vial: 1 g	20-50 mg/kg/dose (maximum: 2 g/dose) IV slow (<50 mg/min) q8hr prn × 3	Cholinesterase reactivator; use after atropine in organophosphate overdose (Chapter 55); oral preparation for prophylaxis
Praziquantel (Biltricide)	See Appendix C-3	
Prazosin (Minipress) Cap: 1, 2, 5 mg	Initial: 5 μg/kg/dose PO; then up to 25 μg/kg/dose q6hr PO Adult: 1 mg q8-12hr PO; may increase slowly to 20 mg/24 hr	Limited experience in children
Prednisolone (Prelone, Orapred) Elix: 15 mg/ml	Asthma: 1-2 mg/kg/24 hr q6hr PO	Liquid steroid preparation; (Orapred "best" tasting; refrigerate)
Prednisone Tab: 5, 10, 20 mg Susp: 5 mg/5 ml	Maintenance: 0.1-0.15 mg/kg/24 hr q12hr PO Asthma: 1-2 mg/kg/24 hr q6hr PO	Table 74-2
Primidone (Mysoline) Susp: 250 mg/5 ml Tab: 50, 250 mg	10-25 mg/kg/24 hr q6-8hr PO; start at 125-250 mg, increase in 125-250 mg increments at 1-wk intervals (adult: initial 250 mg/24 hr PO; maintenance: 750-1250 mg/24 hr q6hr PO)	Therapeutic level: 6-12 μg/ml (or phenobarbital 10-25 μg/ml); Table 81-6 Tox: sedation, nausea, vomiting, diplopia: reduce dosage with renal failure; see Phenobarbital
Probenecid (Benemid) Tab: 500 mg	Load: 25 mg/kg PO; maintenance: 40 mg/kg/24 hr q6hr PO (adult: 2 g/24 hr); 25 mg/kg (adult: 1 g) PO before ampicillin or penicillin treatment of *Neisseria gonorrhoeae*	Not recommended for children <2 yr Tox: GI irritant

Continued

APPENDIX C-1 Common Medications—cont'd

Drugs	Dosages	Comments
Procainamide (Pronestyl) Tab/cap: 250, 375, 500 mg Vial: 100, 500 mg/ml	Load: 2-6 mg/kg/dose IV slow (<50 mg/min) (adult: 100 mg/dose IV slow q10 min prn up to total load of 1 g IV) Maint: 20-80 μg/kg/min IV (adult: 1-3 mg/min IV) or 15-50 mg/kg/24 hr q4-6hr PO (adult: 250-500 mg/dose PO)	IV must be given slowly at concentration <100 mg/ml; do not use with heart block; Table 6-4 Tox: GI irritant, SLE-like syndrome, dysrhythmias
Prochlorperazine (Compazine) Syr: 5 mg/5 ml Tab: 5, 10, 25 mg Supp: 2.5, 5, 25 mg Amp: 5 mg/ml	0.4 mg/kg/24 hr q6-8hr PO, PR (adult: 5-10 mg q6-8hr PO or 25 mg q12hr PR) 0.2 mg/kg/24 hr q6-8hr IM (adult: 5-20 mg/dose IM) (maximum: 40 mg/24 hr)	Only children >2 yr and >10 kg; injectable difficult to obtain Tox: phenothiazine (extrapyramidal, anticholinergic) (Chapter 55)
Promethazine (Phenergan) Syr: 6.25, 25 mg/5 ml Tab: 12.5, 25, 50 mg Supp: 12.5, 25, 50 mg Amp: 25, 50 mg/ml	Nausea, vomiting: 0.25-0.5 mg/kg/dose q4-6hr PO, PR, IM prn (adult: 12.5-25 mg/dose) Sedation: 0.5-1 mg/kg/dose q6hr PO, PR, IM prn (adult: 25-50 mg/dose)	Tox: phenothiazine (sedation, extrapyramidal, anticholinergic) (Chapter 55)
Propantheline (Pro-Banthine)	1-2 mg/kg/24 hr q6hr PO (adult: 15-30 mg QID)	
Propranolol (Inderal) Tab: 10, 20, 40, 80 mg Vial: 1 mg/ml	Dysrhythmias: load: 0.01-0.1 mg/kg/dose (maximum: 1 mg/dose) IV over 10 min (adult: 1 mg/dose IV q5min up to total of 5 mg); maintenance: 0.5-1 mg/kg/24 hr q6hr PO (adult: 10-30 mg/dose q6-8hr PO) Hypertension: 0.5-1.0 mg/kg/24 hr q6-12hr PO (maximum: 320 mg/24 hr PO) Tetralogy spells: 0.1-0.2 mg/kg/dose IV repeated in 15 min prn Migraine prophylaxis: 10-60 mg q8hr PO Thyrotoxicosis: 10-20 mg q6-8hr PO	β-blocker; contraindicated in patient with asthma or CHF; Tables 6-4 and 18-2 Tox: dysrhythmias, hypoglycemia, hypotension, cardiac failure, bronchospasm, weakness; overdose treated with glucagon 0.1 mg/kg/dose IV 1-2 mg/kg/24 hr q6hr PO (adult: 15-30 mg QID)

Many oral drugs may be given 3-4 times/day with more flexibility than implied by the specific intervals noted. Adult dose provided as guideline for maximum dose. *NB*, Newborns <7 days of age; *Pen*, penicillin; *SR*, sustained release; *Tox*, toxicity of drug.

APPENDIX C-1 Common Medications—cont'd

Drugs	Dosages	Comments
Propylthiouracil (PTU)		
Tab: 50 mg	Load: 5 mg/kg/24 hr q6-8hr PO (adult: 300 mg/24 hr); maintenance: ⅓-½ of loading dose once patient is euthyroid (adult: 100-150 mg/ 24 hr)	Tox: blood dyscrasia, hepatic, dermatitis, urticaria, neuritis
Protamine		
Amp: 10 mg/ml	1 mg IV for each 100 units of heparin given concurrently; 0.5 mg IV for each 100 units of heparin given in previous 30 min, and so on; maximum: 50 mg/dose	Heparin antidote Tox: hypotension, bradycardia, flushing
Pseudoephedrine (Sudafed)		
Syr: 30 mg/5 ml Tab: 30, 60 mg	4-6 mg/kg/24 hr q4-6hr PO (adult: 60 mg q4-6hr PO)	Tox: irritability; use with caution in hypertensive patient
Pyrantel (Antiminth)		
Susp: 250 mg/5 ml	11 mg (~0.2 ml)/kg/dose PO once (maximum: 1 g/dose); repeat in 1 wk	Do not use in preexisting liver disease, pregnancy; see Appendix C-3 Tox: nausea, vomiting, hepatic
Quinidine		
Tab: 100, 200, 300, 202 (SR), 300 (SR) mg Cap: 200, 300 mg	15-60 mg/kg/24 hr q6hr PO (adult: 300-400 mg q6hr PO)	Table 6-3 Tox: GI irritant dysrhythmias, hypotension, blood dyscrasia
Racemic epinephrine		
Sol'n: 2.25%	<20 kg: 0.25 ml in 2.5 ml saline nebulizer; 20-40 kg: 0.5 ml; >40 kg: 0.75 ml	Rebound; observe child with croup after treatment; some bronchodilator effect
Ranitidine (Zantac)		
Tab: 150 mg Vial: 25 mg/ml	2-4 mg/kg/24 hr q12hr PO (adult: 150 mg q12hr PO; 50 mg q6-8hr IV; maximum: 400 mg/24 hr IV)	Limited experience in children; similar to cimetidine, fewer drug interactions
Reserpine (Serpasil)		
Elix: 0.25 mg/5 ml Tab: 0.1, 0.25, 0.5, 1 mg	0.02 mg/kg/dose q12hr PO (adult: 0.1-0.25 mg/24 hr)	Usually used in combination with another drug; rarely used; Table 18-2 Tox: severe depression, bradycardia, ulcerogenic

Continued

APPENDIX C-1 Common Medications—cont'd

Drugs	Dosages	Comments
Ribavirin (Virazole) Vial: 6 g/100 ml	20 mg/ml delivered as 190 μg/L in air for 12-18 hr/24 hr × 3 days	Use Viratek Small Particle Aerosol Generator; indicated in hospitalized children at high risk of complications from RSV such as those with underlying heart or lung disease, AIDS, or severe RSV disease
Rifampin (Rimactane, Rifadin) Cap: 150, 300 mg	10-20 mg/kg/24 hr q12-24hr PO (maximum: 600 mg/24 hr) Meningococcal prophylaxis: 10 mg/kg q12hr PO × 2 days (adult: 600 mg q12hr) *H. influenzae* prophylaxis: 20 mg/kg q24hr × 4 days (adult: 600 mg q24hr × 4)	Tox: hepatic, GI irritant, hemolytic anemia; turns urine red; lower dosage in children <1 mo
Rimantadine (Flumadine) Tab: 100 mg Syr: 50 mg/5 ml	5 mg/kg/24 hr q24hr PO (maximum: 150 mg/24 hr) Adult: 100 mg PO q12hr	Begin within 24-48 hr of onset of influenza A and continue for 48 hr after resolution
Rocuronium (Zemuron) Vial: 10 mg/ml	Initial: 0.6-1.2 mg/kg/dose IV; repeat 0.2 mg/kg q20-30min IV, as appropriate	Nondepolarizing neuromuscular blocking agent Tox: hypo/hypertension, dysrhythmia; muscle weakness
Secobarbital (Seconal) Cap: 30, 50, 100 mg Vial: 50 mg/ml	2-6 mg/kg/24 hr q8hr PO (adult: 60-120 mg/24 hr q8-12hr PO)	Short-acting barbiturate; difficult to obtain Tox: drowsiness, respiratory depression
Spectinomycin (Trobicin) Vial: 400 mg/ml	40 mg/kg/dose IM × 1 (adult: 2 g IM × 1)	*N. gonorrhoeae* treatment; not good for syphilis Tox: dizziness, vertigo
Spironolactone (Aldactone) Tab: 25, 50, 100 mg	1-3 mg/kg/24 hr q8-12hr PO (adult: 25-100 mg/24 hr)	Useful adjunctive diuretic to maintain potassium; reduce dosage with renal failure; Table 16-3
Succinylcholine (Anectine) Amp: 20 mg/ml Vial: 0.5, 1 g	1 mg/kg/dose IV (NB: 2 mg/kg/dose IV); maintenance: 0.3-0.6 mg/kg/dose q5-10min IV	Must be able to control airway; optimally, premedicate with atropine
Sulfisoxazole (Gantrisin) Susp: 500 mg/5 ml Tab: 500 mg	Load: 75 mg/kg PO; maintenance: 120-150 mg/kg/24 hr q6hr PO (adult: 500-1000 mg q6hr PO) (maximum: 4-6 g/24 hr)	Do not use in children <2 mo old: maintain good urine flow Tox: rash, Stevens-Johnson, neutropenia; reduce dosage with renal failure

Many oral drugs may be given 3-4 times/day with more flexibility than implied by the specific intervals noted. Adult dose provided as guideline for maximum dose. *NB*, Newborns <7 days of age; *Pen*, penicillin; *SR*, sustained release; *Tox*, toxicity of drug.

APPENDIX C-1 Common Medications—cont'd

Drugs	Dosages	Comments
Sumatriptan (Imitrex) Syringe: 6 mg/0.5 ml Tab: 25, 50 mg	Adult: initial dose 25 mg PO; may give up to 100 mg after 2 hr for maximum daily dose of 200 mg PO; 6 mg initial dose SC and may repeat ≤6 mg SC (at least 1 hr after first dose) up to 12 mg/24 hr SC	Subsequent treatment should reflect initial doses; limited experience in children
Terbutaline (Brethine) Vial: 1 mg/ml	*Parenteral*: 0.01 ml (0.01 mg)/kg/dose (maximum: 0.25 ml/dose) q15-20min SC prn *Aerosol*: 0.03-0.05 mg (0.03-0.05 ml)/kg in 2.5 ml saline given q4hr (adult: 0.5-1.0 mg/dose)	β-Agonist for reactive airway disease; may have more prolonged effect than epinephrine; use parenteral solution for nebulization Tox: sympathomimetic
Tetracycline (Achromycin, Tetracyn) Syr: 125 mg/5 ml Tab/cap: 250, 500 mg Vial: 250, 500 mg (IM has lidocaine)	25-50 mg/kg/24 hr q6hr PO (adult: 250-500 mg q6hr PO) 15-25 mg/kg/24 hr q8-12hr IM (adult: 200-300 mg/24 hr q8-12hr IM) 20-30 mg/kg/24 hr q8-12hr IV over 2 hr (adult: 250-500 mg/dose q8-12hr IV over 2 hr)	Do not use in children <9 yr; parenteral (IM, IV) administration is rarely indicated Tox: GI irritant, hepatic, photosensitization, superinfection
Theophylline (Table 84-1)	Load: 6 mg/kg PO; maintenance: 4-5 mg/kg/dose q6hr PO Load: 5 mg/kg IV slowly: maintenance: 0.6-0.9 mg/kg/hr IV	Therapeutic level: 10-20 μg/ml; Chapter 84 for dosage details Tox: nausea, vomiting, irritability, seizures, dysrhythmias
Thiabendazole (Mintezol)	See Appendix C-3	
Thiopental (Pentothal) Vial: 0.5, 1 g	Sedation: 2 mg/kg/dose IV; 2.5-5 mg/kg/dose PR (adult: 3-5 mg/kg/dose IV)	Respiratory monitoring imperative
Thioridazine (Mellaril) Susp: 25, 100 mg/5 ml Tab: 10, 15, 25, 50, 100 mg	1-2.5 mg/kg/24 hr q8-12hr PO (adult: 75-300 mg/24 hr q8-12hr PO) (maximum: 800 mg/24 hr)	Do not use in children <2 yr; titrate dosage to response Tox: phenothiazine (Chapter 55)
Thiosulfate sodium (25%)	1.35 ml (325 mg)/kg (adult: 12.5 g) IV slowly if Hgb 10 g	
Ticarcillin (Ticar) Vial: 1, 3, 6 g	200-300 mg/kg/24 hr q4-6hr IM, IV (maximum: 18-24 g/24 hr) (NB: 150-225 mg/kg/24 hr q8-12hr)	Similar to carbenicillin; adjust dosage in renal failure; used in combination therapy

Continued

APPENDIX C-1 Common Medications—cont'd

Drugs	Dosages	Comments
Tobramycin (Nebcin) Vial: 10, 40 mg/ml	3-7.5 mg/kg/24 hr q8hr IM, IV (maximum: 300 mg/24 hr) (NB: 4 mg/kg/24 hr q12hr)	Therapeutic peak level: 6-10 μg/ml: caution in renal failure (reduce dosage); slow IV infusion Tox: renal, VIII nerve
Trimethadione (Tridione) Sol'n: 200 mg/5 ml Cap: 300 mg Tab (chew): 150 mg	10-40 mg/kg/24 hr q12hr PO (adult: 900-2400 mg/24 hr q6-8hr PO)	Therapeutic peak level: 600-1000 μg/ml Tox: sedation, vision, headache
Trimethaphan (Arfonad) Vial: 50 mg/ml	50-150 μg/kg/min IV infusion (adult: 0.5-1 mg/min)	Constant monitoring required; tachyphylaxis; Table 18-2 Tox: ganglionic blocker (paralysis of pupils, bladder, bowels)
Trimethobenzamide (Tigan) Supp: 100, 200 mg Vial: 100 mg/ml Cap: 100, 250 mg	15-20 mg/kg/24 hr PO, PR adult: 200 mg/dose q6-8hr PR, IM	IV, IM not recommended; limited experience in children; do not use in patients with acute-onset vomiting; avoid supp in NB
Trimethoprim (TMP)-sulfamethoxazole (SMX) (Bactrim, Septra) Susp: 40 mg TMP/200 mg SMX/5 ml Tab: 80 mg TMP/400 mg SMX: 160 mg TMP/800 mg SMX Amp: 80 mg TMP/400 mg SMX/5 ml	6-12 mg TMP/30-60 mg SMX/kg/24 hr q12hr PO (adult: 80-160 mg TMP/400-800 mg SMX q12hr PO) *Pneumocystis*: 15-20 mg TMP/75-100 mg SMX/kg/24 hr q6-8hr PO, IV *Severe UTI, Shigella*: 8-10 mg TMP/40-50 mg SMX/kg/24 hr q6-8hr PO, IV	Do not use in children <2 mo; rare indications for IV route; reduce dosage in renal failure Tox: bone marrow suppression, GI irritation
Valproic acid or valproate (Depakene) Syr: 250 mg/5 ml Cap: 250 mg Vial: 100 mg/ml (Depacon)	15-60 mg/kg/24 hr q8-24hr PO (adult: 1-3 g/24 hr q8-24hr PO)	Therapeutic level: 50-100 μg/ml; Table 81-6; use in acute management of seizures is controversial; parenteral preparation available Tox: sedation, vomiting, rash, headache, hepatotoxic; increases phenobarbital level (20%) and decreases phenytoin level (50%-100%)

Many oral drugs may be given 3-4 times/day with more flexibility than implied by the specific intervals noted. Adult dose provided as guideline for maximum dose. *NB*, Newborns <7 days of age; *Pen*, penicillin; *SR*, sustained release; *Tox*, toxicity of drug.

APPENDIX C-1 Common Medications—cont'd

Drugs	Dosages	Comments
Vancomycin (Vancocin) Vial: 500 mg Sol'n (oral): 1, 10 g Pulvule: 125, 250 mg	30-40 mg/kg/24 hr q6hr IV (meningitis: up to 60 mg/kg/24 hr q6hr IV) (<500 mg/30 min) (maximum: 2 g/24 hr) (NB: 30 mg/kg/24 hr q12hr IV) For *C. difficile* or pseudomembranous colitis: 40 mg/kg/24 hr q6hr PO	Reduce dosage in renal impairment; also available in oral preparation for staphylococcal enterocolitis and pseudomembranous colitis and *C. difficile* Tox: ototoxic, renal, rash, peripheral neuropathy
Vecuronium (Norcuron) 10 mg/ml	0.08-0.1 mg/kg/dose IV	Nondepolarizing muscle blockade; need to be able to control airway
Verapamil (Isoptin, Calan) Amp: 2.5 mg/ml	0.1-0.2 mg/kg/dose IV over 2 min repeated in 10-30 min prn (adult: 5 mg/dose IV)	Table 6-4; do not use in children less than 1 yr old; largely replaced by adenosine Tox: bradycardia, hypotension
Vitamin K (Aquamephyton) Vial: 2, 10 mg/ml	NB, infant: 1-2 mg/dose IM, IV Child, adult: 5-10 mg/dose IM, IV	May give IV (<1 mg/min) but associated with hypotension and anaphylaxis
Warfarin (Coumadin) Tab: 2, 5, 7.5, 10 mg	0.1 mg/kg/24 hr q24hr PO Adult: 2-10 mg/24 hr q24hr PO after loading with 10-15 mg/24 hr PO × 2-3 days	Adjust dosage to maintain PT at 2 times normal (INR [International Normalized Ratio] 2-3); antidote is vitamin K Tox: dermatitis

APPENDIX C-2 Simplified Schedule for Administration of Pediatric Resuscitation Drugs

Drug (Availability)	Single Dose	Route	DOSE (ML) ADMINISTERED BY WEIGHT									
			5 kg	10 kg	15 kg	20 kg	25 kg	30 kg	35 kg	40 kg	45 kg	50 kg
EPINEPHRINE (1:10,000)* (0.1 mg/ml)	0.01 mg/kg 0.1 ml/kg	IV	0.5	1	1.5	2	2.5	3	3.5	4	4.5	5
SODIUM BICARBONATE (1 mEq/ml)	1 mEq/kg 1 ml/kg	IV	5	10	15	20	25	30	35	40	45	50
ATROPINE (0.1 mg/ml)	0.02 mg/kg 0.2 ml/kg	IV, ET	1	2	3	4	5	6	7	8	9	10
CALCIUM CHLORIDE 10% (100 mg/ml)	20 mg/kg 0.2 ml/kg	IV	1	2	3	4	5	5	5	5	5	5
LIDOCAINE (20 mg/ml)†	1 mg/kg 0.05 ml/kg	IV, ET	0.25	0.5	0.75	1	1.25	1.5	1.75	2	2.25	2.5
FUROSEMIDE (Lasix) (10 mg/ml)	1 mg/kg 0.1 ml/kg	IV	0.5	1	1.5	2	2.5	3	3.5	4	4.5	5
DIAZEPAM (Valium) (5 mg/ml)	0.2 mg/kg 0.04 ml/kg	IV	0.2	0.4	0.6	0.8	1	1.2	1.4	1.6	1.8	2

Before using this schedule, it is essential to be certain that the concentration used is identical to that cited here. Clinical response and patient condition may modify this schedule (see Table 4-2). Drugs can often be administered intraosseously.

* Second dose and ET dose are 0.1 mg/kg or 0.1 ml/kg of 1:1000 solution.

† Also available as 10 mg/ml.

WEIGHT: 10 KG (22 lb)
ET SIZE: 4.0
LARYNGOSCOPE BLADE: 1-2
SUCTION CATHETER: 8 Fr
DEFIBRILLATION: 20 watt-sec
NG TUBE: 8 Fr
FOLEY: 8 Fr

AGE: 1 yr
PULSE: 125 beats/min
RESPIRATORY RATE: 39 ± 11 breaths/min
BP: 96 ± 30 mm hg

Emergency Medications

Drug (Concentration)	Therapy Dose Range	Route*	Comments	Single Dose	Dose Administered
Epinephrine Syringe (1:10,000 = 0.1 mg/ml)	0.01 mg/kg (0.1 ml/kg) initial dose	IV	Maximum dose: 5 ml	0.1 mg	1 ml
Epinephrine (1:1,000 = 1 mg/ml)	0.1 mg/kg (0.1 ml/kg)	Second dose ET	Maximum dose: 5 ml	1 mg	1 ml
Bicarbonate, Sodium (1 mEq/ml)	1 mEq/kg (1 ml/kg)	IV	<1 yr dilute 1:1 with nonbacteriostatic H_2O	10 mEq	10 ml
Atropine (0.1 mg/ml)	0.02 mg/kg (0.2 ml/kg)	IV ET	Minimum dose: 0.1 mg: maximum dose: 2 mg; IV slowly	0.2 mg	2 ml
Calcium Cl 10% (100 mg/ml)	20 mg/kg (0.2 ml/kg)	IV	Maximum dose: 500 mg	200 mg	2 ml
Lidocaine 2% (20 mg/ml)	1 mg/kg (0.05 ml/kg)	IV ET	Maximum total dose: 5 mg/kg	10 mg	0.5 ml
Furosemide (Lasix) (10 mg/ml)	1 mg/kg (0.1 ml/kg)	IV	Maximum dose: 6 mg/kg	10 mg	1 ml
Diazepam (Valium) (5 mg/ml)	0.2 mg/kg (0.04 ml/kg)	IV ET	Maximum total dose: child 10 mg; adult 30 mg	2 mg	0.4 ml
Albuterol (soln: 5 mg/ml)	0.03 ml (0.15 mg)/kg/dose	NEB	May give as often as necessary; monitor	1.5 mg	0.3 ml in 2 ml saline
Naloxone (Narcan) (1 mg/ml)	0.1 mg/kg (0.1 ml/kg)	IV ET	If no response in 10 min may give up to 2 mg IV	1 mg	1 ml
Adenosine (3 mg/ml)	0.1 mg/kg (0.03 ml/kg) (rapid)	IV	May repeat in 2 min; maximum 12 mg initially	1 mg	0.33 ml
Dextrose 50% (0.5 g/ml)	0.5 g/kg (1 ml/kg)	IV	<1 yr dilute to D25W with nonbacterio-static H_2O	5 g	10 ml
Phenytoin (Dilantin)† (50 mg/ml)	Load: (seizure) 15 mg/kg (0.3 ml/kg)	IV PO	Not IM: IV give slowly in saline only: maxi-mum dose: 1250 mg; Dysrhythmia: 5 mg/kg/dose q5-20min prn × 2 IV	150 mg	3 ml
Phenobarbital (65 mg/ml)	Load: 15 mg/kg (0.23 ml/kg)	IV PO	Maximum dose: 300 mg; maintenance: 3-5 mg/kg/day	150 mg	2.3 ml

* Intravenous drugs may commonly be given intraosseously.
† Also available as fosphenytoin (Cerebyx) 50 mg/ml for reduced toxicity and IM administration.

MIXING EMERGENCY DRUGS FOR CONTINUOUS INFUSION

Several alternative approaches to preparing medication for continuous infusion exist, and these are outlined below.

	Rule of 6s	Drug Specific
Dopamine	6 × body wt (kg) equals mg of drug to be added to IV solution to make 100 ml D5W. Infusion of 1 ml/hr will deliver 1 μg/kg/min.	150 mg added to 250 ml D5W (600 μg/ml) Infusion of 1 ml/kg/hr delivers 10 μg/kg/min.
Dobutamine	Same as dopamine.	Same as dopamine.
Nitroprusside	Same as dopamine.	45 mg added to 250 ml D5W (180 μg/ml). Infusion of 1 ml/kg/hr delivers 3 μg/kg/min.
Isoproterenol	0.6 × body wt (kg) equals mg of drug to be added to IV solution to make 100 ml D5W. Infusion of 1 ml/hr will deliver 0.1 μg/kg/min.	1.5 mg added to 250 ml D5W (6 μg/ml). Infusion of 1 ml/kg/hr delivers 0.1 μg/kg/min.

Medication Infusions for 10-kg child

Drug (Concentration)	Therapy Range	Conversion Mixture	Add D5W	Add Drug	Initial Average Dose (Pump Required)
Dopamine (40 mg/ml)	5-20 μg/kg/min IV drip	150 mg in 250 ml D5W = 600 μg/ml; 1 ml/kg/hr =10 μg/kg/min	250 ml	3.75 ml	10 ml/hr
Dobutamine (25 mg/ml when mixed with 10 ml)	2-20 μg/kg/min IV drip	150 mg in 250 ml D5W = 600 μg/ml; 1 ml/kg/hr = 10 μg/kg/min	250 ml	6 ml	10 ml/hr
Nitroprusside (25 mg/ml)	0.5-10 (avg 3 μg) μg/kg/min IV drip	45 mg in 250 ml D5W = 180 μg/ml; 1 ml/kg/hr = 3 μg/kg/min	250 ml	1.8 ml	10 ml/hr
Isoproterenol (Isupel) (0.2 mg/ml)	0.05-1.5 μg/kg/min IV drip	1.5 mg in 250 ml D5W = 6 μg/ml; 1 ml/kg/hr = 0.1 μg/kg/min	250 ml	7.5 ml	10 ml/hr

APPENDIX C-3 Antiparasitic Drugs

Infection	Drug and dosage
AMEBIASIS *(ENTAMOEBA HISTOLYTICA)*	
Asymptomatic carrier	Iodoquinol (previously diiodohydroxyquin) 30-40 mg/kg/24 hr q8hr PO (adult: 650 mg/dose) × 20 days; **or** paromomycin 25-35 mg/kg/24 hr q8hr PO × 7 days; **or** diloxanide furoate (Furamide) (CDC) 20 mg/kg/24 hr q8hr PO (adult: 500 mg/dose) × 10 days
Mild to moderate colitis	Metronidazole (Flagyl) 35-50 mg/kg/24 hr q8hr PO (adult: 750 mg/dose) × 10 days; **plus** iodoquinol, as above, after treatment.
Severe colitis	Metronidazole, as above × 10 days; **plus,** iodoquinol, as above, after treatment
Extraintestinal	Metronidazole, as above × 10 days; **plus,** iodoquinol, as above, after treatment
ASCARIASIS *(Ascaris lumbricoides)*	Mebendazole (Vermox) 100 mg q12hr PO × 3 days (children >2 yr); **or** pyrantel pamoate (Antiminth) 11 mg/kg/dose (maximum: 1 g PO × 1 [one dose only])
BALANTIDIASIS *(Balantidium coli)*	Tetracycline 40 mg/kg/24 hr q6hr PO (children >8 yr only) (adult: 500 mg/dose) × 10 days; **or** iodoquinol 40 mg/kg/24 hr q8hr PO (adult: 650 mg/dose) × 20 days
CUTANEOUS LARVA MIGRANS or **CREEPING ERUPTION** (cutaneous hookworm)	Albendazole 400 mg qd PO × 3 days; **or** Thiabendazole (Mintezol) 50 mg/kg/24 hr (maximum: 1.5 g/dose) q12hr PO × 2-5 days; topical treatment also
CYSTICERCOSIS *(Taenia solium)*	Surgical excision most satisfactory; Praziquantel (Biltricide) 50 mg/kg/24 hr q8hr PO × 15 days (± steroids)
DIENTAMOEBIASIS *(Dientamoeba fragilis)*	Iodoquinol 40 mg/kg/24 hr q8hr PO (adult: 650 mg/dose) × 20 days
FILARIASIS ONCHOCERCIASIS *(Onchocerca volvulus)*	Ivermectin (Mectizan) (CDC) 150 µg/kg once and repeated every 3-12 mo
Other forms **(LOA LOA, TROPICAL EOSINOPHILIA)** *(Wuchereria bancrofti, Brugia malayi)*	Diethylcarbamazine (Hetrazan): *Day 1:* 1 mg PO (adult: 50 mg); *day 2:* 1 mg q8hr PO (adult: 50 mg/dose); *day 3:* 1-2 mg q8hr PO (adult: 100 mg/dose); *days 4-21:* 9 mg/kg/24 hr q8hr PO (adult: 9 mg/kg/24 hr q8hr PO)
FLUKES	
Liver *(Opisthorchis viverrini)* Lung *(Paragonimus westermani)* Chinese liver *(Clonorchis sinensis)*	Praziquantel (Biltricide) 25 mg/kg/dose PO × 3 doses (doses to be taken in 1 day)
GIARDIASIS *(Giardia lamblia)*	Metronidazole (Flagyl) 15 mg/kg/24 hr (adult: 250 mg/dose) q8hr PO × 5 days; **or** Furazolidone (Furoxone) 6 mg/kg/24 hr (adult: 100 mg/dose) q6hr PO × 7-10 days; **or** tinidazole 50 mg/kg (maximum: 2 g) PO once (adult: 2 g PO once)
HOOKWORM *Necator americanus* *Ancylostoma duodenale*	Mebendazole (Vermox) 100 mg q12hr PO (children >2 yr) × 3 days; **or** albendazole 400 mg PO once; **or** pyrantel pamoate (Antiminth) 11 mg/kg/24 hr q24hr (maximum: 1 g/24 hr) PO × 3 days
LEISHMANIASIS *Leishmania donovani* (kala azar) *L. braziliensis* (American mucocutaneous leishmaniasis) *L. mexicana, L. tropica*	Stibogluconate sodium (Pentostam, Tricostam) (CDC) 20 mg/kg/24 hr (maximum: 800 mg/24 hr) q24hr IM, IV × 20-28 days; may need to repeat

Modified from Committee on Infectious Diseases: *Report of the committee on infectious disease*, Elk Grove, Ill, 2000, American Academy of Pediatrics.

CDC: Available from the Centers for Disease Control Parasitic Drug Service, Atlanta; phone: 404-639-3670; for emergencies on nights, weekends, and holidays: 404-639-2888. Other resources include the information system for International Travelers, at 404-639-1410 or 404-332-4555, and the National Center for Infectious Disease (404-488-7760). Consult for recent recommendations.

MALARIA	
Prophylaxis	
For areas without chloroquine resistant *Plasmodium falciparum*	Chloroquine 5 mg base/kg (adult: 300 mg base) qwk PO, beginning 1 wk before potential exposure and continuing for 6 wk after last exposure; **plus** primaquine phosphate 0.3 mg base/kg (adult: 15 mg base) q24hr PO × 14 days after departure from endemic area
For areas with chloroquine resistant *P. falciparum*	Mefloquine: 15-19 kg: ¼ tab; 20-30 kg: ½ tab; 31-45 kg: 3/4 tab; >45 kg: 1 tab; adult: 250 mg PO qwk
Treatment	
P. vivax, P. ovale	Chloroquine phosphate (Aralen, Nivaquine) 10 mg base/kg then 5 mg base/kg at 6 hr, 24 hr, and 48 hr after initial dose (adult: 600 mg base, then 300 mg base at 6 hr, 24 hr, and 48 hr)
P. malariae	Chloroquine, as above
P. falciparum (nonchloroquine-resistant)	Chloroquine, as above
P. falciparum (chloroquine-resistant)	Quinine 25 mg/kg/24 hr (adult: 650 mg/dose) q8hr PO × 3-7 days; **plus** pyrimethamine-sulfaxodoxine <1 yr: ¼ tab; 1-3 yr: ½ tab; 4-8 yr: 1 tab; 9-14 yr: 2 tab; adult: 3 tab at once on last day of quinine **or** tetracycline 20 mg/kg/24 hr q6hr PO × 7 days if >8 yr **or** clindamycin 20-40 mg/kg/24 hr q8hr PO × 3-5 days; parenteral treatment available
PINWORMS *(Enterobius vermicularis)*	Mebendazole (Vermox) 100 mg PO once (children >2 yr) (repeat in 1 wk) **or** pyrantel (Antiminth) 11 mg/kg/dose (maximum: 1 g) PO once (repeat in 1 wk)
PNEUMOCYSTIS PNEUMONIA *(Pneumocystis carinii)*	Trimethoprim (TMP)-sulfamethoxazole (SMX) (Bactrim, Septra) 15 mg TMP, 75 mg SMX/kg/24 hr q6-8hr PO, IV × 14-21 days
SCHISTOSOMIASIS	Praziquantel (Biltricide) 40 mg/kg/24 hr PO × 2 doses in 1 day
Schistosoma haematobium	
S. japonicum	
S. mansoni	
TAPEWORMS	Praziquantel (Biltricide) 5-10 mg/kg PO once
Taenia saginata	
Taenia solium (see Cysticercosis)	
Diphyllobothrium latum	
TOXOPLASMOSIS *(Toxoplasma gondii)*	Pyrimethamine (Daraprim) 2 mg/kg/24 hr (adult: 25 mg/24 hr) q12hr PO × 3 days, then 1 mg/kg/24 hr q12hr PO × 4 wk (supplement with folinic acid 5-10 mg/24 hr) **plus** trisulfapyrimidines or sulfadiazine 100-200 mg/kg/24 hr (adult: 4-6 g/24 hr) q6hr PO × 28 days
TRICHINOSIS *(Trichinella spiralis)*	Mebendazole (Vermox) 200-400 mg/dose (children >2 yr) q8hr PO × 5-10 days; steroids
TRYPANOSOMIASIS, CHAGAS' DISEASE *(Trypanosoma cruzi)*	Nifurtimox (Lampit) (CDC) 1-10 yr: 15-20 mg/kg/24 hr q6hr PO × 90 days; 11-16 yr: 12.5-15 mg/kg/24 hr q6hr PO × 90 days; adult: 8-10 mg/kg/24 hr q6hr PO × 120 days
VISCERAL LARVA MIGRANS *(Toxocara canis)*	Albendazole 400 mg BID PO × 5 days; **or** mebendazole (Vermox) 100-200 mg BID PO × 5 days
WHIPWORM *(Trichuris trichiura)*	Mebendazole (Vermox) 100 mg q12hr PO × 3 days **or** 500 mg PO once

* Associated with serious adverse reactions, including erythema multiforme, Stevens-Johnson syndrome, toxic epidermal necrolysis, and serum sickness. Discontinue if any mucocutaneous lesions develop.

Index

Page numbers followed by f *indicate figures;* t, *tables;* b, *boxes.*

D

E

I

J

K

M

N

O

U

W